Heart Mechanics
Magnetic Resonance Imaging

Mathematical Modeling, Pulse Sequences, and Image Analysis

Heart Mechanics: Magnetic Resonance Imaging—The Complete Guide

Heart Mechanics: Magnetic Resonance Imaging—Mathematical Modeling, Pulse Sequences, and Image Analysis

Heart Mechanics: Magnetic Resonance Imaging—Advanced Techniques, Clinical Applications, and Future Trends

Heart Mechanics
Magnetic Resonance Imaging

Mathematical Modeling, Pulse Sequences, and Image Analysis

El-Sayed H. Ibrahim, PhD

Manager of Cardiac MR R&D
GE Healthcare

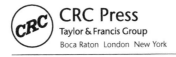

CRC Press
Taylor & Francis Group
Boca Raton London New York

CRC Press is an imprint of the
Taylor & Francis Group, an **informa** business

CRC Press
Taylor & Francis Group
6000 Broken Sound Parkway NW, Suite 300
Boca Raton, FL 33487-2742

First issued in paperback 2019

© 2017 by Taylor & Francis Group, LLC
CRC Press is an imprint of Taylor & Francis Group, an Informa business

No claim to original U.S. Government works

ISBN-13: 978-1-4822-6368-8 (hbk)
ISBN-13: 978-0-367-87117-8 (pbk)

Visit the Taylor & Francis Web site at
http://www.taylorandfrancis.com

and the CRC Press Web site at
http://www.crcpress.com

This book is dedicated to my lovely daughters Nora and Salma, my wife Enas, and my mother Ebtesam.

Contents

Contents (Advanced Techniques, Clinical Applications, and Future Trends)

Foreword

It is my pleasure to write this foreword for El-Sayed Ibrahim's *Heart Mechanics. Magnetic Resonance Imaging—The Complete Guide*. Back in 1987, I worked with colleagues at The Johns Hopkins University Department of Radiology on developing and validating the concept of MRI tagging pulse sequence as the first noninvasive technique for evaluating intramyocardial deformation. Before the invention of the tagging technique, the only way to evaluate regional heart function was through implantation of radiopaque markers, an invasive procedure with limited application to animal models and in open heart surgery. With cardiovascular disease remaining a major cause of death worldwide, it became imperative to find new noninvasive imaging tools that would allow for accurate evaluation of heart function that can be implemented in routine clinical practice. The 1980s witnessed the introduction of MRI in clinical practice with early applications in cardiac imaging. The introduction of the MRI tagging technique opened the door for a new era of cardiac imaging that helped in better understanding and quantifying heart mechanics in both health and disease. This translated into a number of technical developments of the MRI tagging technique, combining tagging with ultrafast cine imaging, and exploring its clinical applications by different groups in the Department of Radiology at Johns Hopkins University as well as from other groups worldwide. After more than a quarter of a century since the introduction of the first tagging sequence, MRI tagging sequences are still being developed and implemented in research and clinical studies to evaluate a wide spectrum of cardiovascular diseases and study the influence of different systemic diseases on cardiac function with unprecedented levels of detail and accuracy. The importance of these techniques stems from their capability of detecting subclinical cardiac dysfunction before deterioration of global heart function, symptoms manifestation, and progression toward heart failure. Therefore, these techniques would allow for early intervention in asymptomatic cardiovascular patients and patients at risk, and potential assessment of novel therapies, especially in heart failure, the growing cause of cardiovascular mortality and morbidity worldwide.

Despite the importance of heart mechanics imaging and the several MRI techniques developed to serve this purpose, a literature gap existed with no scholarly work devoted to cover this field. Therefore, *Heart Mechanics: Magnetic Resonance Imaging—The Complete Guide* nicely fills this gap. With more than 1300 pages covering thousands of references in 24 chapters with about 1400 figures, Sayed managed to provide a comprehensive reference that is a valuable resource for anyone working in the field of cardiac functional imaging with MRI. Not only does the book cover recent MRI techniques for heart mechanics imaging, it also covers the basic building blocks on which these techniques have been built, which provides the reader with the big picture and natural development stages of the different techniques, thus highlighting their similarities, differences, advantages and limitations, and guiding the reader to the technique most suitable for his or her specific application.

With the carefully selected book contributors, who are key experts in their fields from elite institutions all over the world, the reader will appreciate the first-hand experience provided by these investigators on how they developed their techniques and contributed in shaping the field. Furthermore, with the introductory chapters in the book covering basic engineering and medical background materials, *Heart Mechanics: Magnetic Resonance Imaging—The Complete Guide* comes as a self-inclusive reference that provides the reader with a comprehensive resource to master the ideas behind the covered techniques and understand the clinical significance of these quantitative measures of heart function. Finally, with the inclusion of two large chapters devoted to clinical applications of the techniques covered in the book, Sayed managed to provide a balanced coverage that makes the book appealing to both clinicians and scientists. In summary, from his early training at Johns Hopkins University, subsequent research and academic experience, and dedication to excellence, I commend Sayed for this important contribution to the field.

Elias Zerhouni, MD
Director of the National Institutes of Health (NIH),
2002–2008
Executive Vice-Dean, Dean of Research,
and Dean of Clinical Affairs, School of Medicine,
Johns Hopkins University, 1996–2002
Director of the MRI Division,
and Chairman of the Department of Radiology,
Johns Hopkins University, 1988–1996

Preface

MRI RESEARCH AT JOHNS HOPKINS UNIVERSITY

When I started my doctoral program at Johns Hopkins University (JHU) in Baltimore, Maryland, I studied under a joint program between the Department of Electrical and Computer Engineering and the Department of Radiology. This was a perfect niche for me considering my background in computer engineering and research interest, as well as previous research work, in medical imaging. After finishing the coursework at the Homewood Campus and successfully passing the qualifying exam, I moved to the Medical Campus, where I spent the rest of the 5-year PhD program. I was fortunate to work in the Division of Magnetic Resonance Imaging (MRI) Research in the Department of Radiology at JHU. There, I was surrounded by world experts in MRI, with Paul Bottomley, one of the founders (along with Peter Mansfield and Paul Lauterbur) of the early MRI systems in the world, as the division head.

I chose to specialize in cardiac MR (CMR) because of two reasons. The first reason is that CMR imaging was a relatively new area of research, with many challenges because of the respiratory motion, heart motion, air in the lungs surrounding the heart, and many other difficulties. Further, in contrast to other imaging modalities, MRI provides for a large number of cardiac imaging sequences, all combined in one exam. The second reason, or motivation, for choosing to work on CMR is that I was surrounded by world experts in CMR whose developed techniques, especially in heart mechanics, helped shape the field and are being used at major cardiac centers all over the world. This group included Elias Zerhouni, Matthias Stuber, Nael Osman, Dara Kraitchman, Paul Bottomley, Jerry Prince, Ergin Atalar, and Robert Weiss. Of course there are many other key figures in CMR at Hopkins and worldwide, some of whom I had the privilege to work with later in my career, but the ones mentioned here are those in my division with whom I directly worked, or at least worked on projects that they had established.

I hardly overlapped with Elias Zerhouni, as he left Hopkins in 2002 to become the director of the National Institutes of Health (NIH). He is the inventor of the myocardial tagging technique, which allowed for the first time for noninvasive quantification of regional cardiac function and opened the door for a new area of research. Actually, a large number of the techniques covered in this book stemmed from the tagging technique developed by Zerhouni. Matthias Stuber is one of the early investigators who worked on CMR at the Swiss Federal Institute of Technology (ETH) in Zurich in collaboration with the late Stefan Fischer (who invented the famous complementary spatial modulation of magnetization (CSPAMM) tagging technique as well as other important CMR techniques). Matthias also has vast hands-on experience in pulse sequence programming, as he worked with Philips for a number of years supporting clinical research at Harvard University before joining Johns Hopkins University. Dara Kraitchman has both VMD and PhD degrees, which gives her experience in both clinical and basic science in CMR. Dara was of great support for providing the animal models, on which we tested our developed techniques. Paul Bottomley has worked on almost every aspect of MRI, including CMR. Together with Robert Weiss, they established unique projects for studying cardiac metabolism with MR spectroscopy (MRS), one of the most challenging research areas in CMR. Ergin Atalar and Elliot McVeigh worked early on developing cine CMR techniques among many other technical CMR projects. I was lucky to take Ergin's class in MRI, where I learned a lot about MRI physics and mastered the subject such that I was top of the class (~50, mostly grad, students) with A+ grade.

I had two advisors for my PhD program: Jerry Prince from electrical and computer engineering and Nael Osman from radiology. Jerry Prince has a wide expertise in CMR image analysis and data acquisition techniques. Actually, a large number of the famous CMR techniques for measuring heart mechanics have been developed in his lab. My advisor Nael Osman, who is also a former student of Jerry Prince, is known worldwide for the harmonic phase (HARP) analysis and strain encoding (SENC) techniques that he invented at Johns Hopkins. These techniques revolutionized the field of tagging analysis by significantly reducing the image analysis time and presenting the results in an intuitive fashion, which contributed to increasing the popularity of MRI tagging and its implementation on a larger scale.

Besides my mentors, I had the opportunity to interact with a large number of colleagues from prestigious institutions, including Heidelberg University, Berlin Heart Institute, and ETH Zurich, who were in the same lab with me working on CMR. Also, the annual retreat of the MRI Division at JHU was a great gathering opportunity, where I had the chance to meet with everyone at JHU affiliated with MRI research, exchange research ideas, and discuss potential collaboration projects.

MOTIVATION FOR WRITING THIS BOOK

When I started working on CMR, I had no prior knowledge of MRI physics or cardiac imaging, let alone CMR. Taking the MRI class with Dr. Atalar filled the gap for understanding MRI basics from the physics and mathematical perspectives. I augmented the formal coursework by reading as many MRI books as I could to understand the subject from different perspectives: pulse sequence design, signals and systems, etc. At this stage, I discovered a number of valuable books addressing the MRI theory, and I appreciated the different approaches adopted in them. As I started to study the CMR techniques invented by my mentors, based on which I would start off my own research, my task started to become more specific. My advisor Dr. Osman gave me his seminal paper on SENC and asked me to study it and present at the lab's weekly meeting.

When I first read the paper, I started highlighting the words/parts that I did not understand so that I could read more about them. When I finished reading the paper, I only understood the basic concept of SENC, mainly from the illustrating figures, and hardly anything else. The pages' color turned into yellow from too much highlighting. After about three or four weeks of working on the paper, I had enough knowledge to present it on the lab meeting. However, at that time, my CMR knowledge was minimal and I did not grasp the basic CMR concepts quite well.

In the early months of my work on CMR, I worked on building my knowledge by reading key articles about CMR techniques for evaluating heart mechanics as well as articles about MRI pulse sequence design from different groups all over the world. Since then, I kept adding to my CMR knowledge by reading more articles as well as most of the CMR books available in the market. Finally, besides the theoretical knowledge gained from my readings and by attending different seminars and conferences, I received first-hand practical training on machine operation and pulse sequence design and programming. We were fortunate to have Matthias Stuber in our division with his vast experience in pulse sequence programming, but this may not have been a good thing for him as we kept bothering him with our questions!

The reason for explaining my early encounters with CMR is to illustrate the amount of work and efforts I had to make to understand the complete picture necessary for progress in my career. At that time, I wished there were a book dedicated to this area to serve as a complete reference for investigators working on evaluating heart mechanics with MRI, especially those who are in the early stage of their career. After graduation from Johns Hopkins, it came to me that it would be a good idea to write something that would serve this purpose, especially that by that time, I had grasped very good understanding of the basic and advanced applications of heart mechanics with MRI from both theoretical and practical perspectives. Therefore, I started writing a review article about myocardial tagging techniques for the *Journal of Cardiovascular Magnetic Resonance* (JCMR). Although I originally thought that writing such a review paper would be a straightforward task for me, considering my expertise in the field and that I knew what topics to be covered and have already read all key papers related to these topics, it turned out to be a time- and effort-consuming task. Despite my interest in keeping the review article as concise, straightforward, and equation-free as possible, it turned out to be a 40-page article that took me six months to finish!

The encouraging comments I received from the reviewers of my review article as well as the positive feedback from the readers encouraged me to think of something bigger and more comprehensive: to write a book! Another factor that made this idea appealing to me is that I got to know key personnel in the field, mainly from attending annual meetings, especially those of the International Society of Magnetic Resonance in Medicine (ISMRM), Society of Cardiovascular Magnetic Resonance (SCMR), and Institute of Electrical and Electronics Engineers (IEEE). Fortunately,

a number of these experts kindly agreed to contribute to my book, so that chapters about different CMR techniques are coauthored by the scientists who invented and/or developed these techniques themselves, which provides the reader with a first-hand experience of the development stages each of these techniques went through. Furthermore, I was lucky to have my first job as an assistant professor in the Department of Radiology, University of Florida in Jacksonville, with Richard White, an expert in cardiac imaging and one of the few radiologists who investigated the importance and applications of CMR in its early days, as the department chairman, from whom I learnt a lot about different CMR clinical applications.

HOW THIS BOOK WAS WRITTEN

Writing this book was like a second job for me. For more than five years, I would come home from work to start working on the book for 4–6 hours on a daily basis, in addition to working on the weekends and holidays! The more I delved into this project, the more I realized how big it was and how much more work it would take. Nevertheless, the more challenging the project became, the harder I worked and the more determined I became to finish it and see the end product. From the beginning, my goal was clear: I need this book to provide a comprehensive coverage of heart mechanics by MRI and to be useful for anyone working in that field, regardless of the educational background (engineering or medical), experience level (introductory or advanced), or perspective (theoretical or practical).

I followed a number of guidelines in writing this book: (1) Each chapter was written as if it should be the best chapter in the book. Therefore, a lot of time and effort had been spent in writing every chapter, so that the readers would feel that their money was well spent buying this book. My ultimate goal is to see as many scientists and clinicians as possible benefitting from this book. I want this book to save them time and effort and help them in their studies and practice. (2) The book is designed in a modular fashion, such that some chapters can be skipped, based on the reader's experience and interest, without losing track of the main theme of the book. (3) The book provides comprehensive coverage of heart mechanics by MRI, starting from MRI basics all the way to clinical applications and future trends in the field. To ensure meeting this goal, I started working on the book by conducting a detailed literature survey of the different subjects to be covered. Although I have already covered many articles in the JCMR review paper, the larger scope and level of coverage of this book required a detailed literature survey that I had to repeat every few months to make sure that the book's coverage is up to date. In doing so, I ended up with thousands of articles that I read and classified based on the chapters and sections they belong to. This way, I made sure that the book provides a complete coverage of the addressed topics and that the chapters and sections are optimally organized. Furthermore, this strategy allowed me to add preliminary chapters that are necessary for readers lacking certain backgrounds, for example, the heart physiology (Chapter 2) and MRI physics (Chapter 3) chapters for engineers and physicians, respectively.

The second stage of working on the book was to approach experts in the field asking for their contribution, which I really appreciate as I know how busy they are. From that point on, I had two tasks: to write my own chapters and to contribute to and edit the rest of the chapters in the book, which I took care of meticulously. Furthermore, I wanted to avoid a number of caveats in multicontributor books; for example, when (1) the big picture of the covered topic is lost among the foci of the different chapters; (2) the different chapters have different levels of coverage; (3) topics are repeated in different chapters; (4) the authors focus only on their work and do not cover others'; (5) the chapters are almost replicas of a few papers of the authors'; and (6) there is no uniformity in the chapters' design and organization throughout the book. To achieve the book's set up goals, each chapter went through a number of revisions to keep improving it until it reached its final shape. Therefore, I thank all contributors for their flexibility, understanding, and effort that helped make this book come out in this wonderful shape.

One final note is related to the massive amount of literature covered in this book. Although I made every effort to conduct frequent literature searches with different combinations of all possible key words to make this book as comprehensive as possible, which resulted in thousands of articles that are covered in the book, it is possible that I have missed some articles that did not come up in the search results. Therefore, I encourage the readers to contact me and point out potential work to be included in the next edition of the book.

Editor and Author

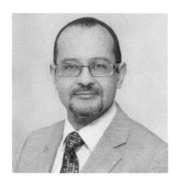

Dr. El-Sayed H. Ibrahim is the manager of Cardiac MR R&D with General Electric Healthcare, based in the headquarters in Wisconsin, USA. Dr. Ibrahim earned his master's and doctoral degrees in computer engineering from Johns Hopkins University under a joint program between the Department of Electrical Engineering and the Department of Radiology. After graduation, he joined the University of Florida as an assistant professor of radiology for five years before moving to Mayo Clinic, University of Michigan, and then switching to Industry. Dr. Ibrahim's research interests include medical imaging and image processing with special emphasis on MRI and cardiovascular imaging. He has more than 150 publications, including books, book chapters, book reviews, journal papers, proceeding papers, and conference abstracts. Dr. Ibrahim is a reviewer for more than 30 international journals, conferences, and grants funding agencies, in addition to being a member of a number of journal editorial boards. He also serves as organizer, moderator, and guest speaker in a number of international meetings/events. Dr. Ibrahim received many awards and nominations for distinguished accomplishments as well as research funding grants for different projects on medical imaging. He is a member of a number of international societies, including the International Society of Magnetic Resonance in Medicine (ISMRM), Society of Cardiovascular Magnetic Resonance (SCMR), and the Institute for Electrical and Electronics Engineers (IEEE). On the educational side, Dr. Ibrahim has been teaching both medical and engineering students at the undergraduate and graduate levels for more than two decades. He also serves as an external expert/committee member for a number of graduate students.

Contributors

Rolf Baumann, MSc
TomTec Imaging Systems
Munich, Germany

Andrew J. Coristine, PhD
Department of Radiology
University of Lausanne
Lausanne, Switzerland

Daniel B. Ennis, PhD
Department of Radiology
University of California
Los Angeles, California

Ahmed S. Fahmy, PhD
Department of Medicine
Harvard University
Boston, Massachusetts

Hélène Feliciano, PhD
Department of Radiology
University of Lausanne
Lausanne, Switzerland

Refaat E. Gabr, PhD
Department of Radiology
University of Texas
Houston, Texas

Edward W. Hsu, PhD
Department of Bioengineering
University of Utah
Salt Lake City, Utah

El-Sayed H. Ibrahim, PhD
GE Healthcare
Waukesha, Wisconsin

Elizabeth R. Jenista, PhD
Department of Medicine
Duke University
Durham, North Carolina

Igor Klem, MD
Department of Medicine
Duke University
Durham, North Carolina

John-Peder E. Kvitting, MD, PhD
Department of Cardiovascular and Thoracic Surgery
Linköping University
Linköping, Sweden

Abbas Nasiraei-Moghaddam, PhD
Faculty of Biomedical Engineering
Amirkabir University of Technology
Tehran, Iran

Davide Piccini, PhD
Department of Radiology
University of Lausanne
Lausanne, Switzerland

Wolfgang G. Rehwald, PhD
Siemens Healthcare
Malvern, Pennsylvania

Frank B. Sachse, PhD
Department of Bioengineering
University of Utah
Salt Lake City, Utah

Brian P. Shapiro, MD
Department of Medicine
Mayo Clinic
Jacksonville, Florida

Andreas Sigfridsson, PhD
Department of Clinical Physiology
Karolinska University
Stockholm, Sweden

Matthias Stuber, PhD
Department of Radiology
University of Lausanne
Lausanne, Switzerland

Christopher L. Welsh, PhD
GE Healthcare
Waukesha, Wisconsin

David C. Wendell, PhD
Department of Medicine
Duke University
Durham, North Carolina

1 Introduction to Heart Mechanics with Magnetic Resonance Imaging

El-Sayed H. Ibrahim, PhD

CONTENTS

LIST OF ABBREVIATIONS

Abbreviation	Meaning
1D	One-dimensional
2D	Two-dimensional
3D	Three-dimensional
4CH	Four-chamber
4D	Four-dimensional
AC	Alternating current
AHA	America Heart Association
C-SENC	Composite SENC
CAD	Coronary artery disease
CMR	Cardiovascular magnetic resonance
CMR-FT	CMR feature tracking
CRT	Cardiac resynchronization therapy
CSPAMM	Complementary SPAMM
CT	Computed tomography
CVD	Cardiovascular disease
DANTE	Delay alternating with nutations for tailored excitation
DC	Direct current
DCM	Dilated cardiomyopathy
DENSE	Displacement encoding with stimulated echoes
DTI	Diffusion tensor imaging
DWI	Diffusion-weighted imaging
ECG	Electrocardiogram
EF	Ejection fraction
EPI	Echo planar imaging
FEM	Finite-element modeling
FOV	Field of view
FT	Fourier transformation
Gd	Gadolinium
GRE	Gradient echo
HARP	Harmonic phase
HCM	Hypertrophic cardiomyopathy
HFNEF	Heart failure with normal EF
HIV	Human immunodeficiency virus
HT	High-tuning
LAX	Long-axis
LISA	Linearly increasing start-up angles
LT	Low-tuning
LV	Left ventricle
LVEF	LV ejection fraction
MESA	Multi-Ethnic Study of Atherosclerosis
MI	Myocardial infarction
MRE	MR elastography
MRI	Magnetic resonance imaging
NMR	Nuclear magnetic resonance
PC	Phase-contrast
PET	Positron emission tomography
RF	Radio-frequency
ROI	Region of interest
RV	Right ventricle
SAR	Specific absorption rate
SAX	Short-axis
SENC	Strain encoding
sf-SENC	Slice-following SENC
sf-fast-SENC	Slice-following fast-SENC
SNR	Signal-to-noise ratio
SPAMM	Spatial modulation of magnetization
SPECT	Single-photon emission computed tomography
SSFP	Steady state with free precession
STE	Speckle-tracking echocardiography
STEAM	Stimulated echo acquisition mode
TE	Echo time
TM	Mixing time
TPM	Tissue phase mapping
TR	Repetition time
VBOF	Variable brightness optical flow

1.1 INTRODUCTION

1.1.1 MRI and Heart Mechanics

Magnetic resonance imaging (MRI) has been established as a valuable modality for measuring heart mechanics. Besides evaluating global heart function, for example, ventricular ejection fraction (EF), it allows for measuring regional myocardial deformation, for example, myocardial strain, strain rate, and torsion. Cine cardiac MRI images have been used for deriving cardiac functional parameters through geometrical, probabilistic, statistical, and mechanical modeling. Further, feature-tracking techniques have been recently implemented for measuring myocardial deformation directly from the cine images. Nevertheless, the invention of MRI tagging in the late 1980s allowed for visualizing transmural myocardial movement for the first time without having to implant physical markers in the heart.

The invention of myocardial tagging opened the door for a series of developments and improvements that continue up to the present day. Different tagging techniques are currently available that are more extensive, improved, and sophisticated than they were 25 years ago. Current MRI techniques for measuring heart mechanics include tagging by magnetization saturation, spatial modulation of magnetization (SPAMM), delay alternating with nutations for tailored excitation (DANTE), complementary SPAMM (CSPAMM), harmonic phase (HARP) analysis, displacement encoding with stimulated echoes (DENSE), strain encoding (SENC), tissue phase mapping (TPM), and MR elastography (MRE). These techniques can generally be classified as either magnitude-based or phase-based techniques, based on the way in which the myocardial deformation information is encoded (either in the MR signal magnitude or phase, respectively).

Although most of the developed techniques have been invented by separate groups and evolved from different perspectives, many of them are in fact closely related to each other, and they represent different sides of the same coin. The development of some of these techniques even followed parallel paths, as illustrated later in the book. Besides, each of these techniques has different versions that provide improved resolution (spatial or temporal), enhanced signal-to-noise ratio

(SNR), three-dimensional (3D) imaging capability, reduced scan time, and composite data acquisition (e.g., myocardial strain and viability). Further, as each technique has its own advantages and limitations, efforts have been made to combine different techniques for improved image quality, 3D coverage, or composite data acquisition.

1.1.2 About This Book and Its Value

Despite the valuable information provided in a number of review articles (Zerhouni 1993, McVeigh 1996, Rademakers and Bogaert 1997, Reichek 1999, Masood et al. 2000, Axel 2002, Castillo et al. 2003, Axel et al. 2005, Petitjean et al. 2005, Gotte et al. 2006, Pai and Axel 2006, Shehata et al. 2009, Ibrahim 2011, 2012) and cardiovascular magnetic resonance (CMR) books (Higgins and de Roos 2002, Nagel et al. 2004, Lee 2005, Pohost and Nayak 2006, Biederman et al. 2007, Kwong 2007, Lardo et al. 2007, Grizzard et al. 2008, McGee et al. 2008, 2015, Manning and Pennell 2010, Bogaert et al. 2012, Myerson et al. 2013, Constantinides 2014, Ordovas 2015), no book has been dedicated to heart mechanics by MRI. This topic is usually covered in one or two chapters at most, despite the breadth and depth of the work that has been done in this field. Although a number of review articles were dedicated to this subject (Zerhouni 1993, McVeigh 1996, Rademakers and Bogaert 1997, Reichek 1999, Masood et al. 2000, Axel 2002, Castillo et al. 2003, Axel et al. 2005, Petitjean et al. 2005, Gotte et al. 2006, Pai and Axel 2006, Shehata et al. 2009, Goergen and Sosnovik 2011, Ibrahim 2011, 2012, Jeung et al. 2012, Simpson et al. 2013, Tee et al. 2013, Jiang and Yu 2014, Modesto and Sengupta 2014, Tavakoli and Sahba 2014, Lorca et al. 2015), these reviews typically focus on certain aspects (e.g., pulse sequences or image analysis) or provide a general overview without delving into detailed mathematical formulation, pulse sequence description, or algorithms analysis or without covering the various clinical applications of the developed techniques. Another point is that current-day techniques for measuring cardiac mechanics are so advanced and complicated that they are hard to comprehend without reviewing the basic blocks on which they have been built and following the incremental developments that led to the present-day techniques. Therefore, this book comes to fill this literature gap. It should be noted that some parts and figures of the tagging review in this chapter are adapted from the review paper by the author (Ibrahim 2011).

This book, together with *Heart Mechanics: Magnetic Resonance Imaging—Advanced Techniques, Clinical Applications, and Future Trends,* covers different techniques and clinical applications for measuring heart mechanics by MRI that have been developed over almost the past three decades. Different developments in MRI pulse sequences and related image processing techniques are described along with the necessities that led to their invention, which ensures smooth flow and easy-to-follow presentation of the covered topics. Besides technical coverage, most of the clinical studies that used these techniques for measuring heart mechanics are also summarized. For each of the covered techniques, the basic pulse

sequence is described along with the improved versions that have been developed based on it. The different versions of each technique are grouped based on the primary development goal, for example, SNR enhancement, scan time reduction, or 3D extension. Different postprocessing algorithms that have been developed for each technique are also covered along with the major applications and studies that have been conducted using these techniques. As different techniques have distinctive advantages and limitations, some efforts have been made to combine different techniques for improved image quality or composite data acquisition. These efforts are also covered along with the similarities and differences between different techniques.

There are a couple of notes about this book. First, I adopted a modular design strategy in this book. So, the reader may find a few topics repeated in different chapters. This was not an oversight or due to the contributions from different people. Rather, I tried to make every chapter as a complete unit, such that the readers familiar with certain chapters can skip them and jump to the chapter of interest without much interruption or the need to go back and forth between different chapters. However, the reader will find that the "repeated" topics are not copied and pasted; they are rather covered at different levels and from different perspectives based on the chapter in which they are covered. So, even the reader who reads the book starting from first chapter onward will find that he or she gains more understanding about the topics that are covered in more than one chapter by looking at them from different angles. The second note is that in the references in the end of each chapter, the reader may find more than one reference for the same work. Again, this was not an oversight; rather, investigators usually publish their work first as a conference abstract or technical paper, followed by a full paper in a clinical journal, technical journal, or both. I therefore included different references such that the reader can get the reference that he or she finds more suitable (or even accessible) to him or her, considering that some publications are freely available on the Internet and others are not.

One advantage of gathering all MRI techniques for measuring the heart mechanics in these two books is that it helps shed the light on their similarities and differences and explore the parallel paths of development that these techniques went through by different research groups. When looking at the big picture, one observes that although some techniques have been separately developed by different investigators whose ideas stemmed from different perspectives, there exist some relationships among many of these techniques. Therefore, these books provide a plethora of ideas and techniques with thousands of references that motivate the reader to think about the future of using MRI for measuring cardiac mechanics in particular and for comprehensively evaluating the heart function in general. Further, the clinical application chapters (Chapters 9 and 10 of *Heart Mechanics: Magnetic Resonance Imaging—Advanced Techniques, Clinical Applications, and Future Trends*) summarize most of the clinical studies that used heart mechanics derived by MRI. This would be a very useful resource for folks who want to start working on any of these applications to know what have been achieved so far and compare the findings from different studies for exploring new ideas, better study planning, and in order not to reinvent the wheel. Finally, although this book is mainly about heart mechanics by MRI, it includes dedicated chapters about heart physiology, MRI physics, cardiovascular MR, myocardial architecture, mechanical modeling, and image processing.

This book is of a great value as it saves the reader thousands of hours and dollars that he or she would had spent searching, purchasing, and summarizing the collection of articles covered in the book with such high level of details and organization. I spent about 5 years continuously working on the two books on a daily basis (including evenings and weekends), an effort that I originally expected to take me about a year or so (this shows how a bad estimator I am!). Seriously, this stemmed from my motivation to generate a valuable piece of work that fills a gap in the literature. Therefore, even for the multiauthor chapters, I worked hand in hand with the coauthors, reviewing and adding to the manuscript they produced and revising (and of course editing) it over and over again to make sure it covers all the topics and studies in that area with optimal chapters' design, illustrations, and figures. Therefore, I ended up writing most of the books, which explains why I spent all this time working on them (this should not underestimate the valuable contributions by different contributors whom additions significantly improved the value of this book). So, I hope the efforts I spent on writing these books would benefit someone working or who wants to work on this career, which would be of a much larger value for me compared to any material benefit I could have obtained using the huge amount of time I dedicated to writing these books in any other investment project. I therefore encourage the readers to contact me with their feedback about the books, so that I can make the next edition even better, as well as for any ideas to discuss, potential collaboration projects, or anything else I can help with (please write "*Heart Mechanics MRI*—Book Feedback" in the e-mail *subject* field to make it easier for me to sort different e-mails).

1.2 CARDIOVASCULAR DISEASE

Cardiovascular disease (CVD) is the leading cause of morbidity and mortality all over the world (Rosamond et al. 2008). In America, an estimated 80 million adults have one or more types of heart diseases, and death from CVD accounts for more than one-third of all global deaths. In addition to its burden on the patients, the management of CVD imposes a huge expense (billions of dollars) on the healthcare system. Further, the increasing population age and patients' survival rate lead to magnifying these costs. It has been shown that the degree of deterioration of the heart function is associated with poorer prognosis. Therefore, the ability to early identify markers of heart failure development would be of tremendous value for addressing this serious health problem.

1.3 HEART PHYSIOLOGY

The cardiovascular system is divided into two distinct circulations, pulmonary and systemic, with the primary purpose of delivering oxygenated blood throughout the body and removing unwanted waste products. To maintain these functions, there is a highly coordinated sequence of cardiac events ranging from electrical stimulation, heart contraction, and blood ejection into the respective circulations. The normal heart has four chambers subdivided into two atria and two ventricles, separated by a septum. The atria are thin-walled structures, which serve as reservoirs and conduits for blood in order to fill the ventricles. The right-sided chambers are part of the pulmonary circulation, which receives deoxygenated blood in the right atrium and circulates it to the lungs through the right ventricle (RV). The oxygenated blood then returns to the left atrium where it is subsequently pumped through the left ventricle (LV) and into the aorta to all body parts.

The myocardial architecture is often considered as a continuum of two helical sheets of fibers that have different orientations within the myocardium. The subendocardial region demonstrates a right-handed myofiber orientation, which gradually changes to a left-handed configuration in the subepicardial layer. During the cardiac cycle, a complex interaction of various myocardial fibers allows the LV to thicken, shorten, and twist. As the subendocardium is largely responsible for longitudinal shortening, these fibers contribute to the ventricular base being pulled toward the apex, thereby shortening the longitudinal axis of the LV. The other myofiber layers (midwall and subepicardium) largely contribute to ventricular twist or torsion. These fibers have greater torque than the subendocardial fibers due to their larger radii, and thus dominate heart motion. Therefore, as depicted by looking from the base toward the apex, these fibers contribute to the clockwise rotation at the apex and counterclockwise rotation of the base during systole and opposite rotation directions during diastole.

1.4 MYOCARDIAL FIBER STRUCTURE

The myocardium consists of myocytes, which are the basic building blocks making up the tissue. In the ventricles, the myocytes follow laminar organization, commonly referred to as sheets. The myofiber structure is an important determinant of the heart function. Knowledge about the myofiber arrangement allows for better understanding of myocardial shortening, lengthening, and twisting, which are important parameters for characterizing regional myocardial deformations and their contribution to the global heart function. Investigations about the myofiber arrangement have provided insights into the heart's function as early as the seventeenth century when Niels Stensen used gross dissection to demonstrate that the heart is a muscle by comparing the myocardial tissue fibers to those of the skeletal muscle.

The distribution of myofiber orientation within the heart wall (Figure 1.1) is the main determinant of stress distribution and myofiber shortening throughout the wall and,

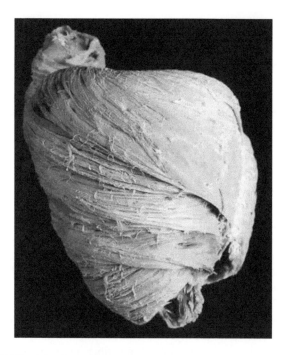

FIGURE 1.1 Organization of the fiber structure revealed by removing the epicardium. (Reproduced from Anderson, R.H. et al., *Clin. Anat.*, 22(1), 64, 2009. With permission.)

therefore, of cardiac perfusion and structural adaptation. The structure–function relationship also applies to cardiac electrophysiology. It is well established that electrical conductivities of the heart tissues are determined by the tissue microstructure, and in particular the local orientation and lamination of the cardiac fibers. These facts are reflected in simulations of electrical propagation in the heart and cardiac electromechanical modeling. In general, anisotropic description of the tissue properties is a crucial component for coupled electromechanical modeling of the heart, which requires integrative modeling of electrical activation, force development, and mechanical deformation based on anisotropic tissue properties.

The myofiber architecture is known to be altered in some cardiac diseases, such as ischemic heart disease and hypertrophic cardiomyopathy. Therefore, an integrated description of the cardiac structure, including fiber, sheet, and band architectures, is thought to provide a unified means for explaining the cardiac electromechanical behavior under different physiological scenarios, which can be used for treatment planning and patient monitoring. In this respect, MR tractography, a recently developed MRI technique, provides a valuable means for visualizing the myocardial fiber structure in health and disease (Figure 1.2).

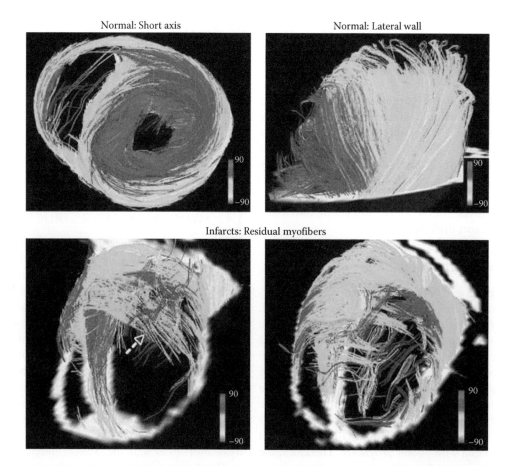

FIGURE 1.2 Comparison of the fiber structure of normal and infarcted rat hearts. Top and bottom rows show normal and infarcted hearts, respectively, both acquired ex vivo, as determined by MR tractography. Note the altered fiber structure in the infarcted region (arrow). (Reproduced from Huang, S. and Sosnovik, D.E., *Curr. Cardiovasc. Imaging Rep.*, 3(1), 26, 2010. With permission.)

1.5 MECHANICAL HEART MODELING

Mechanical heart modeling is important for measuring and understanding myocardial deformation. One fundamental assumption in cardiac mechanical modeling is spatial continuity of the myocardial tissue property. That is, regardless of spatial resolution, the tissue properties and behavior can be represented by a continuous function (Figure 1.3). Theories of continuum mechanics are, therefore, fundamental in modeling the behavior of the myocardium in response to different forces and stresses. In continuum mechanics, the spatial distributions of the applied forces and resulting deformations are represented, and the appropriate relationships between them are established. In addition, continuum mechanics provides a theoretical framework for representing other physical processes and factors attributing to the cardiac contraction–relaxation cycle, such as the distribution of electrical potential, oxygen, temperature, and metabolite concentrations within the myocardium.

1.6 GLOBAL AND REGIONAL MEASURES OF CARDIAC FUNCTION

Although global measures of cardiac function, for example, EF, represent the current clinical standard for evaluating the heart condition, extensive research showed that measures of

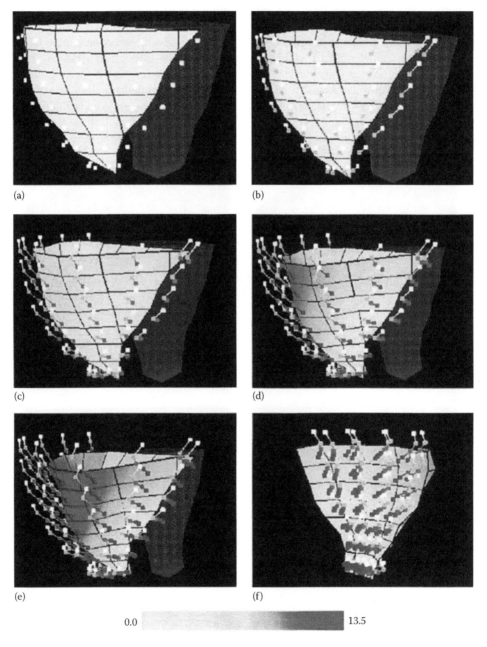

(a)

(b)

(c)

(d)

(e)

(f)

0.0   13.5

FIGURE 1.3 Three-dimensional model showing normal heart displacement. (a–e) Free wall is shown through four phases of systole. Left ventricle (LV) wall drawn shaded for reference. (f) Septal wall at end systole from the vantage point of the LV. (Reproduced from Haber, I. et al., *Med. Image Anal.*, 4(4), 335, 2000. With permission.)

regional myocardial function, for example, strain and strain rate, allow for early identification of cardiac dysfunction, and therefore they are becoming extremely important for diagnosis, risk assessment, treatment planning, and therapeutic efficacy (Figure 1.4). Further, measuring the heart mechanics allows for identifying regions of altered mechanical function and correlating them with other structural, perfusion, electrical, and metabolic properties of the heart.

Myocardial contractility is nonhomogeneous and differs based on location and orientation as well as on time through the cardiac cycle. Besides the spatial and temporal differences in the myocardial contractility patterns in the healthy heart, many pathological conditions do not affect the heart uniformly. This makes global measures of cardiac function insensitive to alterations in regional performance, and even a normal EF may conceal a significant underlying regional dysfunction. For example, significant changes in myocardial strain develop in heart failure with normal EF (HFNEF). Another example is in ischemic heart disease, where ventricular wall stress is a determinant of myocardial oxygen demand and is associated with the risk of ischemic injury. The importance of this association is that identifying abnormal mechanical patterns in the heart could allow for early

detection of individuals with underlying coronary artery disease (CAD) before developing major coronary events. Further, studying the ventricular differences in mechanical activation and time-to-peak contraction is important for evaluating cardiac dyssynchrony, determining optimal myocardial pacing regions, and predicting response to cardiac resynchronization therapy (CRT).

Other examples of regional function alteration can be illustrated in the cases of volume and pressure overloads. In ventricular volume overload, the ventricle remodels by enlarging the cavity size (dilation). An additional mechanism of remodeling involves increasing the amount of contractile material in the cells (hypertrophy). When wall stress continues to increase, the myocytes start to get damaged and the matrix proteins are altered, which increases myocardial stiffness and affects tissue contractility. In pressure overload, the wall stress increases, which triggers ventricular remolding through hypertrophy or through developing force for a longer period of time during systole. Another example of regional function alteration is in cardiac amyloidosis, where the amyloid buildup within the myocardium markedly reduces longitudinal strain, while circumferential and radial strains are partially retained.

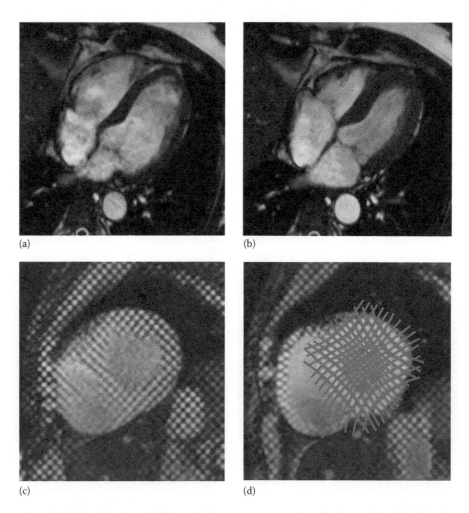

(a)   (b)

(c)   (d)

FIGURE 1.4 Global and regional changes in the heart function. Changes in the ventricular volume between end diastole (a) and end systole (b). (c, d) Intramyocardial deformation at end systole, as depicted by myocardial tagging.

Besides measuring regional function in the LV, there has been a recent interest in measuring strain in the RV, and even in the atria. The RV function plays a significant role in a large number of diseases involving the heart and lung, for example, pulmonary hypertension. On the other hand, as a representative of atrial distensibility, atrial strain is an important factor for determining the transition from hypertension to heart failure.

Despite its importance, measuring regional myocardial deformation is challenging due to the lack of intramyocardial markers that can be tracked through the cardiac cycle. Further, since the heart moves in the through-plane direction during the cardiac cycle, the apparent motion of the inner (endocardium) and outer (epicardium) ventricular borders in the imaging plane has a complex relationship with intramural myocardial deformation.

Originally, the measurement of heart mechanics required implanting physical markers within the myocardium and then tracking the markers' motion during the cardiac cycle using some imaging modality. The implantation of radiopaque markers (Brower et al. 1978, Ingels et al. 1980, Meier et al. 1980, Arts et al. 1993) or ultrasound crystals (Rankin et al. 1976, Myers et al. 1986, Villarreal et al. 1988) into the heart wall allowed for tracking tissue material points within the myocardium and thus measuring local tissue deformation between the tracked markers. However, the implantation process has many limitations: it is an invasive method, it cannot be applied repeatedly, the markers themselves may alter the native motion of the tissue in which they are imbedded, and finally, only a limited number of markers can be implanted and tracked. Thus, the ability to noninvasively and accurately measure myocardial motion would assist in the diagnosis, prognosis, and management of CVD.

1.7 IMAGING MODALITIES FOR EVALUATING CARDIAC FUNCTION

Regular anatomical images show the endo- and epicardium, which upon segmentation provide information about global heart function, for example, EF, stroke volume, and myocardial thickness. Besides MRI, imaging modalities that have been implemented for cardiac imaging include echocardiography, computed tomography (CT), and nuclear imaging.

1.7.1 ECHOCARDIOGRAPHY

Echocardiography is the most widely used modality for cardiac imaging because of its relatively low cost, widespread availability, and portability. Two-dimensional (2D) echocardiography is extensively used for evaluating cardiac morphology, volume, and function. Three-dimensional echocardiography allows for more accurate and reproducible results compared to 2D imaging. Contrast-enhanced echocardiography allows for better quantification of the cardiac function. Doppler echocardiography can be used for measuring blood flow velocity. Tissue Doppler imaging and speckle tracking are two relatively new echocardiographic techniques for measuring myocardial strain. Despite its superior temporal resolution, echocardiography has many limitations, including the need for an adequate acoustic window, operator dependency, geometric assumptions, and low SNR.

1.7.2 COMPUTED TOMOGRAPHY

CT allows for multislice tomographic imaging of the heart with excellent spatial resolution in a short scan time. Cardiac CT is excellent for imaging the coronary artery lumen, plaque, and calcium burden. Contrast-enhanced CT angiography is a prominent application of cardiac CT imaging. The limitations of CT include patient exposure to ionizing radiation, use of iodinated contrast agent, and limited capability of analyzing cardiac function.

1.7.3 NUCLEAR MEDICINE

Nuclear imaging provides valuable information about myocardial perfusion. In contrast to single-photon emission computed tomography (SPECT), which provides only qualitative information, positron emission tomography (PET) permits quantification of the coronary flow reserve. Another important feature of nuclear medicine is its capability of molecular imaging, which allows for analyzing small-scale functional alterations in the heart using specific tracers. Regarding cardiac motion, gated SPECT can be used for quantifying myocardial wall motion and thickening, although it suffers from very poor spatial resolution that affects the measurement accuracy and reproducibility. Another limitation of nuclear imaging is the use of radioactive materials.

1.8 MAGNETIC RESONANCE IMAGING

1.8.1 SCANNER'S HARDWARE AND SOFTWARE

The MRI scanner (Figure 1.5) consists of a very strong tube-shaped magnet and various coils, electronics, and computers. The patient undergoing the MRI exam lies on the scanner table, and coils are attached to the body to receive the MR signal. Afterward, the table is slid into the tunnel inside the magnet and the scan starts. During the scan, various magnetic fields are manipulated in a planned way to interact with the magnetic properties of the tissue and produce the MRI image. A single MRI scan usually takes few minutes (or even seconds), but the whole cardiac MRI exam could take 30–45 minutes depending on the amount of data required and level of details/accuracy sought.

The time sequence of applying the radio-frequency (RF) and gradient pulses required to generate the MR signal is called the MRI pulse sequence. A wide variety of MRI contrast mechanisms can be generated by manipulating the timing and other control parameters of the RF and gradient pulses. The pulse sequence diagram (Figure 1.6) is the timing graph of various RF and gradient pulses applied in different directions. The pulse sequence diagram for the MRI scanner plays the same role as the musical note an orchestra conductor uses to organize the operation of different musical instruments in a concert. Pulse sequences are programmed into

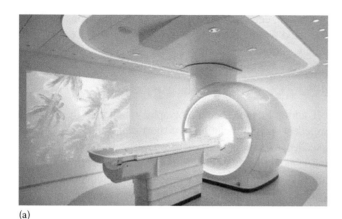

(a)

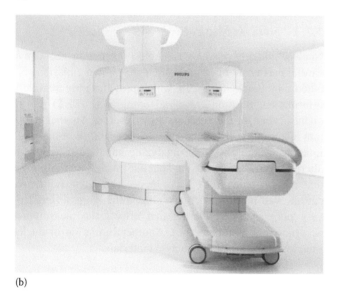

(b)

FIGURE 1.5 Magnetic resonance imaging (MRI) scanners. (a) Conventional and (b) open magnet Philips MRI scanners.

the scanner software, which gives instructions to the scanner hardware elements regarding when and how to run currents in the RF and gradient coils as well as about signal acquisition.

1.8.2   MRI ADVANTAGES AND LIMITATIONS

Achieving good image quality requires careful setting of the scan parameters to optimize the quality metrics relevant to the application at hand. Although image quality is ultimately determined by the imaging goal, in the general sense a good MRI dataset is one that has the highest possible SNR, highest possible spatial and temporal resolutions, and shortest scan time. Nevertheless, changing the scan parameters often results in conflicting effects on these desired features. Therefore, protocol setup always involves some type of a trade-off between SNR, resolution, and scan time. Specifically, accelerating MRI imaging is one of the key development areas in MRI research. Real-time imaging is another area of active MRI research, where fast pulse sequences and smart reconstruction strategies are implemented to improve the temporal resolution (time between two successive image frames). Examples of real-time applications include real-time cardiac imaging, dynamic contrast-enhanced studies, and MRI-guided interventions. Other advanced MRI techniques have been developed for obtaining more information about the scanned organ, for example, fiber structure and elasticity.

MRI is a remarkably safe technique that does not use ionizing radiation and does not require the administration of radioactive isotopes. Generally, the MRI exam does not result in any pain or side effects under normal conditions. Compared to other imaging modalities, MRI stands out as a unique source for providing detailed and quantitative information about cardiac structure and function, blood flow, perfusion, and tissue viability. Since the late 1980s, MRI techniques have been developed for evaluating heart mechanics. Further, advanced

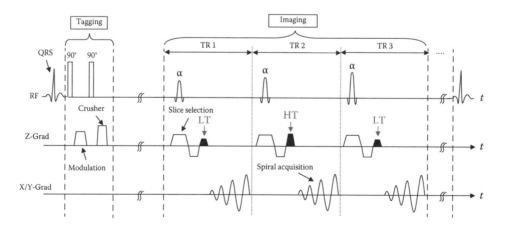

FIGURE 1.6   Magnetic resonance imaging pulse sequence. Strain-encoding pulse sequence with interleaved low-tuning and high-tuning acquisitions and spiral data readout. HT, high tuning; LT, low tuning.

MRI techniques allow for analyzing myocardial microstructure and metabolic activity. MRI has many advantages, including superior tissue contrast, arbitrary selection of the imaging plane, 3D imaging capability, and high resolution. Recent advances in MRI hardware (gradient and coil technology and fast computing workstations) and software (advanced pulse sequences and reconstruction algorithms) are contributing to the modality's widespread adoption in cardiac imaging. In addition to global function analysis, MRI is uniquely capable of quantifying intramyocardial deformation using MRI tagging and other advanced techniques that create virtual myocardial markers. It should be noted that, similar to all imaging modalities, MRI has a number of limitations, including relatively high cost and contraindication with some implanted devices or claustrophobia. Nevertheless, MRI advantages and capabilities far exceed its limitations.

1.9 CARDIOVASCULAR MAGNETIC RESONANCE

In the last 15 years, CMR has emerged as an important clinical tool for evaluating a broad range of heart pathologies. Technical advances have expanded the role of CMR from a primarily tomographic imaging modality to one that is dynamic, allowing for rapid, high-resolution imaging of the myocardial deformation, valve motion, and tissue perfusion. In addition, CMR is a valuable tool for evaluating congenital heart diseases.

CMR offers many advantages over other cardiovascular imaging modalities. Similar to echocardiography and CT, the MRI images are acquired by transmitting and receiving energy from the body, but CMR is uniquely flexible. CMR can provide a variety of tissue contrasts without any changes to the hardware or using contrast agents. The flexibility of CMR imaging results in a large number of imaging options, which can be daunting, but allow the examination to be tailored to the patient's particular clinical question. For example, within the same CMR exam, information can be gathered about cardiovascular morphology, contractile function, viable and nonviable myocardium, valve motion, congenital anomalies, blood flow, and vascular anatomy (Figure 1.7). Furthermore, postprocessing of the CMR images can provide several measures of the heart condition, including ventricular volume, ejection fraction, myocardial strain, fiber orientation, and iron content.

Unique to CMR, the scanner operator can conduct a variety of different medical imaging tests to collect specific physiological information about the heart solely by running different

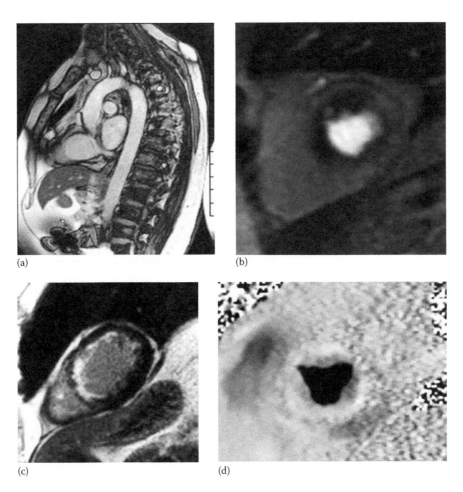

(a)   (b)

(c)   (d)

FIGURE 1.7   (a) Anatomical, (b) perfusion, (c) viability, and (d) flow magnetic resonance imaging images of the heart.

pulse sequences on the same MRI scanner hardware. Each pulse sequence is configured by a large set of scan parameters (a hundred or more) known as an MRI imaging protocol. The protocol tailors the same basic pulse sequence to a specific imaging task. The most important protocol parameters are flip angle, repetition time (TR), echo time (TE), field of view (FOV), spatial resolution, slice thickness, temporal resolution, and selection of magnetization preparation modules. Nomenclature of the parameters is often vendor specific and can be confusing. Different protocol parameters have various degrees of effect on the image properties. Whereas changing TE, TR, or the flip angle can strongly affect the image contrast, and thus the clinical usefulness of an image, modifying other parameters, such as FOV, does not fundamentally alter image characteristics. Protocol optimization is conducted by adjusting the parameters that are relevant to a specific application.

1.10   CINE IMAGING

One of the most important milestones leading to the introduction of CMR in clinical imaging is the robust implementation of the cine sequences. Cine CMR imaging provides high temporal and spatial resolution images of the heart and vasculature, which makes it a highly versatile technique (Figure 1.8). It is used for imaging the heart, pericardium, and great vessels alike. The excellent spatial and temporal resolutions of cine imaging make it an ideal tool for evaluating contractile function. It is a fundamental part of every CMR examination, which can provide a wealth of cardiac functional information, including ventricular volume, EF, myocardial mass, and wall motion. Specifically, cine imaging has become widely accepted as the gold standard for assessment of cardiac volumes, EF, and cardiac mass. Clinical practice guidelines have been set forth by professional radiological and cardiology societies to guide appropriate use of the measured parameters in various clinical indications. LV ejection fraction (LVEF), assessed by cine MRI, is increasingly used in clinical trials, for example, as a surrogate endpoint for drug trials in patients with chronic heart failure or for efficacy testing of stem-cell therapy after myocardial infarction. It has also been used as an endpoint for the evaluation of LV remodeling and as a reference measurement for other imaging techniques. Additionally, cine imaging alone allows for accurate measurement of the RV function and volume, which are used in studies of RV remodeling in patients with complex congenital heart diseases.

Manual, semiautomated, or fully automated techniques for processing the cine images have been developed. These techniques can provide accurate measurements of the ventricular and atrial volumes and diameters, cardiac function, contractility, wall motion, and valve function. However, the simplest and fastest instrument to detect alterations in these parameters may still be the human eye. At the time of image acquisition, changes in the heart function, wall motion, myocardial contractility, and chamber size can be detected visually, and additional scans can be performed on the fly to interrogate the cause. Visual analysis of wall motion and contractile function can be performed on the cine images using the 17-segment America Heart Association (AHA) model, which is the standardized segmentation technique among cardiac imaging societies. In such analysis, each segment is individually analyzed and scored on the basis of its inward wall motion and systolic thickening. Wall motion abnormalities may be indicative of loss of myocytes caused by myocardial infarction, or hibernating or "stunned" myocardium as seen in severe ischemia without loss of myocytes.

1.11   CINE IMAGE ANALYSIS

In cine CMR imaging, a stack of parallel short-axis (SAX) images covering the heart are acquired along with four-chamber, two-chamber, and sometimes three-chamber images (Figure 1.9). Ventricular contours drawn on the cine images during postprocessing are used to generate measures of cardiac volume, mass, and EF. Further, recent efforts have been made to exploit the cine images for evaluating regional heart function, for example, measuring myocardial strain and detecting wall motion abnormalities. Specifically, ventricular wall thickening, defined as the percentage change in wall thickness between end-diastole and end-systole, showed to be a sensitive marker for detecting dysfunctional myocardium. Actually, myocardial radial thickening is easier to measure from the cine images than from tagged images because the tagging pattern sparsely samples the myocardium in the radial direction.

Besides wall thickness measurement, model-based cardiac cine image analysis is an active area of research. Model-based analysis techniques provide a powerful approach for fast and accurate evaluation of the cine images. They have been implemented for evaluating global and regional heart function, and for investigating new descriptors of cardiac function. By customizing anatomical and functional models of the heart

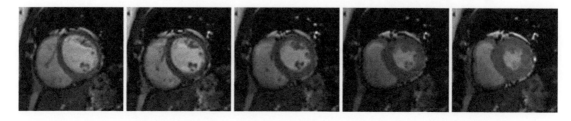

FIGURE 1.8   Short-axis cine images of the heart acquired at different timepoints from end-diastole to end-systole.

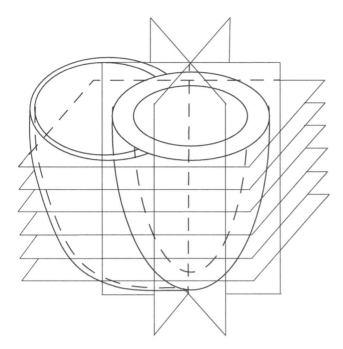

FIGURE 1.9 Stacks of parallel short-axis and radial long-axis planes covering the heart.

to images from an individual subject, information about the heart's shape and function can be obtained, which is helpful for studying normal ranges of variation in the population and differences in pathological cases. Compared to model-free approaches, the model-based techniques have the advantage that they provide information about the expected shapes of the structures of interest, which makes it easier to identify these structures in case of low SNR or in the presence of imaging artifacts. Further, the structures of interest can be described with a small number of parameters, and all image analysis and shape modeling steps can be conducted in a common framework. Despite the useful information they provide, cardiac image analysis techniques that work on images from

an individual timeframe are limited by the data available in that specific timeframe; they do not benefit from the information in the previous and following timeframes. In this respect, temporal characteristics of the heart motion can be incorporated in the designed cardiac models for efficient processing and accurate results.

1.12 MYOCARDIAL FEATURE TRACKING

While the cine CMR images lack the tagging pattern that is used for tracking intramyocardial deformation in the MRI-tagged images, they still have certain features, for example, papillary muscles and septal RV insertion points, which could be tracked to measure regional heart function. CMR feature tracking (CMR-FT) is an image analysis technique that has been recently developed for measuring myocardial contractility patterns from nontagged cine CMR images (Figure 1.10). CMR-FT stemmed from the more established speckle-tracking echocardiography (STE). It should be noted that while the CMR temporal resolution rarely approaches that of echocardiography, the achieved image quality with CMR is superior to that with echocardiography. Basically, CMR-FT is based on defining a relatively small window centered at a certain anatomical pattern (feature) in one image at a certain timeframe and searching for the as-much-as-possible similar local pattern in a window (of the same size and in the vicinity of the original window) in the image at the following time-frame. The displacement found between the two patterns is considered as the local displacement of the tissue.

CMR-FT proceeds in ways broadly comparable to particle image velocimetry and other pattern-tracking approaches, which have been developed over a number of years for fluid dynamics and other engineering and image processing applications. Feature tracking has already been applied in different fields, and although the mathematical kernel is similar, it needs adaptation to the specific application in hand. Specifically, as the heart muscle has distinct characteristics that are not found

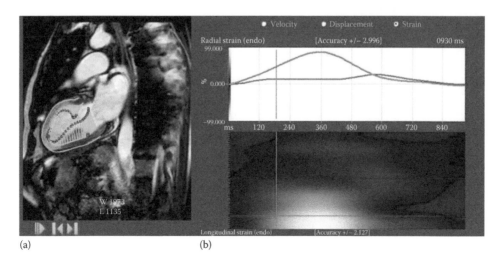

FIGURE 1.10 Feature tracking of a patient with scar. (a) Vector arrows of late systolic velocity tracing, 190 ms after QRS. (b) Radial strain tracing of the entire cardiac cycle. Blue represents the apex showing very low strain values and red is the normal posterior wall. (Reproduced from Maret, E. et al., *Cardiovasc. Ultrasound*, 7, 53, 2009.)

in other applications, optimizing the feature-tracking technology for implementation on the heart is necessary. In this respect, the nature characteristics of cardiac motion are used to optimize the CMR-FT algorithm. Motion periodicity is another characteristic of the heart motion that can be used for CMR-FT optimization, such that any unrealistic movements that might have been caused by artifacts can be detected and excluded.

Compared to CMR tagging, CMR-FT is simpler and faster as it does not require additional tagging sequences or complicated, and sometimes time-consuming, tag analysis techniques. Further, CMR-FT provides both global and regional cardiac functional measures from the same set of cine images; therefore, it can be applied retrospectively on previously acquired datasets that do not include tagged images. Further, CMR-FT has short processing time, which allows for application on a large number of existing datasets. Nevertheless, the accuracy of CMR-FT is suboptimal to CMR tagging as the intrinsic tissue markers in CMR-FT are much less than, and not as uniformly distributed as, the taglines' intersection points in the CMR-tagged images. Therefore, CMR-FT should be used to look at global parameters or parameters in reasonably sized regions and with certain precautions in order to achieve meaningful results.

1.13 MYOCARDIAL MARKER IMPLANTATION

1.13.1 RADIOPAQUE MARKERS AND SONOMICROMETERS

In current clinical practice, noninvasive imaging modalities such as echocardiography and MRI dominate the field for assessment of regional heart function. However, prior to their development, surgically implanted markers (Figure 1.11)

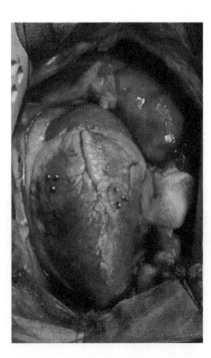

FIGURE 1.11 Markers implanted in the myocardium. (Courtesy of Neil B. Ingels and D. Craig Miller, Department of Thoracic and Cardiovascular Surgery, Stanford University, Stanford, CA.)

provided much of the fundamental knowledge we have today about myocardial motion and deformation. Albeit inherently invasive in nature, surgically implanted markers constitute a valuable tool in experimental animal models, providing the capability for precise tracking of fiducial markers for quantification of myocardial mechanics and valves motion. Nevertheless, the acute nature of these experiments and need for anesthesia might have restricted normal physiological reaction in the studied animals and limited the translational value of these findings to humans.

Prior to the introduction of surgically implanted markers, much of the data on cardiac physiology were obtained from open-chest animals and isolated perfused heart preparations. The radiopaque markers allow for instantaneous determination of the LV size, shape, and volume in the intact heart in both physiological and pathophysiological studies. The radiopaque markers used in different experimental and human studies are in the form of clips, beads, or screws. In this respect, the surgically implanted markers enable tracking a well-defined, albeit limited, number of points of interest in the myocardium that are time resolved in the Lagrangian coordinate system. The early studies provided information on the intact beating heart, confirming the physiological theories associated with the Frank–Starling mechanism and Laplace's law.

Sonomicrometry is the most common marker implantation technique after tantalum makers, wherein piezoelectric crystals, usually made of ceramic material, are implanted in the myocardium. Each implanted crystal has a dual role: transmitting and receiving signals from other crystals. These crystals operate at frequencies of 1 MHz and higher, where the distance between them is continuously measured with high spatial resolution. Based on the data received from the crystals, different cardiac indices, such as volume, wall thickness, and segmental shortening can be measured.

1.13.2 MARKERS' LIMITATIONS AND ADVANTAGES

One of the main reasons for the limited spread of the surgically implanted marker techniques, particularly in human studies, is the highly invasive nature of the method. Further, since the markers need to be surgically implanted, only diseased human hearts have been studied, and therefore, the data obtained may not reflect normal myocardial function, making generalization based on the obtained results difficult. Another limitation of the marker studies is the time-consuming data analysis, which precludes the technique's widespread clinical use. The finite number of implanted markers is also an important limitation. Further, missing or displaced markers are difficult to correct after implantation. An additional limitation of using the radiopaque markers is the need for ionizing radiation, which makes follow-up studies ethically difficult to justify. Finally, it should be noted that the markers themselves might alter normal myocardial function.

Despite their limitations, sonomicrometry remains the gold standard against which new imaging techniques, for example, STE, echocardiographic methods for assessing myocardial work, optical flow techniques, and MRI tagging, have been validated. Further, the high accuracy of the piezo-electric crystals makes them still attractive in the experimental setting for quantifying subtle changes in systolic segmental shortening and wall thickening in diverse settings, such as experimental cardiac surgery and quantification of LV remodeling after myocardial infarction or heart failure. Nevertheless, the use of surgically implanted markers, both radiopaque markers and sonomicrometric crystals, in humans has ceased after the introduction of noninvasive techniques such as MRI tagging.

1.14 MRI TAGGING

MRI tagging was developed to provide detailed spatial information about heart motion, including myocardial strain, strain rate, and torsion. These comprehensive measures of myocardial deformation can be important for clinical risk assessment, which allows for detecting and quantifying regional myocardial abnormalities before the onset of global cardiac dysfunction.

The development of the MRI tagging techniques can be broadly divided into two stages. The first stage (basic techniques) started in 1988 with the invention of tagging by magnetization saturation by Zerhouni et al. (1988) and continued to include SPAMM (Axel and Dougherty 1989), DANTE (Mosher and Smith 1990), and CSPAMM (Fischer et al. 1993) tagging techniques. The second stage (advanced techniques) started in 1999 with the invention of two of today's most widely used techniques HARP (Osman et al. 1999) and DENSE (Aletras et al. 1999b). This stage includes also SENC (Osman et al. 2001), which was subsequently developed in 2001, as well as TPM (Pelc et al. 1994, Zhu et al. 1996, Markl et al. 1999), which was developed in the mid-1990s, but became more popular later with advances in hardware and pulse sequence capabilities. The basic difference between the two categories of tagging techniques is the concept behind motion encoding and implemented postprocessing criterion.

The tagging techniques in the first category (basic techniques) depend on the creation of a visible pattern of saturated magnetization, usually parallel lines, grid pattern, or radial stripes, superimposed on the magnitude-reconstructed images. This allows for immediate visual inspection of the tagline intersections to evaluate myocardial contractility without any postprocessing. Nevertheless, exhaustive postprocessing is needed to quantify myocardial motion. Although different complicated algorithms have been developed for identifying and tracking the taglines, these algorithms consume a long processing time. The techniques in the second category (advanced techniques), on the other hand, depend on k-space analysis or on the signal phase encoded in the acquired data, which allows for faster and more automatic analysis of myocardial motion than with the basic techniques. It should be noted that the images in these advanced techniques may not directly show any tagging pattern (e.g., SENC, DENSE, and TPM), although these techniques are somehow related to the basic tagging techniques. Nevertheless, image processing

results in presenting the motion information in an intuitive and more appealing way. Table 1.1 shows a brief list of the major tagging techniques.

1.15 TAGGING BY MAGNETIZATION SATURATION

1.15.1 Basic Idea

In 1988, Zerhouni et al. (1988) introduced the idea of myocardial tissue tagging, which is based on saturating (or inverting) tissue magnetization to create visible taglines that can be imaged and tracked (Figure 1.12). The developed pulse sequence consists of two consecutive stages: tagging preparation and imaging. During tagging preparation, slice-selective RF pulses are applied perpendicular to the imaging slice to saturate the longitudinal magnetization at specified locations (the intersection of the selected tagging slices and the imaging plane). The rest of the imaging slice is not affected by the tagging pulses and continue to have undisturbed magnetization. During imaging (data acquisition), the tagged areas show darker signal intensity than the nontagged tissues due to the magnetization saturation they have experienced. Because magnetization is an intrinsic property of the underlying tissue, the taglines, being part of the tissue, follow tissue movement. Thus, the acquired image shows visual evidence of tissue deformation that occurred since the time of applying the tagging RF pulses. Typically, tagging is implemented at end-diastole right after the detection of the R-wave of the electrocardiogram (ECG) signal, and imaging takes place at end-systole in order to assess myocardial deformation at maximum heart contraction.

One point, though, has to be taken into consideration, which is the longitudinal relaxation of the tagged magnetization in-between tagging preparation and data acquisition. Longitudinal relaxation has the effect of restoring the tagged magnetization back to the equilibrium condition with exponential rate depending on the tissue longitudinal magnetization relaxivity time constant (T1). Therefore, the longer the time duration between tagging preparation and data acquisition, the lower the contrast between the tagged and nontagged tissues in the acquired image.

1.15.2 Limitations

The tagging technique developed by Zerhouni et al. has been validated in different studies (Lima et al. 1993, Bazille et al. 1994). However, this original tagging technique has a number of limitations: (1) As tagging preparation consists of applying multiple RF pulses, often with 180° flip angles, high specific absorption rate (SAR) may become a problem, thus limiting the number of taglines that can be generated. (2) As multiple RF pulses take a certain time period to perform, different taglines are not created simultaneously, but are rather slightly shifted in time, which results in different relaxation effects on them and different appearance in the tagged image. (3) Since the taglines are created by applying ordinary slice-selective saturation RF pulses, the minimum achievable slice thickness

TABLE 1.1

Evolution of the Tagging Pulse Sequences

Technique	References	Advantages	Limitations
Magnetization saturation	Zerhouni et al. (1988)	Simple idea; first tagging technique	Low resolution; long scan time; high SAR
SPAMM	Axel and Dougherty (1989)	Low SAR; available for clinical applications	Moderate resolution; 2D only; tag fading
Cine SPAMM	McVeigh and Atalar (1992)	Cine capability	Multiple breath-holds
Localized SPAMM	Chandra (1996), Ikonomidou (2002)	Tagging confined to region of interest	Complicated tag preparation
Variable-density SPAMM	McVeigh and Bolster (1998), Ikonomidou and Sergiadis (2003)	Sensitive motion estimation	Long tag preparation time
Radial tagging	Bolster et al. (1990), Bosmans et al. (1996)	Suitable for measuring radial strain and heart rotation	Low resolution for measuring circumferential strain
Ring tagging	Spiegel et al. (2003)	Suitable for measuring circumferential strain	Low resolution for measuring radial strain
DANTE	Mosher and Smith (1990)	High-density pattern of thin tags	Long tag preparation time
CSPAMM	Fischer et al. (1993)	Improved tagging contrast; no tag fading	Double the scan time compared to SPAMM
sf-CSPAMM	Fischer et al. (1994)	Tracks tissue through-plane motion	Lower SNR than CSPAMM
Single BH sf-CSPAMM	Stuber et al. (1999b)	Fast data acquisition; high temporal resolution	EPI possibly causing motion artifacts
HARP	Osman et al. (1999)	Fast tag analysis	Phase errors; low SNR
Real-time HARP	Sampath et al. (2003)	High temporal resolution	Complicated setup
3D HARP	Pan et al. (2005)	3D strain analysis	Long tag analysis time
zHARP	Abd-Elmoniem et al. (2005)	3D tissue tracking; short scan time	Complicated data analysis
fastHARP	Abd-Elmoniem et al. (2007)	Short data acquisition time; 25 fps	Complicated setup
DENSE	Aletras et al. (1999b)	High spatial resolution; black-blood	Low SNR
fast-DENSE	Aletras et al. (1999a)	Single breath-hold	EPI artifacts
meta-DENSE	Aletras and Wen (2001)	High SNR	Long acquisition time
DENSE with CANSEL	Epstein and Gilson (2004)	High SNR; less artifacts	Long scan time
SENC	Osman et al. (2001)	High resolution; simple processing; intuitive view	Low SNR
sf-SENC	Fahmy et al. (2006b)	Through-plane tracking	Low SNR
fast-SENC	Pan et al. (2006)	Real-time imaging	Low resolution
sf-fast-SENC	Ibrahim et al. (2007a)	Real-time imaging with tissue tracking	Low resolution and SNR
C-SENC	Ibrahim et al. (2007b)	Both strain and viability information in one scan	No cine capability

Source: Adapted from Ibrahim, El-S.H., *J. Cardiovasc. Magn. Reson.*, 13, 36, 2011.
BH, breath-hold; C-SENC, composite SENC; EPI, echo planar imaging; SAR, specific absorption rate; sf, slice-following.

is limited by the duration of the RF pulse and gradient strength, with thinner taglines and sharper tag profiles requiring long RF pulses and strong gradients. Nevertheless, despite these limitations, the original slice saturation tagging technique stems its importance from its novelty, which opened the door for a number of advanced tagging techniques that have been developed since then.

1.16 SPAMM

1.16.1 IMPORTANCE

Different MRI tagging techniques have been proposed for measuring myocardial deformation using MRI. Generally, these techniques can be divided into magnitude-based and

phase-based techniques, depending on how the magnetization is manipulated during the MRI scan to capture tissue motion. The SPAMM technique belongs to the first group. SPAMM stands out as the most widely used tagging technique since its introduction in 1989 until the present day.

One year after the introduction of the selective excitation tagging technique by Zerhouni et al., Axel and Dougherty (1989) developed the SPAMM technique, which alleviates the limitations of selective excitation tagging (Figure 1.13). The SPAMM technique's efficiency and short scan time led to its adoption in many clinical studies on different heart diseases. Further, SPAMM was the basis for advanced tagging techniques that were developed later, for example, CSPAMM by Fischer et al. (1993) and HARP analysis by Osman et al. (1999).

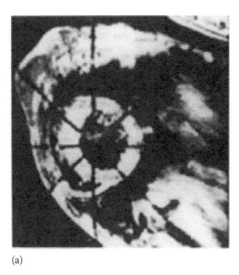 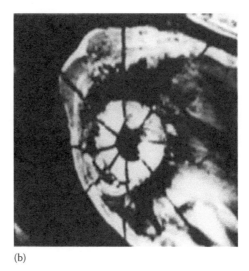

(a) (b)

FIGURE 1.12 Tagging by magnetization saturation. Short-axis tagged images at (a) end diastole and (b) end systole. (Reproduced from Lima, J.A. et al., *J. Am. Coll. Cardiol.*, 21(7), 1741, 1993. With permission.)

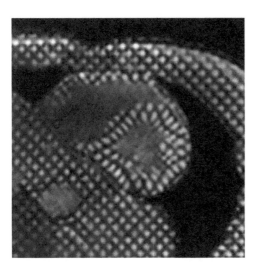

FIGURE 1.13 Spatial modulation of magnetization grid-tagged short-axis image.

1.16.2 BASIC IDEA

The basic SPAMM tagging sequence provides a simple and efficient way for analyzing intramyocardial deformation. The idea behind tags creation with SPAMM is different from that presented by Zerhouni et al. (1988). SPAMM is based on spatially wrapping the magnetization in a periodic fashion by applying only two equal-strength nonselective RF pulses separated by a "wrapping" gradient and followed by a spoiler gradient. These four pulses (two RF pulses and two gradients) comprise the tagging preparation module, which is implemented immediately after the detection of the R-wave of the ECG. Following tagging preparation, a multiphase segmented data acquisition is conducted until the next R-wave, where the tagging/imaging modules are repeated until the data required for constructing all the images are acquired. When the SPAMM images acquired at different heart phases are played

back in a cine loop, myocardial deformation can be tracked, and measures of regional heart function can be quantified (McVeigh and Atalar 1992). SPAMM tagging has been validated in phantom and simulation experiments, where motion measurements from the MRI tags showed excellent agreement with both optical markers (Young et al. 1993, Moore et al. 1994) and analytic solution (Kerwin and Prince 2000).

1.17 DANTE

The DANTE tagging pulse sequence was introduced in 1990 by Mosher and Smith (1990). DANTE consists of a series of short nonselective RF pulses that are played in the presence of a constant modulation gradient (in contrast to SPAMM where the modulation gradient is played in between the RF pulses). DANTE has the advantage that the width and separation of the taglines can be easily modified by controlling the pulse sequence parameters, which allows for optimizing the sequence for different clinical applications (Figure 1.14). Increasing the strength of the modulation gradient or the time separation between the RF pulses results in increasing the tagline density. Increasing the total length of the DANTE pulse train results in thinner taglines.

DANTE is an efficient and flexible tagging sequence. It has the advantages of improved tagging resolution and reduced eddy currents. The short width of the RF pulses minimizes off-resonance artifacts and allows for magnetization excitation in the presence of a continuous modulation gradient. Because the gradients are not rapidly pulsed, smaller eddy currents are generated and the gradient performance (slew rate and stability) is less demanding. Compared to Zerhouni's tagging technique of magnetization saturation, DANTE produces significantly less RF power deposition in the patient; and compared to SPAMM, DANTE can generate sharper taglines with simple control of the taglines' width and spacing.

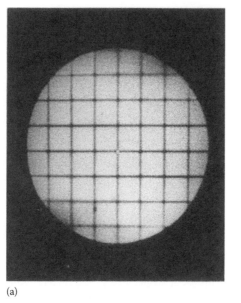
(a)

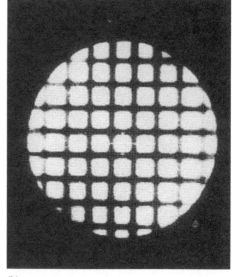
(b)

FIGURE 1.14 Delay alternating with notations for tailored excitation (DANTE) tagging. Comparison of (a) DANTE tagging versus (b) spatial modulation of magnetization in a phantom, showing the high-resolution tagging achieved with DANTE. (Reproduced from Mosher, T.J. and Smith, M.B., *Magn. Reson. Med.*, 15(2), 334, 1990. With permission.)

1.18 CSPAMM

One limitation of the magnetization saturation, SPAMM, and DANTE tagging techniques is the fading of the tagging contrast through the cardiac cycle due to longitudinal magnetization relaxation. The loss of tagging contrast toward the end of the cardiac cycle results in unrecognizable tagging pattern, which precludes the analysis of myocardial motion during diastolic heart phases. It was not until 1993 when Fischer et al. introduced an improved tagging technique, CSPAMM, to resolve this problem (Fischer et al. 1993; Figure 1.15).

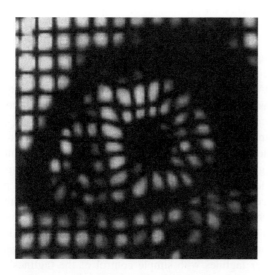

FIGURE 1.15 CSPAMM grid-tagged short-axis image.

1.18.1 Basic Idea

The CSPAMM idea can be easily understood by analyzing the magnetization behavior in the SPAMM sequence. Immediately after tagging application, the whole magnetization is tagged or modulated (90° tagging RF pulses are assumed) and stored in the longitudinal direction. With time, the magnetization experiences longitudinal relaxation, trying to reach the equilibrium state. This has two effects on the stored tagging pattern: (1) introducing a growing nontagged magnetization offset (we call it the DC component, borrowing the term "direct current (DC)" from electrical engineering) and (2) reducing the magnitude of the tagged magnetization component (the peak-to-peak difference of the sinusoidally tagged magnetization). Thus, during the imaging stage, the excited magnetization has two components: DC and tagged (the tagged component can be also referred to as the "alternating current" (AC) component due to the sinusoidal tagging pattern), with the DC overhead impairing the visibility of the (already fading) AC component.

It should also be noted that the multiple application of the imaging RF pulses during data acquisition contributes to reducing the AC magnetization component (each RF pulse consumes part of the tagged magnetization stored in the longitudinal direction). The solution provided in CSPAMM to restore the tagging contrast consists of two parts (1) eliminating the nontagged (DC) magnetization and (2) enhancing the fading tagged (AC) magnetization. The first part is addressed by acquiring two sets of SPAMM images with reversed tagging polarization, such that subtracting the two SPAMM images at any timepoint results in cancelling out the nontagged DC signal (and also doubling the tagged AC signal). The second part of the solution is addressed by applying a ramped imaging flip angle through the cardiac cycle to compensate for the magnetization loss due to longitudinal relaxation and the repeated application of the imaging flip angles at consecutive heart phases. Despite the significant improvement in tagging contrast, CSPAMM has the limitation that it doubles the scan time compared to SPAMM.

1.18.2 SLICE-FOLLOWING CSPAMM

Slice-following CSPAMM is another important contribution by Fischer et al. (1994) to resolve the tissue through-plane motion problem. The heart shows a complicated 3D pattern of contraction through the cardiac cycle. For example, during systole, the myocardium undergoes circumferential and longitudinal shortening, radial thickening, and longitudinal displacement from base to apex (Figure 1.16). In addition, the heart twists as the base and apex rotate counterclockwise and clockwise, respectively (as seen from the base), which is known as the wringing or torsion heart motion during systole. This means that in 2D cine imaging of the heart, the same myocardial tissue is not imaged throughout the cardiac cycle. The imaging plane rather shows whatever tissue lies inside it at the time of data acquisition. This could lead to inaccurate assessment of myocardial motion, for example, an apparent myocardial thickening in a mid-base SAX plane could be in fact due to myocardial basal displacement toward the apex.

The slice-following technique (Fischer et al. 1994) was created as an improvement of CSPAMM to resolve the through-plane motion problem. The technique is based on implementing slice-selective (in the z-direction) tagging instead of the non-selective tagging used in conventional CSPAMM. A thin slice of interest is tagged by switching one (or both) of the tagging RF pulses into a slice-selective pulse, which has the effect of confining the tagging pattern inside the slice of interest without affecting the tissue above and below the tagged slice. During data acquisition, a thicker slice, that encompasses the thin tagged slice, is excited. The excited slice should be thick enough to accommodate the thin tagged slice despite its displacement in the through-plane direction. Because nontagged magnetization is eliminated in CSPAMM, the only source of signal in the acquired image comes from the initially tagged slice, regardless of its displacement in the through-plane direction. This ensures that the same myocardial tissue is imaged during the whole cardiac cycle and that apparent motion illusions are eliminated (Stuber et al. 1999b).

1.19 SPECIAL TAGGING PATTERNS

In MRI tagging, the tagging pattern is created at end-diastole to label the myocardium and as the heart contracts during the cardiac cycle, the tagging pattern deforms accordingly. The motion of the tagging pattern can be observed in the subsequently acquired time-resolved images. The full potential of this advantage, however, is not fulfilled unless the tagging pattern matches both the geometry and motion of the myocardium. In the SAX view, the geometry of both healthy and unhealthy LVs is mainly circular, and the underlying motion pattern can be compactly described in a polar coordinates system. Specifically, it is apparent that, in the SAX view, the heart grossly contracts in the circumferential direction and thickens in the radial direction.

1.19.1 LOCALIZED AND VARIABLE-DENSITY TAGGING

Several attempts have been made to customize the tagging pattern to the gross geometry and motion pattern of the heart. Some investigators (Chandra and Yang 1996, Ikonomidou and Sergiadis 2002) tried to limit tagging only to the location of the heart itself in order to avoid obstructing nearby anatomical details. This so-called "localized" tagging (Figure 1.17a) has been shown in the reported localized-SPAMM and localized-DANTE techniques (Chandra and Yang 1996). Other investigators (McVeigh and Bolster 1998, Ikonomidou and Sergiadis 2003) spatially customized the

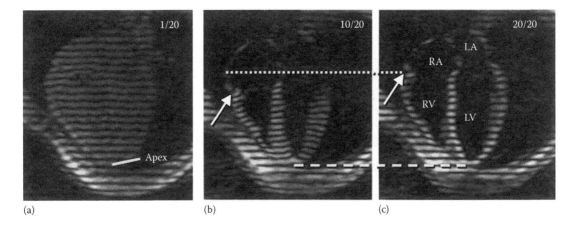

(a)   (b)   (c)

FIGURE 1.16 Longitudinal shortening of the heart during the cardiac cycle. Four-chamber view tagged images at (a) end diastole, (b) systole, and (c) diastole, showing the base movement toward the apex during systole (dotted line and arrows). The frame number in the cardiac cycle (out of 20 total frames) is shown on the top right corner of each image. (Reproduced from Stuber, M. et al., *MAGMA*, 9(1–2), 85, 1999b. With permission.)

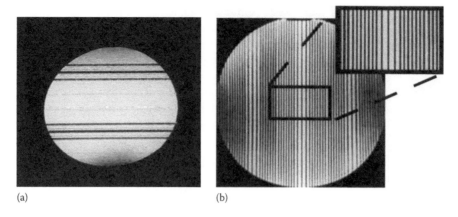

(a)   (b)

FIGURE 1.17   (a) Localized and (b) variable-density tagging. (a: Reproduced from Chandra, S. and Yang, Y., *J. Magn. Reson. B*, 111(3), 285, 1996. With permission; b: Reproduced from McVeigh, E.R. and Bolster, B.D., *Magn. Reson. Med.*, 39(4), 657, 1998. With permission.)

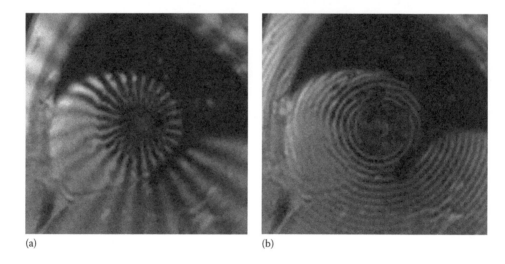

(a)   (b)

FIGURE 1.18   (a) Radial and (b) ring tagging of short-axis slices of the heart.

spacing of the parallel taglines to create variable-density tagging (Figure 1.17b). This approach takes advantage of the fact that during myocardial contraction (in the SAX view), some parts of the heart get closer together, while other parts move farther apart. Therefore, by considering the expected deformation within different regions of the myocardium, a customized tagging pattern can be generated that best captures the underlying deformation. Some investigators described how to produce tagging spots, rather than lines (Kerwin and Prince 2000). This approach produces more discrete features to be tracked during the postprocessing step and obscures less of the underlying anatomy than with conventional taglines.

1.19.2 RADIAL AND CIRCULAR TAGGING

Another category of the tagging techniques aims to closely match the gross geometry of the heart, which is best described in the pseudo-cylindrical coordinate system. This category of tagging techniques includes radial tagging (Bolster et al. 1990, Bosmans et al. 1996; Figure 1.18a), ring tags (Spiegel et al. 2003; Figure 1.18b), and, most recently, polar tagging (Nasiraei-Moghaddam and Finn

2014). These new techniques for generating customized tagging patterns most closely match the annular geometry of the heart (in the SAX view) and directly measure the polar deformation of the heart as it contracts and relaxes.

The main challenges to producing special tagging patterns are the quality of the tagging pattern and efficiency of the corresponding sequence. In fact, these two challenges are very closely related. Creating a perfect tagging pattern requires a lengthy combination of RF pulses and gradients. Therefore, a compromise must be made so that the tagging pattern is acceptable and can be generated in a short period of time. Specifically, for capturing myocardial motion during early systole, this means generating the tagging pattern immediately after the occurrence of the QRS complex of the ECG and before the onset of any measurable heart motion.

1.20   DATA ACQUISITION SEQUENCES

Immediately following tagging preparation, a segmented cine data acquisition is usually implemented over a number of cardiac phases. For breath-hold imaging, the practical limits on temporal and spatial resolutions are determined by the amount of time the patient can hold his or her breath. As a general rule in MRI imaging, the higher the required image quality, the longer the scan time. In myocardial tagging, dense tagging may be required for detailed analysis of regional strain variation across the myocardial wall or in the RV, high temporal resolution may be required for better characterization of the strain–time curves, and/or higher SNR may be required to improve image quality and tagging contrast. Although these improvements result in more accurate strain measurements, they come at the expense of a prolonged breath-hold duration, which may not be tolerable by the patient. There are also other groups of patients who may not even be able to hold their breath during standard scans, for example, patients with respiratory diseases, patients under anesthesia, the elderly, and young children. One solution in these cases is to modify the imaging sequence to include respiratory gating capability, for example, using navigator echoes, which allow the scan to be conducted while the patient is breathing normally. Therefore, the implemented imaging sequence affects the quality and characteristics of the resulting tagged images. Major imaging sequences used in myocardial tagging include GRE, EPI, and SSFP.

1.20.1 Gradient Echo

The gradient echo (GRE) sequence is one of the basic CMR imaging sequences implemented in myocardial tagging (Figure 1.19a). The behavior of the tagged magnetization has been measured in a phantom experiment and was characterized with numerical simulations for conditions used during breath-hold GRE imaging, where the results showed that the magnetization transition into steady state is reproducible after the first heartbeat (Reeder and McVeigh 1994). A segmented

k-space fast GRE pulse sequence has also been developed for high-quality cine imaging of the heart in a short scan time (Epstein et al. 1999).

1.20.2 Echo Planar Imaging

Echo planar imaging (EPI) has been used in myocardial tagging to improve tagging contrast, reduce scan time, and avoid misregistration artifacts from multiple breath-holds. EPI is capable of acquiring the same amount of data as in GRE, but in a much shorter scan time. Furthermore, the tagging contrast in EPI is higher than in GRE and permits tag visualization later in the cardiac cycle during diastole (Tang et al. 1995). Slice-following CSPAMM has been combined with segmented EPI to allow for a single breath-hold scan, where the developed sequence resulted in reliable assessment of both systolic and diastolic phases with high temporal resolution (Stuber et al. 1999b). Further, a hybrid EPI/GRE cardiac tagging sequence has been developed to improve SNR and imaging efficiency (Reeder et al. 1999). Nevertheless, although the hybrid EPI/GRE sequence improves the data acquisition efficiency and tagging contrast, off-resonance and motion artifacts may lead to local phase discontinuities in the raw data when conventional interleaved linear (bottom-up) k-space trajectory is used.

1.20.3 Steady State with Free Precession

The implementation of the balanced steady state with free precession (SSFP) pulse sequence in MRI tagging resulted in improved image quality (Herzka et al. 2003; Figure 1.19b). In SSFP, the remaining transverse magnetization after a certain data readout is not spoiled as in GRE imaging; it is rather reused during the following readouts to contribute to the formation of subsequent timeframes in the cardiac cycle. This is

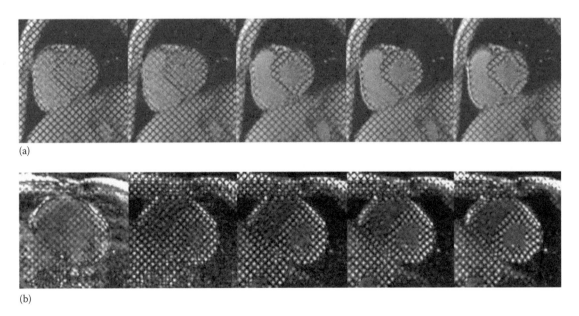

(a)

(b)

FIGURE 1.19 Two series of (a) gradient echo and (b) steady state with free precession short-axis spatial modulation of magnetization–tagged images acquired during early phases in the cardiac cycle. The images show difference in the tissue contrast and signal-to-noise ratio based on the implemented imaging sequence.

achieved by refocusing (balancing) the gradients in all three axes during each TR. SSFP proved to be valuable in cardiac imaging due to its high SNR and excellent myocardium–blood contrast. Nevertheless, the tagging preparation step creates a problem as it interrupts the established steady-state condition and results in severe ghosting artifacts. This problem has been solved using half the flip angle ($\alpha/2$) (Hargreaves et al. 2001, Scheffler et al. 2001) and linearly increasing start-up angles (LISA) (Zwanenburg et al. 2003) magnetization preparation techniques. The tagging fading problem with SSFP has been solved by Ibrahim et al. (2006) in a similar fashion to the ramped flip angle technique developed for the GRE sequence by Fischer et al. (1993). The improved tagging contrast and tag persistence with SSFP facilitate image postprocessing and enable access to the diastolic cardiac phase.

Recently, an SSFP-based phase-sensitive myocardial tagging sequence has been developed to resolve the problem of rectified inverted tags with conventional imaging sequences that leads to the appearance of false taglines in the magnitude-reconstructed images (Derbyshire et al. 2007). Using the phase associated with the tag signal peaks results in improved tagging contrast, which allows for using fully automated algorithms for tracking the taglines.

1.20.4   OTHER DATA ACQUISITION STRATEGIES

An alternative data acquisition strategy is to sample data along radial lines (or spokes) that cross the k-space origin (Peters et al. 2001). Radial sampling is more sensitive to B_0 field inhomogeneity, gradient timing delays, and gradient nonlinearity than Cartesian sampling. However, radial sampling has multiple attractive features for myocardial tagging, including robustness to respiratory motion and flow effects as well as tolerance to the streak-like artifacts in the case of radial undersampling.

Spiral acquisition is another data sampling strategy (Ryf et al. 2004), which has many advantages, including efficient signal sampling with a small number of excitations, reduced sensitivity to flow artifacts (due to the self-refocusing gradients), short TE, and isotropic spatial resolution. Due to its nature, the high-frequency data (k-space periphery) is sufficiently acquired in spiral imaging, which maintains the high spatial resolution needed for visualizing tagging details in the image.

Real-time acquisition of the tagged images is an important area of research, which is based on fast and continuous acquisition, reconstruction, and display of the tagged images with the operator's capability of intervening or altering image acquisition on the fly. Different techniques, including parallel imaging, nonrectilinear data sampling, partial k-space acquisition, reduced FOV, and view sharing, can be implemented to reduce data acquisition and image reconstruction times and improve temporal resolution.

1.21   TAGGING ANALYSIS

In CMR exams with tagging sequences, usually three sets of SAX-tagged images (covering basal, midventricular, and apical locations) and one set of four-chamber (4CH) tagged images are acquired for evaluating LV myocardial contractility. The tagged images are transferred to a computer system for processing and analysis. The basic idea behind all tagging analysis techniques is tracking the taglines and measuring the relative increase or decrease of their in-between distances from one timeframe to another to measure tissue strain. Various strain components are measured from the tagged images: circumferential and radial strains are measured from SAX images, while longitudinal strain is measured from 4CH images. The resulting strain curves show the myocardial contractility pattern during the cardiac cycle. Important cardiovascular parameters can be extracted from the resulting curves, for example, peak strain and its timing, which help in evaluating systolic function. Strain rate could be calculated by differentiating strain with respect to time, which provides useful information about diastolic function. Occasionally, ventricular torsion angle may be obtained by measuring the difference in circumferential tissue rotation between basal and apical SAX slices. Ventricular torsion could be helpful for providing information about the heart efficiency in ejecting blood during systole.

Different postprocessing techniques have been developed for extracting and tracking the taglines from the cine-tagged images (Bankman 2000). Table 1.2 shows a brief list of the major categories of tagging analysis techniques. The amount of postprocessing performed to analyze the tagged images ranges from simple visual inspection of tags deformation to exhaustive calculation of various strain components. Many efforts have been made to facilitate myocardial motion quantification from the tagged images. Semiautomatic methods for tracking tags deformation include active contour models, optical flow analysis, and template-matching techniques. The active contour methods depend on applying spline curves (snakes) that are semiautomatically fitted to the taglines through the implementation of internal and external energy forces. Optical flow analysis depends on tracking the tagging grid intersections, which have signal intensity minima, from one timeframe to another. Finally, template-matching techniques estimate tissue deformation by cross-correlating a predefined tagging pattern with that in the tagged images.

1.21.1   ACTIVE CONTOUR METHODS

As early as 1994, Guttman et al. proposed a template-matching method for detecting the taglines and an active contour method for extracting the myocardial contours (Guttman et al. 1994, Kraitchman et al. 1995). Based on this approach, a software package, called FindTags (Guttman et al. 1997), was created for tagline analysis; however, it required several hours to process one dataset. Another technique has also been developed for spatiotemporal tracking of grid-tagged images (Kumar and Goldgof 1994). Mainly, base (B)-spline curves have been used for representing the taglines (Figure 1.20). B-splines can describe multidimensional tag displacement and characterize myocardial deformation. The use of B-splines for representing the taglines has several advantages, including compact representation, parametric continuity, and local control of

TABLE 1.2

Major Categories of Tagging Analysis Techniques

Method	Characteristics	Advantages	Limitations
Active contour	Uses spline curves that are fitted to the taglines using multiple constraints	Intuitive approach; parametric continuity; local control of the curve shape	Long processing time; sensitive to weights of different constraint forces.
Optical flow	Tracks tagline intersections based on tagging contrast	Possibility for automatic processing; reduced processing time	Sensitive to image quality, especially tagging contrast.
Template matching	Cross correlates a predefined tagging pattern with the resulting images	Reduced processing time	Predefined assumptions must be met.
Sinusoidal analysis	Analyzes data into different frequency components	Decreased sensitivity to noise; high accuracy	Complicated data analysis.
Volumetric modeling	Analyzes a stack of parallel tagged images	3D tagging analysis; more automatic processing	Long processing time.
Finite-element modeling	Creates model tags, which define the taglines in the images	3D tagging analysis; reduced processing time	Measurements are not directly related to clinical understanding.
Statistical modeling	Uses statistical methods for estimating tagline deformation	3D capability; more intuitive and understandable parameters	Predefined assumptions; complicated processing.
3D active contour modeling	Uses 3D spline curves, fitted to the taglines in a set of parallel images	3D capability; high resolution; parametric continuity	Long processing time.

Source: Adapted from Ibrahim, El-S.H., *J. Cardiovasc. Magn. Reson.*, 13, 36, 2011.

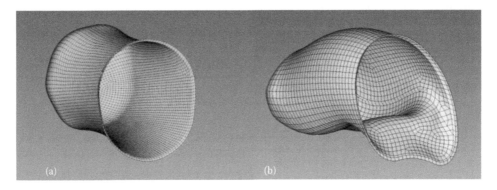

FIGURE 1.20 Example of B-spline approximation of the left ventricle (a) epicardium and (b) endocardium.

the spline shape. In 1998, Amini et al. (1998) used coupled B-spline grids for tracking tag deformations, where they described new techniques for efficient reconstruction of dense myocardial displacement from grid-tagged images. In another study by Ozturk and McVeigh (2000), a method was presented for describing the heart motion using a four-dimensional (4D) tensor product of B-splines on the tagged images.

1.21.2 Optical Flow Analysis

Optical flow techniques have been used in several studies for tracking myocardial tagging (Qian et al. 2006, Carranza-Herrezuelo et al. 2010, Florack and van Assen 2010). Shortly after the development of myocardial tagging, Prince and McVeigh (1992) presented an optical flow method for reconstructing motion from a sequence of MRI-tagged images. The developed method (variable brightness optical flow [VBOF]) was used for motion estimation with compensation for the tagging pattern decay. The developed VBOF method

was markedly superior to standard optical flow techniques for analyzing tagged images with decaying tagging contrast. A few years later, Dougherty et al. (1999) developed an optical flow method for rapid estimation of myocardial displacement from the tagged images. The developed method used a hierarchical estimation technique for computing the motion field that describes tissue displacement from one heart phase to the next one. Another contribution by Prince et al. (2000) came in 2000, where the authors developed a fast, fully automated optical flow method for tracking the tagging pattern by exploiting the Fourier content of the tagged images. The developed method worked by extracting various subband images from the acquired data, and then formulating multiple optical flow constraints for each subband. Another optical flow-based method, developed by Denney et al. (2003), used the maximum likelihood/maximum a posteriori technique for tag detection and strain calculation without applying user-defined contours, which significantly reduces the processing time.

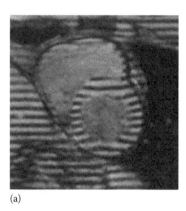
(a)

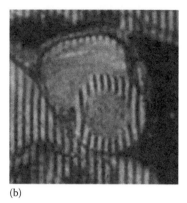
(b)

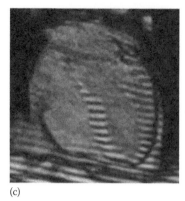
(c)

FIGURE 1.21   Myocardial tagging in three orthogonal orientations: (a) horizontal short-axis (SAX), (b) vertical SAX, and (c) horizontal 4CH tagging.

1.21.3   3D TAGGING ANALYSIS

Three-dimensional analysis of myocardial motion requires the presence of volumetric tagged data (Pipe et al. 1991, O'Dell et al. 1995, Denney and McVeigh 1997, Kuijer et al. 2000, Deng and Denney 2004, 2005). Usually, stacks of orthogonal SAX and long-axis (LAX) slices are combined to allow for tracking tagline deformation in 3D. Different methods have been developed for analyzing 3D myocardial motion. Each method has its advantages and disadvantages with respect to robustness, 3D interaction, computational complexity, and clinical interpretation. Therefore, there is always a trade-off between the temporal and spatial resolutions that each method offers, which makes method selection depend on the application at hand.

One way of measuring 3D myocardial deformation is by combining separate displacement fields fitted to orthogonal one-dimensional (1D) tagged images (Figure 1.21). This approach was adopted by O'Dell et al. (1995), who used three sets of orthogonal tagged images. The first and second sets consist of parallel SAX slices with horizontal and vertical tags, respectively, while the third set consists of 4CH slices with horizontal tags. Other methods for 3D myocardial motion analysis were later proposed (Deng and Denney 2004, 2005). For example, instead of tracking the taglines independently in each slice before reconstructing myocardial deformation, a 3D myocardial deformation model could be directly fitted to all tagged images, which ensures that the tag positions identified in the images are consistent from slice to slice.

1.21.3.1   Active Contours in 3D Tagging Analysis

The active contour techniques (Kerwin and Prince 1998, Huang et al. 1999, Amini et al. 2001, Wang et al. 2001, Tustison et al. 2003) have several advantages for processing 3D tagged images, including immediate generation of tag surfaces, subpixel accuracy of tagline localization, parametric continuity, and the ability to determine the location of a complete tag surface by assigning the location of few control points. Amini et al. (2001) presented several studies that used active contours for 3D analysis of myocardial deformations. For example, in Amini et al. (2001), efficient methods were described for encoding, visualization, and tracking 3D myocardial taglines in the heart from

two sets of orthogonal tagged MRI slices using 3D B-splines. In another study, a method was presented for using 4D B-splines to determine tagline intersections and myocardial strains (Tustison et al. 2003). The developed 4D B-spline model was specified by a 4D grid of control points to interpolate the tag information across space and across all continuous timepoints.

1.21.3.2   Finite-Element Modeling

Finite-element modeling (FEM) (Figure 1.22) is a typical choice for volumetric motion analysis since it analyzes motion throughout the ventricular wall (Young et al. 1996, Young 1999, Hu et al. 2003). Alistair Young (1999) presented the "Model tags" method, which has been developed for direct 3D myocardial tracking from the tagged images without prior identification of the ventricular boundaries or tagline locations. The method utilizes an FEM model to describe the heart shape and motion. Model tags are created as material surfaces, which define the location of the taglines. An objective function, of the difference between the model tags and image stripes, is derived and minimized to allow the model to deform to the taglines in the images. The proposed method significantly reduces the processing time compared to methods that separately track the taglines in each slice.

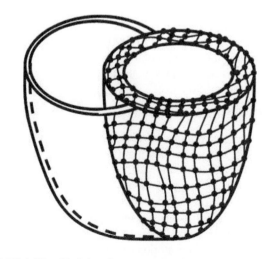

FIGURE 1.22   3D finite-element model of the heart.

1.22   HARP

Most approaches for MR tag analysis implement image processing techniques, for example, deformable models and matched filters, directly on the acquired images to detect and track the tagging pattern deformation during the cardiac cycle. Nevertheless, the long processing time of these techniques and lack of fast quantitative analysis and intuitive visualization mechanisms prevent conventional MRI tagging techniques from being widely adopted in the clinical setting. The HARP technique stands different from the aforementioned tagging analysis techniques as it is based on analyzing the signal in k-space instead of analyzing the image itself (Figure 1.23). HARP allows for rapid analysis and visualization of myocardial strain within few minutes, instead of hours with conventional image-based analysis techniques. Currently, HARP is the most widely used technique for tag analysis. The HARP software is commercially available and has been used worldwide in different research and clinical studies.

1.22.1   Basic Idea

HARP analysis is based on the fact that the tagging pattern modulates the underlying image with spectral peaks in the k-space at multiples of the tagging frequency. The idea in HARP is to isolate the signal peak at the harmonic frequency, which contains the tagging information. After applying Fourier transformation (FT), both harmonic magnitude and phase images can be obtained. The phase image shows intensity gradients interrupted by sharp transitions resulting from phase wrappings every 2π, while the magnitude image shows a blurred anatomical mask of the myocardium. When multiplied together, the phase and magnitude images produce a new image (the harmonic phase image), which is very similar to the original tagged image, as shown in Figure 1.23. As the HARP is a material property of the tagged tissue, the intensity pattern in the HARP image closely follows the tagging pattern in the tagged image. Myocardial motion can be, therefore, estimated by simply tracking (through consecutive time-frames) the phase of the point of interest in a small region of interest (ROI) around it after phase wrapping correction. The analysis criterion implemented in HARP allows for automatic and fast analysis of the tagged images. Since its introduction, HARP underwent a series of improvements, either from the data acquisition or image analysis perspectives, which resulted in enhanced tagline tracking, reduced processing time, real-time image acquisition and analysis (Sampath et al. 2003, Abd-Elmoniem et al. 2007), improved image quality (SNR, spatial resolution, or temporal resolution), increased tagging density, 3D strain analysis capability (Abd-Elmoniem et al. 2005, Pan et al. 2005), and reduced imaging artifacts.

1.22.2   Validation

Different studies have been conducted to evaluate the HARP performance compared to conventional tag analysis techniques

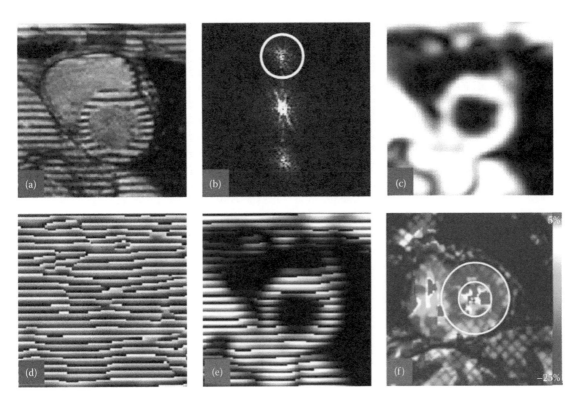

FIGURE 1.23   Harmonic phase (HARP) analysis. (a) Original tagged image. (b) K-space of the image. (c) Magnitude-reconstructed image of the first harmonic peak (inside circle in (b)). (d) Phase-reconstructed image of the first harmonic peak. (e) Harmonic-phase (HARP) image obtained by multiplying the images in (c) and (d). (e) A representative grid-tagged image analyzed with HARP, showing color-coded circumferential strain. (Reproduced from Ibrahim, El-S.H., *J. Cardiovasc. Magn. Reson.*, 13, 36, 2011.)

(Guttman et al. 1994, 1997). Garot et al. (2000) investigated the accuracy of HARP for rapid quantification of myocardial strain in postinfarct patients and volunteers at rest and during dobutamine stress. The results showed that HARP accurately detects subtle changes in myocardial strain under increasing dobutamine doses. As HARP analysis takes only few minutes, it is well suited for studying dynamic changes in regional LV function through consecutive follow-up scans. HARP analysis showed high degree of reproducibility as shown in a study on 441 consecutive exams in the Multi-Center Study of Atherosclerosis (MESA) study (Castillo et al. 2005), where HARP measurements showed excellent inter- and intraobserver agreements for peak systolic strain data and all systolic pooled data.

1.23 DENSE

1.23.1 Basic Idea and Advantages

DENSE provides an assessment of intramyocardial motion similar to other MRI tagging techniques; however, it measures myocardial motion in a fundamentally different way. Instead of visualizing or detecting the taglines or tagging grid, DENSE directly encodes the tissue displacement into the phase of the generated stimulated echo signal and displays the displacement-encoded phase. By encoding tissue displacement directly into the image phase, DENSE obviates the need for tags detection, simplifying quantitation of intramyocardial motion. DENSE reveals motion information on the pixel level by displaying a small vector at each pixel location (Figure 1.24). The vector orientation and length represent the motion direction and magnitude, respectively. One advantage of DENSE is that it is a black-blood sequence due to the disturbance of the modulated magnetization pattern in the blood pool during the mixing time (TM) in-between magnetization modulation and data acquisition, which facilitates myocardial border identification.

1.23.2 Concept of Work

Similar to HARP, DENSE was introduced in 1999 to measure tissue motion from the phase data (Aletras et al. 1999b). However, DENSE evolved as a stimulated echo acquisition mode (STEAM) pulse sequence (Frahm et al. 1985) with displacement encoded in the signal phase in contrast to HARP, which is directly associated with conventional tagging. In fact, although HARP and DENSE were separately developed and presented from different perspectives, they have more similarities than differences, and they represent two sides of the same coin. In their interesting article, Kuijer et al. (2006) evaluated and compared the two techniques as two approaches to phase-based strain analysis.

As a STEAM-based technique, the DENSE pulse sequence consists of three stages: modulation, mixing, and demodulation. During the modulation part of the sequence, the longitudinal magnetization is tipped into the transverse plane, encoded with a modulation gradient, and then stored back into the longitudinal direction until imaging (data acquisition) takes place. Magnetization storage in the longitudinal direction allows for less relaxation and more tagging persistence due to the much longer T1 of the myocardium compared to T2. Tissue displacement occurring during TM is retrieved later in the imaging stage. During imaging, the modulated magnetization is excited (tipped into the transverse plane) and decoded using a gradient with the same magnitude as the modulation gradient. Stationary spins are perfectly rewound and have zero net phase. However, spins that moved (in the direction of the implemented gradient) during TM accumulate phase due to their different spatial positions during modulation and demodulation. By acquiring another DENSE image with different displacement-encoding value and subtracting the two phase images, displacement information in the gradient direction can be obtained.

1.23.3 Developments

The fundamental idea underlying the DENSE method was initially demonstrated by Aletras et al. (1999a,b), when they demonstrated the ability to quantify 2D end-diastolic to end-systolic myocardial displacement from the phase of the stimulated echo signal. Five years later, Epstein and Gilson (2004) presented multiphase, or cine, DENSE, demonstrating for the first time the ability to measure time-varying motion of the heart using serial measurements of the phase of the stimulated echo. Over the subsequent decade, different versions of DENSE have been

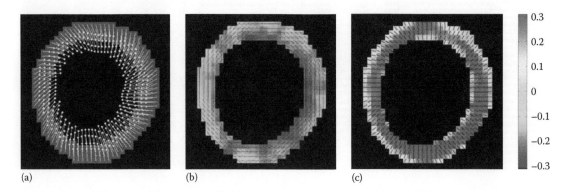

(a)   (b)   (c)

FIGURE 1.24 Displacement encoding with stimulated echoes (DENSE) short-axis images, showing (a) 2D end-diastolic to end-systolic displacement map. (b) Second principal strain. (c) First principal strain. (Reproduced from Epstein, F.H., *J. Nucl. Cardiol.*, 14(5), 729, 2007. With permission.)

developed to increase SNR (Aletras and Wen 2001), reduce artifacts, generate 3D data, and acquire composite data (e.g., simultaneous acquisition of strain and viability or perfusion data). Efforts have been also made to investigate the advantages and disadvantages of different displacement-encoding strategies, develop important postprocessing algorithms for phase unwrapping and motion estimation, and elucidate the physical and mathematical relationships between DENSE, conventional tagging, and HARP techniques. Myocardial and skeletal muscle mechanics measured by DENSE showed to be in good agreement with those from other tagging techniques (Feng et al. 2009), with the advantages that DENSE imaging can be performed with less user intervention and the resulting resolution of the calculated strain map is higher than in conventional tagging.

Presently, DENSE remains predominantly a research method, as studies that may prove the clinical utility of DENSE are underway, but not yet complete. However, the fundamental properties of DENSE coupled with promising, but limited, initial clinical results suggest that DENSE may become a widely used method for quantitative imaging of myocardial function. Promising applications of DENSE, and of quantitative myocardial motion imaging in general, include imaging cardiac dyssynchrony in heart failure patients considered for CRT, detecting ischemia during stress testing, and evaluating the effects of novel experimental therapies for myocardial infarction or heart failure, for example, stem-cell implantation and injectable biomaterials. With continued development and more successful clinical studies, DENSE may soon be available for routine and widespread clinical use.

1.24 SENC

1.24.1 BASIC IDEA AND ADVANTAGES

SENC is a recently developed CMR technique for measuring myocardial strain (Osman et al. 2001). SENC is similar to DENSE in that it is based on a STEAM pulse sequence. However, in contrast to DENSE, the strain information in SENC is obtained from the magnitude images, not from the phase images. SENC has the advantages of measuring

high-resolution strain (on the pixel level) with simple post-processing. A color-coded image is obtained that shows a through-plane strain map. Similar to DENSE, SENC is a black-blood sequence because of the destruction of the tagging pattern in the blood pool during the time in-between tagging application and imaging.

1.24.2 CONCEPT OF WORK

SENC evolved from a tagging perspective, rather than from a STEAM perspective as in DENSE. However, in contrast to conventional tagging sequences, tagging in SENC is applied in the through-plane direction, which creates a stack of magnetization-saturated planes that lie inside, and parallel to, the image plane. During the cardiac cycle, these parallel tagged planes move closer together or further apart based on tissue contraction or stretching, respectively, in the through-plane direction, which affects the tagging (modulation) frequency. At the imaging timepoint, different images are acquired with different demodulation (tuning) values. Usually, two images are acquired, which are called low-tuning (LT) and high-tuning (HT) images. The LT image is acquired at a frequency close to the applied tagging frequency to capture signals from static (noncontracting) tissues. On the other hand, the HT image is acquired at a higher frequency (calculated based on the prescribed slice thickness, applied tagging frequency, and expected strain range) to capture signals from contracting tissues. By a simple combination of the information from the LT and HT images, a color-coded strain map is obtained that shows strain values on the pixel level (Figure 1.25). Because through-plane strain is measured in SENC, SAX and LAX images show longitudinal and circumferential strains, respectively.

1.24.3 DEVELOPMENTS

Similar to HARP and DENSE, SENC underwent several developments. Slice-following SENC (sf-SENC) was created by combining the slice-following technique with SENC imaging (Fahmy et al. 2006b). As in slice-following CSPAMM, a thin slice is tagged (in the z-direction) during

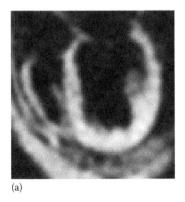 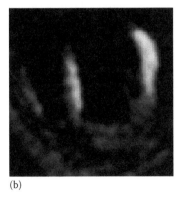 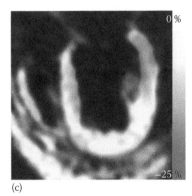

(a)   (b)   (c)

FIGURE 1.25 Strain encoding (SENC) images, showing (a) low-tuning (LT) image (showing noncontracting tissues), (b) high-tuning (HT) image (showing contracting tissues), and (c) SENC color-coded circumferential strain map (note strain loss in the apex). (Reproduced from Ibrahim, El-S.H., *J. Cardiovasc. Magn. Reson.*, 13, 36, 2011.)

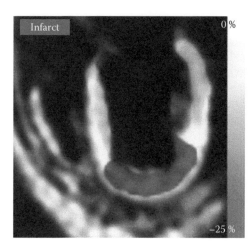

FIGURE 1.26 C-SENC image, showing infarct (in blue), superimposed on a color-coded strain map. (Reproduced from Ibrahim, El-S.H., *J. Cardiovasc. Magn. Reson.*, 13, 36, 2011.)

the modulation stage, followed by excitation of a thicker slice during imaging. The advantage of sf-SENC is that it allows for imaging the same myocardial tissue throughout the cardiac cycle. In another development, the fast-SENC technique was presented, which is a real-time version of SENC (Pan et al. 2006). Fast-SENC allows for real-time strain imaging, which is necessary for certain applications, for example, during contrast injection, dynamic imaging, or intervention CMR. Fast-SENC has been evaluated at 3.0 T and showed that the information derived from the fast-SENC images is equal to that measured from conventional tagging with prolonged breath-holds (Korosoglou et al. 2008). Ibrahim et al. (2007a) combined the features of slice-following and real-time imaging with SENC by developing the slice-following fast-SENC (sf-fast-SENC) technique.

Another contribution by Ibrahim et al. (2007b) is composite SENC (C-SENC), which acquires both myocardial strain and viability information in the same scan. The C-SENC sequence is applied 10–15 minutes after gadolinium (Gd) injection; therefore, it shows bright infarction due to shortened T1, secondary to Gd accumulation in the infarcted tissue. C-SENC results in a composite image that shows both myocardial function and viability information (Figure 1.26). As all information is acquired at approximately the same time, no artifacts are introduced from image misregistration. Another SENC development was presented by Basha et al. (2009) to improve SENC SNR by combining it with SSFP imaging. The results showed that combining SENC with SSFP results in more accurate results than with GRE. Other SENC developments include 3D implementation and combination with other techniques for composite data acquisition (Hess et al. 2009, Sampath et al. 2009).

1.24.4 APPLICATIONS

From the applications point of view, SENC is not only used to image myocardial strain but can also be used to generate black-blood cine images of the heart to estimate global

heart function (Fahmy et al. 2006b). In addition, recent studies showed that SENC is effective for detecting stiff masses (Osman 2003, Fahmy et al. 2006a, Harouni et al. 2011). Garot et al. (2004) compared SENC to conventional 3D tagging for measuring longitudinal strain in healthy volunteers and patients with myocardial infarction. The results showed strong correlation between the strain measurements from the two techniques despite the big difference in postprocessing time and spatial resolution (6–8 hour processing time and 7–8 mm resolution with conventional 3D tagging versus 30 seconds processing time and 2 mm resolution with SENC).

1.25 TISSUE PHASE MAPPING

1.25.1 BASIC IDEA

In the mid-1990s, efforts have been made for measuring myocardial motion based on cine phase-contrast (PC) acquisition (Wedeen 1992, Pelc et al. 1994, 1995, McVeigh 1996, Zhu et al. 1996, 1997). In the last decade, PC-based techniques for measuring myocardial deformation focused on the evaluation of highly time-resolved velocities (Markl et al. 2002, Jung et al. 2006, Petersen et al. 2006, Delfino et al. 2008, Foll et al. 2010). McVeigh (1996) and Masood et al. (2000) published two interesting review articles comparing tagging and PC-based TPM techniques for measuring heart mechanics.

TPM is based on the fact that the generated MR signal is a vector quantity that contains both magnitude and phase. As a consequence, from any acquired MRI dataset, separate magnitude and phase images can be reconstructed. The idea in TPM is to encode velocity in the signal phase by adding a bipolar gradient (in the direction of motion) before data readout, such that the phase image can be used for measuring tissue velocity (Figure 1.27). In order to compensate for unwanted background phase in the image, a separate unencoded reference image is acquired, such that upon subtraction from the velocity-encoded image, true measurement of tissue motion can be estimated. Therefore, 3D velocity-encoding imaging requires at least four scans, the reference scan and velocity-encoded scans with bipolar gradients along the readout, phase-encoding, and slice-selection directions. Therefore, TPM is characterized by relatively long scan times, a typical drawback of PC imaging.

1.25.2 PRACTICAL CONSIDERATIONS

The velocities of myocardial motion are smaller by about an order of magnitude compared to blood flow velocities in the great vessels. Therefore, the velocity-encoding parameter in the scan protocol (*venc*) has to be adapted accordingly. Since longitudinal myocardial motion shows higher velocities than in-plane velocities, the optimal *venc* setting is about 25–30 cm/s in the longitudinal direction and 15–20 cm/s in the in-plane directions. If the *venc* value is set lower than the maximum velocity during the cardiac cycle, aliasing can be observed in the resulting images. Another point to be considered in TPM is that artifacts can occur due to fast-flowing

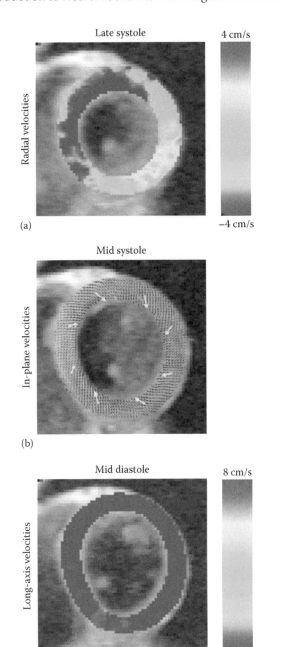

FIGURE 1.27 Tissue phase mapping (TPM) images showing (a) radial, (b) circumferential, and (c) longitudinal strains in a short-axis slice. The arrows' length and orientation in (b) represent transverse velocity's magnitude and direction, respectively, at different segments.

blood within the heart chambers, which may affect the resulting measurements. Therefore, the signal from blood should be suppressed using black-blood imaging or any other technique. As TPM requires a long scan time, temporal and spatial resolutions are limited by the patient's breath-holding capability. To increase the temporal resolution or decrease scan time, several techniques can be implemented, for example, multi-echo imaging, view sharing, and parallel imaging.

Due to the comprehensive nature of the data generated from TPM imaging (different velocity components, temporal domain, imaging of different slices, segmental cardiac analysis, and different velocity parameters), data visualization plays an important role in TPM. The ultimate goal of the postprocessing stage is to provide parameters that can be used for characterizing the functional performance of the heart and improving diagnosis of patients with functional deficits.

1.26 MR ELASTOGRAPHY

MRE is a recently developed noninvasive imaging technique for obtaining in vivo data about biomechanical tissue properties. With manual palpation being an integral part of many diagnostic procedures, it is obvious that elasticity imaging has many interesting and promising potentials in medical imaging. The general concept of MRE is sending low-frequency mechanical waves into the object and imaging those waves via MRI-motion-sensitized sequences (Figure 1.28). This allows for locally solving the stress–strain relationship and measuring the complex-valued shear modulus. Since the viscoelastic tissue properties change strongly with frequency, care must be taken when interpreting the data in terms of elastic and viscous components.

1.26.1 HISTORICAL BACKGROUND

Lewa (1994) was the first to propose using MRI for detecting propagating mechanical waves in tissue. This development accumulated shortly after in a *Science* publication for the visualization of propagating shear waves via MRI (Muthupillai et al. 1995), which triggered the formation of a steadily growing MRE community with different imaging approaches and methods for reconstructing the shear modulus (Plewes et al. 1995, Chenevert et al. 1998, Van Houten et al. 1999, Sinkus et al. 2000). Meanwhile, elastography has been applied to many organs and pathologies, including breast cancer (Sinkus et al. 2000, 2007, McKnight et al. 2002), brain tumors and neurodegenerative diseases (Xu et al. 2007, Wuerfel et al. 2010, Schregel et al. 2012), liver fibrosis (Huwart et al. 2006, 2008, Rouviere et al. 2006), and the heart (Sack et al. 2009). MRE has the advantage of volumetric data acquisition with equal motion sensitivity in all three directions compared to ultrasound elastography. Nevertheless, its disadvantages are the lack of real-time capability and relatively high costs. However, these drawbacks are counterweighted by the high SNR and ability to combine biomechanical information with other physical parameters acquired with other sequences during the MRI exam.

1.26.2 BASIC IDEA

The MRE pulse sequence is similar to a classical MRI diffusion-weighted imaging (DWI) sequence. Nevertheless, the main difference between the two techniques is that in MRE, the acquisition time is controlled by the generation of external waves, in contrast to passively observing the random motion of the water molecules in DWI. Hence, in MRE, the phase data are used for estimating elasticity, which considerably increases the

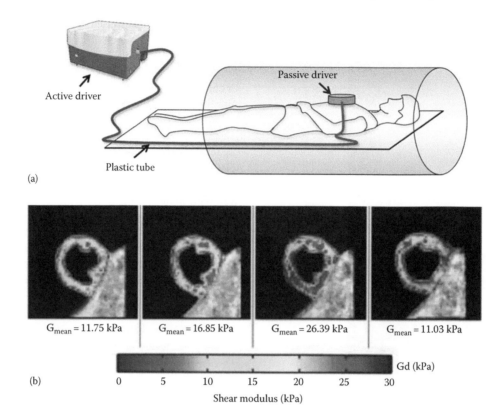

FIGURE 1.28 MR elastography (MRE) setup and results. (a) Experimental setup of an MRE experiment. (Reproduced from Wassenaar, P.A. et al., *Magn. Reson. Med.*, 75(4), 1586, 2016.) (b) Temporal evolution (different time points, 100 ms apart, during diastole) of the shear modulus during the cardiac cycle in a volunteer, as estimated by MRE. Apparently, the myocardium stiffens from the beginning until end diastole and appears to relax just before systole. (Reproduced from Robert, B. et al., Application of DENSE MR-elastography to the human heart: First in vivo results, *Proceedings of the International Society of Magnetic Resonance in Medicine*, Honolulu, HI, 2009b. With permission.)

motion detection sensitivity down to the micron level, depending on the strength of the applied gradients (Muthupillai et al. 1996). Reconstructed MRE shear moduli data have been extensively compared to FEM simulations (Sinkus et al. 2000, Litwiller et al. 2010), phantom data (Ringleb et al. 2005, Sinkus et al. 2005), and data obtained from rheometers (Hamhaber et al. 2003, Vappou et al. 2007, Chatelin et al. 2011). Overall, there is a good agreement for the real part, but to a lesser extent for the imaginary part, as expected from theoretical considerations.

1.26.3 CARDIAC MR ELASTOGRAPHY

MRE in the heart is important because mechanical integrity of the myocardium is a crucial determinant of the overall heart function, where the myocardial mechanical properties are affected by the existence of diseases or changes in the cardiovascular system, especially in the case of heart failure. The symptoms of HFNEF (or the "stiff heart syndrome") represent 35%–55% of the heart failure patients. In this context, the developed diastolic dysfunction is related to changes in the myocardial compliance, and hence to an alteration of its viscoelastic properties (Kitzman et al. 2001). Most probably, the excessively high workload due to the increased myocardial stiffness during the chamber filling is responsible for this condition. Thus, while LVEF remains normal, the required energy for filling the heart is too high and leads at certain point to heart failure. Nevertheless, it should be

noted that adapting the MRE sequences to image the heart raises several challenges. First, TE must be short in order to cope with the short T2 value of the myocardium. Second, due to viscosity, which increases strongly with frequency, it is difficult for the generated waves to reach the heart using externally applied mechanical drivers with high frequencies (>100 Hz), which enforces the implementation of dedicated sequences to cope with these constraints (Rump et al. 2007, Robert et al. 2009a).

In cardiac triggered MRE, the R-wave of the ECG is used to start mechanical vibration with a mechanical transducer pressed against the chest. Either continuous cine-type data acquisitions (Elgeti et al. 2008, Kolipaka et al. 2009a,b) or multiple acquisitions after a fixed delay relative to the R-wave (Robert et al. 2009a) are feasible. The essential, and hence critical, aspect here is the reproducibility of the paradigm. Typically, the induced mechanical vibrations are terminated before systole and then resynchronized with the MRE data acquisition in the next cardiac cycle in order to compensate for the inevitable temporal jitter in the duration of the cardiac cycle.

1.26.4 CURRENT STATUS AND FUTURE DIRECTIONS

In general, MRE is a promising new technique for noninvasive assessment of biomechanical properties. Many research groups worldwide are investigating the diagnostic potential of viscoelastic, poroelastic, nonlinear, and compressional

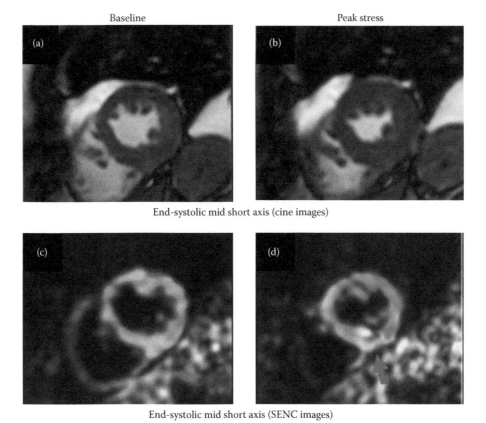

parameters for disease characterization. Compared to strain imaging, MRE has the profound advantage of providing truly intrinsic material parameters. This is possible because in MRE the stress–strain relationship can be solved locally due to the presence of externally imposed low-frequency shear waves. MRE application in the heart is rather challenging due to SNR and resolution issues, rendering the reconstruction process of the complex-valued shear modulus nontrivial. First results with simplified analysis methods demonstrate however a good potential for this method. Different cardiac applications are possible, for example, characterization of fibrosis, evaluation of scar tissue after an infarct, assessment of cardiac viability, and study of myocardial contractility under different conditions. So far, mainly the relationships between nonlinear elastic tissue properties and invasive pressure measurements have been studied. As expected, good correlation is typically found on the individual level between pressure and stiffness. However, many technical challenges still need to be addressed before MRE becomes a clinical tool for cardiac imaging.

1.27 APPLICATIONS OF HEART MECHANICS WITH MRI

Myocardial tagging techniques have been used in several clinical and research studies (Figures 1.29 and 1.30). They have been used for measuring regional LV function (Clark et al.

1991, McKinnon et al. 1991, Rogers et al. 1991, Azhari et al. 1993, Young et al. 1994a, Naito et al. 1995, Matter et al. 1996, Park et al. 1996, Chai et al. 1997, MacGowan et al. 1997, Power et al. 1997, Klein et al. 1998, Clarysse et al. 2000, Moore et al. 2000, O'Dell and McCulloch 2000, Bogaert and Rademakers 2001, Saber and Wen 2004, Rodriguez et al. 2006, Hamdan et al. 2009, Phatak et al. 2009, Cupps et al. 2010), RV contractility pattern (Dong et al. 1995, Naito et al. 1995, Young et al. 1996, Fayad et al. 1998, Klein et al. 1998, Kurotobi et al. 1998, Haber et al. 2000, Hu et al. 2003, Vonk-Noordegraaf et al. 2005, Hamdan et al. 2008, Youssef et al. 2008), heart rotation and torsion (Azhari et al. 1992, Kroeker et al. 1995, Dong et al. 1999, 2001, Stuber et al. 1999a, Lorenz et al. 2000, Nagel et al. 2000, Garot et al. 2002, Sandstede et al. 2002, Setser et al. 2003a, Kanzaki et al. 2006), aging effect on the heart function (Fonseca et al. 2003, Oxenham et al. 2003, Castillo et al. 2005), CAD (Castillo et al. 2005, Edvardsen et al. 2006a, Fernandes et al. 2006), ischemic heart disease (Prinzen et al. 1989, Kroeker et al. 1995, Geskin et al. 1998, Kraitchman et al. 1998, 2003, Sayad et al. 1998, Rogers et al. 1999, Scott et al. 1999, Gerber et al. 2002, Kramer et al. 2002b, Kuijpers et al. 2003, Samady et al. 2004, Paetsch et al. 2005, Bree et al. 2006, Rosen et al. 2006, Soler et al. 2006, Korosoglou et al. 2009, 2010), myocardial infarction (MI) (Gallagher et al. 1982, Kramer et al. 1993, 1996, 2000, Chen et al. 1995, Lima et al. 1995, Marcus et al. 1997, Geskin et al. 1998, Croisille et al. 1999, Gotte et al. 1999, 2001,

FIGURE 1.29 SENC images (c, diastole; d, systole) aid in the detection of inducible myocardial ischemia in the inferior left ventricle wall (arrow), which was missed by conventional cine imaging (a, base line; b, peak stress).

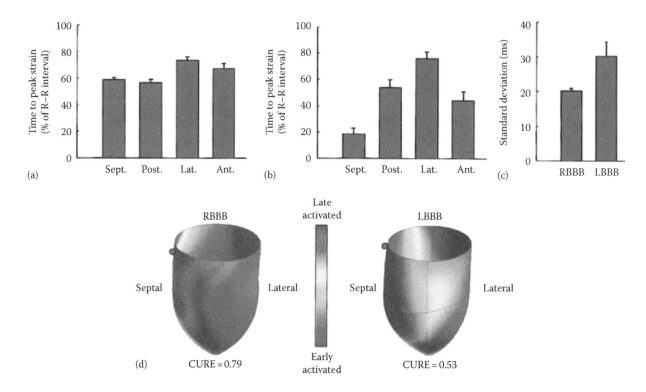

FIGURE 1.30 Comparison of regional and global strain in failing hearts with right bundle branch block (RBBB) and left bundle branch block (LBBB). Time-to-peak strain as percentage of the R–R interval in (a) RBBB heart failure and (b) LBBB heart failure. (c) Standard deviation of time-to-peak strain in RBBB heart failure and LBBB heart failure. (d) Examples of mechanical activation delay maps in RBBB and LBBB. (Reproduced from Byrne, M.J. et al., *J. Am. Coll. Cardiol.*, 50(15), 1484, 2007. With permission.)

Bogaert et al. 2000, Gerber et al. 2000, Nagel et al. 2000, Garot et al. 2002, Heijman et al. 2004, Ashikaga et al. 2005, Gilson et al. 2005, Aletras et al. 2006, Ivancevic et al. 2007, Neizel et al. 2009b, Inoue et al. 2010), dilated cardiomyopathy (DCM) (MacGowan et al. 1997, Curry et al. 2000, Nelson et al. 2000, Young et al. 2001, Setser et al. 2003b, Ashford et al. 2005, Kanzaki et al. 2006), hypertrophic cardiomyopathy (HCM) (Maier et al. 1992, Dong et al. 1994, 1995, Kramer et al. 1994, Young et al. 1994b, Beache et al. 1995, Kurotobi et al. 1998, Mishiro et al. 1999, Bergey and Axel 2000, Haber et al. 2000, Ennis et al. 2003, Edvardsen et al. 2006b, Soler et al. 2006, Kim et al. 2008), interventricular dyssynchrony (McVeigh et al. 1998, Mishiro et al. 1999, Wyman et al. 1999, Curry et al. 2000, Nelson et al. 2000, Pusca et al. 2000, Zwanenburg et al. 2004, 2005, Helm et al. 2005, Lardo et al. 2005, Vonk-Noordegraaf et al. 2005, Hamdan et al. 2009), valvular diseases (Villari et al. 1993, Ungacta et al. 1998, Stuber et al. 1999a, Sandstede et al. 2002), congenital heart diseases (Fogel et al. 1995b, 1996, 1998, Donofrio et al. 1999, Pilla et al. 2002), postsurgery cardiac function evaluation (Donofrio et al. 1999, Wyman et al. 1999, Pusca et al. 2000, Pilla et al. 2002), myocardial elasticity (Osman 2003, Wen et al. 2005, Robert et al. 2009a), and other heart diseases (Kojima et al. 1999, Blom et al. 2000, Kramer et al. 2002a, Rosen et al. 2006, Fernandes et al. 2008, Spottiswoode et al. 2008a, Nasiraei-Moghaddam and Gharib 2009). The following is a brief overview of key studies that implemented MRI techniques for measuring heart mechanics in clinical

applications. Detailed and full coverage of the clinical applications and findings of heart mechanics by MRI is presented in Chapters 9 and 10 of *Heart Mechanics: Magnetic Resonance Imaging—Advanced Techniques, Clinical Applications, and Future Trends*.

1.27.1 REGIONAL LV FUNCTION

As early as 1991, Clark et al. (1991) showed the presence of transmural and longitudinal heterogeneity of circumferential shortening in the normal human LV. Subsequent studies confirmed these results and showed that regional myocardial function is heterogeneous and location dependent in the normal heart (Azhari et al. 1993, Bogaert and Rademakers 2001). In 1995, Naito et al. (1995) showed that the heterogeneity of myocardial contractility is closely correlated with the myocardial fiber architecture. Two years later, MacGowan et al. (1997) measured normal fiber shortening in the LV, where the average value was 15%. In 2000, Clarysse et al. (2000) used MRI tagging to model spatiotemporal myocardial displacement in the normal heart. Other investigators used 3D tagging to study LV regional function (Park et al. 1996, Moore et al. 2000, O'Dell and McCulloch 2000). Advanced tagging techniques have also been used for generating LV myocardial strain maps (Saber and Wen 2004, Hamdan et al. 2009, Phatak et al. 2009). In 2006, Rodriguez et al. (2006) were able to calculate tissue volume change with 1% precision using myocardial tagging. Subsequently, Cupps et al. (2010)

tested the capability of multiparametric strain analysis for optimizing the quantification of regional and transmural myocardial contractile function. Recently, Nasiraei-Moghaddam and Gharib (2009) used MRI tagging to show the presence of helical myocardial architecture in the LV. The aging effect on myocardial LV function has also been studied using MRI tagging (Fonseca et al. 2003, Oxenham et al. 2003, Castillo et al. 2005). Although strain and strain rate are the mostly studied variables using MRI tagging, several studies investigated the wringing (torsion) motion of the heart. In 1993, Azhari et al. (1993) studied myocardial transmural twist using MRI tagging. Another important study came out in 2000, in which Lorenz et al. (2000) studied normal human LV twist throughout systole using MRI tagging.

1.27.2 REGIONAL RV FUNCTION

Despite the complex shape and thin wall of the RV, which make it challenging to study its regional function, RV was the subject of many CMR studies in order to better understand how it works. In 1995, Naito et al. (1995) conducted a study to quantitate the contraction of the RV free wall and identify its normal performance compared to the LV. One year later, Young et al. (1996) used MRI tagging to reconstruct 3D RV motion. A key study then came out in 1998 by Fayad et al. (1998), in which the investigators compared regional variation of the RV free wall and interventricular septum in normal subjects and patients with pulmonary hypertension. Another study was presented 2 years later, in which RV motion was analyzed in normal volunteers and patients with RV hypertrophy (Haber et al. 2000). Recently, two studies were conducted, in which regional RV function was assessed using SENC (Hamdan et al. 2008, Youssef et al. 2008).

1.27.3 ISCHEMIC HEART DISEASE

Out of the importance of studying CAD for better understanding the disease pathophysiology, the MESA study was initiated in 2000 to examine the predominance and advancement of subclinical CVD. Using MRI tagging, different investigators studied the relationship between regional heart function and atherosclerosis risk factors, where important results have been presented (Edvardsen et al. 2006a, Fernandes et al. 2006). Several other studies have been conducted, in which MRI tagging was used to study myocardial function in the presence of ischemia. As early as 1989, Prinzen et al. (1989) used MRI to investigate the relationship between myocardial blood flow and fiber shortening in the ischemic border zone. Later, Kroeker et al. (1995) showed that ischemia has profound effects on the dynamics of apical rotation, a finding that was confirmed later by Garot et al. (2002). In 1998, three articles were published that described the importance of combining tagging with perfusion for evaluating ischemic heart disease (Geskin et al. 1998, Kraitchman et al. 1998, Sayad et al. 1998). In 1999, Scott et al. (1999) used MRI tagging to study the effect of dobutamine on regional LV function. In the same year, Rogers et al. (1999) showed that early

contrast-enhanced CMR predicts late functional recovery after reperfused MI. An important study came out in 2003, in which Kuijpers et al. (2003) showed that stress CMR with myocardial tagging could more reliably detect confirmed new wall motion abnormalities than does stress CMR alone. In the same year, Kraitchman et al. (2003) used HARP for detecting ischemia onset during stress imaging. Later, Samady et al. (2004) showed that electromechanical mapping parameters can identify segments that show improved function and retain contractile reserve early after revascularization. Furthermore, Paetsch et al. (2005) showed that the use of myocardial tagging may reduce the need for high-dose dobutamine stress in stress perfusion scans. Another study showed that lower myocardial flow reserve is related to reduced regional function in asymptomatic individuals (Rosen et al. 2006). Recently, two studies were conducted, in which SENC has been used for detecting inducible ischemia during dobutamine stress scans (Korosoglou et al. 2009, 2010).

1.27.4 MYOCARDIAL INFARCTION

In 2001, Gotte et al. (2001) showed that strain analysis is more accurate than wall thickness analysis for discriminating dysfunctional from functional myocardium. In another study, the investigators showed that LV dilatation and eccentric hypertrophy during remodeling are associated with persistent differences in segmental function between the adjacent and remote noninfarcted regions (Kramer et al. 1993). In 1995, Lima et al. (1995) showed that nonreperfused transmural myocardial infarction is characterized by marked reduction and reorientation of principal strains. In the same year, Chen et al. (1995) used SPAMM tagging for detecting regional MI. More detailed information about myocardial kinematics after MI has been presented by Kramer et al. (1996). An important study then came out in 1997, where the investigators showed that early after MI, regions with dysfunction, normal function, and hyperfunction can be delineated using MRI tagging (Marcus et al. 1997). Two years later, two studies were published, which showed the capability of strain mapping of characterizing ischemic injury (Croisille et al. 1999, Gotte et al. 1999). Regional myocardial function has also been studied in the regions around the infarcted zone (Bogaert et al. 2000, Gerber et al. 2000, Kramer et al. 2000, Inoue et al. 2010). Recently, advanced tagging techniques have been used to examine regional myocardial function in the presence of MI (Ashikaga et al. 2005, Aletras et al. 2006, Ivancevic et al. 2007, Neizel et al. 2009a,b). MRI tagging has also been used to investigate the effect of passive constraints on akinetic area development secondary to acute MI (Pilla et al. 2002). Besides studying human subjects, a number of studies investigated the difference between regional myocardial function in healthy and infarcted animal models (Heijman et al. 2004, Ivancevic et al. 2007).

1.27.5 DILATED AND HYPERTROPHIC CARDIOMYOPATHIES

In 1997, MacGowan et al. (1997) showed that normal fiber shortening is about 15% and this value is markedly reduced in DCM. Two studies came out in 2000 to study mechanical dyssynchrony in DCM (Curry et al. 2000, Nelson et al. 2000). Later, Young et al. (2001) showed that DCM is characterized by a consistent pattern of regional myocardial strain heterogeneity. Two other studies used MRI tagging to examine the systolic torsion pattern in DCM (Setser et al. 2003a, Kanzaki et al. 2006).

In 1992, Maier et al. (1992) observed reduced cardiac rotation in patients with HCM, mainly in the posterior region. Similar results were reported in Kramer et al. (1994) and Young et al. (1994b). In 1994, Dong et al. (1994) reported that the myocardium in patients with HCM is heterogeneously thickened compared to healthy subjects. In 1995, Beache et al. (1995) showed that strain rate characterization provides an objective measure of the disease course in HCM. Later, Mishiro et al. (1999) found that systolic LV wall asynchrony occurs in patients with HCM. In 2000, Bergey and Axel (2000) used MRI tagging to correctly diagnose focal HCM simulating a cardiac mass. Later, two studies confirmed the existence of impaired diastolic function in HCM (Ennis et al. 2003, Edvardsen et al. 2006b). Recently, Kim et al. (2008) showed that impaired circumferential shortening occurs in delayed hyperenhancement areas in HCM.

1.27.6 INTERVENTRICULAR DYSSYNCHRONY

In 1998, McVeigh et al. (1998) used MRI tagging to image asynchronous mechanical activation of the paced heart. In a related work, Wyman et al. (1999) studied the effect of pacing site on mechanical activation pattern using myocardial tagging. In 2000, Pusca et al. (2000) assessed the effect of synchronized direct mechanical ventricular actuation on LV dysfunction. Later, Zwanenburg et al. conducted two interesting studies to map the timing of cardiac contraction with high-temporal-resolution MRI tagging (Zwanenburg et al. 2004) and to study the relationship between peak and onset times of myocardial shortening (Zwanenburg et al. 2005). In 2005, Helm et al. (2005) analyzed cardiac dyssynchrony using circumferential versus longitudinal strain. In the same year, Lardo et al. (2005) presented an important review article about the use of CMR for assessment of ventricular dyssynchrony. Recently, SENC has been used for assessing regional strain and timing of contraction of the LV free wall in healthy individuals (Hamdan et al. 2009).

1.27.7 VALVULAR HEART DISEASE

In 1993, Villari et al. (1993) used MRI tagging to evaluate the LV structure–function interplay in aortic valve disease, where they concluded that changes in the collagen architecture are associated with altered systolic function and passive diastolic properties in aortic valve disease. Later, Ungacta et al. (1998) quantified the differences in regional LV systolic deformation before and after surgery for aortic insufficiency. In 1999, Stuber et al. (1999a) studied the alterations in cardiac torsion and diastolic relaxation of the LV in patients with aortic stenosis. In a similar work, Nagel et al. (2000) evaluated the time course of rotational LV motion in patients with aortic valve stenosis. In another work, changes in the LV systolic rotation and contraction in aortic stenosis were examined before and after surgical valve replacement (Sandstede et al. 2002).

1.27.8 CONGENITAL HEART DISEASE

Fogel et al. (1995a,b, 1996, 1998) presented a series of interesting studies that included the implementation of MRI tagging for evaluating different congenital heart diseases. In 1995, the investigators compared the function of single RVs to systemic RVs in a dual-chamber circulation (Fogel et al. 1995b). In the same year, the changes in systolic regional wall deformation were studied in patients with single ventricle after surgical intervention (Fogel et al. 1995a). In 1996, the investigators used MRI tagging to study the biomechanics of the deconditioned LV (Fogel et al. 1996). Two years later, the same group studied the RV effects on systemic LV mechanics (Fogel et al. 1998). Later, Donofrio et al. (1999) used MRI tagging to measure regional wall motion and strain in the transplanted hearts in pediatric patients.

1.27.9 MYOCARDIAL ELASTICITY

Besides conventional MRE, some studies have been conducted to measure myocardial elasticity with MRI tagging. In 2003, SENC was implemented for detecting stiff masses (Osman 2003), where the results indicated that SENC could be used for assessing myocardial elasticity. A couple of years later, Wen et al. (2005) developed a CMR-based technique that incorporated DENSE and PC velocity mapping to assess regional stress/strain gradients in the LV myocardium during diastole. Recently, Robert et al. (2009a) presented a method based on DENSE for measuring myocardial viscoelastic parameters with the help of an electrodynamic transducer.

1.27.10 OTHER HEART DISEASES

In addition to the studies mentioned earlier, MRI tagging has been used for evaluating the heart condition in other CVD. In 1999, Kojima et al. (1999) investigated the diagnosis of constrictive pericarditis using MRI tagging. In a related work, Spottiswoode et al. (2008b) assessed postoperative systolic septal wall motion abnormality following pericardiectomy. In 2000, Blom et al. (2000) showed that dynamic cardiomyoplasty decreases the myocardial workload. Two years later, Kramer et al. (2002a) studied reverse remodeling and improved regional function after LV aneurysm repair. Later, Setser et al. (2003b) studied the effects of partial left ventriculectomy on myocardial mechanics. In 2005, Ashford et al. (2005) studied the occult cardiac contractile dysfunction in dystrophin-deficient children. Recently, Fernandes et al. (2008) found that arterial stiffness is associated with regional ventricular systolic and diastolic dysfunction.

1.28 BOOK CONTENTS

As previously mentioned, these two books were written to provide a comprehensive and complete coverage of heart mechanics by MRI. In doing so, each chapter in the books serves a specific purpose toward achieving this goal. In this section, the purpose and needs for the different chapters are illustrated along with a brief description of their contents. To ensure comprehensiveness, four chapters were added to this book to cover heart physiology, MRI physics, myocardial architecture, and continuum mechanics.

1.28.1 HEART MECHANICS: MAGNETIC RESONANCE IMAGING—MATHEMATICAL MODELING, PULSE SEQUENCES, AND IMAGE ANALYSIS

1.28.1.1 Preliminary Chapters

Chapter 2 covers heart anatomy, function, and diseases. The chapter provides the basic medical information needed to appreciate the value of the techniques described throughout the book and to understand the way in which these techniques are implemented as well as their clinical applications. This chapter especially addresses readers with nonclinical backgrounds as a reminder of the basics of the cardiovascular system.

Similar to the need for readers with nonclinical backgrounds to learn about the cardiovascular system, it is important for readers without MRI background to learn about MRI physics. The chapter on MRI physics (Chapter 3) covers the basics of MRI in a straightforward fashion, which is very useful for clinicians and those who are new to the field of MRI. The chapter provides the basics of MRI physics needed to understand the advanced topics covered in other chapters and to benefit the most from this book. The chapter starts by explaining the nuclear magnetic resonance (NMR) phenomenon based on classical physics without delving into quantum mechanics details. The chapter then describes image formation and tissue contrast in MRI, followed by description of basic imaging pulse sequences. Fast imaging techniques and other basic and advanced topics are covered in the chapter as well.

Although Chapter 3 covers the basics of MRI physics, it does not focus on cardiac MRI applications. Therefore, Chapter 4 (CMR) comes to serve this purpose. The chapter provides the reader with the big picture of CMR before focusing on the specific area of heart mechanics in later chapters. The chapter succinctly provides general description of CMR, starting from patient preparation and prescription of standard cardiac imaging planes all the way to clinical applications of CMR. Along this journey, the chapter covers special tips and tricks in CMR, including cardiac and respiratory motion compensation techniques, imaging protocols, and data acquisition strategies. The chapter then addresses common CMR techniques, including morphology imaging, perfusion, delayed enhancement, relaxivity mapping, MR angiography, and flow imaging. The chapter then focuses on cine imaging and finally provides a brief introduction to MRI tagging.

1.28.1.2 Myocardial Fiber Structure and Mechanical Heart Modeling

Two other topics were necessary to be covered in this book: myocardial fiber architecture (Chapter 5) and mechanical heart modeling (Chapter 6). As the heart function is affected by its fiber structure, it then makes sense to cover this subject before delving into different techniques for measuring heart mechanics. Chapter 5 fulfills this purpose in addition to providing a comprehensive coverage of cardiac diffusion tensor imaging (DTI), the state-of-the-art technique for measuring the myocardial microstructure. DTI is a key innovation in the field of CMR, which is expected to flourish in the next few years with large effect on our understanding of the myocardial microstructure and its relationship with heart mechanics.

Chapter 6 covers the basics of continuum mechanics and cardiac mechanical models. The importance of this chapter is that it explains different mechanical parameters used to describe the heart function and provides their mathematical representation. This ensures that the reader can correctly interpret the measurements obtained from different imaging techniques and understand the differences among them as well as the assumptions used in different mechanical heart models.

1.28.1.3 Heart Function from Cine Images

Despite of the innovation in MRI tagging, which allowed for noninvasive tracking of intramyocardial deformation, important information about the heart function can still be obtained from conventional nontagged cine images, which are acquired in almost every CMR exam. Further, there is a recent interest in deriving regional parameters of heart mechanics from cine images, thanks to advances in image analysis and mathematical computational techniques. Therefore, the book first covers the cine-based techniques for extracting information about the heart function before focusing on MRI tagging and associated advanced imaging and analysis techniques. Chapters 7 and 8 are devoted to cine image analysis and CMR feature tracking, respectively. Chapter 7 provides a comprehensive coverage of a large number of analytical and model-based techniques for evaluating myocardial wall motion, including techniques based on measuring wall thickening, atlas and geometrical modeling, nonrigid deformation, image intensity analysis, and spatiotemporal filtering.

In contrast to the global heart modeling techniques covered in Chapter 7, Chapter 8 covers the recently developed techniques for extracting parameters of regional myocardial deformation based on tracking the displacement of certain anatomical features in the cine images throughout the cardiac cycle. The chapter describes the CMR-FT technique and its evolution from echo speckle tracking and compares both approaches for measuring heart mechanics. The chapter then discusses different clinical applications of CMR-FT.

1.28.1.4 Basic Tagging Techniques

Chapter 9 introduces the reader to MRI tagging by describing the original tagging technique developed by Zerhouni et al. (1988).

Although this original technique is not currently used in clinical practice, its importance stems from the fact that it introduced for the first time a technique for noninvasive measurement of intramyocardial deformation. Therefore, the innovation of the idea, its technical implementation, and clinical applications deserve a dedicated chapter. The chapter also discusses different approaches for optimizing the performance of the original tagging technique based on numerical simulations. Furthermore, to appreciate the importance of myocardial tagging and validate its results against gold standard methods, the chapter covers the basics of radiopaque and sonomicrometer myocardial marker implantation and tracking techniques. The chapter also covers the importance of these techniques as the only source for analyzing intramyocardial deformation before the introduction of MRI tagging, as well as the basic information obtained about heart mechanics based on these techniques.

Chapter 10 (SPAMM and DANTE) and Chapter 11 (CSPAMM) cover the basic tagging techniques that were developed early on after the introduction of MRI tagging in 1988. The SPAMM tagging technique was developed in 1989 by Axel and Dougherty (1989) 1 year after the introduction of the original tagging technique by Zerhouni et al. (1988). Nevertheless, SPAMM tagging has been in clinical use since then, a testament of its robustness and straightforward implementation. Actually, in many cases, the word tagging is simply used to mean SPAMM tagging. SPAMM tagging is the technique of choice when the radiologist wants to evaluate myocardial contractility and assess the effects of different cardiac diseases on regional heart function. It can be also used in many other applications, for example, the evaluation of constrictive pericarditis. Chapter 10 describes in details the basic SPAMM technique and its validation against other standard techniques. The chapter also covers different SPAMM development stages that took place since its invention, as well as various clinical applications. The chapter also covers the DANTE tagging technique (Mosher and Smith 1990), which was developed at almost the same time as SPAMM. The basic DANTE technique is described in Chapter 10 along with its different developments as well as its advantages and limitations compared to SPAMM.

Chapter 11 covers the CSPAMM technique developed by Fischer et al. (1993). The CSPAMM technique was developed to improve the tagging contrast and address the tags fading limitation in SPAMM. Slice-following CSPAMM (Fischer et al. 1994) is also covered in the chapter along with a description of how the technique allows for imaging the same myocardial tissue despite tissue displacement outside of the imaging plane during the cardiac cycle. The chapter also covers different CSPAMM technical developments, including single breath-hold CSPAMM, high-resolution CSPAMM, off-resonance insensitive (ORI) CSPAMM, orthogonal CSPAMM, and 3D CSPAMM. Clinical applications of CSPAMM are covered in the last section of the chapter.

1.28.1.5 Special Tagging Patterns

Chapter 12 covers special tagging patterns that have been developed to take advantage of the specific heart anatomy, including radial tagging, ring tags, polar tagging, localized tagging, and variable-density tagging. Different aspects of the special tagging patterns are covered in the chapter, including mathematical derivation, pulse sequence design, magnetization analysis, and clinical applications.

The last chapter in *Heart Mechanics: Magnetic Resonance Imaging—Mathematical Modeling, Pulse Sequences, and Image Analysis* (Chapter 13) provides an overview of the advanced tagging and mechanical cardiac analysis techniques covered in *Heart Mechanics: Magnetic Resonance Imaging—Advanced Techniques, Clinical Applications, and Future Trends*, including HARP, DENSE, SENC, TPM, and MRE.

1.28.2 HEART MECHANICS: MAGNETIC RESONANCE IMAGING—ADVANCED TECHNIQUES, CLINICAL APPLICATIONS, AND FUTURE TRENDS

1.28.2.1 Imaging Sequences and Tagging Analysis

Although different tagging chapters in the book discuss the pulse sequence design of the covered techniques, they focus on the tagging preparation part of the pulse sequence, not the imaging (or data acquisition) part. Nevertheless, the setup of the imaging protocol and selection of the imaging parameters affect the resulting image characteristics, including SNR, tagging contrast, tag density, image artifacts, and scan time, which subsequently affect the measurements derived from the tagged images. Therefore, Chapter 1 focuses on the different imaging pulse sequences implemented in MRI tagging and their effects on the results. The chapter covers these topics from both technical and implementation perspectives with results from numerical simulations and in vivo scans. The covered imaging sequences include GRE, SSFP, EPI, radial k-space acquisition, and spiral k-space acquisition. Additional imaging-related topics are covered, including 2D and 3D imaging, parallel imaging, fast data acquisition, real-time imaging, fat suppression, and black-blood imaging.

After covering different tagging techniques and imaging pulse sequences, it is natural to discuss the tagging analysis techniques, which is the purpose of Chapters 2 and 3. In these chapters, a comprehensive coverage of the various tagging analysis methods is provided, including deformable models, optical flow, Gabor filters, meshless models, sinusoidal and harmonic analysis, nonrigid registration, and detagging techniques. The chapters provide a comprehensive coverage of the discussed techniques, including mathematical formulation, illustrations, simulations, comparisons, implementation examples, and analysis results.

1.28.2.2 Advanced Tagging Techniques

The following three chapters in the book (Chapters 4 through 6) cover advanced techniques for measuring heart mechanics, specifically HARP, DENSE, and SENC. Chapter 4 covers the HARP technique from both technical and clinical implementation perspectives. The original HARP technique developed by Osman et al. (1999) is described in details. Improvements of the HARP technique are then discussed, including tagline regeneration, phase unwrapping, backward–forward modeling, HARP with active contours/shortest path analysis, reference tagline restoration, and harmonic peaks combination. Different HARP developments are also covered, including HARP with CSPAMM, TruHARP, FastHARP, real-time HARP, zHARP, and 3D HARP. The chapter then compares HARP to DENSE and discusses different clinical applications of HARP.

Chapter 5 covers the DENSE technique. The basic DENSE technique developed by Aletras et al. (1999b) is discussed in details, including description of the STEAM pulse sequence, based on which DENSE was developed. The different signal echoes in DENSE are described along with different displacement-encoding strategies. The chapter then covers different echo suppression and combination techniques, as well as different DENSE readout strategies. Other DENSE sequence improvements are also discussed, including fat suppression and ramped flip angle. The second section of the chapter covers DENSE image processing techniques, including phase unwrapping, motion recovery, strain estimation, and 3D DENSE. The third section of the chapter compares DENSE to other tagging and MRI techniques, including conventional tagging, HARP, DENSE, TPM, and DWI. This section also covers techniques for combining DENSE with viability, perfusion, elastography, molecular, and SENC imaging. The last section of the chapter discusses different clinical applications of DENSE.

Chapter 6 covers SENC imaging, starting with the original SENC technique developed by Osman et al. (2001) and proceeding to various SENC developments, improvements, and clinical applications that took place since then. The chapter describes the idea behind SENC imaging and its relation to conventional tagging with the help of mathematical formulations and magnetization analysis. The different signals generated in SENC are described along with the image processing and data analysis methods required to measure strain from these signals. SENC improvements are then discussed, including fat suppression, alternating tuning acquisition, localized excitation, fast imaging, and ramped flip angle. The chapter also covers different versions of the SENC technique, including sf-SENC, fast-SENC, slice-following fast-SENC, and C-SENC. Advanced techniques for heart tissue characterization based on SENC imaging are then discussed. Although SENC development stemmed from a tagging perspective, its relationship with the STEAM sequence is discussed in the chapter along with implementation strategies, including correction for through-plane deformation and black-blood imaging. Techniques for combining SENC with HARP and DENSE are then discussed, followed by SENC implementation for measuring tissue elasticity. The final section of the chapter discusses clinical applications of SENC.

1.28.2.3 Tissue Phase Mapping

Chapter 7 covers the TPM technique for measuring myocardial deformation. In contrast to most of the previously covered techniques that retrieve information about myocardial deformation from the magnitude-reconstructed images, TPM depends on encoding the tissue velocity in the phase images, with some advantages compared to magnitude imaging.

Chapter 7 covers the basic principles behind TPM from signal analysis, magnetization behavior, and pulse sequence perspectives. The basic TPM pulse sequence is described in details along with various related technical issues, including blood signal saturation, respiration control, temporal resolution, and parallel imaging. Other topics covered in the chapter include strain rate imaging, acceleration phase mapping, and composite TPM/tagging. The second section of the chapter covers TPM data analysis, including phase error correction, different velocity components, motion tracking, and virtual tagging. The chapter then discusses different TPM-based studies, including those for measuring regional differences of myocardial deformation in the healthy heart, differences based on age and gender, and cardiac dyssynchrony.

1.28.2.4 MR Elastography

Chapter 8 covers recently developed techniques for measuring heart mechanical properties using MRE. The chapter starts by reviewing the theory of mechanical wave propagation in viscoelastic materials, followed by description of different MRE methods and the dependence of the measured complex shear modulus on frequency. The chapter also discusses different MRE transducers, pulse sequences, and methods for reconstructing the viscoelastic parameters. The chapter then discusses cardiac MRE along with the associated challenges and precautions. Finally, the chapter covers applications of cardiac MRE as well as future directions of this technology.

1.28.2.5 Clinical Applications

The next two chapters in the book (Chapters 9 and 10) cover different clinical applications of the techniques described in the book along with clinical findings and implications. The chapters start by covering applications in the healthy heart (both from animal and human studies). A separate section is devoted to applications in the RV and atria due to the challenges of this implementation based on the chambers' thin wall and nonstandard shapes. The studies that evaluated the effects of age and gender on heart mechanics are grouped in another section. The influence of hypertension and diabetes on heart mechanics is then discussed. A large section in the chapters is devoted to cover heart mechanics in ischemic heart disease, including detection of myocardial infarction and tissue viability as well as the management of ischemic heart disease. Applications in heart failure, including HFNEF, are then discussed. The chapters also cover applications in interventricular dyssynchrony and electrophysiological abnormalities. Applications in dilated and hypertrophic cardiomyopathies are then covered, followed by other forms of cardiomyopathies, including Anderson-Fabry disease, Duchenne muscular dystrophy, Emery–Dreifuss muscular dystrophy, arrhythmogenic right ventricular dysplasia (ARVD), and LV noncompaction cardiomyopathy. Applications in valvular heart disease are also discussed, including aortic stenosis, aortic regurgitation, and mitral regurgitation. Pulmonary hypertension is then discussed, followed by pericardial diseases. The chapters also cover heart mechanics in pediatrics and congenital heart diseases, including atrial septal defect, aortic coarctation, tetralogy of Fallot, single ventricles, and transplanted pediatric hearts. The implementation of MRI tagging for measuring flow dynamics is then discussed, as well as heart mechanics in systemic diseases, including human immunodeficiency virus (HIV) and renal diseases. Finally, for completeness, the chapters briefly discuss noncardiac applications of MRI tagging.

Finally, the last chapter in the book (Chapter 11) serves as conclusion and discussion of the topics covered in the book as well as discussion of future trends and challenges in the field.

1.29   SUMMARY AND KEY POINTS

1.29.1   SUMMARY

CMR has evolved as an important imaging modality for studying cardiac function and measuring heart mechanics. Specifically, over the past 25 years, over 10 major MRI techniques have been developed for measuring intramyocardial motion, from which different measures of the heart mechanics, for example, myocardial strain, strain rate, and torsion, can be derived for accurate and early assessment of cardiac dysfunction. The invented techniques underwent development for years, such that a number of different versions exist for each technique, each suitable for certain applications. The capabilities of MRI as an imaging modality along with the advances in the scanners' hardware and pulse sequences resulted in big advancement of the tagging techniques available today than those invented 25 years ago. Despite being invented by different groups in different institutions, many of the developed techniques are somehow related to each other and can be explained following different approaches, which cannot be appreciated unless these techniques are grouped together, as done in these two books. This also allows for studying the advantages and limitations of each technique for better selection of the appropriate technique to use based on the application at hand. Despite the number of available books on CMR in general, there has been a need for a book dedicated to address heart mechanics with MRI along with the large number of developed techniques and clinical applications, which is the purpose of these two books. By providing hundreds of research ideas and reference articles, the books should provide the reader with the motivation to take the next steps in the field.

1.29.2   KEY POINTS

- CVD is the leading cause of morbidity and mortality all over the world.
- Knowledge about the myofiber arrangement allows for better understanding of the heart mechanics.
- Mechanical heart modeling is important for measuring and understanding myocardial deformation.
- Myocardial contractility is nonhomogeneous and differs both spatially and temporally, as well as due to pathology.
- Measures of regional heart function allow for early identification of cardiac dysfunction.

- Despite its wide use for cardiac imaging, echocardiography limitations for measuring heart mechanics include the need for an adequate acoustic window, operator dependency, and geometric assumptions, besides its low SNR.
- MRI has many advantages, including lack of ionizing radiation, superior tissue contrast, arbitrary selection of the imaging plane, 3D imaging capability, and high resolution.
- CMR has emerged as an important clinical tool for evaluating a broad range of CVDs.
- Within the same CMR exam, information can be gathered about cardiovascular morphology, contractile function, viable and nonviable myocardium, valve diseases, congenital anomalies, blood flow, and vascular anatomy.
- Cine MRI imaging is a fundamental part of almost every CMR examination, which can provide useful information about the heart condition, including ventricular volumes and mass, EF, and regional LV and RV wall motion.
- The cine MRI images can be used for wall motion analysis based on different cardiac modeling approaches.
- CMR-FT is used for measuring myocardial deformation based on tracking certain feature points in the cine images during the cardiac cycle.
- Compared to MRI tagging, CMR-FT is simpler and faster, although this comes at the cost of suboptimal measurement accuracy.
- Marker implantation is not a practical method for measuring myocardial contractility due to its invasiveness, which makes it unsuitable for clinical implementation.
- The invention of myocardial tagging opened the door for a series of developments and improvements that continue up to the present day.
- The tagging techniques can be divided in magnitude-based and phase-based techniques based on the criterion used for encoding information about myocardial deformation.
- Tagging by magnetization saturation, developed by Zerhouni et al., was the first tagging technique. It is not currently used in clinical applications. Nevertheless, its importance is that it allowed for the first time for noninvasive measurement of intramyocardial deformation.
- SPAMM tagging is the most widely used tagging technique since its introduction in 1989 until the present day.
- DANTE is an efficient and flexible tagging sequence. It has the advantages of improved tagging resolution and reduced RF power.
- CSPAMM tagging provides improved tagging contrast and access to late phases in the cardiac cycle, although these advantages come at the cost of longer scan time.

- Slice-following CSPAMM allows for measuring the same tissue during the whole cardiac cycle, regardless of tissue through-plane motion.
- Special tagging techniques have been developed to customize the tagging pattern to the gross geometry and motion pattern of the heart. These techniques include radial, circular, polar, localized, and variable-density tagging.
- The data acquisition (imaging) sequence implemented in MRI tagging affects the quality and characteristics of the resulting images and the accuracy of the generated measurements.
- The amount of postprocessing performed to analyze the tagged images ranges from simple visual inspection of tags deformation to exhaustive calculation of various strain components.
- Tagging analysis techniques include active contours, optical flow, template matching, deformable models, Gabor filters, meshless models, sinusoidal and harmonic analysis, and nonrigid registration.
- HARP analysis depends on analyzing the tagged images in the k-space instead of the image itself, which significantly reduces the processing time.
- DENSE directly encodes the tissue displacement into the phase of the generated stimulated echo signal and displays displacement-encoded phase images. DENSE advantages include high resolution and black-blood imaging.
- SENC measures strain in the through-plane direction by applying the tagging planes parallel to (and inside) the imaging slice. SENC advantages include high resolution, simple postprocessing, and intuitive color-coded strain representation.
- The idea of TPM is to encode velocity in the signal phase, such that the phase image can be used for measuring tissue motion and velocity. TPM advantages include high resolution and sensitivity.
- MRE is a noninvasive technique for measuring tissue stiffness. The implementation of MRE on the heart is promising, although a number of difficulties have to be addressed before reliable measurements can be obtained.
- Measuring heart mechanics with MRI has been implemented in a large number of clinical applications covering most CVDs.

REFERENCES

Abd-Elmoniem, K. Z., Sampath, S., Osman, N. F., and Prince, J. L. (2007). Real-time monitoring of cardiac regional function using fastHARP MRI and region-of-interest reconstruction. *IEEE Trans Biomed Eng* **54**(9): 1650–1656.

Abd-Elmoniem, K. Z., Stuber, M., Osman, N. F., and Prince, J. L. (2005). ZHARP: Three-dimensional motion tracking from a single image plane. *Inf Process Med Imaging* **19**: 639–651.

Aletras, A. H., Balaban, R. S., and Wen, H. (1999a). High-resolution strain analysis of the human heart with fast-DENSE. *J Magn Reson* **140**(1): 41–57.

Aletras, A. H., Ding, S., Balaban, R. S., and Wen, H. (1999b). DENSE: Displacement encoding with stimulated echoes in cardiac functional MRI. *J Magn Reson* **137**(1): 247–252.

Aletras, A. H., Tilak, G. S., Natanzon, A., Hsu, L. Y., Gonzalez, F. M., Hoyt, R. F., Jr., and Arai, A. E. (2006). Retrospective determination of the area at risk for reperfused acute myocardial infarction with T2-weighted cardiac magnetic resonance imaging: Histopathological and displacement encoding with stimulated echoes (DENSE) functional validations. *Circulation* **113**(15): 1865–1870.

Aletras, A. H. and Wen, H. (2001). Mixed echo train acquisition displacement encoding with stimulated echoes: An optimized DENSE method for in vivo functional imaging of the human heart. *Magn Reson Med* **46**(3): 523–534.

Amini, A. A., Chen, Y., Curwen, R. W., Mani, V., and Sun, J. (1998). Coupled B-snake grids and constrained thin-plate splines for analysis of 2-D tissue deformations from tagged MRI. *IEEE Trans Med Imaging* **17**(3): 344–356.

Amini, A. A., Chen, Y., Elayyadi, M., and Radeva, P. (2001). Tag surface reconstruction and tracking of myocardial beads from SPAMM-MRI with parametric B-spline surfaces. *IEEE Trans Med Imaging* **20**(2): 94–103.

Anderson, R. H., Smerup, M., Sanchez-Quintana, D., Loukas, M., and Lunkenheimer, P. P. (2009). The three-dimensional arrangement of the myocytes in the ventricular walls. *Clin Anat* **22**(1): 64–76.

Arts, T., Hunter, W. C., Douglas, A. S., Muijtjens, A. M., Corsel, J. W., and Reneman, R. S. (1993). Macroscopic three-dimensional motion patterns of the left ventricle. *Adv Exp Med Biol* **346**: 383–392.

Ashford, M. W., Jr., Liu, W., Lin, S. J., Abraszewski, P., Caruthers, S. D., Connolly, A. M., Yu, X., and Wickline, S. A. (2005). Occult cardiac contractile dysfunction in dystrophin-deficient children revealed by cardiac magnetic resonance strain imaging. *Circulation* **112**(16): 2462–2467.

Ashikaga, H., Mickelsen, S. R., Ennis, D. B., Rodriguez, I., Kellman, P., Wen, H., and McVeigh, E. R. (2005). Electromechanical analysis of infarct border zone in chronic myocardial infarction. *Am J Physiol Heart Circ Physiol* **289**(3): H1099–H1105.

Axel, L. (2002). Biomechanical dynamics of the heart with MRI. *Annu Rev Biomed Eng* **4**: 321–347.

Axel, L. and Dougherty, L. (1989). MR imaging of motion with spatial modulation of magnetization. *Radiology* **171**(3): 841–845.

Axel, L., Montillo, A., and Kim, D. (2005). Tagged magnetic resonance imaging of the heart: A survey. *Med Image Anal* **9**(4): 376–393.

Azhari, H., Buchalter, M., Sideman, S., Shapiro, E., and Beyar, R. (1992). A conical model to describe the nonuniformity of the left ventricular twisting motion. *Ann Biomed Eng* **20**(2): 149–165.

Azhari, H., Weiss, J. L., Rogers, W. J., Siu, C. O., Zerhouni, E. A., and Shapiro, E. P. (1993). Noninvasive quantification of principal strains in normal canine hearts using tagged MRI images in 3-D. *Am J Physiol* **264**(1 Pt 2): H205–H216.

Bankman, I. (2000). *Handbook of Medical Imaging: Processing and Analysis Management.* San Diego, CA: Academic Press.

Basha, T. A., Ibrahim, El-S. H., Weiss, R. G., and Osman, N. F. (2009). Cine cardiac imaging using black-blood steady-state free precession (BB-SSFP) at 3T. *J Magn Reson Imaging* **30**(1): 94–103.

Bazille, A., Guttman, M. A., McVeigh, E. R., and Zerhouni, E. A. (1994). Impact of semiautomated versus manual image segmentation errors on myocardial strain calculation by magnetic resonance tagging. *Invest Radiol* **29**(4): 427–433.

Beache, G. M., Wedeen, V. J., Weisskoff, R. M., O'Gara, P. T., Poncelet, B. P., Chesler, D. A., Brady, T. J., Rosen, B. R., and Dinsmore, R. E. (1995). Intramural mechanics in hypertrophic cardiomyopathy: Functional mapping with strain-rate MR imaging. *Radiology* **197**(1): 117–124.

Bergey, P. D. and Axel, L. (2000). Focal hypertrophic cardiomyopathy simulating a mass: MR tagging for correct diagnosis. *AJR Am J Roentgenol* **174**(1): 242–244.

Biederman, R. W., Doyle, M., and Yamrozik, J. (2007). Cardiovascular MRI tutorial: Lectures and learning. Philadelphia, PA: Lippincott Williams & Wilkins.

Blom, A. S., Pilla, J. J., Pusca, S. V., Patel, H. J., Dougherty, L., Yuan, Q., Ferrari, V. A., Axel, L., and Acker, M. A. (2000). Dynamic cardiomyoplasty decreases myocardial workload as assessed by tissue tagged MRI. *ASAIO J* **46**(5): 556–562.

Bogaert, J., Bosmans, H., Maes, A., Suetens, P., Marchal, G., and Rademakers, F. E. (2000). Remote myocardial dysfunction after acute anterior myocardial infarction: Impact of left ventricular shape on regional function: A magnetic resonance myocardial tagging study. *J Am Coll Cardiol* **35**(6): 1525–1534.

Bogaert, J., Dymarkowski, S., Taylor, A., and Muthurangu, V. (2012). *Clinical Cardiac MRI*. New York: Springer.

Bogaert, J. and Rademakers, F. E. (2001). Regional nonuniformity of normal adult human left ventricle. *Am J Physiol Heart Circ Physiol* **280**(2): H610–H620.

Bolster, B. D., Jr., McVeigh, E. R., and Zerhouni, E. A. (1990). Myocardial tagging in polar coordinates with use of striped tags. *Radiology* **177**(3): 769–772.

Bosmans, H., Bogaert, J., Rademakers, F., Marchal, G., Laub, G., Verschakelen, J., and Baert, A. L. (1996). Left ventricular radial tagging acquisition using gradient-recalled-echo techniques: Sequence optimization. *MAGMA* **4**(2): 123–133.

Bree, D., Wollmuth, J. R., Cupps, B. P., Krock, M. D., Howells, A., Rogers, J., Moazami, N., and Pasque, M. K. (2006). Low-dose dobutamine tissue-tagged magnetic resonance imaging with 3-dimensional strain analysis allows assessment of myocardial viability in patients with ischemic cardiomyopathy. *Circulation* **114**(1 Suppl.): I33–I36.

Brower, R. W., ten Katen, H. J., and Meester, G. T. (1978). Direct method for determining regional myocardial shortening after bypass surgery from radiopaque markers in man. *Am J Cardiol* **41**(7): 1222–1229.

Byrne, M. J., Helm, R. H., Daya, S., Osman, N. F., Halperin, H. R., Berger, R. D., Kass, D. A., and Lardo, A. C. (2007). Diminished left ventricular dyssynchrony and impact of resynchronization in failing hearts with right versus left bundle branch block. *J Am Coll Cardiol* **50**(15): 1484–1490.

Carranza-Herrezuelo, N., Bajo, A., Sroubek, F., Santamarta, C., Cristobal, G., Santos, A., and Ledesma-Carbayo, M. J. (2010). Motion estimation of tagged cardiac magnetic resonance images using variational techniques. *Comput Med Imaging Graph* **34**(6): 514–522.

Castillo, E., Lima, J. A., and Bluemke, D. A. (2003). Regional myocardial function: Advances in MR imaging and analysis. *Radiographics* **23 Spec No.**: S127–S140.

Castillo, E., Osman, N. F., Rosen, B. D., El-Shehaby, I., Pan, L., Jerosch-Herold, M., Lai, S., Bluemke, D. A., and Lima, J. A. (2005). Quantitative assessment of regional myocardial function with MR-tagging in a multi-center study: Interobserver and intraobserver agreement of fast strain analysis with Harmonic Phase (HARP) MRI. *J Cardiovasc Magn Reson* **7**(5): 783–791.

Chai, J. W., Chen, Y. T., and Lee, S. K. (1997). MRI assessment of regional heart wall motion in the longitudinal axis sections of left ventricle by spatial modulation of magnetization. *Zhonghua Yi Xue Za Zhi (Taipei)* **60**(1): 13–20.

Chandra, S. and Yang, Y. (1996). Simulations and demonstrations of localized tagging experiments. *J Magn Reson B* **111**(3): 285–288.

Chatelin, S., Oudry, J., Perichon, N., Sandrin, L., Allemann, P., Soler, L., and Willinger, R. (2011). In vivo liver tissue mechanical properties by Transient Elastography: Comparison with Dynamic Mechanical Analysis. *Biorheology* **48**(2): 75–88.

Chen, M. Y., Tsai, J. W., Chang, M. S., and Yu, B. C. (1995). Assessment of heart wall motion: Modified spatial modulation of magnetization for MR imaging. *Proc Natl Sci Counc Repub China B* **19**(1): 47–53.

Chenevert, T. L., Skovoroda, A. R., O'Donnell, M., and Emelianov, S. Y. (1998). Elasticity reconstructive imaging by means of stimulated echo MRI. *Magn Reson Med* **39**(3): 482–490.

Clark, N. R., Reichek, N., Bergey, P., Hoffman, E. A., Brownson, D., Palmon, L., and Axel, L. (1991). Circumferential myocardial shortening in the normal human left ventricle. Assessment by magnetic resonance imaging using spatial modulation of magnetization. *Circulation* **84**(1): 67–74.

Clarysse, P., Basset, C., Khouas, L., Croisille, P., Friboulet, D., Odet, C., and Magnin, I. E. (2000). Two-dimensional spatial and temporal displacement and deformation field fitting from cardiac magnetic resonance tagging. *Med Image Anal* **4**(3): 253–268.

Constantinides, C. (2014). *Latest Advances in Clinical and Pre-Clinical Cardiovascular Magnetic Resonance Imaging*. Sharjah, United Arab Emirates: Bentham Science Publishers.

Croisille, P., Moore, C. C., Judd, R. M., Lima, J. A., Arai, M., McVeigh, E. R., Becker, L. C., and Zerhouni, E. A. (1999). Differentiation of viable and nonviable myocardium by the use of three-dimensional tagged MRI in 2-day-old reperfused canine infarcts. *Circulation* **99**(2): 284–291.

Cupps, B. P., Taggar, A. K., Reynolds, L. M., Lawton, J. S., and Pasque, M. K. (2010). Regional myocardial contractile function: Multiparametric strain mapping. *Interact Cardiovasc Thorac Surg* **10**(6): 953–957.

Curry, C. W., Nelson, G. S., Wyman, B. T., Declerck, J., Talbot, M., Berger, R. D., McVeigh, E. R., and Kass, D. A. (2000). Mechanical dyssynchrony in dilated cardiomyopathy with intraventricular conduction delay as depicted by 3D tagged magnetic resonance imaging. *Circulation* **101**(1): E2.

Delfino, J. G., Johnson, K. R., Eisner, R. L., Eder, S., Leon, A. R., and Oshinski, J. N. (2008). Three-directional myocardial phase-contrast tissue velocity MR imaging with navigator-echo gating: in vivo and in vitro study. *Radiology* **246**(3): 917–925.

Deng, X. and Denney, T. S., Jr. (2004). Three-dimensional myocardial strain reconstruction from tagged MRI using a cylindrical B-spline model. *IEEE Trans Med Imaging* **23**(7): 861–867.

Deng, X. and Denney, T. S., Jr. (2005). Combined tag tracking and strain reconstruction from tagged cardiac MR images without user-defined myocardial contours. *J Magn Reson Imaging* **21**(1): 12–22.

Denney, T. S., Jr., Gerber, B. L., and Yan, L. (2003). Unsupervised reconstruction of a three-dimensional left ventricular strain from parallel tagged cardiac images. *Magn Reson Med* **49**(4): 743–754.

Denney, T. S., Jr. and McVeigh, E. R. (1997). Model-free reconstruction of three-dimensional myocardial strain from planar tagged MR images. *J Magn Reson Imaging* **7**(5): 799–810.

Derbyshire, J. A., Sampath, S., and McVeigh, E. R. (2007). Phase-sensitive cardiac tagging—REALTAG. *Magn Reson Med* **58**(1): 206–210.

Dong, S. J., Crawley, A. P., MacGregor, J. H., Petrank, Y. F., Bergman, D. W., Belenkie, I., Smith, E. R., Tyberg, J. V., and Beyar, R. (1995). Regional left ventricular systolic function in relation to the cavity geometry in patients with chronic right ventricular pressure overload. A three-dimensional tagged magnetic resonance imaging study. *Circulation* **91**(9): 2359–2370.

Dong, S. J., Hees, P. S., Huang, W. M., Buffer, S. A., Jr., Weiss, J. L., and Shapiro, E. P. (1999). Independent effects of preload, afterload, and contractility on left ventricular torsion. *Am J Physiol* **277**(3 Pt 2): H1053–H1060.

Dong, S. J., Hees, P. S., Siu, C. O., Weiss, J. L., and Shapiro, E. P. (2001). MRI assessment of LV relaxation by untwisting rate: A new isovolumic phase measure of tau. *Am J Physiol Heart Circ Physiol* **281**(5): H2002–H2009.

Dong, S. J., MacGregor, J. H., Crawley, A. P., McVeigh, E., Belenkie, I., Smith, E. R., Tyberg, J. V., and Beyar, R. (1994). Left ventricular wall thickness and regional systolic function in patients with hypertrophic cardiomyopathy. A three-dimensional tagged magnetic resonance imaging study. *Circulation* **90**(3): 1200–1209.

Donofrio, M. T., Clark, B. J., Ramaciotti, C., Jacobs, M. L., Fellows, K. E., Weinberg, P. M., and Fogel, M. A. (1999). Regional wall motion and strain of transplanted hearts in pediatric patients using magnetic resonance tagging. *Am J Physiol* **277**(5 Pt 2): R1481–R1487.

Dougherty, L., Asmuth, J. C., Blom, A. S., Axel, L., and Kumar, R. (1999). Validation of an optical flow method for tag displacement estimation. *IEEE Trans Med Imaging* **18**(4): 359–363.

Edvardsen, T., Detrano, R., Rosen, B. D., Carr, J. J., Liu, K., Lai, S., Shea, S., Pan, L., Bluemke, D. A., and Lima, J. A. (2006a). Coronary artery atherosclerosis is related to reduced regional left ventricular function in individuals without history of clinical cardiovascular disease: The Multiethnic Study of Atherosclerosis. *Arterioscler Thromb Vasc Biol* **26**(1): 206–211.

Edvardsen, T., Rosen, B. D., Pan, L., Jerosch-Herold, M., Lai, S., Hundley, W. G., Sinha, S., Kronmal, R. A., Bluemke, D. A., and Lima, J. A. (2006b). Regional diastolic dysfunction in individuals with left ventricular hypertrophy measured by tagged magnetic resonance imaging—The Multi-Ethnic Study of Atherosclerosis (MESA). *Am Heart J* **151**(1): 109–114.

Elgeti, T., Rump, J., Hamhaber, U., Papazoglou, S., Hamm, B., Braun, J., and Sack, I. (2008). Cardiac magnetic resonance elastography. Initial results. *Invest Radiol* **43**(11): 762–772.

Ennis, D. B., Epstein, F. H., Kellman, P., Fananapazir, L., McVeigh, E. R., and Arai, A. E. (2003). Assessment of regional systolic and diastolic dysfunction in familial hypertrophic cardiomyopathy using MR tagging. *Magn Reson Med* **50**(3): 638–642.

Epstein, F. H. (2007). MRI of left ventricular function. *J Nucl Cardiol* **14**(5): 729–744.

Epstein, F. H. and Gilson, W. D. (2004). Displacement-encoded cardiac MRI using cosine and sine modulation to eliminate (CANSEL) artifact-generating echoes. *Magn Reson Med* **52**(4): 774–781.

Epstein, F. H., Wolff, S. D., and Arai, A. E. (1999). Segmented k-space fast cardiac imaging using an echo-train readout. *Magn Reson Med* **41**(3): 609–613.

Fahmy, A. S., Krieger, A., and Osman, N. F. (2006a). An integrated system for real-time detection of stiff masses with a single compression. *IEEE Trans Biomed Eng* **53**(7): 1286–1293.

Fahmy, A. S., Pan, L., Stuber, M., and Osman, N. F. (2006b). Correction of through-plane deformation artifacts in stimulated echo acquisition mode cardiac imaging. *Magn Reson Med* **55**(2): 404–412.

Fayad, Z. A., Ferrari, V. A., Kraitchman, D. L., Young, A. A., Palevsky, H. I., Bloomgarden, D. C., and Axel, L. (1998). Right ventricular regional function using MR tagging: Normals versus chronic pulmonary hypertension. *Magn Reson Med* **39**(1): 116–123.

Feng, L., Donnino, R., Babb, J., Axel, L., and Kim, D. (2009). Numerical and in vivo validation of fast cine displacement-encoded with stimulated echoes (DENSE) MRI for quantification of regional cardiac function. *Magn Reson Med* **62**(3): 682–690.

Fernandes, V. R., Polak, J. F., Cheng, S., Rosen, B. D., Carvalho, B., Nasir, K., McClelland, R. et al. (2008). Arterial stiffness is associated with regional ventricular systolic and diastolic dysfunction: The Multi-Ethnic Study of Atherosclerosis. *Arterioscler Thromb Vasc Biol* **28**(1): 194–201.

Fernandes, V. R., Polak, J. F., Edvardsen, T., Carvalho, B., Gomes, A., Bluemke, D. A., Nasir, K., O'Leary, D. H., and Lima, J. A. (2006). Subclinical atherosclerosis and incipient regional myocardial dysfunction in asymptomatic individuals: The Multi-Ethnic Study of Atherosclerosis (MESA). *J Am Coll Cardiol* **47**(12): 2420–2428.

Fischer, S. E., McKinnon, G. C., Maier, S. E., and Boesiger, P. (1993). Improved myocardial tagging contrast. *Magn Reson Med* **30**(2): 191–200.

Fischer, S. E., McKinnon, G. C., Scheidegger, M. B., Prins, W., Meier, D., and Boesiger, P. (1994). True myocardial motion tracking. *Magn Reson Med* **31**(4): 401–413.

Florack, L. and van Assen, H. (2010). A new methodology for multiscale myocardial deformation and strain analysis based on tagging MRI. *Int J Biomed Imaging* **2010**: 341242.

Fogel, M. A., Gupta, K., Baxter, B. C., Weinberg, P. M., Haselgrove, J., and Hoffman, E. A. (1996). Biomechanics of the deconditioned left ventricle. *Am J Physiol* **271**(3 Pt 2): H1193–H1206.

Fogel, M. A., Gupta, K. B., Weinberg, P. M., and Hoffman, E. A. (1995a). Regional wall motion and strain analysis across stages of Fontan reconstruction by magnetic resonance tagging. *Am J Physiol* **269**(3 Pt 2): H1132–H1152.

Fogel, M. A., Weinberg, P. M., Fellows, K. E., and Hoffman, E. A. (1995b). A study in ventricular-ventricular interaction. Single right ventricles compared with systemic right ventricles in a dual-chamber circulation. *Circulation* **92**(2): 219–230.

Fogel, M. A., Weinberg, P. M., Gupta, K. B., Rychik, J., Hubbard, A., Hoffman, E. A., and Haselgrove, J. (1998). Mechanics of the single left ventricle: A study in ventricular-ventricular interaction II. *Circulation* **98**(4): 330–338.

Foll, D., Jung, B., Schilli, E., Staehle, F., Geibel, A., Hennig, J., Bode, C., and Markl, M. (2010). Magnetic resonance tissue phase mapping of myocardial motion: New insight in age and gender. *Circ Cardiovasc Imaging* **3**(1): 54–64.

Fonseca, C. G., Oxenham, H. C., Cowan, B. R., Occleshaw, C. J., and Young, A. A. (2003). Aging alters patterns of regional nonuniformity in LV strain relaxation: A 3-D MR tissue tagging study. *Am J Physiol Heart Circ Physiol* **285**(2): H621–H630.

Frahm, J., Merboldt, K. D., Hanicke, W., and Haase, A. (1985). Stimulated echo imaging. *J Magn Reson Imaging* **64**: 81–93.

Gallagher, K. P., Osakada, G., Hess, O. M., Koziol, J. A., Kemper, W. S., and Ross, J., Jr. (1982). Subepicardial segmental function during coronary stenosis and the role of myocardial fiber orientation. *Circ Res* **50**(3): 352–359.

Garot, J., Bluemke, D. A., Osman, N. F., Rochitte, C. E., McVeigh, E. R., Zerhouni, E. A., Prince, J. L., and Lima, J. A. (2000). Fast determination of regional myocardial strain fields from tagged cardiac images using harmonic phase MRI. *Circulation* **101**(9): 981–988.

Garot, J., Lima, J. A., Gerber, B. L., Sampath, S., Wu, K. C., Bluemke, D. A., Prince, J. L., and Osman, N. F. (2004). Spatially resolved imaging of myocardial function with strain-encoded MR: Comparison with delayed contrast-enhanced MR imaging after myocardial infarction. *Radiology* **233**(2): 596–602.

Garot, J., Pascal, O., Diebold, B., Derumeaux, G., Gerber, B. L., Dubois-Rande, J. L., Lima, J. A., and Gueret, P. (2002). Alterations of systolic left ventricular twist after acute myocardial infarction. *Am J Physiol Heart Circ Physiol* **282**(1): H357–H362.

Gerber, B. L., Garot, J., Bluemke, D. A., Wu, K. C., and Lima, J. A. (2002). Accuracy of contrast-enhanced magnetic resonance imaging in predicting improvement of regional myocardial function in patients after acute myocardial infarction. *Circulation* **106**(9): 1083–1089.

Gerber, B. L., Rochitte, C. E., Melin, J. A., McVeigh, E. R., Bluemke, D. A., Wu, K. C., Becker, L. C., and Lima, J. A. (2000). Microvascular obstruction and left ventricular remodeling early after acute myocardial infarction. *Circulation* **101**(23): 2734–2741.

Geskin, G., Kramer, C. M., Rogers, W. J., Theobald, T. M., Pakstis, D., Hu, Y. L., and Reichek, N. (1998). Quantitative assessment of myocardial viability after infarction by dobutamine magnetic resonance tagging. *Circulation* **98**(3): 217–223.

Gilson, W. D., Yang, Z., French, B. A., and Epstein, F. H. (2005). Measurement of myocardial mechanics in mice before and after infarction using multislice displacement-encoded MRI with 3D motion encoding. *Am J Physiol Heart Circ Physiol* **288**(3): H1491–H1497.

Goergen, C. J. and Sosnovik, D. E. (2011). From molecules to myofibers: Multiscale imaging of the myocardium. *J Cardiovasc Transl Res* **4**(4): 493–503.

Gotte, M. J., Germans, T., Russel, I. K., Zwanenburg, J. J., Marcus, J. T., van Rossum, A. C., and van Veldhuisen, D. J. (2006). Myocardial strain and torsion quantified by cardiovascular magnetic resonance tissue tagging: Studies in normal and impaired left ventricular function. *J Am Coll Cardiol* **48**(10): 2002–2011.

Gotte, M. J., van Rossum, A. C., Marcus, J. T., Kuijer, J. P., Axel, L., and Visser, C. A. (1999). Recognition of infarct localization by specific changes in intramural myocardial mechanics. *Am Heart J* **138**(6 Pt 1): 1038–1045.

Gotte, M. J., van Rossum, A. C., Twisk, J. W. R., Kuijer, J. P. A., Marcus, J. T., and Visser, C. A. (2001). Quantification of regional contractile function after infarction: Strain analysis superior to wall thickening analysis in discriminating infarct from remote myocardium. *J Am Coll Cardiol* **37**(3): 808–817.

Grizzard, J., Judd, R., and Kim, R. (2008). *Cardiovascular MRI in Practice: A Teaching File Approach*. New York: Springer.

Guttman, M. A., Prince, J. L., and McVeigh, E. R. (1994). Tag and contour detection in tagged MR images of the left ventricle. *IEEE Trans Med Imaging* **13**(1): 74–88.

Guttman, M. A., Zerhouni, E. A., and McVeigh, E. R. (1997). Analysis of cardiac function from MR images. *IEEE Comput Graph Appl* **17**(1): 30–38.

Haber, I., Metaxas, D. N., and Axel, L. (2000). Three-dimensional motion reconstruction and analysis of the right ventricle using tagged MRI. *Med Image Anal* **4**(4): 335–355.

Hamdan, A., Thouet, T., Kelle, S., Paetsch, I., Gebker, R., Wellnhofer, E., Schnackenburg, B., Fahmy, A. S., Osman, N. F., and Fleck, E. (2008). Regional right ventricular function and timing of contraction in healthy volunteers evaluated by strain-encoded MRI. *J Magn Reson Imaging* **28**(6): 1379–1385.

Hamdan, A., Thouet, T., Kelle, S., Wellnhofer, E., Paetsch, I., Gebker, R., Schnackenburg, B. et al. (2009). Strain-encoded MRI to evaluate normal left ventricular function and timing of contraction at 3.0 Tesla. *J Magn Reson Imaging* **29**(4): 799–808.

Hamhaber, U., Grieshaber, F. A., Nagel, J. H., and Klose, U. (2003). Comparison of quantitative shear wave MR-elastography with mechanical compression tests. *Magn Reson Med* **49**(1): 71–77.

Hargreaves, B. A., Vasanawala, S. S., Pauly, J. M., and Nishimura, D. G. (2001). Characterization and reduction of the transient response in steady-state MR imaging. *Magn Reson Med* **46**(1): 149–158.

Harouni, A. A., Jacobs, M. A., and Osman, N. F. (2011). Finding the optimal compression level for strain-encoded (SENC) breast MRI; simulations and phantom experiments. *Med Image Comput Comput Assist Interv* **14**(Pt 1): 444–451.

Heijman, E., Strijkers, G. J., Habets, J., Janssen, B., and Nicolay, K. (2004). Magnetic resonance imaging of regional cardiac function in the mouse. *MAGMA* **17**(3–6): 170–178.

Helm, R. H., Leclercq, C., Faris, O. P., Ozturk, C., McVeigh, E., Lardo, A. C., and Kass, D. A. (2005). Cardiac dyssynchrony analysis using circumferential versus longitudinal strain: Implications for assessing cardiac resynchronization. *Circulation* **111**(21): 2760–2767.

Herzka, D. A., Guttman, M. A., and McVeigh, E. R. (2003). Myocardial tagging with SSFP. *Magn Reson Med* **49**(2): 329–340.

Hess, A. T., Zhong, X., Spottiswoode, B. S., Epstein, F. H., and Meintjes, E. M. (2009). Myocardial 3D strain calculation by combining cine displacement encoding with stimulated echoes (DENSE) and cine strain encoding (SENC) imaging. *Magn Reson Med* **62**(1): 77–84.

Higgins, C. and de Roos, A. (2002). *Cardiovascular MRI and MRA*. New York: Lippincott Williams & Wilkins.

Hu, Z., Metaxas, D., and Axel, L. (2003). In vivo strain and stress estimation of the heart left and right ventricles from MRI images. *Med Image Anal* **7**(4): 435–444.

Huang, J., Abendschein, D., Davila-Roman, V. G., and Amini, A. A. (1999). Spatio-temporal tracking of myocardial deformations with a 4-D B-spline model from tagged MRI. *IEEE Trans Med Imaging* **18**(10): 957–972.

Huang, S. and Sosnovik, D. E. (2010). Molecular and microstructural imaging of the myocardium. *Curr Cardiovasc Imaging Rep* **3**(1): 26–33.

Huwart, L., Peeters, F., Sinkus, R., Annet, L., Salameh, N., ter Beek, L. C., Horsmans, Y., and Van Beers, B. E. (2006). Liver fibrosis: non-invasive assessment with MR elastography. *NMR Biomed* **19**(2): 173–179.

Huwart, L., Sempoux, C., Vicaut, E., Salameh, N., Annet, L., Danse, E., Peeters, F. et al. (2008). Magnetic resonance elastography for the noninvasive staging of liver fibrosis. *Gastroenterology* **135**(1): 32–40.

Ibrahim, El-S. H. (2011). Myocardial tagging by cardiovascular magnetic resonance: Evolution of techniques—Pulse sequences, analysis algorithms, and applications. *J Cardiovasc Magn Reson* **13**: 36.

Ibrahim, El-S. H. (2012). Imaging sequences in cardiovascular magnetic resonance: Current role, evolving applications, and technical challenges. *Int J Cardiovasc Imaging* **28**(8): 2027–2047.

Ibrahim, El-S. H., Stuber, M., Fahmy, A. S., Abd-Elmoniem, K. Z., Sasano, T., Abraham, M. R., and Osman, N. F. (2007a). Real-time MR imaging of myocardial regional function using strain-encoding (SENC) with tissue through-plane motion tracking. *J Magn Reson Imaging* **26**(6): 1461–1470.

Ibrahim, El-S. H., Stuber, M., Kraitchman, D. L., Weiss, R. G., and Osman, N. F. (2007b). Combined functional and viability cardiac MR imaging in a single breathhold. *Magn Reson Med* **58**(4): 843–849.

Ibrahim, El-S. H., Stuber, M., Schar, M., and Osman, N. F. (2006). Improved myocardial tagging contrast in cine balanced SSFP images. *J Magn Reson Imaging* **24**(5): 1159–1167.

Ikonomidou, V. N. and Sergiadis, G. D. (2002). A rotational approach to localized SPAMM 1-1 tagging. *J Magn Reson* **157**(2): 218–222.

Ikonomidou, V. N. and Sergiadis, G. D. (2003). Multirate SPAMM tagging. *IEEE Trans Biomed Eng* **50**(9): 1045–1051.

Ingels, N. B., Jr., Daughters, G. T., 2nd, Stinson, E. B., and Alderman, E. L. (1980). Evaluation of methods for quantitating left ventricular segmental wall motion in man using myocardial markers as a standard. *Circulation* **61**(5): 966–972.

Inoue, Y., Yang, X., Nagao, M., Higashino, H., Hosokawa, K., Kido, T., Kurata, A. et al. (2010). Peri-infarct dysfunction in post-myocardial infarction: Assessment of 3-T tagged and late enhancement MRI. *Eur Radiol* **20**(5): 1139–1148.

Ivancevic, M. K., Daire, J. L., Hyacinthe, J. N., Crelier, G., Kozerke, S., Montet-Abou, K., Gunes-Tatar, I., Morel, D. R., and Vallee, J. P. (2007). High-resolution complementary spatial modulation of magnetization (CSPAMM) rat heart tagging on a 1.5 Tesla Clinical Magnetic Resonance System: A preliminary feasibility study. *Invest Radiol* **42**(3): 204–210.

Jeung, M. Y., Germain, P., Croisille, P., El ghannudi, S., Roy, C., and Gangi, A. (2012). Myocardial tagging with MR imaging: Overview of normal and pathologic findings. *Radiographics* **32**(5): 1381–1398.

Jiang, K. and Yu, X. (2014). Quantification of regional myocardial wall motion by cardiovascular magnetic resonance. *Quant Imaging Med Surg* **4**(5): 345–357.

Jung, B., Foll, D., Bottler, P., Peterson, S., Hennig, J., and Markl, M. (2006). Detailed analysis of myocardial motion in volunteers and patients using high-temporal-resolution MR tissue phase mapping. *J Magn Reson Imaging* **24**: 1033–1039.

Kanzaki, H., Nakatani, S., Yamada, N., Urayama, S., Miyatake, K., and Kitakaze, M. (2006). Impaired systolic torsion in dilated cardiomyopathy: Reversal of apical rotation at mid-systole characterized with magnetic resonance tagging method. *Basic Res Cardiol* **101**(6): 465–470.

Kerwin, W. S. and Prince, J. L. (1998). Cardiac material markers from tagged MR images. *Med Image Anal* **2**(4): 339–353.

Kerwin, W. S. and Prince, J. L. (2000). A k-space analysis of MR tagging. *J Magn Reson* **142**(2): 313–322.

Kim, Y. J., Choi, B. W., Hur, J., Lee, H. J., Seo, J. S., Kim, T. H., Choe, K. O., and Ha, J. W. (2008). Delayed enhancement in hypertrophic cardiomyopathy: Comparison with myocardial tagging MRI. *J Magn Reson Imaging* **27**(5): 1054–1060.

Kitzman, D. W., Gardin, J. M., Gottdiener, J. S., Arnold, A., Boineau, R., Aurigemma, G., Marino, E. K. et al. (2001). Importance of heart failure with preserved systolic function in patients > or = 65 years of age. CHS Research Group. Cardiovascular Health Study. *Am J Cardiol* **87**(4): 413–419.

Klein, S. S., Graham, T. P., Jr., and Lorenz, C. H. (1998). Noninvasive delineation of normal right ventricular contractile motion with magnetic resonance imaging myocardial tagging. *Ann Biomed Eng* **26**(5): 756–763.

Kojima, S., Yamada, N., and Goto, Y. (1999). Diagnosis of constrictive pericarditis by tagged cine magnetic resonance imaging. *N Engl J Med* **341**(5): 373–374.

Kolipaka, A., McGee, K. P., Araoz, P. A., Glaser, K. J., Manduca, A., and Ehman, R. L. (2009a). Evaluation of a rapid, multiphase MRE sequence in a heart-simulating phantom. *Magn Reson Med* **62**(3): 691–698.

Kolipaka, A., McGee, K. P., Araoz, P. A., Glaser, K. J., Manduca, A., Romano, A. J., and Ehman, R. L. (2009b). MR elastography as a method for the assessment of myocardial stiffness: Comparison with an established pressure-volume model in a left ventricular model of the heart. *Magn Reson Med* **62**(1): 135–140.

Korosoglou, G., Lehrke, S., Wochele, A., Hoerig, B., Lossnitzer, D., Steen, H., Giannitsis, E., Osman, N. F., and Katus, H. A. (2010). Strain-encoded CMR for the detection of inducible ischemia during intermediate stress. *JACC Cardiovasc Imaging* **3**(4): 361–371.

Korosoglou, G., Lossnitzer, D., Schellberg, D., Lewien, A., Wochele, A., Schaeufele, T., Neizel, M. et al. (2009). Strain-encoded cardiac MRI as an adjunct for dobutamine stress testing: Incremental value to conventional wall motion analysis. *Circ Cardiovasc Imaging* **2**(2): 132–140.

Korosoglou, G., Youssef, A. A., Bilchick, K. C., Ibrahim, El-S. H., Lardo, A. C., Lai, S., and Osman, N. F. (2008). Real-time fast strain-encoded magnetic resonance imaging to evaluate regional myocardial function at 3.0 Tesla: Comparison to conventional tagging. *J Magn Reson Imaging* **27**(5): 1012–1018.

Kraitchman, D. L., Sampath, S., Castillo, E., Derbyshire, J. A., Boston, R. C., Bluemke, D. A., Gerber, B. L., Prince, J. L., and Osman, N. F. (2003). Quantitative ischemia detection during cardiac magnetic resonance stress testing by use of FastHARP. *Circulation* **107**(15): 2025–2030.

Kraitchman, D. L., Young, A. A., Bloomgarden, D. C., Fayad, Z. A., Dougherty, L., Ferrari, V. A., Boston, R. C., and Axel, L. (1998). Integrated MRI assessment of regional function and perfusion in canine myocardial infarction. *Magn Reson Med* **40**(2): 311–326.

Kraitchman, D. L., Young, A. A., Chang, C. N., and Axel, L. (1995). Semi-automatic tracking of myocardial motion in MR tagged images. *IEEE Trans Med Imaging* **14**(3): 422–433.

Kramer, C. M., Lima, J. A., Reichek, N., Ferrari, V. A., Llaneras, M. R., Palmon, L. C., Yeh, I. T., Tallant, B., and Axel, L. (1993). Regional differences in function within noninfarcted myocardium during left ventricular remodeling. *Circulation* **88**(3): 1279–1288.

Kramer, C. M., Magovern, J. A., Rogers, W. J., Vido, D., and Savage, E. B. (2002a). Reverse remodeling and improved regional function after repair of left ventricular aneurysm. *J Thorac Cardiovasc Surg* **123**(4): 700–706.

Kramer, C. M., Malkowski, M. J., Mankad, S., Theobald, T. M., Pakstis, D. L., and Rogers, W. J., Jr. (2002b). Magnetic resonance tagging and echocardiographic response to dobutamine and functional improvement after reperfused myocardial infarction. *Am Heart J* **143**(6): 1046–1051.

Kramer, C. M., McCreery, C. J., Semonik, L., Rogers, W. J., Power, T. P., Shaffer, A., and Reichek, N. (2000). Global alterations in mechanical function in healed reperfused first anterior myocardial infarction. *J Cardiovasc Magn Reson* **2**(1): 33–41.

Kramer, C. M., Reichek, N., Ferrari, V. A., Theobald, T., Dawson, J., and Axel, L. (1994). Regional heterogeneity of function in hypertrophic cardiomyopathy. *Circulation* **90**(1): 186–194.

Kramer, C. M., Rogers, W. J., Theobald, T. M., Power, T. P., Petruolo, S., and Reichek, N. (1996). Remote noninfarcted region dysfunction soon after first anterior myocardial infarction. A magnetic resonance tagging study. *Circulation* **94**(4): 660–666.

Kroeker, C. A., Tyberg, J. V., and Beyar, R. (1995). Effects of ischemia on left ventricular apex rotation. An experimental study in anesthetized dogs. *Circulation* **92**(12): 3539–3548.

Kuijer, J. P., Hofman, M. B., Zwanenburg, J. J., Marcus, J. T., van Rossum, A. C., and Heethaar, R. M. (2006). DENSE and HARP: Two views on the same technique of phase-based strain imaging. *J Magn Reson Imaging* **24**(6): 1432–1438.

Kuijer, J. P., Marcus, J. T., Gotte, M. J., van Rossum, A. C., and Heethaar, R. M. (2000). Three-dimensional myocardial strain analysis based on short- and long-axis magnetic resonance tagged images using a 1D displacement field. *Magn Reson Imaging* **18**(5): 553–564.

Kuijpers, D., Ho, K. Y., van Dijkman, P. R., Vliegenthart, R., and Oudkerk, M. (2003). Dobutamine cardiovascular magnetic resonance for the detection of myocardial ischemia with the use of myocardial tagging. *Circulation* **107**(12): 1592–1597.

Kumar, S. and Goldgof, D. (1994). Automatic tracking of SPAMM grid and the estimation of deformation parameters from cardiac MR images. *IEEE Trans Med Imaging* **13**(1): 122–132.

Kurotobi, S., Naito, H., Sano, T., Arisawa, J., Matsushita, T., Takeuchi, M., Kogaki, S., and Okada, S. (1998). Left ventricular regional systolic motion in patients with right ventricular pressure overload. *Int J Cardiol* **67**(1): 55–63.

Kwong, R. Y. (2007). *Cardiovascular Magnetic Resonance Imaging.* Totowa, NJ: Humana Press.

Lardo, A. C., Abraham, T. P., and Kass, D. A. (2005). Magnetic resonance imaging assessment of ventricular dyssynchrony: Current and emerging concepts. *J Am Coll Cardiol* **46**(12): 2223–2228.

Lardo, A. C., Fayad, Z. A., Chronos, N. A., and Fuster, V. (2007). *Cardiovascular Magnetic Resonance.* New York: Martin Dunitz.

Lee, V. S. (2005). *Cardiovascular MR Imaging: Physical Principles to Practical Protocols.* Philadelphia, PA: Lippincott Williams & Wilkins.

Lewa, G. J. (1994). Elastic properties imaging by periodical displacement NMR measurements (EPMRI). *Proceedings of the IEEE Ultrasonics Symposium*, Cannes, France, pp. 691–694.

Lima, J. A., Ferrari, V. A., Reichek, N., Kramer, C. M., Palmon, L., Llaneras, M. R., Tallant, B., Young, A. A., and Axel, L. (1995). Segmental motion and deformation of transmurally infarcted myocardium in acute postinfarct period. *Am J Physiol* **268**(3 Pt 2): H1304–H1312.

Lima, J. A., Jeremy, R., Guier, W., Bouton, S., Zerhouni, E. A., McVeigh, E., Buchalter, M. B., Weisfeldt, M. L., Shapiro, E. P., and Weiss, J. L. (1993). Accurate systolic wall thickening by nuclear magnetic resonance imaging with tissue tagging: Correlation with sonomicrometers in normal and ischemic myocardium. *J Am Coll Cardiol* **21**(7): 1741–1751.

Litwiller, D. V., Lee, S. J., Kolipaka, A., Mariappan, Y. K., Glaser, K. J., Pulido, J. S., and Ehman, R. L. (2010). MR elastography of the ex vivo bovine globe. *J Magn Reson Imaging* **32**(1): 44–51.

Lorca, M. C., Haraldsson, H., and Ordovas, K. G. (2015). Ventricular mechanics: Techniques and applications. *Magn Reson Imaging Clin N Am* **23**(1): 7–13.

Lorenz, C. H., Pastorek, J. S., and Bundy, J. M. (2000). Delineation of normal human left ventricular twist throughout systole by tagged cine magnetic resonance imaging. *J Cardiovasc Magn Reson* **2**(2): 97–108.

MacGowan, G. A., Shapiro, E. P., Azhari, H., Siu, C. O., Hees, P. S., Hutchins, G. M., Weiss, J. L., and Rademakers, F. E. (1997). Noninvasive measurement of shortening in the fiber and cross-fiber directions in the normal human left ventricle and in idiopathic dilated cardiomyopathy. *Circulation* **96**(2): 535–541.

Maier, S. E., Fischer, S. E., McKinnon, G. C., Hess, O. M., Krayenbuehl, H. P., and Boesiger, P. (1992). Evaluation of left ventricular segmental wall motion in hypertrophic cardiomyopathy with myocardial tagging. *Circulation* **86**(6): 1919–1928.

Manning, W. J. and Pennell, D. J. (2010). *Cardiovascular Magnetic Resonance.* London, U.K.: Churchill Livingstone.

Marcus, J. T., Gotte, M. J., Van Rossum, A. C., Kuijer, J. P., Heethaar, R. M., Axel, L., and Visser, C. A. (1997). Myocardial function in infarcted and remote regions early after infarction in man: Assessment by magnetic resonance tagging and strain analysis. *Magn Reson Med* **38**(5): 803–810.

Maret, E., Todt, T., Brudin, L., Nylander, E., Swahn, E., Ohlsson, J. L., and Engvall, J. E. (2009). Functional measurements based on feature tracking of cine magnetic resonance images identify left ventricular segments with myocardial scar. *Cardiovasc Ultrasound* **7**: 53.

Markl, M., Schneider, B., and Hennig, J. (2002). Fast phase contrast cardiac magnetic resonance imaging: Improved assessment and analysis of left ventricular wall motion. *J Magn Reson Imaging* **15**(6): 642–653.

Markl, M., Schneider, B., Hennig, J., Peschl, S., Winterer, J., Krause, T., and Laubenberger, J. (1999). Cardiac phase contrast gradient echo MRI: Measurement of myocardial wall motion in healthy volunteers and patients. *Int J Card Imaging* **15**(6): 441–452.

Masood, S., Yang, G. Z., Pennell, D. J., and Firmin, D. N. (2000). Investigating intrinsic myocardial mechanics: The role of MR tagging, velocity phase mapping, and diffusion imaging. *J Magn Reson Imaging* **12**(6): 873–883.

Matter, C., Nagel, E., Stuber, M., Boesiger, P., and Hess, O. M. (1996). Assessment of systolic and diastolic LV function by MR myocardial tagging. *Basic Res Cardiol* **91**(Suppl. 2): 23–28.

McGee, K. P., Martinez, M. W., and Williamson, E. E. (2015). *Mayo Clinic Guide to Cardiac Magnetic Resonance Imaging.* Oxford, U.K.: Oxford University Press.

McGee, K. P., Williamson, E. E., and Julsrud, P. (2008). *Mayo Clinic Guide to Cardiac Magnetic Resonance Imaging.* Boca Raton, FL: CRC Press.

McKinnon, G. C., Fischer, S. E., and Maier, S. E. (1991). Non invasive measurement of myocardial motion using magnetic resonance tagging. *Austral Phys Eng Sci Med* **14**(4): 189–196.

McKnight, A. L., Kugel, J. L., Rossman, P. J., Manduca, A., Hartmann, L. C., and Ehman, R. L. (2002). MR elastography of breast cancer: Preliminary results. *Am J Roentgenol* **178**(6): 1411–1417.

McVeigh, E. R. (1996). MRI of myocardial function: Motion tracking techniques. *Magn Reson Imaging* **14**(2): 137–150.

McVeigh, E. R. and Atalar, E. (1992). Cardiac tagging with breath-hold cine MRI. *Magn Reson Med* **28**(2): 318–327.

McVeigh, E. R. and Bolster, B. D., Jr. (1998). Improved sampling of myocardial motion with variable separation tagging. *Magn Reson Med* **39**(4): 657–661.

McVeigh, E. R., Prinzen, F. W., Wyman, B. T., Tsitlik, J. E., Halperin, H. R., and Hunter, W. C. (1998). Imaging asynchronous mechanical activation of the paced heart with tagged MRI. *Magn Reson Med* **39**(4): 507–513.

Meier, G. D., Bove, A. A., Santamore, W. P., and Lynch, P. R. (1980). Contractile function in canine right ventricle. *Am J Physiol* **239**(6): H794–H804.

Mishiro, Y., Oki, T., Iuchi, A., Tabata, T., Yamada, H., Abe, M., Onose, Y. et al. (1999). Regional left ventricular myocardial contraction abnormalities and asynchrony in patients with hypertrophic cardiomyopathy evaluated by magnetic resonance spatial modulation of magnetization myocardial tagging. *Jpn Circ J* **63**(6): 442–446.

Modesto, K. and Sengupta, P. P. (2014). Myocardial mechanics in cardiomyopathies. *Prog Cardiovasc Dis* **57**(1): 111–124.

Moore, C. C., Lugo-Olivieri, C. H., McVeigh, E. R., and Zerhouni, E. A. (2000). Three-dimensional systolic strain patterns in the normal human left ventricle: Characterization with tagged MR imaging. *Radiology* **214**(2): 453–466.

Moore, C. C., Reeder, S. B., and McVeigh, E. R. (1994). Tagged MR imaging in a deforming phantom: Photographic validation. *Radiology* **190**(3): 765–769.

Mosher, T. J. and Smith, M. B. (1990). A DANTE tagging sequence for the evaluation of translational sample motion. *Magn Reson Med* **15**(2): 334–339.

Muthupillai, R., Lomas, D. J., Rossman, P. J., Greenleaf, J. F., Manduca, A., and Ehman, R. L. (1995). Magnetic resonance elastography by direct visualization of propagating acoustic strain waves. *Science* **269**(5232): 1854–1857.

Muthupillai, R., Rossman, P. J., Lomas, D. J., Greenleaf, J. F., Riederer, S. J., and Ehman, R. L. (1996). Magnetic resonance imaging of transverse acoustic strain waves. *Magn Reson Med* **36**(2): 266–274.

Myers, J. H., Stirling, M. C., Choy, M., Buda, A. J., and Gallagher, K. P. (1986). Direct measurement of inner and outer wall thickening dynamics with epicardial echocardiography. *Circulation* **74**(1): 164–172.

Myerson, S. G., Francis, J., and Neubauer, S. (2013). *Cardiovascular Magnetic Resonance*. New York: Oxford University Press.

Nagel, E., Stuber, M., Lakatos, M., Scheidegger, M. B., Boesiger, P., and Hess, O. M. (2000). Cardiac rotation and relaxation after anterolateral myocardial infarction. *Coron Artery Dis* **11**(3): 261–267.

Nagel, E., van Rossum, A. C., and Fleck, E. (2004). *Cardiovascular Magnetic Resonance*. Berlin, Germany: Steinkopff.

Naito, H., Arisawa, J., Harada, K., Yamagami, H., Kozuka, T., and Tamura, S. (1995). Assessment of right ventricular regional contraction and comparison with the left ventricle in normal humans: A cine magnetic resonance study with presaturation myocardial tagging. *Br Heart J* **74**(2): 186–191.

Nasiraei-Moghaddam, A. and Finn, J. P. (2014). Tagging of cardiac magnetic resonance images in the polar coordinate system: Physical principles and practical implementation. *Magn Reson Med* **71**(5): 1750–1759.

Nasiraei-Moghaddam, A. and Gharib, M. (2009). Evidence for the existence of a functional helical myocardial band. *Am J Physiol Heart Circ Physiol* **296**(1): H127–H131.

Neizel, M., Lossnitzer, D., Korosoglou, G., Schaufele, T., Lewien, A., Steen, H., Katus, H. A., Osman, N. F., and Giannitsis, E. (2009a). Strain-encoded (SENC) magnetic resonance imaging to evaluate regional heterogeneity of myocardial strain in healthy volunteers: Comparison with conventional tagging. *J Magn Reson Imaging* **29**(1): 99–105.

Neizel, M., Lossnitzer, D., Korosoglou, G., Schaufele, T., Peykarjou, H., Steen, H., Ocklenburg, C., Giannitsis, E., Katus, H. A., and Osman, N. F. (2009b). Strain-encoded MRI for evaluation of left ventricular function and transmurality in acute myocardial infarction. *Circ Cardiovasc Imaging* **2**(2): 116–122.

Nelson, G. S., Curry, C. W., Wyman, B. T., Kramer, A., Declerck, J., Talbot, M., Douglas, M. R., Berger, R. D., McVeigh, E. R., and Kass, D. A. (2000). Predictors of systolic augmentation from left ventricular preexcitation in patients with dilated cardiomyopathy and intraventricular conduction delay. *Circulation* **101**(23): 2703–2709.

O'Dell, W. G. and McCulloch, A. D. (2000). Imaging three-dimensional cardiac function. *Annu Rev Biomed Eng* **2**: 431–456.

O'Dell, W. G., Moore, C. C., Hunter, W. C., Zerhouni, E. A., and McVeigh, E. R. (1995). Three-dimensional myocardial deformations: Calculation with displacement field fitting to tagged MR images. *Radiology* **195**(3): 829–835.

Ordovas, K. G. (2015). *Updates in Cardiac MRI*. Philadelphia, PA: Elsevier.

Osman, N. F. (2003). Detecting stiff masses using strain-encoded (SENC) imaging. *Magn Reson Med* **49**(3): 605–608.

Osman, N. F., Kerwin, W. S., McVeigh, E. R., and Prince, J. L. (1999). Cardiac motion tracking using CINE harmonic phase (HARP) magnetic resonance imaging. *Magn Reson Med* **42**(6): 1048–1060.

Osman, N. F., Sampath, S., Atalar, E., and Prince, J. L. (2001). Imaging longitudinal cardiac strain on short-axis images using strain-encoded MRI. *Magn Reson Med* **46**(2): 324–334.

Oxenham, H. C., Young, A. A., Cowan, B. R., Gentles, T. L., Occleshaw, C. J., Fonseca, C. G., Doughty, R. N., and Sharpe, N. (2003). Age-related changes in myocardial relaxation using three-dimensional tagged magnetic resonance imaging. *J Cardiovasc Magn Reson* **5**(3): 421–430.

Ozturk, C. and McVeigh, E. R. (2000). Four-dimensional B-spline based motion analysis of tagged MR images: Introduction and in vivo validation. *Phys Med Biol* **45**(6): 1683–1702.

Paetsch, I., Foll, D., Kaluza, A., Luechinger, R., Stuber, M., Bornstedt, A., Wahl, A., Fleck, E., and Nagel, E. (2005). Magnetic resonance stress tagging in ischemic heart disease. *Am J Physiol Heart Circ Physiol* **288**(6): H2708–H2714.

Pai, V. M. and Axel, L. (2006). Advances in MRI tagging techniques for determining regional myocardial strain. *Curr Cardiol Rep* **8**(1): 53–58.

Pan, L., Prince, J. L., Lima, J. A., and Osman, N. F. (2005). Fast tracking of cardiac motion using 3D-HARP. *IEEE Trans Biomed Eng* **52**(8): 1425–1435.

Pan, L., Stuber, M., Kraitchman, D. L., Fritzges, D. L., Gilson, W. D., and Osman, N. F. (2006). Real-time imaging of regional myocardial function using fast-SENC. *Magn Reson Med* **55**(2): 386–395.

Park, J., Metaxas, D., and Axel, L. (1996). Analysis of left ventricular wall motion based on volumetric deformable models and MRI-SPAMM. *Med Image Anal* **1**(1): 53–71.

Pelc, L. R., Sayre, J., Yun, K., Castro, L. J., Herfkens, R. J., Miller, D. C., and Pelc, N. J. (1994). Evaluation of myocardial motion tracking with cine-phase contrast magnetic resonance imaging. *Invest Radiol* **29**(12): 1038–1042.

Pelc, N. J., Drangova, M., Pelc, L. R., Zhu, Y., Noll, D. C., Bowman, B. S., and Herfkens, R. J. (1995). Tracking of cyclic motion with phase-contrast cine MR velocity data. *J Magn Reson Imaging* **5**(3): 339–345.

Peters, D. C., Epstein, F. H., and McVeigh, E. R. (2001). Myocardial wall tagging with undersampled projection reconstruction. *Magn Reson Med* **45**(4): 562–567.

Petersen, S. E., Jung, B. A., Wiesmann, F., Selvanayagam, J. B., Francis, J. M., Hennig, J., Neubauer, S., and Robson, M. D. (2006). Myocardial tissue phase mapping with cine phase-contrast mr imaging: Regional wall motion analysis in healthy volunteers. *Radiology* **238**(3): 816–826.

Petitjean, C., Rougon, N., and Cluzel, P. (2005). Assessment of myocardial function: A review of quantification methods and results using tagged MRI. *J Cardiovasc Magn Reson* **7**(2): 501–516.

Phatak, N. S., Maas, S. A., Veress, A. I., Pack, N. A., Di Bella, E. V., and Weiss, J. A. (2009). Strain measurement in the left ventricle during systole with deformable image registration. *Med Image Anal* **13**(2): 354–361.

Pilla, J. J., Blom, A. S., Brockman, D. J., Bowen, F., Yuan, Q., Giammarco, J., Ferrari, V. A., Gorman, J. H., 3rd, Gorman, R. C., and Acker, M. A. (2002). Ventricular constraint using the acorn cardiac support device reduces myocardial akinetic area in an ovine model of acute infarction. *Circulation* **106**(12 Suppl. 1): I207–I211.

Pipe, J. G., Boes, J. L., and Chenevert, T. L. (1991). Method for measuring three-dimensional motion with tagged MR imaging. *Radiology* **181**(2): 591–595.

Plewes, D. B., Betty, I., Urchuk, S. N., and Soutar, I. (1995). Visualizing tissue compliance with MR imaging. *J Magn Reson Imaging* **5**(6): 733–738.

Pohost, G. M. and Nayak, K. S. (2006). *Handbook of Cardiovascular Magnetic Resonance Imaging*. New York: CRC Press.

Power, T. P., Kramer, C. M., Shaffer, A. L., Theobald, T. M., Petruolo, S., Reichek, N., and Rogers, W. J., Jr. (1997). Breath-hold dobutamine magnetic resonance myocardial tagging: Normal left ventricular response. *Am J Cardiol* **80**(9): 1203–1207.

Prince, J. L., Gupta, S. N., and Osman, N. F. (2000). Bandpass optical flow for tagged MRI. *Med Phys* **27**(1): 108–118.

Prince, J. L. and McVeigh, E. R. (1992). Motion estimation from tagged MR image sequences. *IEEE Trans Med Imaging* **11**(2): 238–249.

Prinzen, F. W., Arts, T., Hoeks, A. P., and Reneman, R. S. (1989). Discrepancies between myocardial blood flow and fiber shortening in the ischemic border zone as assessed with video mapping of epicardial deformation. *Pflugers Arch* **415**(2): 220–229.

Pusca, S. V., Pilla, J. J., Blom, A. S., Patel, H. J., Yuan, Q., Ferrari, V. A., Prood, C., Axel, L., and Acker, M. A. (2000). Assessment of synchronized direct mechanical ventricular actuation in a canine model of left ventricular dysfunction. *ASAIO J* **46**(6): 756–760.

Qian, Z., Metaxas, D. N., and Axel, L. (2006). Extraction and tracking of MRI tagging sheets using a 3D Gabor filter bank. *Conf Proc IEEE Eng Med Biol Soc* **1**: 711–714.

Rademakers, F. E. and Bogaert, J. (1997). Left ventricular myocardial tagging. *Int J Card Imaging* **13**(3): 233–245.

Rankin, J. S., McHale, P. A., Arentzen, C. E., Ling, D., Greenfield, J. C., Jr., and Anderson, R. W. (1976). The three-dimensional dynamic geometry of the left ventricle in the conscious dog. *Circ Res* **39**(3): 304–313.

Reeder, S. B., Atalar, E., Faranesh, A. Z., and McVeigh, E. R. (1999). Multi-echo segmented k-space imaging: An optimized hybrid sequence for ultrafast cardiac imaging. *Magn Reson Med* **41**(2): 375–385.

Reeder, S. B. and McVeigh, E. R. (1994). Tag contrast in breath-hold CINE cardiac MRI. *Magn Reson Med* **31**(5): 521–525.

Reichek, N. (1999). MRI myocardial tagging. *J Magn Reson Imaging* **10**(5): 609–616.

Ringleb, S. I., Chen, Q., Lake, D. S., Manduca, A., Ehman, R. L., and An, K. N. (2005). Quantitative shear wave magnetic resonance elastography: Comparison to a dynamic shear material test. *Magn Reson Med* **53**(5): 1197–1201.

Robert, B., Sinkus, R., Gennisson, J. L., and Fink, M. (2009a). Application of DENSE-MR-elastography to the human heart. *Magn Reson Med* **62**(5): 1155–1163.

Robert, B., Sinkus, R., Gennisson, J. L., and Fink, M. (2009b). Application of DENSE MR-elastography to the human heart: First in vivo results. *Proceedings of the International Society of Magnetic Resonance in Medicine*, Honolulu, HI.

Rodriguez, I., Ennis, D. B., and Wen, H. (2006). Noninvasive measurement of myocardial tissue volume change during systolic contraction and diastolic relaxation in the canine left ventricle. *Magn Reson Med* **55**(3): 484–490.

Rogers, W. J., Jr., Kramer, C. M., Geskin, G., Hu, Y. L., Theobald, T. M., Vido, D. A., Petruolo, S., and Reichek, N. (1999). Early contrast-enhanced MRI predicts late functional recovery after reperfused myocardial infarction. *Circulation* **99**(6): 744–750.

Rogers, W. J., Jr., Shapiro, E. P., Weiss, J. L., Buchalter, M. B., Rademakers, F. E., Weisfeldt, M. L., and Zerhouni, E. A. (1991). Quantification of and correction for left ventricular systolic long-axis shortening by magnetic resonance tissue tagging and slice isolation. *Circulation* **84**(2): 721–731.

Rosamond, W., Flegal, K., Furie, K., Go, A., Greenlund, K., Haase, N., Hailpern, S. M. et al. (2008). Heart disease and stroke statistics—2008 update: A report from the American Heart Association Statistics Committee and Stroke Statistics Subcommittee. *Circulation* **117**(4): e25–e146.

Rosen, B. D., Lima, J. A., Nasir, K., Edvardsen, T., Folsom, A. R., Lai, S., Bluemke, D. A., and Jerosch-Herold, M. (2006). Lower myocardial perfusion reserve is associated with decreased regional left ventricular function in asymptomatic participants of the multi-ethnic study of atherosclerosis. *Circulation* **114**(4): 289–297.

Rouviere, O., Yin, M., Dresner, M. A., Rossman, P. J., Burgart, L. J., Fidler, J. L., and Ehman, R. L. (2006). MR elastography of the liver: Preliminary results. *Radiology* **240**(2): 440–448.

Rump, J., Klatt, D., Braun, J., Warmuth, C., and Sack, I. (2007). Fractional encoding of harmonic motions in MR elastography. *Magn Reson Med* **57**(2): 388–395.

Ryf, S., Kissinger, K. V., Spiegel, M. A., Bornert, P., Manning, W. J., Boesiger, P., and Stuber, M. (2004). Spiral MR myocardial tagging. *Magn Reson Med* **51**(2): 237–242.

Saber, N. R. and Wen, H. (2004). Construction of the global lagrangian strain field in the myocardium using DENSE MRI data. *Conf Proc IEEE Eng Med Biol Soc* **5**: 3670–3673.

Sack, I., Rump, J., Elgeti, T., Samani, A., and Braun, J. (2009). MR elastography of the human heart: Noninvasive assessment of myocardial elasticity changes by shear wave amplitude variations. *Magn Reson Med* **61**(3): 668–677.

Samady, H., Choi, C. J., Ragosta, M., Powers, E. R., Beller, G. A., and Kramer, C. M. (2004). Electromechanical mapping identifies improvement in function and retention of contractile reserve after revascularization in ischemic cardiomyopathy. *Circulation* **110**(16): 2410–2416.

Sampath, S., Derbyshire, J. A., Atalar, E., Osman, N. F., and Prince, J. L. (2003). Real-time imaging of two-dimensional cardiac strain using a harmonic phase magnetic resonance imaging (HARP-MRI) pulse sequence. *Magn Reson Med* **50**(1): 154–163.

Sampath, S., Osman, N. F., and Prince, J. L. (2009). A combined harmonic phase and strain-encoded pulse sequence for measuring three-dimensional strain. *Magn Reson Imaging* **27**(1): 55–61.

Sandstede, J. J., Johnson, T., Harre, K., Beer, M., Hofmann, S., Pabst, T., Kenn, W., Voelker, W., Neubauer, S., and Hahn, D. (2002). Cardiac systolic rotation and contraction before and after valve replacement for aortic stenosis: A myocardial tagging study using MR imaging. *AJR Am J Roentgenol* **178**(4): 953–958.

Sayad, D. E., Willett, D. L., Hundley, W. G., Grayburn, P. A., and Peshock, R. M. (1998). Dobutamine magnetic resonance imaging with myocardial tagging quantitatively predicts improvement in regional function after revascularization. *Am J Cardiol* **82**(9): 1149–1151, A10.

Scheffler, K., Heid, O., and Hennig, J. (2001). Magnetization preparation during the steady state: Fat-saturated 3D TrueFISP. *Magn Reson Med* **45**(6): 1075–1080.

Schregel, K., Wuerfel, E., Garteiser, P., Gemeinhardt, I., Prozorovski, T., Aktas, O., Merz, H., Petersen, D., Wuerfel, J., and Sinkus, R. (2012). Demyelination reduces brain parenchymal stiffness quantified in vivo by magnetic resonance elastography. *Proc Natl Acad Sci USA* **109**(17): 6650–6655.

Scott, C. H., Sutton, M. S., Gusani, N., Fayad, Z., Kraitchman, D., Keane, M. G., Axel, L., and Ferrari, V. A. (1999). Effect of dobutamine on regional left ventricular function measured by tagged magnetic resonance imaging in normal subjects. *Am J Cardiol* **83**(3): 412–417.

Setser, R. M., Kasper, J. M., Lieber, M. L., Starling, R. C., McCarthy, P. M., and White, R. D. (2003a). Persistent abnormal left ventricular systolic torsion in dilated cardiomyopathy after partial left ventriculectomy. *J Thorac Cardiovasc Surg* **126**(1): 48–55.

Setser, R. M., White, R. D., Sturm, B., McCarthy, P. M., Starling, R. C., Young, J. B., Kasper, J., Buda, T., Obuchowski, N., and Lieber, M. L. (2003b). Noninvasive assessment of cardiac mechanics and clinical outcome after partial left ventriculectomy. *Ann Thorac Surg* **76**(5): 1576–1585; discussion 1585–1576.

Shehata, M. L., Cheng, S., Osman, N. F., Bluemke, D. A., and Lima, J. A. (2009). Myocardial tissue tagging with cardiovascular magnetic resonance. *J Cardiovasc Magn Reson* **11**: 55.

Simpson, R. M., Keegan, J., and Firmin, D. N. (2013). MR assessment of regional myocardial mechanics. *J Magn Reson Imaging* **37**(3): 576–599.

Sinkus, R., Lorenzen, J., Schrader, D., Lorenzen, M., Dargatz, M., and Holz, D. (2000). High-resolution tensor MR elastography for breast tumour detection. *Phys Med Biol* **45**(6): 1649–1664.

Sinkus, R., Siegmann, K., Xydeas, T., Tanter, M., Claussen, C., and Fink, M. (2007). MR elastography of breast lesions: Understanding the solid/liquid duality can improve the specificity of contrast-enhanced MR mammography. *Magn Reson Med* **58**(6): 1135–1144.

Sinkus, R., Tanter, M., Catheline, S., Lorenzen, J., Kuhl, C., Sondermann, E., and Fink, M. (2005). Imaging anisotropic and viscous properties of breast tissue by magnetic resonance-elastography. *Magn Reson Med* **53**(2): 372–387.

Soler, R., Rodriguez, E., Monserrat, L., Mendez, C., and Martinez, C. (2006). Magnetic resonance imaging of delayed enhancement in hypertrophic cardiomyopathy: Relationship with left ventricular perfusion and contractile function. *J Comput Assist Tomogr* **30**(3): 412–420.

Spiegel, M. A., Luechinger, R., Schwitter, J., and Boesiger, P. (2003). RingTag: Ring-shaped tagging for myocardial centerline assessment. *Invest Radiol* **38**(10): 669–678.

Spottiswoode, B., Russell, J. B., Moosa, S., Meintjes, E. M., Epstein, F. H., and Mayosi, B. M. (2008a). Abnormal diastolic and systolic septal motion following pericardiectomy demonstrated by cine DENSE MRI. *Cardiovasc J Afr* **19**(4): 208–209.

Spottiswoode, B. S., Zhong, X., Lorenz, C. H., Mayosi, B. M., Meintjes, E. M., and Epstein, F. H. (2008b). 3D myocardial tissue tracking with slice followed cine DENSE MRI. *J Magn Reson Imaging* **27**(5): 1019–1027.

Stuber, M., Scheidegger, M. B., Fischer, S. E., Nagel, E., Steinemann, F., Hess, O. M., and Boesiger, P. (1999a). Alterations in the local myocardial motion pattern in patients suffering from pressure overload due to aortic stenosis. *Circulation* **100**(4): 361–368.

Stuber, M., Spiegel, M. A., Fischer, S. E., Scheidegger, M. B., Danias, P. G., Pedersen, E. M., and Boesiger, P. (1999b). Single breath-hold slice-following CSPAMM myocardial tagging. *MAGMA* **9**(1–2): 85–91.

Tang, C., McVeigh, E. R., and Zerhouni, E. A. (1995). Multi-shot EPI for improvement of myocardial tag contrast: Comparison with segmented SPGR. *Magn Reson Med* **33**(3): 443–447.

Tavakoli, V. and Sahba, N. (2014). Cardiac motion and strain detection using 4D CT images: Comparison with tagged MRI, and echocardiography. *Int J Cardiovasc Imaging* **30**(1): 175–184.

Tee, M., Noble, J. A., and Bluemke, D. A. (2013). Imaging techniques for cardiac strain and deformation: Comparison of echocardiography, cardiac magnetic resonance and cardiac computed tomography. *Expert Rev Cardiovasc Ther* **11**(2): 221–231.

Tustison, N. J., Davila-Roman, V. G., and Amini, A. A. (2003). Myocardial kinematics from tagged MRI based on a 4-D B-spline model. *IEEE Trans Biomed Eng* **50**(8): 1038–1040.

Ungacta, F. F., Davila-Roman, V. G., Moulton, M. J., Cupps, B. P., Moustakidis, P., Fishman, D. S., Actis, R. et al. (1998). MRI-radiofrequency tissue tagging in patients with aortic insufficiency before and after operation. *Ann Thorac Surg* **65**(4): 943–950.

Van Houten, E. E., Paulsen, K. D., Miga, M. I., Kennedy, F. E., and Weaver, J. B. (1999). An overlapping subzone technique for MR-based elastic property reconstruction. *Magn Reson Med* **42**(4): 779–786.

Vappou, J., Breton, E., Choquet, P., Goetz, C., Willinger, R., and Constantinesco, A. (2007). Magnetic resonance elastography compared with rotational rheometry for in vitro brain tissue viscoelasticity measurement. *MAGMA* **20**(5–6): 273–278.

Villari, B., Campbell, S. E., Hess, O. M., Mall, G., Vassalli, G., Weber, K. T., and Krayenbuehl, H. P. (1993). Influence of collagen network on left ventricular systolic and diastolic function in aortic valve disease. *J Am Coll Cardiol* **22**(5): 1477–1484.

Villarreal, F. J., Waldman, L. K., and Lew, W. Y. (1988). Technique for measuring regional two-dimensional finite strains in canine left ventricle. *Circ Res* **62**(4): 711–721.

Vonk-Noordegraaf, A., Marcus, J. T., Gan, C. T., Boonstra, A., and Postmus, P. E. (2005). Interventricular mechanical asynchrony due to right ventricular pressure overload in pulmonary hypertension plays an important role in impaired left ventricular filling. *Chest* **128**(6 Suppl.): 628S–630S.

Wang, Y. P., Chen, Y., and Amini, A. A. (2001). Fast LV motion estimation using subspace approximation techniques. *IEEE Trans Med Imaging* **20**(6): 499–513.

Wassenaar, P. A., Eleswarpu, C. N., Schroeder, S. A., Mo, X., Raterman, B. D., White, R. D., and Kolipaka, A. (2016). Measuring age-dependent myocardial stiffness across the cardiac cycle using MR elastography: A reproducibility study. *Magn Reson Med* **75**(4):1586–1593.

Wedeen, V. J. (1992). Magnetic resonance imaging of myocardial kinematics. Technique to detect, localize, and quantify the strain rates of the active human myocardium. *Magn Reson Med* **27**(1): 52–67.

Wen, H., Bennett, E., Epstein, N., and Plehn, J. (2005). Magnetic resonance imaging assessment of myocardial elastic modulus and viscosity using displacement imaging and phase-contrast velocity mapping. *Magn Reson Med* **54**(3): 538–548.

Wuerfel, J., Paul, F., Beierbach, B., Hamhaber, U., Klatt, D., Papazoglou, S., Zipp, F., Martus, P., Braun, J., and Sack, I. (2010). MR-elastography reveals degradation of tissue integrity in multiple sclerosis. *Neuroimage* **49**(3): 2520–2525.

Wyman, B. T., Hunter, W. C., Prinzen, F. W., and McVeigh, E. R. (1999). Mapping propagation of mechanical activation in the paced heart with MRI tagging. *Am J Physiol* **276**(3 Pt 2): H881–H891.

Xu, L., Lin, Y., Han, J. C., Xi, Z. N., Shen, H., and Gao, P. Y. (2007). Magnetic resonance elastography of brain tumors: Preliminary results. *Acta Radiol* **48**(3): 327–330.

Young, A. A. (1999). Model tags: Direct three-dimensional tracking of heart wall motion from tagged magnetic resonance images. *Med Image Anal* **3**(4): 361–372.

Young, A. A., Axel, L., Dougherty, L., Bogen, D. K., and Parenteau, C. S. (1993). Validation of tagging with MR imaging to estimate material deformation. *Radiology* **188**(1): 101–108.

Young, A. A., Dokos, S., Powell, K. A., Sturm, B., McCulloch, A. D., Starling, R. C., McCarthy, P. M., and White, R. D. (2001). Regional heterogeneity of function in nonischemic dilated cardiomyopathy. *Cardiovasc Res* **49**(2): 308–318.

Young, A. A., Fayad, Z. A., and Axel, L. (1996). Right ventricular midwall surface motion and deformation using magnetic resonance tagging. *Am J Physiol* **271**(6 Pt 2): H2677–H2688.

Young, A. A., Imai, H., Chang, C. N., and Axel, L. (1994a). Two-dimensional left ventricular deformation during systole using magnetic resonance imaging with spatial modulation of magnetization. *Circulation* **89**(2): 740–752.

Young, A. A., Kramer, C. M., Ferrari, V. A., Axel, L., and Reichek, N. (1994b). Three-dimensional left ventricular deformation in hypertrophic cardiomyopathy. *Circulation* **90**(2): 854–867.

Youssef, A., Ibrahim, El-S. H., Korosoglou, G., Abraham, M. R., Weiss, R. G., and Osman, N. F. (2008). Strain-encoding cardiovascular magnetic resonance for assessment of right-ventricular regional function. *J Cardiovasc Magn Reson* **10**: 33.

Zerhouni, E. A. (1993). Myocardial tagging by magnetic resonance imaging. *Coron Artery Dis* **4**(4): 334–339.

Zerhouni, E. A., Parish, D. M., Rogers, W. J., Yang, A., and Shapiro, E. P. (1988). Human heart: Tagging with MR imaging—A method for noninvasive assessment of myocardial motion. *Radiology* **169**(1): 59–63.

Zhu, Y., Drangova, M., and Pelc, N. J. (1996). Fourier tracking of myocardial motion using cine-PC data. *Magn Reson Med* **35**(4): 471–480.

Zhu, Y., Drangova, M., and Pelc, N. J. (1997). Estimation of deformation gradient and strain from cine-PC velocity data. *IEEE Trans Med Imaging* **16**(6): 840–851.

Zwanenburg, J. J., Gotte, M. J., Kuijer, J. P., Heethaar, R. M., van Rossum, A. C., and Marcus, J. T. (2004). Timing of cardiac contraction in humans mapped by high-temporal-resolution MRI tagging: Early onset and late peak of shortening in lateral wall. *Am J Physiol Heart Circ Physiol* **286**(5): H1872–H1880.

Zwanenburg, J. J., Gotte, M. J., Marcus, J. T., Kuijer, J. P., Knaapen, P., Heethaar, R. M., and van Rossum, A. C. (2005). Propagation of onset and peak time of myocardial shortening in ischemic versus nonischemic cardiomyopathy: assessment by magnetic resonance imaging myocardial tagging. *J Am Coll Cardiol* **46**(12): 2215–2222.

Zwanenburg, J. J., Kuijer, J. P., Marcus, J. T., and Heethaar, R. M. (2003). Steady-state free precession with myocardial tagging: CSPAMM in a single breathhold. *Magn Reson Med* **49**(4): 722–730.

2 Heart Morphology, Function, and Diseases

Brian P. Shapiro, MD and El-Sayed H. Ibrahim, PhD

CONTENTS

LIST OF ABBREVIATIONS

Abbreviation	Meaning
4-ch	Four-chamber
ADP	Adenosine diphosphate
Ao	Aorta
ARVC	Arrhythmogenic right ventricular cardiomyopathy
ASD	Atrial septal defect
ATP	Adenosine triphosphate
AV	Atrioventricular
CHD	Congenital heart disease
CO	Cardiac output
Cx	Circumflex coronary artery
D-TGA	Complete (dextro) TGA
E-C	Excitation–contraction
ECG	Electrocardiogram
EDP	End-diastolic pressure
EDPVR	End-diastolic pressure–volume relationship
EDV	End-diastolic volume
EF	Ejection fraction
ESP	End-systolic pressure
ESPVR	End-systolic pressure–volume relationship
ESV	End-systolic volume
HFpEF	Failure associated with a preserved ejection fraction
HR	Heart rate
IVC	Inferior vena cava
IVC	Isovolumetric contraction

Abbreviation	Meaning
IVR	Isovolumetric relaxation
LA	Left atrium
LAD	Left anterior descending coronary artery
LAX	Long-axis
LPA	Left pulmonary artery
L-TGA	Congenitally corrected (levo) TGA
LV	Left ventricle
MI	Myocardial infarction
mv	Mitral valve
MVO2	Myocardial oxygen demand
PA	Pulmonary artery
PET	Positron emission tomography
PH	Pulmonary hypertension
pv	Pulmonary valve
P-V	Pressure–volume
RA	Right atrium
RCA	Right coronary artery
RPA	Right pulmonary artery
RV	Right ventricle
RVOT	Right ventricular outflow tract
SA	Sinoatrial
SAX	Short-axis
SV	Stroke volume
SVC	Superior vena cava
TGA	Transposition of the great arteries
TOF	Tetralogy of Fallot
tv	Tricuspid valve
VSD	Ventricular septal defect

2.1 INTRODUCTION

2.1.1 BASICS OF THE CARDIOVASCULAR SYSTEM

In order to fully appreciate the complexity of heart mechanics, one must have a basic understanding of cardiovascular anatomy and physiology. With the technological advancement and sophistication of cardiovascular imaging, there is a renewed interest in the mechanics of heart contraction and relaxation. Newer imaging approaches such as cardiac magnetic resonance imaging (MRI) have made it possible to further explore these mechanisms in various cardiovascular disease states. However, prior to a more in-depth discussion of cardiovascular mechanics, we must first have a basic understanding of cardiovascular morphology and function.

2.1.2 CHAPTER OUTLINE

This chapter provides a basic understanding of the heart structure and function. Further, various heart diseases are discussed along with their relationships with heart mechanics. This chapter serves the purpose of explaining the importance of the different functional measures that will be derived using various MRI techniques in the following chapters.

2.2 CARDIAC ANATOMY

2.2.1 CARDIAC PLANES

There are a number of methods to describe and view the heart, including orthogonal radiographic imaging planes, such as axial, coronal, and sagittal planes (Figure 2.1) and standard echocardiography planes (Figure 2.2) (Edwards et al. 1981, Edwards 1984, Hundley et al. 2010).

Additional methods for viewing the heart include the cardiac long-axis (LAX) imaging in the 2-, 3-, and 4-chamber configurations (Figure 2.3). Further, the left ventricle (LV) and right ventricle (RV) can be subdivided into various short-axis (SAX) sections at the base, mid-ventricle, and apex (Figure 2.4).

2.2.2 ATRIA AND VENTRICLES

The normal heart has four chambers subdivided into two atria and two ventricles, separated by a septum (Figure 2.5).

The atria are thin-walled structures that serve as reservoirs and conduits for blood in order to fill the ventricles. While the majority of ventricular filling is passive and occurs via rapid early filling (i.e., suction), the atria provide some additional mechanical support. For example, during atrial contraction, which occurs as the last cardiac event late in diastole and immediately prior to ventricular contraction, there is an atrial "kick," which provides some additional filling of the ventricle (Ohno et al. 1994). The right atrium (RA) receives systemic venous blood from the inferior and superior vena cava (IVC and SVC), whereas the left atrium (LA) is connected to upper and lower pulmonary veins and receives oxygenated blood from the lungs.

2.2.3 BLOOD CIRCULATIONS

The right-sided chambers are part of the pulmonary circulation, which receives deoxygenated blood from the systemic veins and circulates it in the lungs through the pulmonary arteries (McLaughlin et al. 2009). Due to low pressure and high capacitance, vascular resistance is extremely low in the pulmonary circuit. Deoxygenated blood is passed through a delicate pulmonary capillary network nearby the alveoli where oxygen enters the blood. The oxygenated blood then returns to the left-sided chambers where it is subsequently pumped through the LV and into the aorta where it circulates throughout the body (systemic circulation), which completes the cardiopulmonary circuit (Figure 2.6).

2.2.4 MYOCARDIAL FIBERS

The LV is shaped as a prolate ellipsoid and is tightly woven by distinct muscle fiber layers configured in orthogonal orientations between the epi- and endocardium (Grosberg and Gharib 2009, Bijnens et al. 2012), as shown in Figure 2.7. These various layers form a helical arrangement in order to squeeze and propel the blood forward in a highly coordinated manner.

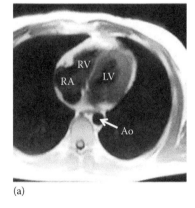 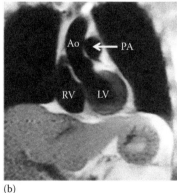 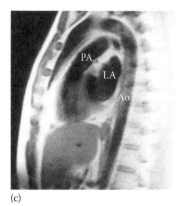

(a) (b) (c)

FIGURE 2.1 Radiographic imaging planes. Typical orthogonal imaging planes ((a) axial, (b) coronal, and (c) sagittal) demonstrated by black-blood scout images using cardiovascular MRI imaging. Ao, aorta; LA, left atrium; LV, left ventricle; PA, pulmonary artery; RA, right atrium; RV, right ventricle.

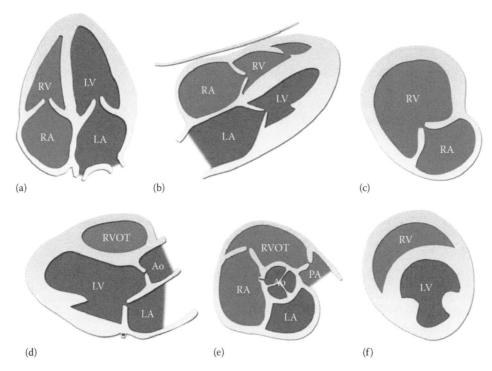

FIGURE 2.2 Echocardiographic imaging planes. (a) Apical 4-chamber. (b) Subcostal. (c) Long-axis inflow tract. (d) Parasternal long-axis. (e) Parasternal short-axis at the basal level. (f) Parasternal short-axis at the papillary muscle level. 4-ch, four-chamber; Ao, aorta; LA, left atrium; LAX, long-axis; LV, left ventricle; PA, pulmonary artery; RA, right atrium; RV, right ventricle; RVOT, RV outflow tract; SAX, short-axis.

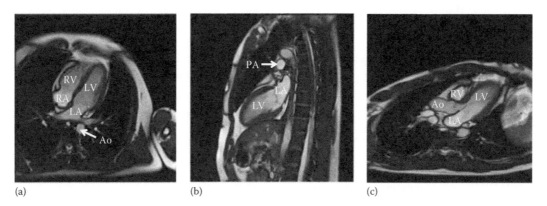

FIGURE 2.3 Cardiac long-axis imaging planes. Steady-state free precession images from an ECG-gated cardiovascular MRI examination demonstrate typical imaging planes, including (a) 4-chamber, (b) 2-chamber, and (3) 3-chamber long-axis views. Ao, aorta; ECG, electrocardiogram; LA, left atrium; LV, left ventricle; PA, pulmonary artery; RA, right atrium; RV, right ventricle.

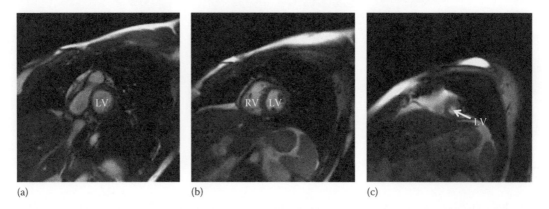

FIGURE 2.4 Cardiac short-axis imaging planes. Images from a normal subject showing short-axis imaging at the (a) base, (b) mid-ventricle, and (c) apex. LV, left ventricle; RV, right ventricle.

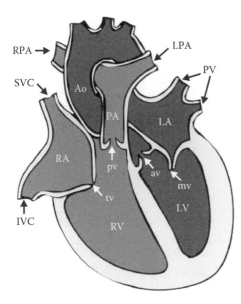

FIGURE 2.5 Heart anatomy. The heart is composed of four chambers: left ventricle (LV), right ventricle (RV), left atrium (LA), and right atrium (RA). Deoxygenated blood enters the RA through the superior vena cava (SVC) and inferior vena cava (IVC), where it moves to the RV through the tricuspid valve (tv). The RV pumps the deoxygenated blood to the lungs though the pulmonary valve (pv) and pulmonary artery (PA), which splits into the left pulmonary artery (LPA) and right pulmonary artery (RPA). Oxygenated blood returns from the lungs through the pulmonary veins (PV), where it enters the LA, and then moves to the LV through the mitral valve (mv). The LV then pumps the oxygenated blood to the whole body through the aortic valve (av) and aorta (Ao).

Myocyte shortening in each respective muscle fiber layer provides the framework for ventricular contraction and is similar to wringing a towel (see detailed discussion in Section 2.4.4).

The ventricular myocytes are surrounded by a connective tissue matrix, which supports the myocytes. Cardiac collagen forms a netlike structure surrounding the myofibers (Figure 2.8), as well as connections linking adjacent myofibers and projections connecting to blood vessels. The abundance, distribution, and type of connective tissue supporting the myocytes are major components to their passive filling properties during diastole.

2.2.5 RIGHT AND LEFT VENTRICLES

While both LV and RV possess similar functions and share morphologic and functional characteristics, there are a number of major differences between them. For example, the RV is a crescent-shaped chamber comprised of inlet, body, and outflow portions (Figure 2.9). The RV body contracts using circumferential fibers predominantly. Yet, the vast majority of contraction is contributed by longitudinal cardiac contraction, whereby the free wall of the ventricle is "pulled" downward toward the apex (Jamal et al. 2003). Thus, the thin-walled, relatively weak RV can eject large amounts of blood into the low-pressure pulmonary circulation (Puwanant et al. 2010).

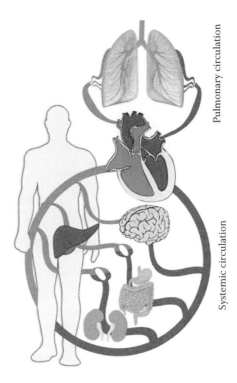

FIGURE 2.6 Blood circulations. Blood circulates through the pulmonary and systemic circulations. In the pulmonary circulation, deoxygenated blood (blue) is pumped from the heart to the lungs through the pulmonary arteries, where it is oxygenated (red) and then returns back to the heart through the pulmonary veins. In the systemic circulation, oxygenated blood is pumped from the heart to the whole body through the aorta, and deoxygenated blood returns from the whole body to the heart through the superior and inferior vena cava. (Courtesy of Dr. Shehab Anwar, National Heart Institute, Cairo, Egypt.)

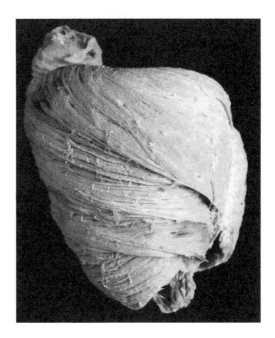

FIGURE 2.7 Myocardial fiber structure. The LV myocardium is peeled at different depths to show fiber orientations from the epi- to endocardium. (Reproduced from Anderson, R.H. et al., *Clin. Anat.*, 22(1), 64, 2009. With permission.)

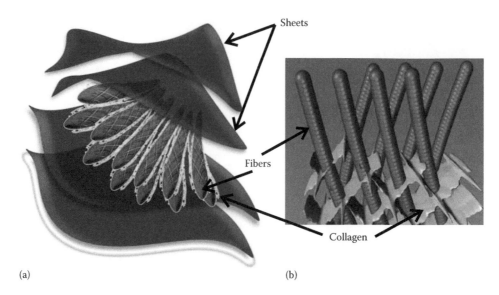

(a)   (b)

FIGURE 2.8   Myocardial sheets and fibers. (a) Sheets and fibers (surrounded by collagen) spatial arrangements. (b) The collagen forms a netlike structure surrounding the fibers and linking them together. (Courtesy of Dr. Shehab Anwar, National Heart Institute, Cairo, Egypt.)

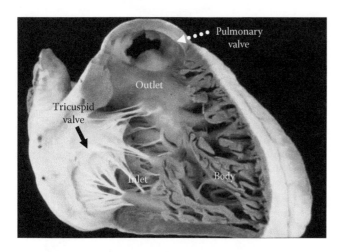

FIGURE 2.9   Right ventricle (RV) structure. A specimen demonstrating the complex nature of the RV. The RV is composed of three distinct areas including the inlet, body, and outlet. Black and white (dashed) arrows represent the tricuspid and pulmonary valves, respectively.

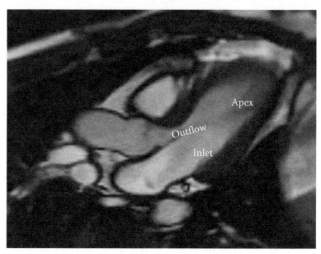

FIGURE 2.10   Left ventricle (LV) structure. Normal cardiovascular MRI image of the LV demonstrating the inlet, apex, and outflow portions.

The LV is spherical and cone shaped. Compared to the low-pressure pulmonary circulation, the systemic circulation has greater pressure and resistance (Sengupta et al. 2006). As such, the LV pumps against a high-pressure system and, thus, is threefold thicker than the RV. Similar to the RV, the LV can be separated into inlet, apex, and outflow portions (Figure 2.10). The LV and RV share a septum, which is further subdivided into the muscular and membranous septum.

2.2.6   PERICARDIUM

The pericardium is the outer layer adjacent to the heart, which acts as a protective barrier. It is composed of two distinct layers including the serous and fibrous pericardium (Figure 2.11). The layer immediately adjacent to the epicardial border, or epicardium, is thin and covers the coronary arteries and

epicardial fat. The outermost layer of this serous pericardium is in direct continuity with the thicker fibrous pericardium. Within this two-layered structure is a small amount of fluid (usually <50 mL), acting as a lubricant (Maisch et al. 2004).

2.2.7   VALVES

The cardiac skeleton anchors four valves, including the valvular rings and annuli (Bonow et al. 2006). The aortic and pulmonary valves, known as the semilunar valves, separate the ventricles from the aorta and pulmonary artery (PA), respectively. They each have similar design, composed of an annulus, commissures, and three cusps (Figure 2.12). Conversely, the atrioventricular (AV) valves include the mitral and tricuspid valves, composed of two and three leaflets, respectively. These valves separate the atria from the ventricles and include

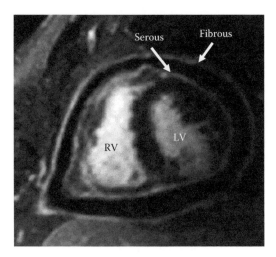

FIGURE 2.11   Pericardium structure. Delayed-enhancement image from a cardiovascular MRI examination in a patient with acute pericarditis and small pericardial effusion. The image depicts the serous and fibrous components of the pericardium, which are typically superimposed. A tiny amount of fluid lubricates the space between them. In this image, a small pericardial effusion is present, thereby providing a more thorough depiction of this sac. LV, left ventricle; RV, right ventricle.

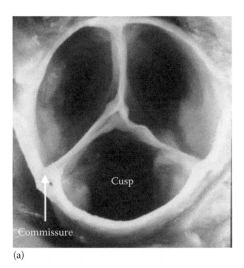

(a)

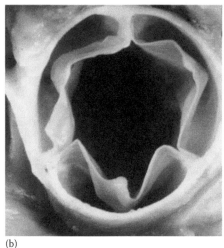

(b)

FIGURE 2.12   Aortic valve structure. A specimen of the aortic valve as seen in (a) diastole and (b) systole.

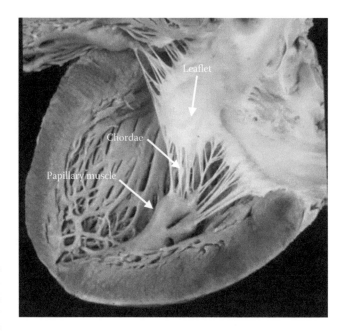

FIGURE 2.13   Mitral valve structure. A specimen of the mitral valve, which is composed of valvular and subvalvular apparatus. The valve is attached to the ventricular wall via chordae tendineae and papillary muscles.

an annulus, commissures, leaflets, chordae tendineae, and papillary muscles (Figure 2.13).

2.2.8   Coronary Arteries

The left and right coronary arteries originate from the aortic sinus, which is located immediately distal to the aortic valve (Sundaram et al. 2009a,b). While variations are not uncommon, these arteries often have a predictable course. The left main artery gives rise to the left anterior descending (LAD) coronary artery, which runs along the anterior interventricular groove and gives rise to diagonal branches as well as septal perforators. This vessel generally supplies the anterior and apical cardiac walls. The circumflex coronary artery (Cx) also arises from the left main, but it courses within the left AV groove and gives rise to obtuse marginal branches. Normally, this territory encompasses the lateral wall of the LV. The right coronary artery arises from the right coronary cusp and runs opposite to the circumflex artery in the right AV groove. This vessel is often dominant and supplies the RV and inferior wall of the LV.

The common coronary regional blood supply is depicted in Figure 2.14. The epicardial coronary arteries course adjacent to the heart, often embedded in the epicardial fat. A dense network of smaller arteries and capillaries provide blood supply within the myocardium. These vessels preferentially supply the endocardium, or innermost layer of the myocardium. Then, the supply spreads toward the epicardium. Thus, in the presence of myocardial ischemia or infarction, the endocardium is injured first, and then the wavefront of injury spreads outward toward the epicardium.

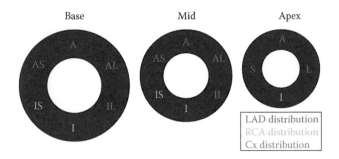

FIGURE 2.14 Coronary territories in the myocardium. Schematic of the LV in a short-axis view from base to apex. The figure shows representative coronary territories for the left anterior descending (LAD), circumflex (Cx), and right coronary arteries (RCA). A, anterior; AL, anterolateral; AS, anteroseptal; I, inferior; IL, inferoseptal; L, lateral; S, septal.

2.2.9 CONDUCTION SYSTEM

The cardiac conduction system provides an electrical signal in order for contraction to occur. The original impulse normally occurs in the sinus node, which is located at the junction of the SVC and RA. Via internodal tracts located within the RA, the AV node is formed, which is adjacent to the tricuspid annulus. The impulse then reaches the His bundle near the membranous ventricular septum, subsequently giving rise to a collection of subendocardial conduction fibers named the right and left bundle branches. The ventricular Purkinje cells are embedded within the myocardium and represent the main source of ventricular contraction.

2.3 CARDIAC PHYSIOLOGY

The cardiovascular system is divided into two distinct circulations, pulmonary and systemic, with the primary purpose to deliver oxygenated blood throughout the body while removing unwanted waste products. To maintain these functions, there is a highly coordinated sequence of events ranging from electrical stimulation, cardiac contraction, and blood ejection into the respective circulations. These complex events and their integration with cardiac mechanics are the focus of this section.

2.3.1 ACTION POTENTIAL

Unlike other muscles in the body that require electrical excitation, the heart is capable of generating its own impulse and beating rhythmically. The action potential is responsible for initiating myocyte activation and is best described by a series of phases (Arnsdorf 1990), as shown in Figure 2.15. Phase 0 begins with rapid depolarization from −90 to +20 mV due to a rapid inward movement of sodium within the cell, and is mainly responsible for cardiac contraction during systole. A slight repolarization of the action potential occurs in phase I from potassium efflux. There is a plateau in the action potential in phase II from inward movement of calcium, which is subsequently followed by

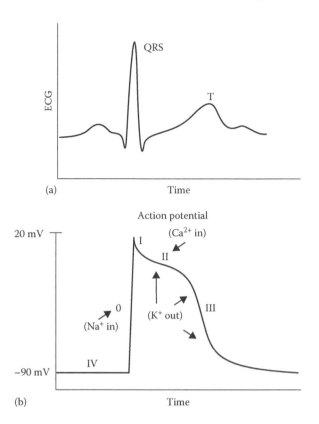

FIGURE 2.15 Action potential. (a) Electrocardiogram (ECG) showing the QRS complex and T wave. (b) Ventricular action potential in the cell showing different phases. Sodium (Na) rapidly enters the cell during phase 0, followed by slight repolarization during phase I. A plateau is reached in phase II associated with calcium (Ca) influx and potassium (K) efflux. Potassium leaves the cell at a higher rate during phase III, reaching phase IV at −90 mV.

phase III when potassium leaves the cell, reaching phase IV at −90 mV. Unique to the heart is the ability of myocytes to display automaticity or the ability to generate an action potential in an "all-or-none" phenomenon when the appropriate electrical threshold is reached. Therefore, particular myocardial cells do possess this automatic trigger, which provides a slight depolarization in order to trigger the subsequent electrical action potential.

2.3.2 EXCITATION–CONTRACTION COUPLING AND MYOCARDIAL CONTRACTION

The coordinated series of events starting with the action potential and ending with cardiac contraction is called excitation–contraction (E-C) coupling (Bers 2002). The action potential leads to calcium inflow from the extracellular space, which then binds to the contractile proteins and brings about the creation of actin–myosin cross-bridges. Myocardial relaxation, conversely, is largely due to calcium efflux and cross-bridge dissolution (Bers and Perez-Reyes 1999). Calcium homeostasis is critical in the regulation of cardiac contraction and relaxation, and it is highly regulated by various ionic channels and exchange proteins.

2.3.2.1 Actin–Myosin Cross-Bridges

The initiation of actin–myosin cross-bridges and cardiac contraction is a complex series of events best understood by a representative schematic (Pollack 1983), as shown in Figure 2.16. The primary contractile unit, or sarcomere, is composed of various myofilaments and proteins (Spotnitz et al. 1979). The outer boundary of the sarcomere is called the Z-line. The thin myofilament, or actin, is attached to this Z-line and includes a variety of regulatory proteins such as troponin and tropomyosin. The myosin thick filament runs in parallel to the actin and contains myosin heads, which interact with actin. A large protein called titin also runs in parallel and acts as a spring and scaffolding structure for the sarcomere. The rapid inflow of calcium activates the regulatory proteins, such as troponin, by binding calcium onto its receptors. This leads to cross-bridge formation and shortening of the sarcomere, which provides the force of cardiac contraction (Hobai and O'Rourke 2001).

2.3.2.2 Factors Affecting Contraction

The force of cardiac contraction and shortening of the sarcomere is highly dependent on the initial sarcomeric length. Maximal overlap (~2.2 μm from respective Z-line or approximate length of a sarcomeric unit) leads to greatest force. However, beyond a certain degree of overlap, force declines as described by the descending limb of the length–tension relationship (Kemp and Conte 2012). Optimal overlap has also been described by the Frank–Starling principle (explained later in the chapter), which highlights the importance of optimal overlap (preload) to cardiac performance (cardiac output [CO]). Indeed, cardiac performance is highly dependent on loading conditions. Preload, or the initial sarcomeric length, is highly dependent on diastolic ventricular pressure and volume. With optimal preload, sarcomeric overlap is optimized, and thus the length–tension relationship is optimized. Afterload, conversely, reflects the load onto the heart following contraction by opposing ejection. Aortic impedance provides an accurate measure of the afterload, where

$$\text{Aortic impedance} = \frac{\text{Aortic pressure}}{\text{Aortic flow}} \quad (2.1)$$

2.3.2.3 Electrocardiogram

Electrical activation of the heart is recorded by placing electrodes on the surface of the body, and it is represented by an electrocardiogram (ECG) (Kligfield et al. 2007), as shown in Figure 2.17. Cardiac electrical conduction begins in the sinoatrial (SA) node and reaches the AV node via internodal pathways. This initial depolarization causes atrial contraction, which is represented by the P wave on the ECG. Ventricular activation then occurs from the spread of this electrical signal through the left and right bundles and within Purkinje cells, causing the QRS complex. Then, ventricular repolarization occurs, which is reflected by the T wave. The ECG contains 12 leads including 6 limb leads (I, II, III, aVR, aVL, aVF) and 6 precordial leads (V1–V6) located at various positions on the body.

2.3.3 Cardiac Cycle

The cardiac cycle and the timing of its events are best understood through plotting pressure, volume, and flow curves over time (Figure 2.18). Cardiac contraction, or systole, begins at the onset of the QRS complex, while diastole (ventricular filling) often occurs from the T wave to the onset of the QRS complex.

2.3.3.1 Systole

Ventricular contraction leads to a rapid rise in pressure, which closes the mitral valve. Initially, the ventricular pressure does not exceed the aortic pressure, and thus, the aortic valve remains closed. During this time, there is a rapid rise in ventricular pressure, while the ventricular volume remains constant (isovolumetric contraction). When the ventricular pressure exceeds the pressure in the aorta, the aortic valve opens and blood is ejected out of the ventricle, leading to a decrease in the ventricular volume.

2.3.3.2 Diastole

When ventricular blood ejection is complete, the LV pressure falls, and thus the aortic valve closes. Ventricular relaxation occurs via active and passive mechanisms. Initially, both the

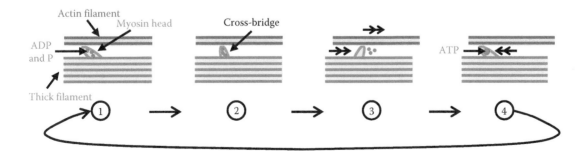

FIGURE 2.16 Actin–myosin interaction and myocardial contraction. (1) Adenosine triphosphate (ATP) is hydrolyzed when the myosin head is not attached to the actin filament. (2) Adenosine diphosphate (ADP) and phosphorus (P) are bound to the myosin filament as the myosin head attaches to actin. (3) After release of ADP and P, the myosin head changes position, which results in movement of the actin filament. (4) The ATP binding causes the myosin head to return to its resting position as in (1).

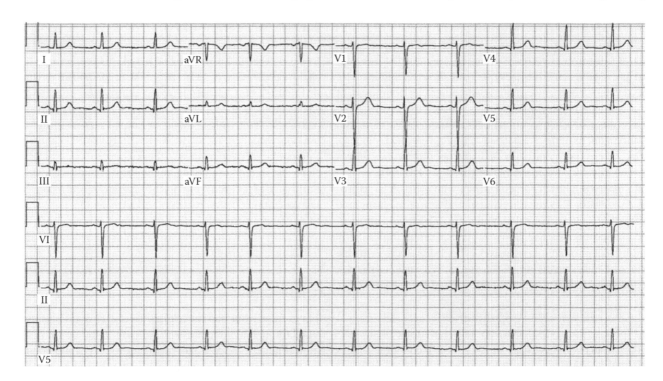

FIGURE 2.17   Electrocardiogram (ECG). Typical ECG demonstrating 12 leads, which represent the cardiac cycle at different positions in the chest cavity.

aortic and mitral valves are closed during diastole, and there is a fall in ventricular pressure, while the volume remains constant (isovolumetric relaxation). During early diastole, as the ventricular pressure continues to fall, the left atrial pressure exceeds the ventricular pressure, and the mitral valve opens causing rapid ventricular filling. At mid-diastole, or diastasis, the ventricular filling slows. At late-diastole, atrial contraction (corresponding with the P wave on the ECG) provides an additional atrial "kick" to further fill the ventricle. The atrial kick accounts for about one-third of LV filling in normal healthy adults. This final event completes the full cardiac cycle. Diastole represents a highly coordinated sequence of events, which includes rapid early filling, untwisting and elongation of the ventricle, and suction of blood from the atrium.

2.4   MEASUREMENTS OF LV CONTRACTILITY

2.4.1   FORCE–VELOCITY RELATIONSHIP

Loading experiments on isolated cardiac muscle bundles provide important insights into contractile patterns and mechanics (Mulieri et al. 1992). If a muscle bundle (i.e., papillary muscle) is stimulated without any load placed on it, then it should have a maximal peak rate of shortening (V_{max}). Isometric shortening refers to a situation whereby no shortening occurs, while isotonic shortening occurs when a contractile force is placed on the muscle bundle. A force–velocity curve is produced during a series of applied conditions including isometric and isotonic contraction, and then load is removed completely to

measure V_{max} (Tomoike 1982). This experiment can only take place in vitro and, therefore, it has minimal application in clinical medicine.

2.4.2   PRESSURE–VOLUME LOOP

The pressure–volume (P-V) loop provides an important means to understand the changes that occur throughout the cardiac cycle and assess contractility in the intact heart (Holubarsch et al. 1996), as shown in Figure 2.19. In addition to describing the timing of events and hemodynamics, information regarding contractility and stiffness indices can also be assessed by simultaneously plotting ventricular pressure and volume.

2.4.2.1   P-V Phases

During phase I, or the ventricular diastolic filling period, the pressure rises incrementally in a nonlinear manner, forming the end-diastolic pressure–volume relationship (EDPVR). The pressure increases out of proportion to the volume due to the stretching of the ventricle and expansion of collagen fibers. As the ventricle stiffens, the EDPVR is shifted leftward and may result in worsened compliance and higher left-sided filling pressures (i.e., diastolic dysfunction) (Ohno et al. 1994, Munagala et al. 2005). Phase II describes isovolumetric contraction whereby the pressure rises without a change in volume. During this stage, contractility can be assessed by the rate of pressure development over time (dP/dt), a sensitive measure for quantifying changes in intrinsic contractile performance. The opening

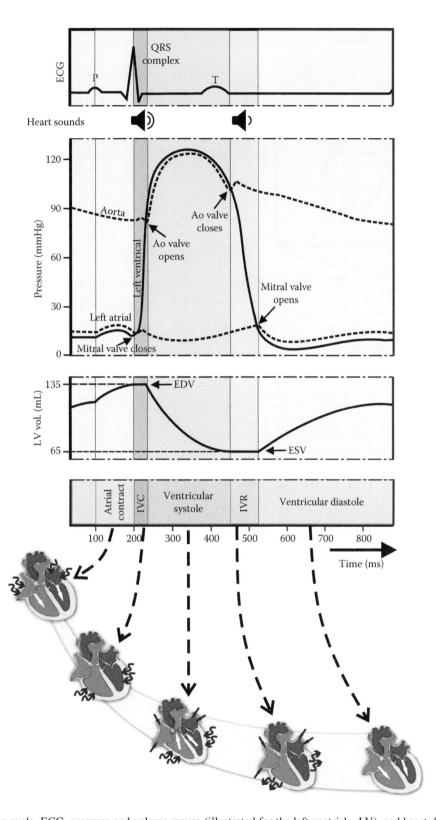

FIGURE 2.18 Cardiac cycle. ECG, pressure and volume waves (illustrated for the left ventricle, LV), and heart deformation during different phases in the cardiac cycle. During the atrial contraction phase, the atrial kick causes the remaining blood in the left atrium (LA) to move to the LV. When the LV pressure exceeds that in the LA, the mitral valve closes and the isovolumetric contraction (IVC) phase starts, where the LV pressure increases without change in its volume. Ventricular systole starts when the LV pressure reaches that in the aorta, which causes the aortic valve to open and blood pumps out of the LV. Isovolumetric relaxation (IVR) starts when the ventricular pressure drops below that in the aorta, which causes the aortic valve to close and the LV pressure to decrease without change in its volume. Finally, ventricular diastole starts when the LV pressure drops below that in the LA. A new cycle starts with another atrial contraction phase. The small curled arrows represent pressure, while the straight black and white arrows show blood flow direction.

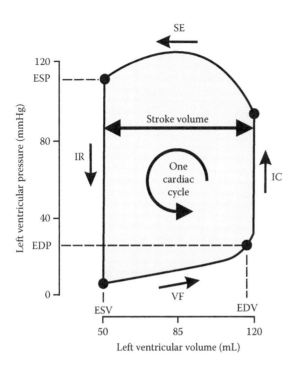

FIGURE 2.19 Pressure–volume (P-V) loop. The loop shows changes in the LV volume and pressure during the cardiac cycle. Different heart phases are shown in the figure (VF, ventricular filling; IC, isovolumetric contraction; SE, systolic ejection; and IR, isovolumetric relaxation). The figure shows change in volume from end-systolic volume (ESV) to end-diastolic volume (EDV) and change in pressure from end-systolic pressure (ESP) to end-diastolic pressure (EDP).

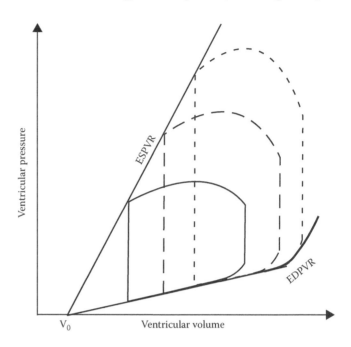

FIGURE 2.20 Changes in the pressure–volume (P-V) loop with preload. Different P-V loops at different preloads. The figure shows the lines representing end-systolic (ES) and end-diastolic (ED) P-V ratios (ESPVR and EDPVR).

of the aortic valve and ejection accounts for phase III, followed by isovolumetric relaxation (phase IV).

2.4.2.2 Cardiac Measures from P-V

The P-V loop can be generated in clinical and experimental settings by using a conductance catheter, which simultaneously measures ventricular pressure and volume (Tomoike 1982, Borlaug and Kass 2009, 2011). Important measurements include end-diastolic (lower right of the P-V loop) and end-systolic (upper left of the P-V loop) pressures. Determination of the EDPVR yields assessment of diastolic stiffness index (E_d). Systolic performance can be measured from the end-systolic pressure–volume relationship (ESPVR) and calculation of systolic elastance (E_{es}), which is the P-V slope at end systole:

$$E = \frac{P}{V - V_0}, \tag{2.2}$$

where V_0 is the volume of the ventricle at zero transmural pressure. Increased slope (i.e., upward shift in the slope) reflects increased systolic contractility and elastance (Figure 2.20).

Arterial stiffness or elastance (E_a) is calculated as the slope generated from the end-systolic and end-diastolic points.

Stroke volume (SV) and ejection fraction (EF) can be derived from the end-diastolic volume (EDV) and end-systolic volume (ESV):

$$SV = EDV - ESV, \tag{2.3}$$

$$EF = \frac{EDV - ESV}{EDV}. \tag{2.4}$$

Various loading conditions can be performed including preload reduction (e.g., balloon catheter inflation of the inferior vena cava), volume expansion (e.g., rapid fluid administration), and increased afterload (e.g., peripheral vasoconstrictor), which enhances understanding of ventricular performance and stiffness.

2.4.3 Measurements of Cardiac Performance

2.4.3.1 Cardiac Output

Cardiac performance can be evaluated via invasive or noninvasive hemodynamic measurements (Swan et al. 1970). In the catheterization lab, thermodilution and Fick's method are the most commonly used techniques for calculating the CO, which is the flow of oxygenated blood to the tissues per unit time. The Fick's method is more precise than thermodilution but requires arterial and venous sampling of blood and direct measurement of oxygen consumption using a tight-fitting mask. The rate of oxygen delivery (analogous to CO) is equal to the amount of oxygen consumption by the tissues. Hence, oxygen consumption is equal to CO times the arteriovenous difference of oxygen. While less accurate, the thermodilution technique is faster and less expensive, wherein cold saline is injected via a catheter (proximal port) into the RA or ventricle, then sampled in the PA (distal port). Thus, the flow or transit through the right heart circulation is equivalent to CO. SV (volume of blood ejected per heartbeat) can be assessed invasively or noninvasively (e.g., using Doppler echocardiography or phase-encoded MRI). If SV is measured, CO, an index that is dependent on contractility, preload, and afterload, can be calculated based on heart rate (HR):

$$CO = SV \times HR. \qquad (2.5)$$

2.4.3.2 Frank–Starling Curve

Cardiac contractility can be expressed by plotting SV against preload, as depicted by the Frank–Starling curve (Sarnoff and Berglund 1954), as shown in Figure 2.21. Diastolic sarcomeric stretch is a reflection of preload. Thus, preload can be defined as the wall stress during end-diastole, which is the maximal resting length of the sarcomere. When end-diastolic pressure (EDP) and/or EDV is higher, the myofilaments are stretched with secondary augmentation of SV. If the stretch is excessive (e.g., >2.2 μm), contractility and SV will decrease (Pieske et al. 1992, Holubarsch et al. 1996). Since chamber volume and sarcomeric lengths are not easily evaluated clinically, pulmonary capillary wedge pressure or left atrial pressure is used as a surrogate for preload. Afterload reflects resistance to ejection, or wall stress to ejection, and represents the total and pulsatile load onto the ventricle.

2.4.3.3 Laplace's Law

Wall stress (S) is a reflection of force, or tension, applied over a defined area. With greater arterial load, ventricular wall tension is higher, and the ventricle hypertrophies (Figure 2.22) to lessen this load based on Laplace's law:

$$S = \frac{P \times r}{2 \times h}, \qquad (2.6)$$

where P, r, and h are pressure, ventricular radius, and wall thickness, respectively.

2.4.3.3.1 Myocardial Hypertrophy

Most commonly, systemic hypertension increases wall tension and is compensated early on by concentric hypertrophy (i.e., inward remodeling) of the LV (James et al. 2000), where the increased wall thickness caused by hypertrophy balances the increased pressure. In general, in accordance with Laplace's law, increased wall thickness decreases wall tension (by distributing it among more muscle fibers) while dilatation increases tension.

2.4.3.3.2 Myocardial Dilation

As the heart dilates, which is the case in a variety of cardiomyopathies associated with reduced EF, wall tension is increased, but this occurs to maintain SV and CO. It should be noted that wall tension is largest in the endocardial surfaces, which have to do more work and are more vulnerable to reductions in coronary blood flow. In general, dilation leads to reduced cardiac efficiency unless hypotrophy is sufficient to normalize wall tension. In heart failure, dilation results in the inability to decrease ventricular radius during contraction, which leads to increased wall tension during systole, an unsteady condition that cannot be maintained for long.

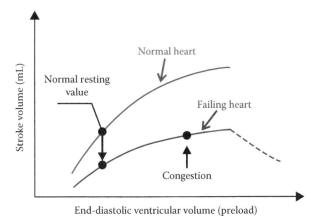

FIGURE 2.21 Frank–Starling curves. Schematic representation of the relationship between ventricular preload and stroke volume for normal (blue curve) and failing (brown curve) hearts. The curves show behaviors for normal volumes and congestion.

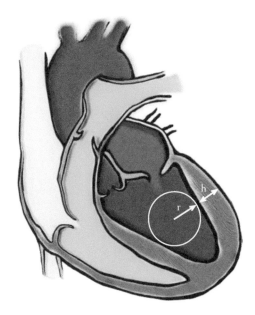

FIGURE 2.22 Laplace's law. The effects of ventricular radius (r) and wall thickness (h) on wall stress illustrated by Laplace's law.

2.4.3.4 Work and Power

Cardiac function can also be assessed via measurement of work and power. Based on analysis from the P-V loop, the mechanical work (W) can be obtained by calculating the area under the curve of the P-V loop (i.e., external work):

$$W = \oint P \, dV, \tag{2.7}$$

where the integration is taken over the P-V loop. Total mechanical work of the LV is composed of external work and dissipated heat during ventricular relaxation. The work done by the LV is about 1 J under resting conditions, which corresponds to a mechanical power of about 1.25 W, and increases to about 8 W during heavy exercise. The three main components that affect work are preload, afterload, and HR. Total work per minute (W_T) can be estimated by oxygen consumption:

$$W_T = BP_S \times SV \times HR, \tag{2.8}$$

where BP_S is systolic blood pressure. Work efficiency is the relationship between performed work and myocardial oxygen uptake. Power is an alternative expression of cardiac contractility, which is expressed as work per unit time, and can be estimated from peak aortic flow and systolic blood pressure.

2.4.4   Cardiac Mechanics

2.4.4.1 Myocardial Helical Structure

Myocardial architecture is often considered as a continuum of two helical sheets of fibers which have different orientations within the myocardium (Ingels 1997). The subendocardial region demonstrates a right-handed myofiber orientation, which gradually changes to a left-handed configuration in the subepicardial layer (Figure 2.23). These layers of myofiber sheets continuously wrap the heart along the longitudinal axis. In reference to the circumferential orientation, the subendocardial fibers are oriented at an angle of approximately 80°. In the midwall of the LV, the fibers are oriented at 0°.

Lastly, the subepicardial fibers are oriented at about −60°. Due to this fiber orientation, the subendocardium is largely responsible for longitudinal motion and deformation, whereas the subepicardium and midwall contribute mostly to rotation (Streeter et al. 1969, Spotnitz 2000).

2.4.4.2 Key Definitions

To better understand deformation and cardiac mechanics, one must review several key terms:

- *Displacement*: distance the tissue moves
- *Strain*: fractional change in tissue length expressed as a percentage of original length
- *Strain rate*: rate of change in strain
- *Rotation*: rotational displacement of tissue, expressed in degrees

2.4.4.3 Myocardial Twisting

During the cardiac cycle, a complex interaction of various myocardial fibers allows the LV to thicken, shorten, and twist (Sonnenblick et al. 1967, Tendulkar and Harken 2006). As the subendocardium is largely responsible for longitudinal shortening, these fibers contribute to the base being pulled toward the apex, thereby shortening the longitudinal axis of the LV. The other myofiber layers (midwall and subepicardium) largely contribute to twist or torsion (Ingels et al. 1989). These fibers have greater torque than the subendocardial fibers due to their larger radii and, thus, dominate motion. Therefore, as depicted by looking from the base toward the apex, these fibers contribute to the clockwise rotation at the apex and counterclockwise rotation of the base during systole, and opposite rotation directions during diastole (Figure 2.24). Together, this causes a "wringing" motion of the heart with preferential electromechanical activation from the apex to the base (Rankin et al. 1976, Olsen et al. 1981). In diastole, the stored force from twisting contributes to suction and ventricular filling during diastole. In general, LV twist is greater with increasing preload and worse in the pressure-overloaded ventricle.

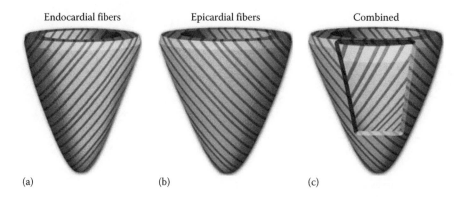

(a)   (b)   (c)

FIGURE 2.23   Fiber orientations in the myocardium. Fiber orientations in the (a) endocardium, (b) epicardium, and (c) both. (Courtesy of Dr. Shehab Anwar, National Heart Institute, Cairo, Egypt.)

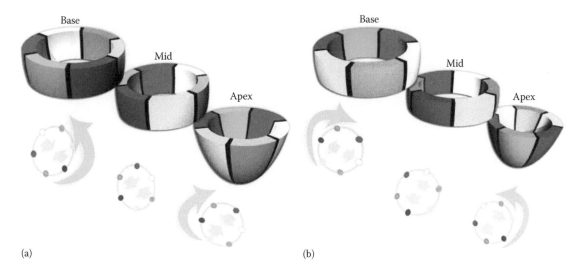

(a)   (b)

FIGURE 2.24 Myocardial twisting. Rotation of different myocardial regions showing (a) myocardial twisting during systole and (b) myocardial untwisting during diastole. (Courtesy of Dr. Shehab Anwar, National Heart Institute, Cairo, Egypt.)

2.5 HEART DISEASES

2.5.1 ISCHEMIC HEART DISEASE AND MYOCARDIAL INFARCTION

The heart is supplied with oxygen via the coronary arteries. It relies on aerobic oxidation, particularly from free fatty acids, and the metabolic requirements are determined by the myocardial oxygen demand (MVO2). Oxygen demand, and thus the degree of coronary vasodilation and blood flow, is highly dependent on contractility, HR, and wall stress. These factors are largely affected by altering loading conditions (i.e., preload and afterload), neurohumoral activation, and activity (i.e., aerobic exercise). Adequate coronary blood flow must meet the metabolic demands of the heart to avoid ischemia or relative insufficient oxygen supply to the myocardium (Kern et al. 2006, Kern and Samady 2010).

2.5.1.1 Ischemia versus Infarction

Myocardial ischemia or injury may cause reversible or irreversible damage to the heart (Thygesen et al. 2007a).

Epicardial obstructive coronary disease leading to significant obstruction (i.e., atherosclerotic plaque, vasospasm) compromises adequate blood flow to the myocardium, whereby the subendocardium is preferentially affected. If there is an adverse "supply–demand mismatch," yet some blood flow is still present, the myocardium is said to be ischemic (Figure 2.25; Bolli and Marban 1999). Thus, when blood flow is restored from revascularization, the myocardium is likely to recover. However, if there is a complete lack of blood flow (i.e., total occlusion from thrombus) or the ischemia is severe, the myocardium may become irreversibly injured or scarred, that is, myocardial infarction (MI), as shown in Figure 2.26.

2.5.1.2 Damage Wavefront

The wavefront of damage in either ischemia or infarction travels from the endocardium toward the epicardium (Reimer and Jennings 1979, Shapiro et al. 2012), as shown in Figure 2.27. The damage severity is highly dependent on coronary distribution as well as duration of injury prior to revascularization. Sudden cardiac death during MI is mainly due to ventricular

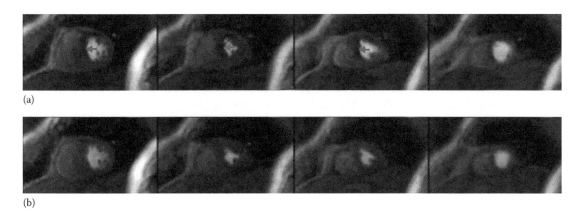

(a)

(b)

FIGURE 2.25 Myocardial ischemia. Perfusion cardiovascular MRI images of different short-axis slices during (a) stress and (b) rest, showing ischemic regions with perfusion deficit in the septal wall (arrows).

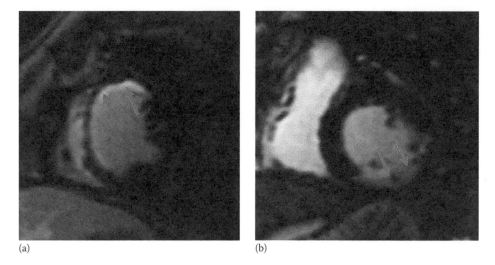

(a)   (b)

FIGURE 2.26   Myocardial infarction. (a) Subendocardial and (b) transmural infarcts, as shown on late gadolinium enhancement (LGE) MRI images.

ST segment changes (i.e., ST segment elevation reflective of myocardial injury or ST segment depression related to ischemia), and chest pain.

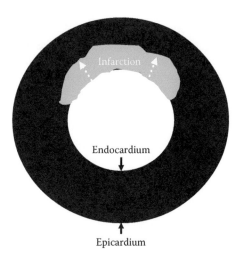

FIGURE 2.27   Myocardial infarction. Cartoon of the LV in a short-axis configuration. Following an infarction, a wavefront of injury travels from endo- to epicardium. Thus, the first injured territory is the endocardial border. With time, the injury extends to the epicardial layer. More transmural extension translates into greater degree of damage.

fibrillation, wherein the damaged myocardial cells trigger an abnormality in impulse conduction.

With myocardial ischemia or infarction, regional and global contractility is typically impaired (Forrester et al. 1976, Boersma et al. 2003, Thygesen et al. 2007b). Myocardial dysfunction may occur within seconds or minutes, as the heart relies heavily on aerobic metabolism and lacks sufficient energy storage. Therefore, LV dysfunction is rapid and typically reflected by worsened contractility and diastolic dysfunction (i.e., rise in LV filling pressures due to poor relaxation and increased stiffness) (Swan et al. 1972). The series of events brought about by ischemia follow a predictable pattern including LV diastolic and systolic dysfunction (including hypokinesia, akinesia, and dyskinesia), electrocardiographic

2.5.1.3   Stunned and Hibernating Myocardium

Following an episode of either complete occlusion causing myocardial injury or severe ischemia, the myocardium may remain "stunned" due to prolonged lack of sufficient blood flow (Shapiro et al. 2012). The hallmark feature of myocardial stunning is that the LV becomes transiently dysfunctional but typically returns to baseline in days to weeks following successful coronary revascularization. "Hibernating" myocardium reflects a different mechanism; but similar to stunning, the myocardium remains alive or viable (Braunwald and Kloner 1982, Braunwald and Rutherford 1986, Camici et al. 2008). When the myocardium is chronically ischemic due to inadequate blood flow, the affected area of muscle compensates via a reduction in systolic performance. Thus, regional and global LV dysfunction ensues. If the affected territory is large, it can cause profound LV dysfunction with drop in EF and symptoms of heart failure (when the heart fails to pump an adequate CO), for example, increased HR even at rest, defective cardiac parasympathetic control, altered baroreceptor function, and reduced cardiac sympathetic activity in response to stimuli. Drop in contractility is a way by which the myocardium tries to match reduced perfusion and low myocardial oxygen consumption (MVO2) and preserve cellular viability (Elsasser 1997). If the myocardium is hibernating, or viable, the affected area typically normalizes following revascularization. In patients with ischemic cardiomyopathy, viability testing can aid in clinical decision-making as it pertains to the need for revascularization. This can be achieved by a variety of testing procedures including positron emission tomography (PET) and cardiac MRI. If the dysfunctional myocardium is viable, then there is high likelihood of deriving benefit from revascularization. Nonviable, or scarred, myocardium may not recover, particularly with severe, that is, transmural, infarction (Schwarz et al. 1996).

2.5.1.4 Contractility Dysfunction

From a cellular perspective, any cessation of blood flow to the myocardium often leads to the inability of the myocytes to adequately shorten (Jennings and Ganote 1974, Virmani et al. 1990). Multiple mechanisms account for this, including damage to the contractile apparatus and inadequate calcium homeostasis. Since the subendocardial layers are preferentially affected first, ischemia typically alters longitudinal motion. If circumferential and twist mechanics are preserved, global EF should be normal. However, in acute MI with transmural involvement, the midwall and subepicardial fibers are also injured, leading to reduction in circumferential and twist mechanics, and thus EF is reduced (Garot et al. 2002a,b, Sengupta et al. 2008b). Therefore, strain imaging may aid in the assessment of injury severity and help predict myocardial viability.

From a global LV function perspective, if transmural injury or infarction is present, there may be regional or global wall motion abnormalities, which can span from hypokinesia to dyskinesia (Eaton et al. 1979). The remainder of myocardial segments may compensate via hyperkinesia. In severe injury, dyssynchrony may also occur, whereby the activation of adjacent myocardial segments is altered, leading to poorly coordinated LV contraction. Following an infarction, particularly if revascularization was late or unsuccessful, the myocytes become injured and necrotic, which leads to their inability to shorten, and adjacent myocytes "slip" past one another. The infarcted zone may then expand and affect adjacent segments. Over time, LV dilatation may occur from a variety of mechanisms including adverse remodeling, neurohumoral activation, and infarct expansion (Pfeffer and Braunwald 1990). This may ultimately lead to marked LV dysfunction, global hypokinesia, myocardial wall thinning, and heart failure, all signs of adverse ventricular remodeling.

2.5.1.5 MI Progression

Over hours to days, the infarcted myocardium undergoes a variety of changes, including edema, cellular infiltration, and replacement fibrosis (Abbate et al. 2005). With hypoxia and abnormal perfusion, regional systolic deformation, and thus strain rate, also declines. Following an MI whereby the underlying myocardium becomes edematous and scarred, the contractile apparatus is affected further, and thus regional deformation is even worse in those particular segments. Nearby regions which were unaffected may become hyperdynamic, and thus their strain rate is higher. Keys to avoid adverse remodeling following an MI are early and complete revascularization and initiation of inhibitors of neurohumoral activation (Pfeffer 1995).

2.5.2 Hypertension and Heart Failure

2.5.2.1 Systemic Hypertension

Systemic hypertension (>140/90 mmHg), often due to increased vascular resistance and/or CO, adds an excessive afterload to the ejecting heart, which can lead to a variety of cardiovascular abnormalities. With excessive afterload, concentric LV hypertrophy typically occurs to maintain near-normal wall tension (Frohlich et al. 1992). Sustained elevated LV pressure is associated with adaptive (myocyte survival) and maladaptive (apoptosis and related degenerative patterns) signals based on the stimulus invoked by the load. Figure 2.28 shows different processes associated with heart remodeling, as previously described (Bonow et al. 2011).

The adaptive changes disperse the tension over a larger surface area of myocytes. However, over time, maladaptive mechanisms occur from this excessive afterload leading to increased fibrosis, neurohumoral activation, and apoptosis (Munagala et al. 2005). This may lead to the syndrome of clinical heart failure associated with a preserved ejection fraction (HFpEF), which often occurs due to increased ventricular stiffness and decreased compliance, that is, reduced ventricular ability to fill adequately at normal diastolic filling pressures (Lam et al. 2007). Thus, ventricular filling occurs at the expense of higher diastolic filling pressures. Some patients may develop an increased ventricular radial dimension, thus increasing wall stress to maintain SV. Over time, with worsening remodeling and neurohumoral activation, the LV can further decompensate with eccentric hypertrophy and systolic dysfunction, characterized by reduced cardiac contractility.

2.5.2.2 Pulmonary Hypertension

Pulmonary hypertension (PH) is a progressive disorder characterized by abnormally increased blood pressure of the pulmonary circulation. The elevated resistance in the pulmonary circulation in PH results in an increased RV afterload, which affects its function. As the RV is more compliant than the LV, it quickly adapts to modified operating conditions. In PH, the RV responds to the elevated afterload by accumulating new sarcomeres in parallel to maintain CO, which leads to RV hypertrophy. In severe PH, the RV has a spherical shape with a larger cross-sectional area than that of the LV (Ibrahim et al. 2011, Ibrahim and White 2012), which impairs the LV function through interventricular cross talk (Figure 2.29). The extra oxygen supply needed by the hypertrophied RV results in a supply–demand mismatch, which compromises the RV systolic function. The pooling blood inside the RV leads to an in-series accumulation of the sarcomeres, which results in RV dilatation. Ultimately, ventricular failure develops, leading to death.

2.5.3 Cardiomyopathies

A cardiomyopathy represents a variety of intrinsic myocardial diseases that compromise either systolic or diastolic function or both, which include dilated, hypertrophic, and restrictive hearts (Maron et al. 2006).

2.5.3.1 Dilated Cardiomyopathy

A dilated cardiomyopathy (Figure 2.30) is often associated with a genetic abnormality (e.g., related to sarcomeric proteins, collagen matrix, or mitochondria), which causes a dilated and weakened heart in susceptible patients. Whereas ischemic cardiomyopathy typically affects a particular region, or vascular

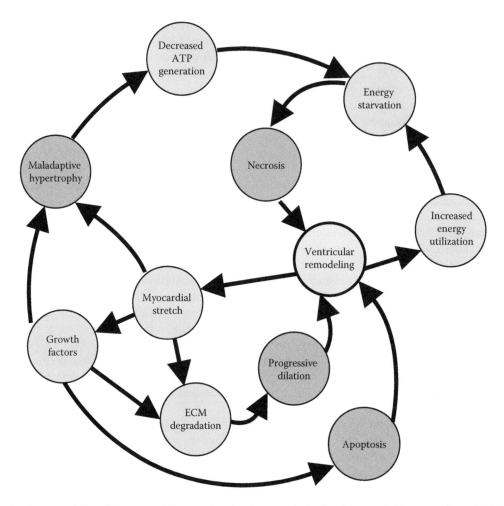

FIGURE 2.28 Cardiac remodeling. Heart remodeling can be adaptive or maladaptive. Myocardial hypertrophy and dilation are forms of remodeling to compensate for changes in the loading conditions. Apoptosis and necrosis appear when the energy demand to sustain cardiac growth exceeds the energy supply. The diagram shows the self-amplifying nature of cardiac remodeling. ATP, adenosine triphosphate; ECM, extracellular matrix.

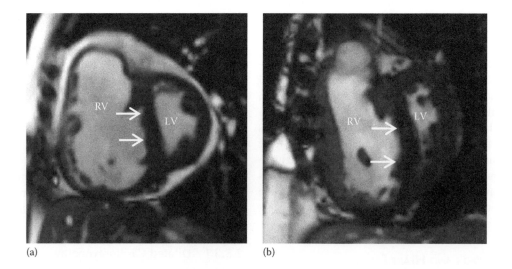

FIGURE 2.29 Pulmonary hypertension (PH). (a) Moderate and (b) severe cases of pulmonary hypertension. The arrows point to ventricular septal deformation due to increased pressure in the right ventricle (RV), which may exceed that in the left ventricle (LV) in severe PH cases.

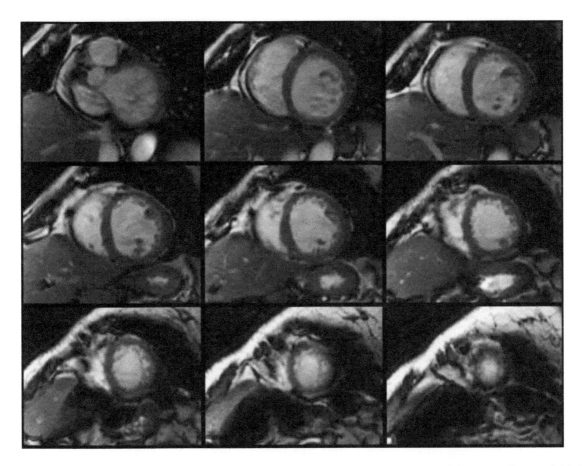

FIGURE 2.30 Dilated cardiomyopathy. A series of short-axis slices covering the LV from base (top left) to apex (bottom right). Note the large size of the heart in the chest, for example, compared to the liver size.

distribution territory, of the myocardium, dilated cardiomyopathies often demonstrate a globally dysfunctional heart, which may be associated with clinical heart failure. Heart mechanics often reflect impaired systolic twist in proportion to the severity of LV dysfunction (Kanzaki et al. 2006).

2.5.3.2 Hypertrophic Cardiomyopathy

Hypertrophic cardiomyopathy (Figures 2.31 and 2.32) is characterized by an inappropriate LV hypertrophy, often asymmetric and involving the septum (Gersh et al. 2011). It occurs due to a genetic abnormality of a sarcomeric protein and is associated with a variety of phenotypes and a wide clinical spectrum. Its clinical diagnosis includes evidence of myocardial hypertrophy (wall thickness ≥15 mm) in the absence of elevated afterload (i.e., hypertension and aortic stenosis).

If the hypertrophy is located in the ventricular basal septum, it may lead to the development of LV outflow obstruction, systolic anterior motion of the mitral valve, and secondary posteriorly directed mitral regurgitation. The obstruction is dynamic, and it is worse in conditions that decrease preload and promote increased contractility. While LV outflow obstruction is the hallmark feature in some patients, many others without obstruction remain symptomatic due to advanced diastolic dysfunction. Additionally, some predisposed patients may be at higher risk for sudden cardiac death, as myocardial disarray leads to replacement or interstitial fibrosis. Given this

substrate, some may develop ventricular tachycardia or fibrillation. Mechanistically, with myocardial disarray and fibrosis, myocardial contractility is quite abnormal in the affected region (Young et al. 1994), which may lead to an absence of systolic deformation in that particular territory. Interestingly, while LV twist is generally preserved, the twist sequence may be altered and absent in the abnormal myocardial territory (i.e., exaggerated rotation at the apex but decreased at the basal septum).

2.5.3.3 Restrictive Cardiomyopathy

A restrictive cardiomyopathy is characterized by an abnormality of the myocardium such that it may become excessively rigid and stiff, leading to abnormal diastolic function (Kushwaha et al. 1997). While there are many underlying causes of restrictive cardiomyopathy, the most common etiology is from cardiac involvement of amyloidosis. In addition to abnormal protein deposition, typical pathologic findings also include hypertrophy and fibrosis, where the myocardium may become firm, rubbery, and thickened. From gross pathologic specimens or advanced cardiovascular imaging, cardiac amyloidosis (Figure 2.33) may cause atrial enlargement (due to elevated LV filling pressures), biventricular hypertrophy, valvular thickening, pericardial effusion, and adverse remodeling of the coronary arteries. In addition to the obvious changes to diastolic function, systolic function may also be affected.

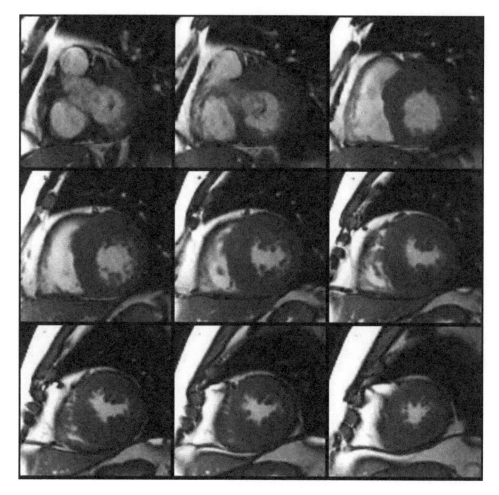

FIGURE 2.31 Hypertrophic cardiomyopathy. A series of short-axis slices covering the LV from base (top left) to apex (bottom right). Note the thick LV wall in all slices.

In fact, cardiac amyloidosis causes deformation inhibition, particularly of the endocardial and epicardial fibers. While longitudinal shortening is abnormal, circumferential and radial shortening is often maintained, and thus, markers of global systolic function such as EF may appear grossly normal (Sengupta et al. 2008a).

2.5.3.4 Arrhythmogenic Right Ventricular Cardiomyopathy

Arrhythmogenic right ventricular cardiomyopathy (ARVC) represents a less common cardiomyopathy, which is due to myocyte apoptosis with secondary fatty and/or fibrous replacement of the myocardium (Gemayel et al. 2001; Figure 2.34). The RV is predominantly affected and may lead to abnormal fat deposition, RV enlargement and dysfunction, as well as outpouchings and dyskinetic segments. The replacement fibrosis may predispose patients to ventricular arrhythmias and sudden cardiac death.

2.5.4 Myocarditis

Certain infections or inflammatory conditions may involve the heart, where myocarditis, or inflammation of the myocardium,

may ensue (Mahrholdt et al. 2006), as shown in Figure 2.35. Most commonly, particular viruses may invade the heart, and then secondarily cause a series of post-inflammatory reactions, as follows: (1) viremia, (2) myocardial viral involvement, (3) myocyte apoptosis and necrosis, (4) edema and inflammatory infiltration, and (5) fibrosis. Depending on severity, myocarditis can lead to LV dilatation and dysfunction as well as heart failure, arrhythmia, and death. Pathologically, the LV may become more spherically shaped, similar to what typically occurs in a dilated cardiomyopathy (Mendes et al. 1999). There may be regional and/or global dysfunction with associated decreased deformation in all directions (i.e., longitudinal, radial, and circumferential). Further, given LV dilatation and poor cardiac contraction, there may also be secondary mitral valve regurgitation due to poor leaflet coaptation.

2.5.5 Valvular Heart Disease

The clinical spectrum of disease and its impact on heart mechanics and loading conditions are quite diverse in valvular heart disease. Ultimately, the cardiac implications depend on which valve is abnormal, severity of damage, and whether the lesion reflects either regurgitation or stenosis. In general,

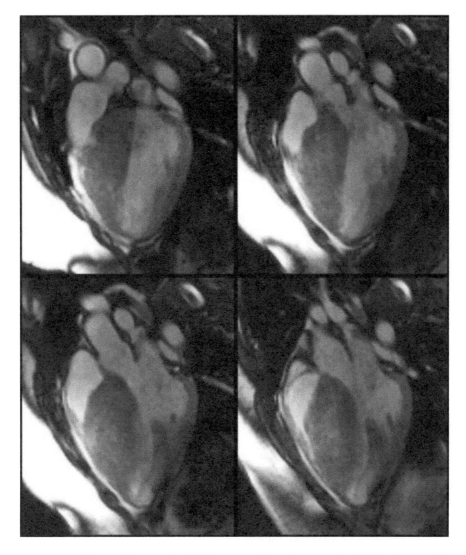

FIGURE 2.32 Reverse curve morphology of the septal wall in hypertrophic cardiomyopathy (HCM). A series of long-axis slices at different time points during systole showing hypertrophied septal wall with reverse curve morphology in HCM.

lesions that cause severe regurgitation lead to increased volume overload, whereas stenosis promotes conditions of pressure overload. Clinical presentation may range from being asymptomatic to having symptoms such as dyspnea, angina, and heart failure.

2.5.5.1 Pressure-Overloaded Ventricle: Aortic Valve Stenosis

Obstruction to outflow can occur at the valvular level (aortic valve stenosis; Figure 2.36) or less commonly at the subvalvular (i.e., hypertrophic obstructive cardiomyopathy) or supravalvular (i.e., aortic narrowing) levels.

Most commonly, valvular stenosis is caused by time-dependent degeneration but can be secondary to congenital (e.g., bicuspid) or rheumatic heart diseases (Freeman and Otto 2005). Over time, as the degree of obstruction worsens, compensatory and concentric LV hypertrophy occurs to decrease wall tension. As the stenosis becomes severe (valve area <1.0 cm^2), the LV becomes more stiff and less compliant

(Nishimura et al. 2008). Increased wall stress leads to replication of sarcomeric proteins, myocyte hypertrophy, and interstitial hypertrophy as predicted by Laplace's law (Stuber et al. 1999). This compensatory mechanism maintains normal or near-normal wall stress early on (Nagel et al. 2000). Increased myocyte hypertrophy may also change the shape of the heart such that it goes from elliptical to spherical. This adaptation causes the LV cavity to be smaller.

With further pressure overload, an afterload mismatch develops, whereby the wall stress overcomes the degree of hypertrophy. As a result, the LV filling pressure becomes higher and LV dysfunction may ultimately occur (Carabello et al. 1980). In general, this may decrease the rate of deformation and lengthen systole (Leonardi et al. 2014). Further, this excessive wall tension preferentially affects the longitudinal fibers, particularly the endocardial fibers (Ozkan et al. 2011). This has a deleterious impact on longitudinal shortening and strain rate, but since twist and circumferential fibers are relatively preserved, there is often normal or

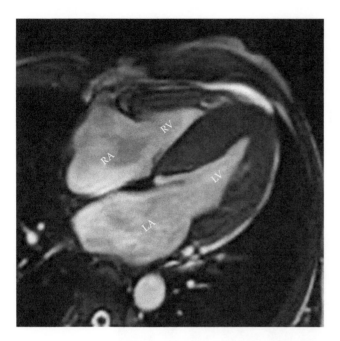

FIGURE 2.33 Cardiac amyloidosis. Four-chamber cardiovascular MRI image of cardiac amyloidosis. There is marked LV and RV hypertrophy, bi-atrial enlargement, and small pericardial effusion.

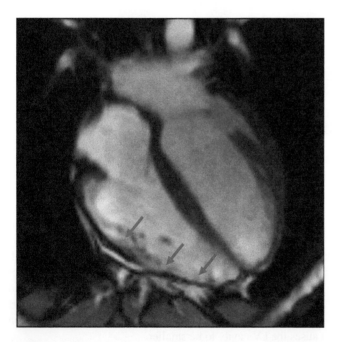

FIGURE 2.34 Arrhythmogenic right ventricular cardiomyopathy (ARVC). Cardiovascular four-chamber MRI image of a patient with ARVC showing infiltrated fatty depositions in the RV (arrows).

hyperdynamic deformation of these fibers (Biederman et al. 2005, van Dalen et al. 2013). While these changes commonly impact the entire ventricle, there are regions of the LV that may have additional wall stress, such as the basal septum, which may have excessive hypertrophy and cause a sigmoid-shaped bulge with worse contractile deformation. In general, these are the changes that occur in the pressure-overloaded

ventricle. However, ultimately the ventricle may begin to fail, and generalized LV dysfunction ensues.

2.5.5.2   Volume-Overloaded Ventricle: Aortic and Mitral Valve Regurgitation

Aortic regurgitation (Figure 2.36), or insufficiency, is typically caused by an intrinsic valvular disease (i.e., degenerative, endocarditis, or bicuspid) or from aortic root dilatation, which causes poor leaflet coaptation (Enriquez-Sarano and Taji 2004). With chronic aortic regurgitation, a proportion of the ejected volume is leaked back into the low-pressure LV during diastole. This leads to excess LV volume, or increased preload, which in turn increases wall tension (Mizariene et al. 2011). In accordance with Laplace's law, and contrary to what occurs in conditions of increased afterload, the ventricle hypertrophies and dilates (Ross et al. 1971). Therefore, there is eccentric remodeling or hypertrophy and myocyte elongation, which in turn compensates for the increased wall tension. If compensated, the degree of LV eccentric hypertrophy and cavity dilatation maintains a normal or near-normal ventricular filling pressure. The increased SV of the LV also predisposes to ventricular enlargement. Early on, as ventricular mass increases and eccentric remodeling occurs, there is actually increased contractile material as well as systolic deformation and strain. Unfortunately, this compensatory mechanism of LV dilatation changes the geometric shape of the heart, ultimately leading to deleterious effects on local wall strain (Borg et al. 2008, Gaasch and Meyer 2008). For example, severe volume-overloaded states are associated with decreased systolic twist, delayed time to peak twist, and reduced diastolic recoil (Tibayan et al. 2004). With severe, progressive aortic regurgitation, eccentric hypertrophy fails to compensate the overloaded ventricle, and thus, wall stress and LV pressure rise. This results in myocyte death and replacement fibrosis, ultimately leading to increased stiffness and worsened regional and global contraction. If progressive and left without repair, a vicious cycle occurs in severe aortic regurgitation, whereby severe LV enlargement and dysfunction ensue. In general, LV dilatation and generalized dysfunction are the hallmark features of the volume-overloaded ventricle as is the case with aortic or mitral valve regurgitation.

2.5.6   Congenital Heart Disease

Congenital heart disease (CHD) represents a highly diverse set of genetic cardiac diseases, which lead to an abnormality in circulatory structure and function. Present at birth and generally due to failure of normal embryonic development, abnormalities can range from simple to complex CHD. Normal cardiac development occurs during the first gestational month, starting with the cardiac tube, which is comprised of the primitive ventricle, bulbus cordis, and truncus. Over the following weeks, the cardiac tube changes configuration, leading to the development of two distinct pumping chambers with their respective conduit arteries (i.e., aorta and PA). The atria form from the sinoatrium, which are separated by the growth

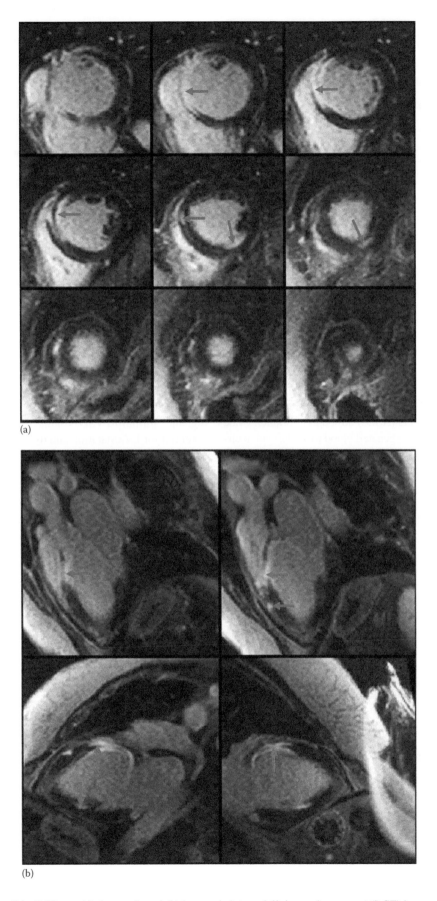

FIGURE 2.35 Myocarditis. Different (a) short-axis and (b) long-axis late gadolinium enhancement (LGE) images of a patient with myocarditis. The arrows point myocardial regions of hyperenhanced signal intensity.

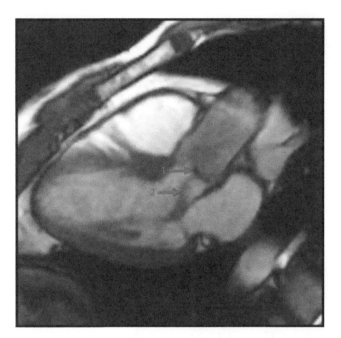

FIGURE 2.36 Aortic stenosis (arrow 1) and regurgitation (jet backward flow; arrow 2).

of the septum primum. The ostium secundum is formed to seal off any atrial septal defects (ASDs) although a foramen ovale persists in order to shunt oxygenated blood to the left-sided circulation during embryonic development. Defects in the atrial or ventricular septa (i.e., ASD and ventricular septal defect [VSD]) cause abnormal shunting of blood during early development. Rotation of the truncus arteriosus causes the normal spiral between the aorta and PA.

2.5.6.1 Atrial and Ventricular Septal Defects

An ASD (Figure 2.37) occurs from a defect in the atrial septum due to abnormal development of the septum. It can be described based on location (primum, secundum, sinus venosus, or coronary sinus), and its severity is dependent on the size and degree of shunting through the defect.

In VSD, there is a left-to-right shunt causing an RV volume overload (Haber et al. 2005). However, these shunts may also lead to right-to-left shunting, particularly in the presence of PH, leading to desaturation of blood and hypoxemia. The ventricular septum consists of inlet, trabecular portion, and outlet. The ventricular defect may occur in the muscular (muscular VSD) or membranous (membranous VSD) septum. A restrictive VSD may cause a large pressure gradient between the LV and RV although the shunt is relatively small. Larger VSDs may lead to hemodynamic derangements with left-to-right shunt. Since this large burden of oxygenated blood then circulates back to the left-sided chambers, it often leads to LV enlargement and generalized dysfunction if not repaired. Pathologically, the LV dilates, becomes spherical, and weakens. The mechanics are similar to volume overloaded LV, as discussed earlier.

2.5.6.2 Patent Ductus Arteriosus

The ductus arteriosus is a small communication from the PA to the descending aorta, which is patent during embryonic development to shunt blood away from the lungs. However, at birth, this duct typically closes due to changes in pulmonary vascular resistance, thereby only leaving a closed remnant. If it remains open, it may cause abnormal left-to-right shunting, and, similar to VSD, volume overload to the LV with the potential for LV dilatation and dysfunction if left unrepaired.

2.5.6.3 Transposition of the Great Arteries

Transposition of the great arteries (TGA) is a rare abnormality in conotruncal development (Figure 2.38). In D-TGA, there is ventriculoarterial discordance and AV concordance such that blood returns to the RA and is pumped into the RV where it is ejected into the systemic aorta (Pettersen et al. 2007). Then, the blood returns to the LA via the pulmonary veins and is pumped into the LV and then to the PA. Unless an additional shunt (i.e., VSD) is present to allow some mixing

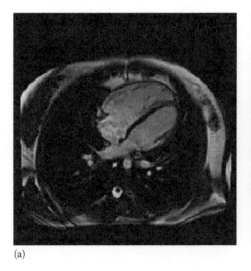
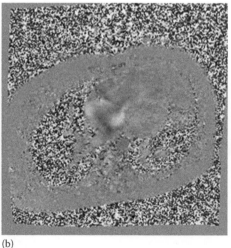

(a)   (b)

FIGURE 2.37 Atrial septal defect (ASD). (a) Magnitude and (b) velocity-encoded phase MRI images of a patient with ASD, showing RV enlargement and shunt flow (asterisk in [b]).

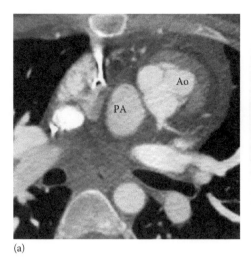
(a)

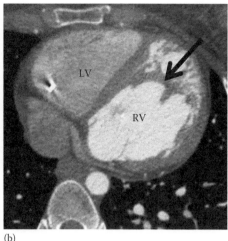
(b)

FIGURE 2.38 Congenitally corrected transposition of the great arteries (TGA). CT images showing the aorta (Ao) arising anterior and to the left of the pulmonary artery (PA) from morphologic right ventricle (RV), showing the moderator band (arrow in [b]). The right-sided ventricle is the morphologic left ventricle (LV). There is atrioventricular and ventriculoarterial discordance and ventricular inversion. (Courtesy of Dr. Prachi Agarwal, University of Michigan, Ann Arbor, MI.)

of blood, this condition is incompatible with life. This CHD is often associated with a large VSD and subpulmonary stenosis. Alternatively, congenitally corrected TGA (L-TGA) is when there are both AV and ventriculoarterial discordance.

2.5.6.4 Tetralogy of Fallot

Tetralogy of Fallot (TOF) is a primary conotruncal abnormality from misalignment with the ventricular septum, which is composed of the following hallmark features: VSD, subpulmonary stenosis, RV hypertrophy, and overriding aorta (Figures 2.39 and 2.40). Severity often depends on the degree of RV outflow obstruction, which is highly variable. In its extreme, pulmonary atresia may restrict appropriate flow into the pulmonary vascular bed and cause excessive right-to-left shunt across the VSD, leading to cyanosis.

2.5.6.5 Ebstein's Anomaly

Ebstein's anomaly consists of apical displacement of the septal tricuspid leaflet and/or valvular dysplasia. The anterior tricuspid leaflet (which is typically adherent to the free wall of the RV) is tethered and, thus, unable to provide adequate coaptation. Thus, severe tricuspid regurgitation occurs, and over time, RV enlargement and dysfunction ensue. This may culminate in findings of right heart failure, such as edema, ascites, pleural effusions, and weight gain. If an ASD or patent foramen ovale is present, it may also lead to right-to-left shunting of deoxygenated blood.

2.5.6.6 Coarctation of the Aorta

An aortic coarctation (Figure 2.41) represents a focal narrowing in the aortic lumen causing varying degrees of obstruction. Often associated with a bicuspid aortic valve or Turner's syndrome, a coarctation may cause severe obstruction to flow in the aorta, leading to the development of collateral vessels. The obstruction also contributes to the pressure-overloaded

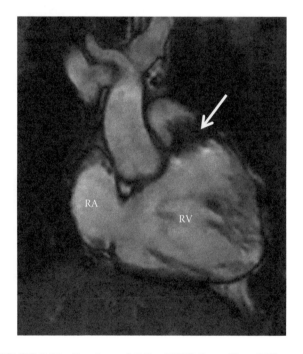

FIGURE 2.39 Tetralogy of Fallot (TOF) Status/Post (S/P) repair and subsequent Melody valve showing a dilated right ventricle (RV) and the artifact (arrow) from the Melody valve. (Courtesy of Dr. Prachi Agarwal, University of Michigan, Ann Arbor, MI.)

ventricle leading to hypertrophy and abnormalities in longitudinal deformation, as discussed earlier.

2.5.7 PERICARDIAL DISEASE

The pericardium is composed of two thin layers of tissue that surround the heart. Since it contains collagen and elastic fibers, if stretched, it can cause decreased compliance and increased stiffness. This may influence the heart in a variety

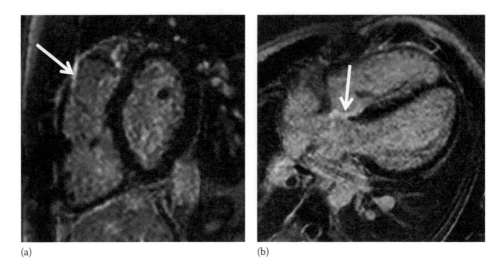

(a)   (b)

FIGURE 2.40   Late gadolinium enhancement MRI in TOF. Typical sites of enhancement (arrows) seen in the right the ventricular outflow tract and region of the ventricular septal defect patch repair. (Courtesy of Dr. Prachi Agarwal, University of Michigan, Ann Arbor, MI.)

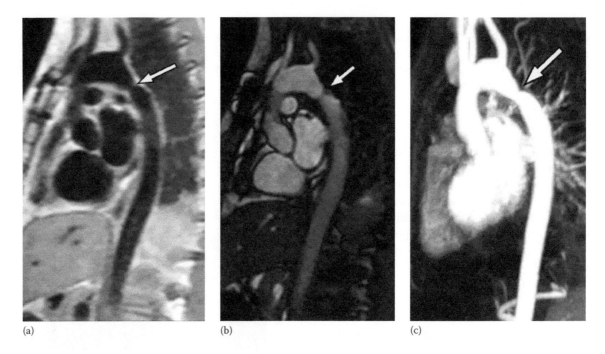

(a)   (b)   (c)

FIGURE 2.41   Aortic coarctation. Focal discrete narrowing (arrow) in the region of isthmus on (a) black blood, (b) SSFP cine, and (c) gadolinium-enhanced MR angiography images. (Reproduced from Stojanovska, J. et al., *Magn. Reson. Imaging Clin. N. Am.*, 23(2), 273, 2015. With permission.)

of ways, such as in enhanced diastolic interaction. Essentially, pericardial constraints may affect diastolic filling and interaction between the ventricles, as discussed in the following text.

2.5.7.1 Constrictive Pericarditis

Excessive pericardial thickening and calcification may occur from a variety of causes, including infectious, postsurgical, radiation, idiopathic, and following prior bouts of acute pericarditis (Spodick 1983). Pathologically, the pericardium becomes more fibrotic and adhesions may encase the heart. As the pericardium stiffens and becomes more fibrotic and adherent, ventricular filling is impeded (Figure 2.42), often leading to increased ventricular filling pressure and accentuated ventricular interaction (Hancock 1980). During early diastole, the ventricle rapidly fills due to enhanced ventricular suction. However, by mid-diastole, ventricular filling is halted abruptly as it abuts the rigid pericardium, which does not provide any further stretch. Therefore, filling is completed prematurely, leading to elevated atrial pressure and venous congestion. Findings of low CO as well as right-sided failure, including systemic venous congestion and effusions, are common in constrictive pericarditis.

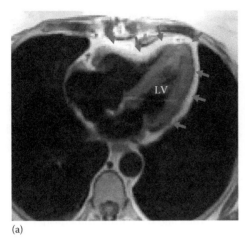 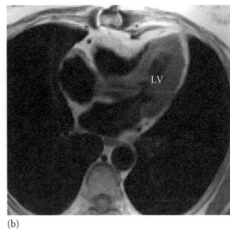

(a)   (b)

FIGURE 2.42 Constrictive pericarditis. Four-chamber images of a patient with constrictive pericarditis (arrows) at (a) end-diastole and (b) end-systole showing ventricular deformity during systole.

The underlying myocardium is normal in constrictive pericarditis, although changes to ventricular geometry and loading conditions are common. Physiologically, the primary abnormalities detected relate to respirophasic changes during the cardiac cycle and accentuation of ventricular interaction (Maisch et al. 2004). For example, during inspiration, the drop in intrathoracic pressure augments venous return to the right-sided chambers. However, this occurs at the expense of left-sided filling for several reasons. First, the interventricular septum shifts leftward, thus decreasing ventricular cavity size and impeding filling. Second, the drop in intrathoracic pressure is not transmitted to the intracardiac chambers as is typically the case. Thus, pulmonary venous and left atrial pressures are lower, but ventricular pressure remains relatively unchanged. Therefore, the transmitral flow, or gradient between LA and LV, is lower. These changes bring about lower LV filling during inspiration. Conversely, with expiration, the opposite occurs. Right-sided filling is reduced at the expense of improved filling of the left-sided chambers. These changes during the respiratory cycle provide diagnostic clues used by echocardiography and hemodynamic invasive catheterization to diagnose constrictive pericarditis.

2.5.7.2 Pericardial Tamponade

While the pathophysiologic mechanisms are somewhat different, the respirophasic changes during the cardiac cycle in pericardial tamponade are quite similar to that discussed with constrictive pericarditis. Increasing volume of the pericardial effusion leads to acute or gradual increase in intra-pericardial pressures. At some point, these intra-pericardial pressures overcome the diastolic filling pressures of the ventricle. Thus, there is impediment of ventricular filling, decline in CO, and ultimately hemodynamic collapse. The heart compensates for drop in CO by tachycardia and hyperdynamic contractility. The hemodynamic effects are largely related to the amount, location, and speed of fluid accumulation.

For example, large pericardial effusions which accumulate gradually are better tolerated than smaller, rapidly developing effusions since the pericardial fibers have longer time to adapt and stretch in the former case.

Occasionally, it may be difficult to clinically differentiate between constrictive pericarditis and restrictive cardiomyopathy. While both lead to diastolic abnormalities, constriction is due to abnormal pericardial compliance while restrictive cardiomyopathy reflects intrinsic myocardial disease. Therefore, in restrictive cardiomyopathy, there is marked endocardial dysfunction with relative sparing of the subepicardium. Thus, longitudinal mechanics are preferentially compromised; nevertheless, EF remains normal as the outer layers are preserved (i.e., circumferential and twist mechanics are relatively preserved). Conversely, constrictive pericarditis causes epicardial dysfunction, which adversely impacts circumferential and twist mechanics. Since the subendocardium is spared, longitudinal motion is preserved if not increased (Sengupta et al. 2008a).

2.6 SUMMARY AND KEY POINTS

2.6.1 SUMMARY

This review chapter highlighted the fundamental principles of cardiac function, including mechanics, hemodynamics, and the underlying principles of contraction. The heartbeat represents a highly coordinated series of events, which can be broken down into cellular and biochemical components. These processes culminate into cardiac contraction, which occurs via longitudinal, circumferential, radial, and rotational deformation. Various disease processes are associated with their own distinct mechanical abnormalities. These changes are readily observed with new imaging techniques such as cardiac MRI and echocardiography. Further understanding of cardiovascular disease mechanisms may be brought about with further imaging studies that evaluate mechanical dysfunction.

2.6.2 Key Points

- Different radiographic and heart-specific imaging planes are used for cardiac imaging.
- The heart is composed of two atria and two ventricles. Blood moves from the atria to the ventricles through the AV (mitral and tricuspid) valves. The LV and RV pump blood to the whole body (systemic circulation) and lungs (pulmonary circulation), respectively, through the aorta and pulmonary arteries.
- The pericardium is the outer layer adjacent to the heart, which acts as a protective barrier.
- The LV myocardium is composed of layers of fibers with varying orientations from the endo- to epicardial surfaces.
- The orthogonal fibers structure between the endo- and epicardial layers results in cardiac deformation during the cardiac cycle.
- The coronary arteries supply the heart with blood, where each artery supplies a specific myocardial region.
- The cardiac conduction system provides an electrical signal in order for contraction to occur. The heart is capable of generating its own impulse and beating rhythmically.
- Cardiac contraction can be explained based on actin–myosin cross-bridges.
- The ECG records the electrical activation of the heart based on electrodes attached to the surface of the body.
- The cardiac cycle and the timing of events are best understood through plotting pressure, volume, and flow over time. The cardiac cycle consists of two main phases: systole (blood ejection from the heart) and diastole (ventricular filling), which are preceded by short isovolumetric contraction (IVC) and isovolumetric relaxation (IVR) phases, respectively.
- The force–velocity relationship provides useful insights into the contractility patterns and mechanics.
- The P-V loop provides important information about changes occurring during the cardiac cycle. The P-V loop can be used to evaluate the heart function, for example, by calculating ESPVR and EDPVR.
- Thermodilution and the Fick's method are the most commonly used techniques for calculating CO.
- Cardiac contractility can be expressed by plotting SV against preload, as depicted by the Frank–Starling curve.
- Laplace's law describes the relationship between wall stress, ventricular pressure, ventricular radius, and wall thickness.
- Myocardial hypertrophy and heart dilation are forms of cardiac remodeling to adapt to changing loading conditions.
- The cardiac function can be assessed from measurement of work and power. Work can be obtained by calculating the area under the curve of the P-V loop. Power is the work performed per unit time.
- Different heart diseases affect cardiac mechanics. Example heart diseases include myocardial ischemia, MI, hypertension (systemic and pulmonary), heart failure (with preserved or reduced EF), cardiomyopathies (including hypertrophic, dilation, restrictive, and ARVC), myocarditis, valvular heart diseases (including valvular stenosis and regurgitation), CHD (including septal defects, patent ductus arteriosus, TGA, TOF, and aortic coarctation), and pericardial diseases (including constrictive pericarditis and pericardial tamponade).

ACKNOWLEDGMENT

The authors would like to thank Dr. Shehab Anwar from the National Heart Institute in Egypt for help with artistic figure design.

REFERENCES

Abbate, A., Bussani, R., Biondi-Zoccai, G. G., Santini, D., Petrolini, A., De Giorgio, F., Vasaturo, F., et al. (2005). Infarct-related artery occlusion, tissue markers of ischaemia, and increased apoptosis in the peri-infarct viable myocardium. *Eur Heart J* **26**(19): 2039–2045.

Anderson, R. H., Smerup, M., Sanchez-Quintana, D., Loukas, M., and Lunkenheimer, P. P. (2009). The three-dimensional arrangement of the myocytes in the ventricular walls. *Clin Anat* **22**(1): 64–76.

Arnsdorf, M. F. (1990). The cellular basis of cardiac arrhythmias. A matrical perspective. *Ann N Y Acad Sci* **601**: 263–280.

Bers, D. M. (2002). Cardiac excitation-contraction coupling. *Nature* **415**(6868): 198–205.

Bers, D. M. and Perez-Reyes, E. (1999). Ca channels in cardiac myocytes: Structure and function in Ca influx and intracellular Ca release. *Cardiovasc Res* **42**(2): 339–360.

Biederman, R. W., Doyle, M., Yamrozik, J., Williams, R. B., Rathi, V. K., Vido, D., Caruppannan, K., et al. (2005). Physiologic compensation is supranormal in compensated aortic stenosis: Does it return to normal after aortic valve replacement or is it blunted by coexistent coronary artery disease? An intramyocardial magnetic resonance imaging study. *Circulation* **112**(9 Suppl.): I429–436.

Bijnens, B., Cikes, M., Butakoff, C., Sitges, M., and Crispi, F. (2012). Myocardial motion and deformation: What does it tell us and how does it relate to function? *Fetal Diagn Ther* **32**(1–2): 5–16.

Boersma, E., Mercado, N., Poldermans, D., Gardien, M., Vos, J., and Simoons, M. L. (2003). Acute myocardial infarction. *Lancet* **361**(9360): 847–858.

Bolli, R. and Marban, E. (1999). Molecular and cellular mechanisms of myocardial stunning. *Physiol Rev* **79**(2): 609–634.

Bonow, R. O., Carabello, B. A., Chatterjee, K., de Leon, A. C., Jr., Faxon, D. P., Freed, M. D., Gaasch, W. H., et al. (2006). ACC/AHA 2006 guidelines for the management of patients with valvular heart disease: A report of the American College of Cardiology/American Heart Association Task Force on

Practice Guidelines (writing Committee to Revise the 1998 guidelines for the management of patients with valvular heart disease) developed in collaboration with the Society of Cardiovascular Anesthesiologists endorsed by the Society for Cardiovascular Angiography and Interventions and the Society of Thoracic Surgeons. *J Am Coll Cardiol* **48**(3): e1–148.

Bonow, R. O., Mann, D. L., Zipes, D. P., and Libby, P. (2011). *Braunwald's Heart Disease: A Textbook of Cardiovascular Medicine*. Philadelphia, PA: Saunders.

Borg, A. N., Harrison, J. L., Argyle, R. A., and Ray, S. G. (2008). Left ventricular torsion in primary chronic mitral regurgitation. *Heart* **94**(5): 597–603.

Borlaug, B. A. and Kass, D. A. (2009). Invasive hemodynamic assessment in heart failure. *Heart Fail Clin* **5**(2): 217–228.

Borlaug, B. A. and Kass, D. A. (2011). Invasive hemodynamic assessment in heart failure. *Cardiol Clin* **29**(2): 269–280.

Braunwald, E. and Kloner, R. A. (1982). The stunned myocardium: Prolonged, postischemic ventricular dysfunction. *Circulation* **66**(6): 1146–1149.

Braunwald, E. and Rutherford, J. D. (1986). Reversible ischemic left ventricular dysfunction: Evidence for the "hibernating myocardium". *J Am Coll Cardiol* **8**(6): 1467–1470.

Camici, P. G., Prasad, S. K., and Rimoldi, O. E. (2008). Stunning, hibernation, and assessment of myocardial viability. *Circulation* **117**(1): 103–114.

Carabello, B. A., Green, L. H., Grossman, W., Cohn, L. H., Koster, J. K., and Collins, J. J., Jr. (1980). Hemodynamic determinants of prognosis of aortic valve replacement in critical aortic stenosis and advanced congestive heart failure. *Circulation* **62**(1): 42–48.

Eaton, L. W., Weiss, J. L., Bulkley, B. H., Garrison, J. B., and Weisfeldt, M. L. (1979). Regional cardiac dilatation after acute myocardial infarction: Recognition by two-dimensional echocardiography. *N Engl J Med* **300**(2): 57–62.

Edwards, W. D. (1984). Anatomic basis for tomographic analysis of the heart at autopsy. *Cardiol Clin* **2**(4): 485–506.

Edwards, W. D., Tajik, A. J., and Seward, J. B. (1981). Standardized nomenclature and anatomic basis for regional tomographic analysis of the heart. *Mayo Clin Proc* **56**(8): 479–497.

Elsasser, A., Schlepper, M., Klovekorn, W. P., Cai, W. J., Zimmermann, R., Muller, K. D., Strasser, R., et al. (1997). Hibernating myocardium: An incomplete adaptation to ischemia. *Circulation* **96**(9): 2920–2931.

Enriquez-Sarano, M. and Tajik, A. J. (2004). Clinical practice. Aortic regurgitation. *N Engl J Med* **351**(15): 1539–1546.

Forrester, J. S., Wyatt, H. L., Da Luz, P. L., Tyberg, J. V., Diamond, G. A., and Swan, H. J. (1976). Functional significance of regional ischemic contraction abnormalities. *Circulation* **54**(1): 64–70.

Freeman, R. V. and Otto, C. M. (2005). Spectrum of calcific aortic valve disease: Pathogenesis, disease progression, and treatment strategies. *Circulation* **111**(24): 3316–3326.

Frohlich, E. D., Apstein, C., Chobanian, A. V., Devereux, R. B., Dustan, H. P., Dzau, V., Fauad-Tarazi, F., et al. (1992). The heart in hypertension. *N Engl J Med* **327**(14): 998–1008.

Gaasch, W. H. and Meyer, T. E. (2008). Left ventricular response to mitral regurgitation: Implications for management. *Circulation* **118**(22): 2298–2303.

Garot, J., Pascal, O., Diebold, B., Derumeaux, G., Gerber, B. L., Dubois-Rande, J. L., Lima, J. A., and Gueret, P. (2002a). Alterations of systolic left ventricular twist after acute myocardial infarction. *Am J Physiol Heart Circ Physiol* **282**(1): H357–H362.

Garot, J., Pascal, O., Diebold, B., Derumeaux, G., Ovize, M., and Gueret, P. (2002b). Changes in left ventricular torsion during ischemia-reperfusion. *Arch Mal Coeur Vaiss* **95**(12): 1151–1159.

Gemayel, C., Pelliccia, A., and Thompson, P. D. (2001). Arrhythmogenic right ventricular cardiomyopathy. *J Am Coll Cardiol* **38**(7): 1773–1781.

Gersh, B. J., Maron, B. J., Bonow, R. O., Dearani, J. A., Fifer, M. A., Link, M. S., Naidu, S. S., et al. (2011). 2011 ACCF/AHA guideline for the diagnosis and treatment of hypertrophic cardiomyopathy: A report of the American College of Cardiology Foundation/American Heart Association Task Force on Practice Guidelines. *Circulation* **124**(24): e783–e831.

Grosberg, A. and Gharib, M. (2009). Modeling the macro-structure of the heart: Healthy and diseased. *Med Biol Eng Comput* **47**(3): 301–311.

Haber, I., Metaxas, D. N., Geva, T., and Axel, L. (2005). Three-dimensional systolic kinematics of the right ventricle. *Am J Physiol Heart Circ Physiol* **289**(5): H1826–H1833.

Hancock, E. W. (1980). On the elastic and rigid forms of constrictive pericarditis. *Am Heart J* **100**(6 Pt 1): 917–923.

Hobai, I. A. and O'Rourke, B. (2001). Decreased sarcoplasmic reticulum calcium content is responsible for defective excitation-contraction coupling in canine heart failure. *Circulation* **103**(11): 1577–1584.

Holubarsch, C., Ruf, T., Goldstein, D. J., Ashton, R. C., Nickl, W., Pieske, B., Pioch, K., et al. (1996). Existence of the Frank-Starling mechanism in the failing human heart. Investigations on the organ, tissue, and sarcomere levels. *Circulation* **94**(4): 683–689.

Hundley, W. G., Bluemke, D. A., Finn, J. P., Flamm, S. D., Fogel, M. A., Friedrich, M. G., Ho, V. B., et al. (2010). ACCF/ACR/AHA/NASCI/SCMR 2010 expert consensus document on cardiovascular magnetic resonance: A report of the American College of Cardiology Foundation Task Force on Expert Consensus Documents. *J Am Coll Cardiol* **55**(23): 2614–2662.

Ibrahim, El-S. H., Shaffer, J. M., and White, R. D. (2011). Assessment of pulmonary artery stiffness using velocity-encoding magnetic resonance imaging: Evaluation of techniques. *Magn Reson Imaging* **29**(7): 966–974.

Ibrahim, El-S. H. and White, R. D. (2012). Cardiovascular magnetic resonance for the assessment of pulmonary arterial hypertension: Toward a comprehensive CMR exam. *Magn Reson Imaging* **30**(8): 1047–1058.

Ingels, N. B., Jr. (1997). Myocardial fiber architecture and left ventricular function. *Technol Health Care* **5**(1–2): 45–52.

Ingels, N. B., Jr., Hansen, D. E., Daughters, G. T., 2nd, Stinson, E. B., Alderman, E. L., and Miller, D. C. (1989). Relation between longitudinal, circumferential, and oblique shortening and torsional deformation in the left ventricle of the transplanted human heart. *Circ Res* **64**(5): 915–927.

Jamal, F., Bergerot, C., Argaud, L., Loufouat, J., and Ovize, M. (2003). Longitudinal strain quantitates regional right ventricular contractile function. *Am J Physiol Heart Circ Physiol* **285**(6): H2842–H2847.

James, M. A., Saadeh, A. M., and Jones, J. V. (2000). Wall stress and hypertension. *J Cardiovasc Risk* **7**(3): 187–190.

Jennings, R. B. and Ganote, C. E. (1974). Structural changes in myocardium during acute ischemia. *Circ Res* **35**(Suppl. 3): 156–172.

Kanzaki, H., Nakatani, S., Yamada, N., Urayama, S., Miyatake, K., and Kitakaze, M. (2006). Impaired systolic torsion in dilated cardiomyopathy: Reversal of apical rotation at mid-systole characterized with magnetic resonance tagging method. *Basic Res Cardiol* **101**(6): 465–470.

Kemp, C. D. and Conte, J. V. (2012). The pathophysiology of heart failure. *Cardiovasc Pathol* **21**(5): 365–371.

Kern, M. J., Lerman, A., Bech, J. W., De Bruyne, B., Eeckhout, E., Fearon, W. F., Higano, S. T., et al. (2006). Physiological assessment of coronary artery disease in the cardiac catheterization laboratory: A scientific statement from the American Heart Association Committee on Diagnostic and Interventional Cardiac Catheterization, Council on Clinical Cardiology. *Circulation* **114**(12): 1321–1341.

Kern, M. J. and Samady, H. (2010). Current concepts of integrated coronary physiology in the catheterization laboratory. *J Am Coll Cardiol* **55**(3): 173–185.

Kligfield, P., Gettes, L. S., Bailey, J. J., Childers, R., Deal, B. J., Hancock, E. W., van Herpen, G., et al. (2007). Recommendations for the standardization and interpretation of the electrocardiogram: Part I: The electrocardiogram and its technology: A scientific statement from the American Heart Association Electrocardiography and Arrhythmias Committee, Council on Clinical Cardiology; the American College of Cardiology Foundation; and the Heart Rhythm Society: Endorsed by the International Society for Computerized Electrocardiology. *Circulation* **115**(10): 1306–1324.

Kushwaha, S. S., Fallon, J. T., and Fuster, V. (1997). Restrictive cardiomyopathy. *N Engl J Med* **336**(4): 267–276.

Lam, C. S., Roger, V. L., Rodeheffer, R. J., Bursi, F., Borlaug, B. A., Ommen, S. R., Kass, D. A., and Redfield, M. M. (2007). Cardiac structure and ventricular-vascular function in persons with heart failure and preserved ejection fraction from Olmsted County, Minnesota. *Circulation* **115**(15): 1982–1990.

Leonardi, B., Margossian, R., Sanders, S. P., Chinali, M., and Colan, S. D. (2014). Ventricular mechanics in patients with aortic valve disease: Longitudinal, radial, and circumferential components. *Cardiol Young* **24**(1):105–112.

Mahrholdt, H., Wagner, A., Deluigi, C. C., Kispert, E., Hager, S., Meinhardt, G., Vogelsberg, H., et al. (2006). Presentation, patterns of myocardial damage, and clinical course of viral myocarditis. *Circulation* **114**(15): 1581–1590.

Maisch, B., Seferovic, P. M., Ristic, A. D., Erbel, R., Rienmuller, R., Adler, Y., Tomkowski, W. Z., Thiene, G., and Yacoub, M. H. (2004). Guidelines on the diagnosis and management of pericardial diseases executive summary; The Task force on the diagnosis and management of pericardial diseases of the European Society of Cardiology. *Eur Heart J* **25**(7): 587–610.

Maron, B. J., Towbin, J. A., Thiene, G., Antzelevitch, C., Corrado, D., Arnett, D., Moss, A. J., Seidman, C. E., and Young, J. B. (2006). Contemporary definitions and classification of the cardiomyopathies: An American Heart Association Scientific Statement from the Council on Clinical Cardiology, Heart Failure and Transplantation Committee; Quality of Care and Outcomes Research and Functional Genomics and Translational Biology Interdisciplinary Working Groups; and Council on Epidemiology and Prevention. *Circulation* **113**(14): 1807–1816.

McLaughlin, V. V., Archer, S. L., Badesch, D. B., Barst, R. J., Farber, H. W., Lindner, J. R., Mathier, M. A., et al. (2009). ACCF/AHA 2009 expert consensus document on pulmonary hypertension a report of the American College of Cardiology Foundation Task Force on Expert Consensus Documents and the American Heart Association developed in collaboration with the American College of Chest Physicians; American Thoracic Society, Inc.; and the Pulmonary Hypertension Association. *J Am Coll Cardiol* **53**(17): 1573–1619.

Mendes, L. A., Picard, M. H., Dec, G. W., Hartz, V. L., Palacios, I. F., and Davidoff, R. (1999). Ventricular remodeling in active myocarditis. Myocarditis Treatment Trial. *Am Heart J* **138**(2 Pt 1): 303–308.

Mizariene, V., Grybauskiene, R., Vaskelyte, J., Jonkaitiene, R., Pavilioniene, J., and Jurkevicius, R. (2011). Strain value in the assessment of left ventricular function and prediction of heart failure markers in aortic regurgitation. *Echocardiography* **28**(9): 983–992.

Mulieri, L. A., Hasenfuss, G., Leavitt, B., Allen, P. D., and Alpert, N. R. (1992). Altered myocardial force-frequency relation in human heart failure. *Circulation* **85**(5): 1743–1750.

Munagala, V. K., Hart, C. Y., Burnett, J. C., Jr., Meyer, D. M., and Redfield, M. M. (2005). Ventricular structure and function in aged dogs with renal hypertension: A model of experimental diastolic heart failure. *Circulation* **111**(9): 1128–1135.

Nagel, E., Stuber, M., Burkhard, B., Fischer, S. E., Scheidegger, M. B., Boesiger, P., and Hess, O. M. (2000). Cardiac rotation and relaxation in patients with aortic valve stenosis. *Eur Heart J* **21**(7): 582–589.

Nishimura, R. A., Carabello, B. A., Faxon, D. P., Freed, M. D., Lytle, B. W., O'Gara, P. T., O'Rourke, R. A., et al. (2008). ACC/AHA 2008 guideline update on valvular heart disease: Focused update on infective endocarditis: A report of the American College of Cardiology/American Heart Association Task Force on Practice Guidelines: Endorsed by the Society of Cardiovascular Anesthesiologists, Society for Cardiovascular Angiography and Interventions, and Society of Thoracic Surgeons. *Circulation* **118**(8): 887–896.

Ohno, M., Cheng, C. P., and Little, W. C. (1994). Mechanism of altered patterns of left ventricular filling during the development of congestive heart failure. *Circulation* **89**(5): 2241–2250.

Olsen, C. O., Rankin, J. S., Arentzen, C. E., Ring, W. S., McHale, P. A., and Anderson, R. W. (1981). The deformational characteristics of the left ventricle in the conscious dog. *Circ Res* **49**(4): 843–855.

Ozkan, A., Kapadia, S., Tuzcu, M., and Marwick, T. H. (2011). Assessment of left ventricular function in aortic stenosis. *Nat Rev Cardiol* **8**(9): 494–501.

Pettersen, E., Helle-Valle, T., Edvardsen, T., Lindberg, H., Smith, H. J., Smevik, B., Smiseth, O. A., and Andersen, K. (2007). Contraction pattern of the systemic right ventricle shift from longitudinal to circumferential shortening and absent global ventricular torsion. *J Am Coll Cardiol* **49**(25): 2450–2456.

Pfeffer, M. A. (1995). Left ventricular remodeling after acute myocardial infarction. *Annu Rev Med* **46**: 455–466.

Pfeffer, M. A. and Braunwald, E. (1990). Ventricular remodeling after myocardial infarction. Experimental observations and clinical implications. *Circulation* **81**(4): 1161–1172.

Pieske, B., Hasenfuss, G., Holubarsch, C., Schwinger, R., Bohm, M., and Just, H. (1992). Alterations of the force-frequency relationship in the failing human heart depend on the underlying cardiac disease. *Basic Res Cardiol* **87**(Suppl. 1): 213–221.

Pollack, G. H. (1983). The cross-bridge theory. *Physiol Rev* **63**(3): 1049–1113.

Puwanant, S., Park, M., Popovic, Z. B., Tang, W. H., Farha, S., George, D., Sharp, J., et al. (2010). Ventricular geometry, strain, and rotational mechanics in pulmonary hypertension. *Circulation* **121**(2): 259–266.

Rankin, J. S., McHale, P. A., Arentzen, C. E., Ling, D., Greenfield, J. C., Jr., and Anderson, R. W. (1976). The three-dimensional dynamic geometry of the left ventricle in the conscious dog. *Circ Res* **39**(3): 304–313.

Reimer, K. A. and Jennings, R. B. (1979). The "wavefront phenomenon" of myocardial ischemic cell death. II. Transmural progression of necrosis within the framework of ischemic bed size (myocardium at risk) and collateral flow. *Lab Invest* **40**(6): 633–644.

Ross, J., Jr., Sonnenblick, E. H., Taylor, R. R., Spotnitz, H. M., and Covell, J. W. (1971). Diastolic geometry and sarcomere lengths in the chronically dilated canine left ventricle. *Circ Res* **28**(1): 49–61.

Sarnoff, S. J. and Berglund, E. (1954). Ventricular function. I. Starling's law of the heart studied by means of simultaneous right and left ventricular function curves in the dog. *Circulation* **9**(5): 706–718.

Schwarz, E. R., Schaper, J., vom Dahl, J., Altehoefer, C., Grohmann, B., Schoendube, F., Sheehan, F. H., et al. (1996). Myocyte degeneration and cell death in hibernating human myocardium. *J Am Coll Cardiol* **27**(7): 1577–1585.

Sengupta, P. P., Korinek, J., Belohlavek, M., Narula, J., Vannan, M. A., Jahangir, A., and Khandheria, B. K. (2006). Left ventricular structure and function: Basic science for cardiac imaging. *J Am Coll Cardiol* **48**(10): 1988–2001.

Sengupta, P. P., Krishnamoorthy, V. K., Abhayaratna, W. P., Korinek, J., Belohlavek, M., Sundt, T. M., 3rd, Chandrasekaran, K., et al. (2008a). Disparate patterns of left ventricular mechanics differentiate constrictive pericarditis from restrictive cardiomyopathy. *JACC Cardiovasc Imaging* **1**(1): 29–38.

Sengupta, P. P., Tajik, A. J., Chandrasekaran, K., and Khandheria, B. K. (2008b). Twist mechanics of the left ventricle: Principles and application. *JACC Cardiovasc Imaging* **1**(3): 366–376.

Shapiro, B. P., Mergo, P. J., Austin, C. O., Kantor, B., and Gerber, T. C. (2012). Assessing the available techniques for testing myocardial viability: What does the future hold? *Future Cardiol* **8**(6): 819–836.

Sonnenblick, E. H., Ross, J., Jr., Covell, J. W., Spotnitz, H. M., and Spiro, D. (1967). The ultrastructure of the heart in systole and diastole. Changes in sarcomere length. *Circ Res* **21**(4): 423–431.

Spodick, D. H. (1983). The normal and diseased pericardium: Current concepts of pericardial physiology, diagnosis and treatment. *J Am Coll Cardiol* **1**(1): 240–251.

Spotnitz, H. M. (2000). Macro design, structure, and mechanics of the left ventricle. *J Thorac Cardiovasc Surg* **119**(5): 1053–1077.

Spotnitz, W. D., Spotnitz, H. M., Truccone, N. J., Cottrell, T. S., Gersony, W., Malm, J. R., and Sonnenblick, E. H. (1979). Relation of ultrastructure and function. Sarcomere dimensions, pressure-volume curves, and geometry of the intact left ventricle of the immature canine heart. *Circ Res* **44**(5): 679–691.

Stojanovska, J., Rodriguez, K., Mueller, G. C., and Agarwal, P. P. (2015). MR imaging of the thoracic aorta. *Magn Reson Imaging Clin N Am* **23**(2): 273–291.

Streeter, D. D., Jr., Spotnitz, H. M., Patel, D. P., Ross, J., Jr., and Sonnenblick, E. H. (1969). Fiber orientation in the canine left ventricle during diastole and systole. *Circ Res* **24**(3): 339–347.

Stuber, M., Scheidegger, M. B., Fischer, S. E., Nagel, E., Steinemann, F., Hess, O. M., and Boesiger, P. (1999). Alterations in the local myocardial motion pattern in patients suffering from pressure overload due to aortic stenosis. *Circulation* **100**(4): 361–368.

Sundaram, B., Patel, S., Agarwal, P., and Kazerooni, E. A. (2009a). Anatomy and terminology for the interpretation and reporting of cardiac MDCT: Part 2, CT angiography, cardiac function assessment, and noncoronary and extracardiac findings. *Am J Roentgenol* **192**(3): 584–598.

Sundaram, B., Patel, S., Bogot, N., and Kazerooni, E. A. (2009b). Anatomy and terminology for the interpretation and reporting of cardiac MDCT: Part 1, Structured report, coronary calcium screening, and coronary artery anatomy. *Am J Roentgenol* **192**(3): 574–583.

Swan, H. J., Forrester, J. S., Diamond, G., Chatterjee, K., and Parmley, W. W. (1972). Hemodynamic spectrum of myocardial infarction and cardiogenic shock. A conceptual model. *Circulation* **45**(5): 1097–1110.

Swan, H. J., Ganz, W., Forrester, J., Marcus, H., Diamond, G., and Chonette, D. (1970). Catheterization of the heart in man with use of a flow-directed balloon-tipped catheter. *N Engl J Med* **283**(9): 447–451.

Tendulkar, A. P. and Harken, A. H. (2006). Mechanics of the normal heart. *J Card Surg* **21**(6): 615–620.

Thygesen, K., Alpert, J. S., and White, H. D. (2007a). Universal definition of myocardial infarction. *Eur Heart J* **28**(20): 2525–2538.

Thygesen, K., Alpert, J. S., White, H. D., Jaffe, A. S., Apple, F. S., Galvani, M., Katus, H. A., et al. (2007b). Universal definition of myocardial infarction. *Circulation* **116**(22): 2634–2653.

Tibayan, F. A., Rodriguez, F., Langer, F., Zasio, M. K., Bailey, L., Liang, D., Daughters, G. T., Ingels, N. B., Jr., and Miller, D. C. (2004). Alterations in left ventricular torsion and diastolic recoil after myocardial infarction with and without chronic ischemic mitral regurgitation. *Circulation* **110**(11 Suppl. 1): II109–II114.

Tomoike, H. (1982). Analysis of in situ heart mechanics. *Jpn Circ J* **46**(10): 1108–1111.

van Dalen, B. M., Tzikas, A., Soliman, O. I., Heuvelman, H. J., Vletter, W. B., Ten Cate, F. J., and Geleijnse, M. L. (2013). Assessment of subendocardial contractile function in aortic stenosis: A study using speckle tracking echocardiography. *Echocardiography* **30**(3):293–300.

Virmani, R., Forman, M. B., and Kolodgie, F. D. (1990). Myocardial reperfusion injury. Histopathological effects of perfluorochemical. *Circulation* **81**(3 Suppl.): IV57–IV68.

Young, A. A., Kramer, C. M., Ferrari, V. A., Axel, L., and Reichek, N. (1994). Three-dimensional left ventricular deformation in hypertrophic cardiomyopathy. *Circulation* **90**(2): 854–867.

3 MRI Basics

El-Sayed H. Ibrahim, PhD and Refaat E. Gabr, PhD

CONTENTS

LIST OF ABBREVIATIONS

Abbreviation	Meaning
1D	One-dimensional
2D	Two-dimensional
3D	Three-dimensional
ADC	Apparent diffusion coefficient; also used for analog-to-digital converter
B_0	Main (static) magnetic field
B_1	Radiofrequency magnetic field
BOLD	Blood oxygen level dependent
bSSFP	Balanced steady-state free precession
BW	Bandwidth
CMR	Cardiac MR
CNR	Contrast-to-noise ratio
CSI	Chemical shift imaging
CT	Computed tomography
DTI	Diffusion tensor imaging
DWI	Diffusion-weighted imaging
ECG	Electrocardiogram
EPI	Echo planar imaging
ETL	Echo train length
FA	Flip angle
FDA	Food and drug administration
FE	Frequency encoding
FFE	Fast field echo
FFT	Fast Fourier transform
FID	Free induction decay
FISP	Fast imaging with steady-state precession
FLAIR	Fluid-attenuated inversion recovery
FLASH	Fast low-angle shot
fMRI	Functional MRI
FOV	Field of view
FSE	Fast spin echo
FT	Fourier transform
GRE	Gradient echo
GMN	Gradient moment nulling
g-factor	Geometry factor
GRAPPA	Generalized auto-calibrating partially parallel acquisition
GRE	Gradient-recalled echo
IF	Intermediate frequency
IR	Inversion recovery
MIP	Maximum intensity projection
MR	Magnetic resonance

MRA	Magnetic resonance angiography
MRI	Magnetic resonance imaging
MRS	Magnetic resonance spectroscopy
MT	Magnetization transfer
NEX	Number of excitations
NMR	Nuclear magnetic resonance
NSA	Number of signal averages
NSF	Nephrogenic systemic fibrosis
PC	Phase contrast
PD	Proton density
PDW	Proton density weighted
PE	Phase encoding
PR	Projection reconstruction
PRESS	Point-resolved spectroscopy
PROPELLER	Periodically rotated overlapping parallel lines with enhanced reconstruction
RARE	Rapid acquisition with relaxation enhancement
REST	Regional saturation
RF	Radiofrequency
SAR	Specific absorption rate
SE	Spin echo
SENSE	Sensitivity encoding
SNR	Signal-to-noise ratio
SPAMM	Spatial modulation of magnetization
SPGR	Spoiled gradient echo
SS	Slice selection
SSFP	Steady-state free precession
STEAM	Stimulated echo acquisition mode
STIR	Short-TI inversion recovery
T_1	Longitudinal (or spin–lattice) relaxation time
T1W	T_1-weighted
T_2	Transverse (or spin–spin) relaxation time
T2W	T_2-weighted
T_2^*	T_2-star: the effective transverse relaxation time
TE	Echo time
TI	Inversion time
TOF	Time of flight
TR	Repetition time
TSE	Turbo spin echo
VENC	Velocity encoding

3.1 INTRODUCTION

Magnetic resonance imaging (MRI) is a medical imaging technique that can *noninvasively* image cross sections and volumes inside the body using the intrinsic magnetic properties of the tissue. Since its discovery, MRI has revolutionized the medical imaging field and has been used in a wide range of clinical applications. With its exquisite soft tissue contrast, MRI is an excellent modality for imaging all body organs including the heart and vascular system. In addition, MRI is a powerful tool in clinical and basic research. There are over 20,000 MRI scanners worldwide performing more than 60 million scans each year. MRI is a multibillion dollar

industry, and it is a diverse field integrating physics, mathematics, engineering, and computer science with medicine and biology to provide valuable information about the status of tissue in health and disease.

3.1.1 DESCRIPTION OF THE MRI SCAN

An MRI scanner (Figure 3.1) consists of a very strong tube-shaped magnet and various coils, electronics, and computers. Depending on the scan type, the patient may be administered a contrast agent before or during the scan. A patient undergoing an MRI exam lies on the scanner table, and coils are attached to the body to receive the MRI signal. Afterward, the table is slid into the tunnel inside the magnet and the scan starts. During the scan, various magnetic fields are manipulated in a planned way to interact with the magnetic properties of the tissue to produce the MRI image. The scan may produce loud noise; therefore, headphones and/or earplugs are used during the scan to protect the patient's hearing. The scan usually takes a few minutes (or even seconds), but it can be as long as an hour depending on the amount of data required and level of detail/accuracy sought (some in vitro scans could last for several hours). A single MRI scan produces a large number of images showing the anatomy and function of the scanned organ. Once the scan is completed, the patient is moved out of the scanner and can leave the room immediately, usually without the need for any recovery time. Example MRI images of the human chest, brain, and spine are shown in Figure 3.2.

3.1.2 MRI PROS AND CONS

MRI imaging is based on the principles of nuclear magnetic resonance (NMR)—a technique that probes the molecular environment using magnetic fields. Because there is no ionizing radiation involved, MRI is a safe imaging modality that can be performed repeatedly or in dynamic studies without concerns about radiation exposure. This is a big advantage for MRI compared to x-ray-based imaging modalities, for example, computed tomography (CT), especially for patients with high sensitivity to radiation exposure like children and pregnant women. MRI is a very flexible and powerful technique that can provide not only anatomical, but also physical, chemical, metabolic, and functional information about the imaged tissue or organ. The main imaging advantage of MRI is its superior soft tissue contrast, making it ideal for imaging many organs and tissues. MRI can image slices in any direction, as well as imaging complete three-dimensional (3D) volumes. The arbitrary slice orientation in MRI allows for easy scan planning and image plane alignment. Furthermore, MRI has numerous contrast mechanisms that can be used to differentiate between different tissues without the administration of contrast agents.

On the other hand, the MRI system is very expensive (~$1 million per Tesla), making it suitable only for hospitals and radiology centers. In addition, MRI is a relatively slow

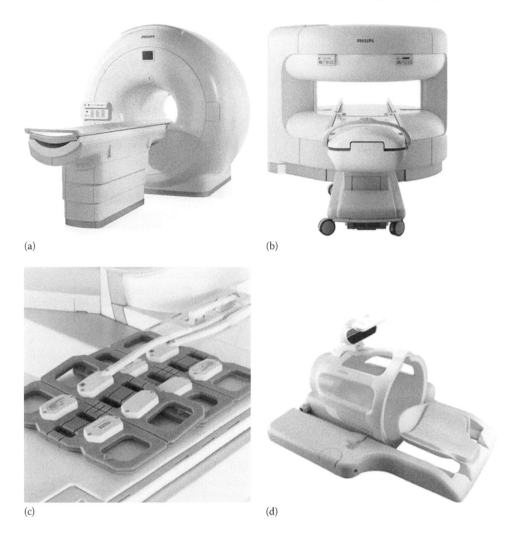

FIGURE 3.1   Magnetic resonance imaging (MRI) scanners and coils. (a) Closed 3 T Philips scanner. (b) Open 1.0 T Philips Panorama system. (c) Siemens phased-array coil. (d) Vivid imaging head coil.

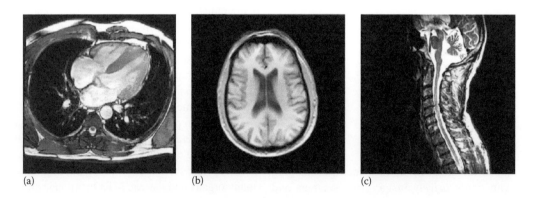

FIGURE 3.2   MRI images. Example MRI images of the human (a) chest, (b) brain, and (c) spine.

imaging technique, which may be problematic if the patient moves during the scan. Further, the tight space inside the MRI scanner and loud noise are problems for claustrophobic patients. Finally, the strong magnetic field involved poses a contraindication for imaging patients with certain metal implants or implanted devices.

3.1.3   HISTORICAL NOTE

In 1938, the NMR phenomenon was described by Isidor Rabi, who was later awarded the Nobel Prize in Physics in 1944 for this discovery. Shortly after, NMR was demonstrated in liquids and solids by two independent research groups lead by Felix

Bloch and Edward Purcell in 1946. Bloch and Purcell received the Nobel Prize in Physics in 1952 for their discoveries. In 1950–1951, "chemical shift" was discovered, based on which NMR spectroscopy was born, where its applications in chemistry and biology expanded rapidly. In 1966, Richard Ernst introduced the Fourier transform NMR, which significantly improved the technique's sensitivity. Ernst earned the 1991 Nobel Prize in Chemistry for his contributions to NMR spectroscopy. In 1973, NMR imaging (now called MRI) was invented by Paul Lauterbur and Peter Mansfield. For this great discovery, the two scientists were awarded the 2003 Nobel Prize in Physiology/Medicine.

3.1.4 CHAPTER OUTLINE

This chapter describes the physical principles of NMR and how MRI images are generated based on these basic principles. Several advanced topics are then briefly introduced. The scanner hardware and safety concerns with MRI imaging are discussed toward the end of the chapter.

3.2 THE NMR PHENOMENON

NMR is the phenomenon in which certain nuclei absorb and reemit electromagnetic energy when placed in a magnetic field and the resonance condition is satisfied. NMR results from the interaction of an external magnetic field with intrinsic magnetic properties of the atoms (specifically the nuclei)

in our bodies. The interaction occurs when the frequency of the excitation magnetic field matches that of the nuclei, a condition known as resonance. Although a full understanding of NMR physics requires a background in quantum physics, classical physics provides an adequate understanding of spin handling in MRI, as detailed in the following text.

3.2.1 SPINS

Elementary subatomic particles like electrons, protons, and neutrons have an intrinsic angular momentum property called *spin*. The word "intrinsic" means that these particles do not have to actually spin in order to have an angular momentum. Associated with this spin property is a small magnetic moment. Nuclei with an odd number of protons or neutrons have a net nuclear magnetic moment and are said to be MR active. These nuclei are classically viewed as current loops that generate magnetic dipoles (Figure 3.3a). They are usually referred to as "spins" and may be viewed as tiny bar magnets (Figure 3.3a). There are many MR active elements such as hydrogen (^{1}H), carbon (^{13}C), fluorine (^{19}F), phosphorus (^{31}P), and sodium (^{23}Na). The hydrogen nucleus, consisting of a single proton, is the most widely used nucleus in MRI because of its abundance in the body. In the absence of external magnetic fields, the magnetic moments of all nuclear spins are subject to thermal motion; therefore, they point in random directions (Figure 3.4a) and do not produce any macroscopic magnetic effect.

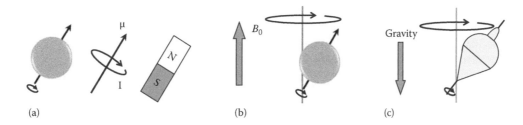

(a)   (b)   (c)

FIGURE 3.3 Nuclear spin and precession. (a) The nuclear spin resembles a current (I) loop that has a magnetic moment (μ) and is presented as a tiny bar magnet. (b) A spin in an external magnetic field precesses around the axis of the external field B_0, similar to a child's top precessing around the gravitational field (c).

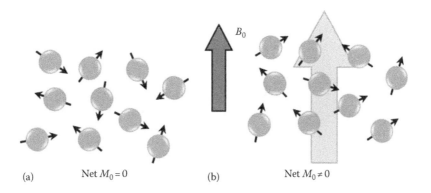

(a)   Net $M_0 = 0$ (b)   Net $M_0 \neq 0$

FIGURE 3.4 Spin polarization. (a) In the absence of an external magnetic field, the spins have an isotropic distribution of orientations, and there is no net magnetic moment. (b) When an external magnetic field is applied, a bias is created along the field direction, resulting in a net magnetic moment (M_0), represented here by the large gray arrow (the bias is exaggerated in the figure for clarity).

3.2.2 Spin Precession

When an external magnetic field B_0 is turned on, the magnetic moment of a spin influenced by this field starts to move around the axis of B_0 in a circular path with a certain angle (Figure 3.3b). This motion is called precession. It is similar to the wobbling motion of a child's top around the axis of the gravity field (Figure 3.3c). The frequency of spin precession (ω_0) is proportional to the strength of the B_0 field (in units of Tesla, T) and is known as the Larmor frequency:

$$\omega_0 = \gamma B_0, \tag{3.1}$$

where

- γ is a constant, known as the gyromagnetic ratio, which is specific to each nucleus
- B_0 is formally the magnetic induction or magnetic flux density, but it is often referred to as the magnetic field

Table 3.1 lists the gyromagnetic ratios of common nuclei used in MRI. For B_0 fields used in clinical MRI, most nuclei have precessional frequencies in the radiofrequency (RF) range of the electromagnetic spectrum.

3.2.3 Spin Polarization

In the presence of an external magnetic field B_0, the spins precess around the direction of B_0 tilted at a constant angle, which depends on the initial position of the spin when B_0 is turned on. The distribution of the angles is random, and thus, no net magnetization is expected. However, the thermal motion of the molecules causes a bias (~0.001%) in the spins orientation, slightly favoring the direction parallel to B_0. The magnetic moments of the precessing spins sum up to a net nonzero magnetization, M_0, also precessing around the axis of B_0 (Figure 3.4b). This process is called spin polarization.

3.2.4 Excitation

The precessing magnetization M_0 has a net nonzero component along the axis of B_0 (called the longitudinal direction) and a zero component in the perpendicular plane (called the

TABLE 3.1
The Gyromagnetic Ratio of Common MR-Active Nuclei

Nucleus	$\gamma/2\pi$ (MHz/T)
^{1}H	42.58
^{13}C	10.71
^{14}N	3.08
^{17}O	−5.77
^{19}F	40.08
^{23}Na	11.27
^{31}P	17.25

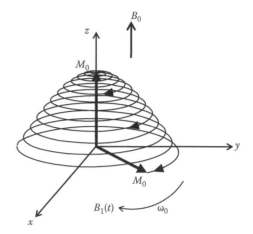

FIGURE 3.5 Magnetization excitation. The application of an external oscillating magnetic field (B_1) perpendicular to the direction of B_0 causes the magnetization vector M_0 to spiral down to the transverse plane.

transverse plane). M_0 is too small relative to B_0 to be directly measured while in the longitudinal direction; therefore, it is better detected if tipped away from the longitudinal direction. This is achieved by the application of a weak RF magnetic field (denoted by B_1) in a direction perpendicular to B_0. The frequency of this RF field is tuned to the Larmor frequency to achieve the resonance condition, enabling efficient energy transfer to the spins. Depending on the coil used, the B_1 field can be linearly polarized (changing along a single direction) or circularly polarized (changing in a circular pattern). A circularly polarized RF field of magnitude B_1 has the form of

$$\hat{B}_1(t) = B_1 \cdot \left[\cos(\omega_0 t)\hat{x} - \sin(\omega_0 t)\hat{y} \right], \tag{3.2}$$

where $\hat{x}$ and $\hat{y}$ are two orthogonal unit vectors in the transverse plane. Nevertheless, a linearly polarized field can be decomposed into two opposing circularly polarized fields, where only the field rotating in the same direction as the precessing spins generates the MR signal. As a result of the combined effect of B_0 and B_1 fields, the spins precess around an axis that is the vector sum of them, eventually spiraling down from the longitudinal direction to the transverse plane, as shown in Figure 3.5. The description of the magnetization excitation may be simplified using a frame of reference that rotates with ω_0 around B_0 as described next.

3.2.4.1 Rotating Frame of Reference

Since the precession frequency is proportional to the strength of the magnetic field, precession is orders of magnitude faster around the direction of B_0 than around the direction of B_1. To simplify the description and visualization of the motion of M_0, it is useful to consider a frame of reference rotating around the axis of B_0 with an angular frequency ω_0. In this *rotating frame of reference*, two simplifications occur: (1) the B_0 field vanishes, and (2) the B_1 field appears pointing in a fixed direction (not rotating). The spins now experience only the B_1 field and, as a result, precess only around the axis of the

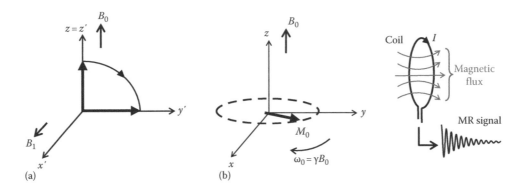

FIGURE 3.6 Rotating frame of reference. (a) In the rotating frame of reference (defined by the axes x' and y' which are rotating clockwise with frequency ω_0), magnetization excitation causes a clockwise rotation of the magnetization vector around the axis of the applied radiofrequency (RF) B_1 field. (b) The precessing magnetization M_0 in the transverse plane (shown in the laboratory (stationary) frame of reference) induces a current (I) in the coil, which is the received MR signal (note that the coil direction is orthogonal to B_0).

B_1 field, tipping into the transverse plane after a 90° rotation (Figure 3.6a). If the observer switches back to the stationary (laboratory) frame of reference, M_0 now lies in the transverse plane, precessing around the longitudinal direction at the Larmor frequency (Figure 3.6b). If a loop of wire (RF coil) oriented orthogonal to B_0 is brought close enough, the precession of the magnetization M_0 induces an electric current in the coil according to the Faraday's law of induction. This current is the MR signal used to construct the MRI image.

3.2.4.2 Flip Angle

The B_1 excitation field (called an RF pulse) is usually applied for a short time period (τ) causing the magnetization to rotate through a certain angle, called the *flip angle*, around the axis of B_1. This flip angle (α) is given by

$$\alpha = \gamma B_1 \tau, \tag{3.3}$$

where τ is the duration of the RF pulse, which is assumed to be constant with magnitude equal to B_1. A flip angle of 90° applied to a magnetization initially aligned along the longitudinal direction (usually taken as the z-axis) tips the magnetization completely into the transverse plane, producing maximum signal. This RF pulse is called an *excitation pulse* (Figure 3.7a). Excitation pulses of smaller flip angles (<90°) are also commonly used to partially rotate the longitudinal magnetization (Figure 3.7b). In this case, the excitation RF pulse, α, creates a transverse magnetization component equal to $M_0\sin(\alpha)$, leaving the longitudinal magnetization at a value of $M_0\cos(\alpha)$.

After the excitation RF pulse is turned off, the magnetization vector starts recovering back toward the equilibrium position (M_0 in the longitudinal direction). This results in exponential decay and exponential recovery of the transverse and longitudinal magnetization components, respectively, which occur independently with time constants T_2 and T_1, respectively. The received signal from the decaying transverse magnetization is called the free induction decay (FID) and is approximately an exponentially decaying sinusoidal function, which carries valuable information about the environment of the excited nuclei. For example, the magnitude of the signal is proportional to the number of nuclei in the excited volume

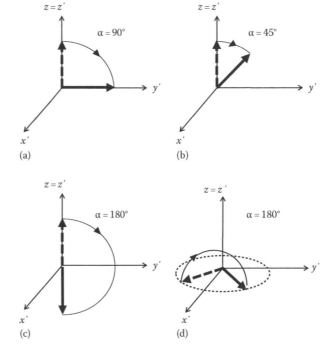

FIGURE 3.7 Flip angle. The final magnetization vector (solid arrow) following the application of different RF pulses applied along the x'-axis, where the initial magnetization vector is represented by the dashed arrow. (a) A 90° excitation pulse. (b) An excitation pulse of 45°. (c) A 180° inversion pulse. (d) A 180° refocusing pulse.

(proton density). This simple MR experiment is illustrated by the pulse diagram in Figure 3.8.

A 180° RF pulse applied to a magnetization initially aligned along the z-axis inverts the magnetization to the negative z-axis (Figure 3.7c). This pulse is called an *inversion pulse*. A 180° flip angle applied to a magnetization initially in the transverse plane causes the magnetization to flip around the pulse axis (assumed to be the x'-axis in Figure 3.7). The magnetization remains in the transverse plane, but its phase is reversed similar to a pancake flip (Figure 3.7d). Such an RF pulse is called a *refocusing pulse* for reasons that will be explained later in the section on *spin echo* (SE).

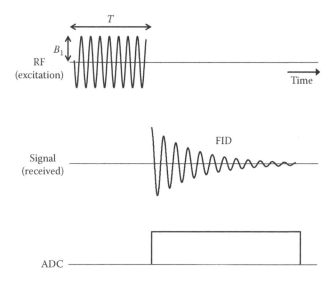

FIGURE 3.8 Simple MRI experiment. An RF excitation tuned to the Larmor frequency produces the MR free induction decay (FID) signal, which is digitized and recorded using an analog-to-digital converter (ADC).

3.2.5 RELAXATION

At equilibrium, M_0 lies in the longitudinal direction. The RF excitation disturbs this equilibrium, tipping M_0 away from the longitudinal direction. At any time point, M_0 is conveniently decomposed into a longitudinal component (along the B_0 direction) and a transverse component (in the transverse plane perpendicular to B_0) denoted by M_z and M_{xy}, respectively (Figure 3.9a). For simplicity, we consider the case of a 90° excitation pulse, which tips the whole magnetization into the transverse plane, resulting in $M_{xy} = M_0$ and $M_z = 0$. Immediately after

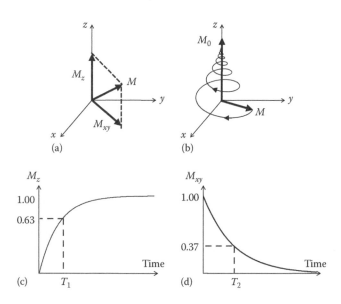

FIGURE 3.9 Magnetization relaxation. (a) The magnetization vector (M) is decomposed into a longitudinal (M_z) and transverse (M_{xy}) components. (b) Following the excitation pulse, the magnetization vector returns to equilibrium. (c) Longitudinal T_1 and (d) Transverse T_2 relaxation curves for a unit magnetization following a 90° RF pulse.

application of the excitation pulse, M_z starts recovering from zero to its equilibrium value M_0 (Figure 3.9b). The recovery process follows an exponential growth and is characterized by the time constant T_1 (Figure 3.9c). T_1 is the time needed for M_z to recover to 63% of its equilibrium value (M_z approximately recovers to M_0 after a time period of $5 \times T_1$). T_1 is called the spin–lattice, or longitudinal, relaxation time constant, which is a tissue-specific characteristic. The recovery process of M_z as a function of time, t, is mathematically formulated as

$$M_z = M_0\left(1 - e^{-t/T_1}\right), \tag{3.4}$$

where $t = 0$ is the time point immediately after the end of the excitation pulse.

In contrast to the growing behavior of M_z during relaxation, M_{xy} experiences an exponential decay during relaxation (Figure 3.9d). Immediately after being tipped into the transverse plane, the different spins composing M_{xy} are aligned in the same direction (in-phase) and sum up to an appreciable M_{xy} signal. Nevertheless, with time (in the order of milliseconds), these spins start to dephase (fan out) and lose coherence due to tiny differences in their molecular environment, which results in different magnetic fields experienced by the spins. Therefore, different spins rotate at slightly different frequencies and accumulate different phase angles (phase out), leading to signal cancellation as time passes. The time constant that characterizes the decay of M_{xy} is called the spin–spin, or transverse, relaxation time, which is a tissue-specific characteristic and is denoted by T_2. It should be noted that T_2 is always less than or equal to the longitudinal relaxation time constant T_1. The decay of the transverse magnetization (in the rotating frame of reference) is mathematically expressed as

$$M_{xy} = M_0 e^{-t/T_2}. \tag{3.5}$$

In practice, two factors contribute to the actual decay of M_{xy}. The first is the natural spin–spin interaction, characterized by the T_2 time constant. The second factor is denoted by T_2' time constant, which is a result of the inhomogeneity in the B_0 field $(1/T_2' = \gamma \Delta B_0)$, which causes differences between the resonance frequencies of the neighboring precessing nuclei. The effective transverse decaying time constant is denoted by T_2^*, given by

$$\frac{1}{T_2^*} = \frac{1}{T_2} + \frac{1}{T_2'}. \tag{3.6}$$

T_2^* is always shorter than T_2. It should be noted that while the T_2 decaying effect is an intrinsic property of the tissue, the T_2' decaying effect is not. In fact, the T_2' effect can be reversed by the application of a 180° RF refocusing pulse, as implemented in the SE sequence. Therefore, while the FID signal decays quickly with T_2^* time constant, the spin echo signal decays at a slower rate with T_2 time constant (Figure 3.10).

Both T_1 and T_2 are field dependent. At higher magnetic (B_0) fields, T_1 becomes longer, whereas T_2 stays approximately the

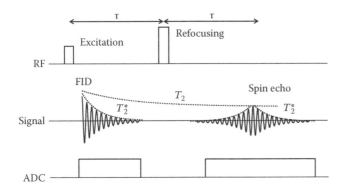

FIGURE 3.10 T_2 and T_2^* decays. A free induction decay (FID) signal and a spin echo (SE) signal are generated by the application of two RF pulses. The time separation between the two RF pulses (τ) is the same as that between the second RF pulse and the peak of the echo signal. The T_2 and T_2^* decays are indicated with dotted lines. ADC, analog-to-digital converter.

TABLE 3.2
Approximate T_1 and T_2 Values for Various Tissues

Tissue	T_1 (ms)		T_2 (ms)	
	1.5 T	3.0 T	1.5 T	3.0 T
Myocardium	900	1300	49	47
Fat	270	375	92	90
Blood	1300	1800	290	275

same. Approximate values for various human tissues at B_0 = 1.5 T are shown in Table 3.2.

3.2.6 BLOCH EQUATION

The dynamics of magnetization precession and relaxation are described by a phenomenological differential equation known as the *Bloch equation*, which relates the rate of change of the macroscopic magnetization (**M**) in the presence of a magnetic field (**B**):

$$\frac{d}{dt}\mathbf{M}(t) = \gamma \mathbf{M}(t) \times \mathbf{B}(t) - \frac{M_x(t)\hat{x} + M_y(t)\hat{y}}{T_2} - \frac{\left(M_z(t) - M_0\right)\hat{z}}{T_1},$$

(3.7)

where

   M and **B** are the vector notations for the magnetization vector and the applied magnetic field, respectively
   × denotes the cross (vector) product

The vector **B** includes the static magnetic field B_0 in addition to any applied RF (B_1) field. The first part in the right-hand side of the Bloch equation describes the precession of the magnetization in the presence of the magnetic field, while the second and third parts describe the magnetization transverse and longitudinal relaxation behaviors, respectively. When relaxation is neglected, the solution of the Bloch equation

produces the basic Larmor precession of the magnetization vector **M** around the direction of **B**. The Bloch equation is also valid in the rotating frame of reference, where in this case **B** (= B_1) is the effective magnetic field seen in the rotating frame of reference. Solving the Bloch equation in the rotating frame yields the T_1 and T_2 relaxation curves in Figure 3.9 (neglecting off-resonance effects).

3.3 MRI CONTRAST MECHANISMS

Image contrast is defined as the difference in signal intensity between two tissues. Contrast results from differences in the characteristics of the two tissues, but it also depends on the imaging sequence. One of the key advantages of MRI over other medical imaging modalities is the large number of control parameters that can be adjusted to change tissue contrast. The most commonly employed contrast mechanisms in MRI are based on differences in tissue relaxation times, as in T_1-weighted (T1W) and T_2-weighted (T2W) images, or differences in the density of spins in the sample, as in proton density (PD)-weighted images. Image contrast can also be based on differences in molecular diffusion, blood flow, temperature, or magnetic susceptibility, to name a few.

3.3.1 MRI PULSE SEQUENCE

To obtain enough data for reconstructing the MRI image, RF excitation and signal recording (during relaxation) are usually repeated multiple times. The series of excitation RF pulses and accompanying gradients (described later) form the MRI pulse sequence. The time duration between two successive RF pulses is called the repetition time (TR), and the time duration between the application of an RF pulse and signal acquisition is called the echo time (TE), as shown in Figure 3.11. While increasing TR allows for more longitudinal magnetization recovery and stronger signals, increasing TE causes more transverse magnetization decay and signal loss. Different MRI pulse sequences are covered in detail later in the chapter.

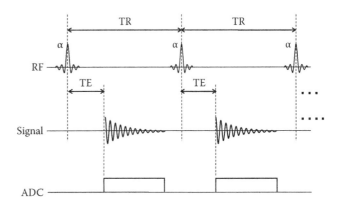

FIGURE 3.11 Repetition time (TR) and echo time (TE) shown in an MRI pulse sequence. RF excitation with flip angle α is repeated. The time duration between successive RF pulses is called the repetition time (TR), and the time duration from the RF pulse to data acquisition is called the echo time (TE). ADC, analog-to-digital converter.

3.3.2 Magnetization Saturation and Steady-State Condition

After the application of a 90° excitation RF pulse, the magnetization is saturated ($M_z = 0$), and further excitation will not produce any detectable signal. The magnetization needs enough time (TR $\geq 5 \times T_1$) to relax to equilibrium ($M_z = M_0$). If TR is made short (compared to T_1) to reduce scan time, the longitudinal magnetization will not have enough time to return to its equilibrium value and is said to be partially recovered. Moreover, for very short values of TR, the transverse magnetization (M_{xy}) may not even completely vanish before the next RF pulse application.

After repeated application of the excitation RF pulses, the longitudinal and transverse magnetizations reach a dynamic steady-state condition such that M_z and M_{xy} attain the same respective values at the same time point in successive TR intervals. This steady-state condition affects the resulting image contrast compared to the case of complete recovery. The number of excitation RF pulses (during the transition period) required to reach the steady-state condition depends on the excitation flip angle, TR, T_1, and T_2 values. Figure 3.12 shows a numerical simulation of the progression of M_z and M_{xy} toward steady state for TR/T_2/T_1 = 600/100/1000 ms. It should be noted that repeated excitations with a very short TR and/or a high flip angle cause significant signal attenuation (saturation effect), which compromises the resulting image quality.

3.3.3 T_1 and T_2 Contrasts

Tissue contrast based on differences in T_1 or T_2 values can be achieved by controlling TR, TE, and the flip angle of the pulse sequence. High T_2 contrast occurs when TE is long (TE ~ T_2), which accentuates the difference between signals received from tissues with different T_2 values (Figure 3.13a). Conversely, a short TE (TE ~ 0) eliminates the T_2 contrast, as there will be insufficient time for the transverse magnetization from different tissues to experience different decay rates based on their T_2 values. On the other hand, a short TR (TR ~ T_1) accentuates T_1 differences, while a long TR (TR $\gg$ T_1) eliminates T_1 contrast, as in the latter case the longitudinal magnetizations from different tissues (which will form the transverse magnetizations after the application of the following RF pulse) will reach the same equilibrium value during the long TR (Figure 3.13b). Therefore, T_2 weighting is achieved with long TR and TE values, while T_1 weighting is achieved with short TR and TE values. In the case of long TR and short TE, the effects of both T_1 and T_2 relaxations are eliminated, thus the signal is merely weighted by the number

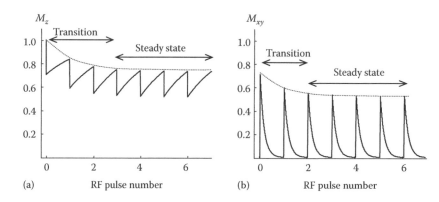

FIGURE 3.12 Magnetization progression toward steady state. Progression of the (a) longitudinal (M_z) and (b) transverse (M_{xy}) magnetizations during the transition to steady state after multiple excitations with a 45° flip angle and TR/T_2/T_1 = 600/100/1000 ms.

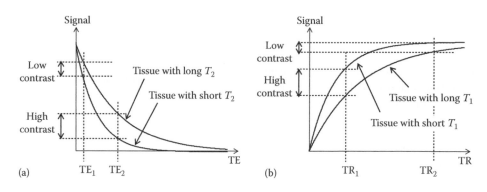

FIGURE 3.13 T_1 and T_2 contrasts. Contrast based on (a) T_2 decay and (b) T_1 recovery of two different tissues. At short TE values (TE$_1$), the signals from the two tissues are hardly distinguishable, while with a long TE (TE$_2$), high T_2 contrast is obtained. Similarly, a long TR value (TR$_2$) attenuates T_1-based differences that are visible at short TR (TR$_1$).

TABLE 3.3
Scan Parameters and Image Contrast

Contrast	TR	TE
T1W	Short (~T_1)	Short ($\ll T_2$)
T2W	Long ($\gg T_1$)	Long (~T_2)
PDW	Long ($\gg T_1$)	Short ($\ll T_2$)

of spins inside the imaged voxel, referred to as proton density weighting (PDW). Table 3.3 summarizes the effects of TR and TE settings on the image contrast. Figure 3.14 shows T1W, T2W, and PDW images of a human brain.

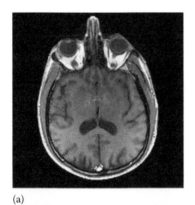

(a)

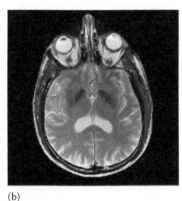

(b)

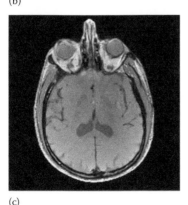

(c)

FIGURE 3.14 T1W, T2W, and proton density weighted (PDW) images. (a) T1W (TR/TE = 450/10 ms), (b) T2W (TR/TE = 3000/80 ms), and (c) PDW (TR/TE = 2000/15 ms) images of an axial human brain slice.

3.4 IMAGE FORMATION

The Larmor equation states that the spin precession frequency is proportional to the external magnetic field strength. MRI employs this simple relation to generate images of the spin distribution by utilizing an external magnetic field that varies (in a predetermined manner) in space. The ability of constructing tomographic images from the NMR signals was a huge breakthrough when it came out in the 1970s. In this section, we describe how this principle is applied to create two-dimensional (2D) and 3D MRI images. The mechanisms of slice selection (SS) and signal localization using the frequency-encoding (FE) and phase-encoding (PE) techniques are described, followed by a description of volumetric 3D imaging. The k-space concept is then described along with signal sampling and readout bandwidth (BW).

3.4.1 SLICE SELECTION

Given that the resonance frequency is proportional to the magnetic field strength, the positions of different spins can be resolved if the external magnetic field is made to vary in space such that there is a one-to-one correspondence between the spin position and its resonance frequency (based on the magnetic field strength at this position). This concept can be used to localize the signal to a single tomographic slice in the body (slice selection technique). This is achieved by applying a linearly varying weak magnetic field gradient pulse, G, in the direction perpendicular to the desired imaging slice, such that M_z varies linearly along that direction. Note that in the absence of any gradient pulses, a uniform magnetic field (= B_0) is experienced by all spins inside the scanner, which means that all spins in the body precess with the same (Larmor) frequency, ω_0, that is, they are indistinguishable. On the other hand, by applying a gradient pulse, $G_u(= \partial B_z/\partial u)$, in a certain direction, u, the net (longitudinal) magnetic field, B_z, varies linearly along that direction, such that

$$B_z(u) = B_0 + G_u u. \tag{3.8}$$

As a consequence, the Larmor frequency varies linearly with position in the u direction. Contrary to other imaging modalities like CT, the orientation of the selected slice in MRI can be selected along any of the three main directions or even at an oblique angle by simple application of the appropriate combination of x-, y-, and z-gradients. Specifically, in the z-direction (head-to-foot direction), the Larmor frequency becomes a function of z:

$$\omega(z) = \gamma(B_0 + G_z z). \tag{3.9}$$

By tuning the center frequency of the excitation RF pulse to match the resonance frequency at a certain z position, a slice is excited at that location. To excite a slice with certain thickness, Δz, the frequency content (BW, $\Delta\omega$) of the RF pulse is adjusted to match the thickness of the required slice (Figure 3.15)

$$\Delta\omega = \gamma G_z \Delta z. \tag{3.10}$$

The frequency content of the pulse also determines the slice profile. It should be noted that the relationship between the shapes

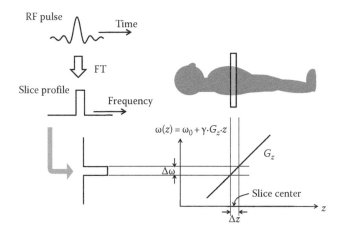

FIGURE 3.15 Slice-selection (SS) concept. The center frequency and bandwidth (BW) of the RF pulse are adjusted to match the center and width of the required slice, respectively. The Fourier transform (FT) of the RF pulse determines the slice profile.

of the RF pulse in the time and frequency domains is governed by a mathematical operator called Fourier transform (FT). For an optimal square slice profile, the excitation RF pulse should have the shape of a sinc function (sinc(x) = sin(x)/x), as shown in Figure 3.15. It should be noted that the signal generated by a slice-selective RF pulse is formed by the sum of the magnetization of all spins inside the excited slice.

3.4.2 FREQUENCY ENCODING

Besides slice selection, the gradient fields can be used to encode different positions inside the slice. For example, to encode spin position in the x-direction, the z-component of the magnetic field is made to vary linearly along the frequency-encoding direction (the x-direction in this case), such that $B_z(x) = \gamma(B_0 + G_x x)$. This is achieved by turning on the magnetic field gradient G_x during the signal readout period (after the slice is already excited), causing different spins along the x-axis to precess with different frequencies. The FT of the signal acquired during the application of this "readout" gradient produces a plot of the energy distribution at each resonance frequency in the signal, and therefore it represents a one-dimensional (1D) projection of the imaged sample along the x-axis (Figure 3.16). It should be emphasized that a single readout signal is not sufficient to reveal the underlying spin distribution in the slice and construct the MRI image; it rather provides partial information about the projection of the spin distribution along the direction of the gradient pulse.

3.4.3 PROJECTION RECONSTRUCTION

The frequency-encoding technique produces a 1D projection of the image along the direction of the applied gradient field. To generate a 2D image, the projection reconstruction (PR) method, borrowed from CT, works by rotating the readout gradient to create projections along different angles. The projections

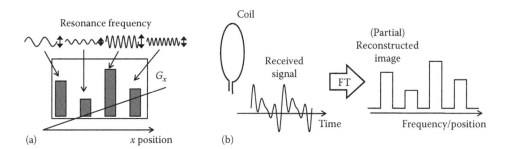

FIGURE 3.16 The frequency-encoding concept. (a) Four objects (rectangles) experience different resonance frequencies proportional to their x-positions (because of the implementation of the G_x gradient). The amplitudes of different sinusoids are determined by their relative spin density (size of the rectangle). (b) Fourier transform (FT) of the received signal produces a 1D projection of the image.

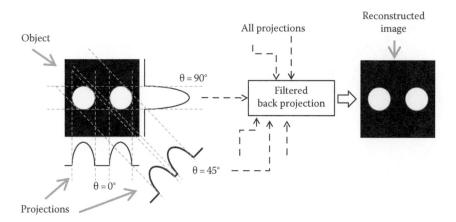

FIGURE 3.17 Projection reconstruction imaging. Frequency encoding along different directions produces projections of the weighted spin density along the gradient directions. The projections are processed by the filtered back projection method to produce the image.

are then used to reconstruct the image using the filtered back-projection method (Figure 3.17). Note that in MRI, the gradient coils are not physically rotated. Instead, rotation of the gradient field is accomplished by simultaneously applying the G_x and G_y gradients, with the field strength of each gradient adjusted to produce the desired projection angle. For example, setting the relative gradients strength as $(G_x, G_y) = (1, 0)$ produces a net gradient and a projection along the x-axis. Similarly, setting $(G_x, G_y) = (\cos(45°), \sin(45°)) = (0.71, 0.71)$ produces a gradient and a projection rotated by 45°. Although PR is an intuitive and straightforward approach for image acquisition and reconstruction, another approach took over in MRI: phase encoding, which is introduced in the next section.

3.4.4 PHASE ENCODING

Similar to frequency encoding, phase encoding uses gradient fields. However, phase encoding uses the gradients to make the *phase* (not the *frequency* as in frequency encoding) of the spins vary linearly with position. The net effect of applying both phase encoding and frequency encoding is modulating the signal in each voxel with a position-dependent phase and frequency. Consider the case where frequency encoding is applied in the x-direction and phase encoding is applied in the y-direction. In this case, a gradient field, G_y, is applied in the y-direction for a short period of time after the excitation RF pulse ends and before the frequency encoding readout gradient starts. During the time period when the phase encoding gradient pulse is on, the spins' frequency variation along the y-axis causes them

to precess with frequencies proportional to their y-positions $(\omega(y))$. When the G_y gradient pulse is terminated after a time period T, the spins have accumulated different phase angles, ϕ, proportional to their y-positions (frequency encoding achieves similar phase rotation at different time points during readout):

$$\phi(y) = \left(\omega(y) - \omega_0\right) \cdot T = \left(\gamma \cdot G_y \cdot T\right) \cdot y. \qquad (3.11)$$

After the phase encoding gradient is switched off, a frequency encoding readout gradient is performed as described earlier. The process of phase encoding/frequency encoding is repeated with different levels of the phase encoding gradient strength in order to resolve the ambiguity of spin distribution in the y-direction. G_y is stepped at least N_y times, where N_y is the image array size (number of pixels) in the y-direction. All signals are then recorded into a 2D data matrix, called k-space. After all data are acquired, the MRI image is obtained by implementing 2D FT on the data matrix. Usually, a modified version of FT, called fast FT (FFT) is implemented for fast image reconstruction. It should be noted that phase encoding can be simultaneously implemented in more than one dimension, as will be explained later. Figure 3.18 illustrates the concept of phase encoding. The weighting factors for a 2×2 matrix are shown in Figure 3.19. The two phase encoding steps rotate the magnetization with 0° and 180° phase angles, resulting in weighting factors of +1 and −1, respectively. The resulting four signals represent different linear combinations of the four image voxels. The linear system of equations can be solved to obtain the unknown voxel values.

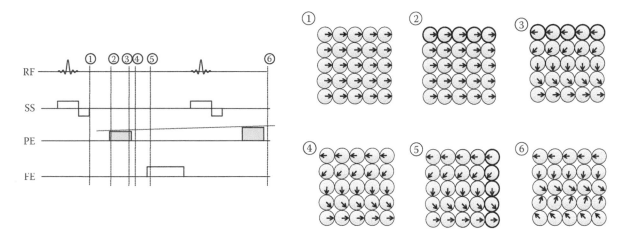

FIGURE 3.18 Frequency-encoding (FE) and phase-encoding (PE) concepts. The PE and FE effects illustrated on a 5 × 5 matrix. PE and FE are performed along the vertical and horizontal axes, respectively. Each spin is represented by a small clock. The phase and frequency of each spin are indicated by the direction of the arrow and thickness of the circle, respectively. Point 1 occurs immediately after the slice-selective (SS) excitation, where all spins are in phase (pointing in the same direction) and precessing with the same (Larmor) frequency (same circle thickness). At point 2, the PE gradient is applied resulting in change in precession frequency along the vertical direction. Toward the end of the PE gradient pulse (point 3), the spins have accumulated different phases (pointing in different directions) proportional to their vertical position. At point 4, the PE gradient is switched off leaving all the spins precessing at the original Larmor frequency; however, spins in different rows are not pointing in the same direction (they have different amounts of accumulated phase). At point 5, the FE gradient is applied, making the spins precess with different frequencies proportional to their horizontal positions. Now, each spin has unique phase (arrow direction) and frequency (circle thickness) based on its positions in the vertical and horizontal directions, respectively. The effect of stepping the phase encoding is shown at point 6, which corresponds to point 4 in the previous PE step. The larger PE gradient causes larger dispersion in the phase of the spins (difference in arrow direction between adjacent vertical spins). It should be noted that all spins contribute to the received signal during the implementation of the FE readout gradient. However, by analyzing the signal based on its frequency (and phase) contents, different signal components can be associated with their relative positions in the image.

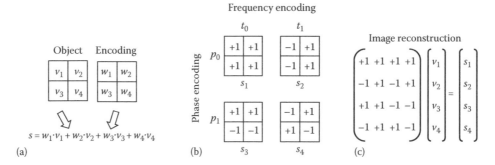

FIGURE 3.19   Example of phase- and frequency-encoding effects in a 2 × 2 image. (a) The image consists of four voxels ($v_1 \ldots v_4$). The encodings have the effect of weighting the voxels with certain weighting factors ($w_1 \ldots w_4$) that determine their contributions in the received signal, s. (b) The weighting factors corresponding to each voxel. Each row corresponds to one PE step (p_0 and p_1), whereas each column corresponds to a sampling timepoint (t_0 and t_1) during the FE readout. The signal values are denoted for the four measurements ($s_1 \ldots s_4$). (c) The weighting factors constitute a linear system of equations that can be solved to obtain the unknown voxel values.

3.4.5   K-SPACE

The MRI acquisition scheme using frequency encoding and phase encoding provides $N_x \times N_y$ signal samples, where all spins in the excited slice contribute to each signal (N_x and N_y represent the image matrix, i.e., the number of pixels in the x- and y-directions, respectively). The collection of all these signals constitute the spatial frequency domain of the image, which is referred to as the k-space (k is the symbol used to denote the spatial frequency variable). The image (I) and k-space (or signal, S) are related by the Fourier transform

$$S(t) = S\left(k_x(t), k_y(t)\right) = \iint_{-\infty}^{\infty} I(x,y) e^{-j2\pi\left(k_x(t)x + k_y(t)y\right)} dxdy,$$

(3.12)

where k_x and k_y are related to the applied gradients by

$$k_x(t) = \frac{\gamma}{2\pi} \int_0^t G_x(\tau) d\tau, \quad k_y(t) = \frac{\gamma}{2\pi} \int_0^t G_y(\tau) d\tau \quad (3.13)$$

The criterion of filling k-space is called the k-space trajectory. For the frequency encoding and phase encoding schemes described earlier, k-space is filled line by line in a rectilinear (Cartesian) fashion. Different rows in k-space represent signals acquired with different phase encoding values, while different points in each row represent successive samples of the resulting signal acquired at different time points during the readout period (Figure 3.20). If the data in k-space lie on a uniform grid, the FFT algorithm is implemented to efficiently reconstruct the MRI image. It should be noted that other k-space trajectories, for example, spiral or radial trajectories, could be implemented for faster filling of k-space, although they necessitate additional processing steps for image reconstruction (described later in the chapter).

It is important to keep in mind a number of k-space properties. The center of k-space contains low-frequency components of the image, which determine the overall image contrast. Conversely, k-space peripheries contain high-frequency information, responsible for the image's fine details or resolution (Figure 3.21). K-space has a very large dynamic range of signal intensities. The signal peak usually occurs at the center of k-space at zero frequency, which is often called the DC signal, borrowed from the term "direct current" used in electrical engineering. The signal intensity then drops rapidly as we move away from the k-space center (Figure 3.22). Therefore, most of the image energy is concentrated at the k-space center (the low-resolution information). Another interesting property is the Hermitian symmetry of

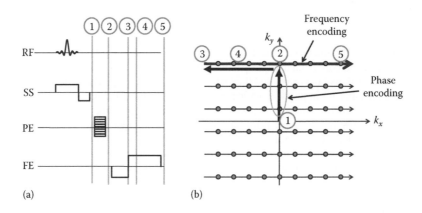

FIGURE 3.20   K-space formation. Phase- and frequency-encodings (a) in the pulse sequence and (b) in k-space. Five different time points are marked to show the path in k-space corresponding to phase- and frequency-encoding.

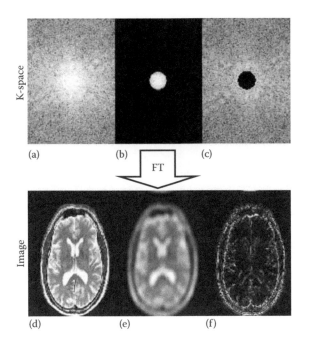

FIGURE 3.21 Image contrast and details. K-space data (top row) and the corresponding images (bottom row). Full k-space data in (a) produces the image shown in (d). Truncation of k-space to the central circular disk in (b) produces a blurred image that displays the low-frequency (coarse) components of the image as shown in (e). Keeping only the periphery of k-space in (c) produces an image with only the high-resolution (fine details) information in (f).

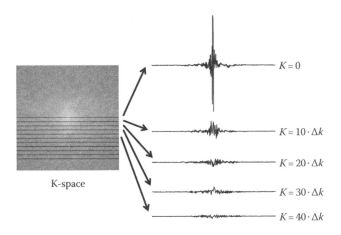

FIGURE 3.22 Data contents in k-space. K-space data (left) and the individual k-space lines (right) at five different positions from low to high frequency. Note the rapid decay in the signal as we move away from the center of k-space in any direction.

k-space. The signal in each half of k-space is a reversed copy of the data in the other half, except for a complex-conjugate operation. This is expressed mathematically as $S(-k_x, -k_y) = S^*(k_x, k_y)$. This property is exploited in fast imaging techniques, where partial k-space acquisition is implemented, as will be described in the section on fast MRI techniques.

3.4.6 3D Imaging

When the purpose of the MRI exam is to study a whole volume rather than a single slice, two approaches can be

followed: multislice imaging and volumetric 3D imaging (Figure 3.23). The first approach is based on acquiring multiple 2D slices covering the volume of interest. Gaps may be introduced in-between the slices to increase the spatial coverage and to reduce the interference (cross talk) between adjacent slices that would result from nonideal slice profiles (Figure 3.23a and c). The multislice approach is simple and straightforward. Furthermore, it allows for efficient use of scan time, as the waiting time for magnetization recovery during TR (after signal acquisition from one slice) can be used for exciting and acquiring signals from other slices—a technique known as *interleaved multislice* imaging (Figure 3.24). The main limitation of 2D imaging is the low resolution in the slice selection direction compared to in-plane resolution, due to the large slice thickness necessary for achieving an acceptable signal-to-noise ratio (SNR). The 3D volumetric imaging approach overcomes this problem by acquiring the signal from the whole volume at the same time, where a nonselective or a thick-slab selective excitation is implemented with phase encoding applied along two of the three spatial dimensions (Figure 3.23b and d). Three-dimensional imaging provides high resolution in all directions (thin slice thickness) with improved SNR. Nevertheless, 3D imaging requires a long scan time, which renders 3D imaging more sensitive to patient motion.

3.4.7 Signal Sampling and Bandwidth

The received analog signal in the coil must be sampled and digitized before processing with digital computers. The sampling must be fast enough to capture the highest frequency components in the signal. Otherwise, high-frequency components will be incorrectly interpreted, leading to overlapping repetition of the imaged object. This repetition is known as *aliasing*, or *wraparound*, artifact. The Nyquist theorem states that the sampling rate (receiver BW) should be at least twice the highest frequency component in the signal (or equal to the signal BW) to prevent aliasing. The sampling interval ΔT is the reciprocal of the receiver BW ($\Delta T = 1/\text{BW}$). To cover a field of view FOV_x along the readout direction, the receiver BW (in Hz) should be set to

$$\text{BW} \geq (\gamma/2\pi) \cdot G_x \cdot \text{FOV}_x. \qquad (3.14)$$

The total sampling time of each signal is $T_s = N_x \times \Delta T$, where N_x is the number of sampling points in the readout direction. The relationship between the sampling interval ΔT and the frequency content in the signal is shown in Figure 3.25. If the object dimension is greater than the prescribed FOV_x, then an anti-aliasing filter must be applied to the signal prior to sampling to eliminate frequencies greater than the sampling frequency, and thus avoiding aliasing. Unfortunately, the same trick cannot be applied along the PE direction; therefore, aliasing occurs in objects extending beyond the prescribed FOV_y. A rectangular FOV in which $\text{FOV}_x \neq \text{FOV}_y$ is a common strategy that, with careful selection of the phase encoding direction, can be used to significantly reduce artifacts in the image.

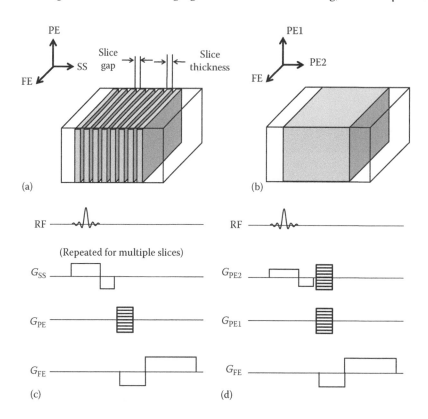

FIGURE 3.23 Multislice and volumetric 3D imaging. (a) Multislice and (b) volumetric 3D imaging with phase encoding implemented along two dimensions. (c) A multislice 2D imaging pulse sequence in which slice selection is performed along the z-direction, phase encoding is performed along the y-direction, and frequency encoding along the x-direction. (d) A 3D pulse sequence, where a thick slab is excited (note small amplitude of the slab-selection gradient) with a selective RF pulse (to prevent signal contamination from outside the volume of interest), followed by phase encoding simultaneously performed in the y- and z-directions. SS, slice selection; PE, phase encoding; FE, frequency encoding.

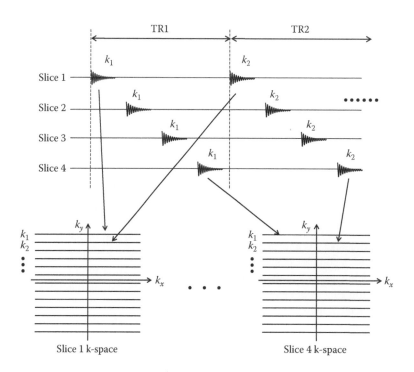

FIGURE 3.24 Interleaved multislice imaging. One k-space line is acquired from multiple slices in the same TR interval, making efficient use of time while waiting for T_1 recovery.

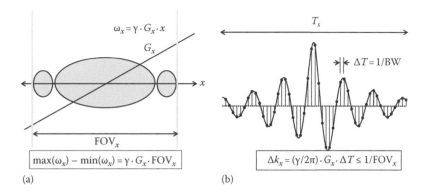

FIGURE 3.25 Data sampling. (a) The frequency-encoding gradient results in a frequency content proportional to the gradient (G_x) and field of view (FOV_x). (b) The time between two samples, ΔT, is equal to the reciprocal of the readout bandwidth (BW). ΔT (and consequently Δk_x) should be chosen such that sampling is fast enough to capture the whole range of frequencies in the sample in order to avoid aliasing.

3.5 PULSE SEQUENCES

The time sequence of the application of the RF and gradient pulses is called the MRI pulse sequence. A wide variety of MRI contrast mechanisms can be generated by manipulating the timing and other control parameters of the RF and gradient pulses. In this section, common MRI pulse sequences are introduced. The *pulse sequence diagram* is the timing graph of various RF and gradient pulses in the slice-selection, phase-encoding, and frequency-encoding directions. The pulse sequence diagram may also show data acquisition blocks, although they are often omitted as it is understood that they occur during frequency encoding. The pulse sequence diagram for the MRI scanner plays the same role as the musical note an orchestra conductor uses to organize the operation of different musical instruments in a concert. Pulse sequences are programmed into the scanner software, which give orders to the scanner hardware elements regarding when and how to run currents in the RF and gradient coils as well as about signal acquisition.

3.5.1 ELEMENTS OF THE PULSE SEQUENCE

A large number of different MRI pulse sequences have been introduced and developed over time. For simplified description of different pulse sequences, it is helpful to first introduce the common building blocks, or modules, of the pulse sequence, namely, RF and gradient pulses. Although pulse sequence modules usually include concurrent application of RF and gradient pulses, the categorization is simplified by describing each of them as either an RF or a gradient module according to its primary function.

3.5.1.1 RF Modules

Figure 3.26 shows different RF and gradient modules that appear in most pulse sequences. The simplest RF module is the *nonselective*, also named "hard" pulse (Figure 3.26a), usually represented by a short rectangular pulse. This short burst of the RF pulse generates a wide BW, thus exciting all spins in the object. The flip angle, given the symbol α, is usually denoted on top of the RF pulse. A second kind of RF pulses is the slice-selective *pulse* (Figure 3.26b). This "soft" pulse is usually modulated with a Gaussian (bell-shaped) or sinc(= $\sin(x)/x$) function to minimize ripples in the slice profile. The

slice-selection pulse is played in the presence of a slice-selection gradient. The second half of the gradient lobe causes phase dispersion along the slice-selection direction leading to significant signal loss. Fortunately, this effect can be avoided by adding an opposite negative gradient lobe, whose area is equal to one-half of the slice-selection gradient area, immediately after the slice-selection pulse. This extra lobe is called a *refocusing lobe* as it refocuses the dispersion in the spins caused by the slice-selection pulse. Both the nonselective and selective RF pulses can be used for signal excitation, inversion, or echo refocusing as previously described in the section about flip angle. *Adiabatic pulses* form another class of RF pulses wherein both the magnitude and frequency of the pulse are modulated to achieve uniform excitation even in the presence of excitation field (B_1) inhomogeneity (Figure 3.26c). Adiabatic pulses can also be used for magnetization inversion or refocusing.

3.5.1.2 Gradient Modules

The gradient fields are used for slice-selection (as described earlier), phase-encoding and frequency-encoding, and many other purposes. The phase-encoding gradient is the gradient that is stepped from one TR interval to another. It is usually represented with an increasing or decreasing sequence of pulse heights, or with a multistep symbol (Figure 3.26d through f). The frequency-encoding (readout) gradient is played out during signal acquisition. Usually, a prephaser lobe is played out immediately before the readout gradient. The prephaser lobe has opposite polarity and half the magnitude of the frequency-encoding gradient (Figure 3.26g), and its purpose is to ensure that a whole k-space line is acquired with the signal peak occurring at the k-space center (center of the readout pulse). If a 180° refocusing RF pulse is played out between the prephasing lobe and readout gradient, as in spin-echo sequences, then the prephasing pulse is performed with the same polarity (sign) as the readout gradient, as shown in Figure 3.26h (in this case, the 180° RF pulse negates the magnetization polarity assuming the role of negative sign). A spoiler (or crusher) gradient is a gradient pulse played after data acquisition to destroy the remaining transverse magnetization before proceeding to acquire more data (Figure 3.26i).

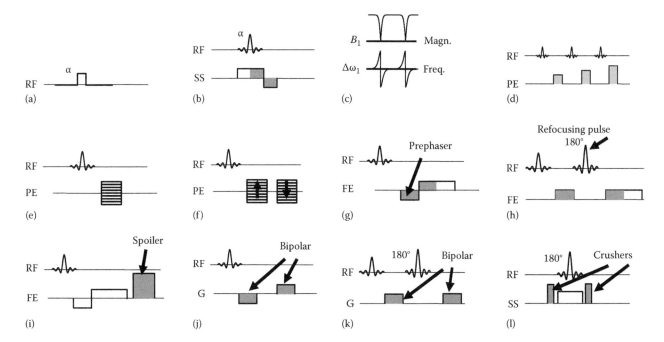

FIGURE 3.26   Common radiofrequency (RF) and gradient modules in MRI pulse sequences. (a) A nonselective (or "hard") RF pulse. (b) A slice-selective (SS) (or "soft") RF pulse. (c) An adiabatic RF pulse where both the amplitude and frequency are modulated. (d) Stepped phase-encoding (PE) gradient between RF pulses. (e) Stepped phase-encoding gradient symbol. (f) Phase-encoding gradient with the arrow showing the direction of gradient stepping. (g) Frequency-encoding (FE) gradient with a prephasing gradient pulse. (h) Frequency-encoding gradient with a refocusing 180° RF pulse separating it from the prephasing pulse. (i) A spoiler gradient (shaded) after data readout to destroy the remaining signal. (j) A bipolar gradient pulse. (k) A bipolar gradient pulse with the two lobes separated by a refocusing RF pulse. (l) Slice-selective refocusing pulse sandwiched between two crusher gradients to dephase the FID resulting from an imperfect 180° pulse.

A bipolar gradient (Figure 3.26j) consists of two gradient lobes of equal areas and opposite polarities. It is used to dephase then rephase the spins to achieve specific goals (e.g., velocity encoding in flow imaging). Similar to the case in Figure 3.26h, if a refocusing RF pulse occurs between the two lobes of a bipolar gradient, then the two gradient lobes are played with the same sign (Figure 3.26k); nevertheless, they still represent a bipolar gradient because their net effect remains the same. Finally, the bipolar gradient may also be used as a crusher gradient to eradicate any FID resulting from an inaccurate 180° RF pulses. In this case the refocusing pulse is sandwiched between two gradient pulses of equal areas to destroy the FID while leaving the echo signal unaffected (Figure 3.26l).

3.5.2 GRADIENT ECHO (GRE) PULSE SEQUENCE

The gradient echo (or gradient recalled echo [GRE]) pulse sequence is a basic imaging sequence in which a gradient pulse along the frequency-encoding direction is used to form an echo. In contrast to spin-echo sequences in which a 180° small RF pulse is used for echo formation, the GRE sequence consists of a single RF pulse with flip angle α ($\leq$90°), followed by phase-encoding and frequency-encoding gradients (Figure 3.27). Short TR is possible to achieve in GRE because the longitudinal magnetization is not significantly altered by the small RF pulses, and thus no long relaxation periods are needed. Therefore, GRE sequences are employed whenever

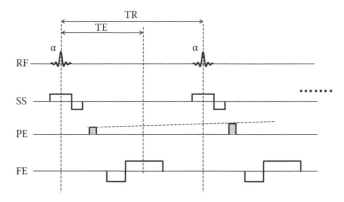

FIGURE 3.27   Gradient echo (GRE) pulse sequence. If needed, a spoiler gradient pulse and/or phase cycling of the RF pulse may be used to destroy the transverse magnetization at the end of the TR period.

speed is necessary as in 3D imaging and cardiac applications. GRE sequences have moderate T_1 and T_2^* weighting. They produce bright-blood images due to the time-of-flight (TOF) effect (discussed later). GRE has the disadvantage of T_2^* weighting, which, compared to T_2 weighting, results in additional signal loss due to field inhomogeneity. However, the T_2^* weighting can be beneficial in susceptibility-based imaging methods. Depending on the manufacturer, the GRE pulse sequence may be referred to by other names. For GRE sequences in which the transverse magnetization is negligible before the application of the next RF pulse, the GRE sequence is known as spoiled gradient echo (SPGR), fast low-angle shot (FLASH), or T_1-weighted fast field echo (FFE).

3.5.3 SPIN ECHO (SE) PULSE SEQUENCE

When an RF pulse flips the magnetization in the transverse plane, the signal starts to decay with T_2^* time constant. The SE sequence (Figure 3.28) elegantly rewinds the field inhomogeneity effect, leaving the signal with pure T_2 weighting (slower rate of decay leading to large signal). This is achieved by applying a refocusing

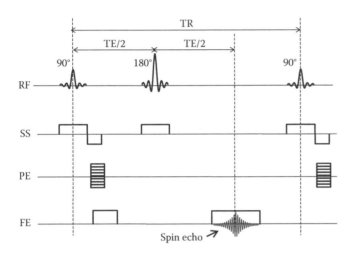

FIGURE 3.28 Spin echo (SE) pulse sequence. A slice-selective refocusing 180° pulse is applied after a time period of TE/2 from the excitation 90° RF pulse to refocus the magnetization at time TE.

180° RF pulse when the magnetization is in the transverse plane after a time period of TE/2. This refocusing pulse reverses the accumulated phase of the individual spins so that after another TE/2 period, all spins become in-phase again.

Figure 3.29 illustrates the spin echo concept: following a 90° excitation RF pulse along the x-axis, the initial longitudinal magnetization (M_0 along the z-axis) is flipped into the transverse plane along the y-axis, where the spins start to dephase. Consider two spins that precess with precession frequencies of $\omega_0 + \Delta\omega_1$ and $\omega_0 + \Delta\omega_2$, respectively (Figure 3.29). At time TE/2, the two spins will have accumulated phase angles of $\Delta\omega_1 \times$ TE/2 and $\Delta\omega_2 \times$ TE/2, respectively, relative to on-resonance spins. When a refocusing 180° RF pulse is applied along the y-axis, the spins flip around the y-axis, effectively reversing the phases of our two spins to be $-\Delta\omega_1 \times$ TE/2 and $-\Delta\omega_2 \times$ TE/2, respectively. The two spins will continue accumulating phase in the same way (direction) they did in the first TE/2 period. Therefore, after another TE/2 period, the spins will have gained additional phases of $\Delta\omega_1 \times$ TE/2 and $\Delta\omega_2 \times$ TE/2, respectively, canceling out the phases accumulated during the first TE/2 period, which brings the spins back in-phase and enhances the received signal.

SE sequences are widely used because they are immune to field inhomogeneity and many other artifacts. They produce images with T_1 or T_2 contrast, and result in images in which the signal from flowing blood is attenuated (black blood). The disadvantages of spin echo imaging include long scan time, which makes it prone to motion artifacts, and high RF power deposition. Fast spin echo (FSE) techniques (discussed later) have dramatically reduced the scan time of the SE sequence.

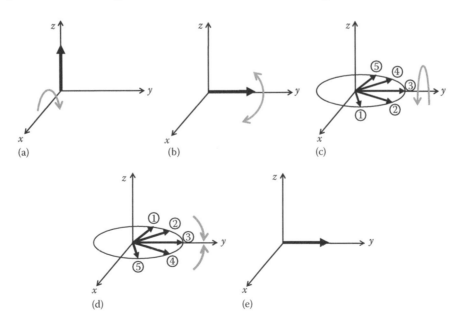

FIGURE 3.29 Spins rephasing in the spin echo pulse sequence. The spin echo pulse sequence rewinds the phase accumulation due to off-resonance using a refocusing RF pulse. The longitudinal magnetization in (a) is flipped to the y-direction with a 90° RF pulse applied along the x-direction. (b) The spins in the transverse plane start to dephase. (c) A 180° refocusing RF pulse is applied along the y-axis at time TE/2 to negate the phases accumulated by the spins. (d) After the refocusing pulse, the spins continue precessing at their off-resonance frequencies, but beginning from the new phase angles to finally come back in-phase at time TE (e). The refocused magnetization in (e) is still smaller than that in (b) due to the intrinsic T_2 decay.

3.5.4 INVERSION RECOVERY (IR) PULSE SEQUENCE

In inversion recovery (IR) pulse sequences, a 180° RF pulse is first applied to invert the magnetization vector M_0 along the z-axis to start with value $= -M_0$ (Figure 3.30). After inversion, the magnetization starts recovering to its equilibrium position ($+M_0$ along the z-axis) with time constant T_1 as

$$M_z(t) = M_0(1 - 2 \cdot e^{-t/T_1}). \qquad (3.15)$$

The signal is created by tipping the magnetization into the transverse plane after a certain time period called inversion time (TI). The IR sequence provides strong T_1 contrast because the T_1 recovery process spans a wide range of magnetization (from $-M_0$ to M_0). IR is considered a preparation sequence and can be used with GRE or SE imaging (a GRE readout module is shown in Figure 3.30).

IR can be used to null the signal from a tissue with known T_1 value by selecting $TI = 0.69 \times T_1$ (Figure 3.31). For example, IR is used for fat suppression in the short-TI inversion recovery (STIR) sequence, for fluid suppression in the fluid-attenuated inversion recovery (FLAIR) sequence, and for attenuating the signal from non-infarcted myocardium in cardiac viability studies.

3.5.5 STIMULATED ECHO (STEAM) PULSE SEQUENCE

The application of two non-180° RF pulses produces a FID signal and a spin echo. When a third RF pulse is applied, a new type of echo is generated, known as the stimulated echo, and the corresponding pulse sequence is known as stimulated echo acquisition mode (STEAM; Figure 3.32). As explained in Figure 3.33, the first RF pulse in the STEAM sequence tips the magnetization into the transverse plane, where it is dephased with the help of a "modulation" gradient. After a time period equal to TE/2, the modulated magnetization is flipped back to the longitudinal direction by a second RF pulse. The remaining magnetization in the transverse plane is then destroyed with the help of a large spoiler gradient to eliminate any signal forming from non-stimulated

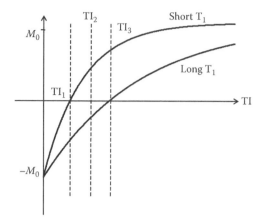

FIGURE 3.31 Inversion time (TI) and tissue suppression. The magnetization recovery curve after an inversion pulse for two tissues with different T_1 time constants. If the image is acquired at TI_1, the short-T_1 tissue (e.g., fat) is effectively suppressed from the image. If imaging occurs at TI_2, the resulting image shows both tissues (no suppression). Finally, imaging at TI_3 eliminates the signal from the long-T_1 tissue (e.g., fluid).

echo sources. After a second period of time (mixing time, TM), a third RF pulse is applied to tip the modulated magnetization back in the transverse plane for imaging. However, before imaging, the modulation effect has to be reversed with the help of a "demodulation" gradient that is applied on the same axis and has the same magnitude as the modulation gradient. The purpose of the demodulation gradient is to bring the modulated (dephased) spins back in-phase to form a measurable signal after a time period of TE/2 (from the application of the third RF pulse).

Two natural questions arise: (1) why modulation and demodulation are needed? and (2) why flip the magnetization back and forth between the transverse and longitudinal directions? The answer to the first question is that the modulation process marks the magnetization at the beginning of the pulse sequence in a certain way, such that it can be distinguished from other magnetization components arising afterward. This unique modulated magnetization then experiences certain effects, for example, motion, during the remaining time until it is demodulated and brought back in the transverse plane for imaging. The answer to the second question is more straightforward. As most tissues in the body have T_2 much shorter than T_1, then the rate of transverse magnetization decay is much faster than longitudinal recovery. As both processes eliminate the effects of any magnetization preparation, "storing" the modulated magnetization in the longitudinal direction during TM saves it from being eliminated by the fast transverse decay. This allows for recording events, for example, motion, during a long period of time (in the order of T_1). Actually, this last feature is the main advantage of STEAM. Nevertheless, a disadvantage of STEAM is that half of the signal is spoiled during the generation of the stimulated echo, causing a 50% signal loss. Due to the application of the modulating/demodulating gradient pair and the echo formation technique, STEAM is very sensitive to motion. STEAM has an important application in tissue motion tracking, as in cardiac tagging, and in MR spectroscopy (MRS) as a localization technique.

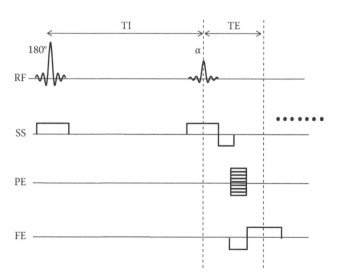

FIGURE 3.30 Inversion recovery (IR) pulse sequence. A GRE reading module is shown in the figure. TI, inversion time.

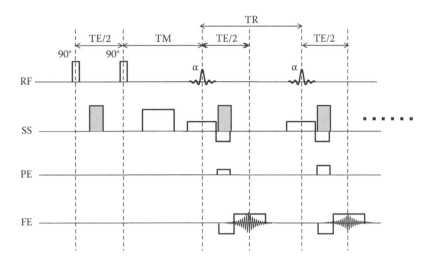

FIGURE 3.32 Stimulated echo acquisition mode (STEAM) pulse sequence. The first 90° RF pulse tips the magnetization into the transverse plane. The (shaded) modulation gradient dephases (modulates) the transverse magnetization in a certain fashion. The second RF pulse "stores" the magnetization in the longitudinal direction, which saves it from being eliminated by transverse relaxation during the mixing time (TM). The spoiler gradient after the second RF pulse eliminates any remaining transverse magnetization after storing the magnetization in the longitudinal direction. The third α° RF pulse (or pulses) tips the magnetization in the transverse plane, where it is refocused (demodulated) using the (shaded) demodulation gradient (which has the same magnitude as the modulation gradient), and is then read out to create an image.

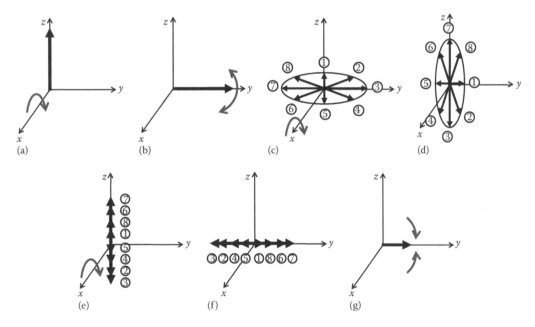

FIGURE 3.33 Signal generation in the stimulated echo (STEAM) pulse sequence. (a) Just before the first RF pulse, the magnetization is at equilibrium along the longitudinal direction. (b) After the first 90° pulse (see Figure 3.32), the magnetization is tipped into the transverse plane. (c) A dephasing (modulation) gradient is applied during the first TE/2 period to modulate the magnetization (dephase the spins in a certain pattern) in the transverse plane. (d) The second 90° RF pulse rotates the magnetization to the x–z plane. (e) The spoiler gradient destroys the transverse magnetization components leaving only the longitudinal components that experience T_1 recovery during the mixing time (TM). (f) A third RF pulse tips the magnetization back into the transverse plane in preparation for imaging. (g) The demodulation gradient reverses the action of the modulation gradient in preparation for imaging (data acquisition). After another TE/2 period, the spins come back in phase, but with half the strength of the initial magnetization (ignoring T_1 and T_2 relaxation).

3.5.6 STEADY-STATE FREE PRECESSION (SSFP) PULSE SEQUENCE

In GRE sequences, the steady-state condition (i.e., when the magnetization has the same magnitude after each TR) is established after a number of repeated excitations. If the transverse magnetization is zero (or close to zero) before the next RF pulse, the GRE sequence is said to be *spoiled* (SPGR). Spoiling can be achieved with long TR (transverse magnetization decays naturally due to transverse relaxation), by applying a dephasing gradient pulse (called crusher or spoiler), or by changing the phase of the excitation RF pulses in a premeditated way—a technique

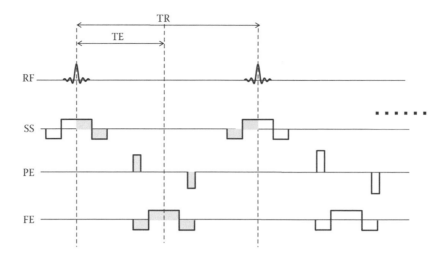

FIGURE 3.34 Balanced steady-state free precession (SSFP) pulse sequence. The net gradient area on any axis in any one TR interval (shaded gradient pulses) is zero.

known as *RF spoiling*. However, if the transverse magnetization does not vanish at the end of one TR, a steady-state free precession (SSFP) condition is achieved, in which the transverse magnetization is refocused between successive RF pulses rather than being spoiled. Therefore, in SSFP the MR signal is enhanced, boosting SNR, and T_2, rather than T_2^*, contrast is achieved. In the balanced SSFP (bSSFP) sequence, the gradients on all axes are balanced during TR, meaning that the net gradient area in any TR interval is zero (Figure 3.34). The T_2^* effects can be eliminated if the echo is made to appear in the middle of the TR period, that is, TE = TR/2. bSSFP is implemented with extremely short TR (TR $\ll T_2 < T_1$) and moderate-to-high flip angles (40°–70°); nevertheless, bSSFP provides a surprisingly high-SNR signal. The images generated with bSSFP are approximately (T_2/T_1)-weighted. However, bSSFP is very sensitive to B_0 inhomogeneity, and the banding artifact (bands of low signal; described later in the chapter) is often seen on bSSFP images. Therefore, a very short TR is used in SSFP to push the banding artifacts away from the region of interest. In addition, good shimming is absolutely necessary for successful application of bSSFP. bSSFP has different names depending on the vendor, such as fast imaging employing steady-state acquisition (FIESTA), true fast imaging with steady-state precession (TrueFISP), or balanced FFE.

3.6 IMAGE CHARACTERISTICS

The downsides of MRI flexibility are its complication and large number of scan parameters to adjust. Achieving good image quality requires careful setting of the scan parameters to optimize the quality metrics relevant to the application at hand. Although image quality is ultimately determined by the imaging goal, in general a good MRI dataset is the one that has the highest possible SNR, highest possible spatial and temporal resolutions, and shortest scan time. Nevertheless, changing the scan parameters often results in conflicting effects on these desired features. Therefore, a protocol setup always involves some type of trade-off between SNR, resolution, and scan time (Figure 3.35). It should be noted that increasing B_0 can

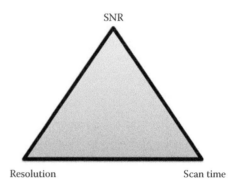

FIGURE 3.35 Image characteristics. The image quality is affected by various trade-offs between SNR, resolution, and scan time.

increase all three metrics together, justifying the trend toward higher magnetic fields. However, as will be detailed later, moving to high field is accompanied by other technical challenges.

3.6.1 FIELD OF VIEW (FOV) AND SPATIAL RESOLUTION

The field of view (FOV) is the spatial area covered by the imaging sequence. Spatial resolution is the distance between two neighboring points in the image (pixels) that can be visually resolved. One reason behind the apparent complexity of MRI is that data acquisition is performed in the spatial frequency domain (k-space) rather than the image domain. Therefore, it is instructive to recognize the relationship between sampling in the k-space and the resolution (Δx, Δy) and FOV in the image space.

Sampling the k-space inevitably causes periodic replication of the object in the image domain at intervals inversely proportional to the sampling interval (Figure 3.36a). If the sampling is not sufficiently dense, the object replicas start to come closer to each other and eventually overlap causing aliasing (Figure 3.36b). By setting the FOV, the user indirectly sets the sampling interval (Δk_x, Δk_y). Therefore, the FOV must be large enough to cover the whole object.

Sampling of the k-space cannot go on without limits. The sampling extent (coverage) of k-space must be limited to a range

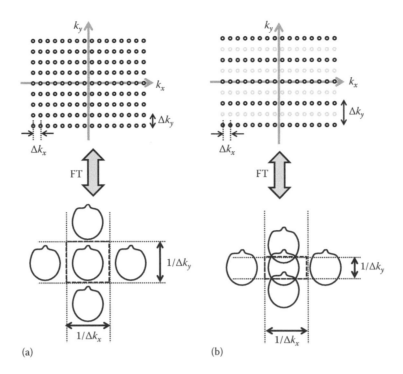

FIGURE 3.36 K-space sampling and image aliasing. (a) Sufficiently high sampling rate (also called full sampling) of k-space pushes all aliasing objects (the head replicas) outside the FOV (dashed square), while (b) undersampling in any direction (vertical direction here, where the light-gray k-space rows are not acquired) causes fold-over of the replicating object (aliasing artifact).

that keeps the scan time short. Nevertheless, the spatial resolution is determined by the finest details in the image, which is determined by the phase-encoding step with the highest spatial frequency (largest gradient area). Therefore, the image resolution is determined by k-space coverage. The following equations summarize the relationship between the image resolution/ FOV and sampling in the k-space (shown in Figure 3.37):

$$\Delta x = \frac{1}{2K_{x,\max}}, \quad \Delta y = \frac{1}{2K_{y,\max}}, \tag{3.16}$$

$$\text{FOV}_x = \frac{1}{\Delta k_x}, \quad \text{FOV}_y = \frac{1}{\Delta k_y}. \tag{3.17}$$

Therefore, higher spatial resolution requires sampling a larger area in k-space, while larger FOV requires dense sampling in the k-space; both result in longer scan times.

If k-space is sampled below the Nyquist rate (the signal frequency BW), it is said to be undersampled, and aliasing occurs. While aliasing in the readout (frequency-encoding) direction can be avoided by increasing the sampling rate (acquisition BW) of the receiver, aliasing in the phase-encoding direction is harder to avoid. One approach to avoid aliasing is by saturating the spins outside the desired small FOV using slice-selective excitation followed by a spoiler gradient. If the scanner software is equipped with multidimensional selective RF pulses, excitation could be restricted to the desired region of interest (selective excitation), avoiding aliasing from magnetization outside the desired anatomy.

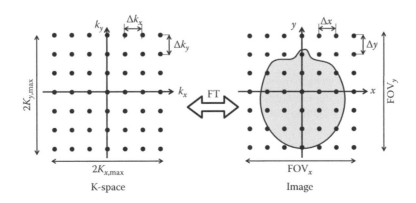

FIGURE 3.37 Image resolution, FOV, and k-space sampling. The relationships between the different variables are given in the text.

3.6.2 SIGNAL-TO-NOISE RATIO (SNR)

SNR is one of the primary indicators of image quality. It quantifies the degree of the "grainy" appearance of the image. The "signal" refers to the true quantity to be measured, while "noise" is any random variation added to this quantity. Randomness is what distinguishes noise from other systematic errors that are referred to as *artifacts*. SNR is defined as the mean value of the signal divided by the noise standard deviation. In MRI, the noise power is proportional to the readout BW.

The MR signal is proportional to the square of the magnetic field strength $(B_0)^2$, while noise is directly proportional to the magnetic field strength B_0. Therefore, SNR is proportional to B_0. The signal in a voxel is proportional to the number of spins inside the voxel, and thus is proportional to the voxel size $\Delta V = \Delta x \times \Delta y \times \Delta z$. In addition, SNR depends on the system hardware (e.g., the RF coil), contrast agents used, and imaging pulse sequence.

To improve SNR, signal averaging is occasionally performed during the MRI scan. Signal averaging improves SNR because the signal is not changed by averaging, while the noise standard deviation decreases by the square root of the number of signal averages (NSA). SNR is therefore proportional to $\sqrt{\text{NSA}}$. In general, SNR is proportional to the square root of the total data acquisition time, which includes the acquisition time in the different phase-encoding and frequency-encoding steps required to reconstruct the image. Note that data acquisition time is the actual duration of data collection and is different from the scan time, where the latter include, besides acquisition time, excitation and encoding times as well as idle time during which the magnetization is allowed to recover. The relationship between SNR and different imaging parameters can therefore be summarized as

$$\text{SNR} \propto B_0 \cdot \text{voxel size} \cdot \sqrt{\text{acquisition time}}. \qquad (3.18)$$

The expression for SNR might be defined in terms of voxel dimensions or in terms of the FOV. Changing one scan parameter can indirectly affect SNR if this parameter affects other parameters used for SNR calculation. It is therefore necessary to keep in mind the basic equation mentioned earlier. For example, the previous formula may be written in terms of the voxel dimensions and total sampling time as

$$\text{SNR} \propto B_0 \cdot \Delta x \cdot \Delta y \cdot \Delta z \cdot \sqrt{(N_x \cdot \Delta T) \cdot N_y \cdot N_z \cdot \text{NSA}}, \qquad (3.19)$$

where

N_x is the number of readout samples
ΔT (=1/BW) is the sampling interval
N_y is the number of phase-encoding steps in the y-direction
N_z is the number of phase-encoding steps in the z-direction in case of 3D imaging ($N_z = 1$ for 2D images)

Alternatively, SNR can be expressed in terms of the FOV dimensions, rather than the voxel size

$$\text{SNR} \propto B_0 \cdot \text{FOV}_x \cdot \text{FOV}_y \cdot \text{FOV}_z \cdot \sqrt{\text{NSA}(N_x \cdot N_y \cdot N_z \cdot \text{BW})}. \qquad (3.20)$$

TABLE 3.4

The Effects of Changing Various Scan Parameters on SNR, Image Resolution, and Scan Time

	SNR	Resolution	Scan Time	Assumptions/Notes
FOV ↑	↑↑	↓↓	—	Same matrix size Increased spatial coverage Reduced fold-over artifacts
NSA ↑	↑	—	↑↑	—
Voxel size ↑	↑↑	↓↓	↓↓	Same FOV
Receiver BW ↑	↓	—	—	Reduced chemical shift effect Shortened minimum TE
TR ↑	↑	—	↑↑	Decreased T_1 weighting More slices in multislice sequences
TE ↑	↓	—	—	Assuming TE ≪ TR Increased T_2 weighting

SNR can thus be improved by increasing the voxel size (lower resolution), averaging more data (longer scan time), or moving to a higher field strength B_0. A lower receiver BW can also improve SNR but results in more chemical shift artifacts. On the other hand, techniques that skip phase-encoding steps (for the sake of faster imaging) sacrifice SNR.

3.6.3 SCAN TIME

The scan time is given by the total number of TR intervals

$$\text{Scan time} = \frac{\text{NSA} \cdot N_y \cdot N_z \cdot \text{TR}}{R}, \qquad (3.21)$$

where R is the undersampling or acceleration factor in parallel imaging. In FSE sequences, R is the echo train length (ETL), described later in the chapter. In interleaved-acquisition multislice imaging, R is the number of slices acquired in a single TR. Table 3.4 shows the effects of various scanning parameters on the three quality metrics discussed in this section.

3.7   FAST MRI TECHNIQUES

One of the main limitations of MRI is its weak sensitivity (low SNR) that prolongs the scan time. Accelerating MRI imaging was, is currently, and most probably will continue to be a main challenge in MRI, hindering the transition of many MRI imaging and spectroscopy techniques to clinical applications. Several methods have been introduced to overcome this problem, which are discussed in this section.

3.7.1 ECHO PLANAR IMAGING

The basic GRE and SE sequences perform a single phase-encoding step after each RF pulse, filling one line in k-space per TR. In echo planar imaging (EPI), the whole k-space is

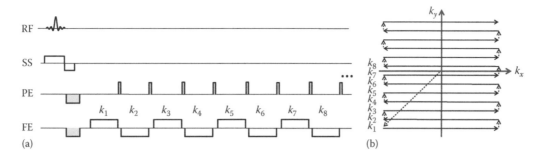
(a)   (b)

FIGURE 3.38 Echo planar imaging (EPI) pulse sequence. (a) Blipped EPI pulse sequence and (b) its k-space trajectory. The prephaser gradients (a: the two large shaded lobes) move the beginning of data acquisition to the corner of k-space (b: dotted line).

acquired in a single shot by rapid switching of the gradients to traverse the entire k-space in less than 100 ms. One variation of EPI is blipped EPI in which the readout direction is sampled in alternating directions (between consecutive k-space lines) with interleaved phase-encoding blips, such that the k-space is traversed in a raster fashion (Figure 3.38). The high acquisition speed of EPI makes it immune to motion artifacts. Nevertheless, EPI is very hardware demanding, requiring gradients with short switching times. Furthermore, the long readout time makes EPI sensitive to off-resonance artifacts resulting from B_0 inhomogeneity, which may cause geometric distortions and image blurring. It should also be noted that the high-speed advantage of the EPI scan comes with concomitant losses in spatial resolution and SNR. One of the primary applications of EPI is functional MRI (fMRI) studies of the brain. To reduce the problems of single-shot EPI, segmented EPI schemes were developed, wherein the k-space is covered in multiple RF shots each covering a subset of k-space lines (e.g., two shots one sampling the odd k-space lines and the other sampling the even lines).

3.7.2 FAST SPIN ECHO (FSE)

FSE (also called turbo spin echo [TSE]) uses multiple refocusing (180°) RF pulses to generate multiple spin echoes. The phase-encoding gradient is stepped for each echo to acquire

one additional k-space line (Figure 3.39). The scan time is reduced by a factor equal to the number of echoes per one TR interval, called the ETL. The contrast in the image is determined by the effective echo time at which the central lines in the k-space are acquired. FSE has largely replaced conventional SE in many clinical applications. The disadvantages of FSE include increased RF power deposition and image blurring that results when a large ETL is used.

3.7.3 NON-CARTESIAN K-SPACE TRAJECTORIES

In theory, k-space can be traversed in infinitely many ways. Despite the straightforward implementation of the standard Cartesian sampling pattern described earlier, it is not the most time-efficient way to collect data. By manipulating the gradient waveforms, many other k-space trajectories can be generated that are more time-efficient or less sensitive to motion and flow artifacts. Spiral, radial, circular, rosette, and Periodically Rotated Overlapping ParallEL Lines with Enhanced Reconstruction (PROPELLER) are few trajectory examples to mention (Figure 3.40).

Figure 3.41 shows a spiral k-space trajectory and the generating gradient waveform. It can be shown that the projection reconstruction method actually samples the k-space in a polar fashion (trajectory shown in Figure 3.40b).

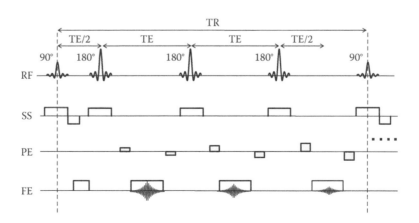

FIGURE 3.39 Fast spin echo (FSE) pulse-sequence. The phase-encoding gradient is stepped for each spin echo to scan a different k-space line (echo train length [ETL] = 3 in this example). The phase-encoding gradient is rewound after each readout. The signal experiences a T_2 decay during the readout.

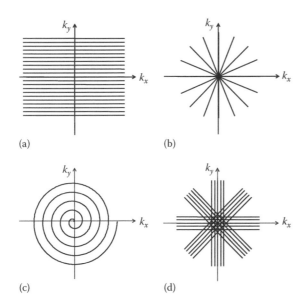

FIGURE 3.40   Nonconventional k-space trajectories. (a) Cartesian, (b) radial, (c) spiral, and (d) PROPELLER k-space trajectories.

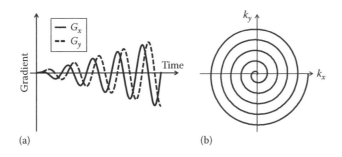

FIGURE 3.41   Spiral imaging. (a) Gradients waveform and (b) k-space trajectory for spiral MRI.

Spiral and radial trajectories are gaining expanding popularity due to their data acquisition efficiency and inherent oversampling of the k-space center making them immune to many artifacts. With non-rectilinear trajectories, however, image reconstruction is not as straightforward as before. To implement the efficient FFT reconstruction, the data must first be interpolated into a rectilinear grid in a process known as "regridding," as shown in Figure 3.42.

3.7.4   REDUCED PHASE ENCODING SCHEMES

Because the scan time is proportional to the number of phase-encoding steps (N_{PE}), reducing N_{PE} is another option for speeding up image acquisition. Reducing N_{PE} below the number necessary for a given FOV and spatial resolution may result in image aliasing artifacts and/or blurring. In this case, additional information is required to fill in the missing data. Partial Fourier and parallel imaging are two widely used techniques that belong to this category of reduced phase-encoding.

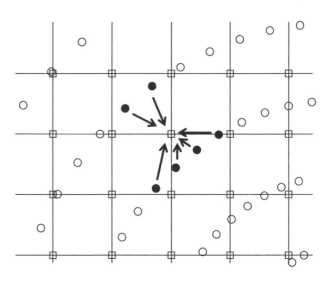

FIGURE 42   Data regridding. Regridding the k-space data acquired using a spiral trajectory (circles). The value at each point on the Cartesian grid (squares) is estimated from the trajectory samples in a small neighborhood around it (solid circles).

3.7.4.1   Partial Fourier Imaging

The weighted spin density of a voxel is a real-valued quantity. A real-valued image has a k-space with Hermitian symmetry, that is, $S(-k_x, -k_y) = S^*(k_x, k_y)$, where the * denotes a complex conjugate. Therefore, in principle, it is sufficient to acquire only one-half of the standard k-space data to be able to construct the image. Although the partial Fourier technique is commonly applied in the phase-encoding direction, it can also be used in the frequency-encoding direction with partial-echo scans.

Unfortunately, in practice, the image is rarely pure real-valued due to field inhomogeneity and other system imperfections. Therefore, to account for phase errors, extra data need to be sampled beyond the k-space center to provide information about phase distribution in the image (Figure 3.43). The central lines in the k-space are then used to estimate a low-resolution phase term that is subsequently used to correct the image. The extra k-space lines may also be included in the final reconstruction process. Because of the reduction in N_{PE}, the speed advantage of partial Fourier imaging comes with a penalty of SNR reduction by a factor of ~$\sqrt{2}$.

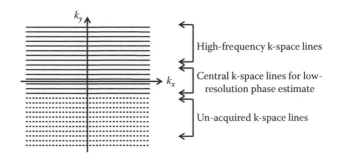

FIGURE 3.43   Partial Fourier imaging. One-half of the k-space is acquired. Few lines are additionally acquired at the center of k-space to correct for phase errors.

3.7.4.2 Parallel Imaging

Standard MRI systems initially consisted of a single receiving coil. Coil arrays (phased arrays) were next introduced consisting of multiple small surface coils (coil elements). Each of the small surface coils "sees" only part of the FOV, and therefore the phased-array coil can produce a high-SNR image because the coil elements do not collect as much noise as would do a large coil. A problem with the surface coils is the reduction in coil sensitivity as the distance from the coil increases. This variation in the sensitivity profile, however, turned out to be a blessing. Parallel imaging combines the information from all coils whose sensitivity profiles overlap to cover the whole object in a short scan time. Because each coil has a different sensitivity at a given location in space, the coil sensitivities provide additional encoding information similar to that achieved with the gradient fields. The speedup in image acquisition is achieved through omitting a number of the phase-encoding steps by undersampling the k-space in the phase-encoding direction. The factor by which k-space is undersampled is called the speedup, acceleration, or data reduction factor, R.

Because undersampling of k-space (using larger Δk value) corresponds to smaller FOV, the reconstructed images will show ghost repetition of the object (called aliasing artifacts). To correctly reconstruct the image from this set of reduced k-space lines, several techniques are available. A group of these techniques (e.g., the sensitivity encoding [SENSE] method) works by unfolding the aliasing in the image domain using the known coil sensitivity maps. As an alternative, k-space methods try to estimate the missing k-space lines from the acquired data before implementing the Fourier transform. The latter approach is adopted in the famous generalized auto-calibrating partially parallel acquisition (GRAPPA) method. Figure 3.44 illustrates SENSE reconstruction in a head image.

Parallel imaging can be used with any pulse sequence to reduce scan time. Nevertheless, the speed advantage of parallel imaging is penalized by a reduction in SNR by a factor of $\sqrt{R}$. In addition, noise in the final image is spatially varying and depends on the coil geometry, which is described by the so-called g-factor map.

3.7.5 Real-Time and Dynamic Imaging

Real-time imaging is an acquisition and image reconstruction strategy that aims to rapidly and continuously acquire images, which is required for some applications, for example, dynamic imaging. Examples of real-time applications include real-time cardiac imaging, dynamic contrast-enhanced studies, and MRI-guided interventions. Real-time imaging uses fast pulse sequences and smart reconstruction strategies to improve the temporal resolution (time between two successive image frames). The reciprocal of the temporal resolution is the frame rate measured in frames per second (fps). Depending on the application, the frame rate of real-time MRI may be as low as multiple seconds for each frame (<1 fps) or as high as tens of frames per second (e.g., 30 fps).

Common pulse sequences used in real-time MRI include SPGR, bSSFP, and FSE, which can be readily combined with partial Fourier reconstruction for faster acquisition. EPI, spiral, and radial k-space trajectories allow for more efficient coverage of the k-space. Single-shot acquisitions usually have low SNR due to the large readout BW; further, the long readout period leads to accumulation of off-resonance errors that ultimately causes geometric distortions and image blurring. Multishot acquisition can improve SNR and image quality in general, but sacrifices the temporal resolution. The invention of parallel imaging added to the capabilities of MRI systems to improve the temporal resolution and to help alleviate some of the image artifacts with EPI or long spiral readout.

Partial k-space filling combined with data sharing is another strategy for real-time imaging of dynamic events. With proper assumptions about the dynamic process, a good-fidelity image can be reconstructed from a small subset of the k-space data. One example of data sharing is the keyhole

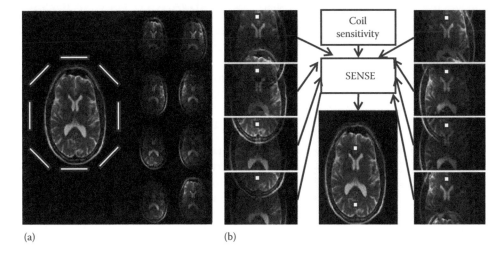

(a)   (b)

FIGURE 3.44 Parallel imaging. (a) A coil array (white bars) simultaneously acquires multiple images, each weighted by the sensitivity of the corresponding coil. (b) Sensitivity-encoding (SENSE) reconstruction for an eight-coil array and a reduction (or acceleration) factor $R = 2$. The marked eight pixels in the undersampled coil images are used along with the known coil sensitivity profiles to estimate the two unknown pixels in the final image. The process is repeated for all pixels in the image.

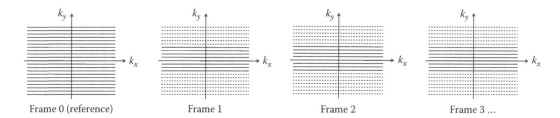

FIGURE 3.45 Keyhole technique. Full sampling of k-space is performed at baseline (reference frame 0), with subsequent low-frequency sampling (only the solid lines around the k-space center) at later frames (frames 1, 2, ...). The acquired high-frequency information from the baseline dataset is combined with the updated low-frequency information to reconstruct the dynamic frames.

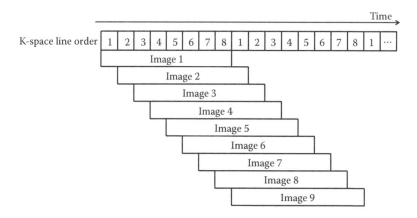

FIGURE 3.46 Sliding-window reconstruction. Only images 1 and 9 are not sharing any views (k-space lines), and they indicate the true temporal resolution. Seven intermediate images (images 2–8) can be reconstructed in-between images 1 and 9 by sharing k-space lines.

technique (Figure 3.45) in which the k-space of a reference image is fully acquired, while only the k-space center is acquired in subsequent frames. The high-frequency information in the reference image is then combined with the low-frequency information in each subsequent frame to reconstruct the dynamic frames. The assumption made here is that the high-frequency information remains largely unchanged.

The keyhole technique described earlier is one example of a family of techniques that can be described as view sharing. View sharing is any technique in which a partial set of the k-space lines is used to reconstruct multiple images, that is, these k-space lines are shared among consecutive images. Another example of view sharing is the sliding-window reconstruction. In this technique, the k-space lines are continuously acquired, as shown in Figure 3.46. However, instead of waiting for a full set of k-space lines to be collected (8 lines in this example), intermediate images are reconstructed midway that combine the previously acquired lines with the new lines. The train of images now has a higher apparent temporal resolution.

Similar to ultrasound, a motion-mode (M-mode) MRI can be obtained. A pencil-beam RF excitation field excites the signal in a narrow column. Because the acquisition time of this single signal is very short, the resulting 1D image can be traced with time, creating the M-mode image. One application of M-mode MRI is to track the motion of the diaphragm to gate data acquisition to the respiratory motion.

K-space segmentation is a technique widely used for cardiac-gated acquisitions. Segmented k-space acquisition is

used to generate cinematic (cine) images of the moving heart by collecting data over multiple cardiac cycles. The R–R interval (time between two consecutive R-waves of the electrocardiogram [ECG] signal) is divided into a number of cardiac phases. An image corresponding to each phase is reconstructed by combining different parts of its k-space from successive cardiac cycles (Figure 3.47).

3.8 ADVANCED TECHNIQUES IN MRI

Since its invention, MRI experienced continuous and increasing developments. A large number of methodological advances have been achieved, and many of them are now used in clinical practice. In this section, we briefly describe important techniques that are in common use.

3.8.1 TISSUE SUPPRESSION METHODS

In many situations, it is desirable to suppress the signal from a certain tissue or signal at a specific location in order to improve contrast, accentuate desired features, or avoid artifacts in the image. Spatial suppression aims at eliminating the signal from inside or outside the region of interest, whereas spectral suppression aims at eliminating the signal in a specific chemical environment (e.g., water or fat).

Tissue suppression strategies may utilize differences in the relaxation times, resonance frequency, or spatial position between tissues to achieve their goal. The most widely used technique for signal suppression is inversion recovery, where

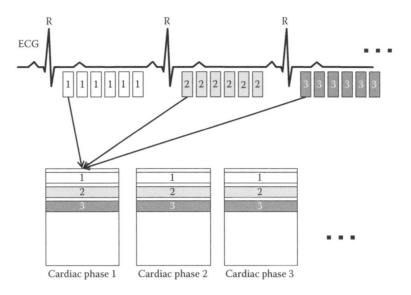

FIGURE 3.47 K-space segmentation in cardiac imaging. In this example, five cardiac phases are assumed. In the first cardiac cycle, the first segment of k-space (labeled 1) is acquired for all cardiac phases (a k-space segment consists of one or more lines). The remaining segments are acquired in the following cardiac cycles until the k-space is fully sampled.

the TI is adjusted to suppress a certain tissue, as described earlier for fat and fluid suppression. Another category of tissue suppression uses *chemical-shift-selective* RF pulses that selectively excite or saturate the signal from water or fat. The third method of tissue suppression eliminates the signal in a certain region of interest (e.g., in a slice adjacent to the imaged slice) using slice-selective pulses followed by spoiler (crusher) gradients, as in *outer volume suppression* techniques.

3.8.2 MR Angiography

MR angiography (MRA) is the application of MRI for imaging the blood vessels. MRI can image the blood vessels using either an exogenous contrast agent, as in *contrast-enhanced* MRA (CEMRA), or with mechanisms that utilize the motion of the blood itself, as in TOF and phase-contrast (PC) techniques.

In CEMRA, a contrast agent is administered intravenously to enhance the blood signal and improve the blood–tissue contrast. The contrast agent works by changing MR parameters like relaxation times (e.g., shortening T_1 or T_2). Most contrast agents used in MRI are based on gadolinium (Gd) chelates (e.g., diethylenetriamine pentaacetic acid [Gd-DTPA] or tetraazacyclododecane tetraacetic acid [Gd-DOTA]). The shortening of T_1 caused by Gd causes the blood signal to recover more quickly, giving a stronger signal relative to other tissues. A word of caution is necessary here: the risk of a serious adverse reaction called nephrogenic systemic fibrosis (NSF) is increased after administration of gadolinium-based contrast agents in patients with severe acute or chronic renal insufficiency and in patients with renal dysfunction due to the hepatorenal syndrome or in the perioperative liver transplantation period.

In TOF-MRA, blood is visualized through signal enhancement or attenuation, attributable to blood motion that brings blood into or carries blood away from the imaging slice, respectively. Flow-related enhancement relies on the inflow of unsaturated "fresh" blood spins, which in contrary to static tissues, have not experienced previous RF pulses, and therefore generate stronger signals in GRE sequences ("bright-blood imaging"; Figure 3.48a). In SE sequences, high-velocity signal loss occurs when blood flows into or out of the slice, causing signal loss (Figure 3.48b). As explained previously in the section on SE, spins have to experience both the 90° excitation and 180° refocusing RF pulses to produce the spin echo. If the blood velocity is so high such that it leaves the slice after the excitation pulse and before the refocusing pulse, then the spins will be out-of-phase by the time of imaging, and they will not produce an echo. On the other hand, the freshly entering spins will experience the 180° pulse, but these spins have never been excited before, and therefore they will not produce an echo either. Therefore, SE produces "black-blood" images.

In PC-MRA (Figure 3.49a), the velocity of the blood is encoded using a bipolar gradient pulse. The bipolar gradient has no effect on static tissues because the phase accumulation during the first gradient lobe is cancelled out by the second lobe. On the other hand, moving blood (with a constant velocity) accumulates a phase proportional to its velocity as a result of the spins changing their location in-between the two lobes of the bipolar gradient. The phase of a reference image (without the bipolar gradient) is required to eliminate non-velocity-related phases in the image. For a bipolar gradient of magnitude G and pulse duration T, blood spins moving with a velocity v accrue a phase difference of

$$\Delta\phi = \gamma G T^2 v. \qquad (3.22)$$

It is crucial when selecting the parameters of the bipolar gradient to make sure that the magnitude of the phase difference

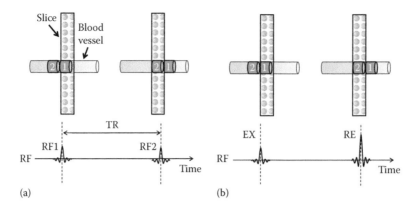

(a)   (b)

FIGURE 3.48 Time-of-flight (TOF) flow imaging. (a) Flow-related signal enhancement. Fresh spins in the flowing blood (denoted by block 2) experience less saturation than the repeatedly excited stationary spins (small balls in the slice) and produce a stronger signal in gradient-echo sequences. (b) High-velocity signal loss in spin-echo sequences. Blood flow out of the slice (block 1) experiences only the excitation pulse (EX), and freshly entering spins (block 2) experience only the refocusing pulse (RE); thus, neither one produces any echoes. Only blood spins that experience both the excitation and refocusing pulses produce an echo.

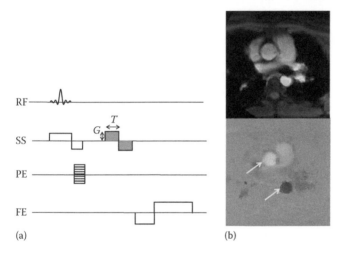

(a)   (b)

FIGURE 3.49 Phase-contrast (PC) flow imaging. (a) Phase-contrast GRE pulse sequence with a phase-encoding bipolar gradient (shaded) of strength G and duration T. The gradient is applied along the slice-selection direction to encode through-plane velocity. (b) A PC magnitude (top) and phase (bottom) images through the heart chambers. The bright and dark vessel cross sections in the phase image show blood velocity in the ascending and descending aortas, respectively (arrows).

does not exceed π; otherwise, phase wrapping occurs, causing velocity aliasing. The velocity for which $\Delta\phi = \pi$ is called the encoding velocity (VENC). The user controls the encoding gradient through the value assigned to the VENC parameter in the imaging protocol. A low value of VENC may result in phase wrapping and quantitative errors in the velocity estimates, whereas high VENC compromises the technique's sensitivity. The optimal value of VENC is slightly above the highest expected velocity. Velocity can be measured along any direction by applying appropriate combination of velocity-encoding gradients. Figure 3.49 shows a PC pulse sequence for through-plane velocity quantification and the resulting PC phase image.

3.8.3 Diffusion MRI

Diffusion is the random microscopic translational motion of molecules. MRI provides elegant techniques to examine this motion, which occurs at a small fraction of a typical MRI voxel size. Using a bipolar gradient pulse of a large gradient area, the MR signal can be sensitized to very small motion, producing diffusion-weighted images (DWIs). Molecular diffusivity is characterized by the apparent diffusion coefficient (ADC)), denoted as D. The diffusion gradient causes signal loss dependent on D. The amount of signal attenuation also depends on a user-defined factor called the "b"-value. The b-value depends on the gradient waveform, and it summarizes the influence of the gradients on the signal. The diffusion-weighted signal is given by

$$S(b) = S_0 \, e^{-b \cdot D}, \qquad (3.23)$$

where S_0 is the reference signal acquired without diffusion weighting. Diffusion is generally anisotropic and is fully described by a diffusion tensor. In diffusion tensor imaging (DTI), multiple DWIs are acquired with the diffusion gradient applied along different directions. At least six directions are required (plus a reference image) to calculate the diffusion tensor at each voxel. DTI can be used to track diffusion pathways, for example, myofiber tracts.

3.8.4 Magnetization Transfer

Magnetization transfer (MT) refers to the application of an RF pulse tuned to the frequency of one species and observing its effect on another species. Magnetization is transferred from the first to the second species through chemical and/or physical interaction. Therefore, MT can provide information about these interactions. MT can also improve the image contrast through signal attenuation of tissues that experience the MT effect.

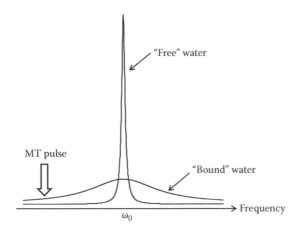

FIGURE 3.50 Magnetization transfer (MT). Magnetization transfer applies off-resonance irradiation (arrow) to protons in large molecules (bound water) and observes the response in the mobile molecules (free water).

The MT application in proton MRI uses RF excitation applied off-resonance from the water peak and observes the response in the water signal (Figure 3.50). Because protons in large molecules (e.g., proteins) as well as water molecules bound to large molecules experience more restricted motion, they have very short T_2 values and a very wide spectrum. Due to their short T_2 (less than 1 ms), bound protons in restricted pools cannot be imaged with conventional MRI. With MT, the magnetization of bound protons can be selectively saturated with off-resonance irradiation without perturbing the free water pool. As the restricted proton pool exchanges magnetization with mobile molecules in free water, it alters the magnetization of free water; therefore the restricted pool can be indirectly probed through its effect on free water. The resulting MT image is weighted by the fraction of bound protons present in the tissue in addition to its exchange dynamics. MT can provide valuable information about the structure integrity of the tissue (e.g., demyelination of neurons). In addition, MT can enhance the image contrast by attenuating signals from the macromolecule-rich tissues relative to the more mobile protons, for example, for the suppression of brain tissue in MR angiography.

3.8.5 MAGNETIC RESONANCE SPECTROSCOPY

MRI produces images of water protons in resonance. However, the human body contains many other organic compounds besides water. MRS is a technique used for probing different chemical compounds in the body, relying on the concept of *chemical shift*. Chemical shift is the change in the resonance frequency according to the chemical environment in different molecules. The difference in the resonance frequency results from the magnetic shielding effects of the orbiting electrons in the molecule. Therefore, chemical shift can be used to resolve different chemical components in much the same way frequency-encoding is used to resolve voxels at different locations. MRS produces a plot of signal intensity versus off-resonance frequency—the MR

spectrum. The MR spectrum consists of multiple peaks corresponding to different molecules. The area under each peak is proportional to the number of spins in a particular molecule, or molecular concentration. The spectra from various voxels can be processed to produce metabolic images (e.g., creatine or choline maps).

The simplest MRS experiment consists of a single RF pulse followed by data acquisition in the absence of any readout gradient (see Figure 3.8). A Fourier transformation of the signal generated from this simple experiment produces an MR spectrum. However, the resulting spectrum is non-localized and is merely an average of the whole sample. There are several methods to localize the spectrum to a specific location of interest in the body based on the local sensitivity of a surface coil, slice-selection RF pulses, phase-encoding gradients, or a combination thereof.

Single-voxel MRS techniques produce a single spectrum which is localized to a single slice, line, or voxel. For example, the application of a single slice-selective RF pulse followed by data acquisition localizes the spectrum to a single slice. The application of two orthogonal slice-selective RF pulses generates a spin echo signal from a column that is the intersection of the two slices. A single voxel is localized by the application of three orthogonal slice-selective pulses. The three pulses are selected to either form a spin echo as in point-resolved spectroscopy (PRESS) or a stimulated echo as in STEAM pulse sequences. Figure 3.51 shows a sample proton spectrum. Single-voxel pulse sequences are simple and easy to implement, but are inefficient when the goal is to obtain spectra from multiple voxels.

Chemical shift imaging (CSI) combines spectroscopy acquisition with phase-encoded localization to generate 1D, 2D, or 3D volumes of spectra. CSI is SNR-efficient, but is rather slow and has poor spatial resolution. CSI can be dramatically accelerated by using EPI and other non-Cartesian k-space trajectories.

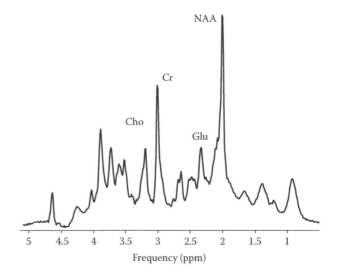

FIGURE 3.51 MR spectroscopy (MRS). A proton spectrum showing various metabolite peaks. NAA, *N*-acetylaspartate; Glu, glutamate; Cr, creatine; Cho, choline.

3.8.6 HIGH-FIELD IMAGING

MRI can be performed at any B_0 field strength, even in the earth's weak magnetic field. However, because SNR is proportional to B_0, using strong magnets is necessary for practical in vivo imaging. Currently, 3 T clinical scanners are common, and 7 T and above scanners are pushing into the market. This high-field trend offers great promise, but it also introduces new technical, safety, and imaging challenges. In this section, the advantages of high-field MRI are introduced, followed by a discussion of the challenges and strategies to address them.

The main motivation behind high-field MRI imaging is the SNR gain with higher B_0. This boost in SNR allows for higher spatial and/or temporal resolution, or could be traded for a shorter scan time. Another advantage is the greater magnetic susceptibility at higher fields, which is beneficial for susceptibility-based imaging methods, such as functional MRI (fMRI) brain studies. Further, in MRS, an additional advantage is the larger separation between spectral peaks, leading to higher spectral resolution.

The technical challenges of high-field MRI include the increased weight of the magnet, increased amount of cryogen needed, and increased rate of cryogen loss. Furthermore, the fringe field of the magnet (the distance beyond which the field drops below 5 G) increases with B_0. The required space and shielding of the scanner room are thus increased with higher field strengths, although self-shielded magnets (with outer superconducting layers) provide a solution to limit the stray field.

Another technical difficulty of high-field imaging is the increased field inhomogeneity, making shimming a more difficult job. Therefore, careful high-order shimming and/or dynamic shim updating may be needed to achieve the desired field uniformity. The most challenging problem with high-field imaging is that the excitation (B_1) field becomes more inhomogeneous at higher field strengths because the signal wavelength becomes comparable to the body size. The shorter wavelength results in destructive interference of the field leading to considerable variations in the flip angle and substantial signal loss across the FOV. This variation in the B_1 field causes inconsistent SNR and contrast throughput image. To reduce this problem, new RF coils with optimized B_1 uniformity are needed. Another remedy that is attracting research is the use of multiple transmitting coils that are individually amplitude- and phase-adjusted to produce a more uniform B_1 field. Image correction strategies are also required to account for field inhomogeneity in quantitative MRI studies.

Safety concerns in high-field imaging include the increased risk of ferromagnetic projectiles and increased torque applied on medical devices and implants (see the section on MRI safety later in the chapter for details). Devices considered MRI-safe at low field may not be safe at higher fields. Faster switching of the gradients may pronounce the effect of nerve stimulation.

Another safety concern when switching to high-field imaging is that the high power deposited in the patient, measured by the specific absorption rate (SAR), which increases with B_0^2. Therefore, SAR is a major limiting factor for many pulse sequences like FSE or bSSFP. Consequently, modifying the pulse sequence design and RF pulses to reduce power deposition is crucial in order to comply with SAR regulations. Parallel imaging could provide a solution, as it reduces the number of RF excitations and consequently reduces power deposition.

The magnetohydrodynamic effect is the phenomenon in which flowing conductive fluids (e.g., blood) inside a magnetic field generate an electric field. The magnetohydrodynamic effect increases at higher fields, distorting the ECG signal and making robust ECG gating more challenging. Vector ECG can help differentiate between the electric signals originating from the heart and those induced by flow based on their spatial orientation.

Finally, relaxation parameters change with increased B_0, altering the contrast of many pulse sequences compared to their contrast at lower field strengths. T_1 increases with field strength, reducing SNR and contrast in T1W images. Therefore, longer TR may be necessary to obtain the same T_1 contrast. The increase in tissue T_1, however, may be advantageous for contrast-enhanced protocols that depend on T_1 reduction, for example, viability delayed-enhancement imaging. Increased T_1 may also be useful for TOF MRA through the stronger saturation of the static tissue relative to the moving blood. In contrast to T_1, T_2 shows slight shortening at higher fields. However, the increased susceptibility at high fields leads to greater T_2^* shortening. Some imaging techniques benefit from this T_2^* shortening including fMRI, which depends on T_2^* shortening resulting from the blood-oxygen-level-dependent (BOLD) effect. Susceptibility-weighted imaging also benefits from the shorter T_2^*. Nevertheless, the drawback of the short T_2^* is the signal loss at relatively long TEs.

3.9 IMAGE ARTIFACTS

Artifacts are undesirable features that appear in the image. Artifacts occur primarily as a consequence of nonideal performance or malfunction of the MRI scanner (e.g., RF interference), but it can also result from the patient motion (e.g., ghost artifact), improper selection of the scan parameters (e.g., aliasing artifact), or it can simply be a fundamental physical limitation (e.g., the truncation artifact). Common MRI artifacts are described in this section along with techniques to avoid or correct for them.

3.9.1 MOTION ARTIFACTS

Patient motion is one of the most common sources of artifacts in MRI. The motion can be voluntary or involuntary, such as chest motion during respiration, cardiac motion, eye motion, swallowing, and blood flow. The motion artifact causes inconsistency in data acquisition and appears as blurring and ghosting in the image along the PE direction. This is a result of the relatively long time separating the acquisition of different k-space lines in the phase-encoding direction compared to the time separation between data samples in the frequency-encoding direction (Figure 3.52).

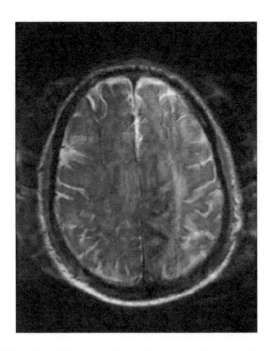

FIGURE 3.52 Motion artifact. Ghosting artifact resulting from head motion. Phase encoding is in the left–right direction.

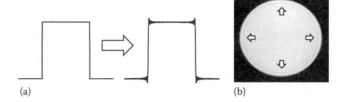

FIGURE 3.53 Ringing (truncation) artifact. (a) Numerical simulation showing the effect of truncating high-frequency components in k-space of a rectangular object (shown). (b) MRI image showing ringing artifact at the sharp edges of the object (arrows).

also called Gibbs artifact or truncation artifact. This artifact results from truncating the coverage of k-space to a small area around the k-space center. The missing high-frequency information manifests at sharp edges in the image. Figure 3.53a shows the results of truncating the k-space of a rectangular object, and Figure 3.53b shows the ringing artifact in an MRI image of a spherical phantom. The ringing artifact can be attenuated by weighting (or windowing) the received MRI signal with a suitable smoothing function or by increasing the image matrix size at the cost of prolonged scan time. Increasing the voxel size is another option for reducing the artifact at the cost of reduced spatial resolution.

3.9.3 Partial Volume Artifact

The partial volume artifact results when the imaging voxel contains more than one type of tissue. For example, a brain voxel that contains both gray matter and white matter, or gray matter and cerebrospinal fluid (see Figure 3.54). A large slice thickness also causes partial volume artifacts, which appear as blurring of the image. The partial volume artifact can be reduced by increasing the image resolution (matrix size) and reducing slice thickness in order to reduce the voxel size. However, this reduces the artifact at the cost of prolonged

Voluntary patient motion can be reduced by instructing the patient to remain still in the magnet during data acquisition. Restraints can be used to further reduce patient motion, and in some cases the patient may be sedated. Involuntary cardiac, eye, and respiratory motion as well as pulsating blood flow is harder to avoid. Nevertheless, synchronizing data acquisition with the patient's ECG and using breath-hold acquisition are common techniques when studying the chest and abdomen, and are also useful for head studies. For long scans that cannot be performed in a single or multiple breath-holds, synchronization of the scan with the respiratory motion may be performed if a respiration monitoring device is available. Alternatively, the respiration motion may be monitored by the MRI sequence itself, offering self-gated acquisition. The motion detection signal in this case is called a *navigator*. Flow artifacts can be reduced using flow compensation techniques, which employ gradient moment nulling (GMN). In GMN, the gradients are designed such that their moments are zeroed at the echo time. A zero zeroth-order moment gradient rewinds the phase of static tissue, while a zero first-order moment gradient rewinds the phase of both static and constant-velocity moving spins.

Simply averaging multiple images is another approach to reduce the motion effect on the image. Additionally, k-space trajectories that oversample the center of k-space (e.g., spiral) naturally average the motion out, because the low-frequency data near the k-space center represent most of the energy in the image.

3.9.2 Ringing Artifact

The ringing artifact appears as alternating bright and dark bands that occur parallel to sharp edges in the image. It is

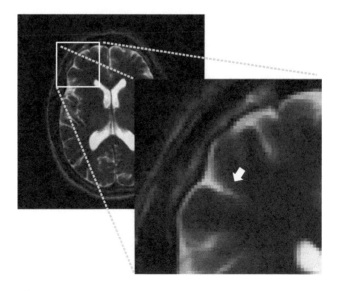

FIGURE 3.54 Partial volume artifact. The partial volume artifact appears at the gray matter/white matter border (arrow).

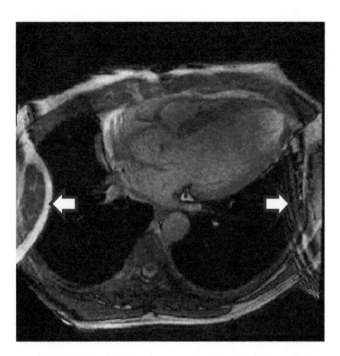

FIGURE 3.55   Aliasing (wrap-around) artifact (arrows). The aliasing artifact is more pronounced in the phase-encoding direction (left–right in this example). In this case, switching the directions of phase- and frequency-encodings can eliminate the artifact.

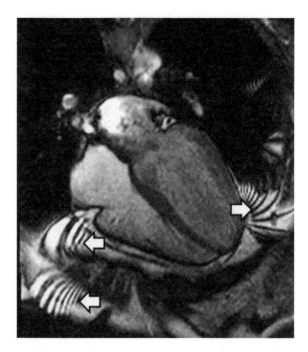

FIGURE 3.56   Off-resonance artifact. Banding artifact (arrows) in an SSFP image.

scan time and/or reduced SNR. Partial volume artifact may also appear in the slice-selection direction due to an imperfect slice profile, known as slice cross talk. Using optimized design of the slice-selection pulses or leaving a small gap between adjacent slices can help reduce the cross talk.

3.9.4   ALIASING ARTIFACT

When the prescribed FOV is smaller than the size of the imaged organ, as seen by the RF receiver coil, the tissues outside the FOV fold back into the FOV where they can obscure other details in the image (Figure 3.55). This is called aliasing, fold-over, or wrap-around artifact, which appears when the prescribed FOV is smaller than the imaged object. This means that the spacing between k-space lines (k-space resolution) is not small enough to unambiguously differentiate between the signals originating from within and outside the FOV. The artifact is more pronounced in the phase-encoding direction. The aliasing artifacts can be minimized by careful choice of the matrix size and orientation (i.e., switching the directions of the phase-encoding and frequency-encoding). Saturation of the signal outside the imaged object may also help reduce aliasing artifacts. Finally, localized excitation with 2D excitation RF pulses could be implemented to avoid aliasing while imaging a small FOV.

3.9.5   OFF-RESONANCE ARTIFACT

Spins precessing with different frequencies are called to be off-resonance. Off-resonance may be an inherent property of the tissue, such as the frequency difference between fat and water, but it also results from B_0 field inhomogeneity

or susceptibility effects. Therefore, off-resonance artifacts take different forms in MRI. One form is the *chemical shift artifact* in which the signals arising from different chemical environments inside the same tissue (e.g., water and fat) appear at different spatial positions in the direction of the readout gradient. The off-resonance artifact may also result in signal void at the boundary between water and fat in the case when the water and fat spins in the voxel are out-of-phase (i.e., have 180° phase difference). The chemical shift artifact can be minimized by increasing the readout BW.

Another manifestation of off-resonance is the banding artifact in which dark bands appear where the spins are 180° out of phase. This is common in SSFP pulse sequences, which are highly sensitive to off-resonance effects (Figure 3.56). Careful B_0 shimming can reduce this artifact; otherwise, frequency shifting could be implemented to move the banding artifacts away from the region of interest.

B_0 field inhomogeneity is also a source of off-resonance artifacts in pulse sequences with long readout windows. For example, EPI and spiral sequences accumulate phase shifts during readout, resulting in geometric distortion and image blurring. Segmenting data acquisition over multiple shots (or interleaves) helps reduce the phase accumulation.

3.10   SCANNER HARDWARE

The MRI scanner consists of multiple components: the main magnet that creates a strong static magnetic field for spin polarization, gradient coils that produce the weak space-varying magnetic field for signal localization, RF coils that excite the magnetization and receive the RF signals, and various electronics and computers (Figures 3.57 and 3.58). The MRI scanner is

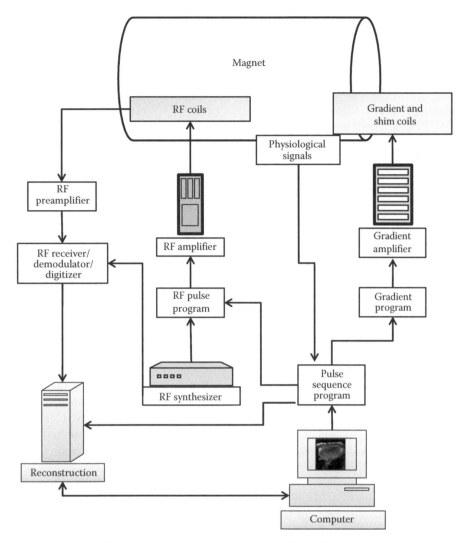

FIGURE 3.57 MRI scanner hardware. The MR system directs the gradient and RF coils based on the pulse sequence program to generate the MR signal. The MR signal goes through the receiver chain and is subsequently used for image reconstruction.

usually distributed in three rooms. The scanner room houses the main magnet, coils, and scanner table. The operator room houses computers for user interaction, protocol preparation, patient databases, image reconstruction, and data visualization. The third room (equipment room) is occupied by the scanner gradient electronics and power amplifiers. There is also additional space for patient preparation.

3.10.1 Main Magnet

The function of the main magnet is to create a stable, strong, and homogeneous magnetic field. The main magnet can be a permanent, resistive, or superconducting magnet. Superconducting magnets are currently the most widely used type of magnets. They make use of certain alloys (e.g., niobium–titanium) that when cooled to a very low temperature (~4 K) lose almost all of their electrical resistance, allowing large electric currents to pass without power dissipation. Once energized, the power source is withdrawn leaving the current circulating in the resistance-free cryogen-cooled coils and producing a very strong magnetic field. To cool the metal

alloys, liquid helium and nitrogen are used. The stray field of the magnet is a real safety hazard in the hospital. Shielding the MRI scanner room with heavy iron helps reduce the stray field. To further reduce the stray field and the required iron shield, self-shielded magnets were developed, which have a much lower stray field. If a magnet fault occurs, the cryogens rapidly boil off and escape the magnet, a condition known as quenching. A quench of the magnet causes the metal alloys to lose their superconductivity. As a result, the magnet quickly loses its strength.

To ensure maximum uniformity of the magnetic field, a process called "shimming" is performed. Following magnet installation, a field map is measured and used to correct for any imperfections that occurred during the magnet manufacturing. The correction can be performed using superconducting shim coils and/or passive ferromagnetic shims. Passive, or fixed, shimming is performed by strategically placing ferromagnetic elements around the magnet in order to render the magnetic field within the bore more homogeneous. A computer program calculates the amounts and locations of the metals to achieve best field homogeneity.

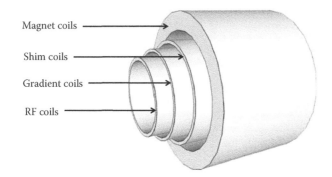

Magnet coils

Shim coils

Gradient coils

RF coils

FIGURE 3.58   The MRI scanner coils.

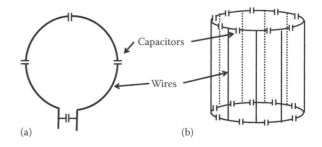

Capacitors

Wires

(a)   (b)

FIGURE 3.59   RF coils. (a) A circular-loop surface coil. (b) A birdcage coil.

When the patient is inside the scanner, however, the magnetic field is again distorted. Therefore, a set of dedicated shim coils are used for "active shimming" to adjust the field from one exam to the next. The scanner determines the electric current required to pass through the shim coils to generate a homogeneous magnetic field. The shim coils provide high-order field correction, with the imaging gradient coils usually providing the first-order (linear) shim. *Dynamic shimming* is the real-time adjustment of the shim coils. Dynamic shim updating is used to improve the shimming in a small region of interest (e.g., a single slice in a stack of slices), where the shim currents are rapidly switched before the imaging pulse sequence starts, and the process is repeated for all slices. Dynamic shimming provides a more uniform B_0 field than shimming the whole volume.

3.10.2   RF Coils

An RF coil consists of one or more loops of wire with distributed capacitors. The RF coil is a resonance circuit (tuned to a certain resonance frequency) that is either used as a transmit-only, receive-only, or transmit/receive (transceiver) probe. In the transmission mode, the current passes in the coil to create the B_1 field required to excite the sample. A good RF transmitter produces a homogeneous B_1 field over a large FOV, with low power losses. The direction of the B_1 field must be perpendicular to the direction of B_0. During reception, the magnetization in the sample induces a current in the coil. A good receiver coil is a low-noise coil with high and spatially uniform sensitivity. RF coils may be classified as volume, surface, or internal coils (Figure 3.59). Volume coils (e.g., the birdcage coil) are large coils that produce and/or detect the signal uniformly from the FOV. The MRI scanner comes with a large built-in volume coil (called the body coil) located inside the scanner housing. A surface coil is usually a small loop of coil placed on the surface of the body. Surface coils are more sensitive to the signal in the vicinity of the coil, and they receive less noise from the body. Therefore, surface coils produce small-FOV images with high SNR. An internal coil goes into the body (e.g., endorectal coil or intravascular catheter) to perform diagnostic imaging or an interventional procedure. Internal coils have the highest SNR. Therefore, they can produce images with very high resolution.

A *quadrature coil* is an RF coil that simultaneously transmits (or receives) the signal using two orthogonal channels, which have 90° phase shift. These coils are referred to as circularly polarized coils. Quadrature coils are efficient excitation coils, because only half the nominal B_1 power is needed for excitation, and hence they reduce power deposition in the patient. They are also good reception coils because they receive the signal through two channels, effectively improving SNR by $\sqrt{2}$. An example of a quadrature coil is the birdcage coil, or the dual surface coil that has two orthogonal loops. A *phased-array coil* is a set of small surface coils each covering a small FOV with high SNR. Signals from all coils are combined to produce a large FOV image with high SNR. Coil arrays are currently widely used for parallel imaging.

Tuning the coil is the adjustment of the tuning capacitors connected to the coil to make the coil resonance frequency equal to the Larmor frequency. *Matching* is the process of adjusting the impedance of the coil circuit to be equal to that of the cable carrying the signal to the preamplifier, usually 50 Ω, for maximum power transfer.

3.10.3   Gradient Coils

Gradient coils are used for slice-selection, phase-encoding, frequency-encoding, flow encoding, diffusion encoding, signal spoiling, field shimming, and many other applications. Gradient coils are designed to produce a magnetic field whose z-component varies linearly along one of the three main axes (Figure 3.60). Linear gradients along oblique directions are obtained by combining the gradients on the three axes with suitable weightings. High-order gradients that produce second- and third-order fields are also available, but are primarily used for shimming purposes. Gradients have certain characteristics that define their performance like the maximum strength, slew rate, linearity, and shielding. The *maximum magnitude* defines the maximum available gradient strength. Gradients with high strength enable shorter pulses, that is, faster scans. The *slew rate* of a gradient is its maximum rate of change (units of T/m/s). Higher slew rates enable faster switching of the gradient, which reduces scan time. A good gradient coil should produce a *linear* gradient over a large FOV. *Shielded gradients* integrate additional coils to reduce field interference.

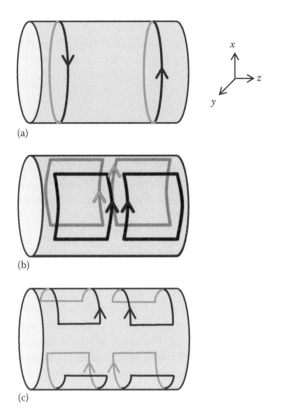

3.10.4 MRI Receiver

The MRI receiver removes the Larmor frequency modulation of the signal and performs the signal conditioning operations necessary for subsequent image reconstruction. Different designs of the MRI receiver are possible, and only the general concepts are discussed here. The MR signal detected by the RF coil is too weak for reliable processing. Therefore, a low-noise preamplifier is necessary to boost the signal. The amplified MR signal is then transmitted to the receiver, which may apply more amplification and then demodulates (changes the frequency) the signal to an intermediate frequency (IF) lower than the RF frequency (Figure 3.61). Using phase-sensitive (quadrature) detection, the receiver generates real and imaginary signal components. Next, the signal is filtered by a band-limiting (anti-aliasing) filter to remove frequencies outside the desired BW. Finally, the signal is digitized with an ADC and digitally filtered before being passed to the computer for image reconstruction.

3.11 MRI SAFETY

MRI is a remarkably safe technique that does not use ionizing radiation and does not require the administration of radioactive isotopes. Generally, the MRI exam does not result in any pain or side effects under normal conditions. However, MRI is not hazard-free. The main hazards in MRI are the force acting on ferromagnetic objects and the potential heating/burns due to excessive power deposition. In addition, MRI can have other limitations, such as the loud noise caused by the gradient coils and the tight bore space of the magnet that may cause anxiety in some patients. The main hazards in MRI are discussed in this section along with some precautions for safe operation of the scanner.

3.11.1 Field Strength and Magnetic Projectiles

The MRI scanner uses a very strong magnetic field that is thousands of times the earth's magnetic field. Very high magnetic fields are under development. The Food and Drug Administration (FDA) regulations in the United States require that B_0 be less than 8 T for adults, children, and infants older than 1 month old. Neonates (less than 1 month old) are restricted to fields no stronger than 4 T.

FIGURE 3.60 Gradient coils. (a) The z-gradient coil is a Maxwell coil. (b) The y-gradient and (c) x-gradient coils are saddle coils. The arrows on the wires show the direction of current flow in the coils.

When the gradients are rapidly switched during a pulse sequence, electric currents (called *eddy currents*) are induced in the conducting structures in the magnet. Eddy currents circulating in the magnet structures generate an opposing field that distorts the original gradient field, causing image artifacts. Active shielding of the gradient coils reduces the fringe field of the gradients and significantly reduces eddy currents. Eddy currents can also be reduced through "preemphasis" of the gradient waveforms. Preemphasis means that the gradient driving current is modified such that when the eddy current field is added, the result is close to the desired ideal waveform.

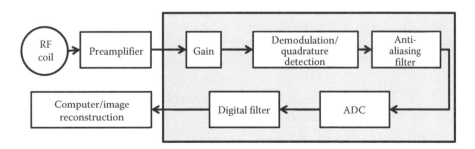

FIGURE 3.61 MRI receiver. The received signal from the RF coil is preamplified and then transmitted to the MRI receiver (shaded region), where more amplification could be applied. The MRI receiver then demodulates the signal, removes frequencies outside the desired bandwidth, and applies analog-to-digital conversion (ADC) and digital filtering before the signal is used for image reconstruction.

In addition to field strength, the field rapidly drops outside the magnet creating a strong magnetic field gradient. Similar to the force that a pressure gradient exerts on water to cause flow, the magnetic field gradient exerts a tremendous translational force on magnetic objects. The force is proportional to the product of the field gradient and field strength. Ferromagnetic objects brought close to the MRI scanner are pulled toward the magnet with great force and could fly at a high-speed heading to the scanner center. These deadly projectiles can cause serious injury or death to the patient inside the scanner or to staff members who happen to be on the projectile's path. For example, in a horrible accident, a child was killed with a metal oxygen tank brought close to the scanner. The projectiles may also cause significant harm to the magnet, RF coils, or gradients coils. It must be remembered that the magnet is always on. Therefore, careful inspection of all materials brought inside the scanner room is a must at all times to prevent such dangerous accidents. All equipments brought into the scanner room should be MRI compatible, including wheelchairs, oxygen tanks, trolleys, and cleaning tools. In addition, the scanner room should be locked if not in use to prevent accidents.

3.11.2   Medical Devices and Implants

Another hazard of the strong magnetic field of the MRI scanner is the interaction with implantable devices. In addition to the attracting forces described earlier, the strong static magnetic field exerts a torque on magnetic and metallic objects, which tries to rotate the objects to align them with the field's direction. This torque is a hazard for implanted medical devices such as prostheses, intracranial aneurysm clips, cardiac pacemakers, or defibrillators. The magnetic interaction with these devices can damage the device, potentially causing damage to the tissue or even patient death. Therefore, patients must be screened to assure that there is no potential hazard and that all devices and implants are MRI compatible.

3.11.3   Nerve Stimulation

When a gradient field is rapidly switched on and off, the changing magnetic field induces a voltage in nearby electrical conductors. This effect may result in electrical nerve stimulation, causing discomfort and/or pain to the patient. The FDA guidance limits the rate of change of the magnetic field (dB/dt) to levels that do not result in painful peripheral nerve stimulation. An upper dB/dt limit of 20 T/s is suggested in the literature. However, the scanner software should automatically constrain the pulse sequence from producing rapid changes in the field.

3.11.4   Local Heating and Burns

The RF fields may interact with the cables and electrodes (e.g., ECG leads) during the scan, producing a heating hazard. The heated metallic pieces, cables, and contact electrodes may result in skin heating or even burns. Metallic objects such as those in the clothes should be removed or kept off the patient skin. Cables and electrodes used for imaging should be MRI compatible. The electrodes must be in good contact with the skin to prevent localized current paths. The cables should not form loops, and they should be kept off the skin using a blanket.

3.11.5   Power Deposition

Power deposition is measured by the SAR, which is the power deposited in the patient in watts per kilogram (W/kg). SAR of 1 W/kg would increase the temperature of an insulated slab by about 1°C/h. SAR increases with the square of the magnitude of the B_0 and B_1 fields. The FDA regulates the maximum SAR, as shown in Table 3.5.

3.11.6   Acoustic Noise

During the MRI exam, rapid switching of the gradient coils inside the strong magnet causes the MRI scanner to act as a giant speaker. The frequency of gradient switching lies in the audible range, producing annoying loud noise when a pulse sequence is played out. The noise is particularly high with fast sequences like EPI, and the noise level becomes higher at higher B_0 field. Gradient acoustic noise can reach high and dangerous levels that can cause damage to the patient's hearing. For protection, the scan noise should not exceed certain regulatory limits. The patient is strongly recommended to wear hearing protection like earplugs or headphones during the exam. The FDA regulates the limits on the sound pressure level, mandating the peak unweighted sound pressure level to be no greater than 140 dB; and the A-weighted root mean square (rms) sound pressure level to be no greater than 99 dB$_A$ with hearing protection in place.

3.11.7   Claustrophobia

Claustrophobia is the excessive fear of tight or enclosed spaces. The tight bore space of the narrow and long MRI magnet may trigger a claustrophobic reaction in the patient in the form of severe anxiety or panic attacks. Therefore, preparing the patient and educating him/her about the MRI system, imaging procedure, and what to expect during the exam (like loud noise) may help mitigate the effects of the confined space. To further reduce the claustrophobic effects of MRI, it is recommended to keep audio and visual contact with the patient, use bright light in the bore, and use mirrors to change the patient's visual field. Relaxation techniques and even sedation may be necessary in some cases.

TABLE 3.5
FDA Regulations on SAR Limits

Site	Dose	Time (min)	SAR (W/kg)
Whole body	Averaged over	15	4
Head	Averaged over	10	3
Head or torso	Per gram of tissue	5	8
Extremities	Per gram of tissue	5	12

In order to reduce the feeling of the confined space, new generations of MRI have shorter and wider bores. Also, open MRI systems, which use vertical magnets, have been developed. Although the open systems have rather low B_0 field strength, they often produce acceptable image quality for many procedures. Another option that totally eliminates the confined-space problem of MRI is the development of MRI systems dedicated to certain organs (e.g., the extremities).

3.12 SUMMARY AND KEY POINTS

3.12.1 SUMMARY

MRI is a safe and powerful imaging technique for imaging anatomical, physiological, and functional information. MRI operation is based on the NMR phenomenon. The hydrogen nucleus is the most imaged nucleus due to its abundance in the body, although other nuclei, for example, sodium and phosphorus, are also used for imaging. After RF excitation, the magnetization returns to equilibrium with independent longitudinal (T_1) and transverse (T_2) relaxations, which are tissue-specific parameters that are used, along with proton density, to differentiate between different tissues. MRI is made possible with the implementation of the imaging gradients, which are used to localize the signal in space. The acquired signal samples are used to construct the k-space, which upon applying Fourier transformation, provides the required MRI image. GRE, SE, IR, STEAM, and SSFP are famous imaging sequences. EPI, FSE, non-rectilinear k-space trajectories, parallel imaging, and partial k-space acquisition are examples of fast MRI techniques. Although MRI has been developed by leaps and bounds since its introduction for clinical use in the early 1980s, there is still a long way to go to exploit all its features. Advanced MRI applications continue to emerge, especially with ongoing developments in hardware and software capabilities. Multiscale and multimodality imaging are particular areas of interest, especially with potential roles in key applications such as regenerative medicine and tissue engineering.

3.12.2 KEY POINTS

- MRI is a noninvasive medical imaging modality with no ionizing radiation or radioactive materials involved.
- MRI has plethora of imaging and control parameters, which make it a powerful imaging modality with anatomical, physiological, and functional imaging capabilities.
- MRI operation is based on the NMR phenomenon, in which certain nuclei absorb and reemit electromagnetic energy when placed in a magnetic field and the resonance condition is satisfied.
- Nuclei with an odd number of protons or neutrons have a net nuclear magnetic moment, and they are referred to as spins.

- The hydrogen nucleus, containing one proton, is the most widely used nucleus in MRI.
- The main magnetic field polarizes the spins, such that their nonzero net magnetization points in the direction of the main magnetic field.
- The magnetization field is tipped into the transverse direction (excited) with the help of an external weak RF magnetic field (RF pulse).
- The RF pulse could be an excitation, inversion, or refocusing pulse.
- After the excitation RF pulse is turned off, the magnetization returns to its equilibrium position with independent T_1 and T_2 relaxations.
- The Bloch equation describes the dynamics of magnetization precession and relaxation.
- After repeated application of the excitation RF pulses, the magnetization reaches a dynamic steady-state condition.
- T_1-weighted images are acquired by using short TE and short TR.
- T_2-weighted images are acquired by using long TE and long TR.
- PD-weighted images are acquired by using short TE and long TR.
- Slice selection is achieved by applying a linearly varying weak magnetic field gradient in the direction perpendicular to the desired imaging slice during the application of a BW-limited excitation RF pulse.
- Frequency encoding (readout) is implemented to encode the spin positions in the x-direction.
- Projection reconstruction is implemented by rotating the readout gradient to create projections along different angles, from which the image is reconstructed using the filtered back-projection technique.
- Phase encoding is implemented to encode the spin positions in the y-direction.
- K-space is the matrix formed by the signal samples acquired at different FE and PE values.
- The MRI image is constructed by applying Fourier transform to the k-space.
- K-space does not have one-to-one correspondence with the image space.
- The k-space center and periphery contain low-resolution and high-resolution information, respectively, which determine the image's contrast and resolution, respectively.
- 3D imaging can be achieved by performing multislice imaging or 3D volumetric imaging, where the latter includes the implementation of two nested loops of phase-encodings in the y- and z-directions.
- The data sampling rate should be high enough to avoid aliasing artifacts.
- The pulse sequence diagram is the timing graph of various RF and gradient pulses in the SS, PE, and FE directions.
- The RF pulses could be either nonselective (hard) or selective (soft).

- Key pulse sequences include GRE, SE, IR, STEAM, and SSFP.
- GRE is a bright-blood robust imaging sequence with T_1 or T_2^* weightings.
- SE is a black-blood imaging sequence with T_1 or T_2 weightings.
- IR is used to attenuate the signal from certain tissues or flowing blood.
- STEAM modulates the magnetization and allows for recording events, such as motion.
- SSFP is a modification of the GRE sequence, where all gradients are balanced in all channels. SSFP has remarkably high SNR.
- There is a trade-off between SNR, resolution, and scan time. The only way to boost all of them is to image at a higher magnetic field strength.
- The FOV in the image space is equal to one over the resolution in the k-space, and vice versa.
- SNR is proportional to the magnetic field strength, voxel size, and square root of total data acquisition time.
- EPI is a very fast imaging technique, although it is sensitive to off-resonance artifacts.
- FSE is a fast imaging technique, whose speed and contrast are determined by the echo train length (ETL).
- Spiral, radial, and PROPELLER are examples of unconventional k-space trajectories. They are fast and more suitable for certain applications than the Cartesian trajectory.
- Parallel imaging accelerates scan time at the cost of SNR. SENSE and GRAPPA are famous parallel imaging techniques.
- Partial k-space acquisition is feasible due to the Hermitian property of k-space.
- Partial k-space acquisition and data sharing techniques allow for real-time and dynamic imaging applications. Example techniques include keyhole, view sharing, and sliding window reconstruction.
- Segmented k-space acquisition is implemented in cardiac imaging by synchronizing data acquisition with the cardiac cycle.
- Spatial- and spectral-selective RF pulses are used for tissue suppression.
- MR angiography is used for imaging blood vessels with the help of exogenous contrast agents, for example, gadolinium, or intrinsic contrast mechanisms, for example, with TOF and phase-contrast techniques.
- Diffusion-weighted imaging is used for measuring microscopic translational motion of molecules.
- Magnetization transfer accentuates the image contrast through signal attenuation of certain tissues in the image.
- MR spectroscopy (MRS) is used for probing different chemical compounds in the body based on the concept of chemical shift.
- High-field imaging allows for improved image quality and shorter scan time, but it is associated with technical challenges.
- MRI artifacts include motion, ringing, partial volume, aliasing, and off-resonance artifacts.
- The scanner hardware includes the main magnet, RF coils, gradient coils, shim coils, electronics, and computers.
- MRI is a safe imaging modality, although some issues have to be considered, including ferromagnetic projectile objects, medical devices/implants contraindications, nerve stimulations, local heating/burns, acoustic noise, and claustrophobia.

BIBLIOGRAPHY

Bernstein, M. A., King, K. E., et al. (2004). *Handbook of MRI Pulse Sequences*. Burlington, MA: Academic Press.

Bottomley, P. A. (2008). Turning up the heat on MRI. *Journal of the American College of Radiology: JACR* **5**(7): 853–855.

de Graaf, R. A. (2007). *In Vivo NMR Spectroscopy: Principles and Techniques*. Chichester, U.K.: John Wiley & Sons.

Haacke, E. M., Brown, R. W., et al. (1999). *Magnetic Resonance Imaging: Physical Principles and Sequence Design*. New York: Wiley-Liss.

Hashemi, R. H., Bradley, W. G., et al. (2010). *MRI: The Basics*. Philadelphia, PA: Lippincott Williams & Wilkins.

Ibrahim, El-S. H. and Osman, N. F. (2010). Chap. 28: Magnetic resonance imaging. In *Handbook of Physics in Medicine and Biology*, R. Splinter (ed.). Boca Raton, FL: CRC Press/ Taylor & Francis Group, pp. 28-18–28-21.

Levitt, M H. (1999). *Spin Dynamics: Basics of Nuclear Magnetic Resonance*. Chichester, U.K.: John Wiley & Sons.

Liang, Z. P. and Lauterbur, P. C. (1999). *Principles of Magnetic Resonance Imaging: A Signal Processing Perspective*. Piscataway, NJ: Wiley-IEEE Press.

McRobbie, D. W., Moore, E. A., et al. (2007). *MRI from Picture to Proton*. Cambridge, U.K.: Cambridge University Press.

Nishimura, D. G. (2010). *Principles of Magnetic Resonance Imaging*. Stanford, CA: Stanford University.

Schenck, J. F. (2005). Physical interactions of static magnetic fields with living tissues. *Progress in Biophysics and Molecular Biology* **87**(2–3): 185–204.

Stafford, R. J. (2005). High field MRI: Technology, applications, safety, and limitations. *Medical Physics* **32**: 2077.

Vlaardingerbroek, M. T., Boer, J. A., et al. (2004). *Magnetic Resonance Imaging*. New York: Springer.

Westbrook, C., Roth, C. K., et al. (2011). *MRI in Practice*. Chichester, U.K.: Wiley-Blackwell.

4 Introduction to Cardiovascular Magnetic Resonance Imaging

Elizabeth R. Jenista, PhD; David C. Wendell, PhD; Igor Klem, MD; El-Sayed H. Ibrahim, PhD; and Wolfgang G. Rehwald, PhD

CONTENTS

LIST OF ABBREVIATIONS

Abbreviation	Meaning
1D	One-dimensional
2D	Two-dimensional
3D	Three-dimensional
ACCF	American College of Cardiology Foundation
AHA	America Heart Association
ARVD	Arrhythmogenic RV dysplasia
ASD	Atrial septal defects
CAD	Coronary artery disease
CEMRA	Contrast-enhanced MRA
CEST	Chemical exchange saturation transfer
CHD	Congenital heart disease

CNR	Contrast-to-noise ratio
CSI	Chemical shift imaging
CSPAMM	Complementary SPAMM
CT	Computed tomography
DANTE	Delays alternating with nutations for tailored excitation
DE	Delayed enhancement
DENSE	Displacement encoding with stimulated echoes
DWI	Diffusion-weighted imaging
ECG	Electrocardiogram
EDD	End-diastolic diameter
EF	Ejection fraction
EPI	Echo planar imaging
ESD	End-systolic diameter
FAB	Antigen-binding fragment
FDA	Food and Drug Administration
FLASH	Fast low-angle shot
FOV	Field of view
GFR	Glomerular filtration rate
GRAPPA	Generalized autocalibrating partially parallel acquisition
GRE	Gradient echo
HARP	Harmonic phase
HASTE	Half-Fourier acquisition single-shot TSE
HCM	Hypertrophic cardiomyopathy
ICD	Implantable cardioverter defibrillator
IQ	Image quality
IR	Inversion recovery
IRA	Infarct-related artery
LGE	Late gadolinium enhancement
LV	Left ventricle
LVEF	LV ejection fraction
LVOT	LV outflow tract
MI	Myocardial infarction
MIP	Maximum intensity projection
MRA	Magnetic resonance angiography
MRS	Magnetic resonance spectroscopy
NSF	Nephrogenic systemic fibrosis
PARACEST	paramagnetic CEST
PC	Phase contrast
PET	Positron emission tomography
PRESS	Point-resolved spectroscopy
ROI	Region of interest
RV	Right ventricle
SAR	Specific absorption rate
SCMR	Society of Cardiovascular Magnetic Resonance
SE	Spin echo
SEM	Standard error of the mean
SENC	Strain encoding
SENSE	Sensitivity encoding
SNR	Signal-to-noise ratio
SPAMM	Spatial modulation of magnetization
SPECT	Single photon emission computed tomography
SR	Saturation recovery
SSFP	Steady-state free precession
STEAM	Stimulated echo acquisition mode
STIR	Short TI inversion recovery
T2W	T2-weighted
TE	Echo time
TI	Inversion time
TR	Repetition time
TSE	Turbo spin echo
UI	User interfaces
USPIO	Ultrasmall superparamagnetic iron oxides
VENC	Velocity encoding
VRT	Volume rendering technique

4.1 INTRODUCTION

4.1.1 CARDIOVASCULAR MAGNETIC RESONANCE IMAGING

Since the first chest x-ray images visualizing enlarged cardiac structures, cardiovascular imaging has played a vital role in patient diagnosis and management. Today, a variety of different techniques are available to clinicians to evaluate cardiovascular morphology and function. For example, with its relatively compact size, affordable cost, and portability, echocardiography has become a valuable first-line tool in clinical cardiac care. Various x-ray-based techniques, like fluoroscopy and computed tomography (CT), are used on a daily basis in the diagnosis and care of patients with cardiovascular disease. Over the last two decades, the versatility of cardiovascular magnetic resonance (CMR) imaging has allowed it to become the gold standard for myocardial viability and functional imaging. CMR has the advantages of high tissue contrast and spatial resolution, capability of modifying the plane orientation without the need to move the patient or scanner hardware, three-dimensional (3D) imaging capability, lack of ionizing radiation, and the plethora of physical and control parameters that can be adjusted to image various measures of cardiac function. CMR applications are increasingly growing in parallel with improvements in the scanners' hardware and software capabilities. CMR imaging not only provides anatomical information, but also provides functional, perfusion, viability, and metabolic information about the heart muscle as well as angiography, vessel wall characteristics, and flow hemodynamics in the vasculature.

4.1.2 CHAPTER OUTLINE

This chapter presents the CMR techniques used in a typical clinical examination, with specific emphasis on measuring global cardiac function. Both technical details and practical clinical information are provided to give the reader a glimpse into the role of CMR in clinical practice. This chapter covers image acquisition as well as quantitative, semiquantitative, and qualitative methods for cardiac functional assessment from CMR images.

This chapter starts by introducing a brief overview of different cardiac imaging modalities, followed by the advantages, capabilities, and safety profile of CMR imaging. The basics of a CMR examination are then provided, including patient setup. This chapter then addresses different types of motion encountered in cardiovascular imaging as well as different techniques to compensate for them. The concepts of pulse sequence, imaging protocol, and scan parameters are then described, followed by description of different data acquisition strategies and CMR-related artifacts. The chapter then addresses different CMR imaging techniques, including morphology, perfusion, delayed-enhancement (DE), magnetization relaxation, MR angiography, and flow velocity imaging techniques. The chapter then focuses on cine imaging and its implementations, especially for evaluating cardiac morphology and function. Finally, the chapter briefly summarizes different tagging techniques, followed by discussing advanced technology in CMR imaging. It should be noted that some of the basic MRI imaging aspects were briefly covered in Chapter 3; however, they are covered here in more details from a CMR perspective; not from the general MRI perspective as in Chapter 3.

4.2 CARDIOVASCULAR IMAGING

4.2.1 ECHOCARDIOGRAPHY

Echocardiography creates images of cardiac structure and function based on reflection of the sound waves at tissue interfaces, such as at the interface between blood and myocardium. High temporal resolution movies of cardiac motion and valve function can be created using M-mode echocardiography, and two-dimensional (2D) images can be created using B-mode echocardiography to provide measurements such as myocardial thickness and chamber diameter. In addition, Doppler echocardiography can be used to visualize and quantify blood flow velocities.

While echocardiography has become an important first-line tool for clinical cardiac care, it has several drawbacks, specifically limited spatial resolution, low image quality, poor penetration depth, and high dependency on sonographer's skills (Kremkau and Taylor 1986). Additionally, the quantification of ventricular and atrial volumes, blood flow, and pressure gradients are highly dependent on image quality, and the LV volume measurements often underestimate those calculated by other techniques (Kim et al. 2008). Furthermore, the large difference in density between the lungs and surrounding tissues results in a limited number of usable cardiac imaging windows. The size of these cardiac windows narrows in adults and is usually more constrained in obese patients, resulting in increased examination time.

4.2.2 COMPUTED TOMOGRAPHY AND NUCLEAR IMAGING

Another standard cardiac imaging modality is CT, which uses high-energy x-rays that are attenuated according to the density of bone or tissue through which they pass, and are then incident on a detector array. The emitter/detector array rotates around the patient, acquiring projections through the body from multiple angles, where these projection data are reconstructed to create high spatial resolution images of cardiac anatomy. Cardiac CT imaging requires a slow heart rate, which is established by administering beta-blocker medication prior to scanning. Detailed information on coronary artery patency and calcification can be obtained with the administration of an iodinated contrast agent (Shaw et al. 2003, Vliegenthart et al. 2005, Detrano et al. 2008). Atrial and ventricular volumes, but no true functional data, can also be obtained with this CT imaging. In recent years, there have been attempts to acquire both systolic and diastolic frames in CT imaging, but this approach exposes the patient to higher radiation dose than in standard CT. A common CT dose for a chest CT is 700 versus 200 mrem for a head CT, and the dose increases further with coronary CT angiography (CTA): 2000 mrem versus 500 mrem for head CTA. Despite radiation exposure, CT is particularly useful for diagnosis in emergency medicine because of its short scan time compared to other modalities.

Nuclear imaging-based techniques for the evaluation of cardiac function use either single photon emission computed tomography (SPECT) or positron emission tomography (PET). In these examinations, the patient receives an intravenous injection of a radioactive isotope, where the distribution of this tracer within the myocardium is used as an indication of myocardial perfusion. These studies look for stress-induced ischemia by obtaining identical image series at rest and stress. The stress-induced vasodilation can be achieved either pharmacologically or by physical exercise on a treadmill next to the scanner. In the stress test, the tracer is injected at peak exercise, which is taken up by the cells based on regional perfusion and remains elevated within nonischemic tissue. The patient is imaged later once the tracer has been cleared from the blood, but not from the myocardium. The radioactive decay of the isotope is localized within the tissue by the detector array surrounding the patient. Myocardial perfusion assessment by nuclear imaging can be challenging due to the low spatial resolution of these techniques, which can miss small perfusion defects. Despite this limitation, PET stress testing is still the first-line procedure for assessing exercise-induced ischemia. This test is commonly ordered when a subclinical stenosis is suspected after a CT scan or a fluoroscopic catheterization.

4.2.3 CARDIOVASCULAR MAGNETIC RESONANCE (CMR)

4.2.3.1 CMR Advantages and Capabilities

In the last decade, CMR has emerged as an important clinical tool that can be used to evaluate a broad range of cardiovascular pathologies. Technical advances have expanded the role of CMR from a primarily tomographic imaging modality to one that is dynamic, allowing for rapid and high-resolution imaging of ventricular function, valve motion, myocardial perfusion, and viability. In addition, CMR is now considered the gold standard for evaluation of regional and global systolic function, myocardial infarction and viability, as well as assessment of congenital heart disease (CHD).

CMR offers many potential advantages over other cardiovascular imaging modalities. Similar to echocardiography and CT, the CMR images are acquired by transmitting and receiving energy from the body, but CMR is uniquely flexible. CMR can provide a variety of tissue contrasts without any changes to hardware and without ionizing radiation. The flexibility of CMR results in a large variety of imaging options, which can be daunting, but also allows the examination to be tailored to the patient's particular clinical question. For example, within the same CMR examination, information can be gathered about cardiovascular morphology, contractile function, viable and nonviable myocardium, valve disease, congenital anomalies, blood flow, and vascular anatomy. Furthermore, post-processing of the CMR images provides several measures of the heart condition, including ventricular volumes and mass, ejection fraction (EF), cardiac strain, fiber orientation, and iron content.

Conducting an efficient clinical CMR examination depends on appropriate choice of the imaging techniques, known as pulse sequences, and configuration of the sequence (imaging) parameters. The assembly of imaging parameters is simply called a "protocol," and while there are protocol-specific parameters, many parameters are general and are present in virtually all protocols.

4.2.3.2 CMR Safety

The CMR environment can potentially inflict serious injury on patients and staff. Injuries may result from the static magnetic field (projectile impact injuries), very rapid gradient field switching (induction of electric currents leading to peripheral nerve stimulation), radiofrequency (RF) energy deposition (heating of the imaged portion of the body), and acoustic noise. The institution of access policies to the magnet room minimizes the risk of projectile injuries. Patients are extensively screened for metal prior to imaging, and all facility personnel undergo dedicated MR safety training. This risk can be further reduced through clear labeling of the devices as "MR safe," "MR conditional," or "MR unsafe." An item is termed "MR safe" if it poses no known hazards in the magnetic environment. An "MR conditional" device has no known hazards in a specified MR environment. However, it must be used only under the conditions provided on the device label; for example, the leads of a neurostimulator must be placed according to the label to ensure that it meets the "MR conditional" safety requirement. An "MR unsafe" device, for example, a ferromagnetic item such as a pair of scissors, is hazardous in all MR environments.

The Food and Drug Administration (FDA) has placed limits on the rate of change of the magnetic gradient fields (slew rate), and the amount of RF energy that can be transmitted into the patient (specific absorption rate; SAR). All clinical scanners monitor the slew rate and calculate the SAR level to prevent nerve stimulation and heating, respectively. Acoustic noise of 100 dB or more can be generated from vibration of the gradient coils during image acquisition. Protective hearing devices, such as headphones or earplugs, reduce the noise level to prevent hearing impairment and increase patient comfort. In practice, continuous voice communication between the scanner operator and the patient throughout the examination is important for patient comfort and safety. The patient is also provided with a squeeze ball to alert the scanner operator that he/she needs an immediate help.

Patients with medical devices or implants may face additional hazards, including device and lead heating, induction of electrical currents, and device movement or malfunction. Ferromagnetic aneurysm clips and electronic medical devices such as neural stimulators, insulin pumps, or implantable cardioverter defibrillators (ICDs) were traditionally considered as a strict contraindication to MRI. However, there is a growing subset of metallic implants and electronic devices that may safely undergo MRI examinations. A comprehensive list of MRI safe implants and devices can be found elsewhere (Shellock and Crues 2014, Shellock 2016). Prosthetic valves and coronary artery stents are now considered safe for MRI scanning (Shellock and Crues 2014, Patel et al. 2006, Shellock 2016), and recently, the FDA approved the use of MRI immediately after implantation of paclitaxel and sirolimus drug-eluting stents. Also, preliminary reports suggest that MRI can be safely performed in some patients with modern pacemakers and ICDs and that the benefits of the MRI examination often outweigh its risk (Roguin et al. 2004, 2005, Nazarian et al. 2006, Sommer et al. 2006, Naehle et al. 2009). Very recently, MRI-compatible pacemakers have been manufactured and approved by the FDA for noncardiac imaging at 1.5 T, and FDA approval for cardiac imaging in the presence of these devices is forthcoming. This push for more MRI-compatible cardiac devices shows the expanding role of CMR in cardiac patient management, and the need for MRI-safe devices.

4.2.3.3 Gadolinium-Based Contrast Agents and Nephrogenic Systemic Fibrosis (NSF)

It has been reported that a small subset of patients with end-stage renal disease may be at risk for developing nephrogenic systemic fibrosis (NSF) after receiving a gadolinium-based contrast agent (Kanal et al. 2007, Wertman et al. 2008, Altun et al. 2009, Kribben et al. 2009). NSF is characterized by an increased tissue deposition of collagen, often resulting in thickening and tightening of the skin, predominantly involving the distal extremities. NSF may also affect other organs including skeletal muscles, lungs, pulmonary vasculature, heart, and diaphragm. Thus, such contrast agents should be used cautiously, and noncontrast CMR tests should be considered for patients with severe chronic renal disease (glomerular filtration rate [GFR] < 30 mL/min/1.73 m^2), particularly in those undergoing peritoneal dialysis or hemodialysis. Other risk groups include patients with acute renal failure (where the estimated GFR may not accurately reflect renal function), patients with hepatorenal syndrome, and patients in the peritransplant period after liver transplantation. A policy regarding the use of gadolinium contrast agents in the setting of renal disease has been published by the American College of Radiology (ACR) (Kanal et al. 2007).

4.3 CMR IMAGING PROTOCOLS

4.3.1 Patient Setup and Preparation

In order to perform a successful CMR examination, two simple patient preparation steps are required. First, the patient needs to be screened for metal to determine if he/she has any metal implants, metallic debris (e.g., from welding), or devices that might interact with the strong magnetic field. This step protects the patient from possible injury due to metal interaction with the magnetic field. Second, the chest needs to be prepared for electrocardiogram (ECG) electrode placement in order to improve the ECG signal quality needed for proper cardiac synchronization.

4.3.1.1 ECG Electrodes Placement

A high-quality ECG signal is necessary for acquiring artifact-free MR images. The most effective method for synchronizing the image acquisition to the heartbeat is to use a three- or four-lead ECG signal. Missing ECG triggers (mistriggering) can result in image artifacts such as blurring and ghosting. While ECG synchronization is well established, it can be challenging to have adequate ECG signal quality within the MRI environment. Electrode and lead placement is an important factor in obtaining a good signal, and it is different from electrode positioning for a standard diagnostic ECG. Only MRI-safe electrodes should be used and the leads should not form loops to reduce the risk of burns resulting from the build-up of current induced by the magnetic fields. Before attaching the ECG electrodes, hair should be removed by shaving the respective skin locations. These locations should be cleaned from oil with a special abrasive and conductive gel. Also, the leads must be appropriately spaced to minimize interference from voltage differences between the leads.

4.3.1.2 ECG Signal Quality Optimization

The ECG signal quality often deteriorates when the patient is placed inside the magnet due to two effects: the magnetohydrodynamic effect and rapidly switching currents in the gradient coils. The magnetohydrodynamic effect (Dimick et al. 1987) reduces ECG quality in the magnet due to the flowing magnetized blood, which induces voltages that are then superimposed on the heart's electrical activity, thus distorting the ECG signal. This effect is proportional to static field strength and is therefore worse at 3 T than at 1.5 T. The second potential source of ECG signal interference is due to the rapidly switching currents in the gradient coils, which likewise induces interfering signals. Scanner manufacturers have addressed these issues by designing more robust four-lead vector ECGs and implementing pattern detection algorithms to reliably determine the R-wave occurrence even in the presence of interference. If the ECG signal is still too low, or if the magnetohydrodynamic effect is too strong, the scanner operator can acquire a stack of scout images to determine the orientation of the heart. Using these images, the leads can be repositioned to improve the ECG signal strength.

As a rule of thumb, the signal strength and waveform fidelity are always better in the absence of the magnetic field. Therefore, if the signal quality is already poor outside the magnet, an unusable signal can be expected once the patient is moved inside the MRI scanner.

4.3.2 Accounting for Physiological Motion

4.3.2.1 Types of Motion

Like most medical imaging modalities, CMR can be affected by physiological motion, primarily the cardiac and respiratory motion. High-quality images can be obtained in most patients through the combination of breath-holding and synchronizing image acquisition to the ECG. A poor ECG signal, and thus improper synchronization, or an imperfect breath-holding leads to characteristic image artifacts which can be minimized by the scanner operator. Slowing down the heart rate using beta-blockers, as is done in cardiac CT (de Graaf et al. 2010), is not common in CMR. Instead, the operator can find the quiescent period of the cardiac cycle (typically during mid-diastole) and move the data readout time accordingly. The motion sensitivity of the image is dependent on the type of implemented data readout. Whereas gradient-echo (GRE) and steady-state free precession (SSFP) sequences are relatively motion robust, the turbo-spin echo (TSE) readout is much more susceptible to motion artifacts and must be carefully implemented. Interestingly, even imaging stationary vessels, such as the aorta, benefits from ECG synchronization by minimizing artifacts from periodic vessel pulsations. For scans that exceed the typical patient's breath-hold capability, respiratory navigators could be used to track the position of the patient's diaphragm while the patient breathes freely (Stuber and Weiss 2007). The following section details the main techniques used to minimize the negative effects of cardiac and respiratory motion.

4.3.2.2 Cardiac Motion and Sequence Synchronization

Synchronization of the pulse sequence to the cardiac cycle is necessary, and it is most commonly achieved by detecting the R-wave of the ECG signal. The advantage of ECG triggering is that it provides not only the duration of the cardiac cycle (the RR interval), but also the time when the R-wave occurs indicating the beginning of heart contraction. Pulse oximetry signal ("pulse ox") can be also used for cardiac synchronization. This signal also monitors the RR duration, but its trigger is delayed relative to the R-wave. This delay differs between patients and can vary within the same patient depending on heart rate, blood pressure, etc. Therefore, it is cumbersome to set up a cardiac-gated CMR acquisition using pulse ox triggering. However, it may be the only available option in case of unreliable ECG.

An alternative cardiac synchronization technique that may be available in the future is called self-gating. This technique does not require an ECG signal; it is rather based on an artificial physiological signal derived from the raw data acquired during each cardiac cycle. The technique is based on the periodical signal intensity variation with the size of the blood pool according to the cardiac phase. Plotting this information versus time delivers a substitute for the ECG signal (Larson et al. 2004). This method is wireless and therefore can be applied to fetal MRI where the ECG signal cannot differentiate the fetal heart rate from that of the mother. Another novel cardiac synchronization approach uses a phonocardiogram, which works well even at the ultrahigh field of 7 T, where a standard ECG signal is severely distorted due to the magnetohydrodynamic effect (Frauenrath et al. 2010).

4.3.2.3 Respiratory Motion and Sequence Synchronization

As discussed in the beginning of this chapter, in some scans, respiratory motion causes image artifacts such as blurring and ghosting in the phase-encoding direction due to changes in the heart position and shape with the respiratory phase. In clinical practice, the effects of respiratory motion can be reduced or eliminated using different strategies. The simplest and most common technique is breath-holding. However, this strategy limits the maximum scan time to the breath-holding capability of the patient. Further, sometimes, the reproducibility of breath-holding can vary, causing differences in the position of the heart. End-expiratory breath-holding, rather than end-inspiratory, has been shown to reduce the variability in the diaphragm position (Holland et al. 1998).

Another approach for reducing breathing artifacts is to acquire multiple signal averages while the patient is breathing. With this technique, ghosting is reduced, but scan time is increased and effective spatial resolution is degraded. While this tradeoff is often acceptable for 2D imaging, it is not recommended or 3D imaging due to prohibitively long scan times and loss of spatial resolution.

A respiratory navigator (Ehman and Felmlee 1989), which is integrated into some pulse sequence, provides an alternative strategy for reducing breathing artifacts. Such sequences continually acquire a localized spin echo (one-dimensional (1D) technique) or a low-resolution image (2D technique) to monitor the position of the diaphragm while the patient is freely breathing. Only while the diaphragm position is within a predefined range, known as the "acceptance window," around the end-expiratory position, data acquisition can resume. 2D navigators are more robust than 1D techniques, but image acquisition and processing takes longer (Stuber et al. 2002), and thus their primary application is in body MRI. The 1D methods include the "crossed-pair" (Stuber and Weiss 2007) and "pencil-beam" (Stuber et al. 2002) navigators. The crossed-pair navigator combines a 90° excitation slice and a crossed 180° refocusing slice to create a spin echo along a thin beam of the intersection of the two slices. The pencil-beam navigator uses a 2D RF-pulse to excite spins along a cylindrical beam. For either type of 1D navigators, the signal is read out along the beam to monitor motion in one direction. The beam is usually positioned perpendicular to the diaphragm–lung interface at the dome of the right lobe of the liver and parallel to the direction of respiratory motion.

Figure 4.1 shows a typical setup of a crossed-pair navigator on a commercial scanner's user interface. In this example of navigator scouting, about three respiratory cycles were captured, where the longer and flat end-expiratory position appears on the top, and the brief end-inspiratory position appears on the bottom of the interface line in the figure. The navigator detects the lung (dark) and liver (bright) interface within the search region (rectangle in the figure) using an edge detection algorithm. Data acquisition resumes only when the respiratory position is within the acceptance window.

4.3.2.4 Limits of Respiratory Navigation and Potential Solutions

While navigators are often an effective method for monitoring respiration, they have limited acquisition efficiency, resulting in long scan times. Respiratory gating limits data acquisition to a small fraction of the respiratory cycle. Acceptance rates of less than 40% are not uncommon (Piccini et al. 2012). Additionally, if the breathing pattern is irregular or there is respiratory drift over the course of the scan, the navigator efficiency drops (Taylor et al. 1999) and scan time increases, or the scan never completes. In current navigator methods, adjustment of the search and acquisition windows is done automatically with "motion adaptive gating" (Wang and Ehman 2000) or "drift correction," which partially resolves this issue.

The size of the acceptance window affects the image quality and scan duration. A narrow acceptance window (e.g., 1 mm) potentially improves image quality by reducing the effect of motion but comes at the expense of decreased scan efficiency. An increased scan time tends to degrade the overall image quality, partially due to small patient shifts in non-monitored directions. Therefore, an acceptance window of 1.5–2.5 mm is typically chosen. The drift in the diaphragm position results in a corresponding shift in the position of the heart. While a correction factor linking the shift of the diaphragm to that of the heart is commonly used, the same factor is used for all patients, ignoring interpatient variability and causing suboptimal image quality (Danias et al. 1997).

Self-navigated techniques have recently been introduced to overcome these drawbacks (Stehning et al. 2005, Lai et al. 2008, Piccini et al. 2012). In these techniques, the cardiac motion due to respiration is directly assessed at the heart rather than indirectly at the diaphragm, eliminating the need for a correction factor. Motion is compensated for directly in the k-space using a single reference line acquired at the beginning of each acquisition segment, and therefore the technique has a 100% scanning efficiency. Nevertheless, these methods are still in development and are not yet available in commercial cardiac imaging packages.

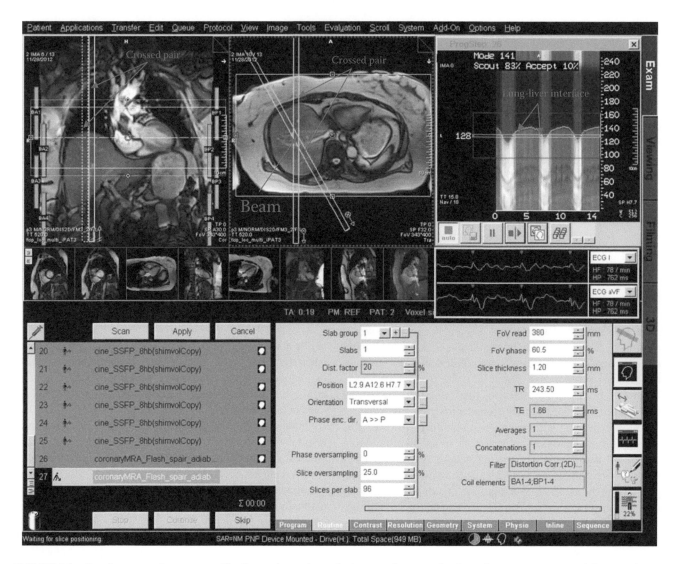

FIGURE 4.1   Respiratory navigator setup. The figure shows the typical setup of a crossed-pair navigator on a commercial scanner's user interface.

4.3.3   CMR PROTOCOL, DATA ACQUISITION STRATEGIES, AND IMAGE ARTIFACTS

4.3.3.1   Pulse Sequences, Imaging Protocols, and Scan Parameters

4.3.3.1.1   Basic Definitions

The MRI scanner acquires images by running pulse sequences, which are software programs that control the gradient coil switching, activation of transmitter and receiver coils, and recording of the MR signal. Unique to MRI, the scanner operator can conduct a variety of different medical imaging tests to collect specific physiological information purely by running different pulse sequences on the same MRI scanner hardware. Each pulse sequence is configured by a large set of scan parameters (a hundred or more) known as an MRI protocol. The protocol tailors the same basic pulse sequence to a specific imaging task. The most important protocol parameters are flip angle, repetition time (TR), echo time (TE), field of view (FOV), spatial resolution, temporal

resolution, number of segments, and selection of preparation modules. Nomenclature of the parameters is often vendor specific and can be confusing. Figure 4.2 shows part of a scanner's user interface with typical and frequently used protocol parameters.

4.3.3.1.2   Protocol Optimization

Different protocol parameters have various degrees of effect on the image properties. Whereas changing TE, TR, or flip angle can strongly affect the image contrast, and therefore its clinical usefulness, modifying other parameters, such as FOV, do not fundamentally alter image characteristics. Protocol optimization is conducted by adjusting the parameters that are relevant to a specific application. For example, if high spatial resolution is necessary for clarifying anatomical details, then reducing FOV and increasing the imaging matrix are viable options. On the other hand, if high temporal resolution is necessary for capturing fast motion, then TR and TE should be minimized, and the acquisition bandwidth should

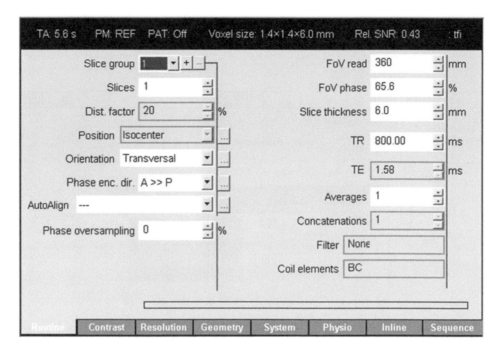

FIGURE 4.2 Typical MRI protocol parameters. The figure shows part of a scanner's user interface with typical and frequently used protocol parameters.

be increased. Other special parameter adjustments should be made for specific-purpose sequences. Also, it should be noted that some imaging parameters may need to be adjusted based on the imaging field strength. For example, when imaging at a lower magnetic field strength, the pixel size, flip angle, and TR may be increased to improve signal-to-noise ratio (SNR) at the cost of lower spatial resolution.

4.3.3.1.3 Parameter Classification

The sequence parameters can be loosely divided into three groups, depending on how frequently the parameters are used:

1. The first group represents the parameters that are set up once during protocol building, and are not usually modified during the scan time. These typically include TE, readout type (GRE or SSFP), readout bandwidth, and activation of preparation pulses. This type of parameters defines the sequence's basic properties, such as image contrast, and therefore is not changed at scan time.

2. The second parameter group is modified on a per-scan basis, for example, the readout duration (temporal resolution) and readout position within the cardiac cycle (e.g., systole vs. diastole). The field of view is also modified for each patient according to the patient's body habitus. Many more parameters are commonly edited by the scanner operator, but they are beyond the scope of this chapter.

3. A third parameter group consists of field strength-dependent parameters with some overlap with groups 1 and 2. For example, at higher field strength, longer T1 values require a reduction of the flip angle to

maximize the readout signal for given TE and TR according to the Ernst angle equation (Pelc 1993). Readout SNR increases proportionally with field strength and decreases with larger readout bandwidths. Therefore, faster readouts are possible at 3 T because higher readout bandwidths can be used while maintaining similar SNR levels to those at 1.5 T.

4.3.3.2 CMR-Specific Protocol Parameters

4.3.3.2.1 Synchronization with the Cardiac Cycle

As previously discussed, synchronization of the pulse sequence to the cardiac cycle is critical. It requires additional parameters beyond those used for imaging other parts of the body. Figure 4.3 shows common CMR parameters and values for controlling the sequence acquisition relative to the cardiac cycle. Important parameters are the physiological signal source and synchronization mode. The signal source is usually the ECG or the pulse ox signal, and the mode can be "triggering" or "gating," as will be described later.

The parameters that control the timing of data acquisition within the cardiac cycle are shown in Figure 4.3. The parameters necessary for ECG synchronization are signal source, acquisition window, trigger pulse, trigger delay, TR, and segments. Modifying these parameters allows the scanner operator to control the readout timing within the cardiac cycle. The trigger signal source (ECG or pulse ox) is determined by the first signal/mode parameter. This also defines the method of ECG synchronization, in this case "ECG/Trigger." The Trigger delay is the time between the recognized trigger, commonly the R-wave, and the start of acquisition. The TR used here is defined as the time from the end of the trigger delay to the end of data acquisition. The definition of TR is vendor-dependent

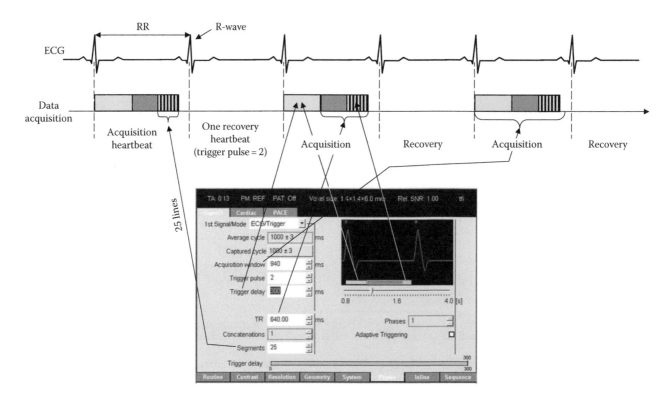

FIGURE 4.3 CMR protocol parameters related to the physiological signal. The figure shows common CMR parameters and values for controlling the sequence acquisition relative to the cardiac cycle.

and may deviate from its textbook definition as the time between acquiring two consecutive lines of data in the k-space. Next, the acquisition window is set, which defines the accepted timeframe in which the sequence can run. This is normally set to 10% below the RR interval, where the minimum value of the acquisition window is the TR + Trigger delay. The Trigger pulse (2 in this case) describes the number of detected cardiac triggers required for the sequence to resume.

4.3.3.2.2 Parameter Dependencies

Most CMR parameters have a direct or indirect effect on other parameters. While some parameters can be changed in isolation, others are inherently linked. For example, changes in FOV can result in changes in the bandwidth, TE, and TR. The relationship between the parameters can be complicated, so the software behind the scanner user interface (UI) automatically adjusts the values of affected parameters and displays the ranges of acceptable values for them. The UI, therefore, provides the necessary framework for widespread use of clinical MRI examinations.

4.3.3.3 Data Acquisition Strategies

4.3.3.3.1 Segmented and Single-Shot Acquisitions

In MRI, the duration of data acquisition depends on many factors such as spatial resolution, TR, TE, and heart rate. There are a variety of acquisition methods that can be used depending on the patient's breath-holding capability and the type of imaging sequence. The two most common acquisition strategies are segmented acquisition and single-shot acquisition. Segmented acquisitions distribute data collection over

multiple heartbeats, while single-shot acquisition is done during only one heartbeat.

In segmented imaging, data acquisition is split up into multiple parts and multiple heartbeats. Each part, or segment, only collects a small portion of the entire dataset. In the example of Figure 4.4, a total of 160 lines are acquired in 8 segments of 20 lines per segment. Each segment is acquired in the same cardiac phase for eight consecutive heartbeats. During segmented acquisition, the patient must hold his or her breath to ensure that all data are collected from exactly the same anatomical location. Otherwise, respiratory motion between heartbeats would result in image blurring.

Single-shot, also called snapshot techniques (Sievers et al. 2007), and real-time imaging are widely available and are becoming faster and more popular. Acquiring all the data at once in a single shot delivers poorer temporal and spatial resolutions compared to segmented acquisition, but in a fraction of the scan time. Moving structures may appear blurred if the temporal resolution is too low, analogous to camera shake in the realm of photography.

4.3.3.3.2 Competing Constraints of Temporal and Spatial Resolutions and Their Effect on Breath-Hold Duration

Ideally, an MR image would have the best possible spatial resolution and would be acquired in a photography-like snapshot for excellent temporal resolution. Unfortunately, the acquisition of high spatial and/or temporal resolution CMR images requires significantly more data, and therefore cannot be acquired in a single shot within a fraction of a single

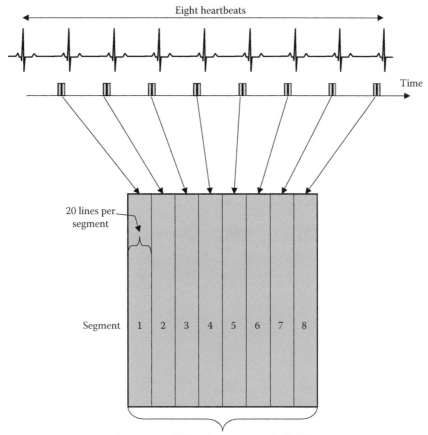

FIGURE 4.4   Segmented acquisition and data sorting. The figure shows an 8-heartbeat acquisition with 20 lines per segment.

heartbeat. Rather, high-resolution acquisitions must be spread out over multiple heartbeats using segmented acquisition.

For example, the data in Figure 4.5a were acquired with a total of 160 k-space lines over 8 heartbeats, with 20 lines per heartbeat. Each line took 3 ms to acquire yielding a temporal resolution of 20×3 ms = 60 ms. Assuming an FOV of 320 mm, the spatial resolution is 320 mm/160 pixels = 2 mm. For an RR of 1000 ms, the breath-hold would have taken 8 s. If the breath-hold is too long for the patient, it can be reduced by sacrificing either spatial or temporal resolution. In Figure 4.5b, temporal resolution was sacrificed by doubling the number of lines per segment. Therefore, 40 lines were acquired per heartbeat yielding a total of 160 lines in only four heartbeats with a temporal resolution of 120 ms, while maintaining the spatial resolution. Alternatively, as shown in Figure 4.5c, the breath-hold can be reduced by decreasing the spatial resolution to only 80 lines. As FOV remains the same, the spatial resolution is 320 mm/80 pixels = 4 mm. This demonstrates the possible trade-offs between temporal resolution, spatial resolution, and breath-hold duration.

4.3.3.4   CMR Image Artifacts

The large number of available CMR imaging sequences leads to a large variety of image artifacts. Most artifacts are sequence-specific and depend on the patient's physiology. Pinpointing the artifact source can be tricky, as the location

of the artifact in the image does not necessarily correspond to the physical location of the artifact source. Also, the artifact appearance, location, and intensity are affected by the sampling order of the raw data. For all these reasons, eliminating or reducing CMR artifacts can be difficult, but is essential for obtaining clinically unambiguous information. A working knowledge of artifact types is therefore indispensable for the MRI technologist as well as the reading clinician (Saremi et al. 2008). Examples of common CMR artifacts are included in this section, along with approaches to remedy them. Other general MRI artifacts were covered earlier in Chapter 3.

The three major sources of CMR artifacts originating from the patient are (1) poor breath-holding capability, (2) poor synchronization of imaging with the cardiac cycle, and (3) metal artifacts, for example, from prosthetic valves, stents, or fenestration patches. These artifacts result in ghosting throughout the image, blurriness of important structures, and signal dropout and flow-related artifacts from blood passing near the metal part. Recognizing the type of artifact and finding its source allows the scanner operator to apply an artifact-specific solution, which usually leads to a significant image quality improvement.

4.3.3.4.1   Breathing Artifacts

Breathing artifacts are common in CMR, especially in patients with compromised lung function or heart failure. In some types of acquisition, poor breath-holding appears as blurring

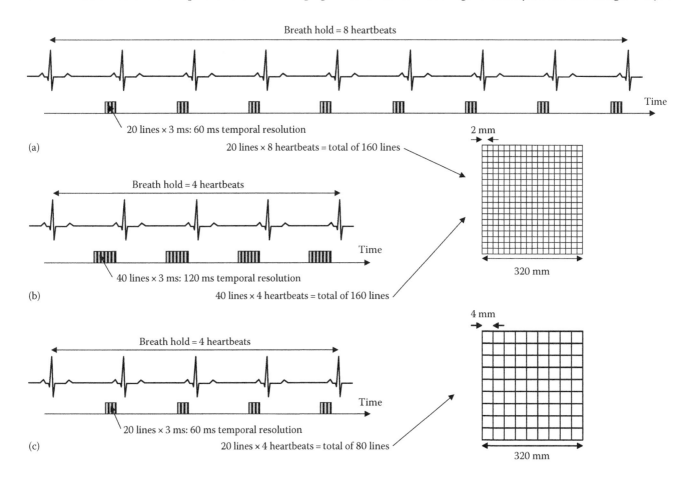

FIGURE 4.5 Segmented acquisition and the competing constraints of spatial resolution, temporal resolution, and scan time. (a) High spatial resolutions; high temporal resolution; and long scan time. (b) High spatial resolutions; low temporal resolution; and short scan time. (c) Low spatial resolutions; high temporal resolution; and short scan time.

of the image or as discrete ghosting, as shown in Figure 4.6a. These artifacts can be corrected by shortening the breath-hold duration for the patient, or by simply emphasizing the need for consistent breath-holding. Figure 4.6b shows the image quality (IQ) improvement achieved with proper breath-holding.

4.3.3.4.2 Cardiac Synchronization Artifacts

Artifacts caused by poor synchronization of image acquisition with the ECG signal normally occur in patients with arrhythmia, such as in atrial fibrillation, premature ventricular contractions, or dyssynchrony between the atria and ventricles or between the left ventricle (LV) and right ventricle (RV). Poor synchronization is reflected as blurry myocardial borders, as shown in Figure 4.7a. The low IQ seen in panel Figure 4.7a is improved with proper cardiac synchronization, as shown in Figure 4.7b. While such artifacts may prohibit the quantification of LV volume assessment by automated methods, visual scoring can still be used.

4.3.3.4.3 Metal Artifacts

Metallic structures near the heart can cause signal loss that may obscure the anatomy of interest. The signal voids adjacent to the metallic structure can also influence the phase of nearby spins, propagating the artifact across the image.

Additionally, blood passing near metallic structures can experience the same effects and show signal voids downstream. These artifacts are especially problematic in SSFP imaging compared to GRE imaging. These artifacts can obscure valve function, as seen in Figure 4.8a. IQ can be significantly improved by altering the readout scheme from SSFP to a GRE readout such as the Fast Low Angle Shot (FLASH) acquisition, as shown in Figure 4.8b. GRE is less sensitive to magnetic field inhomogeneities, which reduces the appearance of the metallic artifact. The lower SNR of GRE relative to SSFP is an acceptable tradeoff in this case. Figure 4.8c shows a low-quality SSFP cine image in a different patient with prosthetic mitral and tricuspid valves, and Figure 4.8d shows the improvement obtained by switching to GRE.

4.3.4 Plane Scouting

4.3.4.1 Scouting for Standard Cardiac Views

Plane scouting is the first and simplest scan of every CMR examination, which is conducted to determine standard cardiac views that can be used throughout the scan. Scout images are single-shot SSFP images acquired in diastole with ECG triggering, usually during free breathing. Synonyms for "scout scans" are "localizers" or "plan scans," depending on

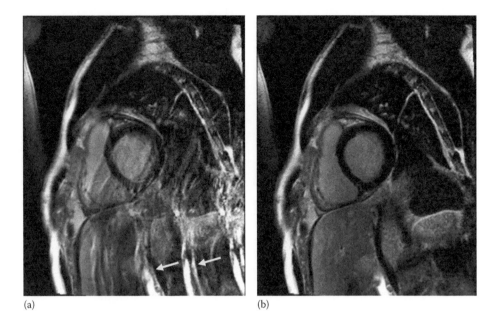

(a)   (b)

FIGURE 4.6 Breathing artifacts. (a) Breathing during data acquisition causes ghosting artifacts of the chest wall (yellow arrows). (b) Artifacts are eliminated using the appropriate breath-holding technique. Both images were acquired using a segmented inversion recovery GRE sequence.

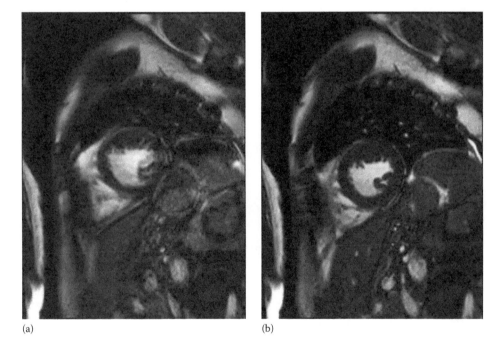

(a)   (b)

FIGURE 4.7 Cardiac synchronization artifacts. (a) Artifacts present as inconsistent image intensity and blurry boundaries of the myocardium. (b) The artifacts are eliminated using proper cardiac synchronization. Both images were acquired at the same slice location and time in the cardiac cycle, and with the same temporal resolution.

the scanner manufacturer. Scout images are used to establish the short- and long-axis views of the heart and confirm the optimal position of the anterior and posterior receiver coil arrays placed around the thorax. Scout images allow the scanner operator to position the heart at the magnet's isocenter where the magnetic field is most homogeneous. The first scout images are acquired as parallel stacks in the sagittal, coronal,

and axial orientations, as shown in Figure 4.9(1A-1C). Because of patient-to-patient anatomical variations, both the short- and long-axis cardiac views lie at arbitrary, "double-oblique" angles with respect to the coronal, sagittal, and axial planes.

Once the images along the scanner coordinates have been acquired, they can be used to prescribe a single-oblique view. A two-chamber view (panel 2) can be obtained by going

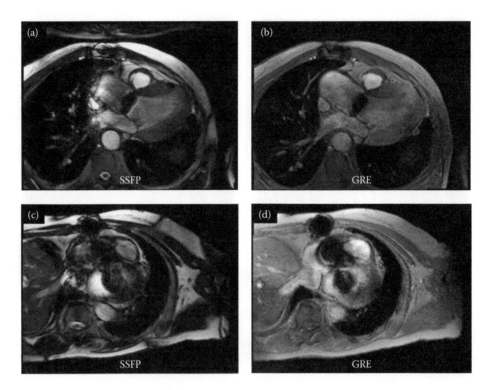

FIGURE 4.8 Metal artifacts. (a) Through-plane SSFP image of mechanical aortic valve. (b) GRE image at the same slice location as in (a). (c) En-face SSFP image of prosthetic mitral and tricuspid valves in a different patient. (d) GRE image at the same slice location as in (c). Note reduced metal artifacts and improved image quality in GRE compared to SSFP.

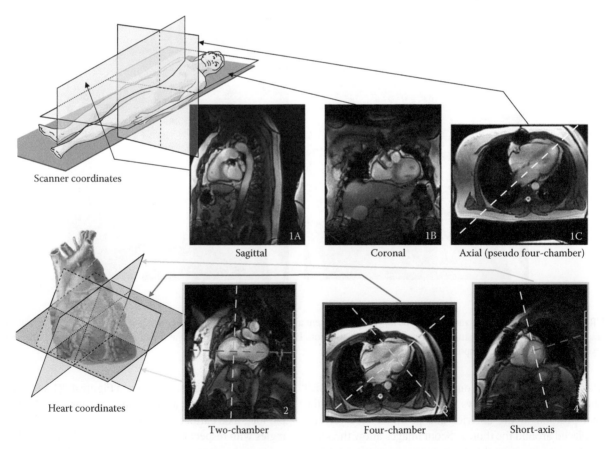

FIGURE 4.9 Scouting of standard cardiac views. The figure outlines the typical order of scouting steps. Additionally, the color-coded dashed lines and solid boundary lines show the relative orientations of the planes, where the dashed lines are perpendicular to the image on which they are plotted.

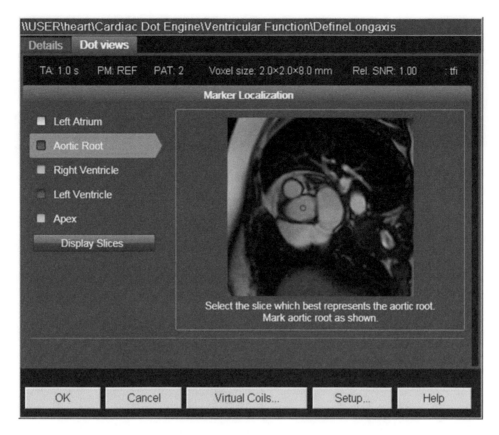

FIGURE 4.10   Automated scouting on a typical user interface. The scanner displays the calculated reference points to allow the scanner operator make adjustments if necessary.

perpendicular to panel 1C, through the LV apex and middle of the mitral annulus while staying parallel to the interventricular septum (dashed white line in 1C). From this view, a four-chamber view (panel 3) can be obtained (red dashed line) by going perpendicular to the two-chamber view, again going through the mitral annulus and the LV apex. From the four-chamber view, the short-axis view (panel 4) is obtained by cutting along the blue dashed line that is perpendicular to both the four-chamber and two-chamber views. Other scouting orders are also possible. For example, a short-axis view could be acquired based on panel 2 (dashed blue line) and then used to obtain true four-chamber and two-chamber views.

4.3.4.2   Automated Scouting

Recently, some manufacturers have automated the scouting procedure to simplify and accelerate this task. The scanner automatically identifies reference cardiac structures, such as the left atrium, aortic root, RV, LV, and LV apex (see Figure 4.10) and establishes the standard cardiac views based on this information. The scanner displays the calculated reference points to allow the scanner operator make adjustments if necessary.

4.4   COMMON CMR TECHNIQUES

This section provides an overview of different imaging sequences in the CMR examination (Table 4.1). The following sections focus on cine imaging and derived measures of heart function.

4.4.1   MORPHOLOGY IMAGING

Structural and anatomical information can be obtained through the use of common morphology imaging protocols. In general, morphology images are acquired as a stack of parallel slices cutting through the anatomical region of interest. There are two main types of morphology imaging sequences: bright-blood and black-blood sequences. Morphology images are usually recorded in single-shot mode allowing for rapid and substantial anatomical coverage.

4.4.1.1   Bright-Blood Imaging

Bright-blood morphology sequences commonly use SSFP readouts without any preparation pulses. SSFP produces images in which blood appears bright and muscle appears dark. The contrast generated, to first order, is T2/T1 weighted (Simonetti et al. 2001). Figure 4.11 shows clinical examples of such images in the three main planes along the scanner axes. Table 4.1 specifies typical protocol parameters of a bright-blood SSFP sequence.

4.4.1.2   Dark-Blood Imaging

Morphology can also be imaged with a turbo-spin echo (TSE) readout, where flowing blood appears relatively dark. However, intrinsic blood signal suppression is often incomplete and flow and motion artifacts are common. Therefore, TSE is always combined with a dark-blood preparation (DB-prep) module to null the blood signal and minimize

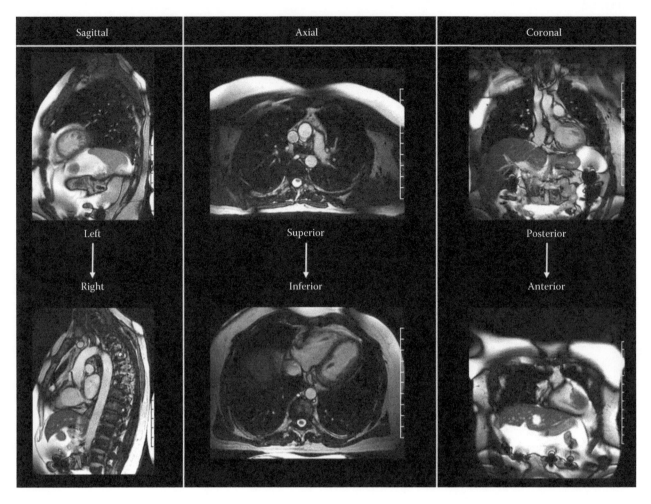

FIGURE 4.11 Bright-blood morphology images. The figure shows clinical images in the sagittal (left and right), axial (superior and inferior), and coronal (posterior and anterior) planes.

artifacts (Edelman et al. 1991). The single-shot version of TSE that is often used in CMR is the "half-Fourier acquisition single-shot TSE" (HASTE) sequence, which incorporates TSE imaging with fast partial raw data acquisition and DB-prep. Figure 4.12 shows typical HASTE images using imaging parameters similar to those in Table 4.1.

4.4.1.3 Which Sequence to Use?

The choice between bright-blood SSFP and dark-blood HASTE imaging depends on the clinical question. With bright-blood imaging, smaller brighter structures within the blood pool may be obscured, but dark structures are easy to identify. In dark-blood imaging, stagnant blood flow can cause incomplete black-blood preparation, resulting in blood appearing bright adjacent to stationary structures.

Since both scans can cover the entire thorax in less than 2 minutes, it is usually best to use both techniques to prevent any ambiguity in the findings. Additionally, if it is necessary to acquire higher spatial resolution images of certain key views, segmented imaging can be performed during a breath-hold scan. Dark-blood sequences should be performed before administration of a gadolinium-based contrast agent since the shortened blood T1 will impair suppression of the

blood signal. Bright-blood sequences can be performed before or after contrast agent administration.

4.4.2 Perfusion Imaging

4.4.2.1 Myocardial Perfusion at Stress and Rest

Over the last decade, a series of MRI technical and clinical advancements have led to the growing use of myocardial perfusion CMR imaging for the detection of coronary artery disease (CAD) (Rehwald et al. 2010). The American College of Cardiology Foundation (ACCF) Appropriateness Criteria Working Group has determined that, in patients with intermediate risk of CAD, the use of perfusion CMR is appropriate for evaluating chest pain and for determining the physiological significance of indeterminate coronary artery lesions (Hendel et al. 2006).

Perfusion CMR acquires a temporal series of single-shot images that are later played as a movie showing the transit of a gadolinium-based contrast media during its first pass through the myocardium, as shown in Figure 4.13a. Stress perfusion is performed during pharmacological vasodilation, usually with adenosine, which is administered at a dose of 140 μg/kg/min. While adenosine can cause some minor side effects such as

TABLE 4.1
Different Cardiac CMR Imaging Sequences and Parameter Settings

Imaging Type	Example Images	Important Protocol Parameters
Cine	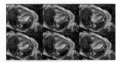	Segmented, breath hold, SSFP readout, TE = 1.27 ms, TR = 2.54 ms, flip angle = 55–90°, segments = 13, calculated phases = 25, trigger pulse = 1, slice thickness = 6 mm, bandwidth = 1302 Hz/pixel, matrix size = 256 × 190
Morphology (bright blood)		Single shot, free breathing, SSFP readout, TE = 1.14 ms, TR = 2.7 ms, flip angle = 60°, segments = 65, trigger pulse = 1, slice thickness = 6 mm, bandwidth = 1149 Hz/pixel, matrix size = 256 × 184
Morphology (HASTE, black blood)		Single shot, free breathing, TSE readout, TE = 55 ms, echo spacing = 4.2, flip angle = 90°, segments = 65, trigger pulse = 3, slice thickness = 8 mm, bandwidth = 751 Hz/pixel, darkblood preparation module, matrix size = 256 × 161
Stress perfusion imaging		Single shot, breath hold during first pass, GRE readout, TE = 1.17 ms, TI = 100–120 ms, flip angle = 12°, segments = 60, trigger pulse = 1, slice thickness = 8 mm, bandwidth = 849 Hz/pixel, matrix size = 256 × 176
Delayed enhancement (T1-weighted imaging)	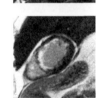	*Single shot*: Free breathing, SSFP readout, TE = 1.17 ms, echo spacing = 2.8 ms, TI = 300–400 ms, (or 800–900 ms for thrombus imaging), flip angle = 55°, segments = 63, trigger pulse = 2, slice thickness = 6 mm, bandwidth = 1028 Hz/pixel, matrix size = 256 × 208 *Segmented GRE*: Breath hold, GRE readout, TE = 1.86 ms, echo spacing = 5 ms, flip angle = 19°, segments = 35, trigger pulse = 2, slice thickness = 6 mm, bandwidth = 332 Hz/pixel, matrix size = 320 × 240 *Segmented SSFP*: Breath hold, SSFP readout, TE = 1.17 ms, echo spacing = 2.8 ms, flip angle = 55°, segments = 13, trigger pulse = 2, slice thickness = 6 mm, bandwidth = 1028 Hz/pixel matrix size = 320 × 240
T2-weighted imaging (turbo spin echo)	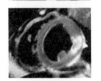	Segmented, breath hold, TSE readout, TE = 68 ms, echo spacing 3.38, flip angle = 90°, turbo factor = 25, trigger pulse = 2, slice thickness = 6 mm, bandwidth = 888 Hz/pixel, matrix size = 256 × 192, black blood prep, SPAIR fat suppression
T2* imaging	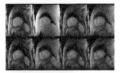	Single shot with multiple measurements (8), breath hold, GRE readout, TEs = 1.9, 3.8, 6.1, 8.4, 10.7, 13.0, 15.2, and 17.5 ms, flip angle = 20°, segments = 7, trigger pulse = 1, slice thickness = 10 mm, bandwidth = 1300 Hz/pixel, matrix size = 192 × 124
Contrast-enhanced MR angiography		Segmented, breath hold, ECG gated, GRE readout, TE = 1.04 ms, echo spacing = 3.72 ms, flip angle = 25°, trigger pulse = 1, bandwidth = 650 Hz/pixel, matrixsize = 320 × 280 × 230
Flow velocity imaging		Segmented, breath hold, GRE readout, TE = 2.25 ms, flip angle = 15°, segments = 4, calculated phases = 30, slice thickness = 6 mm, bandwidth = 574 Hz/pixel, matrix size = 256 × 200, VENC = 80 cm/s (pulmonary veins), 200 cm/s (aortic valve), 150 cm/s (pulmonic valve)

Abbreviations: SPAIR, spectral attenuated with adiabatic inversion recovery; TI, inversion time; TSE, turbo spin echo; VENC, velocity encoding.

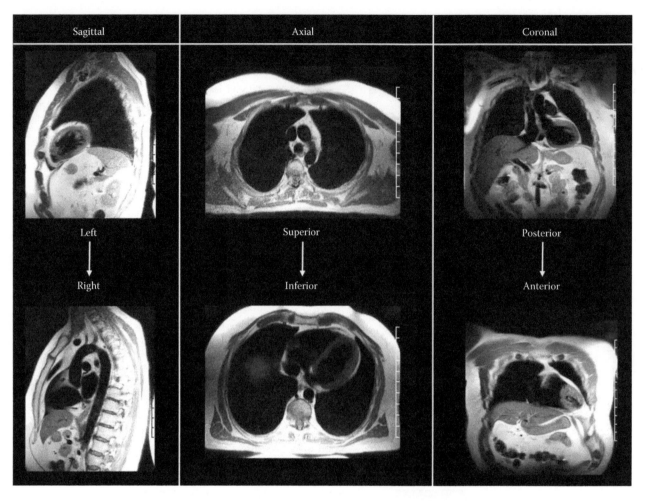

FIGURE 4.12   Black-blood morphology images. The figure shows clinical images in the sagittal (left and right), axial (superior and inferior), and coronal (posterior and anterior) planes.

chest discomfort, serious side effects such as bronchospasm or atrio-ventricular block are rare. Due to its short half-life of less than 10 seconds, side effects can be quickly resolved by turning off the adenosine infusion. Adenosine causes vasodilation and, in normal coronary arteries, can increase coronary blood flow four- to fivefold relative to baseline (Wilson et al. 1990). However, in the presence of a significant coronary artery stenosis, these large increases in blood flow are not possible. This results in blood flow difference between the territories supplied by the stenosed vessels showing little or no flow increase, and the territories supplied by normal arteries exhibiting a multifold increase in blood flow. Different local blood flow causes different amounts of the contrast agent to be delivered regionally, which is reflected as different myocardial signal intensities in the T1-weighted perfusion images. A perfusion defect is typically represented by a "hypoenhanced," darker area, as shown in the region of interest (ROI) highlighted by the red arrow in the four right images in Figure 4.13a. In Figure 4.13b, the myocardial signal intensity in the red and blue ROIs in the precontrast image in Figure 4.13a is plotted versus time. The dotted blue curve, representing normally perfused myocardium, peaks earlier and at a higher level than the red dashed curve, representing the perfusion defect.

As a last step of a CMR examination, the same perfusion scan is repeated at rest, meaning in absence of a stress agent. Comparison of stress and rest scans and of delayed-enhancement images at the same slice locations allows for identifying reversibly and irreversibly injured myocardium (Klem et al. 2006).

4.4.2.2   Data Acquisition

The perfusion data readout strategy that is most commonly employed uses an ECG-triggered, single-shot, spoiled GRE sequence with the vendor-specific names FLASH (Siemens), Spoiled Grass (SPGR; GE), and T1 Fast Field Echo (T1-FFE; Philips). The image contrast is T1-weighted, which is typically implemented by a saturation-recovery (SR) preparation pulse plus time delay applied prior to each readout. In order to visualize the perfusion defect during the contrast agent wash-in, the acquired images must have sufficient temporal resolution. Here, temporal resolution stands for the time between two consecutive single shots at the same slice location, and not for the time per shot. In clinical practice, every slice location is typically scanned once per heartbeat resulting in a temporal resolution equal to the RR interval, which is sufficient to pick up perfusion defects. This temporal resolution

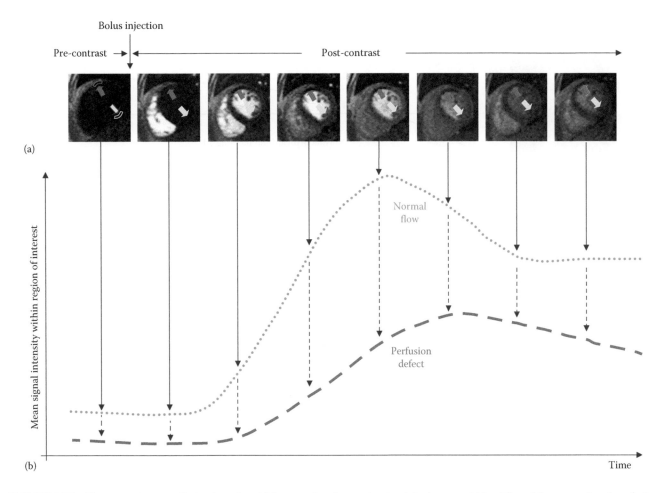

FIGURE 4.13 First-pass stress perfusion imaging. (a) Images showing contrast uptake in normal blood flow (blue arrows) and perfusion defect (red arrows). (b) Signal intensity in normal blood flow and perfusion defect.

limits the total number of slices that can fit within a single RR interval. In general, the total scan time per image must be at least 100 ms to ensure adequate spatial resolution, SNR, and contrast-to-noise ratio (CNR); but should not exceed 200 ms to allow for a reasonable slices coverage. A longer time delay between the SR pulse and readout results in better image contrast and SNR, while a shorter delay allows for more slices per RR interval. A compromise between image contrast and the number of slices is achieved at the scan time, considering the patient's heart rate as well as the number of slices needed to cover the entire ventricle (heart size). Perfusion imaging is typically performed for 40–60 heartbeats, during which 40–60 images are collected at 4–6 different short-axis slice locations.

4.4.3 Delayed Enhancement

4.4.3.1 Myocardial Viability

Delayed enhancement (DE-CMR), also called late gadolinium enhancement (LGE), is a method that can simultaneously evaluate myocardial infarction (MI) and viability (Kim et al. 1999, Fieno et al. 2000, Ricciardi et al. 2001, Simonetti et al. 2001, Wagner et al. 2003). DE-CMR can identify the presence, extent, and location of both chronic and acute MI

(Ricciardi et al. 2001, Simonetti et al. 2001, Wu et al. 2001), which has shown to provide improved detection of subendocardial MI relative to SPECT (Wagner et al. 2003).

Following intravenous administration of gadolinium contrast agent, DE-CMR differentiates abnormal myocardial tissue in which there is an excess accumulation of the contrast agent relative to normal tissue. The optimal image contrast between abnormal tissue and normal myocardium is acquired using a segmented GRE or SSFP acquisition with an inversion recovery (IR) pulse that provides heavy T1 weighting (Kim et al. 1999, Fieno et al. 2000, Simonetti et al. 2001, Wu et al. 2001, Wagner et al. 2003). Figure 4.14 shows a typical DE-CMR image on the left and the normal-myocardium and infarct T1-relaxation curves (after applying the inversion recovery pulse) on the right. Data are acquired when the signal of the T1-recovery curve of normal myocardium is about zero. This is commonly known as "nulling" of normal myocardium. The time of data acquisition relative to the inversion pulse is controlled by the "inversion time" (TI), which is a protocol parameter on every scanner UI. The infarct has shorter T1, secondary to preferential accumulation of the gadolinium contrast agent in it, and thus its signal has substantially recovered at TI, and thus it appears bright in the CMR image, whereas normal myocardium appears dark (nulled).

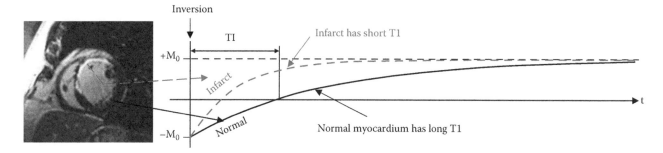

FIGURE 4.14 An example DE-CMR image and the T1-relaxation curves of normal and infarcted myocardium. Inversion time (TI) is adjusted such that the normal myocardium signal crosses zero (is "nulled") at the time of data readout.

The DE-CMR contrast is optimal approximately 10–15 minutes after a one time intravenous injection of a gadolinium chelate dose of 0.1–0.20 mmol/kg. This time delay allows for both adequate distribution of the contrast agent throughout different tissues, and for reduction of the contrast agent concentration in the blood pool. If images are acquired too soon after contrast agent injection, as shown in the top image of Figure 4.15a, it can be difficult to identify subendocardial infarcts. Data are acquired on every other heartbeat to ensure adequate recovery of the longitudinal magnetization between the inversion pulses. If bradycardia is present, imaging can occur on every heartbeat (Kim et al. 2003). It is also possible to use a single-shot, real-time version of DE-CMR to acquire lower resolution images without breath-holds (Li et al. 2004,

Sievers et al. 2007). This technique provides complete LV coverage in less than 30 seconds. It can be considered the preferred approach in acutely ill patients, patients unable to breath-hold, or those with irregular heart rhythms.

4.4.3.2 Nonischemic Cardiomyopathies

DE-CMR can be also used for the evaluation of nonischemic cardiomyopathies, such as hypertrophic cardiomyopathy (Choudhury et al. 2002, Moon et al. 2003a,b, Shah et al. 2005), dilated cardiomyopathy (McCrohon et al. 2003, Bellenger et al. 2004, Assomull et al. 2006), sarcoidosis (Patel et al. 2004), and arrhythmogenic RV dysplasia (ARVD). Typical examples of DE-CMR nonischemic cardiomyopathies are shown in Figure 4.15b.

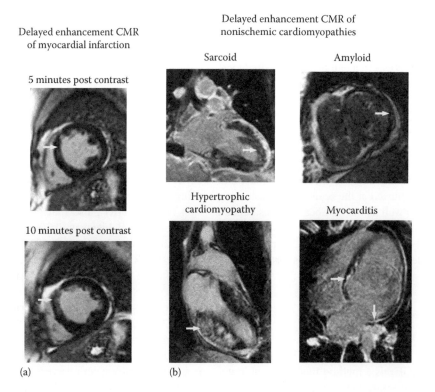

FIGURE 4.15 Examples of DE-CMR images. (a) DE-CMR images should be acquired more than 10 minutes after contrast is administered so there is sufficient contrast between the myocardium, infarct, and blood pool (arrows). (b) DE-CMR can be also used to diagnose a range of nonischemic cardiomyopathies (arrows), as shown by example images of sarcoid, amyloid, hypertrophic cardiomyopathy, and myocarditis.

4.4.4 T1, T2, and T2* Imaging

Multi-contrast imaging is useful for tissue characterization, for example, differentiating acute from chronic myocardial infarction, as well as inflammation, as in myocarditis. In plaque imaging, multi-contrast imaging is used to identify different plaque components, for example, lipid core, fibrous tissue, and fibrous cap. Multi-contrast imaging is also used to investigate the presence of edema or cystic fluid.

4.4.4.1 T1-Weighted Imaging

T1-weighted (T1W) imaging is widely used in CMR. The most common applications are DE-CMR and myocardial perfusion imaging, as already discussed in the previous sections. Additional applications include detection of thrombus and characterization of cardiac masses. In general, T1-weighting is provided by either an IR or saturation recovery (SR) pulse. Depending on the application, different data readouts can be used to provide additional T1-weighting. For example, a GRE readout with a short TR increases T1-weighting. In triggered TSE imaging, T1-weighting is achieved by setting short effective TE and short TR (trigger pulse of 1).

4.4.4.2 T2-Weighted Imaging

T2-weighted (T2W) imaging has shown promise for assessing acute, inflammatory processes (Abdel-Aty et al. 2004), such as in the setting of myocardial necrosis, acute MI, or active myocarditis. In these cases, the myocardial tissue becomes edematous as its water content increases measurably within the region of necrosis (Whalen et al. 1974). As a result, edematous myocardium has a longer intrinsic T2, for example, between 60 and 65 ms in acute infarct, but only 45–50 ms in normal myocardium (Kellman et al. 2007).

There are two main approaches for acquiring T2W images of the heart: TSE with a long effective TE, and T2-prepared SSFP, as shown in Figure 4.16. TSE images are usually acquired with a DB-prep and T2-weighting is achieved by using a long effective TE of 50–80 ms. T1-weighting and fat suppression can be added through the application of a third inversion pulse, known as short TI inversion recovery (STIR)

imaging. The third inversion pulse suppresses the fat signal and, additionally, may improve the contrast between edematous and normal areas by providing some T1-weighting. The choice of other parameters, including slice thickness, preferred receiver coil, and analysis method, are often institution specific, and there is no consensus protocol for their settings. With appropriate settings, T2W-TSE or STIR-TSE can depict edematous regions as bright or "hyperintense" (red arrow in Figure 4.16a), whereas nonedematous regions appear gray (yellow arrow in Figure 4.16a).

One disadvantage of TSE imaging is that it is highly sensitive to motion. Motion artifacts can be minimized by carefully selecting the TSE readout timing, but this is difficult for high heart rates, and it is almost impossible to prevent artifacts in the presence of arrhythmias (Kellman et al. 2007). Single-shot T2-prepared SSFP imaging provides an alternative to the dark-blood TSE for T2-weighted imaging. T2-prepared SSFP uses a T2-preparation module played prior to the SSFP readout. A T2-preparation module (Brittain et al. 2005) consists of a 90° flip angle, followed by a train of two to four refocusing pulses, and a final flip-back pulse. The refocusing pulses impart T2-weighting on the transverse magnetization, and the flip-back pulse returns the T2-prepared magnetization to the longitudinal direction, ready for imaging. By increasing the time between the refocusing pulses (T2-prep time), more T2-weighting can be generated. For edema imaging, T2-preparation times of about 60 ms are used. This method has several advantages: no breath-holds, less motion sensitivity, and higher diagnostic accuracy than dark-blood TSE with respect to determining the coronary artery distribution and differentiation of acute from chronic MI (Kellman et al. 2007). Figure 4.16b shows a T2-prepared SSFP image of the same slice as in Figure 4.16a. The tissue with elevated signal intensity matches between the two images.

4.4.4.3 T2* Imaging

T2* imaging can be used in patients with known or suspected hemolytic anemia and/or iron overload pathologies to exclude the presence of cardiac siderosis (Anderson et al. 2001).

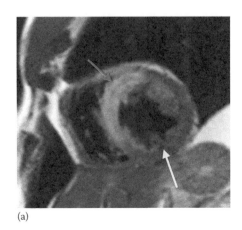
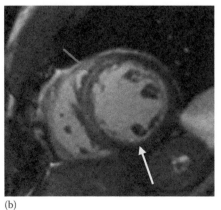

(a)   (b)

FIGURE 4.16 T2-weighted imaging of myocardial edema. The figure shows (a) black-blood T2W-TSE and (b) bright-blood T2-prepared SSFP images. The red arrows indicate edematous regions due to acute MI. The normal myocardium appears gray (yellow arrow).

Similar to the T2 transverse relaxation time, T2* describes the decay of the magnetization vector in the transverse plane, but the T2* time constant also incorporates reversible dephasing effects caused by magnetic field inhomogeneities and susceptibility effects. Iron accumulation in tissue causes both magnetic field inhomogeneities and susceptibility effects. By determining the T2* value of the tissue, the amount of myocardial iron can be estimated (Anderson et al. 2001).

T2* mapping is performed by acquiring a series of single-shot GRE images with different TE values. The TE values range from a minimum, dictated by the scanner hardware, to a maximum of approximately 20 ms. TE values longer than 20 ms result in very low SNR and do not improve the calculation of T2*. For every pixel, an exponential decay curve is fitted to the signals obtained at the different TEs, and the T2* value is extracted from the fitted curve (Anderson et al. 2001).

While T2* imaging is used at some imaging centers, it is not yet part of a standard clinical CMR examination. More clinical information about iron imaging will be provided in the section about cutting-edge CMR techniques at the end of this chapter.

4.4.5 MR Angiography (MRA) and Coronary Imaging

4.4.5.1 Contrast-Enhanced Angiography

When combined with morphological imaging, contrast-enhanced magnetic resonance angiography (CEMRA) can be used to fully define arterial or venous structures (Maki et al. 1998, Neimatallah et al. 1999, Carr et al. 2002). Angiograms are particularly useful for determining vascular anatomy in patients with congenital defects (Hartnell et al. 1996). An angiography scan is quite frequently combined with velocity-encoding (VENC) imaging to examine abnormal flow patterns and measure blood flow velocity.

In a CEMRA examination, two high-resolution 3D datasets of the vasculature of interest are acquired. First, the angiography sequence is run in the absence of a contrast agent. The acquisition is then repeated during a bolus injection of contrast agent. The use of a T1 shortening contrast agent, such as a gadolinium-based agent, allows for the generation of high signal intensity within the vascular bed relative to the surrounding tissues. The two datasets are post-processed to remove the surrounding tissue by subtracting the dataset acquired before contrast agent injection from that acquired during contrast injection. The removal of the surrounding tissue allows for a clean 3D reconstruction of the vasculature. The data are often displayed as a maximum intensity projection (MIP), where multiple MIPs from all view directions can be combined into a rotating 3D movie of the vasculature. It is also possible to reconstruct the data using a volume rendering technique (VRT), which allows for the visualization of the vasculature from any angle.

When acquiring images of structures that move either due to cardiac motion or pulsatile flow, ECG-triggering is critical to minimize blurring artifacts. For highly dynamic structures such as the ascending aorta, it is important to acquire the images during diastole, and also to take into account the time at early diastole, during which there is passive relaxation of the aorta due to elastic recoil. This short period of "diastolic vessel relaxation" leads to appreciable vascular motion that can blur the edges of the angiogram and compromise its quality. Figure 4.17 shows an example of an ECG-triggered, contrast-enhanced angiogram after routine post-processing. The MIP in Figure 4.17a demonstrates subclavian artery stenosis. In this example, the aortic arch demonstrates a bovine branching pattern. This is a normal variant wherein the innominate artery and left common carotid artery (1) have a common origin. The right common carotid artery arises at an acute angle from the right innominate artery causing a kink in the vessel, which appears in the image as signal void (2). The image in Figure 4.17b is an example from a different

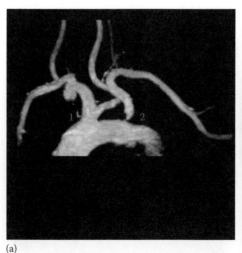 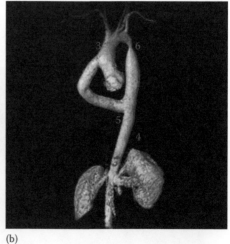

(a)   (b)

FIGURE 4.17 Example of MIP-constructed contrast-enhanced angiograms in patients with (a) subclavian artery stenosis and (b) aortic graft. (a) Subclavian artery stenosis showing the innominate artery and left common carotid artery having a common origin (1), and the right common carotid artery arising at an acute angle from the right innominate artery, shown as signal void (2). (b) Aortic graft between the ascending thoracic aorta (3) and descending thoracic aorta (4) (at the level of the base of the left atrium (5)), bypassing an aortic coarctation (6).

patient with an aortic graft between the ascending thoracic aorta (3) and descending thoracic aorta (4). The graft extends rightward then wraps around the heart and reconnects into the descending aorta at the level of the base of the left atrium (5). This graft bypasses the coarctation of the aorta (6).

4.4.5.2 Coronary Imaging

Coronary MRA may be used to directly visualize coronary anatomy and morphology. Coronary MRA images are acquired using a 3D, navigated sequence (Stuber and Weiss 2007) with an SSFP or GRE readout and with magnetization preparation (T2-preparation or magnetization transfer) implemented prior to each readout to differentiate the lumen from myocardium (Ehman and Felmlee 1989, Brittain et al. 2005). Coronary MRA is technically demanding due to the combined effects of cardiac motion and small size of the coronary arteries (3–5 mm), leading to vessel blurring. The precise assessment of stenosis severity and visualization of distal segments is difficult, leading to intermediate sensitivity and specificity values for the detection of CAD in validation studies (Kim et al. 2001). Currently, the only clinical indication that is considered appropriate for coronary MRA is evaluation of patients with suspected coronary anomalies (Hendel et al. 2006).

4.4.6 Flow Velocity Imaging

4.4.6.1 Idea of Operation

Velocity-encoding CMR (VENC-CMR) employs a segmented cine sequence with GRE readout, breath-holding, and ECG triggering. The sequence is similar to standard GRE, but includes a matched pair of gradients with identical areas and opposite polarities (bipolar gradient) that causes moving spins, such as flowing blood, to acquire a phase shift (Pelc et al. 1992, Debatin et al. 1994, Saloner 1999). The first gradient pulse dephases the spins based on their spatial location, where in the absence of motion or flow, the second gradient pulse reverses this dephasing so that no net phase is acquired. If the spins are moving while experiencing both gradients, then they are refocused by the second gradient with a phase shift relative to the stationary case. This phase shift is proportional to the velocity and direction of the motion, so that speed and travel direction can be calculated.

VENC-CMR is also called phase-contrast CMR (PC-CMR) and can be used for quantification of flow and motion, similar to Doppler echocardiography. Two sets of images must be acquired to account for phase shifts due to other factors. The first image (with the bipolar gradient) contains phase due to flow as well as background phase due to other unknown effects, while the second image (without the bipolar gradient) is independent of flow or "flow-compensated," but still contains the same background phase. Subtracting the flow-compensated image from the velocity-encoded image results in a phase difference image that contains flow information only.

There are important differences between VENC-CMR and Doppler echocardiography. With VENC-CMR, blood flow through an orifice is directly measured en-face with "through-plane" velocity encoding, while Doppler echocardiography measures the blood flow profile indirectly, which has uniform velocity across the vessel. This allows VENC-CMR for directly imaging structures that are difficult to visualize by echocardiography, for example, baffles, sinus venosus, and atrial septal defects (ASDs). A disadvantage of VENC-CMR is that it is usually not performed in real time, and requires breath-holding to minimize respiratory motion artifacts. Consequentially, it is difficult to measure changes in flow that occur with respiration.

4.4.6.2 VENC and Velocity Aliasing

The velocity-encoding value (VENC) is set by the scanner operator, which is optimized when set to the highest anticipated velocity. In this case, the largest encoded velocity produces a phase shift of +180°. Figure 4.18a shows the acquired phase shift as a function of blood flow velocity for a VENC of 100 cm/s. If the VENC value is set lower than the maximum velocity found in the imaged vessel, then spins moving faster than the VENC value will accumulate a phase shift larger than 180°. For example, spins that create a phase shift of +185° are interpreted as having phase shift of −175° and appear to have the opposite polarity, which is referred to as aliasing. In panel Figure 4.18b, the red arrow points out a region of aliasing in the phase-contrast image; it is the dark region within the otherwise bright vessel. Figure 4.18c shows an analogous example where the VENC was correctly set. Note that this panel shows reverse flow, which is represented by a dark color.

4.4.6.3 Flow Patterns

The assumption that velocity is uniform across the vessel lumen is not true in all cases. The type of blood flow depends on many factors including vessel diameter and flow velocity. In long, large vessels (e.g., aorta and pulmonary arteries), the flow is usually laminar, with a parabolic velocity profile having almost zero velocity at the walls and maximal velocity in the center of the vessel, as shown in the first and last profiles of Figure 4.19a. Flowing blood around a curve, for example, in the aortic arch, tends to skew toward the outer wall of the aorta due to the viscous and inertial properties of blood, as shown in Figure 4.19a (Kilner et al. 1993b). In branch vessels, distal to a bifurcation, for example, the iliac or carotid bifurcation, the parabolic profile skews toward the inner edges of the bifurcated vessels, which then develops back into a parabolic profile downstream of the bifurcation, as shown in Figure 4.19b (Zarins et al. 1983). A stenosis causes an increase in velocity through the narrow region, and centrally distal to the stenosis, with nonlaminar (possibly turbulent) flow surrounding the centralized jet, as shown in Figure 4.19c (Menon et al. 2012). In certain areas of the body where flow is not fully developed, for example, near the aortic valve, the velocity profile is more blunted (pluglike), because the parabolic profile has not had time to fully develop due to high acceleration when the valve first opens. In large arteries throughout the cardiac cycle, a fully developed, pulsatile flow can be described as a Womersley profile, as shown in Figure 4.19d. The profile is drawn for time points A through E, where the deceleration of flow at point C causes a W-shaped profile across the vessel. Arterial blood flow is pulsatile in nature,

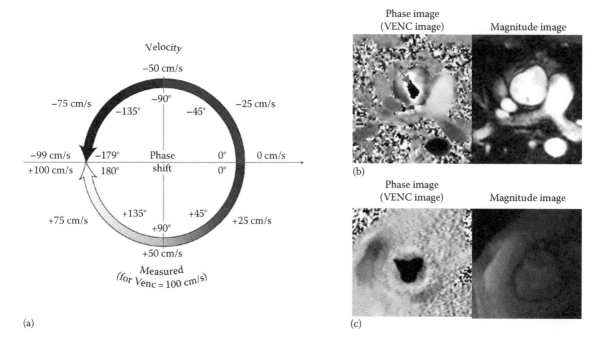

FIGURE 4.18   Description and examples of velocity-encoded imaging. (a) VENC is the velocity at which the phase angle is ±180°. Max velocity in one direction is white, while max velocity in the opposite direction is black. (b) Too low VENC causing aliasing (black pixels in the center of the white signal). (c) Correctly selected VENC eliminates the aliasing artifact (flow direction here is encoded in the opposite direction, i.e., appears black; not bright).

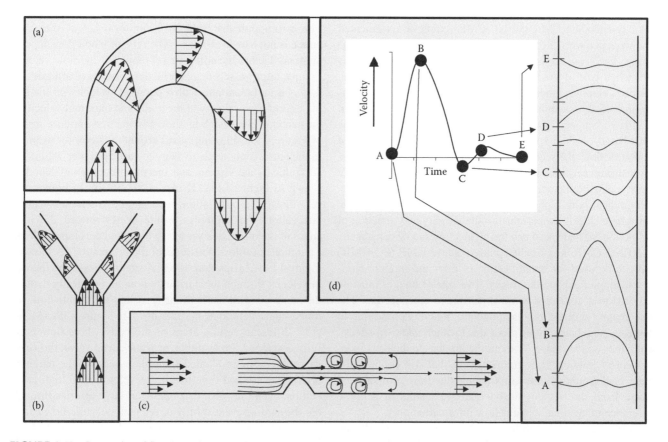

FIGURE 4.19   Properties of flow in various vessels. (a) Thoracic aorta showing inertial forces skewing the velocity profile toward the outer wall. (b) Bifurcating vessel showing skewing toward the inner wall nearest the flow divider. (c) Influence of stenosis on downstream flow characteristics. (d) Womersley velocity profile of pulsatile flow in large arteries throughout the cardiac cycle.

with a period defined by the cardiac cycle. VENC-CMR can visualize velocities within the vessel providing a more sensitive measure of velocity than Doppler echocardiography.

4.4.6.4 Applications

Commonly used clinical measures from blood flow imaging are the absolute maximum, or peak, systolic velocity in units of m/s or cm/s to assess aortic stenosis, average flow (total, forward, and reverse) to assess valve regurgitation, and cardiac output. Shunts between pulmonary and systemic circulation are evaluated by measuring pulmonary flow (Q_P) and systemic blood flow (Q_S), and calculating the Q_P/Q_S flow ratio.

4.5 CINE IMAGING

The excellent spatial and temporal resolutions of cine CMR makes it an ideal tool for imaging cardiac contractile function. It is a fundamental part of almost every CMR examination and has become widely accepted as the noninvasive gold standard for contractile function assessment. Cine CMR provides a wealth of cardiac functional parameters, including global function, regional LV and RV wall motion, ventricular volume, ejection fraction, and mass measurements. It has been used as an endpoint for the evaluation of LV remodeling (Lamb et al. 2002, Friedrich et al. 2003, Bellenger et al. 2004) and as a

reference method for other imaging techniques (Ioannidis et al. 2002, Kjaergaard et al. 2006, Fischbach et al. 2007).

4.5.1 BASICS OF CINE CMR

4.5.1.1 Imaging the Heart Function

4.5.1.1.1 Heart Coverage

The cine CMR sequence provides a movie of the beating heart, visualizing its contractile function. The standard protocol acquires images using segmented acquisition with ECG synchronization and breath-holding. For patients with severely impaired breathing or arrhythmia, real-time cine techniques are available that allow for free breathing and do not require an ECG signal.

Typically, a stack of multiple closely spaced (contiguous or with 1–2 mm gaps) short-axis slices of 6–8 mm thickness is acquired to provide full coverage of the left and right ventricles. Short-axis views, perpendicular to the long-axis views, can be planned on long-axis scout images, as described earlier. In addition, cine images can be obtained in multiple long-axis orientations, such as the two-chamber, three-chamber, or four-chamber views.

Figure 4.20 shows cine images where the cardiac phases are individually displayed, instead of being combined into one

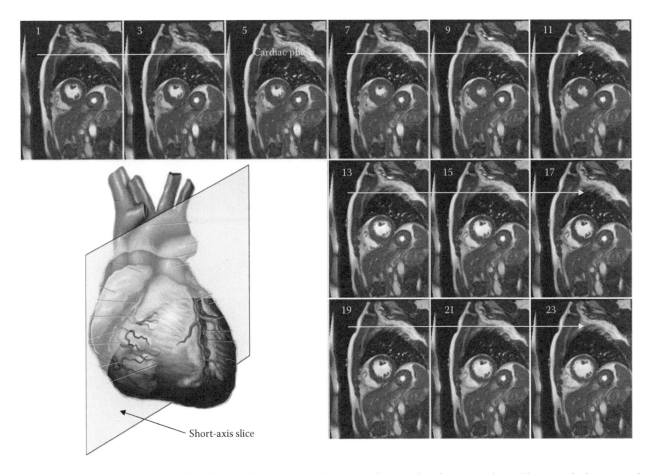

FIGURE 4.20 Individual frames (cardiac phases) of a cine movie. Twelve out of twenty-four frames are shown. Note ventricular contraction and thickening during systole (cardiac phases 1–9).

moving image. In this example, a single mid-ventricular short-axis slice with 24 images representing 24 cardiac phases was acquired. Cardiac phase (cine frame) number 1 corresponds to the first phase after the R-wave, frame 9 to peak-systole, and frame 23 to late diastole. Typically, 20–30 cine frames are acquired with 30–50 ms temporal resolution.

4.5.1.1.2 GRE and SSFP Sequences

Originally, cine images were acquired using a GRE readout, which is largely T1-weighted. Due to the long T1 of blood, blood-myocardium contrast depends on the inflow of fresh (bright) blood. Slow blood exchange, as common in long-axis slices or with reduced cardiac function, combined with short TR, results in saturation of the blood signal, thus reducing the image contrast (Finn et al. 2006). Therefore, currently, images are routinely acquired with SSFP due to its high SNR, fast speed, less flow dependency, and excellent blood-to-myocardium contrast.

In the majority of patients, SSFP provides excellent image quality and blood-myocardium contrast, but in the case of high velocity jets or in the presence of metallic prosthetic valves, SSFP can exhibit severe flow artifacts and signal dropout. Under these circumstances, switching to GRE yields better image quality despite its lower SNR. The loss of SNR and CNR can be overcome to some extent by acquiring the images after the administration of contrast agent. The contrast agent

significantly shortens T1 of blood, reducing the saturation of the blood signal.

To date, 2D imaging is still the clinical method of choice in CMR cine imaging. Nevertheless, with improvement in acquisition speed powered by recent advances in parallel acquisition (Sodickson and Manning 1997, Pruessmann et al. 1999, Griswold et al. 2002), parallel transmission (Katscher and Bornert 2006), and higher field strength, 3D cine acquisition of an entire short-axis stack within a single breath-hold may replace 2D cine imaging in the future.

4.5.1.2 Segmented Data Acquisition and Data Sorting

Segmented image acquisition is the primary acquisition strategy for cine imaging. Briefly, segmented acquisition refers to distributing the acquisition of raw data over many heartbeats in order to improve spatial and temporal resolutions. As the acquisition of one segment occupies only a small fraction of the cardiac cycle, then multiple segments can be acquired throughout the cardiac cycle. Each segment contains the same lines of k-space, but is acquired at a different time within the RR interval, and thus represents a different cardiac phase. Figure 4.21 illustrates this concept with typical imaging parameters of 20 lines per segment, 25 cardiac phases, and 8 heartbeats needed to collect all the data. During each heartbeat, a different segment (different lines of k-space) is acquired. In the first heartbeat, the first segment (lines 1–20) is acquired

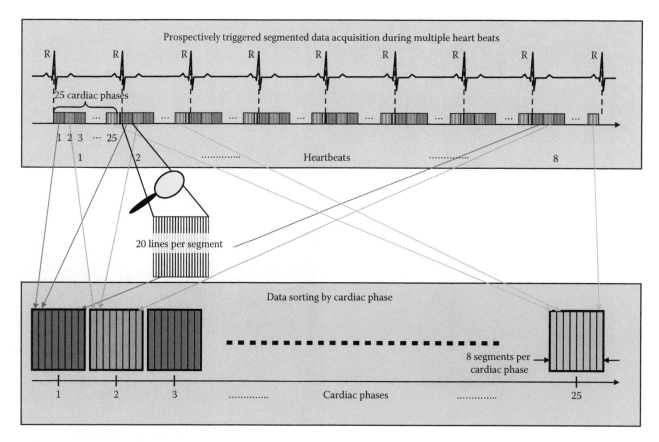

FIGURE 4.21 Data acquisition and sorting in a prospectively triggered segmented cine sequence. The 1st segment acquired after the R-wave is colored in red, the 2nd in orange, the 3rd in blue, and the 25th in green. Assume that the small gray region after each green segment is a dead time of about 10% of the RR.

for all cardiac phases. In the second heartbeat, the second segment (lines 21–40) is acquired for all cardiac phases, and this pattern is repeated until all the lines of k-spaces are acquired. Note that in Figure 4.21, the color-coding refers to the cardiac phase of the segment, not the heartbeat during which a segment was acquired. After 8 heartbeats, all 8 segments for all 25 cardiac phases are collected, with 160 k-space lines per phase (20 lines per segment × 8 heartbeats = 160 lines). A total of 4000 lines (160 lines per phase × 25 phases = 4000 lines) are acquired. After acquisition, the raw data are sorted according to its cardiac phase, as shown by the colored arrows. The resulting images can be displayed as frames of a movie depicting the beating heart.

When cine imaging was first introduced, data segmentation had not been invented yet (Lenz et al. 1989). Instead, only the first raw data line (k-space line number 1) was acquired throughout the first heartbeat, then the second line during the second heartbeat, and so on. The acquisition of an entire cine dataset therefore took $RR \times N_L$, where N_L is the number of lines per cardiac phase. For example, for RR of 800 ms and N_L of 160 lines, a total of 128 seconds (2 minutes, 8 seconds) of data acquisition is required, which is beyond breath-holding capability. Therefore, the scans were performed during free breathing and multiple averages were acquired to reduce breathing artifacts, further increasing scan time. With the introduction of segmented acquisition, the acquisition time could be dropped to $RR \times N_L/N_{LPS}$, where N_{LPS} is the number of lines per segment. Using $N_{LPS} = 20$, data acquisition in this scenario takes about 6.4 seconds, which is well within most patients' breath-holding capability.

4.5.1.3 Data Acquisition Strategies

4.5.1.3.1 Prospective Triggering

The previously described data acquisition strategy uses a synchronization method known as "prospective triggering." In this approach, the assignment of the acquired lines to different cardiac phases is already known ahead of time, "prospectively," and is based solely on the acquisition time after R-wave detection. The R-waves serve as sequence "triggers," shown as vertical black dashed lines in Figure 4.21. The triggers prompt the sequence to run, starting with acquisition of the red segment. The acquisition is generally interrupted near end-diastole in order to wait for the next R-wave, causing about 10% of the RR interval to be spent waiting for the next trigger. The problem with this approach is that T1 recovery occurs during the dead time so that the magnetization is no longer at the steady-state condition. As a consequence, the first cardiac phase has significantly more signal than the last phase. When played as a cine loop, the abrupt change in image intensity between the last and consecutive first phase is visible as "lightning artifact" (Lenz et al. 1989). Additionally, ghosting artifacts can occur due to the varying RR duration, resulting in signal intensity fluctuations between segments. This effect occurs with both GRE and SSFP readouts, but the artifacts are much worse with SSFP, as establishing steady-state is the underlying condition for SSFP to function without major

artifacts. For all these reasons, maintaining a steady-state condition is very important for cine imaging. In prospectively triggered sequences, "dummy readouts" (or "dummy pulses" or "dummy excitations") have been introduced to maintain steady-state magnetization. The exact number of dummy readouts depends on the length of each RR.

4.5.1.3.2 Retrospective Gating

A more recent synchronization technique is called "retrospective gating" (Lenz et al. 1989) or "retro-gating," which forms the basis of the "retrospectively gated cine sequence." In this approach, the sequence is not triggered, but runs asynchronous to the ECG signal. Each recorded line receives a time stamp relative to the previous R-wave, allowing "gating" to the ECG signal after data acquisition is complete, "retrospectively." While gating and triggering are often mistakenly used synonymously, gating refers to the asynchronous data acquisition with later data sorting by timestamp to establish synchrony with the ECG, whereas triggering refers to synchronized data acquisition with the ECG signal. In retrospective gated sequences, interpolation is used to reconstruct the acquired data into a fixed number of equally-spaced cardiac phases. Fluctuations in the RR interval during the acquisition can potentially lead to more blurring than in prospective triggered sequence. In general, retrospective gating is a more robust synchronization method, with the advantages that it has more uniform signal intensity over time. To satisfy this condition in the case of fluctuations in the RR interval, each set of segments (e.g., the set of first segments) is acquired for about 120% of the average RR interval. As a result, each segment is asynchronously acquired over two RR intervals with varying data amounts from the first and second heartbeats; therefore image acquisition is about 20% longer than in the prospectively triggered case. Any number of cardiac phases can be reconstructed by temporally interpolating the data from time points before and after the desired time points.

4.5.1.3.3 Triggered Retro-Gating

The current clinical method of choice, called "triggered retro-gating," is a combination of prospective triggering and retrospective gating, which provides improved data acquisition compared to either technique. This method is also colloquially referred to as "retro-gated cine sequence," even though it combines triggering and gating. Similar to retrospective gating, the acquisition is continuous, but the switch to the next segment is triggered by the R-wave, as shown in Figure 4.22a. Image reconstruction is identical to that of the retrospectively gated sequence. Figure 4.22b shows data sorting and reconstruction for 20 lines per segment and about 25 cardiac phases acquired over 8 heartbeats. Because the recording is continuous and no two consecutive RR intervals are alike, after the 25th cardiac phase (green), a varying number of lines (pink) are recorded, 10 in the first RR of this example. Usually, more cardiac phases are reconstructed than acquired, and data are obtained using interpolation. Weighted averaging and nearest-neighbor interpolation are two obvious choices, and the selection is vendor-dependent.

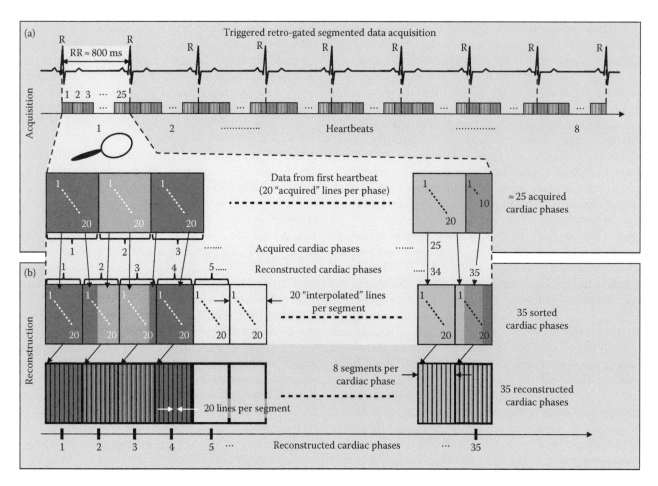

FIGURE 4.22 Triggered retro-gating cine acquisition. (a) Acquisition, and (b) data sorting in a triggered retro-gating segmented cine sequence. This example uses the same parameters and the same color scheme as in Figure 4.21. The area highlighted in light gray shows the line sorting of the first segment.

The example in Figure 4.22b (top panel) uses nearest-neighbor interpolation to sort the data of about 25 acquired phases into 35 reconstructed phases.

The time points of the reconstructed data can be calculated using the RR interval and number of reconstructed phases. The RR interval of 800 ms is divided into 35 reconstructed cardiac phases of about 23 ms each, centered at 11.5 ms (#1), 34.5 ms (#2), 57.5 ms (#3), 80.5 ms (#4), and so forth. The time points of the acquired (not interpolated) data are centered at 16 ms (#1), 48 ms (#2), 80 ms (#3), 112 ms (#4), etc. The acquired lines that are closest to the time point of the reconstructed cardiac phase are used to create the reconstructed phase. For example, the lines for the first reconstructed phase (centered at 11.5 ms) are taken from the first acquired phase, as they are closest to the 11.5 ms. However, the lines for the second phase (at 34.5 ms) are taken partly from the first and second acquired phases. The exact sorting depends on the time stamp of each acquired line and the desired time point of the reconstructed cardiac phase.

4.5.1.3.4 Challenges with Arrhythmia

Arrhythmias pose the most significant challenge to cine imaging. Arrhythmias appear in cine images as choppy cardiac contraction or altered contraction pattern. In cine images, this is due to combining raw data lines from systolic and diastolic phases into the same raw data space (k-space), falsely assuming that they stem from the same cardiac phase. In situations where cine imaging is obscured by true arrhythmia, prospective triggering or real-time imaging may be employed leading to appreciable IQ improvement.

There are a variety of gating and triggering options for cine imaging. While the triggered retro-gated cine sequence is the most commonly used method for clinical practice, there are some instances, such as arrhythmias, that necessitate the use of a different triggering scheme. By understanding the principles behind each method, the scanner operator can choose the most appropriate method for the individual patient.

4.5.2 CINE CMR PARAMETERS AND ADVANCED TECHNICAL TOPICS

4.5.2.1 Lines per Segment, Temporal Resolution, and Scan Duration

Temporal resolution, number of segments, spatial resolution, and breath-hold duration are all interrelated in cine CMR and are controlled by a variety of physiological parameters.

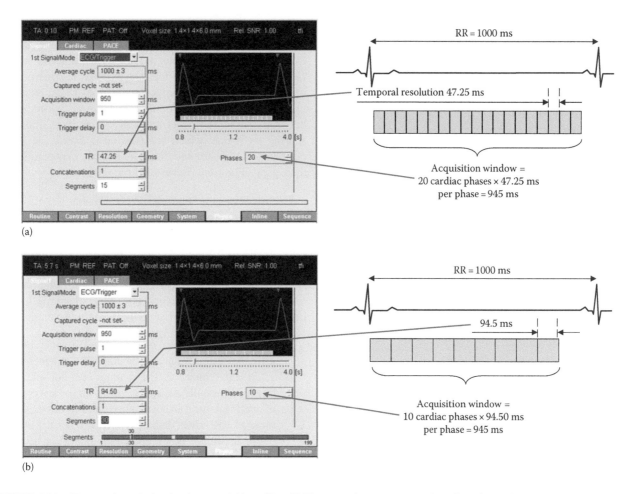

FIGURE 4.23 Temporal resolution in cine acquisition. Cine CMR protocol parameters and cardiac phases showing (a) high and (b) low temporal resolutions. Note the difference in the "Segments" parameters between the two cases.

Figure 4.23 shows the relationship between acquisition window, number of cardiac phases, and duration per phase for a prospectively gated cine sequence. The duration per phase is commonly referred to as temporal resolution and is sometimes abbreviated as repetition time (TR), but it must not be confused with the textbook definition of TR. For a fixed acquisition window, increasing the number of cardiac phases leads to a shorter duration per phase, and thus better temporal resolution, as shown in Figure 4.23a. On the other hand, decreasing the number of cardiac phases results in a longer duration per cardiac phase and poorer temporal resolution, as shown in Figure 4.23b. Adjusting the parameter "segments" can modify the temporal resolution. The relationship between the parameters "temporal resolution," "number of cardiac phases," and "lines per segment" is thus relatively simple, which is frequently handled by the scanner UI.

To reiterate, reducing the "lines per segment," also called "segments" or "views per segment" by some manufacturers, improves temporal resolution by shortening the time per cardiac phase, but extends the scan time. Improving the spatial resolution by acquiring more lines for a fixed FOV requires the acquisition of more segments which likewise increases the

scan time. Conversely, using poorer temporal or spatial resolution reduces the scan time.

Adjustments to temporal resolution can be made on the fly depending on the patient's breath-hold capability. For prospectively triggered sequences, the scanner operator does not directly manipulate the number of acquired cardiac phases; instead, the scanner operator must adjust the acquisition window and lines per segment in order to change the number of cardiac phases acquired.

The relationship between temporal resolution and acquired cardiac phases is not as simple for retro-gated and triggered retro-gated sequences. In these sequences, the scanner operator can directly modify the number of reconstructed cardiac phases, but the changes in the number of reconstructed cardiac phases must be done cautiously. By choosing a large number of reconstructed cardiac phases, one can seemingly achieve excellent temporal resolution, yet these are only interpolated data. Analogous to prospective sequences, the true temporal resolution in retro-gated sequences depends only on the number of lines per segment. Often, increased temporal resolution is desired to improve visualization of subtle wall motion abnormalities. By artificially inflating the apparent temporal resolution without acquiring more data, these anatomical subtleties will not be seen. Therefore, it is not recommended to artificially inflate the reconstructed cardiac phases as it does not lead to actual improvement in temporal resolution.

4.5.2.2 Advanced Technical Topics

4.5.2.2.1 Echo Sharing/View Sharing/Shared Phases

"Echo sharing" or "view sharing" allows for increasing the number of reconstructed cardiac phases in prospectively triggered cine sequences. Because the data are shared between cardiac phases, the method is also called "shared phases" (Rehwald et al. 2001). One example of view sharing is to only acquire the odd-numbered raw (k-space) data lines for odd-numbered cardiac phases, and only the even-numbered lines for the even-numbered phases. Using nearest-neighbor interpolation or averaging, one can calculate the missing odd- or even-numbered lines for each cardiac phase. With this method, it is possible to reconstruct twice as many cardiac phases compared to conventional prospectively triggered cine imaging. However, with the proliferation of retro-gated cine sequences, this approach is less commonly used.

4.5.2.2.2 Fast Imaging

The echo planar imaging (EPI) sequence allows for acquiring all k-space lines in a raster fashion after only one excitation RF pulse in 50–100 ms, despite its sensitivity to off-resonance and motion artifacts (Ibrahim 2012). Otherwise, nonrectilinear k-space trajectories, for example, radial and spiral acquisitions, could be adopted for faster data acquisition with the necessary data regridding operation before image reconstruction. Partial k-space acquisition is another strategy for reducing scan time, which is based on exploiting the symmetrical properties of k-space for acquiring only half the k-space with 50% reduction in scan time (although this comes at the expense of reduced SNR) (Ibrahim 2012). Localized excitation is another technique that allows for acquiring less data while avoiding aliasing artifacts. Finally, compressed sensing techniques have been considered for reconstructing images from sparse raw data, which is well suited for CMR imaging. Compressed sensing has been successfully implemented in different CMR applications, including single breath-hold whole-heart imaging (Santos et al. 2006).

4.5.2.2.3 Parallel Imaging

Parallel imaging is another way of reducing scan time, where a number of adjacent small coils (coil elements) are used to acquire the MR signal. Each coil element "sees" only part of the imaged object, and the resulting small-FOV images are combined to form an image of the whole object. Sensitivity encoding (SENSE) (Pruessmann et al. 1999) and generalized autocalibrating partially parallel acquisition (GRAPPA) (Griswold et al. 2002) are common parallel imaging techniques that are based on reconstructing the data in the image space and k-space, respectively. Nevertheless, it should be noted that both techniques require prior knowledge about individual coil sensitivities in the phased-array matrix.

4.5.2.2.4 Real-Time Imaging

Certain cardiovascular applications need real-time imaging, for example, dynamic imaging. Besides implementation of fast and parallel imaging techniques, data sharing could be implemented to further reduce scan time. These techniques are based on the assumption that images are slightly changed between consecutive timeframes. Key hole is a famous data sharing technique, which is based on updating the k-space periphery at a slower rate than the k-space center to save on data acquisition time (Bernstein et al. 2004).

4.5.2.2.5 Imaging Strategies in the Presence of Arrhythmia

Cardiac arrhythmia severely degrades cine image quality. For patients with frequent ectopic heartbeats, retro-gating is problematic because the data sorting and interpolation algorithm combines data from RR intervals of different lengths, resulting in poor image quality. The practical approach to cine imaging in the presence of arrhythmia is three-tiered.

Strategy 1: In the case of occasional ectopic beats, arrhythmia rejection can be implemented in retro-gated cine sequences. The scanner operator selects a target RR, usually the average RR over the last couple of heartbeats, and an acceptance window defining the range of RR values that are considered normal (without arrhythmia). When an ectopic heartbeat occurs, the data collected before and after the erratic R-wave are discarded and are recollected in a later normal heartbeat. Scan time will be slightly increased, but remains within breath-holding capability.

Strategy 2: Another option is to use prospectively triggered, rather than retro-gated, cine imaging. For atrial arrhythmia, such as atrial fibrillation, where the duration of systole is relatively constant, prospective triggering from the detection of the R-wave to early diastole is used. The acquisition window is set to the length of the shortest RR interval, which allows regional and global systolic function to be visualized with acceptable image quality.

Strategy 3: If the cardiac rhythm is completely random or unreliable (e.g., bigeminy), then the scanner operator can switch to a real-time sequence. Real-time cine does not require any physiological triggering and consists of very fast consecutive single-shot acquisitions with relatively low temporal resolution (typically 50–60 ms). Usually, multiple heartbeats are recorded to visualize both regular and arrhythmic beats. Real-time images have lower spatial resolution, larger slice thickness, and lower SNR than segmented cine images. High acquisition speed is achieved using parallel acquisition techniques combined with real-time reconstruction (Hansen et al. 2008) and high readout bandwidth to shorten the repetition time, both leading to an SNR reduction. Radial sampling is also an option as it allows for smaller FOVs without introducing folding artifacts that would be observed with Cartesian sampling.

4.6 CLINICAL APPLICATIONS OF CINE CMR

Cardiac contraction is 3D and its pattern is a complex combination of translation and rotation (Herman and Gorlin 1969). In brief, during systolic contraction of the healthy heart, the squeezing action of the cardiac muscle causes the myocardium to thicken and perform translational and rotational movements according to the myocardial fibers orientation. The ventricular volume decreases and the base moves toward the apex. Heart diseases can affect the contraction pattern and strength, either globally or regionally, resulting in hypokinesia or dyskinesia (reduced or absent contraction of the ventricular wall, respectively) and impaired blood exchange. Local dyskinesia, for instance, can occur in a chronically infarcted territory such as a transmural myocardial scar. Assessment of cardiac contractile function and wall motion is therefore of highest clinical value.

One of the most important milestones leading to the introduction of CMR in clinical imaging was the robust implementation of SSFP cine sequences. Cine CMR imaging provides high temporal and spatial resolution images of the heart and vasculature, which make it a highly versatile technique. It is used for imaging the heart, pericardium, and great vessels alike.

Manual, semiautomated, or fully automated quantification techniques have been developed. These methods can provide accurate measurements of the ventricular and atrial volumes, diameters, cardiac function, contractility, wall motion, and valve function. However, the simplest and fastest instrument to detect alterations in these parameters may still be the human eye. At the time of acquisition, changes in the heart function, wall motion, myocardial contractility, and chamber size can be detected visually, and additional scans can be performed to interrogate the cause. In this section, we discuss visual scoring as well as quantitative techniques that can be applied to cine images to evaluate cardiac morphology and function.

4.6.1 CARDIAC MORPHOLOGY AND FUNCTION

4.6.1.1 Left Ventricular Volumes, Mass, and Function

Cine MRI has become widely accepted as the gold standard for the assessment of cardiac volumes, ejection fraction (EF), and cardiac mass (Pennell et al. 2004). Clinical practice guidelines have been set forth by imaging and cardiology professional societies to guide appropriate use in various clinical indications (Hendel et al. 2006). Cine CMR measurements of LV ejection fraction (LVEF) are increasingly used in clinical trials, for example, as a surrogate endpoint for drug trials in patients with chronic heart failure (Bellenger et al. 2004, Kjekshus et al. 2009) or for efficacy testing of stem-cell therapy after myocardial infarction (Surder et al. 2010, Heeger et al. 2012). Additionally, CMR alone allows for accurate measurements of RV function and volume, which are used in studies on RV remodeling in patients with complex congenital heart disease (Giardini et al. 2007, van der Bom et al. 2013).

The Society of Cardiovascular Magnetic Resonance (SCMR) has established standardized protocols for the assessment of LV mass and volume, which are measured from a stack of short-axis images through planimetry of the myocardial borders (Kramer et al. 2008). Absolute and normalized reference values exist for the LV parameters, stratified by age and gender (Maceira et al. 2006b). The major advantage of 3D imaging (3D echo, CMR, and CT) compared to M-mode or 2D echocardiography is that no geometric modeling is required to calculate cardiac volumes. This is of particular importance in nonuniform ventricles with distorted geometry such as in patients with cardiomyopathy or after myocardial infarction.

CMR assessment of the LV mass has been validated using postmortem hearts (Bottini 1975). The reproducibility of LV mass measurement is excellent with average standard error of the mean (SEM) of 7.8, 4.8, and 9.0 g for interstudy, intraobserver, and interobserver reproducibility, respectively (Myerson et al. 2002). LV volume measurement with CMR has also been validated against human cadaver heart casts (Rehr et al. 1985), which showed an excellent reproducibility (Kim et al. 2009). In one study, the reproducibility of CMR was directly compared to 2D echocardiography, which was previously the standard method for analysis of LV volume and LVEF. The SEMs for end-diastolic volume (EDV), end-systolic volume (ESV), and LVEF by CMR in normal subjects were 4.3 mL, 2.8 mL, and 1.7%, and in heart failure patients were 7.6 mL, 7.4 mL, and 2.4%, respectively. The errors in 2D echocardiography were higher, at 6.4 mL, 7.0 mL, and 5.6% in normal subjects, and at 17.6 mL, 19.7 mL, and 7.0% in heart failure patients (Grothues et al. 2002). 3D echocardiography interstudy reproducibility was better than 2D echocardiography, with averaged SEM for EDV, ESV, and EF of 8.2 mL, 7.4 mL, and 4.4%, respectively (Jenkins et al. 2004, Kuhl et al. 2004), which are closer to CMR repeatability.

4.6.1.2 Visual Assessment of Ventricular Morphology and Function

Regional and global systolic function can be assessed by visual inspection of the stack of short-axis and standard long-axis (two-chamber, three-chamber, and four-chamber views) images, as shown in Figure 4.9. Visual LVEF estimation as a global parameter of systolic function is commonly reported, yet some clinicians consider quantification techniques as the preferred method. However, quantification is time-consuming and requires experience with the analysis tool and clinical knowledge to verify that the calculations are in accordance with visual assessment.

Visual analysis of wall motion and contractile function is reported using the 17-segment America Heart Association (AHA) model, which is the standardized segmentation technique among cardiac imaging societies (Cerqueira et al. 2002). Each segment should be analyzed individually and scored on the basis of its inward wall motion and systolic thickening. Segments are scored as follows: normal or hyperkinesis = 1, hypokinesis = 2, akinesis (negligible thickening and inward motion) = 3, dyskinesis (paradoxical systolic outward motion or thinning) = 4. Figure 4.24a shows a commercial vendor's reading sheet using the 17-segment model. Figure 4.24b shows the CMR report of a typical patient generated from the reading sheet. The other columns relate to hyperenhancement observed in DE-MR images, as discussed later.

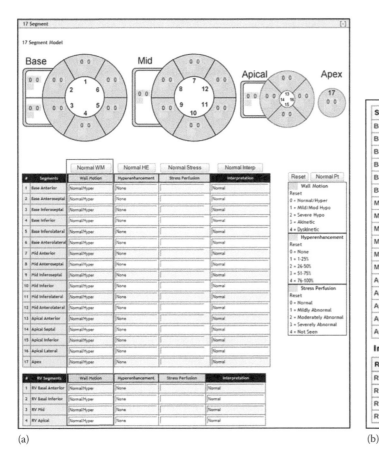

(a)   (b)

FIGURE 4.24 Visual assessment of myocardial function. (a) Reading sheet with 17-segment model. Note that the wall motion column is within the red rectangle. (b) Part of a report created by filling out the reading sheet in a typical cardiac patient. Wall motion columns are within the red rectangle. (Courtesy of Heart Imaging Technologies, Durham, NC.)

Wall motion abnormalities may be indicative of a loss of myocytes caused by myocardial infarction, or hibernating or "stunned" myocardium as seen in severe ischemia without loss of myocytes (Braunwald and Kloner 1982, Conti 1991). Figure 4.25 shows an example of wall motion scoring. For each patient, only two frames of a series of cine images are shown. Figure 4.25a shows the mid-diastolic frame, and Figure 4.25b shows the peak systolic frame of a normal patient. Figure 4.25c and d shows images of diastolic and systolic phases in a patient with wall motion abnormality. The arrows highlight a dyskinetic septum. Correlating cine images with wall motion abnormalities to delayed-enhancement images (Figure 4.25e) and perfusion images acquired at the same slice location is important for discriminating dysfunctional, yet viable, regions from those that are irreversibly damaged. The arrow in Figure 4.25e highlights a hyperenhanced region indicating myocardial infarction.

4.6.1.3 Quantitative Assessment of Left Ventricular Dimensions

Left ventricular dimensions and myocardial wall thickness are assessed by 2D measurement of septal and inferolateral wall thickness at end-diastole, at the level of the mitral leaflet tips. These measurements are shown as red and blue lines, respectively, in a normal heart (Figure 4.26a), a heart with a chronic thinned septal infarct (Figure 4.26b), and a heart with hypertrophic cardiomyopathy (HCM) (Figure 4.26c). The internal LV diameter is measured at the same location at both end-diastole and end-systole, specifically the end-diastolic diameter (EDD) and end-systolic diameter (ESD), which are shown as green lines in the figure. These measurements can be performed on the three-chamber view, which requires the reader to be certain that this imaging plane was acquired though the center of the LV cavity. If this is not known, a short-axis slice can be used instead. Both methods are depicted in Figure 4.26a. Care has to be taken that the moderator band at the RV side of the septum and the trabeculations at the inferolateral wall are avoided. For 2D measurements, the reference values used are the same as those for echocardiography (Lang et al. 2005).

Systolic wall thickening is calculated from the myocardial wall thickness. Systolic thickening is defined as systolic wall thickness minus diastolic wall thickness, divided by diastolic wall thickness, expressed as a percentage. For example, a thickness increase from 8 mm at end-diastole to 12 mm at end-systole corresponds to a 50% systolic wall thickening.

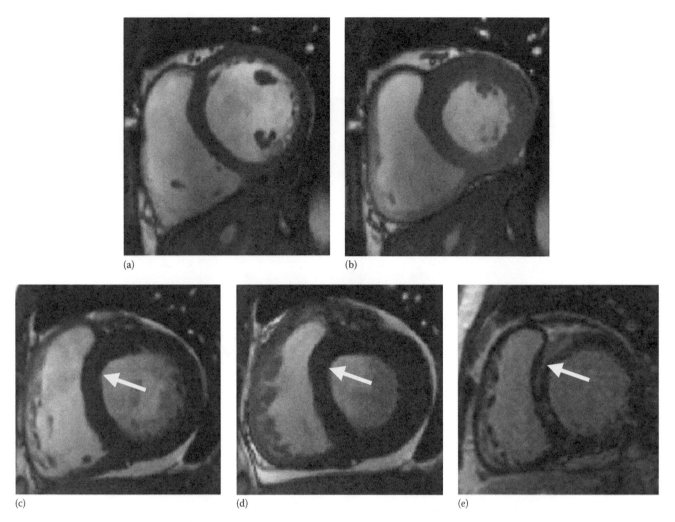

(a)

(b)

(c)

(d)

(e)

FIGURE 4.25 Wall motion abnormality in cine imaging. (Top) Normal patient wall motion in (a) diastole and (b) systole; (bottom) Patient with reduced wall motion and thickening in (c) diastole and (d) systole, which correspond to the delayed-enhancement pattern in (e), as shown by the arrows.

4.6.1.4 Quantitative Assessment of Ventricular Morphology and Function by Myocardial Contouring

Left ventricular volumes are quantitatively determined by delineating the endocardial borders at end-diastole and end-systole on a complete stack of short-axis images that covers the entire LV from base to apex. Figure 4.27 shows an example of a midventricular short-axis slice with endocardial contours in red. For LV mass quantification, the epicardial border is outlined as well, at end-diastole only (the green contour). The Simpson's method is used to calculate the volume by multiplying the area inside the delineated contour by the slice thickness (plus gap thickness if present). LV mass is measured by multiplying the myocardial volume (= epicardial volume – endocardial volume) by the myocardial density of 1.05 kg/m^3.

4.6.1.4.1 Manual Contouring

While manual contouring is more time-consuming, it is still the standard approach. Automated and semiautomated methods are available, but are hardly used in routine clinical practice (Angelie et al. 2005, Kwong 2008). All major MRI

vendors now provide dedicated evaluation software for quantification and evaluation of the cardiac function (Figure 4.28). In addition, there are several platform-independent software tools that are commercially available.

Three key points need to be considered during image acquisition and analysis in order to have reproducible and accurate results with quantitative CMR volume analysis:

Key point 1: The end-systolic frame has to be chosen correctly unless contours are outlined on all frames. This is usually done by visual inspection of all frames. It is important to note that some semiautomated software tools may automatically select a frame that is not the correct one. Importantly, an adequate temporal resolution of 45 ms or less (Miller et al. 2002) is required to avoid overestimation of the end-systolic volume, and hence underestimation of LVEF.

Key point 2: In the most basal short-axis slice of the stack, longitudinal displacement of about 13 ± 4 mm and twist of the mitral valve plane during systole may cause LV to move out of the imaging plane, causing

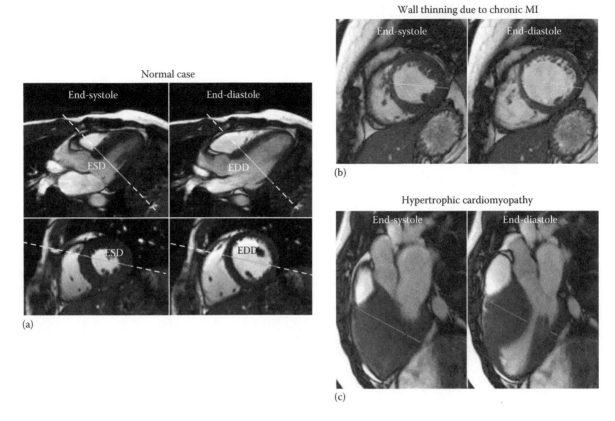

FIGURE 4.26 Quantitative assessment of left ventricular dimensions. Measurement of the LV diameter (green line) and myocardial septal (red) and lateral (blue) wall thickness in (a) normal volunteer; (b) patient with chronic MI; and (c) patient with hypertrophic cardiomyopathy.

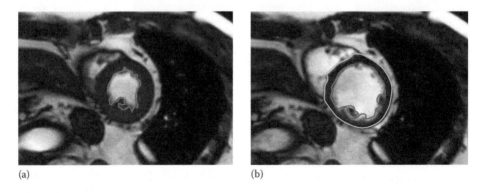

FIGURE 4.27 Endocardial (red) and epicardial (green) contours in a short-axis slice. Contouring of a mid-ventricular short-axis slice at (a) end-systole and (b) end-diastole.

the atrium to be imaged in systole. Figure 4.29a shows a typical basal short-axis slice (bottom) during end-diastole relative to a four-chamber view (top). In the ideal case shown in Figure 4.29b, the LV is visualized at end-diastole, and the entire contour contains only left atrium at end-systole, and is therefore not included in end-systolic volume measurement (no contour is drawn). However, typically the systolic frame includes portions of both the atrium and ventricle, as illustrated in Figure 4.29c; therefore, the operator has to decide how much of the basal slice area to include. Software tools exist that track the valve motion on long-axis

images to correct for the LV volume loss due to the atrioventricular ring descent (Maceira et al. 2006b). Another option is to select the most basal slice as the one where at least 50% of the blood volume is surrounded by the myocardium (Hudsmith et al. 2005). A practical approach depicted in Figure 4.29c is drawing a line halfway through the blood pool, including the ventricle-blood border, but excluding the atrium-blood border. There is no consensus on which method is best. Nevertheless, it is important that only one of these methods is consistently applied in the imaging center to avoid reporting changes in serial measurements.

1. Draw circle for approximate
   endocardium— LV blood pool border:

3. Repeat for all slices in end-diastole and end-systole:

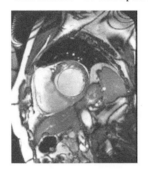

2. Nudge contour to follow actual
   endocardium—LV blood pool border:

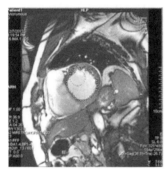

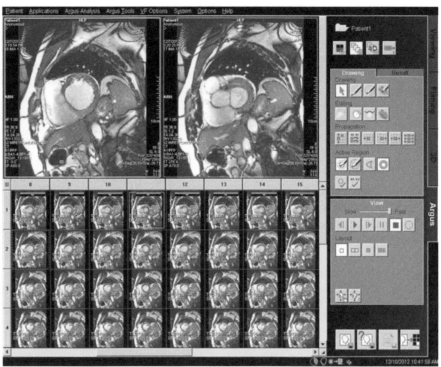

FIGURE 4.28 Manual contouring of the left ventricle. The figure shows three steps for drawing the contours using a commercial image analysis software.

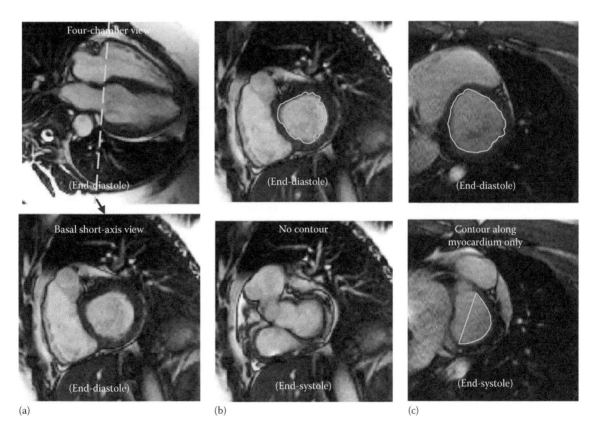

(a)   (b)   (c)

FIGURE 4.29 Displacement of the basal short-axis slice during the cardiac cycle. (a) Basal slice at end-diastole. (b) Ideal case, where the basal slice disappears from the imaging plane at end-systole. (c) Typical case, where part of the basal slice (inside the green contour) appears in the imaging plane at end-systole.

Key point 3: The papillary muscles are often seen detached from the wall within the blood pool. The logical rule is to include them in the LV mass but exclude from the LV chamber volumes. Notably, some reference studies have however included papillary muscles into the LV volumes (Salton et al. 2002), which is important to know when using results from these studies as reference normal values. Note that inclusion or exclusion of the papillary muscles results in significant differences in LV mass and volume measurements (Janik et al. 2008).

4.6.1.4.2 Semiautomatic Contouring

Most commercially available contouring software packages have features that enable faster contouring of the myocardium. Some semiautomatic features include automatic identification of the end-diastolic and end-systolic timeframes, contour propagation into other slices and cardiac phases, interactive border definition, or manual adjustment of automatically created contours. By reducing the number of images that require manual contouring and the time required for drawing the contours, these tools resulted in increased efficiency for quantification of the ventricular function.

4.6.1.4.3 Automatic Contouring (Computer-Assisted Ventricular Modeling)

Automatic methods have the potential to further increase the speed of quantitative analysis. A wide range of algorithms and tools are available for automatic and semiautomatic segmentation of cine images. Automatic segmentation methods require little to no user input and rely on image processing algorithms to define the endocardial and epicardial borders. Nevertheless, over 15 years of research on the topics of LV and RV segmentation have not resulted in a definitive solution (Petitjean and Dacher 2011).

Accurate segmentation algorithms require consistent delineation of both the epicardium and endocardium. The segmentation of each border has its own set of challenges: the epicardium is surrounded by fat and lung tissues, which have dramatically different signal intensities, while the endocardium-blood pool border has small trabeculations and papillary muscles that have identical signal intensity to the

---

TABLE 4.2

Ranges for Normal and Increasing Degrees of Severity for CMR Cine Cardiac Measurements in Men and Women, with and without Indexing to Body Surface Area

	Men	Women		Men	Women
LV End-Diastolic Diameter (mm)			**Anteroseptal Thickness (mm)**		
Normal	<62	<55	Normal	<12	<10
Mildly increased	62–69	55–64	Mildly increased	12–14	10–13
Moderately increased	70–79	65–74	Moderately increased	15–18	14–17
Severely increased	>79	>74	Severely increased	>18	>17
LV End-Diastolic Diameter Index (mm/m²)			**Inferolateral Thickness (mm)**		
Normal	<32	<33	Normal	<11	<9
Mildly increased	32–35	33–36	Mildly increased	11–14	9–13
Moderately increased	36–40	37–40	Moderately increased	15–18	13–17
Severely increased	>40	>40	Severely increased	>18	>17
LV End-Diastolic Volume (mL)			**LV Mass Index (g/m²)**		
Normal	<196	<143	Normal	<80	<60
Mildly Increased	196–229	143–179	Mildly increased	80–99	60–74
Moderately increased	230–270	180–220	Moderately increased	100–120	75–90
Severely increased	>270	>220	Severely increased	>120	>90
LV End-Diastolic Volume Index (mL/m²)			**RV Volume Index (mL/m²)**		
Normal	<95	<78	Small	<55	<47
Mildly increased	95–115	78–100	Normal	58–114	47–103
Moderately increased	116–135	101–120	Mildly increased	115–171	104–153
Severely increased	>135	>121	Moderately increased	172–228	154–206
			Severely increased	>228	>206
LV Ejection Fraction (%)			**RV Ejection Fraction (%)**		
Normal	>54	>56	Normal	>46	>49
Mildly depressed	40–54	40–56	Mildly depressed	36–46	37–49
Moderately depressed	30–39	30–39	Moderately depressed	24–35	25–36
Severely depressed	<30	<30	Severely depressed	<24	<25

endocardium. While there are many automatic methods for LV contouring, many of these methods fail in the RV due to its thin wall, trabeculations, and complex shape.

4.6.1.5 Normal Values for Ventricular Volume and Function

Quantitative measurements can be used to determine the severity and progression of heart diseases. Values and ranges for many common metrics are listed in Table 4.2. Briefly, the measurement ranges can be broken down into normal, mild, moderate, and severe. The measurements can be interpreted directly as raw numbers, or can be indexed to the body surface area in m², as shown in Table 4.2, or to the body height in m. For example, in men, an LV end-diastolic diameter below 62 mm is considered normal, from 62 to 69 mm is mildly increased, from 70 to 79 mm is moderately increased, and >79 mm is severely increased. These ranges vary slightly between men and women. Normal values for SSFP- and GRE-based cine images have been published (Lorenz et al. 1999, Marcus et al. 1999, Salton et al. 2002, Alfakih et al. 2004, Grebe et al. 2004, Hudsmith et al. 2005, Maceira et al. 2006a,b). Professional athletes have to be evaluated separately as their values are often outside the normal distribution range (Abergel et al. 2004).

4.6.2 APPLICATIONS OF CINE CMR FOR VARIOUS CLINICAL INDICATIONS

4.6.2.1 Tissue Characterization

Assessment of wall thickness and thickening by cine CMR can provide clinically useful details about myocardial viability,

and can aid in the diagnosis of HCM. Wall thickness and LV diameter measurements were discussed in Section 4.6.1.3.

Evaluating end-diastolic wall thickness in combination with systolic wall thickening by cine MRI during dobutamine stress was helpful for detecting irreversible myocardial damage due to chronic infarction, when compared to a healthy control group (Baer et al. 1998, Sandstede 2003). In one study, myocardial viability was predicted with sensitivity of 92% and specificity of 56% (Baer et al. 1998). Importantly, wall thinning is only observed in chronic infarctions (older than 4 months). Thus, end-diastolic wall thickness can only be used as a criterion for viability in chronic MI with high sensitivity, but low specificity.

Cine CMR is also clinically useful in combination with other CMR imaging tests such as DE-CMR and myocardial perfusion at stress and rest. The combination of these CMR imaging tests allows the clinician to differentiate between viable, reversibly injured "at-risk" myocardium (viable, but not normally contracting), and irreversibly injured (not viable and akinetic) tissue in acute and chronically infarcted (scar) states (Wilke et al. 1997, Klocke et al. 2001, Epstein et al. 2002, Kim and Shah 2004, Lee et al. 2004). Figure 4.30 shows two examples of patients, in whom the combination of cine CMR and DE-CMR provided better diagnosis than any of the tests alone. Figure 4.30a, before revascularization, shows poor wall thickening in the cine MR images, but no irreversibly injured myocardium by DE-CMR. The absence of irreversible injury prompted the clinician to perform revascularization of the infarct-related artery (IRA). As a result, contractile function and wall thickening improved markedly as shown on the right in the end-systolic cine frame. The patient in Figure 4.30b

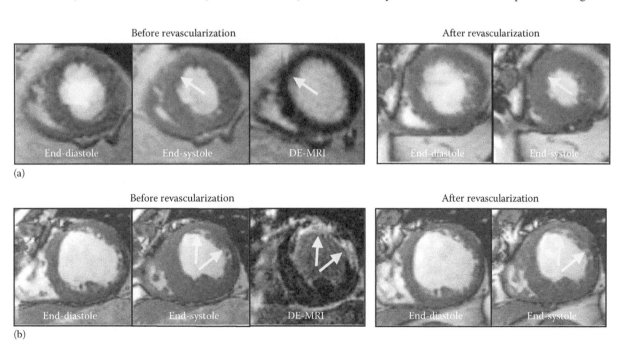

FIGURE 4.30 Cine and delayed-enhancement (DE) images showing reversible and irreversible ventricular dysfunction. Cine and DE images from a patient with (a) reversible ventricular dysfunction and (b) irreversible dysfunction. (a) The arrows point to an area that was not hyperenhanced in the DE image before revascularization; therefore, contractility improved after revascularization. (b) Hyperenhancement was present in the DE image prior to and post revascularization, and there was no contractility improvement after revascularization.

had poor wall thickening prior to revascularization, as well as a large myocardial infarction in the same area. As expected from these initial findings, revascularization of the IRA did not improve contractile function, as shown in the two cine frames on the right, because the tissue was already irreversibly injured.

4.6.2.2 Constrictive Pericarditis

CMR offers techniques for assessing both pericardial morphology and hemodynamic effects of constrictive physiology. Concerning pericardial thickness and calcification, most published images for morphological characterization of the pericardium were obtained with spin echo (SE) imaging, wherein a pericardial thickness of 2 mm or smaller was considered normal, and a thickness larger than 4 mm considered abnormal (Masui et al. 1992). These thresholds were helpful for confirming the diagnosis of constrictive pericarditis, particularly in cases of extreme pericardial thickening above 5 mm. Nevertheless, these older SE protocols were limited by long acquisition times (in the range of minutes), which prohibited breath-holding. Thus, despite a spatial resolution of 1.5 mm, respiratory motion may have degraded the effective resolution on the order of 4 mm. Therefore, the 4 mm cutoff value may have been a reflection of technical limitations of the technique; not of true pericardial dimension. The faster SSFP sequence can be performed in a single breath-hold and it allows for an in-plane resolution of less than 2 mm. Studies with SSFP imaging showed that normal pericardium is usually a very delicate structure of only 1–2 mm in thickness. Therefore, nowadays, pericardial thickness is best assessed by a combination of SSFP cine MRI and turbo spin echo (TSE), as shown in Figure 4.31a and b. The advantage of TSE compared to SE is that it can be performed within a breath-hold duration, but its disadvantage is that motion-induced blurring must be minimized by acquiring the data during mid-diastole. SSFP cine imaging is useful for evaluating the pericardium as it can provide high spatial resolution morphology images as well as dynamic functional information.

To diagnose the hemodynamic effects of constrictive pericarditis, it is helpful to study the LV motion during respiration while running a real-time SSFP cine sequence, as shown in Figure 4.31c through e. During the first filling period in inspiration, the septum moves toward the LV side ("septal bounce") as a consequence of preferential RV filling due to increased ventricular interdependence, a hemodynamic hallmark of pericardial constriction (Francone et al. 2006), as shown in Figure 4.31d and e. Although the number of studied patients is quite

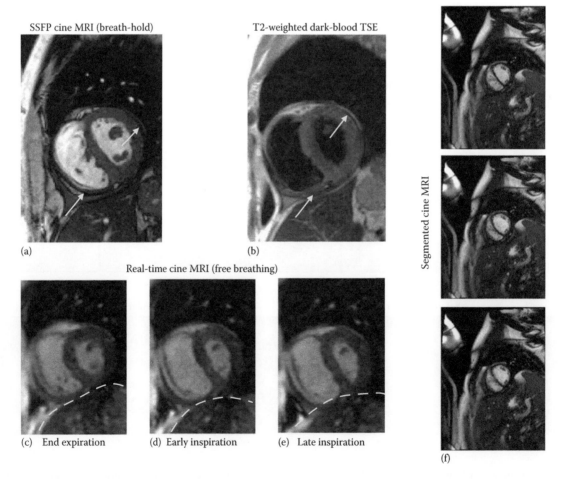

FIGURE 4.31   Constrictive pericarditis assessed by cine CMR images. (a, b) Constrictive pericarditis causes thickening of the pericardium (arrows). (c–e) Real-time cine CMR showing ventricular interdependence during early inspiration. (f) Constrictive pericarditis causes flattening of the ventricular septum and a characteristic "double bounce" in cine CMR images.

small, constrictive pericarditis and restrictive cardiomyopathies appear to be distinguishable with this test. Another characteristic of constrictive pericarditis is the brief rapid bounce during early diastole, which can be appreciated using breath-hold segmented cine CMR imaging, as shown in Figure 4.31f.

In addition to conventional cine imaging, tagged cine imaging can provide supplementary information about the heart function. Normally, tagging gridlines at the interface between the pericardium and epicardium should shear during systole as the two surfaces move independently and slide during contraction. Conversely, in the setting of pericardial adhesions, gridlines at the interface would remain intact, as the motion of the two surfaces is concordant.

4.6.2.3 Valvular Diseases, Lesions, and Stenosis

Cine CMR can be used to visualize valve morphology, function, and accelerated flow as seen in stenotic valves or valvular insufficiency. Valvular morphology images provide insight into the cause of regurgitation (e.g., prolapse or lack of coaptation) and to some extent can visualize vegetations and calcifications. It is noteworthy that the valves' erratic motion and small size may limit the visualization of valvular lesions with segmented cine sequences. Flow jets appear as signal voids on cine CMR images due to intravoxel dephasing of spins associated with nonlaminar flow. The cine images through the valve plane in Figure 4.32a show aortic valve insufficiency or aortic regurgitation, as dark flow jet (arrows)

from the aorta into the LV. Figure 4.32b shows aortic stenosis as flow jet (arrows) into the aorta due to the restricted opening of the aortic valve. The severity of the regurgitation can be estimated by measuring the extent of the regurgitant flow jet into the LV cavity, flow reversal in the descending aorta, LV size, and quantitative regurgitant volume and fraction measurements with VENC-CMR. The en-face view of the aortic valve in Figure 4.32c shows the regurgitant orifice during diastole, and the restricted opening during systole (Figure 4.32d). Figure 4.32e and f shows normal aortic valve in its closed and open states, respectively.

The severity of aortic stenosis can be also assessed by performing an area measurement of the valve opening, known as valve planimetry, and by measuring the peak velocity of the flow jet. Good agreement has been shown between valve area by planimetry on cine CMR images, measurements from transesophageal and transthoracic echocardiography, and invasive hemodynamic measurements via catheterization (Friedrich et al. 2002, John et al. 2003, Kupfahl et al. 2004, von Knobelsdorff-Brenkenhoff et al. 2009). Peak velocity measurements by VENC-MRI correlate well with Doppler echocardiography measurements (Kilner et al. 1993a, Caruthers et al. 2003). To accurately planimeterize the valve opening and measure peak velocity, it is important to image the aortic valve across the leaflet tips. This is performed by obtaining two orthogonal cine long-axis views of the flow jet and one short-axis view, orthogonal to both long-axis views,

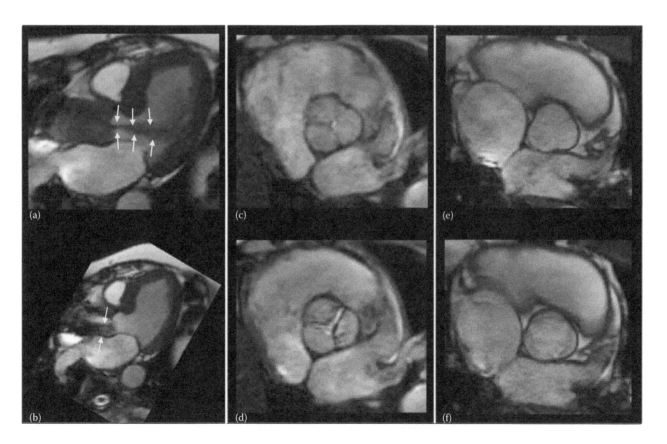

FIGURE 4.32 Aortic regurgitation and stenosis. Aortic valve disease exhibiting both (a) aortic valve insufficiency and (b) stenosis. (c–f) En-face views showing (c) regurgitant orifice and (d) restricted opening, compared to (e,f) normal opening of the valve.

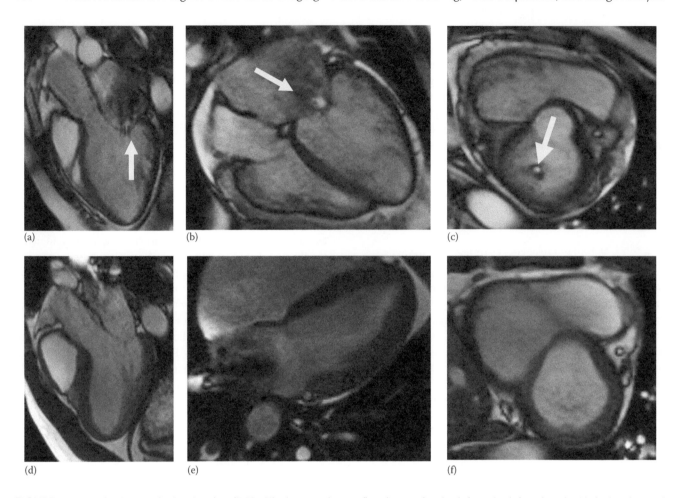

FIGURE 4.33 Mitral regurgitation by cine CMR. The images show a flow jet moving back into the left atrium in (a) 3-chamber and (b) 4-chamber views; (c) lack of coaptation of the mitral valve leaflets. (d–f) show the same views in a normal heart.

at the origin of the jet. Ideally, a stack of images is obtained through the valve to determine optimal slice location for planimetry, which is then performed using cine CMR images due to their higher temporal resolution compared to VENC-MRI.

Pulmonic and mitral valve stenosis are evaluated similar to aortic stenosis. Figure 4.33a through c depicts a heart with mitral valve regurgitation as indicated by the arrows, which is caused by a lack of coaptation of the mitral valve leaflets. For comparison, Figure 4.33d through f shows the same views in a normal heart.

Quantitative assessment of regurgitation, specifically the forward and reverse volumes and the resulting regurgitant fraction, can be directly derived from a single through-plane VENC-CMR image (if peak flow is laminar). In valves with higher velocities such as the aortic or mitral valve, nonlaminar flow causes intravoxel dephasing resulting in signal loss, and thus flow underestimation, in the VENC-CMR images. In these cases, regurgitation can be quantified using an indirect approach. For example, mitral regurgitation can be obtained by subtracting the forward flow in the proximal ascending aorta from the diastolic inflow across the mitral valve. To minimize signal loss, TE should be always minimized.

Cine CMR can also be useful for visualizing accelerated flow not caused by valve stenosis, for example, in HCM.

In its severe form, the ventricular septum is so thickened that it obstructs the blood flow in the LV outflow tract (LVOT). Figure 4.34a and b shows a normal heart at diastole and systole. Figure 4.34c and d shows the same views in a heart with LVOT obstruction. The obstruction causes blood flow below the aortic valve to accelerate, which can be visualized with cine CMR (arrow in Figure 4.34e) and appears similar to aortic valve stenosis in the resulting image.

Besides identifying flow obstruction in HCM, cine CMR can improve the detection of HCM by assessing myocardial wall thickness. For example, it was reported that in 6% of patients with suspected or known HCM, cine CMR imaging established the diagnosis of HCM, while no hypertrophy was seen on echocardiography (Rickers et al. 2005). Moreover, echocardiography appeared to underestimate the magnitude of hypertrophy compared to cine CMR imaging (Missouris et al. 1996, Stewart et al. 1999). This finding may be of clinical relevance since extreme hypertrophy (wall thickness ≥ 30 mm) is recognized as an important risk factor for sudden cardiac death. Compared to the normal thickness shown in Figure 4.34a, a much increased ventricular wall thickness can be appreciated in the heart of the HCM patient, as shown in Figure 4.34c.

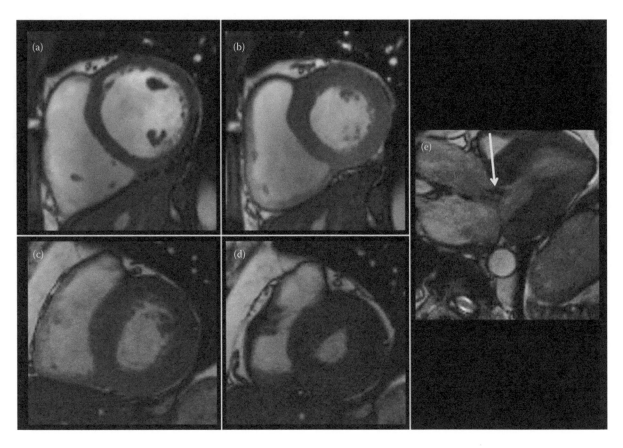

FIGURE 4.34 Myocardial wall thickening in the absence and presence of LVOT obstruction. Wall thickness of a normal heart during (a) diastole and (b) systole. The same views in the presence of LVOT obstruction in an HCM patient during (c) diastole and (d) systole showing ventricular hypertrophy. (e) Three-chamber view of the hypertrophic ventricle showing LVOT obstruction and accelerated flow below the aortic valve (arrow).

4.6.2.4 Cardiac Masses

Most publications on CMR for the evaluation of cardiac masses characterize them by comparing their signal intensities on T1, T2, and proton-density weighted images, and by determining their mobility with cine MRI (Lund et al. 1989, Kaminaga et al. 2003, Pennell et al. 2004). However, differentiating between benign and malignant masses by image intensities alone is usually difficult, and the results can be poor (Hoffmann et al. 2003). A comprehensive protocol for clinical evaluation of cardiac masses consists of multiple pulse sequences to assess morphology, mobility, vascularity, and necrosis of the mass, in addition to inherent differences in T1 and T2 values (Fuster and Kim 2005). For instance, the mobility of an atrial myxoma can be determined by cine CMR to evaluate interference with the atrioventricular valve, which would result in regurgitation or damage of the valve. Increased vascularity prominent in malignancies, such as angiosarcoma, can be demonstrated with CMR perfusion. Tissue necrosis within the core of a malignant tumor can be identified by DE-CMR as a hyperenhanced region. Fat can be verified by imaging the same slice with and without a fat-saturation technique. Figure 4.35 illustrates this comprehensive approach in a patient with a mass in the left atrium: morphology using a dark-blood HASTE sequence,

mobility of the mass using cine CMR, vascularity using a perfusion sequence, and necrosis by contrast agent uptake with DE-CMR. This comprehensive approach enables the physician to determine whether a conspicuous structure in the CMR image is truly a cardiac mass, or whether it is merely a rare, but benign, morphological variant, for example, Eustachian valve, lipomatous hypertrophy of the intra-atrial septum, or Coumadin ridge.

4.6.2.5 Thrombus

Left ventricular thrombus represents an important subset of cardiac masses. While it is most commonly found in the LV apex, thrombus may occur elsewhere, with predilection for locations with stagnant blood flow, for instance, adjacent to an akinetic wall. The presence of LV thrombus may be apparent on cine CMR images if the thrombus is clearly intracavitary and mobile. However, layered mural thrombi can be difficult to detect since the image intensity difference between the thrombus and normal myocardium is minimal (Mollet et al. 2002, Srichai et al. 2006, Weinsaft et al. 2008, 2009). An emerging technique for diagnosing thrombus is DE-CMR performed immediately after contrast agent administration (Mollet et al. 2002, Srichai et al. 2006). It is based on avascularity of the thrombus, which

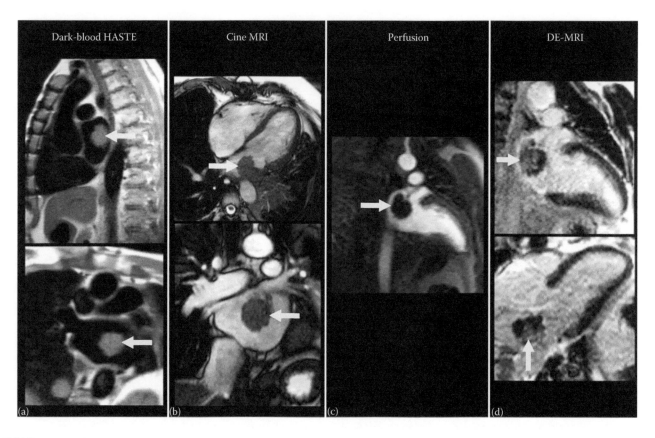

FIGURE 4.35 Cardiac masses assessed by CMR (arrows). Evaluation of cardiac mass using (a) HASTE sequence to show morphology, (b) cine images to visualize motion, (c) perfusion imaging to determine vascularity, and (d) delayed-enhancement CMR to accentuate differences in contrast uptake between the mass and myocardium, and between different regions within the mass itself.

prevents it from taking up any contrast agent. Thus, on DE-CMR images, thrombus can be identified as a nonenhancing structure surrounded by bright ventricular blood and gray (partially enhancing) myocardium. Image contrast between the thrombus and myocardium/blood can be maximized by running the DE-CMR sequence with a long TI between 500 and 600 ms, where the signal from the thrombus is nulled, causing its dark appearance in the CMR image. Thrombus delineation is thus improved relative to the myocardium, which is particularly useful for diagnosing mural thrombi. Atrial thrombi are frequently observed in patients with atrial fibrillation, which causes blood stagnation within the atria, specifically in the atrial appendage. Cine CMR images of the atria that include the atrial appendage can show the moving thrombi, which can help determine the risk of embolization.

4.6.2.6 Congenital Heart Disease

Quantitative results from CMR can greatly facilitate the diagnosis of congenital heart disease (CHD). Cardiac morphology as well as abnormal motion and flow patterns specific to congenital defects can be simultaneously visualized using cine CMR. Surgical correction for CHD often results in anomalous cardiovascular anatomy, which can be confusing, especially in subsequent follow-up examinations. In this case, 3D images from contrast-enhanced CMR angiography (CEMRA) allow the physician to obtain an accurate picture of the vascular anatomy.

Combined with cine CMR, CEMRA is also useful for visualizing abnormal communications between the left and right chambers, known as shunts. Cine CMR images can directly depict flow jets through the shunts. Ventricular and atrial volumes can be measured to determine if abnormal volumes exist, which can be indicative of a shunt across the atrial or ventricular septum. Examples of abnormal chamber volumes include an enlarged right atrium due to left-to-right shunting through an atrial septal defect (ASD), or due to anomalous pulmonary veins draining into the right atrium. The flow through the shunt can be quantified analogous to the echocardiographic "Q_P/Q_S" method that measures the systemic flow through the aortic valve (Q_S) and the pulmonary flow through the pulmonic valve (Q_P) and expresses them as ratio Q_P/Q_S (Beerbaum et al. 2001). A Q_P/Q_S ratio >1.0 indicates a left-to-right shunt, and a ratio >2.0 indicates a large shunt. Whereas this shunt assessment is indirect, CMR can also directly quantify ASD severity by imaging it en-face and by measuring its size and blood flow velocity using VENC-CMR images. Figure 4.36a and b shows four-chamber and short-axis views used to localize the ASD shown in the en-face view in Figure 4.36c. Size measurements can be obtained from the magnitude images of the VENC-CMR data on the left, and velocity flow data from the phase difference map on the right. To measure true velocity of the flow through the ASD, it is important to position the imaging plane as perpendicular to the flow as possible, accounting for the double-oblique nature

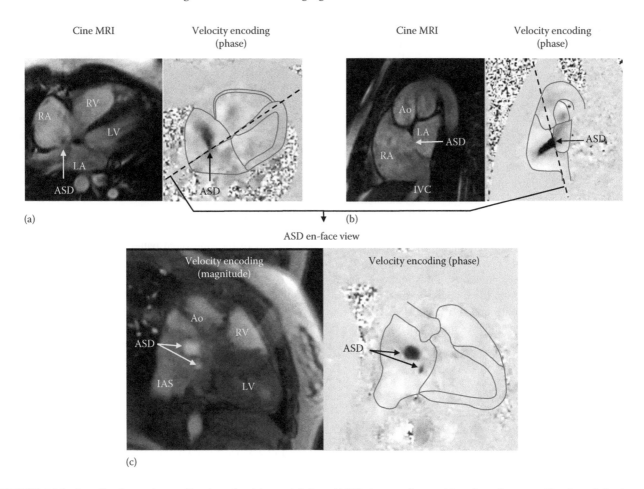

FIGURE 4.36 Localization and quantification of atrial septal defects (ASD) size, number, and location using a combination of cine imaging and VENC-CMR. (a) Four-chamber and (b) short-axis views used to prescribe (dashed black lines) a double-oblique VENC-CMR slice through the ASD, as shown in (c). Ao, aorta; IAS, interatrial septum; IVC, inferior vena cava.

of the atrial septum, septal motion throughout the cardiac cycle, and direction of ASD flow, which may not be exactly perpendicular to the septum.

More details on slice orientation for ASD assessment can be found elsewhere (Beerbaum et al. 2003). ASDs can be of irregular shape, which is why it is important to measure its anterior–posterior as well as its cranial–caudal diameter to obtain the most accurate clinical assessment (Thomson et al. 2008). Recent publications suggest that direct en-face VENC-CMR imaging correlates better with invasive oximetry than the indirect Q_P/Q_S method (Thomson et al. 2008), provided that the imaging plane is optimally oriented. Additionally, the presence of multiple ASDs can be determined from the VENC-CMR image, and the characteristics of the surrounding tissue can serve to determine if the patient should undergo percutaneous or surgical closure.

4.7 EVALUATION OF CARDIAC FUNCTION WITH CMR TAGGING

Regional abnormalities in myocardial contractility can allow for early detection of cardiovascular diseases. While CMR techniques such as cine imaging allow for visual and semiquantitative analysis of myocardial function, detailed quantitative description of myocardial dysfunction is difficult to obtain. The myocardial tagging technique was developed to overcome this limitation by providing detailed spatial information about myocardial deformation parameters, including strain, strain rate, and torsion. These comprehensive measures of myocardial deformation can be important for clinical risk assessment, which allows for detecting and quantifying regional myocardial abnormalities. Although these techniques will be covered in more details throughout the book, this section provides a brief overview of them.

Both in-plane and through-plane CMR tagging methods exist. In-plane tagging techniques were developed first, in which a periodic stripe pattern or 2D grid of dark lines, termed "tags," is created in the myocardium. These tags are tracked over time to display myocardial deformation during the cardiac cycle, allowing for immediate visual interpretation of motion abnormalities. Techniques for automated fast analysis of the tagged images are available, which are based on changes in the k-space due to tags deformation. Through-plane tagging methods were developed later, which are based on the realization that tagging creation in the slice-selection direction causes characteristic changes in the k-space that can be used to assess through-plane tissue deformation. As the images created with through-plane tagging techniques often have no visible tags, simple and fast post-processing techniques can be used to provide motion information (Ibrahim 2011).

4.7.1 MAGNETIZATION SATURATION

The first tagging technique was introduced by Zerhouni et al. (1988) in 1988, who used a preparation module in which slice-selective pulses are applied perpendicular to the imaging plane to create saturation bands at specified locations in the myocardium, as shown in Figure 4.37a. As magnetization is an intrinsic tissue property, the saturation bands (taglines) move during the cardiac cycle following myocardial deformation, such that the resulting tagged images show the intramyocardial motion that occurs between tag application and data readout. There are several limitations to this method, including long tagging preparation time, nonuniform tag intensity as the taglines are created sequentially, high SAR, and low spatial resolution. While Zerhouni's method is not commonly used in clinical practice, it provided the framework upon which all subsequent tagging sequences were built.

4.7.2 SPATIAL MODULATION OF MAGNETIZATION (SPAMM)

An important extension to Zerhouni's method is the Spatial Modulation of Magnetization (SPAMM) tagging method developed by Axel and Dougherty (1989a,b). SPAMM generates a tagging pattern of parallel lines or a 2D tagging grid by applying the tagging module on one or two orthogonal directions, respectively, before data acquisition. SPAMM preparation is typically applied after detection of the R-wave of the ECG, followed by a multi-heartbeat segmented cine acquisition (McVeigh and Atalar 1992). SPAMM creates periodic spatially modulated magnetization through the application of two equally strong nonselective RF pulses separated by a wrapping, or modulation, gradient (Figure 4.37b). The first RF pulse tips the magnetization into the transverse plane, where the gradient pulse is applied along the desired tagging direction to establish a sinusoidal pattern of the magnetization. The second RF pulse tips the modulated magnetization back to the longitudinal axis. Remaining transverse magnetization is then eliminated using a crusher or spoiler gradient. To construct a grid tagging pattern, tagging preparation is implemented consecutively in two orthogonal directions (not shown in Figure 4.37b). During cardiac contraction, the taglines are deformed, allowing for precise visualization of regional heart function. An improved SPAMM method was shortly introduced, which uses a binomial number of pulses to create sharper tag lines (Axel and Dougherty 1989a), thus improving the tagging profile without sacrificing the efficiency of SPAMM. The development of SPAMM allowed myocardial tagging to become part of standard clinical CMR examinations for evaluating the heart function. Its major limitation, though, is the T1 decay of the taglines that is apparent in the later phases of the cardiac cycle and interferes with automatic tag analysis.

4.7.3 COMPLEMENTARY SPAMM (CSPAMM)

Complementary SPAMM (CSPAMM) (Fischer et al. 1993) was developed to overcome the magnetization relaxation limitation in SPAMM. CSPAMM consists of two separate SPAMM-prepared scans, one with a sinusoidal tagging pattern and the other with an inverted sinusoidal pattern, as shown in Figure 4.37c. Immediately after the application of the tagging preparation module, the taglines in the two scans have zero unmodulated magnetization, and thus undergo the same T1 magnetization recovery process. Therefore, when subtracting the two images at any time point, the recovered unmodulated magnetization (due to T1 relaxation) is subtracted out, resulting in a sharp tagging pattern with nulled magnetization at the troughs of the sinusoidal pattern. The subtraction process also results in doubling the signal of the tagged magnetization, which is translated into 40% increase in SNR than in SPAMM (similar to acquisition of two averages), but at the expense of doubling the scan time. Another improvement in CSPAMM was the implementation of ramped readout flip angles to compensate for tag fading during the cardiac cycle (secondary to T1 relaxation), which results in uniform tagging contrast (signal difference between the tagged and un-tagged myocardium) throughout the cardiac cycle for better analysis of diastolic cardiac phases. CSPAMM tagging was further improved by combining it with slice-following capability (Fischer et al. 1994) to ensure tracking the same tissue during the cardiac cycle regardless of tissue displacement outside of the imaging plane.

4.7.4 DELAYS ALTERNATING WITH NUTATIONS FOR TAILORED EXCITATION (DANTE)

Delays Alternating with Nutations for Tailored Excitation (DANTE) (Mosher and Smith 1990) creates a high-density pattern of thin tags by means of a continuous gradient pulse and a train of RF pulses with equal interpulse delays (Morris and Freeman 1978), as shown in Figure 4.37d. DANTE has some advantages over SPAMM, including larger flexibility for adjusting tags spacing and thickness, which can be achieved by changing the magnitude of the gradient pulse or the duration between the RF pulses. The limitations of DANTE are similar to SPAMM, which include the dependence of the tagging contrast on T1 relaxation and fading of the taglines with time. Further, DANTE preparation is time-consuming due to the time delay between tagging preparation and the beginning of data readout.

4.7.5 HARMONIC PHASE (HARP) ANALYSIS

Harmonic phase (HARP) was developed as a rapid analysis technique for extracting myocardial motion information from the tagged images (Osman et al. 1999), as shown in Figure 4.37e. The periodic tagging pattern in the image causes modulation of the central signal peak in k-space. The distance between the modulated (harmonic) peaks and central peak in k-space is a function of tag spacing; the closer the taglines, the larger the distance between the harmonic peaks in k-space. The peak at the first harmonic frequency contains the tag displacement information. Therefore, using only this peak (via k-space filtering),

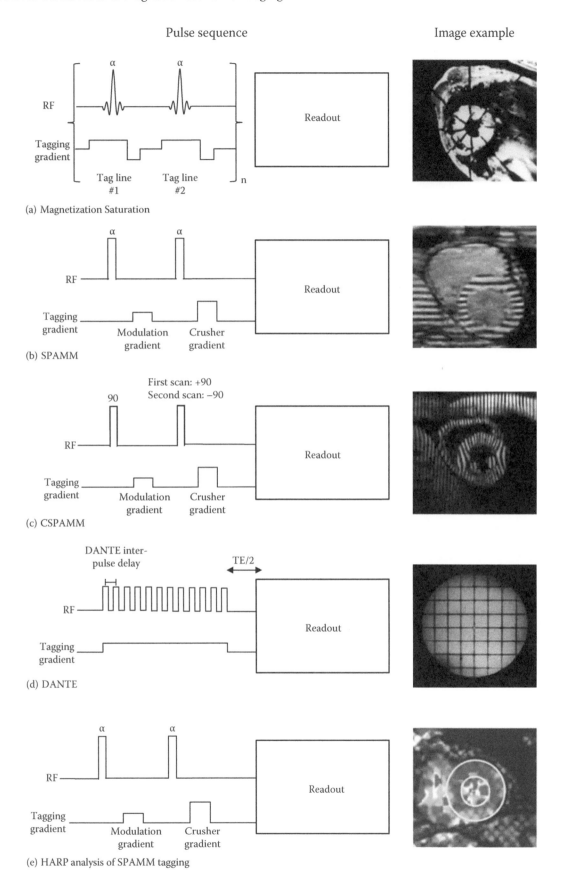

FIGURE 4.37 Tagging techniques. (a) Magnetization saturation. (Reproduced from Lima, J.A. et al., *J. Am. Coll. Cardiol.*, 21(7), 1741, 1993. With permission.) (b) SPAMM. (c) CSPAMM. (d) DANTE. (Reproduced from Mosher, T.J. and Smith, M.B., *Magn. Reson. Med.*, 15(2), 334, 1990. With permission.) (e) HARP. *(Continued)*

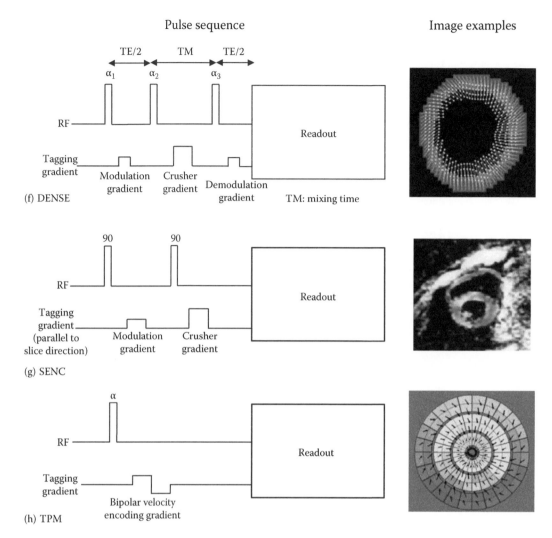

FIGURE 4.37 (Continued) Tagging techniques. (f) DENSE. (Reproduced from Epstein, F.H., *J. Nucl. Cardiol.*, 14(5), 729, 2007. With permission.) (g) SENC. (h) TPM.

harmonic magnitude and phase images can be obtained. The magnitude image shows a blurred anatomical image, while the harmonic phase image shows intensity gradients with sharp transitions due to the wrapped phase created by tagging. The phase can be unwrapped and subsequently tracked at specific points of interest. By tracking the tissue phase from one timeframe to the next one, myocardial displacement can be estimated.

HARP provides fast and automatic analysis of the tagged images, which allowed the tagging techniques to become more frequently used in clinical practice. HARP, as with any 2D imaging method, can have errors due to through-plane motion. However, the combination of HARP analysis with CSPAMM imaging allows for improved HARP analysis (Kuijer et al. 2001).

4.7.6 DISPLACEMENT ENCODING WITH STIMULATED ECHOES (DENSE)

Displacement Encoding with Stimulated Echoes (DENSE) was developed as an imaging method for detecting myocardial motion using phase changes as a function of tissue displacement, similar to PC imaging (Aletras et al. 1999),

as shown in Figure 4.37f; therefore, DENSE combines the advantages of tagging and PC imaging. DENSE is based on the Stimulated Echo Acquisition Mode (STEAM) imaging sequence, which consists of three stages: modulation, mixing, and demodulation. First, the longitudinal magnetization is tipped into the transverse plane and modulated with a modulation gradient, then tipped back into the longitudinal direction. Later at the imaging time point, the modulated magnetization is excited and unwrapped using a demodulation gradient with the same magnitude as the modulation gradient. Stationary spins are perfectly unwrapped with the second gradient and thus have accumulated zero phase, while spins that have moved between modulation and demodulation have accumulated nonzero phase due to their spatial displacement. A second DENSE image can be acquired with no modulation to serve as a reference. When subtracting the two images, extraneous phase not related to motion is removed, and therefore the information about myocardial displacement along the gradient direction is obtained. By applying the modulation gradient on different axes, displacement information can be derived in any spatial direction, for example, in the readout, phase-encoding, and slice-selection directions. Therefore, DENSE can assess in-plane as well as through-plane motion.

DENSE provides highly detailed motion information. After post-processing, motion information is often displayed as a vector where the vector length and orientation represent the magnitude and direction, respectively, of myocardial displacement at each pixel in the image. An additional advantage of DENSE is its inherent black-blood property due to spin dephasing of the flowing blood, which allows for easy detection of the endocardial border. A disadvantage of DENSE is low SNR, although this limitation can be overcome with newer variations of the technique and by imaging at higher field strength (Aletras and Wen 2001, Epstein and Gilson 2004).

4.7.7 STRAIN ENCODING (SENC)

Strain encoding (SENC) was developed to measure myocardial through-plane strain (Osman et al. 2001), that is, longitudinal and circumferential strains are measured from the short-axis and long-axis SENC images, respectively (Figure 4.37g). SENC uses a tagging preparation similar to SPAMM, but the tag planes are oriented parallel to (and inside) the imaging slice (i.e., SENC applies tags in the through-plane direction). During the cardiac cycle, these tagged planes move closer together or further apart (in the through-plane direction) depending on tissue deformation, which affects their tagging frequency. Usually, two images are acquired at different "tuning" frequencies, which are called the low-tuning and high-tuning images. Usually, the low-tuning image is acquired at the applied tagging frequency, which captures signals from static tissues that did not deform, while the high-tuning image is acquired at a higher frequency to capture signals from contracting tissues. By combining information from both images, a color-coded strain map can be obtained. SENC provides high resolution (on the pixel level), intuitive colored strain maps, and requires relatively simple post-processing. It has similar limitations to DENSE, including SNR reduction.

4.7.8 TISSUE PHASE MAPPING (TPM)

Tissue phase mapping (TPM) imaging is based on detecting phase changes in velocity-encoded images, as shown in Figure 4.37h. Its underlying physics are similar to VENC-CMR. When combined with cine imaging, multiple images can be produced depicting cardiac motion throughout the cardiac cycle. Unlike conventional tagging, the resolution of motion detection is not dependent on tag separation, as there is no tagging pattern involved. However, it should be noted that encoding slow velocities (as in the myocardium compared to flowing blood) requires large first-order gradient moments, which results in long echo times (scan time). In addition, TPM imaging is sensitive to phase errors due to eddy currents, susceptibility effects at tissue interfaces (such as at the posterior LV wall), and phase distortions due to cardiac motion. Therefore, a reference image has to be obtained to correct for the background phase. Finally, the TPM images require post-processing to show motion parameters (Lingamneni et al. 1995).

4.8 CUTTING-EDGE CMR TECHNIQUES

Whereas the previously described CMR sequences can be considered as established clinical imaging techniques, the following CMR methods have a lot of potential, but are not yet frequently used in clinical practice.

4.8.1 INTERVENTIONAL CMR

Interventional CMR refers to catheter-based therapeutic procedures using CMR rather than conventional radiographic guidance. Catheter-based procedures conducted without x-rays are very attractive since ionizing radiation is avoided, which is especially important for pediatrics, pregnant women, and patients who need frequent imaging. To accurately place and guide an intravascular catheter, interventional CMR relies on real-time imaging with frame rates of 1–10 fps (Lederman 2005). Catheters developed for interventional CMR and MR-compatible surgical tools are commercially available. To localize the catheter in the MRI image, the catheter acts as an imaging coil sensitive to, and thus highlighting only, its immediate environment. Another approach is to use small RF coils that mark the catheter's tip. Such catheters are navigated through the cardiac chambers to obtain invasive measurements of blood pressure, oxygenation (Schalla et al. 2003), and local blood flow (Volz et al. 2004). Interventional CMR techniques could be also used for guided cell delivery, valve replacement, balloon angioplasty, and repair of different cardiovascular complications. One ideal future application of interventional CMR would be the administration of contrast agent via the catheter directly into the coronary artery to determine vessel patency analogous to diagnostic x-ray angiography. Another application is intracoronary administration of adenosine to investigate exercise-induced ischemia in different coronary artery territories (Lederman et al. 2002). MRI-guided electrophysiology procedures, for example, tissue ablation to interrupt symptomatic atrial or ventricular arrhythmia (Susil et al. 2002), will hopefully become another advantageous application of interventional CMR. Delayed-enhancement CMR could be performed immediately after the procedure to visualize the regions of necrotic tissue created during the ablation. Last, but not least, MRI-guided placement of devices, such as artificial valves, stents, and ASD closure devices (Buecker et al. 2002, Rickers et al. 2003, Schalla et al. 2005), may be a future use of interventional CMR. For instance, the optimal positioning of an aortic stent-valve in relation to the coronary arteries and aortic root would be possible without exposure to radiation.

4.8.2 DIFFUSION CMR

Diffusion-weighted imaging (DWI) is based on the realization that molecules prefer to flow along the main fiber direction of tissue. The first application of DWI was white-matter tractography in the brain and spine, but recently the same idea has been applied to the heart. In histological studies, Streeter et al. (1969) and Streeter and Hanna (1973) demonstrated that cardiomyocytes form myofiber tracts with a crossing helical architecture. These myofiber tracts have a right-handed helix angle in the subendocardium, are oriented circumferentially in the mid-myocardium, and have a left-handed helix angle subepicardially. The assumption underlying the utility of diffusion CMR is that heart diseases perturb this regular pattern of the myofibers, and thus diffusion imaging techniques can detect these changes. Specifically, in healthy myocardium, one would expect the myofibers to be highly anisotropic (directional), resulting in anisotropic diffusion (Sosnovik et al. 2009). Conversely, in diseased myocardial regions, the loss of myofibril integrity results in more isotropic diffusion, which could be seen by diffusion CMR, for example, diffusion tensor imaging (DTI). Provided that diffusion CMR is sufficiently sensitive to slow diffusion, small regional changes in the myocardial structure could be imaged. This is especially important for pathologies where no macroscopic effects (e.g., fibrosis or cell death) are present, but only microscopic changes (e.g., myofibril disorganization) are present, which requires a very sensitive technique to pick up these minute changes. The reader is referred to Chapter 5 for more details on cardiac DTI.

Diffusion CMR is still in its infancy stages. Studies have validated cardiac diffusion images with histology. For these studies, most images were acquired in ex vivo hearts with specialized RF coils, and the translation into clinical practice is not expected in the immediate future.

4.8.3 Cardiac MR Spectroscopy (MRS)

Magnetic resonance spectroscopy (MRS) allows for the measurement of molecular and chemical changes within the human body, and it can be viewed as one of the original forms of molecular imaging. While the majority of imaging studies have been performed on the hydrogen nucleus, that is, the proton, there are many other nuclei that can be probed with MRS. For example, sodium (^{23}Na) spectroscopy can be used to obtain information on myocardial viability (Jansen et al. 2004), phosphorous (^{31}P) spectroscopy provides information on cellular high-energy metabolism (Weiss et al. 1990), and oxygen (^{17}O) spectroscopy can assess mitochondrial respiration (Lu et al. 2012). Different MRI sequences have been developed for voxel localization in spectroscopy, including point-resolved spectroscopy (PRESS), STEAM, and chemical shift imaging (CSI). In vivo cardiac MRS is technically very demanding, and thus it is not commonly used clinically, because of two main reasons. First, in vivo MRS must be able to resolve closely spaced characteristic spectral peaks, which requires excellent magnetic field homogeneity that can be only achieved with shimming, a time-consuming procedure that is further complicated in the heart by cardiac and respiratory motions. Second, the signal of nonproton nuclei is much lower than the proton signal. The exact value depends on their gyromagnetic ratio and natural abundance in the tissue, which is much lower than the natural abundance of hydrogen. Further, in order to obtain a spectrum with adequate SNR, it is necessary to acquire the same spectrum multiple times and average the data, causing

a significantly extended scan time. Finally, the cardiac MRS scan needs to be ECG-triggered and respiratory-triggered or navigated (Kozerke et al. 2002, Schär et al. 2004), because the shimming quality can be only optimized for a small portion of the respiratory and cardiac cycles at a time. MRS also requires suppression of the water peak in proton spectroscopy.

4.8.4 Molecular and Cellular CMR

With the development of new contrast agents, for example, ultrasmall superparamagnetic iron oxides (USPIO), and contrast mechanisms, for example, chemical exchange saturation transfer (CEST) and paramagnetic CEST (PARACEST), the field of molecular/cellular CMR imaging is expected to play a potential role in the future of cardiovascular imaging. These imaging techniques would allow for evaluating and improving state-of-the-art cardiac medical research, including tissue engineering, stem cell implantation, and regenerative medicine for "repairing" diseased myocardium, enhancing myocardial contractility, and improving heart function in general.

Much attention has been given to the development of new, targeted, and theranostic contrast agents for molecular CMR imaging. These contrast agents are designed to target specific cellular structures to provide tissue-specific contrasts. For example, one contrast agent is monocrystalline iron oxide nanoparticles, which is designed to specifically attach to the antimyosin antigen-binding fragment (FAB). It permits immunospecific CMR imaging of myocardial infarction (Weissleder et al. 1992). Another agent is designed to specifically target collagen, which is a principal component of myocardial remodeling occurring as a response to infarction (Caravan et al. 2007). While these compounds have shown promising results in animal models, they have not been yet demonstrated in humans.

The development of hyperpolarization techniques has allowed for imaging and spectroscopic analysis of previously inaccessible molecules and molecular pathways. Hyperpolarized carbon (^{13}C) has been used for a wide variety of imaging targets, including intracellular pH (Schroeder et al. 2010), cardiac metabolism of pyruvate, and inhibition of carbohydrate oxidation after brief ischemia (Merritt et al. 2008, Tyler et al. 2008, Hu et al. 2009, Schroeder et al. 2009, Lau et al. 2010, Moreno et al. 2010). While these methods and compounds are very promising, they are technically challenging. Hyperpolarized magnetization is destroyed by a 90° RF pulse as it does not naturally recover. Hence, special care in pulse sequence design must be taken. The hyperpolarized state also decays with T1, meaning that the hyperpolarized contrast agents need to be used within at most five times the T1 of the hyperpolarized nucleus, usually between 1 and 2 minutes after hyperpolarization.

Finally, fluorine imaging is gaining popularity due to its high sensitivity and lack of background signal. Fluorine atoms in the perfluorocarbon core of nanoparticles have been used for identifying areas of vascular stenosis due to their sensitivity to oxygen content (Morawski et al. 2004).

4.8.5 Tissue Iron Imaging

Blood disorders, for example, thalassemia, sickle-cell disease, and hereditary hemochromatosis, lead to myocardial iron overload. Elevated tissue iron levels are toxic and can cause endocrine, cardiac, and hepatic dysfunction. Iron levels can be assessed with T2*-weighted CMR, since iron shortens T2* in the tissue due to its paramagnetic properties. T2*-weighted CMR can also depict hemorrhage and calcification. By acquiring multiple images with different echo times, the T2* relaxation curve can be determined on the pixel level, where T2* values can be calculated using exponential curve fitting, and plotted as a T2* map.

Monitoring T2* as a measure of myocardial iron content is of vital importance for patient diagnosis and management, as elevated iron levels are cardiotoxic and can lead to diastolic and systolic dysfunction, cardiomyopathy, and ultimately heart failure (Pennell 2006). In addition to identifying iron overload, T2* imaging CMR can also track the effectiveness of the chelation therapy on lowering myocardial iron concentration (Anderson et al. 2004, Pennell 2006, Modell et al. 2008). Most research on T2* imaging is concerned with thalassemia (Pennell 2006). For this disease, T2* imaging has been validated against standard invasive iron quantification techniques (Anderson et al. 2001). Its reproducibility across different MRI scanner models and vendors has been also shown (Westwood et al. 2003).

In normal subjects at 1.5 T, T2* is larger than 35–40 ms (Anderson et al. 2001, Leonardi et al. 2008, Kirk et al. 2009). A T2* value that is smaller than 20 ms (at 1.5 T) is considered diagnostic for myocardial iron overload. Heart failure is usually not observed unless T2* is below this cutoff value. A cardiac T2* value smaller than 10 ms is associated with severe iron overload with high risk for developing symptomatic heart failure and/or arrhythmia in thalassemia major (Kirk et al. 2009). While normal and abnormal values for T2* are established at 1.5 T, few studies investigated the capabilities of T2* imaging at 3 T for evaluating iron overload. It has been shown that through careful parameter optimization and shimming, imaging at 3 T allows for higher sensitivity for detecting lower iron concentrations with the clinical significance of prompt initiation of chelation therapy for higher chances of reversing iron overload before heart failure ensues (Ibrahim et al. 2012).

4.9 SUMMARY AND KEY POINTS

4.9.1 Summary

This chapter provided a condensed overview of basic CMR techniques, illuminating the technical principles underlying image acquisition and contrast formation. The major focus of this chapter was cine CMR imaging for cardiac function and morphology assessment and how to clinically interpret the images. Available physiological signal synchronization methods were discussed. Guidelines on the use of synchronization method and readout type for specific cardiac pathophysiology were given. Analysis tools were presented for quantitative, semiquantitative, and qualitative assessment of cardiac function, myocardial viability and ischemia, and flow. We attempted to comprehensively present techniques used for CMR research studies as well as efficient methods commonly favored in clinical routines. Practical tips on how to remedy common CMR image artifacts and improve ECG signal quality were provided to help troubleshoot common CMR image quality issues. A brief overview of the myocardial tagging techniques was provided. At last, we discussed upcoming CMR techniques with potentially large clinical benefit.

In summary, CMR offers the broadest range of imaging tests performed by a single modality. The operator has a huge, and thus often confusing, choices among different CMR methods. The field is still evolving, creating even more techniques of potential clinical use. For CMR to be practical and easy-to-use, much simpler user interfaces, standardized image acquisition methods, and automated data analysis and quantification software have to be developed. Some vendors have realized this need and are now providing so-called optimization engines to simplify, standardize, and accelerate MRI of specific body parts, including the heart.

The future of CMR imaging is very promising. MRI is undergoing continuous developments in both hardware (fast gradients, powerful amplifiers, and coil design) and software (pulse sequences, reconstruction algorithms, and user interface modules) techniques. These developments will help improve CMR imaging with its challenging needs. Interventional CMR is rapidly growing with the advantage of saving the patient from the x-ray radiation associated with traditional fluoroscopy. Another promising area is high-field CMR. 7 T scanners are being installed worldwide, and started to be used for clinical service, which will result in improved image quality, reduced scan time, and emerging of new applications. Finally, multimodality imaging using composite PET-MRI scanners will open the door for advanced molecular imaging for better understanding of the heart function in health and disease.

4.9.2 Key Points

- CMR offers many potential advantages over other cardiovascular imaging modalities.
- A high-quality ECG signal is necessary for acquiring artifact-free CMR images.
- Synchronization of the pulse sequence to the cardiac cycle is necessary, which is most commonly achieved by detecting the R-wave of the ECG signal.
- Breath-holding is the simplest and most commonly used technique for avoiding respiratory motion artifacts.
- A respiratory navigator, which is integrated into the imaging pulse sequence, provides an alternative strategy for reducing breathing artifacts.
- Self-navigated techniques have recently been introduced for respiratory motion compensation.
- Each pulse sequence is configured by a large set of scan parameters, known as the MRI protocol.

- Different protocol parameters have various degrees of effects on the image characteristics.
- Most MRI parameters have a direct or indirect effect on other parameters.
- The two most common data acquisition strategies are segmented and single-shot acquisition.
- Segmented acquisition distributes data collection over multiple heartbeats, while single-shot acquisition is done during only one heartbeat.
- There are competing effects among spatial resolution, temporal resolution, and scan time.
- CMR-related artifacts include those related to breathing, cardiac synchronization, and metallic devices/implants.
- Scouting is the first and simplest scan of every CMR examination, which is conducted to determine standard cardiac views that can be used throughout the scan.
- Morphology images are acquired as a stack of parallel slices cutting through the anatomical region of interest.
- The choice between bright-blood GRE and dark-blood SE imaging depends on the clinical question.
- Perfusion CMR acquires a temporal series of single-shot images that are later played as a movie showing the transit of a gadolinium-based contrast media during its first pass through the myocardium.
- Delayed-enhancement CMR is a method that can simultaneously evaluate myocardial infarction and viability.
- Multi-contrast imaging is useful for tissue characterization.
- T1-weighted imaging is widely used in CMR, including perfusion and delayed-enhancement imaging.
- T2-weighted imaging has shown promise for assessing acute, inflammatory processes.
- T2* imaging can be used in patients with known or suspected hemolytic anemia and/or iron overload pathologies.
- When combined with morphological imaging, contrast-enhanced MRA can be used to fully define arterial or venous structures.
- Coronary MRA may be used to directly visualize the coronary anatomy and morphology.
- Velocity-encoded PC imaging is used for quantification of flow and motion, similar to Doppler echocardiography.
- Cine imaging is a fundamental part of almost every CMR examination, which has become widely accepted as the noninvasive gold standard for contractile function assessment.
- Segmented data acquisition is the primary acquisition strategy for cine imaging.
- Cardiac synchronization strategies include prospective triggering, retrospective gating, and triggered retro-gating.
- Advanced techniques that could enhance data acquisition efficiency in cine CMR include echo sharing, fast k-space trajectories, parallel imaging, and real-time techniques.
- Cine images are used for evaluating the heart volumes, mass, and function, using either a qualitative or quantitative approach.
- Ventricular contouring, for providing quantitative measures of the heart function, could be implemented using manual, semiautomated, and automated approaches.
- Cine CMR imaging could be used in different applications, including tissue characterization, constrictive pericarditis, valvular diseases, cardiac masses, thrombus, and congenital heart diseases.
- The tagging techniques provide detailed information about regional myocardial contractility.
- The tagging techniques include selective magnetization saturation, SPAMM, CSPAMM, DANTE, HARP, DENSE, SENC, and TPM.
- Advanced CMR techniques include interventional CMR, cardiac DTI, cardiac MRS, and molecular imaging.

REFERENCES

Abdel-Aty, H., Zagrosek, A., Schulz-Menger, J., Taylor, A.J., Messroghli, D., Kumar, A., Gross, M., Dietz, R., and Friedrich, M.G. (2004). Delayed enhancement and T2-weighted cardiovascular magnetic resonance imaging differentiate acute from chronic myocardial infarction. *Circulation* **109**(20): 2411–2416.

Abergel, E., Chatellier, G., Hagege, A.A., Oblak, A., Linhart, A., Ducardonnet, A., and Menard, J. (2004). Serial left ventricular adaptations in world-class professional cyclists: Implications for disease screening and follow-up. *J Am Coll Cardiol* **44**(1): 144–149.

Aletras, A.H., Ding, S., Balaban, R.S., and Wen, H. (1999). DENSE: Displacement encoding with stimulated echoes in cardiac functional MRI. *J Magn Reson* **137**(1): 247–252.

Aletras, A.H. and Wen, H. (2001). Mixed echo train acquisition displacement encoding with stimulated echoes: An optimized DENSE method for in vivo functional imaging of the human heart. *Magn Reson Med* **46**(3): 523–534.

Alfakih, K., Reid, S., Jones, T., and Sivananthan, M. (2004). Assessment of ventricular function and mass by cardiac magnetic resonance imaging. *Eur Radiol* **14**(10): 1813–1822.

Altun, E., Martin, D.R., Wertman, R., Lugo-Somolinos, A., Fuller, E.R., and Semelka, R.C. (2009). Nephrogenic systemic fibrosis: Change in incidence following a switch in gadolinium agents and adoption of a gadolinium policy—Report from two US universities. *Radiology* **253**(3): 689–696.

Anderson, L., Holden, S., Davis, B., Prescott, E., Charrier, C., Bunce, N., Firmin, D., Wonke, B., Porter, J., and Walker, J. (2001). Cardiovascular T2-star (T2*) magnetic resonance for the early diagnosis of myocardial iron overload. *Eur Heart J* **22**(23): 2171–2179.

Anderson, L.J., Westwood, M.A., Holden, S., Davis, B., Prescott, E., Wonke, B., Porter, J.B., Malcolm Walker, J., and Pennell, D.J. (2004). Myocardial iron clearance during reversal of siderotic cardiomyopathy with intravenous desferrioxamine: A prospective study using T2* cardiovascular magnetic resonance. *Br J Haematol* **127**(3): 348–355.

Angelie, E., De Koning, P., Danilouchkine, M., van Assen, H., Koning, G., Van Der Geest, R., and Reiber, J. (2005). Optimizing the automatic segmentation of the left ventricle in magnetic resonance images. *Med Phys* **32**: 369.

Assomull, R.G., Prasad, S.K., Lyne, J., Smith, G., Burman, E.D., Khan, M., Sheppard, M.N., Poole-Wilson, P.A., and Pennell, D.J. (2006). Cardiovascular magnetic resonance, fibrosis, and prognosis in dilated cardiomyopathy. *J Am Coll Cardiol* **48**(10): 1977–1985.

Axel, L. and Dougherty, L. (1989a). Heart wall motion: Improved method of spatial modulation of magnetization for MR imaging. *Radiology* **172**(2): 349–350.

Axel, L. and Dougherty, L. (1989b). MR imaging of motion with spatial modulation of magnetization. *Radiology* **171**(3): 841–845.

Baer, F.M., Theissen, P., Schneider, C.A., Voth, E., Sechtem, U., Schicha, H., and Erdmann, E. (1998). Dobutamine magnetic resonance imaging predicts contractile recovery of chronically dysfunctional myocardium after successful revascularization. *J Am Coll Cardiol* **31**(5): 1040–1048.

Beerbaum, P., Körperich, H., Barth, P., Esdorn, H., Gieseke, J., and Meyer, H. (2001). Noninvasive quantification of left-to-right shunt in pediatric patients: Phase-contrast cine magnetic resonance imaging compared with invasive oximetry. *Circulation* **103**(20): 2476–2482.

Beerbaum, P., Körperich, H., Esdorn, H., Blanz, U., Barth, P., Hartmann, J., Gieseke, J., and Meyer, H. (2003). Atrial septal defects in pediatric patients: Noninvasive sizing with cardiovascular MR imaging. *Radiology* **228**(2): 361–369.

Bellenger, N.G., Rajappan, K., Rahman, S.L., Lahiri, A., Raval, U., Webster, J., Murray, G.D., Coats, A.J., Cleland, J.G., and Pennell, D.J. (2004). Effects of carvedilol on left ventricular remodelling in chronic stable heart failure: A cardiovascular magnetic resonance study. *Heart* **90**(7): 760–764.

Bernstein, M.A., King, K.F., and Zhou, X.J. (2004). *Handbook of MRI Pulse Sequences*. Burlington, MA: Elsevier.

Bottini, E. (1975). Abortion: A hypothesis on the role of ABO blood groups and placental alkaline phosphatase. *Soc Biol* **22**(3): 221–228.

Braunwald, E. and Kloner, R. (1982). The stunned myocardium: Prolonged, postischemic ventricular dysfunction. *Circulation* **66**(6): 1146–1149.

Brittain, J.H., Hu, B.S., Wright, G.A., Meyer, C.H., Macovski, A., and Nishimura, D.G. (2005). Coronary angiography with magnetization-prepared T2 contrast. *Magn Reson Med* **33**(5): 689–696.

Buecker, A., Spuentrup, E., Grabitz, R., Freudenthal, F., Muehler, E.G., Schaeffter, T., van Vaals, J.J., and Günther, R.W. (2002). Magnetic resonance–guided placement of atrial septal closure device in animal model of patent foramen ovale. *Circulation* **106**(4): 511–515.

Caravan, P., Das, B., Dumas, S., Epstein, F.H., Helm, P.A., Jacques, V., Koerner, S., Kolodziej, A., Shen, L., and Sun, W.C. (2007). Collagen-targeted MRI contrast agent for molecular imaging of fibrosis. *Angew Chem* **119**(43): 8319–8321.

Carr, J.C., Laub, G., Zheng, J., Pereles, F.S., and Finn, J.P. (2002). Time-resolved three-dimensional pulmonary MR angiography and perfusion imaging with ultrashort repetition time. *Acad Radiol* **9**(12): 1407–1418.

Caruthers, S.D., Lin, S.J., Brown, P., Watkins, M.P., Williams, T.A., Lehr, K.A., and Wickline, S.A. (2003). Practical value of cardiac magnetic resonance imaging for clinical quantification of aortic valve stenosis comparison with echocardiography. *Circulation* **108**(18): 2236–2243.

Cerqueira, M.D., Weissman, N.J., Dilsizian, V., Jacobs, A.K., Kaul, S., Laskey, W.K., Pennell, D.J., Rumberger, J.A., Ryan, T., and Verani, M.S. (2002). Standardized myocardial segmentation and nomenclature for tomographic imaging of the heart. A statement for healthcare professionals from the Cardiac Imaging Committee of the Council on Clinical Cardiology of the American Heart Association. *Int J Cardiovasc Imaging* **18**(1): 539–542.

Choudhury, L., Mahrholdt, H., Wagner, A., Choi, K.M., Elliott, M.D., Klocke, F.J., Bonow, R.O., Judd, R.M., and Kim, R.J. (2002). Myocardial scarring in asymptomatic or mildly symptomatic patients with hypertrophic cardiomyopathy. *J Am Coll Cardiol* **40**(12): 2156–2164.

Conti, C.R. (1991). The stunned and hibernating myocardium: A brief review. *Clin Cardiol* **14**(9): 708–712.

Danias, P.G., McConnell, M.V., Khasgiwala, V.C., Chuang, M.L., Edelman, R.R., and Manning, W.J. (1997). Prospective navigator correction of image position for coronary MR angiography. *Radiology* **203**(3): 733–736.

de Graaf, F.R., Schuijf, J.D., van Velzen, J.E., Kroft, L.J., de Roos, A., Sieders, A., Jukema, J.W., Schalij, M.J., van der Wall, E.E., and Bax, J.J. (2010). Evaluation of contraindications and efficacy of oral beta blockade before computed tomographic coronary angiography. *Am J Cardiol* **105**(6): 767–772.

Debatin, J.F., Ting, R.H., Wegmuller, H., Sommer, F.G., Fredrickson, J.O., Brosnan, T.J., Bowman, B.S., Myers, B.D., Herfkens, R.J., and Pelc, N.J. (1994). Renal artery blood flow: Quantitation with phase-contrast MR imaging with and without breath holding. *Radiology* **190**(2): 371–378.

Detrano, R., Guerci, A.D., Carr, J.J., Bild, D.E., Burke, G., Folsom, A.R., Liu, K., Shea, S., Szklo, M., and Bluemke, D.A. (2008). Coronary calcium as a predictor of coronary events in four racial or ethnic groups. *N Engl J Med* **358**(13): 1336–1345.

Dimick, R.N., Hedlund, L.W., Herfkens, R.J., Fram, E.K., and Utz, J. (1987). Optimizing electrocardiograph electrode placement for cardiac-gated magnetic resonance imaging. *Invest Radiol* **22**(1): 17–22.

Edelman, R., Chien, D., and Kim, D. (1991). Fast selective black blood MR imaging. *Radiology* **181**(3): 655–660.

Ehman, R.L. and Felmlee, J.P. (1989). Adaptive technique for high-definition MR imaging of moving structures. *Radiology* **173**(1): 255–263.

Epstein, F.H. (2007). MRI of left ventricular function. *J Nucl Cardiol* **14**(5): 729–744.

Epstein, F.H. and Gilson, W.D. (2004). Displacement-encoded cardiac MRI using cosine and sine modulation to eliminate (CANSEL) artifact-generating echoes. *Magn Reson Med* **52**(4): 774–781.

Epstein, F.H., London, J.F., Peters, D.C., Goncalves, L.M., Agyeman, K., Taylor, J., Balaban, R.S., and Arai, A.E. (2002). Multislice first-pass cardiac perfusion MRI: Validation in a model of myocardial infarction. *Magn Reson Med* **47**(3): 482–491.

Fieno, D.S., Kim, R.J., Chen, E.L., Lomasney, J.W., Klocke, F.J., and Judd, R.M. (2000). Contrast-enhanced magnetic resonance imaging of myocardium at risk: Distinction between reversible and irreversible injury throughout infarct healing. *J Am Coll Cardiol* **36**(6): 1985–1991.

Finn, J.P., Nael, K., Deshpande, V., Ratib, O., and Laub, G. (2006). Cardiac MR imaging: State of the technology. *Radiology* **241**(2): 338–354.

Fischbach, R., Juergens, K.U., Ozgun, M., Maintz, D., Grude, M., Seifarth, H., Heindel, W., and Wichter, T. (2007). Assessment of regional left ventricular function with multidetector-row computed tomography versus magnetic resonance imaging. *Eur Radiol* **17**(4): 1009–1017.

Fischer, S.E., McKinnon, G.C., Maier, S.E., and Boesiger, P. (1993). Improved myocardial tagging contrast. *Magn Reson Med* **30**(2): 191–200.

Fischer, S.E., McKinnon, G.C., Scheidegger, M.B., Prins, W., Meier, D., and Boesiger, P. (1994). True myocardial motion tracking. *Magn Reson Med* **31**(4): 401–413.

Francone, M., Dymarkowski, S., Kalantzi, M., Rademakers, F., and Bogaert, J. (2006a). Assessment of ventricular coupling with real-time cine MRI and its value to differentiate constrictive pericarditis from restrictive cardiomyopathy. *Eur Radiol* **16**(4): 944–951.

Frauenrath, T., Hezel, F., Renz, W., d'Orth Tde, G., Dieringer, M., von Knobelsdorff-Brenkenhoff, F., Prothmann, M., Schulz Menger, J., and Niendorf, T. (2010). Acoustic cardiac triggering: A practical solution for synchronization and gating of cardiovascular magnetic resonance at 7 Tesla. *J Cardiovasc Magn Reson* **12**: 67.

Friedrich, M.G., Dahlof, B., Sechtem, U., Unger, T., Knecht, M., Dietz, R., and TELMAR Investigators. (2003). Reduction (TELMAR) as assessed by magnetic resonance imaging in patients with mild-to-moderate hypertension—A prospective, randomised, double-blind comparison of telmisartan with metoprolol over a period of six months rationale and study design. *J Renin Angiotensin Aldosterone Syst* **4**(4): 234–243.

Friedrich, M.G., Schulz-Menger, J., Poetsch, T., Pilz, B., Uhlich, F., and Dietz, R. (2002). Quantification of valvular aortic stenosis by magnetic resonance imaging. *Am Heart J* **144**(2): 329–334.

Fuster, V. and Kim, R.J. (2005). Frontiers in cardiovascular magnetic resonance. *Circulation* **112**(1): 135–144.

Giardini, A., Lovato, L., Donti, A., Formigari, R., Gargiulo, G., Picchio, F.M., and Fattori, R. (2007). A pilot study on the effects of carvedilol on right ventricular remodelling and exercise tolerance in patients with systemic right ventricle. *Int J Cardiol* **114**(2): 241–246.

Grebe, O., Kestler, H.A., Merkle, N., Wöhrle, J., Kochs, M., Höher, M., and Hombach, V. (2004). Assessment of left ventricular function with steady-state-free-precession magnetic resonance imaging. *Z Kardiol* **93**(9): 686–695.

Griswold, M.A., Jakob, P.M., Heidemann, R.M., Nittka, M., Jellus, V., Wang, J., Kiefer, B., and Haase, A. (2002). Generalized autocalibrating partially parallel acquisitions (GRAPPA). *Magn Reson Med* **47**(6): 1202–1210.

Grothues, F., Smith, G.C., Moon, J.C., Bellenger, N.G., Collins, P., Klein, H.U., and Pennell, D.J. (2002). Comparison of inter-study reproducibility of cardiovascular magnetic resonance with two-dimensional echocardiography in normal subjects and in patients with heart failure or left ventricular hypertrophy. *Am J Cardiol* **90**(1): 29–34.

Hansen, M.S., Atkinson, D., and Sorensen, T.S. (2008). Cartesian SENSE and k-t SENSE reconstruction using commodity graphics hardware. *Magn Reson Med* **59**(3): 463–468.

Hartnell, G., Cohen, M., Meier, R., and Finn, J. (1996). Magnetic resonance angiography demonstration of congenital heart disease in adults. *Clin Radiol* **51**(12): 851–857.

Heeger, C.H., Jaquet, K., Thiele, H., Zulkarnaen, Y., Cuneo, A., Haller, D., Kivelitz, D. et al. (2012). Percutaneous, transendocardial injection of bone marrow-derived mononuclear cells in heart failure patients following acute ST-elevation myocardial infarction: ALSTER-Stem Cell trial. *EuroIntervention* **8**(6): 732–742.

Hendel, R.C., Patel, M.R., Kramer, C.M., Poon, M., Carr, J.C., Gerstad, N.A., Gillam, L.D., Hodgson, J.M.B., Kim, R.J., and Lesser, J.R. (2006). ACCF/ACR/SCCT/SCMR/ASNC/NASCI/SCAI/SIR 2006 Appropriateness criteria for cardiac computed tomography and cardiac magnetic resonance imaging: A report of the American College of Cardiology Foundation Quality Strategic Directions Committee Appropriateness Criteria Working Group, American College of Radiology, Society of Cardiovascular Computed Tomography, Society for Cardiovascular Magnetic Resonance, American Society of Nuclear Cardiology, North American Society for Cardiac Imaging, Society for Cardiovascular Angiography and Interventions, and Society of Interventional Radiology. *J Am Coll Cardiol* **48**(7): 1475–1497.

Herman, M.V. and Gorlin, R. (1969). Implications of left ventricular asynergy. *Am J Cardiol* **23**(4): 538–547.

Hoffmann, U., Globits, S., Schima, W., Loewe, C., Puig, S., Oberhuber, G., and Frank, H. (2003). Usefulness of magnetic resonance imaging of cardiac and paracardiac masses. *Am J Cardiol* **92**(7): 890–895.

Holland, A.E., Goldfarb, J.W., and Edelman, R.R. (1998). Diaphragmatic and cardiac motion during suspended breathing: Preliminary experience and implications for breath-hold MR imaging. *Radiology* **209**(2): 483–489.

Hu, S., Chen, A.P., Zierhut, M.L., Bok, R., Yen, Y.F., Schroeder, M.A., Hurd, R.E., Nelson, S.J., Kurhanewicz, J., and Vigneron, D.B. (2009). In vivo carbon-13 dynamic MRS and MRSI of normal and fasted rat liver with hyperpolarized 13 C-pyruvate. *Mol Imaging Biol* **11**(6): 399–407.

Hudsmith, L.E., Petersen, S.E., Francis, J.M., Robson, M.D., and Neubauer, S. (2005). Normal human left and right ventricular and left atrial dimensions using steady state free precession magnetic resonance imaging. *J Cardiovasc Magn Reson* **7**(5): 775–782.

Ibrahim, El-S.H. (2011). Myocardial tagging by cardiovascular magnetic resonance: Evolution of techniques—Pulse sequences, analysis algorithms, and applications. *J Cardiovasc Magn Reson* **13**(1): 1–40.

Ibrahim, El-S.H. (2012). Imaging sequences in cardiovascular magnetic resonance: Current role, evolving applications, and technical challenges. *Int J Cardiovasc Imaging* **28**(8): 2027–2047.

Ibrahim, El-S.H., Rana, F.N., Johnson, K.R., and White, R.D. (2012). Assessment of cardiac iron deposition in sickle cell disease using 3.0 Tesla cardiovascular magnetic resonance. *Hemoglobin* **36**(4): 343–361.

Ioannidis, J.P., Trikalinos, T.A., and Danias, P.G. (2002). Electrocardiogram-gated single-photon emission computed tomography versus cardiac magnetic resonance imaging for the assessment of left ventricular volumes and ejection fraction: A meta-analysis. *J Am Coll Cardiol* **39**(12): 2059–2068.

Janik, M., Cham, M.D., Ross, M.I., Wang, Y., Codella, N., Min, J.K., Prince, M.R. et al. (2008). Effects of papillary muscles and trabeculae on left ventricular quantification: Increased impact of methodological variability in patients with left ventricular hypertrophy. *J Hypertens* **26**(8): 1677–1685.

Jansen, M.A., Van Emous, J.G., Nederhoff, M.G.J., and Van Echteld, C.J.A. (2004). Assessment of myocardial viability by intracellular 23Na magnetic resonance imaging. *Circulation* **110**(22): 3457–3464.

Jenkins, C., Bricknell, K., Hanekom, L., and Marwick, T.H. (2004). Reproducibility and accuracy of echocardiographic measurements of left ventricular parameters using real-time three-dimensional echocardiography. *J Am Coll Cardiol* **44**(4): 878–886.

John, A.S., Dill, T., Brandt, R.R., Rau, M., Ricken, W., Bachmann, G., and Hamm, C.W. (2003). Magnetic resonance to assess the aortic valve area in aortic stenosis: How does it compare to current diagnostic standards? *J Am Coll Cardiol* **42**(3): 519–526.

Kaminaga, T., Takeshita, T., and Kimura, I. (2003). Role of magnetic resonance imaging for evaluation of tumors in the cardiac region. *Eur Radiol* **13**(6): L1–L10.

Kanal, E., Barkovich, A.J., Bell, C., Borgstede, J.P., Bradley, W.G., Froelich, J.W., Gilk, T., Gimbel, J.R., Gosbee, J., and Kuhni-Kaminski, E. (2007). ACR guidance document for safe MR practices: 2007. *Am J Roentgenol* **188**(6): 1447–1474.

Katscher, U. and Bornert, P. (2006). Parallel RF transmission in MRI. *NMR Biomed* **19**(3): 393–400.

Kellman, P., Aletras, A.H., Mancini, C., McVeigh, E.R., and Arai, A.E. (2007). T2-prepared SSFP improves diagnostic confidence in edema imaging in acute myocardial infarction compared to turbo spin echo. *Magn Reson Med* **57**(5): 891–897.

Kilner, P.J., Manzara, C.C., Mohiaddin, R.H., Pennell, D.J., Sutton, M., Firmin, D.N., Underwood, S.R., and Longmore, D.B. (1993a). Magnetic resonance jet velocity mapping in mitral and aortic valve stenosis. *Circulation* **87**(4): 1239–1248.

Kilner, P.J., Yang, G., Mohiaddin, R., Firmin, D., and Longmore, D. (1993b). Helical and retrograde secondary flow patterns in the aortic arch studied by three-directional magnetic resonance velocity mapping. *Circulation* **88**(5): 2235–2247.

Kim, H.W., Farzaneh-Far, A., and Kim, R.J. (2009). Cardiovascular magnetic resonance in patients with myocardial infarction: Current and emerging applications. *J Am Coll Cardiol* **55**(1): 1–16.

Kim, H.W., Farzaneh-Far, A., Klem, I., Rehwald, W.G., and Kim, R.J. (2008). Magnetic resonance imaging of the heart. In *Hurst's the Heart*, V. Fuster and R.A. O'Rourke (eds.), McGraw-Hill Medical, New York, vol. 2, pp. 631–667.

Kim, R. and Shah, D. (2004). Fundamental concepts in myocardial viability assessment revisited: When knowing how much is alive is not enough. *Heart* **90**(2): 137–140.

Kim, R.J., Fieno, D.S., Parrish, T.B., Harris, K., Chen, E.L., Simonetti, O., Bundy, J., Finn, J.P., Klocke, F.J., and Judd, R.M. (1999). Relationship of MRI delayed contrast enhancement to irreversible injury, infarct age, and contractile function. *Circulation* **100**(19): 1992–2002.

Kim, R.J., Shah, D.J., and Judd, R.M. (2003). How we perform delayed enhancement imaging. *J Cardiovasc Magn Reson* **5**(3): 505–514.

Kim, W.Y., Danias, P.G., Stuber, M., Flamm, S.D., Plein, S., Nagel, E., Langerak, S.E., Weber, O.M., Pedersen, E.M., and Schmidt, M. (2001). Coronary magnetic resonance angiography for the detection of coronary stenoses. *N Engl J Med* **345**(26): 1863–1869.

Kirk, P., Roughton, M., Porter, J.B., Walker, J.M., Tanner, M.A., Patel, J., Wu, D., Taylor, J., Westwood, M.A., and Anderson, L.J. (2009). Cardiac T2* magnetic resonance for prediction of cardiac complications in thalassemia major. *Circulation* **120**(20): 1961–1968.

Kjaergaard, J., Petersen, C.L., Kjaer, A., Schaadt, B.K., Oh, J.K., and Hassager, C. (2006). Evaluation of right ventricular volume and function by 2D and 3D echocardiography compared to MRI. *Eur J Echocardiogr* **7**(6): 430–438.

Kjekshus, J.K., Torp-Pedersen, C., Gullestad, L., Kober, L., Edvardsen, T., Olsen, I.C., Sjaastad, I. et al. (2009). Effect of piboserod, a 5-HT4 serotonin receptor antagonist, on left ventricular function in patients with symptomatic heart failure. *Eur J Heart Fail* **11**(8): 771–778.

Klem, I., Heitner, J.F., Shah, D.J., Sketch, M.H., Jr., Behar, V., Weinsaft, J., Cawley, P. et al. (2006). Improved detection of coronary artery disease by stress perfusion cardiovascular magnetic resonance with the use of delayed enhancement infarction imaging. *J Am Coll Cardiol* **47**(8): 1630–1638.

Klocke, F.J., Simonetti, O.P., Judd, R.M., Kim, R.J., Harris, K.R., Hedjbeli, S., Fieno, D.S., Miller, S., Chen, V., and Parker, M.A. (2001). Limits of detection of regional differences in vasodilated flow in viable myocardium by first-pass magnetic resonance perfusion imaging. *Circulation* **104**(20): 2412–2416.

Kozerke, S., Schär, M., Lamb, H.J., and Boesiger, P. (2002). Volume tracking cardiac 31P spectroscopy. *Magn Reson Med* **48**(2): 380–384.

Kramer, C.M., Barkhausen, J., Flamm, S.D., Kim, R.J., and Nagel, E. (2008). Standardized cardiovascular magnetic resonance imaging (CMR) protocols, society for cardiovascular magnetic resonance: Board of trustees task force on standardized protocols. *J Cardiovasc Magn Reson* **10**: 35.

Kremkau, F.W. and Taylor, K.J. (1986). Artifacts in ultrasound imaging. *J Ultrasound Med* **5**(4): 227–237.

Kribben, A., Witzke, O., Hillen, U., Barkhausen, J., Daul, A.E., and Erbel, R. (2009). Nephrogenic systemic fibrosis: Pathogenesis, diagnosis, and therapy. *J Am Coll Cardiol* **53**(18): 1621–1628.

Kuhl, H.P., Schreckenberg, M., Rulands, D., Katoh, M., Schafer, W., Schummers, G., Bucker, A., Hanrath, P., and Franke, A. (2004). High-resolution transthoracic real-time three-dimensional echocardiography: Quantitation of cardiac volumes and function using semi-automatic border detection and comparison with cardiac magnetic resonance imaging. *J Am Coll Cardiol* **43**(11): 2083–2090.

Kuijer, J., Jansen, E., Marcus, J.T., van Rossum, A.C., and Heethaar, R.M. (2001). Improved harmonic phase myocardial strain maps. *Magn Reson Med* **46**(5): 993–999.

Kupfahl, C., Honold, M., Meinhardt, G., Vogelsberg, H., Wagner, A., Mahrholdt, H., and Sechtem, U. (2004). Evaluation of aortic stenosis by cardiovascular magnetic resonance imaging: Comparison with established routine clinical techniques. *Heart* **90**(8): 893–901.

Kwong, R. (2008). *Cardiovascular Magnetic Resonance Imaging*. Humana Press, Totowa, New Jersey.

Lai, P., Larson, A.C., Bi, X., Jerecic, R., and Li, D. (2008). A dual-projection respiratory self-gating technique for whole-heart coronary MRA. *J Magn Reson Imaging* **28**(3): 612–620.

Lamb, H.J., Beyerbacht, H.P., de Roos, A., van der Laarse, A., Vliegen, H.W., Leujes, F., Bax, J.J., and van der Wall, E.E. (2002). Left ventricular remodeling early after aortic valve replacement: Differential effects on diastolic function in aortic valve stenosis and aortic regurgitation. *J Am Coll Cardiol* **40**(12): 2182–2188.

Lang, R.M., Bierig, M., Devereux, R.B., Flachskampf, F.A., Foster, E., Pellikka, P.A., Picard, M.H. et al. (2005). Recommendations for chamber quantification: A report from the American Society of Echocardiography's Guidelines and Standards Committee and the Chamber Quantification Writing Group, developed in conjunction with the European Association of Echocardiography, a branch of the European Society of Cardiology. *J Am Soc Echocardiogr* **18**(12): 1440–1463.

Larson, A.C., Kellman, P., Arai, A., Hirsch, G.A., McVeigh, E., Li, D., and Simonetti, O.P. (2004). Preliminary investigation of respiratory self-gating for free-breathing segmented cine MRI. *Magn Reson Med* **53**(1): 159–168.

Lau, A.Z., Chen, A.P., Ghugre, N.R., Ramanan, V., Lam, W.W., Connelly, K.A., Wright, G.A., and Cunningham, C.H. (2010). Rapid multislice imaging of hyperpolarized 13C pyruvate and bicarbonate in the heart. *Magn Reson Med* **64**(5): 1323–1331.

Lederman, R.J. (2005). Cardiovascular interventional magnetic resonance imaging. *Circulation* **112**(19): 3009–3017.

Lederman, R.J., Guttman, M.A., Peters, D.C., Thompson, R.B., Sorger, J.M., Dick, A.J., Raman, V.K., and McVeigh, E.R. (2002). Catheter-based endomyocardial injection with real-time magnetic resonance imaging. *Circulation* 105(11): 1282–1284.

Lee, D.C., Simonetti, O.P., Harris, K.R., Holly, T.A., Judd, R.M., Wu, E., and Klocke, F.J. (2004). Magnetic resonance versus radionuclide pharmacological stress perfusion imaging for flow-limiting stenoses of varying severity. *Circulation* 110(1): 58–65.

Lenz, G.W., Haacke, E.M., and White, R.D. (1989). Retrospective cardiac gating: A review of technical aspects and future directions. *Magn Reson Imaging* 7(5): 445–455.

Leonardi, B., Margossian, R., Colan, S.D., and Powell, A.J. (2008). Relationship of magnetic resonance imaging estimation of myocardial iron to left ventricular systolic and diastolic function in thalassemia. *JACC Cardiovasc Imaging* 1(5): 572–578.

Li, W., Li, B.S.Y., Polzin, J.A., Mai, V.M., Prasad, P.V., and Edelman, R.R. (2004). Myocardial delayed enhancement imaging using inversion recovery single-shot steady-state free precession: Initial experience. *J Magn Reson Imaging* 20(2): 327–330.

Lima, J.A., Jeremy, R., Guier, W., Bouton, S., Zerhouni, E.A., McVeigh, E., Buchalter, M.B., Weisfeldt, M.L., Shapiro, E.P., and Weiss, J.L. (1993). Accurate systolic wall thickening by nuclear magnetic resonance imaging with tissue tagging: Correlation with sonomicrometers in normal and ischemic myocardium. *J Am Coll Cardiol* 21(7): 1741–1751.

Lingamneni, A., Hardy, P.A., Powell, K.A., Pelc, N.J., and White, R.D. (1995). Validation of cine phase-contrast MR imaging for motion analysis. *J Magn Reson Imaging* 5(3): 331–338.

Lorenz, C.H., Walker, E.S., Morgan, V.L., Klein, S.S., and Graham, T.P. (1999). Normal human right and left ventricular mass, systolic function, and gender differences by cine magnetic resonance imaging. *J Cardiovasc Magn Reson* 1(1): 7–21.

Lu, M., Atthe, B., Mateescu, G.D., Flask, C.A., and Yu, X. (2012). Assessing mitochondrial respiration in isolated hearts using (17)O MRS. *NMR Biomed* 25(6): 883–889.

Lund, J.T., Ehman, R.L., Julsrud, P.R., Sinak, L.J., and Tajik, A.J. (1989). Cardiac masses—Assessment by MR imaging. *Am J Roentgenol* 152(3): 469–473.

Maceira, A., Prasad, S., Khan, M., and Pennell, D. (2006a). Normalized left ventricular systolic and diastolic function by steady state free precession cardiovascular magnetic resonance. *J Cardiovasc Magn Reson* 8(3): 417–426.

Maceira, A.M., Prasad, S.K., Khan, M., and Pennell, D.J. (2006b). Reference right ventricular systolic and diastolic function normalized to age, gender and body surface area from steady-state free precession cardiovascular magnetic resonance. *Eur Heart J* 27(23): 2879–2888.

Maki, J.H., Prince, M.R., and Chenevert, T.C. (1998). Optimizing three-dimensional gadolinium-enhanced magnetic resonance angiography. *Invest Radiol* 33(9): 528–537.

Marcus, J., DeWaal, L., Götte, M., Van der Geest, R., Heethaar, R., and Rossum, A.C.V. (1999). MRI-derived left ventricular function parameters and mass in healthy young adults: Relation with gender and body size. *Int J Card Imaging* 15(5): 411–419.

Masui, T., Finck, S., and Higgins, C. (1992). Constrictive pericarditis and restrictive cardiomyopathy: Evaluation with MR imaging. *Radiology* 182(2): 369–373.

McCrohon, J.A., Moon, J.C., Prasad, S.K., McKenna, W.J., Lorenz, C.H., Coats, A.J., and Pennell, D.J. (2003). Differentiation of heart failure related to dilated cardiomyopathy and coronary artery disease using gadolinium-enhanced cardiovascular magnetic resonance. *Circulation* 108(1): 54–59.

McVeigh, E.R. and Atalar, E. (1992). Cardiac tagging with breath-hold cine MRI. *Magn Reson Med* 28(2): 318–327.

Menon, A., Wendell, D.C., Wang, H., Eddinger, T.J., Toth, J.M., Dholakia, R.J., Larsen, P.M., Jensen, E.S., and LaDisa, J.F. (2012). A coupled experimental and computational approach to quantify deleterious hemodynamics, vascular alterations, and mechanisms of long-term morbidity in response to aortic coarctation. *J Pharmacol Toxicol Methods* 65(1):18–28.

Merritt, M.E., Harrison, C., Storey, C., Sherry, A.D., and Malloy, C.R. (2008). Inhibition of carbohydrate oxidation during the first minute of reperfusion after brief ischemia: NMR detection of hyperpolarized $^{13}CO_2$ and $H^{13}CO_3^-$. *Magn Reson Med* 60(5): 1029–1036.

Miller, S., Simonetti, O.P., Carr, J., Kramer, U., and Finn, J.P. (2002). MR Imaging of the heart with cine true fast imaging with steady-state precession: Influence of spatial and temporal resolutions on left ventricular functional parameters. *Radiology* 223(1): 263–269.

Missouris, C.G., Forbat, S.M., Singer, D.R., Markandu, N.D., Underwood, R., and MacGregor, G.A. (1996). Echocardiography overestimates left ventricular mass: A comparative study with magnetic resonance imaging in patients with hypertension. *J Hypertens* 14(8): 1005–1010.

Modell, B., Khan, M., Darlison, M., Westwood, M.A., Ingram, D., and Pennell, D.J. (2008). Improved survival of thalassaemia major in the UK and relation to T2* cardiovascular magnetic resonance. *J Cardiovasc Magn Reson* 10(1): 42.

Mollet, N.R., Dymarkowski, S., Volders, W., Wathiong, J., Herbots, L., Rademakers, F.E., and Bogaert, J. (2002). Visualization of ventricular thrombi with contrast-enhanced magnetic resonance imaging in patients with ischemic heart disease. *Circulation* 106(23): 2873–2876.

Moon, J.C.C., McKenna, W.J., McCrohon, J.A., Elliott, P.M., Smith, G.C., and Pennell, D.J. (2003a). Toward clinical risk assessment in hypertrophic cardiomyopathy with gadolinium cardiovascular magnetic resonance. *J Am Coll Cardiol* 41(9): 1561–1567.

Moon, J.C.C., Sachdev, B., Elkington, A.G., McKenna, W.J., Mehta, A., Pennell, D.J., Leed, P.J., and Elliott, P.M. (2003b). Gadolinium enhanced cardiovascular magnetic resonance in Anderson-Fabry disease. Evidence for a disease specific abnormality of the myocardial interstitium. *Eur Heart J* 24(23): 2151–2155.

Morawski, A.M., Winter, P.M., Yu, X., Fuhrhop, R.W., Scott, M.J., Hockett, F., Robertson, J.D., Gaffney, P.J., Lanza, G.M., and Wickline, S.A. (2004). Quantitative magnetic resonance immunohistochemistry with ligand-targeted (19)F nanoparticles. *Magn Reson Med* 52(6): 1255–1262.

Moreno, K.X., Sabelhaus, S.M., Merritt, M.E., Sherry, A.D., and Malloy, C.R. (2010). Competition of pyruvate with physiological substrates for oxidation by the heart: Implications for studies with hyperpolarized [1–13C] pyruvate. *Am J Physiol Heart Circ Physiol* 298(5): H1556–H1564.

Morris, G.A. and Freeman, R. (1978). Selective excitation in Fourier transform nuclear magnetic resonance. *J Magn Reson* (1969) 29(3): 433–462.

Mosher, T.J. and Smith, M.B. (1990). A DANTE tagging sequence for the evaluation of translational sample motion. *Magn Reson Med* 15(2): 334–339.

Myerson, S.G., Bellenger, N.G., and Pennell, D.J. (2002). Assessment of left ventricular mass by cardiovascular magnetic resonance. *Hypertension* 39(3): 750–755.

Naehle, C.P., Strach, K., Thomas, D., Meyer, C., Linhart, M., Bitaraf, S., Litt, H., Schwab, J.O., Schild, H., and Sommer, T. (2009). Magnetic resonance imaging at 1.5-T in patients with implantable cardioverter-defibrillators. *J Am Coll Cardiol* **54**(6): 549–555.

Nazarian, S., Roguin, A., Zviman, M.M., Lardo, A.C., Dickfeld, T.L., Calkins, H., Weiss, R.G., Berger, R.D., Bluemke, D.A., and Halperin, H.R. (2006). Clinical utility and safety of a protocol for noncardiac and cardiac magnetic resonance imaging of patients with permanent pacemakers and implantable-cardioverter defibrillators at 1.5 tesla. *Circulation* **114**(12): 1277–1284.

Neimatallah, M.A., Ho, V.B., Dong, Q., Williams, D., Patel, S., Song, J.H., and Prince, M.R. (1999). Gadolinium-enhanced 3D magnetic resonance angiography of the thoracic vessels. *J Magn Reson Imaging* **10**(5): 758–770.

Osman, N.F., Kerwin, W.S., McVeigh, E.R., and Prince, J.L. (1999). Cardiac motion tracking using CINE harmonic phase (HARP) magnetic resonance imaging. *Magn Reson Med* **42**(6): 1048–1060.

Osman, N.F., Sampath, S., Atalar, E., and Prince, J.L. (2001). Imaging longitudinal cardiac strain on short-axis images using strain-encoded MRI. *Magn Reson Med* **46**(2): 324–334.

Patel, M., Cawely, P., and Heitner, J. (2004). Improved diagnostic sensitivity of contrast enhanced cardiac MRI for cardiac sarcoidosis. *Circulation* **108**: 645.

Patel, M.R., Albert, T.S., Kandzari, D.E., Honeycutt, E.F., Shaw, L.K., Sketch, M.H., Jr., Elliott, M.D., Judd, R.M., and Kim, R.J. (2006). Acute myocardial infarction: Safety of cardiac MR imaging after percutaneous revascularization with stents. *Radiology* **240**(3): 674–680.

Pelc, L.R., Pelc, N.J., Rayhill, S.C., Castro, L.J., Glover, G.H., Herfkens, R.J., Miller, D.C., and Jeffrey, R.B. (1992). Arterial and venous blood flow: Noninvasive quantitation with MR imaging. *Radiology* **185**(3): 809–812.

Pelc, N.J. (1993). Optimization of flip angle for T1 dependent contrast in MRI. *Magn Reson Med* **29**(5): 695–699.

Pennell, D.J. (2006). T2* magnetic resonance and myocardial iron in thalassemia. *Ann N Y Acad Sci* **1054**(1): 373–378.

Pennell, D.J., Sechtem, U.P., Higgins, C.B., Manning, W.J., Pohost, G.M., Rademakers, F.E., van Rossum, A.C., Shaw, L.J., and Yucel, E.K. (2004). Clinical indications for cardiovascular magnetic resonance (CMR): Consensus Panel report. *Eur Heart J* **25**(21): 1940–1965.

Petitjean, C. and Dacher, J.N. (2011). A review of segmentation methods in short axis cardiac MR images. *Med Image Anal* **15**(2): 169–184.

Piccini, D., Littmann, A., Nielles-Vallespin, S., and Zenge, M.O. (2012). Respiratory self-navigation for whole-heart bright-blood coronary MRI: Methods for robust isolation and automatic segmentation of the blood pool. *Magn Reson Med* **68**(2): 571–579.

Pruessmann, K.P., Weiger, M., Scheidegger, M.B., and Boesiger, P. (1999). SENSE: Sensitivity encoding for fast MRI. *Magn Reson Med* **42**(5): 952–962.

Rehr, R., Malloy, C., Filipchuk, N., and Peshock, R. (1985). Left ventricular volumes measured by MR imaging. *Radiology* **156**(3): 717–719.

Rehwald, W.G., Kim, R.J., Simonetti, O.P., Laub, G., and Judd, R.M. (2001). Theory of high-speed MR imaging of the human heart with the selective line acquisition mode. *Radiology* **220**(2): 540–547.

Rehwald, W.G., Wagner, A., Albert, T.S.E., Sievers, B., Dyke, C.K., Elliott, M.D., Grizzard, J.D., Kim, R.J., and Judd, R.M. (2010). Clinical cardiovascular magnetic resonance imaging techniques. In *Cardiovascular Magnetic Resonance*, W. Manning and D. J. Pennell (eds.), Saunders/Elsevier, Philadelphia, PA.

Ricciardi, M.J., Wu, E., Davidson, C.J., Choi, K.M., Klocke, F.J., Bonow, R.O., Judd, R.M., and Kim, R.J. (2001). Visualization of discrete microinfarction after percutaneous coronary intervention associated with mild creatine kinase-MB elevation. *Circulation* **103**(23): 2780–2783.

Rickers, C., Jerosch-Herold, M., Hu, X., Murthy, N., Wang, X., Kong, H., Seethamraju, R.T., Weil, J., and Wilke, N.M. (2003). Magnetic resonance image-guided transcatheter closure of atrial septal defects. *Circulation* **107**(1): 132–138.

Rickers, C., Wilke, N.M., Jerosch-Herold, M., Casey, S.A., Panse, P., Panse, N., Weil, J., Zenovich, A.G., and Maron, B.J. (2005). Utility of cardiac magnetic resonance imaging in the diagnosis of hypertrophic cardiomyopathy. *Circulation* **112**(6): 855–861.

Roguin, A., Donahue, J.K., Bomma, C.S., Bluemke, D.A., and Halperin, H.R. (2005). Cardiac magnetic resonance imaging in a patient with implantable cardioverter-defibrillator. *Pacing Clin Electrophysiol* **28**(4): 336–338.

Roguin, A., Zviman, M.M., Meininger, G.R., Rodrigues, E.R., Dickfeld, T.M., Bluemke, D.A., Lardo, A., Berger, R.D., Calkins, H., and Halperin, H.R. (2004). Modern pacemaker and implantable cardioverter/defibrillator systems can be magnetic resonance imaging safe: In vitro and in vivo assessment of safety and function at 1.5 T. *Circulation* **110**(5): 475–482.

Saloner, D. (1999). Flow and motion. *Magn Reson Imaging Clin N Am* **7**(4): 699–715.

Salton, C.J., Chuang, M.L., O'Donnell, C.J., Kupka, M.J., Larson, M.G., Kissinger, K.V., Edelman, R.R., Levy, D., and Manning, W.J. (2002). Gender differences and normal left ventricular anatomy in an adult population free of hypertension: A cardiovascular magnetic resonance study of the Framingham Heart Study Offspring cohort. *J Am Coll Cardiol* **39**(6): 1055–1060.

Sandstede, J.J. (2003). Assessment of myocardial viability by MR imaging. *Eur Radiol* **13**(1): 52–61.

Santos, J.M., Cunningham, C.H., Lustig, M., Hargreaves, B.A., Hu, B.S., Nishimura, D.G., and Pauly, J.M. (2006). Single breath-hold whole-heart MRA using variable-density spirals at 3T. *Magn Reson Med* **55**(2): 371–379.

Saremi, F., Grizzard, J.D., and Kim, R.J. (2008). Optimizing cardiac MR imaging: Practical remedies for artifacts. *Radiographics* **28**(4): 1161–1187.

Schalla, S., Saeed, M., Higgins, C.B., Martin, A., Weber, O., and Moore, P. (2003). Magnetic resonance–guided cardiac catheterization in a swine model of atrial septal defect. *Circulation* **108**(15): 1865–1870.

Schalla, S., Saeed, M., Higgins, C.B., Weber, O., Martin, A., and Moore, P. (2005). Balloon sizing and transcatheter closure of acute atrial septal defects guided by magnetic resonance fluoroscopy: Assessment and validation in a large animal model. *J Magn Reson Imaging* **21**(3): 204–211.

Schär, M., Kozerke, S., and Boesiger, P. (2004). Navigator gating and volume tracking for double-triggered cardiac proton spectroscopy at 3 Tesla. *Magn Reson Med* **51**(6): 1091–1095.

Schroeder, M.A., Atherton, H.J., Cochlin, L.E., Clarke, K., Radda, G.K., and Tyler, D.J. (2009). The effect of hyperpolarized tracer concentration on myocardial uptake and metabolism. *Magn Reson Med* **61**(5): 1007–1014.

Schroeder, M.A., Swietach, P., Atherton, H.J., Gallagher, F.A., Lee, P., Radda, G.K., Clarke, K., and Tyler, D.J. (2010). Measuring intracellular pH in the heart using hyperpolarized carbon dioxide and bicarbonate: A 13C and 31P magnetic resonance spectroscopy study. *Cardiovasc Res* **86**(1): 82–91.

Shah, D.J., Judd, R.M., and Kim, R.J. (2005). Technology insight: MRI of the myocardium. *Nat Clin Pract Cardiovasc Med* **2**(11): 597–605.

Shaw, L.J., Raggi, P., Schisterman, E., Berman, D.S., and Callister, T.Q. (2003). Prognostic value of cardiac risk factors and coronary artery calcium screening for all-cause mortality. *Radiology* **228**(3): 826–833.

Shellock, F.G. (2016). *Reference Manual for Magnetic Resonance Safety, Implants, and Devices*. Los Angeles, CA: Biomedical Research Publishing Group.

Shellock, F.G. and Crues, J.V. (2014). *Magnetic Resonance: Bioeffects, Safety, and Patient Management*. Los Angeles, CA: Biomedical Research Publishing Group.

Sievers, B., Elliott, M.D., Hurwitz, L.M., Albert, T.S.E., Klem, I., Rehwald, W.G., Parker, M.A., Judd, R.M., and Kim, R.J. (2007). Rapid detection of myocardial infarction by subsecond, free-breathing delayed contrast-enhancement cardiovascular magnetic resonance. *Circulation* **115**(2): 236–244.

Simonetti, O.P., Kim, R.J., Fieno, D.S., Hillenbrand, H.B., Wu, E., Bundy, J.M., Finn, J.P., and Judd, R.M. (2001). An improved MR imaging technique for the visualization of myocardial infarction. *Radiology* **218**(1): 215–223.

Sodickson, D.K. and Manning, W.J. (1997). Simultaneous acquisition of spatial harmonics (SMASH): Fast imaging with radiofrequency coil arrays. *Magn Reson Med* **38**(4): 591–603.

Sommer, T., Naehle, C.P., Yang, A., Zeijlemaker, V., Hackenbroch, M., Schmiedel, A., Meyer, C. et al. (2006). Strategy for safe performance of extrathoracic magnetic resonance imaging at 1.5 tesla in the presence of cardiac pacemakers in non-pacemaker-dependent patients: A prospective study with 115 examinations. *Circulation* **114**(12): 1285–1292.

Sosnovik, D.E., Wang, R., Dai, G., Reese, T.G., and Wedeen, V.J. (2009). Diffusion MR tractography of the heart. *J Cardiovasc Magn Reson* **11**(1): 1–15.

Srichai, M.B., Junor, C., Rodriguez, L.L., Stillman, A.E., Grimm, R.A., Lieber, M.L., Weaver, J.A., Smedira, N.G., and White, R.D. (2006). Clinical, imaging, and pathological characteristics of left ventricular thrombus: A comparison of contrast-enhanced magnetic resonance imaging, transthoracic echocardiography, and transesophageal echocardiography with surgical or pathological validation. *Am Heart J* **152**(1): 75–84.

Stehning, C., Bornert, P., Nehrke, K., Eggers, H., and Stuber, M. (2005). Free-breathing whole-heart coronary MRA with 3D radial SSFP and self-navigated image reconstruction. *Magn Reson Med* **54**(2): 476–480.

Stewart, G.A., Foster, J., Cowan, M., Rooney, E., McDonagh, T., Dargie, H.J., Rodger, R.S.C., and Jardine, A.G. (1999). Echocardiography overestimates left ventricular mass in hemodialysis patients relative to magnetic resonance imaging. *Kidney Int* **56**(6): 2248–2253.

Streeter, D.D. and Hanna, W.T. (1973). Engineering mechanics for successive states in canine left ventricular myocardium I. Cavity and wall geometry. *Circ Res* **33**(6): 639–655.

Streeter, D.D., Spotnitz, H.M., Patel, D.P., Ross, J., Jr., and Sonnenblick, E.H. (1969). Fiber orientation in the canine left ventricle during diastole and systole. *Circ Res* **24**(3): 339–347.

Stuber, M., Botnar, R.M., Fischer, S.E., Lamerichs, R., Smink, J., Harvey, P., and Manning, W.J. (2002). Preliminary report on in vivo coronary MRA at 3 Tesla in humans. *Magn Reson Med* **48**(3): 425–429.

Stuber, M. and Weiss, R.G. (2007). Coronary magnetic resonance angiography. *J Magn Reson Imaging* **26**(2): 219–234.

Surder, D., Schwitter, J., Moccetti, T., Astori, G., Rufibach, K., Plein, S., Lo Cicero, V. et al. (2010). Cell-based therapy for myocardial repair in patients with acute myocardial infarction: Rationale and study design of the SWiss multicenter Intracoronary Stem cells Study in Acute Myocardial Infarction (SWISS-AMI). *Am Heart J* **160**(1): 58–64.

Susil, R.C., Yeung, C.J., Halperin, H.R., Lardo, A.C., and Atalar, E. (2002). Multifunctional interventional devices for MRI: A combined electrophysiology/MRI catheter. *Magn Reson Med* **47**(3): 594–600.

Taylor, A.M., Jhooti, P., Firmin, D.N., and Pennell, D.J. (1999). Automated monitoring of diaphragm end-expiratory position for real-time navigator echo MR coronary angiography. *J Magn Reson Imaging* **9**(3): 395–401.

Thomson, L.E.J., Crowley, A.L., Heitner, J.F., Cawley, P.J., Weinsaft, J.W., Kim, H.W., Parker, M., Judd, R.M., Harrison, J.K., and Kim, R.J. (2008). Direct en face imaging of secundum atrial septal defects by velocity-encoded cardiovascular magnetic resonance in patients evaluated for possible transcatheter closure. *Circ Cardiovasc Imaging* **1**(1): 31–40.

Tyler, D., Emmanuel, Y., Cochlin, L., Hudsmith, L., Holloway, C., Neubauer, S., Clarke, K., and Robson, M. (2008). Reproducibility of 31P cardiac magnetic resonance spectroscopy at 3 T. *NMR Biomed* **22**(4): 405–413.

van der Bom, T., Winter, M.M., Bouma, B.J., Groenink, M., Vliegen, H.W., Pieper, P.G., van Dijk, A.P. et al. (2013). Effect of valsartan on systemic right ventricular function: A double-blind, randomized, placebo-controlled pilot trial. *Circulation* **127**(3): 322–330.

Vliegenthart, R., Oudkerk, M., Hofman, A., Oei, H.-H.S., van Dijck, W., van Rooij, F.J., and Witteman, J.C. (2005). Coronary calcification improves cardiovascular risk prediction in the elderly. *Circulation* **112**(4): 572–577.

Volz, S., Zuehlsdorff, S., Umathum, R., Hallscheidt, P., Fink, C., Semmler, W., and Bock, M. (2004). Semiquantitative fast flow velocity measurements using catheter coils with a limited sensitivity profile. *Magn Reson Med* **52**(3): 575–581.

von Knobelsdorff-Brenkenhoff, F., Rudolph, A., Wassmuth, R., Bohl, S., Buschmann, E.E., Abdel-Aty, H., Dietz, R., and Schulz-Menger, J. (2009). Feasibility of cardiovascular magnetic resonance to assess the orifice area of aortic bioprostheses. *Circ Cardiovasc Imaging* **2**(5): 397–404.

Wagner, A., Mahrholdt, H., Holly, T.A., Elliott, M.D., Regenfus, M., Parker, M., Klocke, F.J., Bonow, R.O., Kim, R.J., and Judd, R.M. (2003). Contrast-enhanced MRI and routine single photon emission computed tomography (SPECT) perfusion imaging for detection of subendocardial myocardial infarcts: An imaging study. *Lancet* **361**(9355): 374–379.

Wang, Y. and Ehman, R.L. (2000). Retrospective adaptive motion correction for navigator-gated 3D coronary MR angiography. *J Magn Reson Imaging* **11**(2): 208–214.

Weinsaft, J.W., Kim, H.W., Shah, D.J., Klem, I., Crowley, A.L., Brosnan, R., James, O.G., Patel, M.R., Heitner, J., and Parker, M. (2008). Detection of left ventricular thrombus by delayed-enhancement cardiovascular magnetic resonance: Prevalence and markers in patients with systolic dysfunction. *J Am Coll Cardiol* **52**(2): 148–157.

Weinsaft, J.W., Kim, R.J., Ross, M., Krauser, D., Manoushagian, S., LaBounty, T.M., Cham, M.D., Min, J.K., Healy, K., and Wang, Y. (2009). Contrast-enhanced anatomic imaging as compared to contrast-enhanced tissue characterization for detection of left ventricular thrombus. *JACC Cardiovasc Imaging* **2**(8): 969–979.

Weiss, R.G., Bottomley, P.A., Hardy, C.J., and Gerstenblith, G. (1990). Regional myocardial metabolism of high-energy phosphates during isometric exercise in patients with coronary artery disease. *N Engl J Med* **323**(23): 1593–1600.

Weissleder, R., Lee, A., Khaw, B., Shen, T., and Brady, T. (1992). Antimyosin-labeled monocrystalline iron oxide allows detection of myocardial infarct: MR antibody imaging. *Radiology* **182**(2): 381–385.

Wertman, R., Altun, E., Martin, D.R., Mitchell, D.G., Leyendecker, J.R., O'Malley, R.B., Parsons, D.J., Fuller, E.R., and Semelka, R.C. (2008). Risk of nephrogenic systemic fibrosis: Evaluation of gadolinium chelate contrast agents at four American universities. *Radiology* **248**(3): 799–806.

Westwood, M.A., Anderson, L.J., Firmin, D.N., Gatehouse, P.D., Lorenz, C.H., Wonke, B., and Pennell, D.J. (2003). Interscanner reproducibility of cardiovascular magnetic resonance T2* measurements of tissue iron in thalassemia. *J Magn Reson Imaging* **18**(5): 616–620.

Whalen, D.A., Jr., Hamilton, D.G., Ganote, C.E., and Jennings, R.B. (1974). Effect of a transient period of ischemia on myocardial cells: I. Effects on cell volume regulation. *Am J Pathol* **74**(3): 381.

Wilke, N., Jerosch-Herold, M., Wang, Y., Huang, Y., Christensen, B.V., Stillman, A.E., Ugurbil, K., McDonald, K., and Wilson, R.F. (1997). Myocardial perfusion reserve: Assessment with multisection, quantitative, first-pass MR imaging. *Radiology* **204**(2): 373–384.

Wilson, R.F., Wyche, K., Christensen, B.V., Zimmer, S., and Laxson, D.D. (1990). Effects of adenosine on human coronary arterial circulation. *Circulation* **82**(5): 1595–1606.

Wu, E., Judd, R.M., Vargas, J.D., Klocke, F.J., Bonow, R.O., and Kim, R.J. (2001). Visualisation of presence, location, and transmural extent of healed Q-wave and non-Q-wave myocardial infarction. *Lancet* **357**(9249): 21–28.

Zarins, C.K., Giddens, D.P., Bharadvaj, B., Sottiurai, V.S., Mabon, R.F., and Glagov, S. (1983). Carotid bifurcation atherosclerosis. Quantitative correlation of plaque localization with flow velocity profiles and wall shear stress. *Circ Res* **53**(4): 502–514.

Zerhouni, E.A., Parish, D.M., Rogers, W.J., Yang, A., and Shapiro, E.P. (1988). Human heart: tagging with MR imaging—A method for noninvasive assessment of myocardial motion. *Radiology* **169**(1): 59–63.

CONTENTS

ABBREVIATIONS

Abbreviation	Meaning
1D	One-dimensional
2D	Two-dimensional
3D	Three-dimensional
ADC	Apparent diffusion coefficient
BH	Breath-hold
DED	Diffusion-encoding directions
DENSE	Displacement-encoding
DHE	Delayed hyperenhancement
DKI	Diffusion kurtosis imaging
DSI	Diffusion spectrum imaging
DTI	Diffusion tensor imaging
DWI	Diffusion-weighted imaging
EPI	Echo-planar imaging
FA	Fractional anisotropy
FACT	Fiber assignment by continuous tracking
FAM	Fiber architecture matrix

FLASH	Fast low-angle shot
FSE	Fast spin echo
GRAPPA	Generalized autocalibrating partially parallel acquisitions
GRE	Gradient-recalled echo
HA	Helix angle
HARDI	High angular-resolution diffusion imaging
HCM	Hypertrophic cardiomyopathy
IVM	Intravoxel incoherent motion
LV	Left ventricle
MD	Mean diffusivity
NAV	Navigator-echo
NED	Number of encoding directions
NEX	Number of excitations
NSA	Number of signal averages
ODF	Orientation distribution function
PA	Propagation angle
PC	Phase contrast
PCATMIP	Principal component analysis with temporal maximum intensity projection
PROPELLER	Periodically rotated overlapping parallel lines with enhanced reconstruction
PSS	Prolate spheroidal system
QBI	Q-ball imaging
RA	Relative anisotropy
RV	Right ventricle
SE	Spin echo
SENSE	Sensitivity encoding
SMS	Simultaneous multislice
SNR	Signal-to-noise ratio
SSFP	Steady-state free precession
STEAM	Stimulated-echo acquisition mode
VR	Volume ratio

5.1 INTRODUCTION

5.1.1 MYOFIBER STRUCTURE AND HEART FUNCTION

Myofiber structure is an important determinant of the heart function (Waldman et al. 1988). The distribution of myofiber orientation within the heart wall is the main determinant of stress distribution and myofiber shortening throughout the wall (Bovendeerd et al. 1992), and therefore, of cardiac perfusion (Garrido et al. 1994) and structural adaptation (Arts et al. 1994, Geerts et al. 2002). Myofiber structure also plays a key role in electrical propagation inside the heart (Chen et al. 1993). Myofiber architecture is known to be altered in some cardiac diseases, such as ischemic heart disease and ventricular hypertrophy (Scollan et al. 1998). Therefore, detailed knowledge of the myocardial fiber microstructure promises to lead to better understanding of the heart function in health and disease.

Anisotropy is one of the most consistent observations in studies of cardiac structure. It is present in cardiac material and functional properties at essentially all scales. This includes the arrangement of collagen fibers and actin–myosin contractile structures at the subcellular level, arrangement of myocytes with respect to their neighbors at the cellular level,

and observable texture of the cardiac muscle at the organ level. For this reason, fiber orientation is an intrinsic part of cardiac structure, which affects its local material properties, mechanical and electrical behaviors, and other functions of the heart. Therefore, the ability to extract fiber structure information from the heart as an organ or samples of its tissues is vital to explain these effects. Over time, many studies have presented mathematical and theoretical models for different aspects of the cardiac structure as technological advances make fiber structure information available. Notable examples in biomechanics include constitutive characterization of cardiac tissues and its subsequent use in functional modeling of the whole heart (Humphrey 2002, Fung 2010). Experimental observations, like mechanical testing of the myocardial tissue, have shown that mechanical properties of the heart are dependent on the tissue microstructure, such as fiber orientation, sheetlike formation of fibers (i.e., lamination), and associated arrangement of the extracellular matrix. Nevertheless, information on both organ geometry and tissue anisotropy is necessary to reach meaningful results from the application of these models (McCulloch 2000, Guccione et al. 2010).

The structure–function relationships also apply to cardiac electrophysiology (Clayton et al. 2011), where it is well established that the electrical conductivities of the cardiac tissues also exhibit anisotropy (Clerc 1976, Roberts et al. 1979) and that they are determined by tissue microstructure, in particular, the local orientation and lamination of cardiac fibers. Therefore, this information should be reflected in simulations of electrical propagation and coupled electromechanical modeling (Sachse 2004), which requires integrative modeling of the heart electrical activation, force development, and mechanical deformation based on anisotropic tissue properties. For example, the anisotropic cardiac tissue properties could be used to produce comprehensive models seeking to provide explanations of the basic mechanisms of ventricular contraction, expansion, and torsion (Hunter et al. 1998). For these reasons, mapping of the myofiber structure is a key for the implementation and quantitative analysis of cardiac functional behaviors, and to gain new understanding of the heart mechanics.

5.1.2 CHAPTER OUTLINE

This chapter discusses the methods and practical challenges for elucidating fiber structure from the myocardial tissues, with special emphasis on magnetic resonance diffusion tensor imaging (MR-DTI or DTI for short). The chapter first presents a brief review of current and traditional methods for fiber structure analysis and their applications. The fundamental theory behind DTI is then introduced, including its experimental design strategy, followed by practical applications of the technology in cardiac tissues. Considerations about DTI implementation in practice, parameters selection effects on the results, and other technical challenges are then discussed. Finally, the chapter covers advanced cardiac MRI tractography topics, including scan time optimization, advanced postprocessing, and visualization techniques. It should be noted that although this chapter focuses on the heart microstructure using DTI, the reader is referred to Chapter 6 for basic definition of tensors.

5.2 MYOCARDIAL FIBER STRUCTURE AND ORIENTATION

An integrated description of the cardiac structure describing identifiable features, including fiber, sheet, and band architecture, is thought to provide a unified means to explain cardiac electromechanical behavior under different physiological scenarios, which can be used for treatment planning or monitoring of the heart condition (Greenbaum et al. 1981, Spotnitz 2000, Gilbert et al. 2007). Knowledge of the myofiber arrangement allows us to better understand myocardial shortening, lengthening, and twisting (Sengupta et al. 2008a,b), which are important parameters for characterizing regional deformations within the myocardium and their contribution to global heart function. Investigations of myofiber arrangement have provided insights into the heart function as early as the seventeenth century when Niels Stensen used gross dissection to demonstrate that the heart is a muscle by comparing myocardial tissue fibers to those of the skeletal muscle (Tubbs et al. 2012).

The myocardium consists of myocytes, which are the basic building blocks making up the tissue. The myocytes vary in shape and size. Typical length and diameter of ventricular myocytes are 120 and 20 μm, respectively. In the ventricles, the myocytes follow laminar organization, commonly referred as "sheets," about four cells in thickness (Costa et al. 1999).

5.2.1 HYPOTHESES OF MYOCARDIAL STRUCTURE

Dissection and visual observation of the principal fiber orientation in the ventricular muscle was a major tool throughout the twentieth century to develop and evaluate different structural hypotheses, such as the myocardial bundles (Robb and Robb 1942), ventricular myocardial band (Torrent-Guasp 1957), and others (Rushmer et al. 1953, Streeter and Hanna 1973a). At least two different perceptions are represented by these hypotheses: the ventricular muscle comprising discrete bundles versus the muscle is a continuous tissue. The myocardial bundle hypothesis suggests that the ventricular muscle is developed from four distinct muscle bundles, whereas the ventricular myocardial band hypothesis proposes that both ventricles are formed from a continuous muscle band, arranged as basal and apical loops, as shown in Figure 5.1 (Torrent-Guasp et al. 2001). While various functional and structural studies support the ventricular myocardial band hypothesis (Gao et al. 2009), it remains controversial (Buckberg 2005, Buckberg et al. 2006b, Anderson et al. 2007, Lunkenheimer et al. 2013). Histological sections have been also used to quantitatively describe and model cardiac fiber arrangement in various species, including canine (Streeter 1969, Armour and Randall 1970, Streeter and Hanna 1973b, Streeter et al. 1979, Freeman et al. 1985, LeGrice et al. 1995a), primate (Ross and Streeter 1975), porcine (Tezuka et al. 1990, Lunkenheimer et al. 2006), ovine (Ennis et al. 2008), murine (McLean and Prothero 1991), and also in humans (Armour and Randall 1970, Pearlman et al. 1981, 1982).

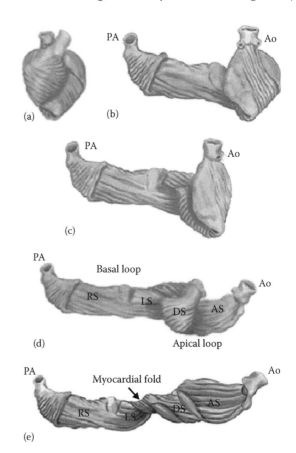

FIGURE 5.1 Sketch of Torrent-Guasp's ventricular myocardial band. (a) The ventricles are formed from a band, which extends between the pulmonary artery (PA) and the aorta (Ao). (b–e) The band can be unwound in several steps. The myocardial band can be divided into four segments: right segment (RS), left segment (LS), descending segment (DS), and ascending segment (AS). (Reproduced from Buckberg, G. et al., *Circulation*, 118(24), 2571, 2008. With permission.)

5.2.2 HEART DISSECTION FOR STUDYING MYOCARDIAL STRUCTURE

Several studies found that the myocardial fiber orientation varies during ventricular contraction and relaxation (Streeter and Hanna 1973b, Freeman et al. 1985, Waldman et al. 1988, Hales et al. 2012). Further studies revealed that the ventricular fiber orientation is dependent on the spatial location in the heart as well as the species from which the heart is obtained. Commonly, large, but smooth, changes in the fiber orientation were found in the ventricular wall (Streeter et al. 1969), as shown in Figure 5.2 and illustrated in Figure 5.3. For instance, in canine left ventricular (LV) free wall, the fibers orientation ranged from approximately 50° to 80° at the subendocardium, to 0° at the mid myocardium, to approximately −60° to −80° at the subepicardium (Streeter and Hanna 1973b, Streeter 1979), where an angle of +90° or −90° corresponds to an apical-base orientation and 0° corresponds to an equatorial orientation.

A series of histological studies revealed that the ventricular myocardial fibers follow circumferential, longitudinal, and oblique organization, akin to helical spirals starting at

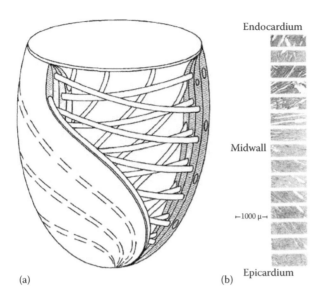

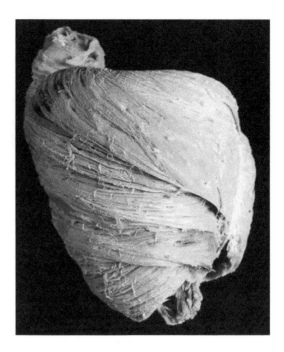

FIGURE 5.2 Sketch of Streeter's model of left ventricular fiber orientation and the underlying histological sections. (a) The model describes the canine LV as a nested set of fiber shells. Fiber orientation in each shell is helical and locally homogeneous. (b) Histological sections through the LV free wall. Fiber orientation ranged from approximately 60° at the subendocardium myocytes, to 0° at the mid-myocardium, to approximately −75° at the subepicardium. (Reproduced from Streeter, D.D., Jr. and Hanna, W.T., *Circ. Res.*, 33(6), 639, 1973a. With permission.)

FIGURE 5.4 Organization of the fiber structure revealed by the technique of peeling. (Reproduced from Anderson, R.H. et al., *Clin. Anat.*, 22(1), 64, 2009. With permission.)

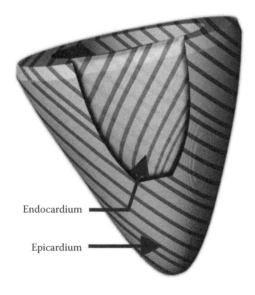

FIGURE 5.3 Schematic of the fiber orientations in the endo- and epicardial layers of the myocardium. (Courtesy of Dr. Shehab Anwar, National Heart Institute, Cairo, Egypt.)

the cardiac base toward the apex (Hort 1960, Streeter 1979, Torrent-Guasp 1980, Wu et al. 2006). The subendocardial helix ascends from apex to base counterclockwise (as seen from the base), while the subepicardial fiber ascends in a clockwise manner (Lunkenheimer et al. 2006). Mathematical modeling showed that the double-helical arrangement of the LV myocardial fibers is beneficial for distributing strain

uniformly and expending energy efficiently (Vendelin et al. 2002, Wu et al. 2007b). When different layers of the heart wall were revealed by the technique of peeling (Anderson et al. 2006, 2009), a unique ventricular structure was observed (Figure 5.4), although aggregated myocytes and the layers isolated by supporting connective tissue do not form separable fibers.

5.2.3 Quantification of Fiber Orientation

5.2.3.1 Helix Angle

For quantification of fiber orientation, the helix and transverse angles have been introduced by Streeter and Hanna (1973a,b). The helix angle (HA) represents the longitudinal component of the fiber orientation, whereas the transverse angle represents the transmural component, as shown in Figure 5.5. The ventricular architecture is intimately related to force generation at different spatiotemporal scales (Kocica et al. 2007). In fact, the timing of contraction, in particular between the left- and right-handed helices, has been proposed to govern the efficiency of apical untwisting, determining ventricular suction, which challenges the concept of passive dilatation as the sole cause of changing the ventricular volume before filling. Instead, both systolic and diastolic myocardial dynamics possess some level of active contraction, which disappears or becomes limited according to contraction of local helix segments (Buckberg et al. 2008). Thus, three-dimensional (3D) reconfiguration of the ventricular cavities is the net result of an efficient arrangement of forces from one-dimensional (1D) sarcomere shortening (Kocica et al. 2007). It should be noted that although this complex architecture of the ventricular mass creates electrical

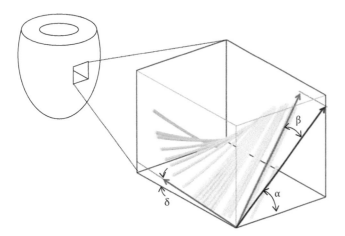

FIGURE 5.5 Schematic of myocardial angular fiber and sheet orientation. Fibers (green) from a single myocardial sheet are shown inside a block whose sides coincide with parallel radial (short axis), neighboring axial (long axis), and opposed tangent planes. Within this geometry, a local coordinate system with components running parallel to the edges of the block can be used to frame the local fiber direction (red arrow) by means of two angles: the helix angle, α, and the imbrication (also known as transverse, or intrusion) angle, β. The sheet angle, δ, is used to define the local sheet orientation.

and mechanical inhomogeneities at the microscopic level; at the macroscopic level, these stochastic events are averaged and appear consistent with a homogeneous medium.

5.2.3.2 Imbrication Angle

Recent studies indicated that the principal axis of cardiac myocytes is not strictly aligned with the epicardial surface (Lunkenheimer et al. 2006, Smerup et al. 2013a). In approximately 60% of the porcine LV myocardium, the myocyte fibers exhibit a transverse angle of 7.5°–37.5° from the epicardial surface, which has been subsequently referred to as the imbrication or intrusion angle, as shown in Figure 5.5

(Geerts et al. 2002, Anderson et al. 2007, Weiss et al. 2007). This arrangement is able to optimize ventricular ejection by controlling regional wall thickening in a way that minimizes the ventricular cavity resistance to flow (Lunkenheimer et al. 2006). Therefore, the ventricular structure provides an explanation to the complex pattern of heart motion based on the interaction among opposing forces: (1) the forces produced by myocytes tangential to the walls, which serve as spatial constraints to the ventricular cavities, and (2) the secondary forces resulting from a combination of obliquely oriented myocytes (running from epicardium to endocardium) and the connective tissue supporting matrix (Anderson et al. 2008).

5.2.3.3 Sheet Angle

While there have been abundant studies on fiber orientation, less is known about the lamination of the cardiac fibers, or myocardial sheet structure (Tseng et al. 1997). The proposed reason for lamination is discontinuity of tissue microstructure, in particular the extensive cleavage planes between muscle layers, which have been proposed following interpretations of an electron microscopy study on canine ventricular myocardium (Hunter et al. 1992, LeGrice et al. 1995a), where the laminae were observed to have a thickness of 48.4 ± 20.4 μm, corresponding to the width of 4 ± 2 myocytes. Similar to the myocardial fiber orientation, the laminae are angled with respect to the epicardial surface (Figure 5.6), where the sheet angle (Figure 5.5) varies as a function of the anatomical location (Scollan et al. 1998, Cheng et al. 2005). Measurements during contraction of canine hearts showed that the laminae deform by thinning and extending transversely to the muscle fibers, depending on their location (Costa et al. 1999). Further, there were large interlaminar transverse shear strains in addition to the sheets deformation during systole; both mechanisms are important for normal regional ventricular function (Costa et al. 1999). This shows that the same mechanisms that are responsible

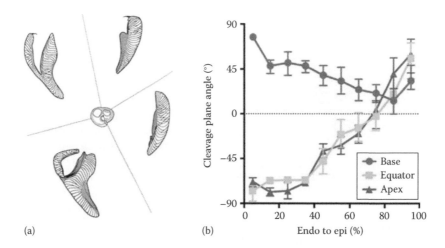

(a)   (b)

FIGURE 5.6 Lamination of cardiac fibers in the ventricles. Transmural sections at different circumferential sites were extracted from canine hearts and manually annotated. (a) Sketch of laminae. (b) The lamination was quantitatively described by a cleavage angle. Lamination varies transmurally and at different ventricular sites. (a: Reproduced from Hunter, P.J. et al., An anatomical heart model with applications to myocardial activation and ventricular mechanics, in: Pilkington, T.C., Loftis, B., Thompson, J.F. et al., eds., *High Performance Computing in Biomedical Research*, CRC Press, Boca Raton, FL, 1992. With permission.)

for wall thickening during systole also operate in reverse to account for wall thinning during diastole (Takayama et al. 2002, Buckberg et al. 2006a).

5.2.3.4 Alternative System for Defining Fiber Orientation

Besides the fiber angles defined in Figure 5.5, the fiber structure could be defined with respect to the radial, longitudinal, and circumferential directions, as shown in Figure 5.7.

5.2.4 MYOCARDIAL STRUCTURE AND FUNCTION

Arrangement of the ventricular myocardium as a unique myocardial band or as a collection of radial sheets is currently being hypothesized, though no comprehensive validation supports either of the proposed explanations (Anderson et al. 2008). Recent studies even point out seeming contradictions within the cardiac structure as the helical fibers exhibit symmetry and the laminae follow a regular arrangement, whereas the anisotropic fibers branch asymmetrically and the laminae merge without following a regular pattern (Gilbert et al. 2007). In the past, the Torrent-Guasp hypothesis has been dominating, but recently the discussion has been widened to a more general view of cardiac structure (Criscione et al. 2005) that indicates regional specializations of the myocardial architecture within a continuum meshwork. The original structural hypotheses may therefore represent a simplification of these more comprehensive views.

It should be noted that the arrangement of the myocytes affects the cumulative force and shortening attained. While the net maximum force is proportional to the number of myocytes arranged in parallel, the net maximum shortening is proportional to the myocytes coupling in series (Anderson et al. 2006). During ventricular contraction, each myocyte shortens by less than 15% of its length. Individual shortening, therefore, appears to undercapitalize wall thickness (which is appreciably more than 15%) and ventricular volume changes. Therefore, it remains to be explained how this limited

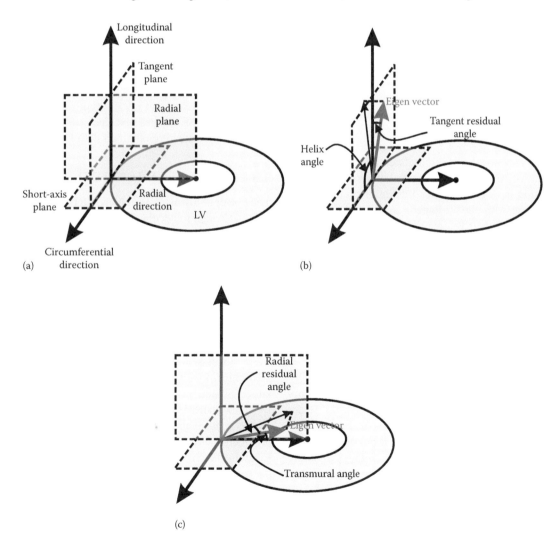

FIGURE 5.7 Schematics of the cylindrical coordinate system for defining the myocardial structure. (a) The main directions (longitudinal, radial, and circumferential) and planes (tangent, radial, and short-axis) defining the coordinate system. (b) The helix and tangential residual angles characterize the primary and tertiary eigenvectors of the diffusion tensor. (c) The transmural and radial residual angles characterize the secondary eigenvector.

shortening of the individual myocytes results in a significant ventricular wall thickening. This could be partly attributed to the coupling between individual myocytes and the supporting collagenous network (Anderson et al. 2008), or due to substantial local reorientation of the laminar architecture with varying loads across the cardiac cycle (Helm et al. 2005b). For example, it has been suggested that the myocytes realign themselves within the ventricular wall thickness during systole, creating an effective reallocation that increases mid-wall myocyte count by about 40% compared to diastole (Anderson et al. 2008).

5.2.5 MYOCARDIAL STRUCTURE IN THE RIGHT VENTRICLE AND ATRIA

In contrast to the LV wall, the right ventricle (RV) wall lacks a central layer of circumferentially aligned myocytes (Anderson et al. 2009). Commonly, the helical angulation of the RV myocytes undergoes a continuous change. Exceptions include the myocytes making up the epicardial layers, which are aligned parallel to the atrioventricular groove, and the circularly aligned myocytes in the outflow portion of the RV.

Compared to the fiber arrangements in the ventricles, those in the atria are more complex (Sachse 2004). The atria are comprised of muscle bundles, including the crista terminalis and Bachmann bundle, both of which have longitudinal fiber orientations. The atrial tissues in regions adjacent to blood vessels, such as inferior vena cava, superior vena cava, and pulmonary veins, have circumferential fiber orientations. In contrast, in the region of the sinoatrial node, the fiber orientation is more difficult to define, largely because the myocytes are irregularly shaped, do not follow a common orientation, and their volume ratio is reduced (compared to the atrial working myocardium). Based on histology and mathematical interpolation approaches, several models of the atrial fiber orientation have been developed, primarily for simulation of atrial electrical conduction (Seemann et al. 2006, Dossel et al. 2012).

5.2.6 NONINVASIVE APPROACHES FOR EVALUATING MYOCARDIAL STRUCTURE

Despite the fact that histology remains the commonly accepted gold standard for characterizing myocardial structures, it is preferable in many cases to employ alternative techniques that circumvent the known limitations of histology. For example, noninvasive techniques are useful for evaluating unique or difficult-to-obtain specimens and for the possibility of doing so in vivo. Techniques that are less labor-intensive or do not require the use of external stains or contrast agents would also be beneficial. Noninvasive approaches include radiological techniques such as x-ray diffraction and contrast-enhanced micro-computed tomography (CT), which have been used to assess myocardial orientation (Sowerby et al. 1994, Yagi et al. 2004, Aslanidi et al. 2013). Nevertheless, the most promising radiological technique is perhaps MRI,

which offers unparalleled soft tissue contrast, diverse native contrast mechanisms, and does not utilize ionizing radiation. MRI has been used to characterize fiber orientation through susceptibility mapping (Vignaud et al. 2006) and DTI (Hsu et al. 1998, Scollan et al. 1998). Because DTI has the desirable feature of using water molecular motion as the endogenous contrast, it has emerged as the preferred radiological technique and viable alternative to histology for characterizing myocardial structures.

Besides DTI, which is the main topic of this chapter, the feasibility of other MRI techniques has been examined for detecting fiber architecture in the heart. For example, Kohler et al. (2003) used high-resolution (78 μm pixel size, 1 mm slice thickness) T2* mapping to determine myocardial fiber structure and compared the results to diffusion-weighted images of isolated rat hearts imaged at 11.75 T. The results showed that the distribution of the field inhomogeneities within the tissue in the T2* images provides very similar information about myocardial fiber structure to those obtained from diffusion imaging. In a similar study, Gilbert et al. (2012b) used a high-resolution fast low-angle shot (FLASH) MRI sequence to image rat hearts on a 9.4 T scanner. The resulting images provided useful information about the myoarchitecture compared to those from DTI images. Finally, Nasiraei-Moghaddam and Gharib (2009) used displacement-encoding (DENSE) MRI to confirm the existence of myocardial helical bands, where the resulting DENSE images revealed strong resemblance to the heart fiber architecture obtained with DTI.

5.3 FUNDAMENTALS OF DTI

The power of diffusion-weighted MRI is derived from its sensitivity to water molecular dynamics, which closely follows the tissue microstructure. For example, diffusion MRI is capable of detecting the neuronal size changes during early stages of acute cerebral ischemia (Moseley et al. 1990). By generalizing the principles of diffusion MRI to describe anisotropic diffusion in 3D space, DTI can be used to characterize tissue fiber structure (Le Bihan et al. 2001). In the heart, although the exact biophysical mechanism is incompletely understood, it has been suggested that water diffusion anisotropy arises from the combined effects induced by the cardiomyocyte membrane, extracellular connective tissue, and microvasculature (Schmid et al. 2005).

Mathematical descriptions of the macroscopic and microscopic consequences of molecular diffusion were originally provided by Fick and Einstein, respectively (Fick 1855, Einstein 1956). Torrey (1956) then incorporated anisotropic translational diffusion in the MRI Bloch equations as an additional source of signal attenuation. About a decade later, Stejskal and Tanner (1965) solved the Bloch–Torrey equation for the case of free anisotropic diffusion in the principal frame of reference. The pioneering work on combining MRI and diffusion anisotropy came from the rigorous formalism of the diffusion tensor by Basser et al. (1994a,b). In this section, the physical basis of DTI and its experimental design strategy will be discussed.

5.3.1 DIFFUSION MR IMAGING

5.3.1.1 Diffusion and Statistical Random Motion

In general, there are two types of diffusion that are of interest in MRI: movement of molecules from regions of higher to lower concentrations and the random or Brownian motion of molecules due to thermal energy. For distinction, the latter is often referred to as self-diffusion. For the sake of simplicity, from this point forward, the term "diffusion" will be used to refer to self-diffusion, particularly water self-diffusion.

In statistical mechanics, the average displacement along a given axis, say, the x-axis, $\langle x \rangle$, of diffusing water molecules is related to the diffusion coefficient, D, via the Einstein's equation:

$$\langle x \rangle = \sqrt{2D\Delta}, \qquad (5.1)$$

where Δ is the diffusion time (e.g., time between leading edges of the diffusion-encoding gradient pulses in the MRI sequence). In biological tissues, D decreases (compared to free water) due to microstructure obstructions (e.g., cell membranes, fibers). These obstruction effects are generally anisotropic (i.e., not uniform in all directions), which gives rise to a preferred direction of water diffusion because, intuitively, the water molecules diffuse fastest in the direction parallel to tissue fibers, as shown in Figure 5.8. DTI can be therefore implemented in the heart to characterize its fiber structure, that is, the fiber organization and orientation.

5.3.1.2 Diffusion Gradients and Phase Accumulation

In MRI, linearly varying magnetic field gradients (or simply gradients) are used to manipulate the resonance frequencies of the individual magnetic moments, or spins, that contribute to the detected MR signal. Specifically, the relative frequency with which a spin located at position $\boldsymbol{r}$ precesses (with respect to a spin located at the origin) can be expressed as

$$\omega(\boldsymbol{r}, t) = \gamma \, \boldsymbol{G}(t) \cdot \boldsymbol{r}(t), \qquad (5.2)$$

where
γ is the gyromagnetic ratio (for ^{1}H)
$\boldsymbol{G}$ is the applied 3D gradient field (in the x, y, and z directions)

Now, consider the scenario in Figure 5.9, where a spin is first subjected to a gradient pulse of $+G$ amplitude, followed by an equal but opposite gradient, $-G$.

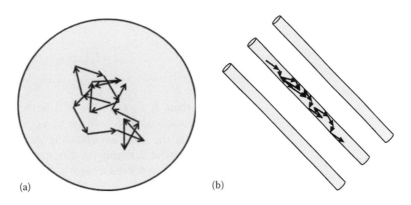

(a)   (b)

FIGURE 5.8 There are two different types of diffusion environments: unordered (or isotropic) and ordered (or anisotropic) diffusions. (a) In isotropic diffusion, the barriers to diffusion are the same in all directions, so diffusion is equal in all directions, such as in the brain gray matter. (b) In anisotropic diffusion, the barriers to diffusion are highly ordered; therefore, diffusion has a "preferred" or faster direction. This is observed in highly ordered tissue such as brain white matter.

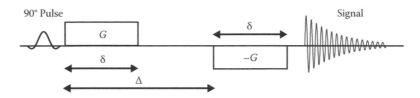

FIGURE 5.9 Diffusion synthesizing gradients. A pair of gradient pulses are used to sensitize MRI to diffusion. An individual spin is tagged with a given phase during the first gradient pulse (with amplitude = G), depending on its spatial location. The second gradient pulse (with amplitude = $-G$) undoes the phase tagging for stationary spins. For spins that move or diffuse between the two gradient pulses, the resulting phase after the second pulse is proportional to the distance moved between the two gradients.

Suppose that during the first gradient pulse, the spin is located at position r_1, and as such, it would acquire a phase of

$$\phi_1 = \gamma\, \boldsymbol{G} \cdot \boldsymbol{r}_1\, \delta, \tag{5.3}$$

where δ is the duration of the diffusion gradient pulse. Furthermore, suppose the spin has moved during the time between the two gradient pulses, such that it is located at position r_2 during the second gradient. The spin would then acquire an additional phase of

$$\phi_2 = -\gamma\, \boldsymbol{G} \cdot \boldsymbol{r}_2\, \delta. \tag{5.4}$$

Consequently, the cumulative (or net) phase accumulated by the spin after it experienced the two gradient pulses is

$$\begin{aligned}
\phi_{net} &= \phi_2 + \phi_1 \\
&= -\gamma\, \boldsymbol{G} \cdot \boldsymbol{r}_2\, \delta + \gamma\, \boldsymbol{G} \cdot \boldsymbol{r}_1\, \delta \\
&= -\gamma\, \boldsymbol{G} \cdot (\boldsymbol{r}_2 - \boldsymbol{r}_1)\delta.
\end{aligned} \tag{5.5}$$

The phase accumulated by the spin is, therefore, proportional to the distance the spin has moved from r_1 to r_2. If a spin has not moved, the cumulative phase will be zero.

5.3.1.3 MR Signal in the Presence of Diffusion

The effect of diffusion in the presence of a sensitizing gradient on the MR signal can be found by solving for the expected value of the phase dispersion for an individual spin, which is a random process, according to the signal equation:

$$I = I_0 \int \exp(-i\phi_{net}) P(\boldsymbol{r}_2|\boldsymbol{r}_1)\, d\phi, \tag{5.6}$$

where

I_0 is the diffusion-independent signal
$P(\cdot)$ is the probability density function of the diffusion, which, in the case of free (or unrestricted) diffusion, has a Gaussian distribution with a standard deviation specified by Equation 5.1, $\sigma = \sqrt{2D\Delta}$.

It can be shown that when diffusion is encoded using a pair of rectangular gradient pulses of opposite polarity with magnitudes equal to $G = |\boldsymbol{G}|$, like those shown in Figure 5.9, the Stejskal–Tanner expression for diffusion can be derived as

$$I = I_0 \exp\left(-\gamma^2 G^2 \delta^2 \left(\Delta - \frac{\delta}{3}\right) D\right) = I_0 \exp(-bD), \tag{5.7}$$

where $b = \gamma^2 G^2 \delta^2 (\Delta - \delta/3)$ is the so-called diffusion-weighting factor. Therefore, diffusion manifests itself in the acquired image as signal loss or attenuation. In turn, the diffusion coefficient D, better known in MRI as the apparent diffusion coefficient (ADC), can be computed from the MR signals acquired with and without the diffusion-encoding gradients, I and I_0, respectively, according to

$$D = \left(\frac{-1}{b}\right) \ln\left(\frac{I}{I_0}\right). \tag{5.8}$$

To illustrate the effect of diffusion encoding and the underlying myocardial fiber structure, Figure 5.10 shows a non-diffusion-weighted image, I_0, along with a diffusion-weighted image, I, of a human heart sample. Because the amount of diffusion-induced MR signal attenuation is dependent on the rate of diffusion along the encoding direction, the fact that different regions of the LV have different intensities is an indication that the underlying myocardial fibers are oriented in different directions.

5.3.2 MRI of Anisotropic Diffusion

The orientation dependence of the effect of anisotropic diffusion on the MR signal can be more easily explained by first considering a special system in which the principal axes of diffusion coincide with the laboratory gradient axes. Specifically, suppose diffusivities are D_1, D_2, and D_3 along the principal axes aligned with the laboratory x-, y-, and z-axes, respectively. The combined signal attenuation is given by the superposition of Equation 5.7 applied to each axis, or

$$I = I_0 \exp(-b_x D_1 - b_y D_2 - b_z D_3), \tag{5.9}$$

where $b_i = \gamma^2 G_i^2 \delta^2 (\Delta - \delta/3)$ is the diffusion-weighting factor associated with each $i = x$-, y-, or z-axis. Moreover, provided that the diffusion-encoding gradients in different axes are identical in timing but differ in only their relative amplitudes, Equation 5.9 reduces to

$$I = I_0 \exp\left(-b\, \boldsymbol{u}^T \begin{bmatrix} D_x & 0 & 0 \\ 0 & D_y & 0 \\ 0 & 0 & D_z \end{bmatrix} \boldsymbol{u}\right), \tag{5.10}$$

where $\boldsymbol{u}$ is the unit vector denoting the composite gradient direction (e.g., $\boldsymbol{u} = \begin{bmatrix}100\end{bmatrix}^T$, $\begin{bmatrix}010\end{bmatrix}^T$, and $\begin{bmatrix}001\end{bmatrix}^T$ for the x-, y-, and z-directions, respectively). Note that implicit in Equation 5.10 is that $G = \sqrt{G_x^2 + G_y^2 + G_z^2}$ should be used for computing the diffusion-weighting factor.

The obvious limitation of Equation 5.10 is that, more often than not, the principal diffusion axes do not coincide with the laboratory axes. In the general case when the coordinate systems are not aligned, Equation 5.10 can be modified by mapping the laboratory axes onto the diffusion coordinate system via the transformation $\boldsymbol{u} = \boldsymbol{R}\boldsymbol{g}$, resulting in

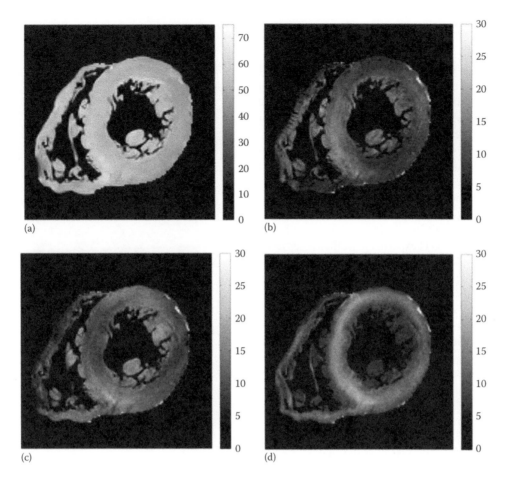

FIGURE 5.10 The diffusion effect on MR signal intensity. (a) Non-diffusion-weighted MRI image of a cardiac sample, shown alongside diffusion-weighted images of the same sample encoded in the (b) x-direction, (c) y-direction, and (d) z-direction with a b-value of 2000 s/mm^2.

$$I = I_0 \exp\left(-b\, \boldsymbol{g}^T \boldsymbol{R}^T \begin{bmatrix} D_1 & 0 & 0 \\ 0 & D_2 & 0 \\ 0 & 0 & D_3 \end{bmatrix} \boldsymbol{R}\, \boldsymbol{g} \right) = I_0 \exp\left(-b\, \boldsymbol{g}^T \boldsymbol{D}\, \boldsymbol{g}\right),$$
(5.11)

where $\boldsymbol{g}$ is the directional unit vector (in laboratory coordinates) of the diffusion-encoding gradient, and

$$\boldsymbol{D} = \boldsymbol{R}^T \begin{bmatrix} D_1 & 0 & 0 \\ 0 & D_2 & 0 \\ 0 & 0 & D_3 \end{bmatrix} \boldsymbol{R} = \begin{bmatrix} D_{xx} & D_{xy} & D_{xz} \\ D_{xy} & D_{yy} & D_{yz} \\ D_{xz} & D_{yz} & D_{zz} \end{bmatrix}$$
(5.12)

is the rank-2 tensor that characterizes the diffusion in 3D space—otherwise known as the diffusion tensor. Since diffusion cannot physically be negative, the principal diffusivities (i.e., the diagonal terms of the diffusion tensor) must be nonnegative, which results in the diffusion tensor being positive semidefinite. Many diffusion tensor-fitting algorithms incorporate the positive definiteness constraint in their fitting (Basser and Jones 2002). It can be seen from Equations 5.11 and 5.12 that the major task in DTI is to use the choices of encoding gradient directions $\boldsymbol{g}$ to selectively probe the elements of the diffusion tensor.

Following similar derivations as described earlier, the signal attenuation due to anisotropic diffusion in the presence of time-varying gradient waveforms can be expressed as (Mattiello et al. 1994)

$$I = I_0 \exp\left(-\sum_{i=1}^{3} \sum_{j=1}^{3} b_{ij} D_{ij} \right),$$
(5.13)

where b_{ij} (i, j belongs to x, y, z) corresponds to individual entries of the "$\boldsymbol{b}$-matrix," $\boldsymbol{b}$. For the gradient waveform shown in Figure 5.9, $\boldsymbol{b}$ is given by

$$\boldsymbol{b} = \gamma^2 \int_0^{TE} \boldsymbol{F}(t)\boldsymbol{F}(t)^T \, dt,$$
(5.14)

where

$$\boldsymbol{F}(t) = \int_0^t \boldsymbol{G}(t')\, dt',$$
(5.15)

$$\boldsymbol{G}(t) = \left[G_x(t), G_y(t), G_z(t) \right]^T,$$
(5.16)

and TE is the echo time.

5.3.3   THE DTI EXPERIMENT

5.3.3.1   Anisotropic Diffusion and Diffusion Ellipsoid

Regardless of whether the approach described by Equation 5.11 or Equation 5.13 is used, a typical DTI experiment consists of acquiring a series of diffusion-weighted MRI images encoded with one or more *b*-values along at least six noncollinear gradient directions (since the diffusion tensor is a rank-2 symmetric tensor, as shown in Equation 5.12) and an estimation of the diffusion tensor, usually on a pixel-by-pixel basis, via appropriate curve fitting of the observed signals to the signal attenuation equation. Given that a non-diffusion-weighted image (commonly referred to as a b_0 image) is needed to estimate the diffusion-independent signal I_0, the minimum scan time for a DTI experiment is, therefore, seven times longer than a conventional scan of the same anatomy. Nevertheless, alternative techniques for tensor reconstruction from a reduced number of measurements have been investigated. For example, Gullberg et al. (2001) developed a 3D inversion technique for the reconstruction of second-order tensor fields from Radon planar projections and showed that the developed technique is capable of imaging diffusion in the myocardial fibers using fewer number of measurements than in conventional DTI.

Directly, the estimated diffusion tensor bears little use for inferring the tissue microstructure since the relevant information is embedded in the tensor elements. Mathematically, the surface of equal probability (at a given time) for finding water molecules, which are initially located at the origin but subject to anisotropic diffusion governed by a diffusion tensor, is an ellipsoid. As an ellipsoid is described by the length and orientation of its major and minor axes, the diffusion tensor is related to the magnitudes and directions of the underlying principal diffusion processes, represented by eigenvalues and eigenvectors, respectively. Consequently, by applying linear algebraic eigenvalue decomposition, the diffusion tensor can be converted into a product of a diagonal matrix of its eigenvalues and a transformation (or rotation) matrix of its eigenvectors. According to Equation 5.12, the eigenvalues and eigenvectors of the diffusion tensor correspond to the diffusivities (observed along the principal axes of diffusion) and the orientations of the axes, respectively, as shown in Figure 5.11. The central premise of DTI is that the direction in which water diffusion is the fastest, that is, along the eigenvector with the largest eigenvalue, coincides with the local tissue fiber orientation.

5.3.3.2   DTI-Derived Diffusion Parameters

To make the derived parameters even more intuitive in cardiac DTI, the fiber orientations are often reported in terms of their helical angles and, to a less extent, imbrication angles (see Figure 5.5 for definitions). On the other hand, the diffusion tensor eigenvalues are commonly used to compute mean diffusivity (MD) and fractional anisotropy (FA) as follows:

$$MD = \frac{(D_1 + D_2 + D_3)}{3}, \quad (5.17)$$

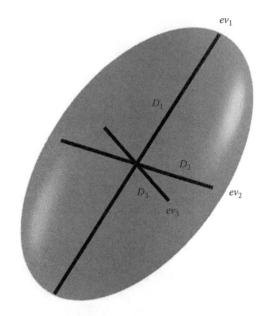

FIGURE 5.11   Diffusion ellipsoid. The magnitude of diffusion in the three principal axes is proportional to the eigenvalues D_1, D_2, and D_3. The orientations of the three principal axes are indicated by the eigenvectors ev_1, ev_2, and ev_3.

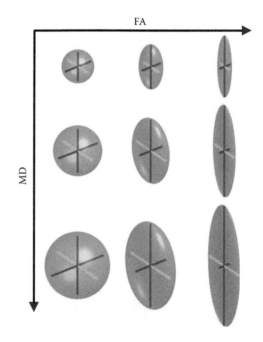

FIGURE 5.12   Visualization of the diffusion profiles with different fractional anisotropy (FA) and mean diffusivity (MD) values.

$$FA = \sqrt{\frac{3}{2}} \sqrt{\frac{(D_1 - MD)^2 + (D_2 - MD)^2 + (D_3 - MD)^2}{D_1^2 + D_2^2 + D_3^2}}, \quad (5.18)$$

where D_1, D_2, and D_3 represent the eigenvalues of the system. To a first-order approximation, MD is proportional to the size of the diffusion tensor, whereas FA is analogous to the standard deviation of its eigenvalues (Figure 5.12). FA is a normalized quantity, with FA of zero and unity denoting no and

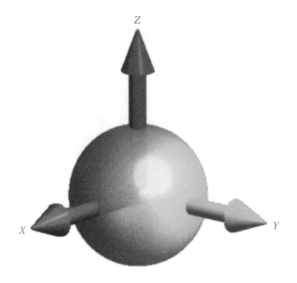

FIGURE 5.13 Red, green, and blue are used to color-code the fiber orientations in the three main axes.

infinite anisotropy, respectively. Red, green, and blue colors are usually used to color-code the fiber orientation in different orthogonal directions, as shown in Figure 5.13.

Alternative, but less frequently used, indices of anisotropy, such as relative anisotropy (RA) and volume ratio (VR)

(Basser and Pierpaoli 1996, Bammer 2003), are calculated as follows:

$$RA = \frac{\sqrt{(D_1 - D_2)^2 + (D_2 - D_3)^2 + (D_3 - D_1)^2}}{(D_1 + D_2 + D_3)}, \quad (5.19)$$

$$VR = \frac{D_1 D_2 D_3}{MD^3}. \quad (5.20)$$

FA, RA, and VR are similar in that they are all quantitative measures of the degree of diffusion anisotropy, but they differ in their sensitivity to different types of anisotropy. FA is more sensitive to lower anisotropy values, VR is sensitive to large anisotropy values, and RA is linearly dependent on different levels of anisotropy (Bammer 2003). In practice, not only are the aforementioned indices convenient quantities that capture the overall magnitude of diffusion (MD) and degree of anisotropy (FA, RA, and VR), but they also have the nice feature of being rotationally invariant (i.e., they do not depend on the orientations of the diffusion principal axes). The fiber orientation (HA) and the scalars MD and FA for the specimen shown in Figure 5.10 are illustrated in Figures 5.14 and 5.15.

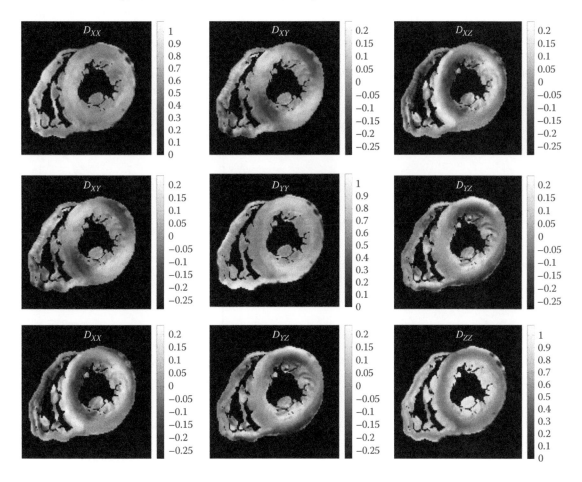

FIGURE 5.14 Maps representing the diffusion tensor parameters derived from the diffusion data. The parameters are derived from the images shown in Figure 5.10. The rows and columns correspond to the 3 × 3 diffusion tensor as explained in Equation 5.12.

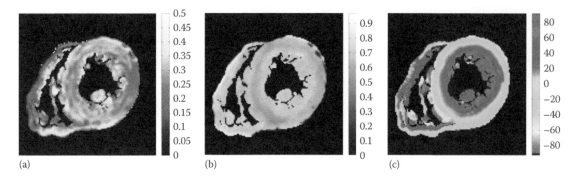

FIGURE 5.15 DTI parameters derived from the diffusion tensor. The parameters are derived from the images shown in Figure 5.14. (a) Fractional anisotropy (FA). (b) Mean diffusivity (MD). (c) Helix angle (HA).

5.4   CARDIAC DTI IN PRACTICE

DTI has been used to characterize tissue structure in a number of applications, including studies of the myocardium and its function. This section offers a brief survey of these applications, which include validations of DTI, tissue specimen characterization, DTI of cardiac pathophysiology, examples of clinical applications of DTI, and biomechanical modeling using DTI data.

5.4.1   Validation of Myocardial DTI

5.4.1.1   DTI Results Compared to Histology

As with any newly introduced imaging technique, the extent to which DTI is useful, in the current case for characterizing myocardial structures, requires it to be validated against the commonly accepted gold standard for obtaining the same

measurements, which is histology. Early applications of DTI in the myocardium were soon followed by studies that directly correlated DTI-measured myocardial fiber orientations with histology, including separate studies performed on freshly excised canine RV samples (Hsu et al. 1998), as well as perfused (Scollan et al. 1998) and formalin-fixed whole rabbit LV (Holmes et al. 2000). Using diffusion MR imaging, these studies have helped establish DTI as a valid alternative to histology for measuring myocardial fiber orientation. Because the studies were performed on differently prepared myocardial samples, they also suggest that DTI, at least for fiber orientation mapping, is immune to the effects of tissue preparation (e.g., fixation). In a study performed on a freshly excised canine ventricular sample (Figure 5.16), the fiber orientation HA measured by DTI and histology were found to differ on average by 2°–5° (Hsu et al. 1998). A similar study was performed on porcine hearts and the results are shown in Figure 5.17 (Schmid et al. 2005).

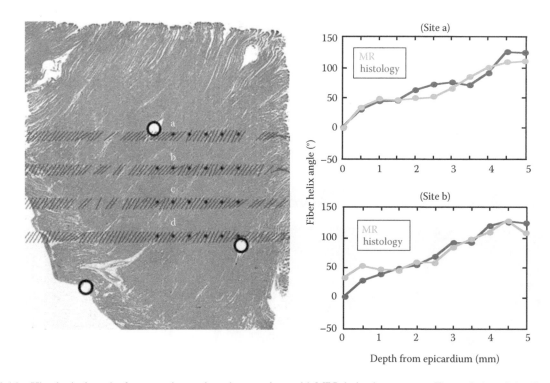

FIGURE 5.16   Histological results from a canine study and comparison with MRI-derived parameters. The variation of the fiber orientation across the myocardium agrees with the HA measured with MRI.

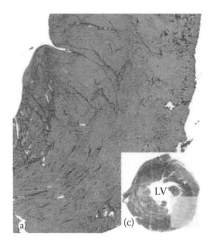
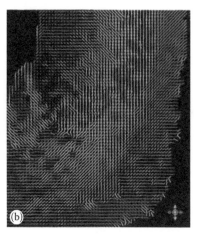

FIGURE 5.17 Comparison of histological and DTI results in the LV of a porcine heart. (a) Histology, (b) fiber direction derived from DTI, and (c) reference anatomy. (Reproduced from Schmid, P. et al., *Eur. J. Cardiothorac. Surg.*, 27(3), 468, 2005. With permission.)

5.4.1.2 The Effect of Tissue Preparation Technique

Although previous studies provided similar results from the heart tissues regardless of the preparation technique, recent studies pointed out some differences, especially in FA, depending on tissue preparation. In one study, Eggen et al. (2012) showed that the delay in tissue fixation after death, if no proper preservation using organ transplantation techniques is performed, compromises the measurement of fiber orientations because diffusion becomes less restricted in the myocardium as it decomposes. The authors recommended that hearts should be recovered as soon as possible, preferably within 3 days postmortem, for accurate measurement of fiber orientations with DTI (Figure 5.18).

In another study, Mazumder et al. (2013) found slight differences in FA between fresh and formalin-fixed porcine hearts as formalin fixation resulted in more isotropic diffusion pattern of the cardiac muscle fibers (Figure 5.19).

5.4.1.3 Myocardial Laminar Structure

5.4.1.3.1 Roles of Second and Third Eigenvalues

Being a noninvasive technique, DTI may be uniquely suited to help address the controversy over the existence of myocardial laminar or sheet structure. The concern here is that the laminar structure may not be an intrinsic property of the myocardium, but rather an artifact introduced during the tissue preparation steps, for example, fixation and sectioning

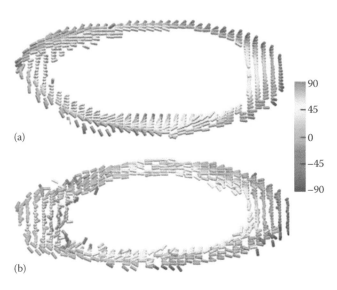

FIGURE 5.18 3D visualization of fiber orientations in a short-axis slice of a fixed heart based on time of imaging postmortem. (a) Imaging immediately postmortem. (b) Imaging 6.4 days postmortem. (Reproduced from Eggen, M.D. et al., *Magn. Reson. Med.*, 67(6), 1703, 2012. With permission.)

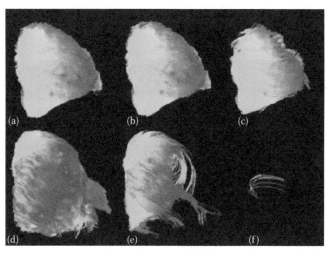

FIGURE 5.19 3D fiber tractography in the entire LV in fresh and formalin-fixed hearts. (a–c) show results in a fresh heart, while (d–f) show results in a formalin-fixed heart. FA was set to [0.1, 1] in (a, d); [0.2, 1] in (b, e); and [0.3, 1] in (c, f). (Reproduced from Mazumder, R. et al., Diffusion tensor imaging of fresh and formalin fixed porcine hearts: A comparison study of fiber tracts, *Proceedings of International Society for Magnetic Resonance in Medicine*, Salt Lake City, UT, 2013. With permission.)

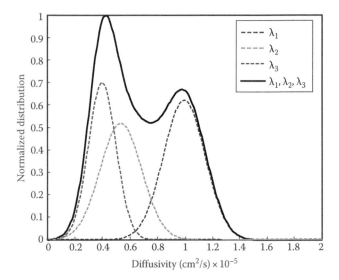

FIGURE 5.20 Example histograms showing grouped eigenvalue populations.

(Legrice et al. 1997, Gilbert et al. 2012a). In DTI, one would intuitively expect myocardial sheets to make water molecules diffuse more freely within rather than across any laminar structure. Consequently, the existence of myocardial sheets would manifest in that (1) there exist distinct second and third eigenvalues in the myocardium (see the example in Figure 5.20) and (2) the eigenvectors associated with the second and third eigenvalues exhibit nonrandom organization. Indeed, distinct populations of the second and third eigenvalues (within statistical confidence levels) were observed in the canine myocardium (Helm et al. 2005a,b). Further, nonrandom second eigenvector fields were reported in fixed mouse hearts (Figure 5.21) (Jiang et al. 2004). The organized appearance of the second eigenvector was also observed in ex vivo human myocardial specimens (Rohmer et al. 2007). Moreover, similar organized appearance was observed in fresh excised (Hsu et al. 1998) and perfused unfixed myocardium (Scollan et al. 1998).

The link between the DTI second eigenvector and myocardial laminar structure is further supported by findings from a subsequent study comparing DTI and cut-face ink blots of the bovine myocardium (Tseng et al. 2003), showing a parallel relationship between the eigenvectors and symmetry axes of the myocardial architecture. Specifically, the first, second, and third eigenvectors corresponded to the fiber, sheet, and sheet normal directions, respectively. The use of cut-face ink blots provided a method by which the fiber and sheet orientations could be measured under the same conditions when using different imaging modalities (e.g., optical vs. MRI) through minimizing the possibility of tissue alterations between data acquisitions.

5.4.1.3.2 Fiber Architecture Matrix

The fiber architecture matrix (FAM) was recently introduced by Mekkaoui et al. (2013b) to fully characterize myofiber dynamics in vivo. The FAM is a function of the complete tensor eigensystem. It encodes the myofiber architecture by presenting the projections of all three eigenvectors with respect to the radial, circumferential, and longitudinal cardiac planes (Figure 5.22).

Based on these findings, sheet tractography in the heart was extended (Mekkaoui et al. 2013a) to include trajectories of the secondary and tertiary eigenvectors, and the resulting information was used to reconstruct ribbonlike tracts of myolaminar sheets in normal and infarcted hearts. Figure 5.23 shows that the torsion angle in the remote zone of the infarcted hearts is significantly reduced, which may account for the contractile dysfunction in this zone.

5.4.1.3.3 Distinct Sheet Populations

While the original description of the myolaminar sheet structure illustrated a single sheet population, biomechanical studies (Arts et al. 2001) and histological examination (Harrington et al. 2005) suggested that there exist not only one, but two distinct sheet populations in the myocardium. Further, a recent study comparing DTI and histology results showed that there might be two distinct sheet populations, oriented orthogonal to each other (Figure 5.24), which contribute to wall thickening during contraction (Kung et al. 2011).

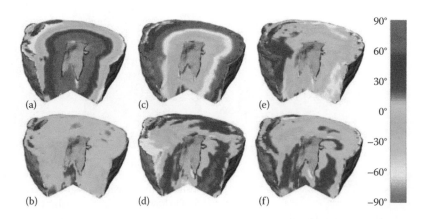

FIGURE 5.21 Left ventricles of mouse hearts rendered in 3D and false-colored based on different diffusion parameters. (a) Helix angle (HA) of the first eigenvector. (b) Tangential residual angle of the first eigenvector. (c) HA of the third eigenvector. (d) Tangential residual angle of the third eigenvector. (e) Transmural angle of the second eigenvector. (f) Radial residual angle of the second eigenvector. (Reproduced from Jiang, Y. et al., *Magn. Reson. Med.*, 52(3), 453, 2004. With permission.)

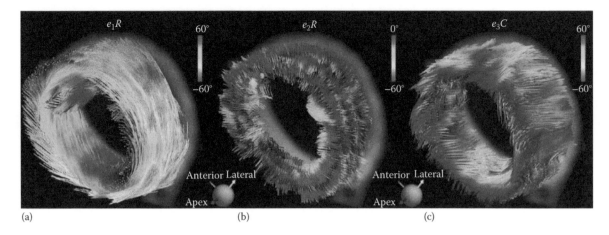

FIGURE 5.22 3D fiber tracts calculated from the fiber architecture matrix. (a) The projection of the primary eigenvector onto the radial direction shows the myofibers colored based on the helix angle (HA). (b) The projection of the secondary eigenvector onto the radial direction shows the myofiber sheets colored based on the sheet angle. (c) The projection of the tertiary eigenvector onto the circumferential direction shows the myofiber orientation from base to apex. (Reproduced from Mekkaoui, C. et al., Dynamics of the fiber architecture matrix in the human heart in vivo, *Proceedings of International Society for Magnetic Resonance in Medicine*, Salt Lake City, UT, 2013b. With permission.)

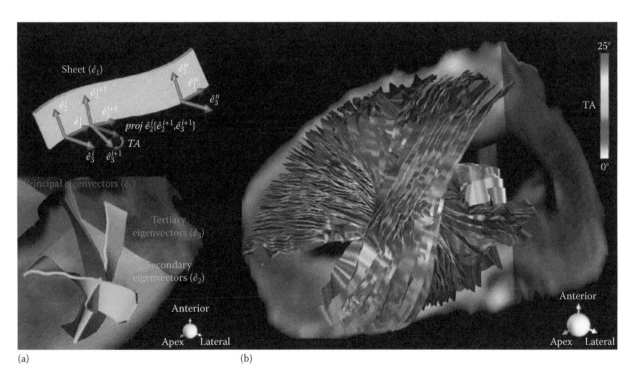

FIGURE 5.23 Ribbonlike sheet representation tractography based on eigen analysis. The sheet's major and minor axes are determined by the primary and secondary eigenvectors, respectively, while the sheet thickness is determined by the tertiary eigenvalue. (a) The sheet torsion angle is determined by changes in the orientation of the minor axis between adjacent segments of the tract. (b) Sheet tractography in the lateral wall of the LV in a normal human heart. The tracts are oriented by the HA and color-coded by the sheet torsion angle along the tract. (Reproduced from Mekkaoui, C. et al., Sheet tractography provides a multi-dimensional representation of architecture in normal and infarcted hearts, *Proceedings of International Society for Magnetic Resonance in Medicine*, Salt Lake City, UT, 2013a. With permission.)

In a recent study by Hales et al. (2012), the authors suggested that myocardial tissue layers in alternating sheet populations align toward a short-axis orientation during systole, which, combined with inter-sheet slippage, contribute to ventricular deformation during contraction. In a similar study, Toussaint et al. (2013b) showed that the laminae are organized parallel to the myocardial wall during diastole and spread to a chevron pattern during systole, where the sheet planes align almost parallel to the short-axis plane in mid-wall regions (Figure 5.25).

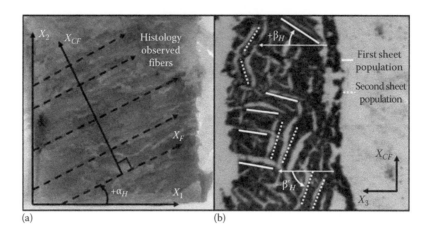

FIGURE 5.24 Fiber and sheet orientations observed from histology. (a) Fiber orientations. (b) Sheet orientations, showing two distinct sheet populations. (Reproduced from Kung, G.L. et al., *J. Magn. Reson. Imaging*, 34(5), 1080, 2011. With permission.)

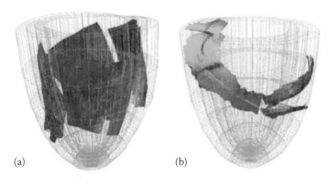

FIGURE 5.25 3D visualization of laminae plane tractography. (a) During diastole. (b) During systole. (Reproduced from Toussaint, N. et al., Cardiac laminae structure dynamics from in-vivo diffusion tensor imaging, *Proceedings of International Society for Magnetic Resonance in Medicine*, Salt Lake City, UT, 2013b. With permission.)

5.4.1.3.4   High-Resolution DTI

High-resolution DTI (100 μm resolution) was introduced in mouse hearts, which allowed for more detailed characterization of the myocardial microstructure (Jiang et al. 2004). Cardiac studies using high-resolution DTI were consequently performed to illustrate microstructural changes in the myocardium following dyssynchronous heart failure in canines (Helm et al. 2006) and myocardial infarction in sheep (Walker et al. 2005a). Another high-resolution DTI study linking cardiac microstructure to its function was performed on rats, which found that wall thickening during contraction is related to changes in the fiber and sheet structure configurations (Chen et al. 2005). Three-dimensional high-resolution DTI has been recently implemented for imaging porcine (Pashakhanloo et al. 2013) and murine (Angeli et al. 2013) hearts.

5.4.1.3.5   DTI and 3D Imaging

DTI and 3D MRI imaging created the possibility of characterizing the organization of myocytes in 3D space rather than in a 2D plane as in histology. Studies using alternative methods to DTI suggested that not all myocardial fibers are

oriented circumferentially, but there are intruding fibers that are oriented radially (Lunkenheimer et al. 2006). Other studies using histology (Omens et al. 1994) and confocal microscopy (Young et al. 1998) found evidence that the organization of myocytes vary in 3D space. Studies using DTI on postmortem porcine hearts found that the ventricular mass is arranged as a mesh of tangential and intruding fibers and that there is no support for a unique myocardial band, as shown in Figure 5.26 (Schmid et al. 2005, 2007, Smerup et al. 2009).

5.4.1.3.6   Fast and Slow Diffusion Components

In an interesting study, a non-exchanging, two-component diffusion tensor model was fitted to diffusion-weighted images obtained in rat hearts ex vivo (Hsu et al. 2001). The results suggested the existence of at least two distinct components of anisotropic diffusion, characterized by a "fast" component and a "slow" component, which exhibited highly similar orientations (Figure 5.27). It was suggested that the fast and slow components correspond to the vasculature and cellular components, respectively, of the myocardium.

5.4.2   Applications of Cardiac DTI

5.4.2.1   DTI and Heart Function

The DTI data have been used within the realm of cardiac biomechanics in a wide variety of studies. Some of these studies aim to improve our understanding of the overall structure/function of the heart (Anderson et al. 2007, Lunkenheimer et al. 2008, Axel et al. 2014) (Figure 5.28). For example, Lohezic et al. (2014) used DTI and diffusion spectrum imaging (DSI) to study isolated rat hearts during diastole, volume overload, and peak systole. The results showed significant decrease in mean FA and decrease in rightward shift in HA during systole, associated with decrease and increase of the proportions of left-handed and right-handed fibers, respectively. Ventricular overload, on the other hand, was associated with more decrease and less increase in the proportions of left-handed and right-handed fibers, respectively. DSI was used to resolve intravoxel diffusion orientations and non-Gaussian

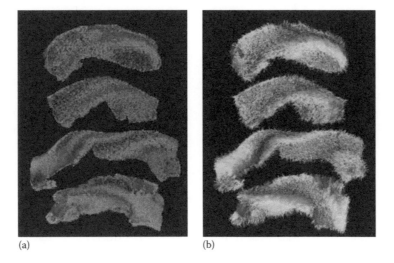

FIGURE 5.26 3D visualization of the first eigenvectors derived from porcine hearts fixed in gel. (a) Color-coded map. (b) The results of localized fiber tracking. (Reproduced from Schmid, P. et al., *Anat. Rec. (Hoboken)*, 290(11), 1413, 2007.)

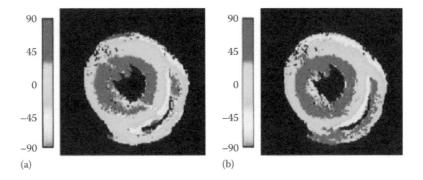

FIGURE 5.27 Fast and slow helix angle (HA) maps. (a) Fast and (b) slow compartments of diffusion. (Reproduced from Hsu, E.W. et al., *Magn. Reson. Med.*, 45(6), 1039, 2001a. With permission.)

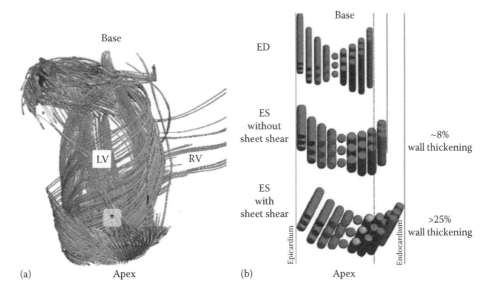

FIGURE 5.28 DTI for probing myocardial microstructure. (a) Diffusion tensor "fiber" tracking of a canine heart reveals large-scale connectivity of the end-to-end anastomoses of continuously branching myocytes. With sufficiently high spatial resolution (especially required at the apex and base) the principal eigenvector can be tracked from asterisk (*) to asterisk (*) while tracing out aspects of the base, apex, endocardium, and epicardium. (b) A representative sheetlet structure comprised of three myocyte layers. Incompressible myocyte shortening of ~15% gives rise to only ~8% radial wall thickening when sheet-shear is absent. In the presence of sheet shear, which is accommodated by the sheetlets, radial wall thickening increases to >25%. (Reproduced from Axel, L. et al., *J. Cardiovasc. Magn. Reson.*, 16, 89, 2014.)

diffusion, which showed decrease in both generalized FA and mean kurtosis compared to the slack state.

Other studies seek to measure stress, strain, and other biomechanical parameters by constructing finite element models of myocardial infarction (Kramer 2009, Vadakkumpadan et al. 2010, Wenk et al. 2011), as well as computational representations of cardiomyopathy (Campbell and McCulloch 2011) and cardiac growth (Bovendeerd 2012). Researchers are also using DTI data to characterize the effects of fiber structure remodeling in animal disease models (Chen et al. 2003, Ripplinger et al. 2007, Strijkers et al. 2009) and to quantify differences across species (Healy et al. 2011) or during the cardiac cycle (Wu and Wu 2009).

A number of studies suggested that ventricular fiber orientation is a result of mechanical feedback (Bovendeerd et al. 1992, Arts et al. 1994, Rijcken et al. 1996, 1999). These studies applied biomechanical simulation and optimization approaches to derive fiber orientations leading to, for instance, uniform mechanical load. A study on ovine LV, however, reported difficulties for predicting fiber orientations based on mechanical feedback (Ennis et al. 2008), where it was suggested that detailed geometrical information is required for prediction of fiber orientation.

5.4.2.2   Structure Variability Based on Site and Species

Since its advent, DTI has been used to characterize the normal myocardium in vitro and ex vivo across several species. In one study on healthy goat hearts (Geerts et al. 2002, Toussaint et al. 2013a), HA was found to vary transmurally across the LV, with the steepest slope found in the anterior and septal sites. Similar variability of the HA slope was also observed in rabbit (Scollan et al. 2000) and mouse hearts (Jiang et al. 2004). The heterogeneity of the anisotropy index, FA, was measured, where it was found that it varies transmurally across the myocardium (Jiang et al. 2007; see Figure 5.29).

The variability of cardiac microstructure has been studied across different species which showed significant fiber structural differences between any pair of the examined species (Figure 5.30) (Healy et al. 2011). DTI has been also

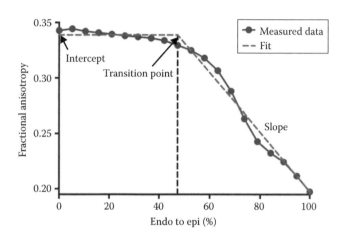

FIGURE 5.29   Variation of fractional anisotropy (FA) across the myocardial thickness, and a profile fit to an ideal step-ramp function.

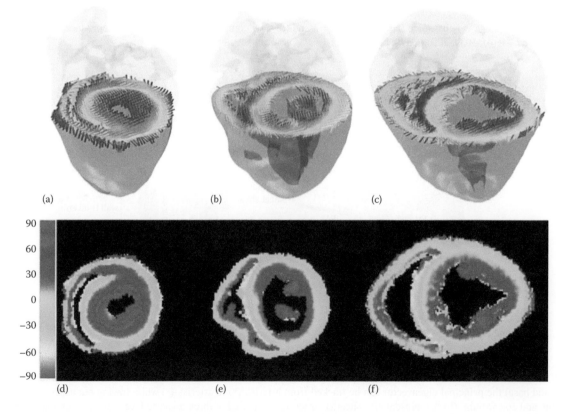

FIGURE 5.30   Myocardial fiber orientation maps from different species. (a, d) Mouse. (b, e) Rabbit. (c, f) Sheep. (a–c) Cylindrical rods representation. (d–f) False-colored HA maps. (Reproduced from Healy, L.J. et al., *J. Cardiovasc. Magn. Reson.*, 13, 74, 2011. With permission.)

implemented for studying the influence of subject characteristics on DTI parameters in the normal heart, where the results suggested that FA and MD are independent of physical characteristics in healthy subjects, although there was an association between the epicardial HA and age (McGill et al. 2014).

5.4.2.3 Fiber Structure in the RV

DTI has been used for imaging fiber structure in the RV. For example, Nielsen et al. (2009) used DTI to show that the RV 3D architecture is preserved during experimentally induced RV hypertrophy (Figure 5.31). In another study by Mekkaoui et al. (2014b), the authors showed that DTI of both the LV and RV can be simultaneously performed in vivo. Recently, Hammer et al. (2013b) used DTI for in vivo imaging of a patient with systemic RV, which provided more information about myofiber architecture adaptation in these patients (Figure 5.32).

In a recent study, Mekkaoui et al. (2015b) used DTI to evaluate the LV and RV responses to pressure overload. The results showed that, compared to the LV that contains a large number of circumferential myofibers, the RV contains only few circumferential myofibers. Therefore, instead of undergoing a rightward shift in fiber structure in response to pressure overload as in the LV, the RV architecture remains unchanged, unable to adapt to the overload (Figure 5.33).

5.4.2.4 Fetal Heart Development

5.4.2.4.1 Human Studies

Recently, DTI has been implemented to study fetal and neonatal heart development, which could have a potential impact on treatment of congenital heart diseases at an early stage. Mekkaoui et al (2013d,e) used DTI to characterize the evolution of fiber architecture in the developing human fetal heart (Figures 5.34 and 5.35). The results showed that the human

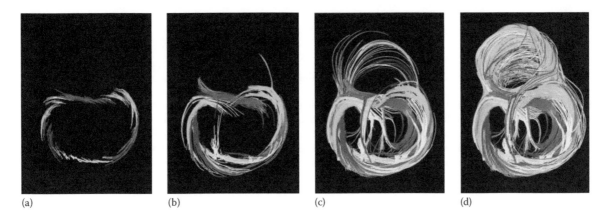

(a)   (b)   (c)   (d)

FIGURE 5.31 Intrusion and extrusion of the fiber tracks through the RV wall. The tracks progress (a–d) from around the short-axis of the RV endocardium. Intrusion is shown in the clockwise direction in the superior aspect of the RV and in the counter-clockwise direction in the inferior part. (Reproduced from Nielsen, E. et al., *Anat. Rec. (Hoboken)*, 292(5), 640, 2009. With permission.)

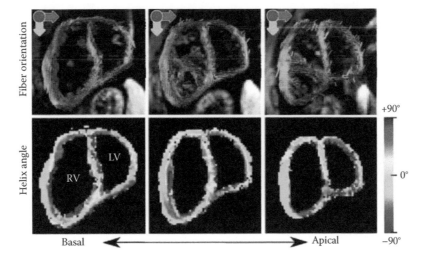

FIGURE 5.32 Color-coded fiber orientation and helix angle (HA) in both LV and RV in a patient with systemic RV. The circumferential pattern is clearly visible throughout both ventricles, as shown in the fiber orientation images. The HA maps show lower angles in the RV. (Reproduced from Harmer, J. et al., In-vivo diffusion tensor imaging of the systemic right ventricle at 3T, *Proceedings of International Society for Magnetic Resonance in Medicine*, Salt Lake City, UT, 2013b. With permission.)

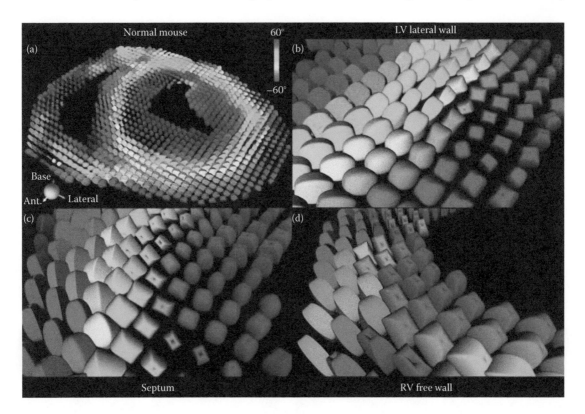

FIGURE 5.33 Myofiber structure in the LV and RV. (a) Supertoroidal glyph field of the short axis of a normal mouse heart color-coded by the helix angle (HA). The LV myocardium has a large number of circumferential myofibers, some of which extend a short distance into the RV. However, the bulk of the RV free wall has few circumferential myofibers. (b–d) Magnified view of fiber architecture in the (b) lateral wall and (c) septum of the LV, and (d) in the RV free wall. Supertoroidal glyphs are color-coded by HA and show paucity of circumferential myofibers in the RV free wall and, in contrast, their abundance in both the septum and lateral wall of the LV. (Reproduced from Mekkaoui, C. et al., *J. Cardiovasc. Magn. Reson.*, 17(Suppl 1), O3, 2015b.)

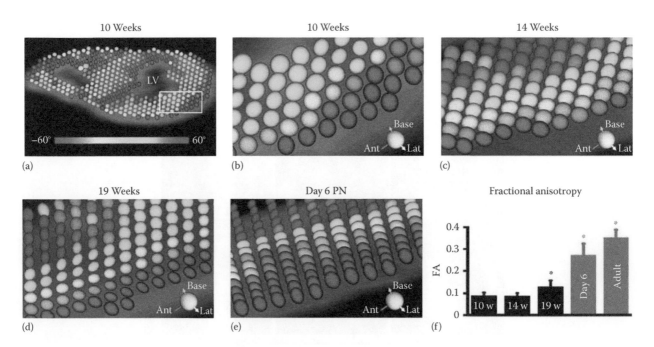

FIGURE 5.34 Transition from tissue isotropy to anisotropy in the developing human fetal heart. (a, b) At 10 weeks, the diffusion glyphs are disordered and spherical. (c) At 14 weeks, the glyphs' orientations are similar to those seen in adult hearts but they remain highly spherical. (d) At 19 weeks of gestation, the glyphs are now somewhat elliptical in shape. (e) At day 6 postnatal (PN), the orientation and elliptical shape of the glyphs is very similar to that seen in adult hearts. (f) Fractional anisotropy at 10, 14, and 19 weeks of gestation remains very low. (Reproduced from Mekkaoui, C. et al., *PLoS One*, 8(8), e72795, 2013e.)

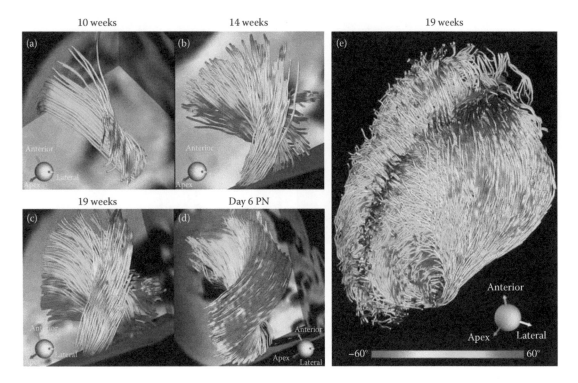

FIGURE 5.35 Tractography of myofiber tracts in the LV, color-coded by the helix angle (HA), during fetal development. (a) At 10 weeks, few tracts are present. (b) By 14 weeks, the tract density has increased and the crossing helical pattern of the subendocardial and subepicardial fibers can be seen. (c) At 19 weeks, the fiber tracts resemble the pattern seen after birth. (d) At 6 days postnatal (PN). (e) Tractography of the entire heart at 19 weeks. (Reproduced from Mekkaoui, C. et al., *PLoS One*, 8(8), e72795, 2013e.)

fetal heart remains highly isotropic until 14–19 weeks of gestation. The arrangement of myofibers into a crossing helical pattern develops within 14–19 weeks of gestation before the beginning of cardiac contraction, which may be necessary for cardiomyocytes' maturation and alignment. The process of myofibers' arrangement into dense sheets then begins and the process evolves further after birth. In another study, Pervolaraki et al. (2013) used high-resolution DTI on postmortem human fetal hearts to visualize different cardiac structures, for example, cleavage planes, HA, and fiber organization, during different heart developmental stages.

5.4.2.4.2 Animal Studies

In a couple of other studies, the development of the heart structures in fetal pig hearts was studied using DTI (Chen et al. 2013, Zhang et al. 2013). Zhang et al. (2013) used DTI to study the cardiomyocytes' architectural plasticity in fetal, neonatal, and adult pig hearts at mid-gestation, preborn, postnatal days 1, 5, and 14, and adulthood. The results showed that the myocytes' helical architecture formation started at midgestation. Postnatal changes in the cardiomyocytes' architecture occurred between days 1 and 14—primarily in the septum and RV free wall. The balanced volume ratio of the LV to RV cardiomyocytes rapidly changed at birth toward an LV-dominant pattern by postnatal day 14. At the same time, the subendocardium HA in the RV free wall decreased by about 30° between postnatal days 1 and 14. These adaptive postnatal changes in the heart's architecture reflect a significant developmental plasticity in the cardiomyocytes' structure

and function in response to the new demands of the LV and RV functions after birth (Chen et al. 2013, Zhang et al. 2013).

5.4.3 DTI AND CARDIAC PATHOPHYSIOLOGY

The presence of heart diseases often involves multiscale myocardial structure remodeling, which is reflected by variations of some DTI parameters. Despite the lack of comprehensive understanding of the mechanisms governing these variations, their correlations with health and pathology have shown promise as potential tools for diagnosis, computational modeling, and progression monitoring of disease. DTI studies on multiple animal models suggest sensitivity to pathology. Therefore, DTI may be clinically useful for locating areas of fiber disarray accompanying diseases, such as myocardial infarction and hypertrophic cardiomyopathy, which may be useful for determining the disease extent or for treatment follow-up.

5.4.3.1 Myocardial Infarction

5.4.3.1.1 Changes in the Myocardial Structure

In ischemic heart disease, reduction of tissue diffusivity was observed in isolated ischemic rabbit hearts (Scollan et al. 1998). The same observation was confirmed in another study performed on excised hearts of infarcted porcine, which also associated infarction with flatter HA (Wu et al. 2006). The effects of infarction on the border and remote zones have also been studied using DTI. In another study where the fiber structure of excised rat hearts was visualized in 3D, it was shown that the infarct areas change from a normal fiber distribution

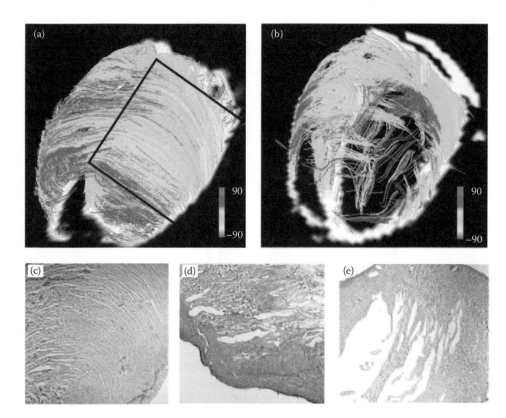

FIGURE 5.36   DTI and histology results showing fiber structure in normal and infarcted myocardium. 3D visualization of (a) normal and (b) infarcted rat hearts. Histology sections of the (c) normal and (d, e) infarcted heart are shown for comparison. (Reproduced from Sosnovik, D.E. et al., *Circ. Cardiovasc. Imaging*, 2(3), 206, 2009b. With permission.)

pattern to mesh-like orthogonally intersecting networks, which extend across the infarcted area to the border zones, as shown in Figure 5.36 (Sosnovik et al. 2009b). A similar study on porcine models of infarction showed that the infarct border zone, delineable by DTI, contains viable myocardial strands, which may have an effect on post-infarct electrophysiology (Figure 5.37) (Zhang et al. 2010).

Structural changes were also observed during the progression of LV myocardial infarction (Strijkers et al. 2009, Winklhofer et al. 2014) and following surgical restoration (Walker et al. 2005a). For example, the double helix myocardial structure shifted more leftward around the infarcted myocardium, and the redistribution of fiber architecture correlated with the infarct size and LV function, as shown in Figure 5.38 (Wu et al. 2007a, Huang and Sosnovik 2010). These changes were measured predominately in terms of fiber angles, showing that the local fiber structure may not be fully altered despite the use of some surgical interventions, which may be rendered unnecessary (Walker et al. 2005a).

5.4.3.1.2   Changes in DTI parameters

The effects of infarction on FA, apparent diffusion coefficient (ADC), and HA have also been studied. When compared to its healthy state in pigs, the infarcted myocardium exhibits decreased FA, increased ADC, and flatter HA (Wu et al. 2006, 2007a). These changes insinuate fiber disarray, which is observed accompanying fibrosis formation (Wu et al. 2007a,b).

5.4.3.2   Heart Remodeling Postmyocardial Infarction

A detailed knowledge of the ventricular fiber structure is important for understanding the nature of cardiac electromechanics in health and disease. During post-infarct healing, the fibers rearrange parallel to the fibers outside the border zone (Walker et al. 2005b). Also, local fiber aggregation is disturbed by increasing or decreasing the fiber density due to edema, which may be affected by increased fibrosis. Tissue structure becomes irregular, or discontinuous, which may promote electrical function anomalies or mechanical failure (Walker et al. 2005a,b, 2008). Generally, the alteration of fiber structure in most cases is a dynamic process that accompanies healing or remodeling, and varies over time.

In a study on a mouse model, the infarcted region showed lower ADC than the remote region, and the low values of the DTI parameters increased with time subsequent to infarction. Increased FA peaked after 28 days, which may be associated with the observed development of structured collagen fibers in this region (Strijkers et al. 2009). At the molecular level, FA was found to be associated with decreased induction of endothelin-1 (ET-1) and caspase-3, improved adenosine triphosphate (ATP) storage in the myocardium, as well as enhanced functional recovery after global warm ischemia (Collins et al. 2007). Another study on infarcted sheep hearts revealed significant reorganization of the 3D aggregation of adjacent fibers in the remote zone of remodeled hearts, as shown in Figure 5.39 (Mekkaoui et al. 2012). Regardless of

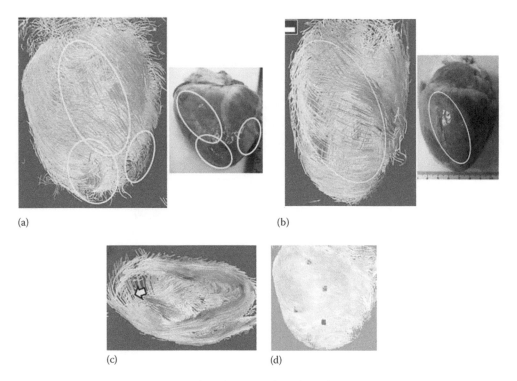

FIGURE 5.37 3D visualization of fiber structure derived from DTI in infarcted hearts. The yellow ellipsoids indicate the regions of (a) heart #1 and (b) heart #2 that experience fiber disruption in the DTI results and show infarction in the explanted hearts. A cross-sectional view of heart #2 is shown in (c), with fiber disruption below the surface indicated with the yellow arrow. (d) Selected disrupted regions inside the infarct in heart #1. (Reproduced from Zhang, S. et al., *Ann. Biomed. Eng.*, 38(10), 3084, 2010. With permission.)

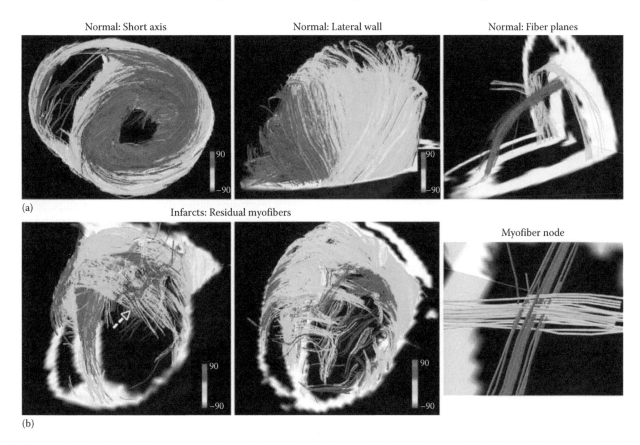

FIGURE 5.38 Comparison of fiber structure of normal and infarcted rat hearts. (a) and (b) show normal and infarcted hearts, respectively, both acquired ex vivo. Note the altered fiber structure in the infarcted hearts. Also, the residual fibers in infarcted myocardium often exhibit orthogonal orientations, which create nodes. (Reproduced from Huang, S. and Sosnovik, D.E., *Curr. Cardiovasc. Imaging Rep.*, 3(1), 26, 2010b. With permission.)

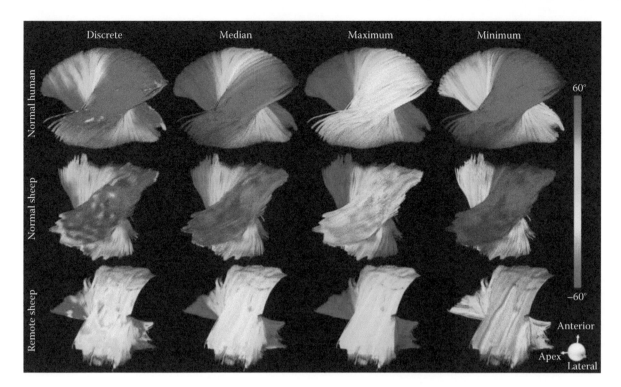

FIGURE 5.39   3D visualization of the helix angle (HA) in human and sheep (normal and infarcted) hearts. The first, second, and third rows show results from normal human heart, normal sheep heart, and remote zone of infarcted (anteroseptal infarct) sheep hearts, respectively, using discrete, median, maximum, and minimum classifications for HA. Fiber tracts are located in the lateral wall. (Reproduced from Mekkaoui, C. et al., *J. Cardiovasc. Magn. Reson.*, 14, 70, 2012.)

angle classification, a positive (rightward) shift in myocardial HA is observable in all layers of the remote zone, particularly in the subepicardium. In a recent study by Sosnovik et al. (2014), the authors used DTI to monitor the response of mice hearts to bone marrow-derived cell injection after 3 weeks of coronary ligation. The results showed positive response, translated into decreased MD, increased FA, and appearance of new myofiber tracts with correct orientation (Figure 5.40).

5.4.3.3   Hypertrophic Cardiomyopathy

DTI has been used for studying hypertrophy (Tseng et al. 2006, Ferreira et al. 2014a). In conjunction with strain imaging, DTI has been used to study hypertrophic cardiomyopathy (HCM) in humans, establishing a relationship between myofiber disarray, mainly measured by FA, and hypokinesis, measured by tissue deformation (Tseng et al. 2006). HCM showed locally reduced FA, which indicates myofiber disarray (Figure 5.41). The same areas also showed decreased myocardial strain, especially in the direction perpendicular to the fibers within the local sheet structure, which showed the highest correlation between FA and hypokinesis. An increase in the imbrication (or intrusion) angle was observed in hypertrophic mouse hearts (Schmitt et al. 2009). In another study, MR DSI showed that the decrease in the voxel-to-voxel fiber orientation coherence is associated with ablation of myosin binding protein-C (MyBP-C) (Wang et al. 2010). Orientational coherence of the fibers, mainly located in the mid-myocardium–subendocardium, leads to the development

of abnormal torsion, an anomaly that is observed in congenital HCM in knockout mouse models.

Recently, Ferreira et al. (2014b) used in vivo cardiac DTI to analyze the cross-myocyte components of diffusion and gain insight into mean intravoxel sheetlet orientations and their change between diastole and systole in normal and HCM subjects. The results showed that the hypertrophic regions in HCM are associated with systolic hypercontraction and diastolic failure of relaxation. Specifically, in contrast to normals who showed myocardial sheetlet and shear layer transition from more wall-parallel orientation during diastole to more wall-perpendicular orientation during systole, HCM was associated with impaired sheetlet reorientation during diastole (Figure 5.42).

5.4.3.4   Other Heart Diseases

Additional observations as well as multiple speculative explanations have been made in studies of other heart diseases. For example, FA has been suggested as an indicator of functional recovery following heart transplantation in dogs (Collins et al. 2007). In another study, myocardial architecture showed to be linked to initiation and maintenance of reentrant arrhythmias (Chen et al. 1993) as well as to mechanical coupling during systolic wall thickening (LeGrice et al. 1995b, Hsu et al. 1998). In a study by Cheng et al. (2013), DTI has been used to study progressive myocardial sheet dysfunction from 3 to 16 months in Duchene Muscular Dystrophy Mice (mdx), where the results delineated the micro-anatomical structure of the mdx heart muscle and showed that calcium regulates the sheet function.

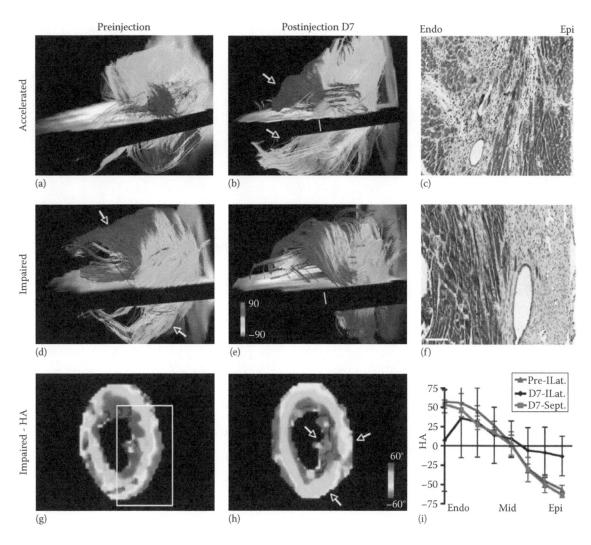

FIGURE 5.40 Serial diffusion tensor magnetic resonance imaging tractography in BL6-BL6 mice showing (a–c) an accelerated healing response after bone marrow mononuclear cell injection and (d–f) an impaired response. (a) Only a few subendocardial and subepicardial tracts are seen in the apical half of the left ventricle pre-injection. (b) After injection, coherent tracts (arrows) are seen in both the subepicardium and subendocardium. (c) Masson's trichrome (short-axis plane, ×10) at the level of the white line in (b) confirms the presence of correctly oriented myofibers in the subendocardium and subepicardium. (d) Pre-injection image shows coherent tracts in the subendocardium and subepicardium (arrows). (e) After bone marrow mononuclear cell injection, fewer tracts are present in the anterolateral subendocardium, and tracts in the subepicardium of the inferolateral wall have been completely lost. (f) Masson's trichrome (×10, short-axis section at level of white line in (e)) confirms the disorganization of fibers in the subendocardium and the complete loss of fibers in the subepicardium. White bar, 100 μm. (g–i) Helix angle (HA) maps of the heart shown in (d–f). Before injection, HA transitions smoothly from the endocardium to epicardium (white box, g). After injection, HA, particularly in the subendocardium and subepicardium (arrows, h), is highly disordered. (i) The transmural evolution of HA in the inferolateral (ILat) wall is relatively normal pre-injection (blue) but severely perturbed at day 7 (D7) after injection (black). The plot of HA in the septum at day 7 (red) is shown for comparison. Endo, endocardial; Epi, epicardial; and Sept., septal. (Reproduced from Sosnovik, D.E. et al., *Circulation*, 129(17), 1731, 2014. With permission.)

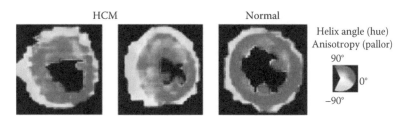

FIGURE 5.41 Fractional anisotropy (FA)-weighted helix angle (HA) maps of two cases of human hypertrophic cardiomyopathy (HCM) and a normal human heart. Disruptions of normal fiber structure and decreased FA are observed in the HCM cases. (Reproduced from Tseng, W.Y. et al., *J. Magn. Reson. Imaging*, 23(1), 1, 2006. With permission.)

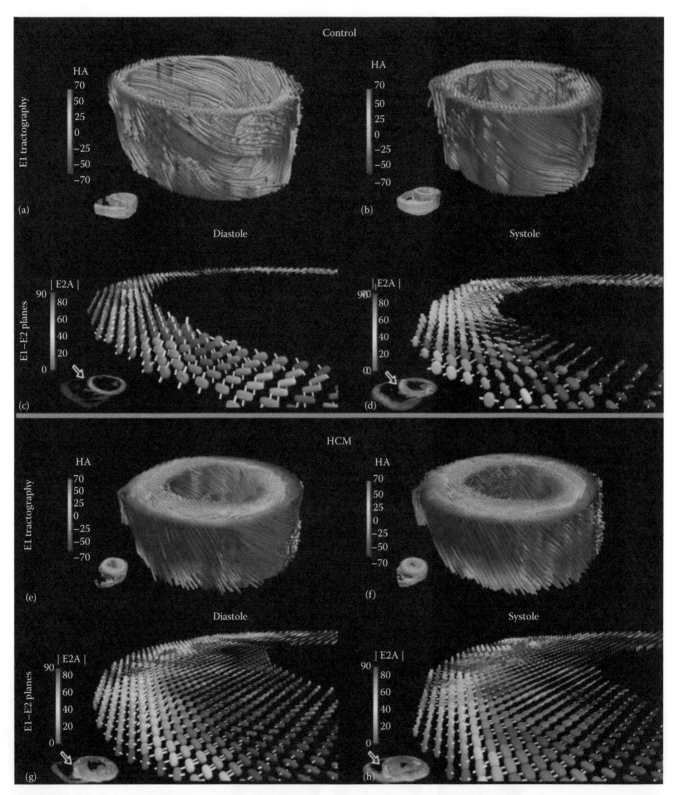

FIGURE 5.42   Three-dimensional visualization of the principal myocyte-parallel (helix angle; HA) and cross-myocyte (secondary eigen-vector; E2) directions of diffusion in hypertrophic cardiomyopathy (HCM). (a, b, e, f) Principal eigenvector tractography for (a,b) a control and (e,f) an HCM patient in (a,e) late-diastole and (b,f) end-systole. Scale bars show color coding for the helix angle. The poor quality of the tracts in the diastolic control example is due to the reduced spatial resolution available. (c, d, g, h) The diffusion tensor represented by super-quadric glyphs superimposed with cylinders representing the E2 direction of each tensor only. The superquadric glyphs are color-coded according to the absolute E2 angle as shown in the scale bars: blue toward wall-parallel and red toward wall-perpendicular orientations. The glyphs typically re-orientate from blue to red in the control, but in the hypertrophic septal regions in HCM, are aligned in what would normally be a relatively systolic, more wall-perpendicular orientation, in both diastole as well as systole. (Reproduced from Ferreira, P.F. et al., *J. Cardiovasc. Magn. Reson.*, 16, 87, 2014b.)

In a recent study by Abdullah et al. (2014), the authors showed that diffuse fibrosis in heart failure is associated with decreased FA and increased mean, secondary, and tertiary diffusivities. In another study, Mekkaoui et al. (2015a) used DTI with a supertoroidal model to detect diffuse fibrosis in vivo. The results showed the capability of the supertoroidal model and derived toroidal volume of detecting subtle changes in the tissue microstructure in LV hypertrophy better than the traditional indices of MD and FA. Recently, Wu et al. (2015) used DTI to study situs inversus and situs solitus mutant mouse hearts. The results showed that both mutant hearts have much lower FA, but much higher ADC, axial diffusivity, and radial diffusivity, which reflect less fibers coherence and sheet integrity compared to normal hearts.

5.4.4 In Vivo Cardiac DTI

5.4.4.1 Initial Studies

The noninvasive nature of DTI provided hope that it could be used to characterize myocardial structures in vivo in both animals and humans, which would be desirable to better understand both healthy heart function and disease progression. The earliest studies of in vivo cardiac DTI were performed simply to demonstrate the feasibility of the technique, which is not trivial due to the complications arising from the beating motion of the heart, or to document its sensitivity to myocardial remodeling in diseases. Initial studies performed on perfused rat hearts (Garrido et al. 1994) and on human hearts in vivo (Edelman et al. 1994, Reese et al. 1995) showed not only that diffusion MRI on the beating heart to be technically feasible, but also showed fiber myocardial architecture imparted on anisotropy of water diffusion. Subsequent studies revealed that tissue strain in the beating myocardium had effects on the observed diffusion signal, which could be eliminated by either retrospective corrections (Reese et al. 1996) or

averaging during acquisition (Tseng et al. 1999) (strain effects in DTI are discussed in more detail later in the chapter).

5.4.4.2 Fiber Structure and Heart Function

One natural application of in vivo cardiac DTI is to investigate the structure–function relationship in the same heart (Nguyen et al. 2015). Studies have shown that myocardial fiber orientations obtained with DTI map well with fiber shortenings obtained by velocity-encoded MRI measurements (Tseng et al. 2000) and that the myocardial sheets contribute to ventricular wall thickening during cardiac contraction (Dou et al. 2003).

5.4.4.2.1 DTI and Myocardial Strain

In Tseng et al. (2000), DTI was implemented to obtain images of fiber orientation in vivo in eight healthy subjects for comparison with strain images. The comparison showed that fiber shortening, as measured by DTI, was more uniform over the myocardium than the measured radial, circumferential, longitudinal, or cross-fiber strain. It was also found that fiber orientation corresponded with the direction of maximum contraction in the epicardium and with the direction of minimum contraction in the endocardium and varied linearly in-between (Tseng et al. 2000).

5.4.4.2.2 DTI and Myocardial Strain Rate

In Dou et al. (2003), DTI and phase-contrast (PC) MRI were used to acquire myocardial sheet structure and strain rate, respectively (Figure 5.43). The involvement of myocardial sheets in ventricular radial thickening during contraction was studied by registering the results of DTI and strain rate data. The sheet function in normal subjects was found to be heterogeneous throughout the ventricular myocardium, as opposed to the contribution of fiber shortening to wall thickening, which was found to be uniform and symmetric.

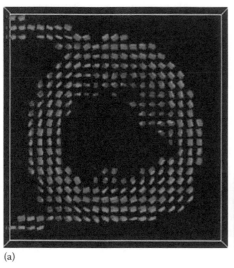 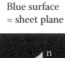 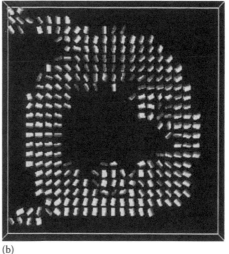

Blue surface = sheet plane

Eigensystem = box axes

Yellow normal = 1° shortening

Blue normal = 1° thickening

(a) (b)

FIGURE 5.43 Registered results from DTI and strain rate measurements. (a) DTI measurements. (b) Strain rate measurements. The fiber orientation is indicated by the red surface and the sheet normal orientation is indicated by the blue surface in the DTI results. In the strain rate results, the box length is proportional to the stretch in each direction. The yellow, pink, and blue surfaces correspond to the directions of maximum shortening, minimum shortening, and maximum thickening, respectively. (Reproduced from Dou, J. et al., *Magn. Reson. Med.*, 50(1), 107, 2003. With permission.)

The strain rate results showed that the sheet shear and extension were most prominent in the anterior free wall and that the sheet-normal thickening was prominent near the RV insertions (Dou et al. 2003).

5.4.4.3   Studying Cardiac Pathology In Vivo

The feasibility of in vivo imaging paved the way for DTI to be possibly used as a tool for detecting or diagnosing cardiac pathology. To date, DTI has been utilized to evaluate the effects of several cardiac diseases and exploit remodeling of the myocardial microstructure as a marker of these diseases. In myocardial infarction, the microstructural remodeling was evident in increased MD, decreased FA, and altered HA in the adjacent zones (Wu et al. 2006, 2009a). In hypertrophic cardiomyopathy, the myocardial fiber disarray manifested in a decreased FA, which correlated with intramural myocardial strain hypokinesis (Tseng et al. 2006). In a study by Sosnovik et al. (2009b), changes in the 3D myocardial fiber architecture, as a result of ischemic heart disease, were visualized via diffusion tractography (discussed later in the chapter). Although in vivo applications of DTI are still in their infancy and the biophysics linking microstructural alterations to DTI observations need to be better understood, DTI has already been shown to be a valuable tool for evaluating cardiac pathology, with the potential to be used for monitoring myocardial remodeling during recovery.

5.4.5   DTI and Computational Cardiac Modeling

5.4.5.1   Fiber Structure in Cardiac Biomodeling

Computational studies of cardiac physiology are useful not only to perfect our overall understanding of the heart function, but also to provide investigations involving computerized experiments that can be used as a complement to traditional experimentation by providing a versatile and highly controlled environment. The potential role of DTI in computational biomechanics and electrophysiology was quickly realized when it became apparent that DTI presents a noninvasive alternative to conventional histology for characterizing myocardial fiber structures. Even when performed on ex vivo specimens after the in vivo experiments, DTI adds subject-specific and morphologically accurate structural information to help model and interpret the experimental functional data. The spatial definition of anisotropic material orientation, made available by the directional information in DTI, has been used in biomechanical (McCulloch 2000, O'Dell and McCulloch 2000, Guccione et al. 2010, Zhang et al. 2012), electrical (Winslow et al. 2000, Muzikant et al. 2002), and coupled electromechanical (Sachse 2004, Nordsletten et al. 2011, Kuijpers et al. 2012) models.

5.4.5.2   Modeling Isotropic and Orthotropic Materials

Information from DTI has been used to define directional parameters in two ways: to define local fiber orientation in transversely isotropic (axially symmetric, or axisymmetric) materials and to represent both fiber and sheet orientation in orthotropic material models. In transversely isotropic materials, like those used to represent fiber reinforcement and some active contraction models (Guccione and McCulloch 1993, Guccione et al. 1993, Tang et al. 2010), directionality is usually represented by a unit vector parallel to the first eigenvector of the diffusion tensor, which has been correlated to the local fiber direction. In orthotropic materials (Walker et al. 2005b), the first eigenvector is used in conjunction with the second or third eigenvectors, which follow secondary cardiac microstructural arrangement (sometimes interpreted as sheet structures) (Helm et al. 2005a).

In a recent study, DTI has been used to introduce a theoretical model of anatomy and fiber orientation of the LV (Pravdin et al. 2013). In that study, the Torrent-Guasp approach was adopted to build cardiac anatomical models of increasing complexity, which allowed for representing anisotropic properties of the heart, such as fiber rotation, spiraling, and maximal angle of torsion. The simulated fiber orientations showed good agreement with the experimental data of LV anisotropy. In another study, a method was presented to analyze the helix and transverse angles between the fibers and the myocardial wall (Munoz-Moreno et al. 2010). The developed method automatically computed the theoretical value of these angles at each voxel, as well as the real value based on DTI data.

5.4.5.3   Fiber Structure and Mechanical Efficiency

It has been suggested that regulation of the ventricular wall function requires a level of heterogeneity in structure and function (Brutsaert 1987, McGill et al. 2015). Some studies have investigated these regulatory relationships, for instance, by applying mathematical models of the myocyte macroscopic alignment and observing their effect on ventricular contraction (Dorri et al. 2010). The results showed that LV function is robust to small-to-moderate rotational variations in the myocyte alignment, up to 14°, which could be found in normal hearts. Severe deterioration of LV function occurred only when deviations in alignment exceeded 30°.

In another study, a 3D finite element model of LV mechanics has been used to prove that the myofibers locally adapt their orientation to achieve minimal fiber-cross fiber shear strain during the cardiac cycle (Rijcken et al. 1999). The adapted structure was relatively more efficient and able to generate more pump work with the same amount of mass. Conversely, rearrangement of the connections would lead to reduction of the forces between the myofibers and extracellular matrix.

Recently, Smerup et al. (2013b) presented a geometrical model to establish the mechanical link between cardiomyocyte shortening and systolic deformation of the LV. The study showed that continuous transmural distribution of HA is necessary for smooth shortening of the cardiomyocytes, although changes in torsional and transmural angulations are required for systolic thickening while maintaining the cardiomyocyte shortening within its normal range. Nevertheless, techniques for analyzing living subjects can be somewhat limited because, as discussed earlier, in vivo DTI is still being developed. Nevertheless, it is possible to use a tensor field from a representative sample, or population of samples, by registering the data to patient-specific geometry using advanced mathematical interpolation techniques (Vadakkumpadan et al. 2012).

5.4.5.4 Electromechanical Modeling

5.4.5.4.1 Fiber Structure and Electrical Conductivity

Information from studies of fiber orientation and lamination has been integrated into coupled electromechanical models of the whole heart and its compartments. These integrated models constitute the basis for computational simulation of cardiac electrophysiology as well as mechanics. For simulations of electrophysiology, the information about fiber arrangement is applied to define conductivity tensors. The anisotropy of these macroscopic conductivity tensors reflects the microscopic arrangement of cells and extracellular space. For instance, the bi-domain model of cardiac conduction requires definition of local intracellular and extracellular electrical conductivity tensors. These interactions are integrated with mechanical modeling to provide a more complete interactive examination of the fiber structures. Species for which integrated models have been developed include dogs (Nielsen et al. 1991, Legrice et al. 1997, Bayer et al. 2012), rabbits (Vetter and McCulloch 1998, Bishop et al. 2010), rats (Plank et al. 2009, Hales et al. 2012), and humans (Sachse et al. 2000, Seemann et al. 2006, Dorri et al. 2007).

5.4.5.4.2 Propagation Angle and Myocardial Voltage

Recently, Mekkaoui et al. (2014a) correlated changes in the tractographic propagation angle (PA), a topographic measure of fiber architecture, with changes in myocardial voltage on electro-anatomical maps of infarcted sheep hearts (Figure 5.44). As narrow range of PA exists in normal hearts, PA could be used to differentiate between normal

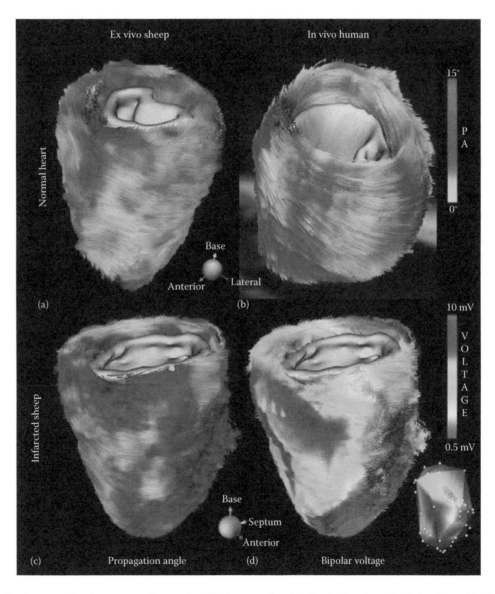

FIGURE 5.44 Tractograms showing propagation angle (PA) in normal and infarcted hearts and relationship with bipolar voltage. PA values in (a) a normal sheep heart (ex vivo) are similar to those in (b) a normal human heart (in vivo) during systole. (c) Tracts of an infarcted sheep heart, color-coded by PA show that PA is significantly increased in the infarct zone. (d) Tractograms color-coded by bipolar voltage show that regions of low voltage correlate well with regions of high PA. The inset displays the original bipolar voltage map and measurement locations. (Reproduced from Mekkaoui, C. et al., *J. Cardiovasc. Magn. Reson.*, 16(Suppl 1), O68, 2014a.)

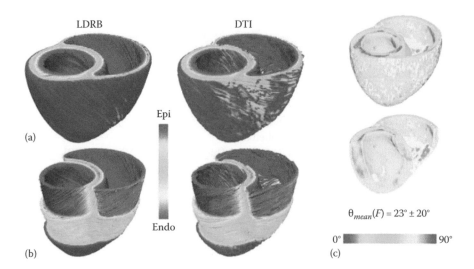

FIGURE 5.45 Comparison of fiber orientation estimation using the Laplace–Dirichlet rule-based (LDRB) algorithm and traditional DTI fitting in a healthy, ex vivo canine heart. (a) 3D visualized fiber tracts in canine ventricles. (b) 3D visualized fiber tracts with parts of the epicardium digitally peeled away. (c) Mean difference angle between LDRB and DTI fiber orientation estimates. (Reproduced from Bayer, J.D. et al., *Ann. Biomed. Eng.*, 40(10), 2243, 2012. With permission.)

myocardium, heterogeneous scar, and dense scar. Typically, myocardium with PA > 10° does not support electrical conduction, while PA between 4° and 10° shows good correlation with bipolar voltage values in heterogeneous and arrhythmogenic scars, which reflects the importance of PA for identifying patients with risk for sudden cardiac death (Mekkaoui et al. 2014a).

5.4.5.5 Regularization Techniques and Modeling Noisy Data

Although fiber orientation is typically assigned to heart models based on DTI data, alternative methodologies could be used if the DTI data are noisy or absent. For example, in Bayer et al. (2012), a Laplace–Dirichlet rule-based algorithm has been used to perform this task with speed and precision, which ensured smooth and continuous transmural and apex-basal direction changes throughout the myocardium (Figure 5.45). In another study, Lekadir et al. (2016) used Markov Random Field for dense 3D reconstruction of cardiac fiber orientations from sparse DTI slices. The developed method included statistical constraints to relate missing data to known fibers as well as a consistency term to ensure local fiber continuity.

5.5 TECHNICAL CONSIDERATIONS

Although the general strategy for the DTI experiment is straightforward—acquire diffusion-weighted images in multiple encoding directions and then fit the data to the diffusion tensor signal equation to characterize the underlying diffusion anisotropy—several factors make its implementation in practice technically challenging. Issues to consider include low signal-to-noise ratio (SNR), long scan time, hardware limitation, and image distortion. Many methodological developments have been undertaken, and significant progress has been achieved in addressing practical challenges of DTI,

albeit most of the efforts have been targeted for DTI studies of the brain. This section, not intended to be an exhaustive review, but as a background, describes in general terms some of these technical challenges and discusses the special considerations needed for performing cardiac DTI.

5.5.1 DTI Pulse Sequences

As explained earlier in the chapter, translational diffusion can be encoded into the MR signal using a pair of equal, but of opposite polarity, gradient pulses. Therefore, by incorporating such a pair, an MRI pulse sequence can be turned into a diffusion-weighted sequence for obtaining diffusion-weighted images (DWI).

5.5.1.1 Gradient Echo and Spin Echo Sequences

Figure 5.46 shows examples of diffusion-weighted gradient-recalled echo (GRE) and spin echo (SE) sequences with the diffusion-encoding parts of the sequences shaded in gray. Note that due to the refocusing 180° RF pulse in the spin echo sequence, the diffusion-encoding gradient pair should have the same polarity. By placing diffusion-encoding gradient pulses in all imaging axes, the pulse sequence can be made sensitive to diffusion along any given direction in 3D space as specified by the relative amplitudes of the encoding gradient pulses. Regardless of the pulse sequence used to realize diffusion encoding, one immediate consequence of diffusion encoding is that the minimum TE of the sequence is lengthened (e.g., an extra 40 ms is required to generate diffusion-weighting b-value of 1000 s/mm² using a 40 mT/m gradient), which can aggravate the SNR challenge in DTI experiments.

Because the GRE sequence is more prone to susceptibility or distortion artifacts, the SE sequence is preferred over the GRE sequence for acquiring diffusion-weighted images.

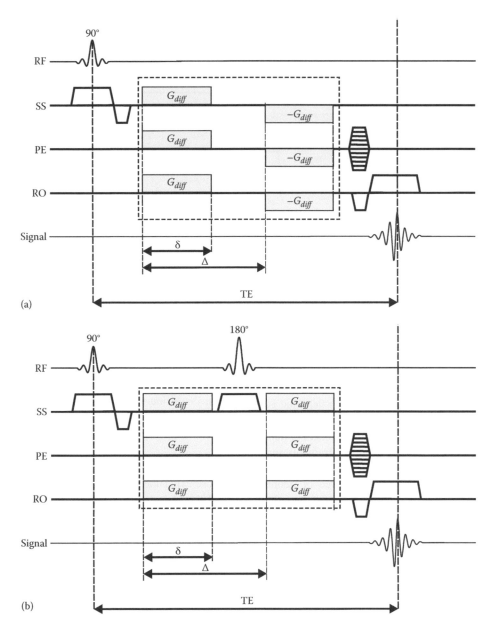

FIGURE 5.46 Diffusion-weighted gradient-echo and spin-echo pulse sequences. (a) Diffusion-weighted gradient-recalled echo (GRE) sequence. (b) Diffusion-weighted spin echo (SE). The gray-shaded rectangles mark the diffusion-sensitizing gradients. PE, phase encoding; RF, radiofrequency; RO, readout; SS, slice selection; TE, echo time.

However, SE acquisitions suffer from long scan times, which are further exacerbated by the need to signal average or encode diffusion in a large number of directions to improve the accuracy of the DTI experiment.

5.5.1.2 Echo-Planar Imaging

5.5.1.2.1 Pulse Sequence

To make the DTI scan time practically acceptable, especially for in vivo applications, the diffusion-weighted spin-echo echo-planar imaging (EPI) has been used (Figure 5.47), and to date it remains the sequence of choice for most DTI studies, at least for brain applications. The typical scan time of an EPI acquisition is in the order of 100 ms, which is especially advantageous when hundreds or thousands of

images are desired (e.g., in high angular-resolution diffusion imaging). Although the issue with scan time is alleviated, the diffusion-weighted EPI sequence has its own set of technical challenges, including blurring arising from signal decay, and image distortions at tissue-air boundaries due to susceptibility effects. However, the most notable challenge is image distortion generated by eddy currents associated with the use of large diffusion-encoding gradient pulses. These distortions vary in both appearance and magnitude as different diffusion-encoding gradient directions and levels are used. If left uncorrected, these distortions cause inconsistent tissue borders in the resulting images, which are characterized by artificially high FA values observed at the tissue edges.

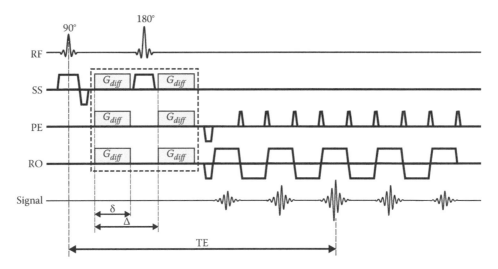

FIGURE 5.47   Spin-echo echo-planar imaging (EPI) pulse sequence with diffusion gradient pulses. PE, phase encoding; RF, radiofrequency; RO, readout; SS, slice selection; TE, echo time.

5.5.1.2.2   Eddy Currents and Correction Techniques

Eddy currents are generated in the electrically conductive elements of the MRI scanner when there is a rapidly changing magnetic field (i.e., when the gradient is switching on or off), and they act to oppose the very same magnetic field that generated them. In effect, eddy currents produce time-dependent magnetic field gradients that oppose the gradients applied in the pulse sequence. These unwanted added gradients make the k-space path (during signal sampling) deviate from its intended trajectory, which is the main source of geometric distortions in the image and, to a less conspicuous manner, differences between the prescribed and actual b-value (Tournier et al. 2011).

Eddy current distortion correction is an active area of research in DTI. Several techniques have been introduced, which can be categorized into three general approaches. The first approach is based on analytical modeling of the eddy current-induced gradients and their effects. For example, when eddy currents induced by diffusion gradients in the phase-encoding direction generate a constant offset to the phase-encoding pulse, the effect is geometric scaling in that direction (Haselgrove and Moore 1996). By determining similar effects in each imaging gradient axis, the distortions can be predicted and corrected in all gradient directions. Clearly, the analytic approach performs best when the eddy current effects are both proportional and predictable. Otherwise, an alternative approach based on retrospective image registration can be used (Andersson and Skare 2002, Mistry and Hsu 2006). The second approach for eddy current correction involves designating some undistorted reference image, which is typically the non-diffusion-weighted or b_0 ($b \approx 0$) scan, and using image-processing techniques to correct the distortions via image registration. The performance of this correction technique depends on the sophistication of the image registration algorithm (e.g., degree of freedom of the corrected distortion) and the image similarity metric used (cross correlation, mutual information, etc.). In contrast to the first two approaches that involve post-processing correction, a third approach takes advantage of the pulse sequence, such that the eddy current effects are reduced or eliminated during acquisition, for example by employing twice-refocused echoes to obtain distortion-free diffusion-weighted scans (Reese et al. 2003) or by using pre-distorted pulses, such that after the eddy current effect, they produce distortion-free images.

5.5.1.3   Fast Spin Echo

Because experimental requirements as well as pulse sequence performances vary, in addition to SE, GRE and EPI, many other pulse sequences have been used for acquiring diffusion MRI or DTI data. For example, diffusion-encoding gradients have been used in conjunction with fast spin echo (FSE) pulse sequences (Figure 5.48). On one hand, the FSE sequences offer the advantages of speed (compared to conventional spin echo sequence) and being free of geometric distortions that are synonymous with EPI. On the other hand, FSE can be hampered by elevated RF power deposition (specific absorption rate [SAR]) associated with the use of multiple RF pulses, as well as ghosting and T2 blurring artifacts when the precise RF conditions (especially for the refocusing 180° pulses) are not met.

5.5.1.4   Other Pulse Sequences

In addition to FSE, DWI or DTI experiments have been performed using advanced MRI sequences such as spiral (Li et al. 1999, Liu et al. 2004) (Figure 5.49), steady-state free precession (SSFP) (Le Bihan et al. 1989, McNab and Miller 2008) (Figure 5.50), periodically rotated overlapping parallel lines with enhanced reconstruction (PROPELLER) (Pipe et al. 2002, Skare et al. 2006) (Figure 5.51), and stimulated-echo acquisition mode (STEAM) (Merboldt et al. 1992) (Figure 5.52) sequences. Further, parallel imaging techniques, for example, sensitivity encoding (SENSE) (Pruessmann et al. 1999, Bammer et al. 2002) and generalized autocalibrating partially parallel acquisitions (GRAPPA) (Griswold et al. 2002, Holdsworth et al. 2009),

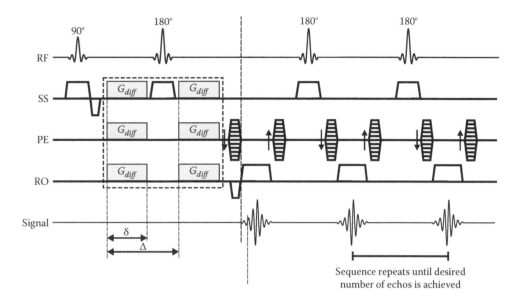

FIGURE 5.48 Diffusion-weighted fast spin echo (FSE) pulse sequence with diffusion-weighted gradients. The sequence is characterized by one excitation and multiple echo generations. PE, phase encoding; RF, radiofrequency; RO, readout; SS, slice selection.

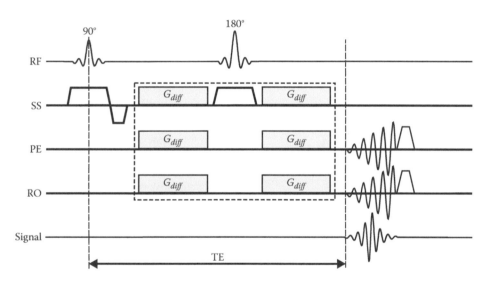

FIGURE 5.49 Diffusion-weighted spin-echo spiral pulse sequence. Data readout is conducted by applying simultaneous sinusoidal gradients on the RO and PE directions to generate the spiral readout trajectory. Data readout is followed by crusher gradients to dissipate remaining transverse magnetization. PE, phase encoding; RF, radiofrequency; RO, readout; SS, slice selection.

have been implemented in diffusion imaging. Needless to say, each pulse sequence has its own set of challenges and limitations, and the reader is referred to elsewhere (Bernstein et al. 2004, Bammer et al. 2009) for a more exhaustive review of technical considerations associated with these pulse sequences. The large number of pulse sequences that have been used for DWI or DTI is a testament to the robustness of the DTI methodology and the flexibility with which it can be implemented.

5.5.1.5 Advanced 3D Sequences

A number of 3D high-resolution DTI pulse sequences have been recently proposed. Harmer et al. (2013b) presented a 3D STEAM-based high-resolution DTI sequence with fat saturation

capability. When combined with respiratory navigation, the developed technique enabled high-quality in vivo DTI of both the LV and RV (Figure 5.53). In another study, Stoeck et al. (2013) developed a single-shot spin echo-based high-resolution DTI using asymmetric Stejskal–Tanner diffusion-encoding and 3D tensor reconstruction. With single-shot acquisition, the developed sequence was not affected by respiratory motion, which holds a potential for in vivo cardiac DTI.

5.5.2 DTI EXPERIMENTAL STRATEGY

5.5.2.1 Factors Affecting DTI

Besides the pulse sequence used, the design of the DTI experiment (e.g., size of the dataset and number of

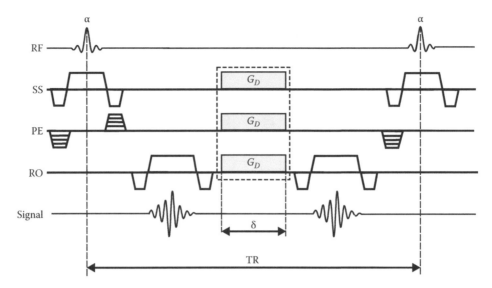

FIGURE 5.50 Diffusion-weighted steady-state free precession (SSFP) pulse sequence. The figure shows one repetition time (TR) period in the sequence, where all gradients, except for the diffusion gradients, are balanced during TR. PE, phase encoding; RF, radiofrequency; RO, readout; SS, slice selection.

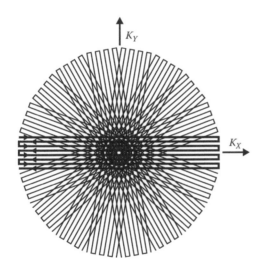

FIGURE 5.51 PROPELLER k-space trajectory. k-space is traversed using a few parallel lines that are rotated in a radial fashion to cover the whole k-space. The PROPELLER sequence is highly immune to motion artifacts.

diffusion-encoding directions) can also have profound effects on the accuracy of the results of the DTI experiments. For example, in the worst-case scenario when a DTI experiment fails to include the minimum number of noncollinear diffusion-encoding gradient directions, it would yield indeterminable diffusion tensors and be useless. The DTI experiment consists of one (or more) b_0 image and a series of diffusion-weighted scans encoded in different sensitizing directions. Therefore, factors that naturally affect the accuracy of the obtained diffusion tensors, and the information therein (e.g., fiber orientations), include the SNR of the individual images, number of diffusion-encoding directions, distribution of the encoding directions, and number and placement of the b-values to be used. As with the

diffusion-weighted pulse sequences discussed in the previous section, much efforts have been taken to understand the impact of each of these parameters on the quality of DTI, as will be explained in the following sections.

5.5.2.2 DTI and Striving for SNR

5.5.2.2.1 Factors Affecting SNR in DTI

The main strategic consideration in experimental DTI is to address its low SNR, which is due to the nature of both diffusion encoding (i.e., via signal attenuation) and T2 relaxation during the prolonged TE necessary to accommodate the diffusion-encoding pulses. Moreover, the SNR issue is aggravated by the tradeoff among scan time (necessitated by the large dataset size), resolution, and SNR. Similar to any quantitative MRI experiment, insufficient SNR can be detrimental to DTI. Low SNR can manifest in directly proportional random errors in the DTI results, for example, as determined by the mean deviation angle from the true value in the estimated fiber orientation (Chen and Hsu 2005). Noise can also result in systematic bias of the DTI parameters, including overestimation of FA, where sorting of noisy DTI eigenvalues gives rise to the artificial appearance of anisotropy (Basser and Pajevic 2000). Not surprisingly, in one way or another, all considerations in the DTI experimental strategy are related to boosting the effective SNR.

5.5.2.2.2 Signal Averaging

Perhaps the simplest way to improve the DTI accuracy is to signal average and improve SNR of the individual diffusion-weighted scans. The relationships among signal averaging, scan time, and the resulting image SNR are well established: scan time is directly proportional to the number of signal averages and SNR is proportional to the square root of the number of signal averages. However, causes of inaccuracy in DTI include not only image noise but also factors such

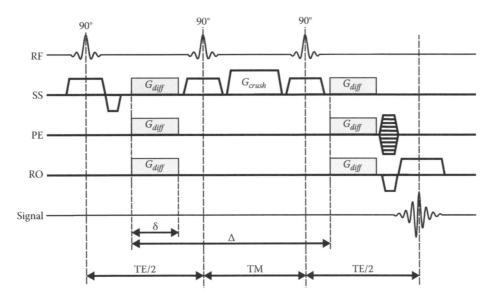

FIGURE 5.52 Stimulated-echo acquisition mode (STEAM) pulse sequence with diffusion-weighted gradients. The STEAM pulse sequence is unaffected by the rapid transverse magnetization relaxation due to magnetization storage in the longitudinal direction during the mixing time, TM. PE, phase encoding; RF, radiofrequency; RO, readout; SS, slice selection.

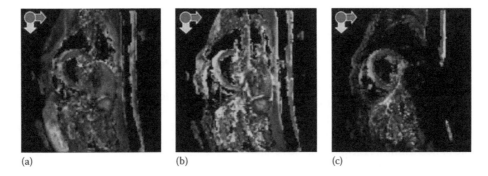

FIGURE 5.53 High-resolution fractional anisotropy (FA) maps, color-coded by the direction of the principal eigenvector of the diffusion tensor, with and without fat suppression. (a) No fat suppression is implemented. (b) Fat suppression with SPIR (spectral presaturation with inversion recovery). (c) Fat suppression with SSGR (slice-selective gradient reversal). (Reproduced from Harmer, J. et al., In-vivo high resolution diffusion tensor imaging of the human heart at 3T: Fat suppression in the presence of b_0 field inhomogeneities, *Proceedings of International Society for Magnetic Resonance in Medicine*, Salt Lake City, UT, 2013a. With permission.)

as directional sampling and tensor estimation. Therefore, accounting for these latter factors can improve the DTI accuracy beyond what is achievable by only signal averaging individual diffusion scans. In a recent study by Scott et al. (2015b,c), the authors showed that averaging the complex data in DTI improves the results accuracy compared to just averaging the magnitude data. However, it should be noted that averaging the complex data is not straightforward as the diffusion-weighting process introduces a spatially varying phase in the image. However, this phase variation can be corrected during image reconstruction to compensate for the noise floor effects at high b-values.

5.5.2.2.3 The Number of Encoding Directions

Indeed, in the context of acquisition of a whole DTI dataset, increasing the number of diffusion-encoding directions is actually a form of signal averaging. Employing more

noncollinear gradient directions has the additional benefit of reducing the directional sampling error and is generally preferred over signal averaging in the same encoding directions. For a given scan time (i.e., combination of the number of individual diffusion-weighted scans and number of averages), the most efficient means to improve DTI accuracy is to acquire diffusion-weighted scans in as many different encoding directions as possible and to distribute the encoding direction unit vectors as evenly spread out as possible on a unit sphere (Jones et al. 1999a). Techniques such as tessellation of icosahedrons (Frank 2001, Tuch et al. 2002) (see Figure 5.54) and electrostatic repulsion on a unit sphere (Jones et al. 1999a) have been proposed and showed to be effective for optimizing the selection of the encoding directions. In general, because of the finite number of variables in diffusion tensor fitting (i.e., seven, including the diffusion-independent magnetization term) and the square root nature

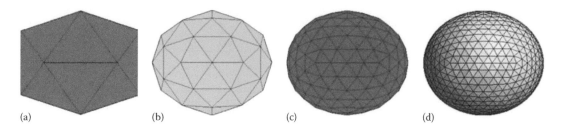

(a)   (b)   (c)   (d)

FIGURE 5.54 Schemes for choosing diffusion-sensitizing directions by uniformly covering a unit sphere. (a–d) show the unit sphere covered with increasing number of directions.

of averaging, DTI quality improvement by increasing the number of diffusion-encoding directions is most pronounced when the number of directions is relatively small.

5.5.2.2.4 *Signal Averaging and b_0 Scan*

In increasing the number of diffusion-encoding directions, it should be also noted that since in tensor computation the same b_0 image is used for estimating the effective diffusivity in each encoding direction, the b_0 image has disproportional impact on the accuracy of the whole DTI experiment. Therefore, the use of a high number of diffusion-encoding directions must be balanced by proportional increase in signal averaging of the b_0 scan (Xing et al. 1997, Jones et al. 1999a).

5.5.2.2.5 *Comparative Examples*

To demonstrate the dependence of DTI quality on the number of encoding directions, Choi et al. (2010) obtained DTI images with 6, 15, and 32 diffusion-sensitizing gradient directions at a mid-ventricular level of an excised porcine heart on a 3 T MRI scanner (b-value of 800 s/mm^2). As expected, the results show that by increasing the number of diffusion-sensitizing gradient directions, the bias in FA was significantly reduced, and the number and length of visualized coherent fibers were significantly increased.

In a recent study, Mazumder et al. (2014) studied the effects of optimizing the number of encoding directions (NED) and the number of signal averages (NSA or NEX) on estimating HA with minimum acquisition time (Figure 5.55). The results showed that an NED/NSA combination of 12/6, 30/3, or 64/2 results in robust estimation of HA in 9.76, 11.72, and 16.27 minutes, respectively; therefore, NED/NSA of 12/6 is the combination that results in the shortest possible acquisition time.

5.5.2.3 **The Effect of b-Value on DTI**

5.5.2.3.1 *Small versus Large b-Values*

Besides the number of diffusion-encoding directions, the choice of the diffusion-weighting b-factor (or b-value) can also have an impact on the accuracy of the DTI experiment. Intuitively, the DTI experiment is akin to measuring the decay constant of an exponentially attenuating signal, or the slope of the signal on a semi-logarithmic plot, with the b-value as the independent variable. If the b-value used is too large (i.e., too much attenuation), the diffusion-weighted scans would contain

more image noise than tissue information, although increasing the b-value in cardiac DTI results in smoother MD and FA maps (Scott et al. 2014, 2015, 2015a) (Figure 5.56). In contrast, if too small b-value is used, even a small amount of noise in the image would have disproportionally large impact on the fitted slope or decay constant. Therefore, diffusion-weighted scans acquired with different b-values do not contribute equally to the accuracy of the DTI experiment.

Recently, Wu et al. (2013) studied the effect of b-value on revealing post-infarct myocardial microstructure. The authors used b-value ranging from 500 to 2500 s/mm^2 for imaging ex vivo heart samples 1, 3, 5, and 7 days after infarction (Figure 5.57). The results showed that MD and FA decrease gradually with b-values in all studied regions and that the optimal b-value depends on the generated map; specifically, moderate b-values of 1500 or 2000 s/mm^2 resulted in the most sensitive FA for detection of fiber integrity degradation, while small b-values less than 1500 s/mm^2 resulted in the greatest ability of MD for monitoring diffusivity alterations during the necrotic and fibrotic phases.

5.5.2.3.2 *Optimal b-Value*

The implications of the DTI experimental design are two-fold. First, there exists an optimal b-value to be used in DTI scans. Empirical experience and studies (Xing et al. 1997, Jones et al. 1999a, Alexander and Barker 2005) have shown that diffusion-weighted scans that achieve a factor of $e^{-1} \approx 0.4 - 0.5$ attenuation of the signal contribute the most to the accuracy of the DTI experiment. Combined with considerations for the number and distribution of encoding directions, it is preferable to use the DTI scan time to repeat the same b-value meeting the optimal attenuation criterion at different additional encoding directions (note that the single b-value criterion does not apply to experiments fitting models other than the diffusion tensor). Second, because of the unequal contribution of the images toward the accuracy of DTI, a weighted curve fitting technique would yield more accurate diffusion tensor estimations than one that weighs all signal data equally (Koay et al. 2006). It should be noted that using diffusion-weighted reference images helps isolate diffusion from the effects of microvascular perfusion, which reduces the dependence of MD and FA on the implemented b-value (Scott et al. 2014).

Besides b-value optimization, the diffusion time has also an effect on DTI-derived parameters and fiber tractography, as

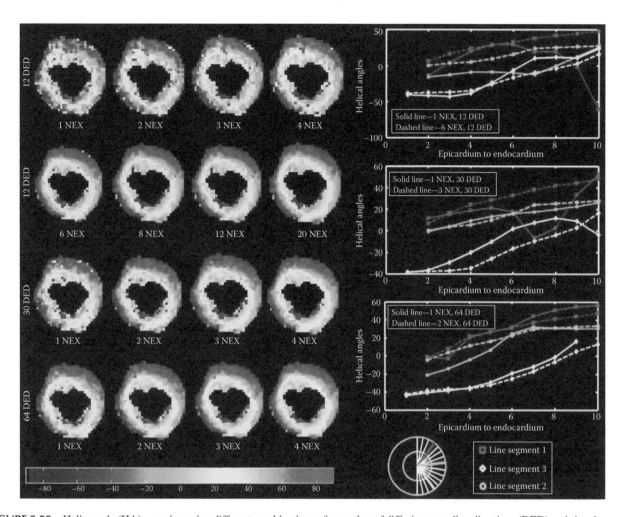

FIGURE 5.55 Helix angle (HA) mapping using different combinations of a number of diffusion-encoding directions (DED) and signal averages (NEX). DED values of 12, 30, and 64 were used with 1, 2, 3, and 4 NEXs. The curves on the right side show line profiles from three transmural line segments drawn on the free wall of the LV. (Reproduced from Mazumder, R. et al., *J. Cardiovasc. Magn. Reson.*, 16(Suppl 1), P359, 2014.)

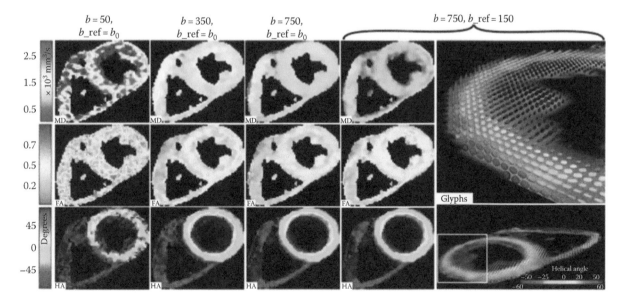

FIGURE 5.56 DTI maps of mean diffusivity (MD), frcational anisotropy (FA), and helix angle (HA) for different b-values. The first, second, and third rows show MD, FA, and HA maps. Three pairs of b-values were selected: $b = 50$, $b = 350$, $b = 750$. Superquadratic glyphs is shown for the b-values selected as optimal ($b = 750$, $b\_ref = 150$ s/mm^2). (Reproduced from Scott, A.D. et al., *J. Cardiovasc. Magn. Reson.*, 16(Suppl 1), O27, 2014.)

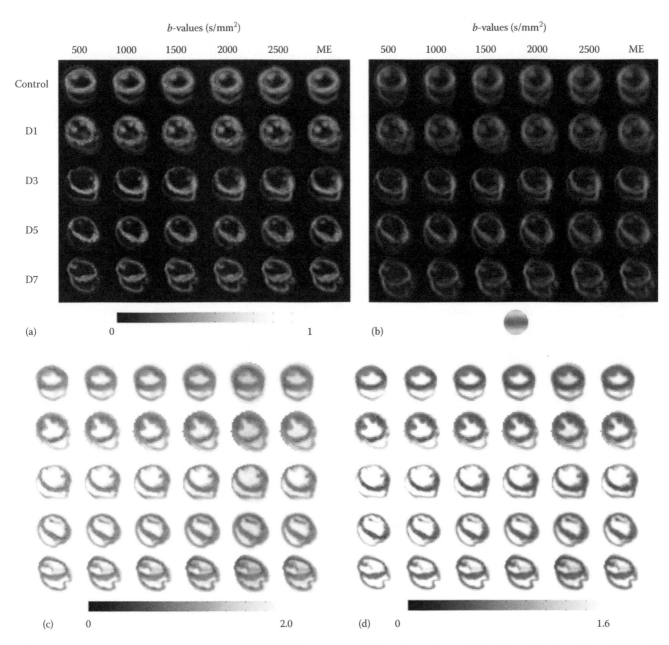

FIGURE 5.57 Fractional anisotropy (FA) maps and diffusivities in normal and infarcted hearts imaged with different *b*-values. Maps of (a) FA, (b) color-coded FA, (c) axial diffusivity ($\lambda_\parallel$), and (d) radial diffusivity ($\lambda_\perp$) computed from diffusion imaging using five different *b*-values (500, 1000, 1500, 2000, and 2500 s/mm²; *b*_ref = 0 s/mm² for all cases) in control and infarcted (days (D) 1, 3, 5, and 7 post-infarction) hearts. The unit of diffusivity is ×10⁻³ mm²/s. ME, monoexponential fitting. (Reproduced from Wu, Y. et al., *Magn. Reson. Imaging*, 31(6), 847, 2013. With permission.)

shown in Figure 5.58. In the study by Froeling et al. (2014a), it has been shown that the two-tensor fit results in two compartments with different diffusion properties; most probably the slower diffusion compartment represents the actin and myosin filaments within the muscle fiber, whereas the faster diffusion compartment represents the space surrounding the sarcomeres.

5.5.2.4 Gradient Settings

5.5.2.4.1 Physical Limitations

Although optimal strategies for DTI acquisition are known, their practical implementation can be hampered by instrumentation limitations. More often than not, the optimal diffusion-weighting *b*-value cannot be achieved due to the low or finite gradient strength available, especially in clinical whole-body scanners. As a work around, one way to boost the effective *b*-value is to employ multiple gradients at the same time. For example, turning on two gradients simultaneously boosts the *b*-value by a factor of $\sqrt{2}$ compared to when a single gradient is used. In this regard, while both {(1, 0, 0), (0, 1, 0), (0, 0, 1), (1, 1, 0), (1, 0, 1), (0, 1, 1)} and {(1, 1, 0), (1, −1, 0), (0, 1, 1), (0, 1, −1), (1, 0, 1), (1, 0, −1)} sets contain six noncollinear directions and thus satisfy the criterion for minimal DTI encoding directions, the latter always employs two-gradient directions, which is better for practical use. It is worth noting that using multiple gradients simultaneously to increase the *b*-value must be weighed against the fact that

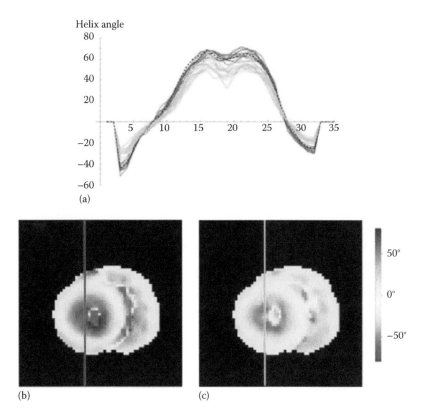

FIGURE 5.58 Helix angle (HA) based on different diffusion times. (a) HA for a cross-sectional line as indicated in parts (b) and (c). (b) HA map for diffusion time of 52 ms. (c) HA map for diffusion time of 322 ms. (Reproduced from Froeling, M. et al., *J. Cardiovasc. Magn. Reson.*, 16(Suppl 1), P77, 2014a.)

practice also dictates feasible gradient directions, which may interfere with the gradient optimization settings.

5.5.2.4.2 Gradients Infidelity

Implicit in the earlier discussion on encoding direction and *b*-value optimization is that the gradient waveforms of the pulse sequence are precisely known, which can be difficult in practice. For example, even with the best shimming effort, background gradient is inevitable. Unaccounted for background gradient not only sets the DTI encoding scheme off its optimal conditions but also causes erroneous DTI estimations from errors in computing the *b*-matrix elements (e.g., using Equation 5.14) due to the associated cross-terms, which can be of a bigger concern (Basser and Jones 2002). Fortunately, the effects of the cross-terms are multiplicative in both amplitude and polarity, and a simple, yet effective, means to eliminate them is to acquire diffusion-weighted scans with the same magnitude, but opposite polarity, encoding gradients, and take the geometric average (i.e., square root of the product of the two image intensities) of the scans (Hsu et al. 1998). The drawback of this strategy, obviously, is that the scan time is doubled. This is yet another example that the optimization of the DTI experimental strategy often involves addressing not a single consideration, but weighting and trading-off among multiple counter-opposing factors.

5.5.2.5 Post-Processing Algorithms

In addition to the aforementioned measures for optimizing the DTI experiment, the accuracy of DTI can also be improved in the post-processing stage (Hasan et al. 2011). For example, by recognizing that a properly estimated diffusion tensor should bear certain characteristics of the physical entity (e.g., having only real, positive eigenvalues), appropriate numeric estimation algorithms (e.g., Cholesky factorization) can be applied to avoid bad tensor fittings produced in noisy pixels (Koay et al. 2006).

By recognizing that noise tends to produce more variability than the underlying tissue structure in the tensors estimated for neighboring pixels, denoising or other *a priori* information-based regularization techniques could be used to boost the DTI quality, often without requiring additional scans (Frindel et al. 2009). The common idea behind regularization is to introduce *a priori* information about the solution in order to smooth the diffusion images while preserving relevant details (Hsu and Henriquez 2001, Frindel et al. 2007). Denoising is in effect a form of image smoothing, which can be achieved by techniques as simple as low-pass filtering of the images. Different denoising techniques have been evaluated on both simulated and empirical DW and DTI images (Chen and Hsu 2005), including cardiac scans (Bao et al. 2007, 2009). For DTI, it has been found that vector- or tensor-based denoising is better than image-based treatment, since in the former case deviations introduced after acquisition (e.g., during tensor fitting and diagonalization) are also removed (Chen and Hsu 2005).

Separately, sparse representation-based techniques, which effectively randomize the noise effects, have been used for denoising cardiac DTI images while preserving the image's useful coherent structures (Bao et al. 2009). Because of their estimation nature, these regularization techniques offer the benefit of being able to capture the essential DTI information from only a small subset of the original dataset, which has the potential for accelerating DTI scan times. One example of such techniques is using the compressed sensing methodology in DTI (Welsh et al. 2013), which is described in more detail later in the chapter.

5.5.3 SPECIAL CONSIDERATIONS FOR IN VIVO CARDIAC DTI

Besides the same challenges facing all DTI applications, in vivo cardiac DTI requires at least three additional technical considerations, all of which stem from the physiology of the heart: motion artifacts, myocardial strain, and tissue perfusion. It is clear that the specific heart physiology adds technical challenges that need to be considered for performing in vivo cardiac DTI. Despite technological advances that have made most of the known issues tractable, complete understanding and compensating for motion effects in cardiac DTI remain works in progress. In the meantime, caution is warranted when interpreting in vivo cardiac DTI results.

5.5.3.1 Motion Artifacts

Compared to other organs, the heart undergoes large, but relatively periodic, beating motion, such that unattended motion can lead to pronounced ghosting and streaking artifacts along the phase-encoding axis of the MRI image. Because of the large diffusion-encoding gradients used, motion artifacts in diffusion-weighted MRI are orders of magnitude worse than in regular anatomical scans. This issue has recently been studied by Wei et al. (2013b) with the aid of ground-truth data from polarized light imaging and simulated diffusion-weighted images and based on motion information derived from displacement-encoding (DENSE) imaging. The results showed that the heart motion causes significant signal loss in diffusion-weighted images, which leads to overestimation of MD and FA, and reduced range of fiber angles between the endo- and epicardium.

5.5.3.1.1 DTI with Free Breathing

In a recent study, Wei et al. (2013a) demonstrated the feasibility of in vivo free-breathing cardiac DTI in healthy volunteers using the principal component analysis with temporal maximum intensity projection (PCATMIP) method to minimize the motion-induced signal loss, despite the time-consuming limitation of PCATMIP. The PCATMIP method could be also combined with shifted trigger delay acquisitions and image registration to improve the quality of in vivo DTI (Wei et al. 2013c). In a subsequent study, the same research group added the wavelet-based image fusion technique to the PCATMIP method to provide a clinically compatible and robust technique for studying 3D cardiac fiber architecture properties from free-breathing DTI images (Wei et al. 2015).

5.5.3.1.2 Cardiac and Respiratory Gating

Motion artifacts from periodically moving organs or objects can be greatly reduced by employing gated acquisition (e.g., dual cardiac and respiratory-gated imaging). Indeed, cardiac gating

at the time point when bulk systolic motion is minimal has been shown effective in improving the quality of cardiac DTI (Rapacchi et al. 2011). Another way to address motion is to employ navigator echoes (de Crespigny et al. 1995), which are additional echoes formed by the MRI signal in the absence of phase encoding, to estimate motion and compensate for its effects via post-processing correction. A high-resolution, cardiac DTI study using a prospective navigator echo showed potential for in vivo DTI in humans, with results shown in Figure 5.59 (Nielles-Vallespin et al. 2013b). In another study, the navigator echo technique was improved by Ferreira et al. (2013b) for high-quality free-breathing cardiac DTI. The developed technique, combined with robust post-processing, showed to be capable of producing in vivo DTI images of the heart comparable to those obtained with breath-hold.

5.5.3.1.3 Signal Averaging to Reduce Motion Effects

Signal averaging could be implemented to improve image quality and mitigate motion effects. In a study by Ferreira et al. (2013a), the authors showed an increase in the quality of diffusion measurements (HA, FA, and MD) with the number of signal averages, where measurement changes became relatively small when the number of signal averages exceeded five (Figure 5.60).

5.5.3.1.4 Spatiotemporal Motion Correction

In multiple breath-hold scans, motion effects could be minimized through motion correction among different frames and slices. This approach was adopted by Mekkaoui et al. (2013c), who showed that motion correction over space and time using rigid registration can significantly reduce the motion displacement produced by multiple breath-holds and improve DTI quality (Figure 5.61).

5.5.3.1.5 Bipolar Diffusion Gradients

It may be possible to reduce the sensitivity to motion in diffusion MRI by replacing the conventional unipolar diffusion-encoding gradient pulses with bipolar pulses, which cancel first gradient moments (hence reduces motion sensitivity), albeit that the achievable diffusion-weighting b-value by bipolar gradient pulses is also expected to be significantly reduced. One method to attain higher b-values while minimizing the effects of motion is to use stimulated-echo acquisition mode (STEAM) acquisition in conjunction with double cardiac gating, where the excitation and re-excitation (i.e., first and third) RF pulses are synchronized to the cardiac cycle (Edelman et al. 1994), as shown in Figure 5.62. Even with the halved SNR associated with STEAM, the approach has been found effective in mitigating motion, and is increasingly used in DTI studies in humans and large animals (Dou et al. 2002, Wu et al. 2009a, Nielles-Vallespin et al. 2013b). Regardless of the means implemented for motion compensation, the increased sensitivity of diffusion MRI makes motion extremely challenging to correct for and leaves very little room for uncorrected instrument imperfections.

Recently, Stoeck et al. (2015a,b,c) showed that second-order motion-compensated diffusion gradients significantly reduce DTI sensitivity to bulk heart motion compared to first-order

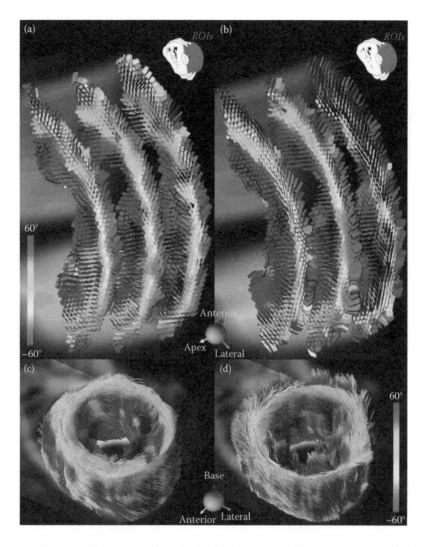

FIGURE 5.59 Visualization of tensor solutions from data obtained in vivo in a healthy human subject using breath-holds and prospective navigator to reduce sensitivity to motion. (a) Breath-hold and (b) navigator echo-based superquadratic glyph fields of the lateral wall in three contiguous short-axis slices. (c) Breath-hold and (d) navigator echo-based 3D fiber tractograms of the LV. (Reproduced from Nielles-Vallespin, S. et al., *Magn. Reson. Med.*, 70(2), 454, 2013b. With permission.)

motion-compensated gradients. In another study, Welsh et al. (2015) employed the principles of gradient moment nulling to develop a diffusion-encoding scheme designed to compensate for higher-order motion components, including acceleration and jerk. The authors used the developed sequence for in vivo imaging of rats, and concluded that compensation for acceleration and other lower-order motion components can be an effective alternative to high-performance gradients for improved in vivo DTI in the heart.

5.5.3.2 Strain Memory Effects in DTI

Even if the images are free from motion artifacts, motion of the heart can lead to erroneous estimates due to the strain-memory effect of the diffusion constants. Strain alters the relative distance between any two given points of the tissue. Because the diffusion-weighted MR signal is derived in part based on the probability of spatial displacement, strain can add or subtract from the displacement and lead to over- or

underestimation of the diffusion measurements. The effects of strain on in vivo cardiac DTI measurements have long been documented (Reese et al. 1996). Because myocardial strain can be separately quantified via, for example, tagged MRI, its effects can be subtracted to obtain pure diffusion and fiber orientation measurements from in vivo cardiac DTI data (Reese et al. 1996). Moreover, because the strain effects depend on the average strain across the cardiac cycle, it has been shown possible to obtain strain-free in vivo cardiac DTI measurements by selecting the right timing (trigger) delay in gated cardiac acquisitions (Tseng et al. 1999). In a recent study by Stoeck et al. (2014), the authors used a dual-phase (systole and diastole) STEAM-based DTI technique that includes correction for myocardial strain based on 3D myocardial tagging. The results showed small effect of strain correction on HA; however, larger differences were observed between the strain-corrected and uncorrected measurements in the transverse and sheet angles (Figure 5.63).

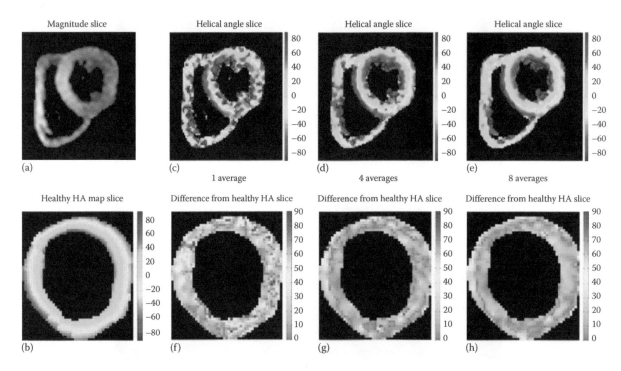

FIGURE 5.60 Helix angle (HA) maps with different number of averages. Examples from a basal slice of a volunteer. (a) Magnitude image. (b) Healthy statistical average (HSA) map of HA. (c–e) HA maps using 1, 4, and 8 averages, respectively. (f–h) Difference (in degrees) between the HAS and HA maps for 1, 4, and 8 averages, respectively. (Reproduced from Ferreira, P. et al., Helix angle (HA) healthy statistical average technique for HA quantification in vivo cardiac diffusion tensor imaging, *Proceedings of International Society for Magnetic Resonance in Medicine*, Salt Lake City, UT, 2013a. With permission.)

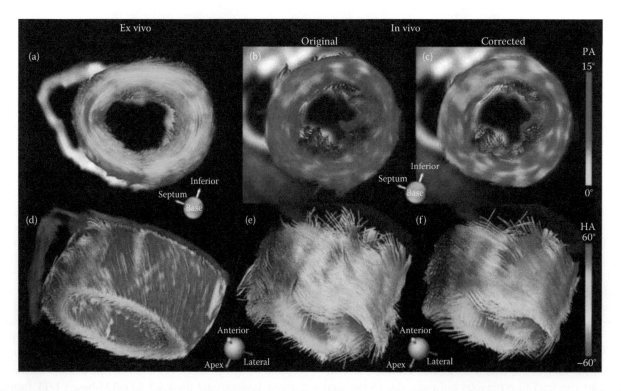

FIGURE 5.61 MR tractography with and without motion correction. MR tractography of a human heart (a, d) ex vivo, (b, e) in vivo before, and (c, f) in vivo after motion correction. Fiber tracts are color-coded by (a–c) propagation angle (PA) and (d–f) helix angle (HA). PA is significantly reduced after motion correction and becomes similar to ex vivo results. The HA map shows more coherent fibers in the subepicardium after motion correction. (Reproduced from Mekkaoui, C. et al., Improved tractography of the human heart in vivo by motion correction of multi-breathold diffusion tensor MRI, *Proceedings of International Society for Magnetic Resonance in Medicine*, Salt Lake City, UT, 2013c. With permission.)

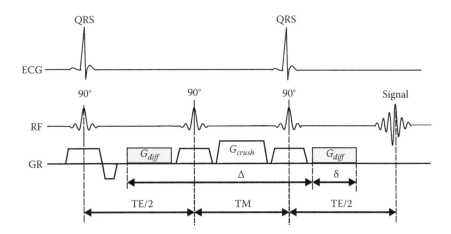

FIGURE 5.62 Stimulated-echo acquisition mode (STEAM) pulse sequence with incorporated diffusion-sensitizing gradients. The first and third RF pulses are synchronized to occur at the same time point in the cardiac cycle (see ECG signal at the time of applying the first and third RF pulses). STEAM allows for higher b-values given a fixed gradient strength, but at the cost of losing half of the acquired signal due to using a stimulated echo. ECG, electrocardiogram; GR, gradient echo; RF, radiofrequency; TE, echo time; TM, mixing time.

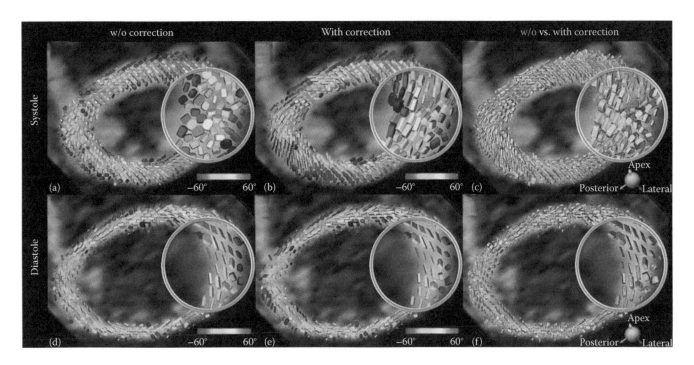

FIGURE 5.63 Systolic and diastolic tensor maps with and without strain correction. Diffusion tensor fields acquired in (a, b) systole and (d, e) diastole are represented by superquadric glyphs and color-coded by the helix angle (a, d) before and (b, e) after strain correction. The diffusion tensor fields before and after strain correction are merged in (c, f) to visualize its impact. (a–c) Insets demonstrate a major realignment of the tensor field into the typical helical pattern upon strain correction in systole. (d–f) In diastole, strain correction effects are characterized mainly by small changes in the principal diffusivities. (Reproduced from Stoeck, C.T. et al., *PLoS One*, 9(9), e107159, 2014.)

5.5.3.3 Perfusion Effects in DTI

Recent advances in gradient hardware technology have made high-strength gradients available (up to 80 mT/m in whole-body scanners and 1500 mT/m or more in small animal systems), which in turn made it practically feasible to employ bipolar encoding gradient pulses capable of generating moderate, but sufficient, b-values for diffusion MRI and DTI, especially for cardiac applications (Gamper et al. 2007). Bipolar diffusion pulses offer not only reduced motion sensitivity but also have decreased memory effects of strain (Dou et al. 2002). However, besides the impact on accuracy as previously explained, using relatively low b-values associated with bipolar gradient pulses can also inadvertently introduce effects from tissue perfusion and lead to additional errors in DTI measurements.

Perfusion, in this case blood flow in the capillary bed, has long been known for causing additional spin phase dispersion and leading to overestimated diffusion coefficients via the so-called intravoxel incoherent motion (IVIM) effect (Le Bihan et al. 1988) in highly vascularized organs such as the liver (Luciani et al. 2008). Because the capillary flow is faster than the diffusion of water, the flow-mediated perfusion effect can be eliminated from diffusion measurements by employing sufficiently high diffusion weighting ($b > 200$ s/mm^2). The perfusion dependence of diffusion MRI has been studied (Le Bihan et al. 1988, Le Bihan and Turner 1992) and recently demonstrated empirically on a perfused heart (Abdullah et al. 2013).

5.6 ADVANCED METHODS AND APPLICATIONS

Despite the advances that have been achieved in addressing the limitations and challenges facing DTI, room for improvement remains. This section discusses some of the areas and methods that are being developed to further improve the overall utility of DTI, including means to better characterize diffusion and the underlying tissue structures, accelerate data acquisition, and visualize the derived myocardial fiber architecture.

5.6.1 BEYOND DTI

5.6.1.1 DTI and Complex Fiber Structures
Since its advent, DTI has rapidly become the method of choice for characterizing ordered tissue structures. Because of the unique advantages of MRI for brain imaging, most DTI studies and related technological developments have focused on imaging the brain white matter. In the formulation of the underlying principles (described earlier in the chapter), DTI necessarily assumes that the principal axes of the anisotropic diffusion system are orthogonal and that there exists only one orientation of anisotropy. Although these assumptions are adequate, for example in areas of brain white matter where axonal fibers are uniformly oriented, they create a pitfall for regions such as the optic chiasm where the fibers cross, merge, or branch (Figure 5.64). Much work has been done to improve the ability of DTI, or more generally diffusion MRI, to resolve "complex" fiber structures, which is beginning to be applied and benefit the characterization of myocardial structures.

Ironically, much of the limitation of DTI originates from the intrinsic properties of the diffusion tensor that are forced upon the observed diffusion-weighted signal during the estimation process. Because the distances resolved by MRI are far larger than the diffusion scale, each voxel represents many distinct diffusional environments (Wedeen et al. 2005). The presence of distinct diffusion microenvironments (e.g., fiber populations of different orientations) provides a complicated, voxel-averaged diffusion signal that is underspecified by the six degrees of freedom of the conventional DTI model. Forcibly fitting the heterogeneous diffusion signal to the diffusion tensor equation results in ambiguous fiber orientation and degree of anisotropy estimation (Roberts and Schwartz 2007). In order to resolve this ambiguity, alternative methods to characterize the diffusion signal have been introduced, which include both nonparametric and parametric approaches. Most of these techniques have been developed for characterizing white matter structure in the brain, and have just begun to be applied to the myocardium.

5.6.1.2 Nonparametric Diffusion Techniques
The strategy in nonparametric approaches is to observe diffusion along a large number of directions and directly identify the orientations of anisotropy (e.g., via the degree of attenuation of the signal) without fitting the observed data to the DTI signal equation. Diffusion MRI techniques that follow this general approach include high angular-resolution diffusion imaging (HARDI) (Frank 2001, Tuch et al. 2002) and diffusion spectrum imaging (DSI) (Wedeen et al. 2005).

DSI requires data to be acquired on a 3D Cartesian grid in q-space (where a point in q-space is defined by a diffusion-weighting magnitude, or b-value, and a diffusion-encoding directional vector), from which the 3D Fourier transform can be easily performed. For each voxel, the inverse Fourier transform of q-space produces the 3D diffusion probability density function (PDF), whose peaks correspond to the orientations of the fiber populations, as shown in Figure 5.65 (Tournier et al. 2011). Since DSI utilizes diffusion data with high angular and spatial resolution, the myofiber tracings, or tractograms (explained later in the chapter), are considered more accurate. DSI tractography results from an ex vivo rat heart are shown in Figure 5.66 (Sosnovik et al. 2009a).

Because the accuracy of the estimated fiber orientations depends on the angular sampling resolution, HARDI and DSI generally require diffusion to be observed in a high number, typically hundreds, of encoding directions. Although these high angular-resolution diffusion techniques are capable of resolving multiple fiber populations that may be present in a single voxel, their main limitation is that the required scan time can be prohibitive.

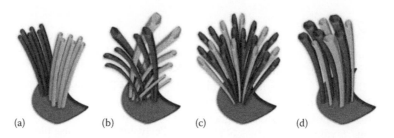

(a)   (b)   (c)   (d)

FIGURE 5.64 Examples of complex fiber configurations within a single voxel. (a) Adjacent fiber populations with different orientations. (b) Interdigitating fibers crossing at different orientations. (c) Fanning fibers. (d) Bending fibers.

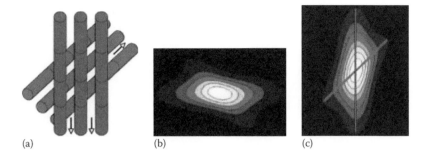

FIGURE 5.65 Visualization of fiber crossings detection in DSI. (a) Schematic of two crossing-fiber populations within a single imaged voxel. (b) Simulation of the resulting q-space from applying diffusion imaging to (a). Each point in the q-space is equal to the signal intensity of the given voxel when the corresponding diffusion- or q-vector is applied. (c) Resulting probability distribution function (PDF) from taking the Fourier transform of the q-space in (b). The orientation of the dominant fiber populations can be derived by finding the peaks of the resulting PDF, as shown by the blue and red lines. (Reproduced from Sosnovik, D.E. et al., *J. Cardiovasc. Magn. Reson.*, 11, 47, 2009a.)

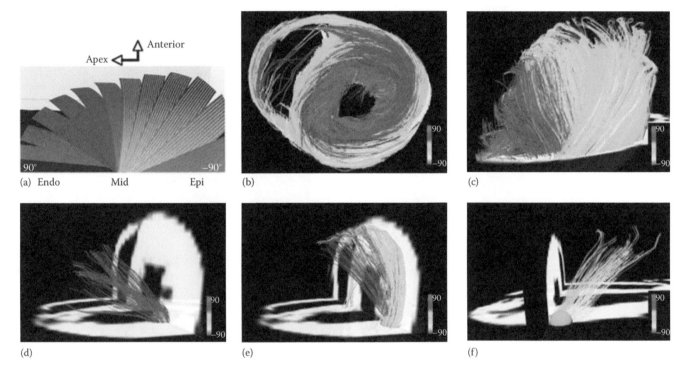

FIGURE 5.66 Fiber tractography performed on DSI data acquired from a normal, ex vivo rat heart. The results are shown (a, c–f) from the lateral wall and (b) in the short axis. Only fibers intersecting a spherical region of interest are shown in (d–f). (Reproduced from Sosnovik, D.E. et al., *J. Cardiovasc. Magn. Reson.*, 11, 47, 2009a.)

5.6.1.3 Q-Ball Imaging

The second approach to address the limitation of the DTI formalism is to employ parametric descriptions or models of diffusion that are more sophisticated than the simple diffusion tensor. For example, Q-ball imaging (QBI) is a truncated version of DSI in which the diffusion images are acquired in one shell of q-space (i.e., single diffusion-weighting b-value and multiple diffusion-encoding directions) (Tuch 2004). In QBI, spherical harmonic basis functions obtained by, for example, the Funk–Radon transform of the DW signal provide an approximation to the radial integral of the 3D diffusion PDF, or the so-called diffusion orientation distribution function (ODF) (Tournier et al. 2011). Similar to DSI,

the fiber orientations are obtained by identifying the peaks of the derived ODF. QBI has been applied and compared to DTI (Figures 5.67 through 5.69) for characterizing myocardial structures in recent studies that detected the presence of complex fiber structures in localized regions such as insertions of the RV and bases of the papillary muscles (Shi et al. 2007, Dierckx et al. 2009). However, QBI appears not to offer additional benefit to DTI, for example, for quantifying the myofiber orientation in the bulk of the ventricular myocardium. Therefore, additional QBI studies need to be performed to validate whether QBI provides higher quality or more accurate characterization of the myocardium (Hagmann et al. 2006).

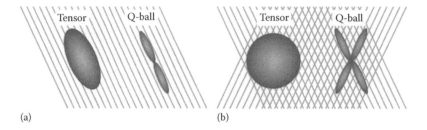

(a)   (b)

FIGURE 5.67   Comparison of diffusion tensor ellipsoid and Q-ball orientation distribution function in single-fiber population and cross-ing-fiber environments. (a) If a single fiber population is present within a voxel, then the diffusion tensor solution is sufficient. (b) If two crossing-fiber populations are present, the diffusion tensor solution yields a result that underestimates the diffusion anisotropy and makes it impossible to discern the orientation of the crossing fibers. The QBI yields a result that is robust to the two environments.

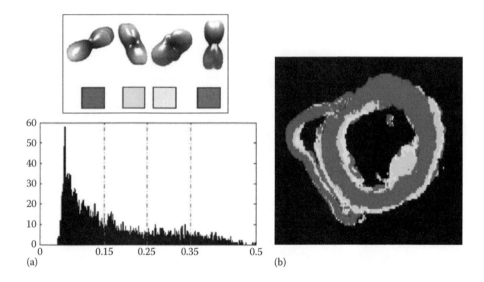

(a)   (b)

FIGURE 5.68   Q-ball imaging performed in a canine heart. (a) Relative frequency of different fiber configurations. (b) False-colored map showing the spatial location of the different fiber configurations shown in (a).

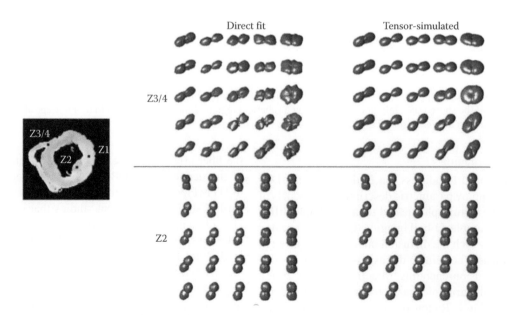

FIGURE 5.69   Comparison of DTI and Q-ball fitting of diffusion data acquired in a healthy canine heart. Different regions of interest (small black squares) are indicated on the myocardium in the image on the left. The results of the DTI and Q-ball fitting methods are most different in the Z3/4 region at the insertion point between the right and left ventricles. The results are almost identical in the Z2 region.

5.6.1.4 High-Order Parametric Diffusion Techniques

Other parametric diffusion models that have been introduced include higher-order diffusion tensors (Ozarslan and Mareci 2003) and kurtosis (Jensen et al. 2005). These techniques are mathematically related and rely on modeling the diffusion signal from HARDI acquisitions to obtain the ODF. Higher-order diffusion tensors essentially incorporate extra terms into the diffusion tensor to describe the additional diffusion features, whereas diffusion kurtosis imaging (DKI) quantifies the non-monoexponential behavior of the diffusion signal using a fourth-order diffusion tensor. Because of the use of models (i.e., parametric fitting), the modeled approaches generally require fewer number of diffusion-encoding directions than unmodeled HARDI experiments, thus reducing the potentially prohibitive scan time.

5.6.2 ACCELERATING DTI ACQUISITION

5.6.2.1 DTI and Compressed Sensing Reconstruction

5.6.2.1.1 Benefits of Using Compressed Sensing

Because of its minimum dataset requirement of seven acquisitions, and the frequent use of signal averaging (including increasing the number of encoding gradient directions) to improve its accuracy, practical applications of DTI have been hampered by long scan times. Due to the repetitive nature of DTI experiments, reduction or elimination of data redundancies has been explored as a potential means to accelerate data

acquisition (Hsu and Henriquez 2001). Compressed sensing is an advanced technique that reconstructs MRI images from partially sampled data (Donoho 2006, Lustig et al. 2007). The relative benefits of compressed sensing are demonstrated in the images in Figure 5.70. Conventional reconstructions (e.g., using direct inverse Fourier transform) of partially sampled k-space data often lead to structured artifacts such as blurring and ringing in the resulting images. One key feature of compressed sensing is randomized k-space sampling, which turns the effects of partial k-space sampling into incoherent, noise-like artifacts. The effects of these artifacts are then minimized to yield images close to what the fully sampled k-space would have achieved, but using data that was acquired in a fraction of the time.

5.6.2.1.2 Problem Formulation

The ideal experiment for applying compressed sensing is one where some knowledge about the images to be reconstructed already exists. In general, compressed sensing reconstruction can be formulated as the minimization of some cost function given in the form of

$$C(m) = \left\| \vec{F}(m) - \vec{y} \right\|_2^2 + \alpha \left\| \psi(m) \right\|_1, \qquad (5.21)$$

where

$\left\| \vec{F}(m) - \vec{y} \right\|_2^2$ is the data fidelity term

$\left\| \psi(m) \right\|_1$ is the image sparsifying term

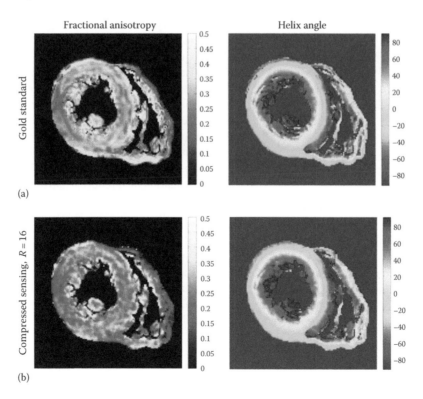

FIGURE 5.70 Fractional anisotropy and helix angle (HA) maps using compressed sensing (CS). The figure shows results (a) using all acquired data or the "gold-standard" traditionally reconstructed case, and (b) using 1/16th of the acquired data, reconstructed using model-based compressed sensing reconstruction. Note similarity between gold-standard and CS-reconstructed images despite the significant reduction in scan time with CS.

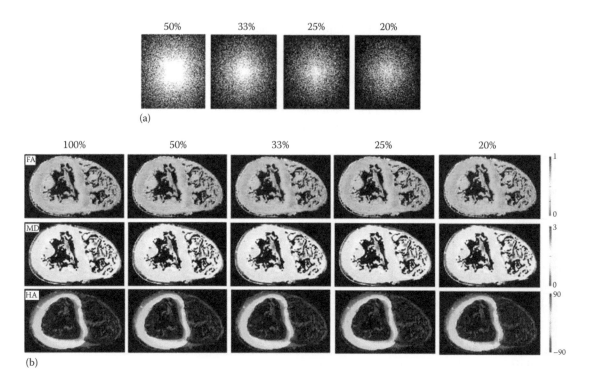

FIGURE 5.71 DTI parameter maps with data undersampling using the fast composite splitting algorithm (FCSA). (a) Sampling patterns and (b) fractional anisotropy (FA)/mean diffusivity (MD)/helix angle (HA) DTI maps acquired with full sampling as well as 50%, 33%, 25%, and 20% sampling ratios. Note similarity between maps acquired with different sampling ratios. (Reproduced from Giannakidis, A. et al., *J. Cardiovasc. Magn. Reson.*, 16(Suppl 1), W5, 2014.)

The fidelity term is akin to least squares fitting between the acquired signal, y, and estimated image, m, transformed into the measurement domain, or k-space, by the undersampled Fourier operator $F(\cdot)$. The image sparsifying term is used to drive the estimated image, m, to have desired features, such as smoothness (absence of noise) or sparsity, using a transform, ψ. Common examples of image sparsifying transforms are the total variation (TV) and wavelet transforms. The estimated image, m, is reconstructed by minimizing Equation 5.21 with respect to m

$$\hat{m} = \min_{m}\left(\left\| \vec{F}(m) - \vec{y} \right\|_2^2 + \alpha \left\| \psi(m) \right\|_1 \right), \qquad (5.22)$$

which is performed using a numerical method such as gradient descent or conjugate gradient. The relative contributions from the data fidelity and image sparsifying terms are controlled by the regularizing term, α.

DTI lends itself well to compressed sensing because of the redundancies across the diffusion-weighted images (e.g., same organ size and shape with only diffusion contrast differences). The general cost function in Equation 5.21 can be altered to include the series of diffusion-weighted images (Adluru et al. 2007)

$$C(m_n) = \sum_{n=1}^{N}\left(\left\| \vec{F}(m_n) - \vec{y} \right\|_2^2 + \alpha \left\| \psi(m_n) \right\|_1 \right). \qquad (5.23)$$

The reconstructed individual diffusion-weighted images, m_n, can then be used to obtain the diffusion tensors similar to the standard DTI experiment.

5.6.2.1.3 Modified Compressed Sensing Techniques

Recently, Giannakidis et al. (2013, 2014) presented two variations of compressed sensing for cardiac DTI. The first technique is called fast composite splitting algorithm (FCSA) (Giannakidis et al. 2014), which showed to outperform conventional compressed sensing reconstruction by providing more accurate results in less processing time (Figure 5.71). The second technique is called circular Cartesian undersampling (CIRCUS) (Giannakidis et al. 2013), which is a combination of 3D Cartesian undersampling scheme and compressed sensing reconstruction (Figure 5.72). CIRCUS-based DTI of the heart helped reduce acquisition time without affecting the measurement accuracy.

5.6.2.2 Model-Based Partial Data Reconstruction

A model-based approach has been recently proposed (Welsh et al. 2013) in which the diffusion tensor is directly reconstructed from partially sampled k-space data. This is done by replacing the diffusion images, m_n, with the diffusion model defined in Equation 5.11:

$$m_n = I_0 e^{-b\,g_n^T Dg_n} e^{i\phi_n}, \qquad (5.24)$$

with an explicit term for the image phase ϕ_n to help correct affine distortions commonly found in diffusion-weighted images. The reference image, I_0, is fully sampled under the proposed scheme and the image phase, ϕ_n, is generally estimated using the fully sampled low-order data in k-space.

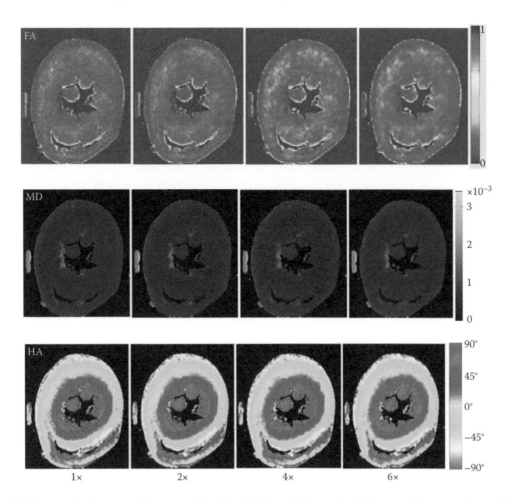

FIGURE 5.72 DTI fractional anisotropy (FA), mean diffusivity (MD), and helix angle (HA) maps with data undersampling (acceleration rates of 1, 2, 4, and 6) using the circular Cartesian undersampling (CIRCUS) method. (Reproduced from Giannakidis, A. et al., Fast-track cardiac diffusion tensor imaging with compressed sensing based on a novel circular cartesian undersampling, *Proceedings of International Society for Magnetic Resonance in Medicine*, Salt Lake City, UT, 2013.)

Therefore, the cost function becomes a function of only the unknown diffusion tensor, D:

$$C(D) = \sum_{n=1}^{N} \left(\left\| \vec{F}\left(I_0 e^{-b\, g_n^T D g_n} e^{i\phi_n}\right) - \vec{y} \right\|_2^2 + \alpha \left\| \psi\left(I_0 e^{-b\, g_n^T D g_n}\right) \right\|_1 \right). \tag{5.25}$$

The advantage of this model-based approach is that the number of unknowns (to be solved) is greatly reduced. Because there are fewer unknowns, noise or undersampling artifacts have less impact on the reconstructed tensor. Also, fewer steps in the reconstruction result in fewer propagation errors. In addition, setting up the cost function as in Equation 5.25 forces the acquired signal, y, to fit or explain itself according to the diffusion tensor model. Since the minimization of the cost function is an iterative process, a more accurate tensor solution is expected.

5.6.2.3 Other Techniques for Accelerating DTI

5.6.2.3.1 Intravoxel Incoherent Motion

Besides compressed sensing, other conventional approaches have been developed for accelerating in vivo cardiac DTI.

Froeling et al. (2014b) developed a cardiac diffusion MRI protocol for obtaining whole-heart DTI and intravoxel incoherent motion (IVIM) data within 15 minutes. The authors used a spin echo sequence with bipolar diffusion-weighting gradients and flow compensation. A reduced FOV was obtained using outer volume suppression. The images were acquired with 200 ms cardiac triggering delay and free breathing on a 3 T scanner (Figure 5.73). In another study, Moulin et al. (2015) used DTI and IVIM for whole-heart in vivo imaging using a real-time slice-following SE-EPI sequence with navigator echo.

5.6.2.3.2 Localized Excitation and Partial K-Space Acquisition

The reduction in scan time could be also used to cover more of the cardiac cycle. Nielles-Vallespin et al. (2013a) adopted this approach for performing in vivo DTI acquisitions of the heart over the whole cardiac cycle. To achieve this goal, the authors used a STEAM single-shot EPI sequence applied on a 3 T scanner. Localized excitation and partial k-space acquisition techniques were implemented to minimize the readout time. The developed technique allowed for obtaining

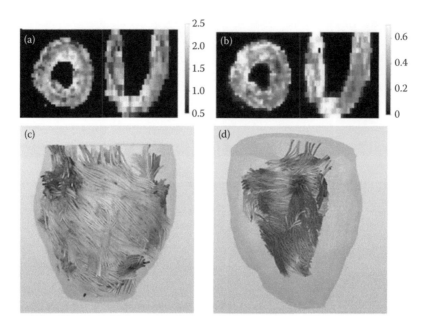

FIGURE 5.73 DTI parameter maps based on the intravoxel incoherent motion (IVIM) fit. (a) Mean diffusivity (MD) map. (b) Fractional anisotropy (FA) map. (c, d) 3D fiber tractography based on the IVIM tensor fit, color-coded for the helix angle (HA) of the whole heart and inside the myocardial wall, respectively. (Reproduced from Froeling, M. et al., *J. Cardiovasc. Magn. Reson.*, 16(Suppl 1), O15, 2014b. With permission.)

MD, FA, HA, and superquadric glyph maps over seven heart phases throughout the cardiac cycle.

5.6.2.3.3 *Multislice Imaging*

von Deuster et al. (2013) adopted a different approach for improving the efficiency of in vivo DTI by a factor of two using dual-slice imaging. Specifically, a concurrent dual-slice single-shot EPI sequence was implemented using multi-band STEAM acquisition and parallel imaging. Nevertheless, it should be noted that, compared to sequential single-slice acquisition, dual-slice imaging requires perfect B_0 homogeneity over a larger volume to avoid off-resonance artifacts.

Recently, simultaneous multislice (SMS) excitation using blipped controlled aliasing (CAIPI) readout was combined with diffusion-weighted STEAM sequence for simultaneous acquisition of diffusion data from three short-axis slices in the heart (Lau et al. 2015). The results showed no differences in ADC or HA measurements obtained with the developed technique versus standard single-slice acquisitions, although a 10% mean bias was observed in FA between the two imaging schemes. However, the capability of reducing scan time is a great potential of SMS imaging, especially for in vivo DTI. In another study, Mekkaoui et al. (2015c) used a navigator-echo blipped-CAIPI STEAM sequence with SMS excitation rate of 3 and spatiotemporal registration for whole-heart DTI in under 25 minutes (Figure 5.74).

5.6.3 MR DTI TRACTOGRAPHY

Visualizing directional information from DTI is useful to verify the results and interpret structural data. The so-called DTI tractography, which deals with computational reconstruction and rendering of the tissue fibers based on DTI data,

has been used to visualize spatial connectivity in diffusion tensor fields. Since its introduction (Jones et al. 1999b, Mori et al. 1999), DTI tractography has been used for visualizing the structural connectivity of the brain white matter and was more recently adapted in the heart (Hagmann et al. 2006, Rohmer et al. 2007, Mukherjee et al. 2008).

5.6.3.1 Basics of DTI Tractography

In general, tractography involves calculating continuous lines representative of the fibers by selecting initial seed points, marching according to the local diffusion directions, and stopping the process when some termination criteria are met (Figure 5.75). Starting at an arbitrary location inside the myocardium, the first eigenvector of the diffusion tensor is assumed to provide a suitable estimate of the fiber orientation within each imaging voxel (Lin et al. 2001). An initial technique, called fast march, consists of connecting pixels by straight lines continuing over a given total distance (Stieltjes et al. 2001). Such a basic approach is an efficient way to generate results, but may be sensitive to noise and divergences due to fiber crossing. Another simple method to obtain orientation estimates uses nearest-neighbor interpolation, where the orientation at the new location is estimated and the next step is taken along that direction until the track is terminated. A new linear-invariant tensor interpolation method has been recently introduced to linearly interpolate components of the tensor shape without introducing spurious changes in the tensor shape (Gahm et al. 2012, Choi et al. 2013).

5.6.3.2 Complementary Information for DTI Tractography

The resulting virtual fiber length is subject to indicators of continuity, user assumptions, and sometimes interpretation

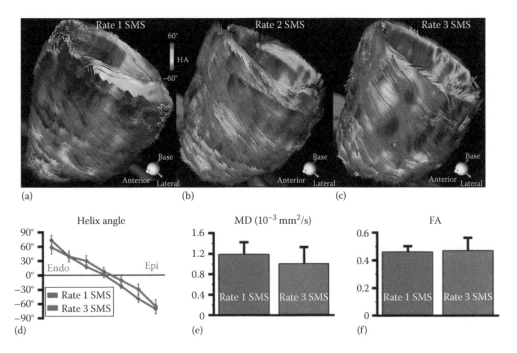

FIGURE 5.74 DTI using simultaneous multislice excitation. Breath-hold DTI of the same volunteer with (a) rate 1, (b) rate 2, and (c) rate 3 simultaneous multislice (SMS) imaging. The resolved tracts are color-coded by the helix angle (HA). Tract coherence remains high with both rate 2 and rate 3 SMS. No significant differences were seen between rate 1 and rate 3 acquisitions ($n = 7$) in (d) the transmural slope of HA, (e) mean diffusivity (MD) (10^{-3} mm²/s), and (f) fractional anisotropy (FA). (Reproduced from Mekkaoui, C. et al., Free-breathing diffusion tensor MRI of the entire human heart in vivo using simultaneous multislice excitation and spatiotemporal registration, *Proceedings of International Society for Magnetic Resonance in Medicine*, Toronto, Ontario, Canada, 2015c. With permission.)

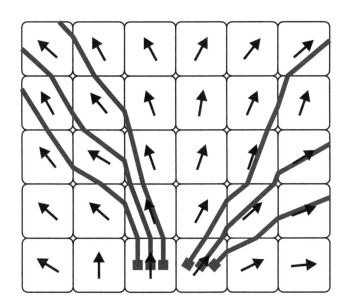

FIGURE 5.75 Schematic of how to perform tractography on DTI data. A path is traced along the direction of the principal eigenvector until the boundary of the voxel is reached, after which the direction of tracing is changed according to the principal eigenvector of the new voxel. This is continued until the stopping condition is reached.

of histological sections (Song et al. 2010, Mekkaoui et al. 2012). Therefore, common termination criteria include placing a limit on the propagation steps, a logic measure on the local anisotropy measures, and an angular distance on the propagation nodes (Masutani et al. 2003). Also, *a priori*

conditions, such as anatomical knowledge, are applied to the termination criteria to refine the tracking results with respect to the physiology under investigations (Tournier et al. 2011). For example, in a recent study, Choi et al. (2013) studied the effects of FA threshold and minimum fiber length on the tractography results (Figure 5.76). As shown later in this section, more sophisticated techniques continue to be developed to address data quality limitations, reduce computational cost, and improve visualization (Westin et al. 2002).

5.6.3.3 Fiber Tracking Algorithms

DTI fiber tracking algorithms can be divided into deterministic and probabilistic methods (Mukherjee et al. 2008, Sosnovik et al. 2009a).

5.6.3.3.1 Deterministic Tractography Algorithms

In general, deterministic tractography algorithms use line propagation techniques for calculating the fiber pathways (Tournier et al. 2011). Some techniques calculate the trajectories using a series of automatic decision-making schemes based on user-defined initial locations or seeds (Zhukov and Barr 2003, Poveda et al. 2012). For instance, the deterministic fiber assignment by continuous tracking (FACT) method uses user-defined voxels (Mori et al. 1999, Mukherjee et al. 2008), where the direction of fiber trajectories (referred to as streamlines) corresponds to the first eigenvector of the DTI field at each voxel. When the virtual fiber crosses the voxel, the first eigenvector of the next voxel becomes the new direction. The method can be augmented with smoothing, turning

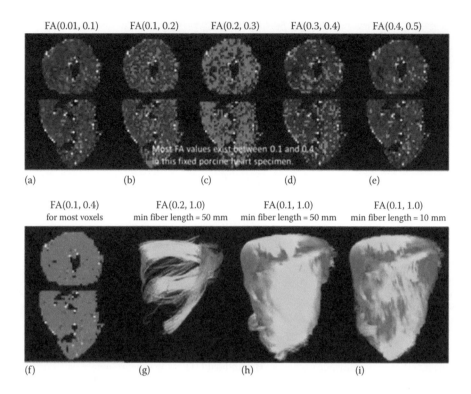

FIGURE 5.76 (a–e) Fractional anisotropy (FA) distribution and (f–i) MR tractography for varying FA thresholds (inside the parentheses). (Reproduced from Choi, S. et al., Potential of diffusion tensor imaging as a virtual dissection tool for cardiac muscle bundles: A pilot study, *Proceedings of International Society for Magnetic Resonance in Medicine*, Salt Lake City, UT, 2013. With permission.)

angle limits, and termination criteria based on FA to control streamline propagation (Mukherjee et al. 2008).

5.6.3.3.2 Probabilistic Tractography Algorithms

While deterministic tractography algorithms provide only a single estimate of the fibers' path, probabilistic algorithms provide their results in the form of a probability distribution (Frindel et al. 2010). Most probabilistic approaches are based on deterministic streamline techniques. To obtain an estimate of the distribution of possible connections, a large number of probabilistic paths are generated from the same seed point (Tournier et al. 2011). A key element of these methods is accurate characterization of the fiber orientation PDF, which can be estimated based on FA, Bayesian modeling, or bootstrap statistics (Mukherjee et al. 2008). The probabilistic DTI fiber tracking techniques, though more dependent on the diffusion tensor image quality and user-defined methods (e.g., the form and method to obtain the PDFs), they have a greater dispersion capability than the deterministic methods, which translates into potentially less accurate but longer fiber tracking ability.

5.6.3.4 Tractography Validation

Results validation is an important issue in DTI tractography. Therefore, tractography is sometimes integrated with methods to visualize the diffusion tensor itself, which can include confidence information (Vilanova et al. 2005, Toussaint et al.

2010). Sometimes, fiber crossing, a critical though challenging aspect for determining the propagation direction at fiber crossings, is also included (Masutani et al. 2003). Fiber crossings are characterized by low anisotropy and lack of correspondence between the eigenvectors and the underlying crossing tracts. Additional uncertainty could be also attributed to low SNR as well as motion and imaging artifacts (Mukherjee et al. 2008).

5.6.3.5 Tractography Visualization

The tools used to visualize tractography data extend well beyond lines representing fibers. Colors, thicknesses, volumetric rendering, lighting, and shading are also used to reduce ambiguity and help the assimilation of volumetric data (Peeters et al. 2006). For example, coloring can be used to visualize local properties, for example, anisotropy mapping, by letting the local fiber color components be proportional to the eigenvalues length according to 1, D_2/D_1, D_3/D_1 for red, green, and blue, respectively (Masutani et al. 2003). An example of tractography applied to the LV is shown in Figure 5.77, which includes basic results from a fiber tracking algorithm in a single color, the same results with the aid of directional coloring and lighting effects, and the composite of 3D rendering of the fibers and surrounding tissue. Figure 5.78 shows high-definition rendering aimed to simulate the fibers in a realistic background (Giannakidis et al. 2012).

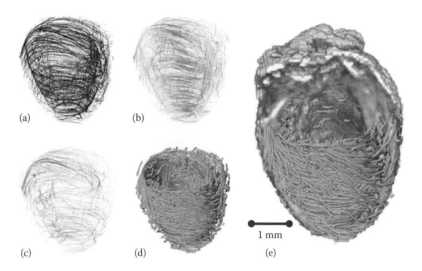

FIGURE 5.77 Visualization of high-resolution DTI tractography. (a) Typical lines resulting from a tractography algorithm. (b) Coloring of the lines based on direction. (c) Adding lighting effects on the colored lines. (d) 3D rendering of the tracks as circular extrusions along the lines. (e) Composite view of volumetric rendering of the heart, combined with the tractography results.

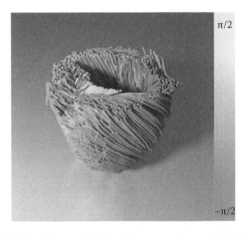

FIGURE 5.78 The application of tractography combined with 3D rendering of a mouse LV. Tractography is used to define a virtual fiber field based on diffusion imaging data. These virtual fibers are sometimes interpreted as longitudinally connected myocytes. (Courtesy of Dr. Grant Gullberg, Lawrence Berkeley National Laboratory, Berkeley, CA.)

5.6.3.6 Multiscale Tractography Visualization

Recently, Poveda et al. (2012, 2013) introduced a multiscale technique for simplified tractography visualization by retaining the main geometric features of the fiber tracts (Figures 5.79 and 5.80), making it easier to display the main architectural organization of the heart, for example, the Torrent-Guasp helical structure. The developed technique is based on pyramid representation of the information, which applies Gaussian filtering and exponential reduction on the data.

5.6.3.7 Advanced Tractography Techniques

5.6.3.7.1 Boolean-Weighted Undirected Graphs

Advanced tractography techniques have been proposed, for example, setting tracking as finding a path in a Boolean-weighted undirected graph where each voxel is defined as a vertex and an edge connects each pair of neighboring voxels (Frindel et al. 2010). By implementing this technique, the results become more robust to modeling errors and noise, and the resulting (virtual) fiber bundle density is optimized

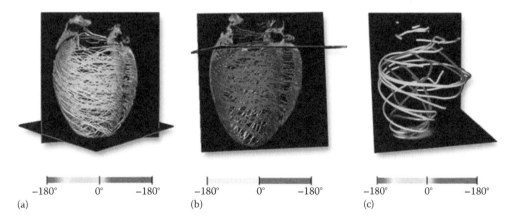

FIGURE 5.79 Simplified tractography reconstruction. (a) Tractography reconstruction with nearly 350 seeds, represented by a full-color scheme determining the orientation of the fibers. (b) Two-color scheme, which increases the difference between counter-directional helical fiber tracts. (c) Simplified tractography. (Reproduced from Poveda, F. et al., *JACC Cardiovasc. Imaging*, 5(7), 754, 2012. With permission.)

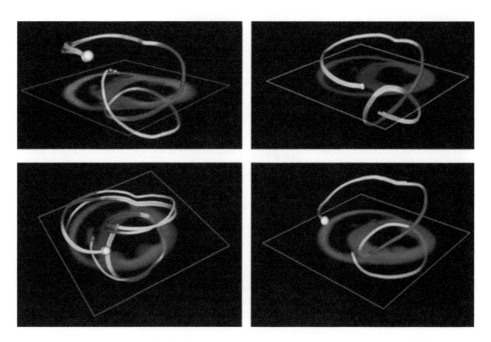

FIGURE 5.80   Selected tractography paths highlighting the helical myocardial structure using simplified reconstruction. Four examples of tracts reconstructed with manually picked seeds, always chosen near the pulmonary artery, on simplified tractography. (Reproduced from Poveda, F. et al., *JACC Cardiovasc. Imaging*, 5(7), 754, 2012. With permission.)

because the fibers' start- and endpoints are automatically calculated from the volumetric data, and seed points are not required. Therefore, this algorithm is particularly well suited for cardiac imaging.

5.6.3.7.2   Feature-Based Interpolation

Another example of advanced tractography techniques is formulating a feature-based interpolation framework from the cardiac DTI data by extracting specific tensor features like eigenvalues and orientations to generate a new, tractography-specific tensor (Yang et al. 2012). This way, the tensor's symmetry and positive-definiteness are preserved along with FA and MD monotonicity, while at the same time FA collapse and, thus, artificial fiber crossing are eliminated.

5.6.3.7.3   Tractography from Sparse DTI Data

Lastly, a recently proposed method produced 3D LV fiber architecture from sparse in vivo DTI data by using an idealized prolate spheroidal geometry and interpolating with anisotropic Gaussian regression (Toussaint et al. 2010). The main advantages of this approach are the integration of the object's curvilinearity in the analysis and approximation of cardiac DTI information, which are important steps when the data are sparsely distributed across the ventricle (Toussaint et al. 2013a).

5.7   SUMMARY AND KEY POINTS

5.7.1   SUMMARY

Considering that the heart is active since before birth and for the most part throughout a person's life, myocardial

microstructure changes by orders of magnitude in both time and space, making structural measurements rather challenging. The short contextual survey of cardiac structural measurements with DTI in this chapter illustrates the versatile response to this challenge. It is worth mentioning that there are some promising examples of the future of cardiac fiber structure imaging, and how it can have a positive effect on the way we understand cardiac structure and function. Despite its complexity, the myofiber structure is intimately linked to diagnosing, monitoring, and treating cardiovascular diseases, the largest causes of death in the world. For this reason, many researchers and clinicians recognize the value of applying the newly gained information about heart function on personalized medicine. This ideal scenario includes two fundamental stages: characterization of functional and material parameters in health and disease, and predicting the outcome of an intervention in a patient. The first stage involves gathering large databases of relevant information, including anatomical and diffusion tensor imaging, and establishing analysis criteria useful for classifying phenotypes and recognizing diseases (Tu et al. 2003, Fonseca et al. 2011). Such an approach would provide clinicians with information-age diagnostic tools never seen before (Trayanova et al. 2012).

Much of the statistical work, for example, the ability to merge large amounts of tensor images, has been already applied on the brain for classification of adult and developing structures (Huang 2010, Cui et al. 2013), and their cardiac counterparts are underway. Furthermore, thanks to advances in computational cardiology, the ability of predicting the outcomes of treatment is no longer a dream. Computational models are becoming an important tool for treatment planning and for the prevention of treatment side effects (Lonyai et al. 2010,

McDowell et al. 2012). With the advent of more comprehensive approaches, like electromechanical models of the whole heart and the ability to acquire fiber structure information in vivo, predicting the outcome of surgical procedures should be feasible. Despite all technical and scientific difficulties, the hope for improving the quality of life of millions of cardiovascular patients is the goal of researchers and clinicians working to answer relevant questions in cardiac biomechanics, including the characterization of cardiac fiber structure.

5.7.2 KEY POINTS

- The myocardium consists of myocytes, which are the basic building blocks making up the tissue.
- An integrated description of the cardiac structure describing identifiable features, including fibers, sheets, and band architectures, provide an important means to explain cardiac mechanics.
- The myocardial fiber orientation varies during contraction and relaxation of the ventricles. The ventricular fiber orientation is dependent on the spatial location in the heart and the species from which the heart is obtained.
- The ventricular myocardial fibers follow circumferential, longitudinal, and oblique organization, akin to helical spirals starting at the cardiac base toward the apex.
- The subendocardial helix ascends from apex to base counterclockwise (as seen from the base), while the subepicardial fiber ascends in a clockwise manner.
- The double-helical arrangement of the LV myocardial fibers is beneficial for distributing strain uniformly and expending energy efficiently.
- The myocyte fibers exhibit a transverse (imbrication) angle from the epicardial surface. This arrangement optimizes the ventricular ejection power by controlling regional wall thickening in a way that minimizes the ventricular cavity resistance to flow.
- Similar to the myocardial fiber orientation, the laminae are angled with respect to the epicardial surface, where the sheet angle varies as a function of the anatomical location.
- Diffusion MRI is used to describe anisotropic diffusion in 3D space. DTI can then be used to characterize the tissue fiber structure.
- A typical DTI experiment consists of acquiring a series of diffusion-weighted MRI scans encoded with one or more b-values along at least six noncollinear gradient directions.
- The diffusion tensor is related to the magnitudes and directions of the underlying principal diffusion processes, represented by the tensor's eigenvalues and eigenvectors, respectively.
- The fiber orientations are often reported in terms of their helix angles and, to a less extent, imbrication angles. On the other hand, the diffusion tensor eigenvalues are commonly used to compute the mean diffusivity and fractional anisotropy.

- The excellent correspondence between DTI and histology results supports the hypothesis that the first eigenvector of the MR diffusion tensor coincides with the orientation of the local myocardial fibers.
- Distinct populations of second and third eigenvalues were observed on the DTI of the heart, which supports the existence of myocardial laminar or sheet structure.
- DTI started to be implemented for in vivo cardiac imaging, albeit the limitation of long scan time. One natural application of in vivo cardiac DTI is to investigate the structure–function relationship in the same heart and to provide a tool for detecting or diagnosing cardiac pathology.
- The myocardial fiber orientations obtained with DTI map well with fiber shortenings, and the myocardial sheets contribute to ventricular wall thickening during cardiac contraction.
- High-resolution DTI has been recently introduced, which allows for more detailed characterization of the myocardial microstructure.
- Recently, DTI has been implemented for studying fetal and neonatal heart development, which could have a potential impact on treatment of congenital heart diseases at an early stage.
- DTI may be clinically useful for locating areas of fiber disarray in different diseases, such as myocardial infarction and hypertrophic cardiomyopathy.
- A reduction of tissue diffusivity was observed in ischemic hearts.
- Compared to healthy hearts, the infarcted myocardium exhibits decreased FA, increased ADC, and flatter HA. Further, the double helix myocardial structure showed more leftward shift around the infarcted myocardium, and the redistribution of fiber architecture correlated with the infarct size and LV function.
- Hypertrophic cardiomyopathy showed locally reduced diffusion FA, which indicates myofiber disarray. Further, an increase in the imbrication angle was observed in hypertrophic hearts.
- Myocardial architecture showed to be linked to initiation and maintenance of reentrant arrhythmias as well as to mechanical coupling during systolic wall thickening.
- The potential role of DTI in computational biomechanics and electrophysiology was quickly realized when it became apparent that DTI presents a noninvasive alternative to conventional histology for characterizing myocardial fiber structures.
- Issues to be considered when conducting cardiac DTI include low SNR, long scan time, hardware limitations, and image distortion.
- The main strategic consideration in experimental DTI is to address its low SNR, which is due to the nature of both diffusion encoding and T2 relaxation during the prolonged TE necessary to accommodate the diffusion-encoding pulses.

- Because the GRE sequence is more prone to susceptibility or distortion artifacts, SE imaging is preferred over GRE for acquiring diffusion-weighted images.
- The diffusion-weighted SE-EPI has been implemented to make the DTI scan time practically acceptable, especially for in vivo applications.
- Different pulse sequences, including FSE, SSFP, STEAM, spiral, and PROPELLER, have been implemented for diffusion-weighted imaging.
- For a given scan time, the most efficient means to improve DTI accuracy is to acquire diffusion-weighted scans in as many different encoding directions as possible and to distribute the encoding direction unit vectors as evenly spread out as possible on a unit sphere.
- The choice of the diffusion-weighting b-value has an impact on the accuracy of the DTI experiment.
- The heart motion causes significant signal loss in diffusion-weighted images. Therefore, the effects from respiratory motion, tissue perfusion, and myocardial strain have to be addressed for accurate measurements of the DTI parameters in in vivo imaging.
- Navigator-echo free breathing has been implemented to minimize respiratory motion artifacts in DTI.
- Nonparametric high angular-resolution diffusion imaging (HARDI) and diffusion spectrum imaging (DSI) observe diffusion in a high number, typically hundreds, of encoding directions to solve the ambiguity in determining myofiber orientations inside a voxel.
- Complicated parametric diffusion models, like Q-ball imaging (QBI), could be implemented to resolve ambiguity in fiber orientations.
- Compressed sensing has been implemented to accelerate DTI data acquisition without introducing imaging artifacts.
- Tractography is used to visualize spatial connectivity in the diffusion tensor fields. It is based on calculating continuous lines, representative of the fibers, by seeding initial points, marching according to the local diffusion directions, and stopping the process when some termination criteria are met. DTI fiber tracking algorithms can be divided into deterministic and probabilistic methods.
- The tools used to visualize the tractography data extend well beyond lines representing fibers. Colors, thicknesses, volumetric rendering, lighting, and shading effects can be also used to reduce ambiguity and help display volumetric data.

ACKNOWLEDGMENTS

The authors would like to thank Dr. Tamer Basha from Harvard University for help with design of line-art figures.

REFERENCES

Abdullah, O., Gomez, A.D., Merchant, S., Stedham, O., Heidinger, M., Poelzing, S., and Hsu, E.W. (2013). Effects of perfusion on cardiac MR diffusion measurements. *Proceedings of International Society for Magnetic Resonance in Medicine*, Salt Lake City, UT.

Abdullah, O.M., Drakos, S.G., Diakos, N.A., Wever-Pinzon, O., Kfoury, A.G., Stehlik, J., Selzman, C.H. et al. (2014). Characterization of diffuse fibrosis in the failing human heart via diffusion tensor imaging and quantitative histological validation. *NMR Biomed* **27**(11): 1378–1386.

Adluru, G., Hsu, E.W., and Dibella, E.V. (2007). Constrained reconstruction of sparse cardiac MR DTI data. *Lect Note Comput Sci* **4466**: 91–99.

Alexander, D.C. and Barker, G.J. (2005). Optimal imaging parameters for fiber-orientation estimation in diffusion MRI. *Neuroimage* **27**(2): 357–367.

Anderson, R.H., Ho, S.Y., Sanchez-Quintana, D., Redmann, K., and Lunkenheimer, P.P. (2006). Heuristic problems in defining the three-dimensional arrangement of the ventricular myocytes. *Anat Rec A Discov Mol Cell Evol Biol* **288**(6): 579–586.

Anderson, R.H., Sanchez-Quintana, D., Niederer, P., and Lunkenheimer, P.P. (2008). Structural-functional correlates of the 3-dimensional arrangement of the myocytes making up the ventricular walls. *J Thorac Cardiovasc Surg* **136**(1): 10–18.

Anderson, R.H., Sanchez-Quintana, D., Redmann, K., and Lunkenheimer, P.P. (2007). How are the myocytes aggregated so as to make up the ventricular mass? *Semin Thorac Cardiovasc Surg Pediatr Card Surg Annu* 76–86.

Anderson, R.H., Smerup, M., Sanchez-Quintana, D., Loukas, M., and Lunkenheimer, P.P. (2009). The three-dimensional arrangement of the myocytes in the ventricular walls. *Clin Anat* **22**(1): 64–76.

Andersson, J.L. and Skare, S. (2002). A model-based method for retrospective correction of geometric distortions in diffusion-weighted EPI. *Neuroimage* **16**(1): 177–199.

Angeli, S., Befera, N., Cofer, G., Johnson, G.A., and Constantinides, C. (2013). Construction of a fiber atlas of the murine heart. *Proceedings of International Society for Magnetic Resonance in Medicine*, Salt Lake City, UT.

Armour, J.A. and Randall, W.C. (1970). Structural basis for cardiac function. *Am J Physiol* **218**(6): 1517–1523.

Arts, T., Costa, K.D., Covell, J.W., and McCulloch, A.D. (2001). Relating myocardial laminar architecture to shear strain and muscle fiber orientation. *Am J Physiol Heart Circ Physiol* **280**(5): H2222–H2229.

Arts, T., Prinzen, F.W., Snoeckx, L.H., Rijcken, J.M., and Reneman, R.S. (1994). Adaptation of cardiac structure by mechanical feedback in the environment of the cell: A model study. *Biophys J* **66**(4): 953–961.

Aslanidi, O.V., Nikolaidou, T., Zhao, J., Smaill, B.H., Gilbert, S.H., Holden, A.V., Lowe, T. et al. (2013). Application of micro-computed tomography with iodine staining to cardiac imaging, segmentation, and computational model development. *IEEE Trans Med Imaging* **32**(1): 8–17.

Axel, L., Wedeen, V.J., and Ennis, D.B. (2014). Probing dynamic myocardial microstructure with cardiac magnetic resonance diffusion tensor imaging. *J Cardiovasc Magn Reson* **16**: 89.

Bammer, R. (2003). Basic principles of diffusion-weighted imaging. *Eur J Radiol* **45**(3): 169–184.

Bammer, R., Auer, M., Keeling, S.L., Augustin, M., Stables, L.A., Prokesch, R.W., Stollberger, R., Moseley, M.E., and Fazekas, F. (2002). Diffusion tensor imaging using single-shot SENSE-EPI. *Magn Reson Med* **48**(1): 128–136.

Bammer, R., Holdsworth, S.J., Veldhuis, W.B., and Skare, S.T. (2009). New methods in diffusion-weighted and diffusion tensor imaging. *Magn Reson Imaging Clin N Am* **17**(2): 175–204.

Bao, L., Zhu, Y., Liu, W., Robini, M., Pu, Z., and Magnin, I. (2007). Analysis of cardiac diffusion tensor magnetic resonance images using sparse representation. *Conf Proc IEEE Eng Med Biol Soc* **2007**: 4516–4519.

Bao, L.J., Zhu, Y.M., Liu, W.Y., Croisille, P., Pu, Z.B., Robini, M., and Magnin, I.E. (2009). Denoising human cardiac diffusion tensor magnetic resonance images using sparse representation combined with segmentation. *Phys Med Biol* **54**(6): 1435–1456.

Basser, P.J. and Jones, D.K. (2002). Diffusion-tensor MRI: Theory, experimental design and data analysis—A technical review. *NMR Biomed* **15**(7–8): 456–467.

Basser, P.J., Mattiello, J., and LeBihan, D. (1994a). Estimation of the effective self-diffusion tensor from the NMR spin echo. *J Magn Reson B* **103**(3): 247–254.

Basser, P.J., Mattiello, J., and LeBihan, D. (1994b). MR diffusion tensor spectroscopy and imaging. *Biophys J* **66**(1): 259–267.

Basser, P.J. and Pajevic, S. (2000). Statistical artifacts in diffusion tensor MRI (DT-MRI) caused by background noise. *Magn Reson Med* **44**(1): 41–50.

Basser, P.J. and Pierpaoli, C. (1996). Microstructural and physiological features of tissues elucidated by quantitative-diffusion-tensor MRI. *J Magn Reson B* **111**(3): 209–219.

Bayer, J.D., Blake, R.C., Plank, G., and Trayanova, N.A. (2012). A novel rule-based algorithm for assigning myocardial fiber orientation to computational heart models. *Ann Biomed Eng* **40**(10): 2243–2254.

Bernstein, M.A., King, K.F., and Zhou, X.J. (2004). *Handbook of MRI Pulse Sequences*. Academic Press, Burlington, MA.

Bishop, M.J., Plank, G., Burton, R.A., Schneider, J.E., Gavaghan, D.J., Grau, V., and Kohl, P. (2010). Development of an anatomically detailed MRI-derived rabbit ventricular model and assessment of its impact on simulations of electrophysiological function. *Am J Physiol Heart Circ Physiol* **298**(2): H699–H718.

Bovendeerd, P.H. (2012). Modeling of cardiac growth and remodeling of myofiber orientation. *J Biomech* **45**(5): 872–881.

Bovendeerd, P.H., Arts, T., Huyghe, J.M., van Campen, D.H., and Reneman, R.S. (1992). Dependence of local left ventricular wall mechanics on myocardial fiber orientation: A model study. *J Biomech* **25**(10): 1129–1140.

Brutsaert, D.L. (1987). Nonuniformity: A physiologic modulator of contraction and relaxation of the normal heart. *J Am Coll Cardiol* **9**(2): 341–348.

Buckberg, G., Hoffman, J.I., Mahajan, A., Saleh, S., and Coghlan, C. (2008). Cardiac mechanics revisited: The relationship of cardiac architecture to ventricular function. *Circulation* **118**(24): 2571–2587.

Buckberg, G.D. (2005). Architecture must document functional evidence to explain the living rhythm. *Eur J Cardiothorac Surg* **27**(2): 202–209.

Buckberg, G.D., Castella, M., Gharib, M., and Saleh, S. (2006a). Active myocyte shortening during the 'isovolumetric relaxation' phase of diastole is responsible for ventricular suction; 'systolic ventricular filling'. *Eur J Cardiothorac Surg* **29**(Suppl 1): S98–S106.

Buckberg, G.D., Castella, M., Gharib, M., and Saleh, S. (2006b). Structure/function interface with sequential shortening of basal and apical components of the myocardial band. *Eur J Cardiothorac Surg* **29**(Suppl 1): S75–S97.

Campbell, S.G. and McCulloch, A.D. (2011). Multi-scale computational models of familial hypertrophic cardiomyopathy: Genotype to phenotype. *J R Soc Interface* **8**(64): 1550–1561.

Chen, B. and Hsu, E.W. (2005). Noise removal in magnetic resonance diffusion tensor imaging. *Magn Reson Med* **54**(2): 393–401.

Chen, J., Liu, W., Zhang, H., Lacy, L., Yang, X., Song, S.K., Wickline, S.A., and Yu, X. (2005). Regional ventricular wall thickening reflects changes in cardiac fiber and sheet structure during contraction: Quantification with diffusion tensor MRI. *Am J Physiol Heart Circ Physiol* **289**(5): H1898–H1907.

Chen, J., Song, S.K., Liu, W., McLean, M., Allen, J.S., Tan, J., Wickline, S.A., and Yu, X. (2003). Remodeling of cardiac fiber structure after infarction in rats quantified with diffusion tensor MRI. *Am J Physiol Heart Circ Physiol* **285**(3): H946–H954.

Chen, J., Zhang, L., Allen, J.S., Hu, L., Caruthers, S.D., Lanza, G.M., and Wickline, S.A. (2013). Diffusion tensor MRI revealed developmental changes of cardiomyocyte architecture in pig hearts. *Proceedings of International Society for Magnetic Resonance in Medicine*, Salt Lake City, UT.

Chen, P.S., Cha, Y.M., Peters, B.B., and Chen, L.S. (1993). Effects of myocardial fiber orientation on the electrical induction of ventricular fibrillation. *Am J Physiol* **264**(6 Pt 2): H1760–H1773.

Cheng, A., Langer, F., Rodriguez, F., Criscione, J.C., Daughters, G.T., Miller, D.C., and Ingels, N.B., Jr. (2005). Transmural sheet strains in the lateral wall of the ovine left ventricle. *Am J Physiol Heart Circ Physiol* **289**(3): H1234–H1241.

Cheng, Y.J., Chen, J., Caruthers, S.D., and Wickline, S.A. (2013). Progressive myocardial sheet dysfunction from 3 to 16 months in duchene muscular dystrophy mice (mdx) defined by diffusion tensor MRI (DTI). *Proceedings of International Society for Magnetic Resonance in Medicine*, Salt Lake City, UT.

Choi, S., Mazumder, R., Schmalbrock, P., Knopp, M.V., White, R.D., and Kolipaka, A. (2013). Potential of diffusion tensor imaging as a virtual dissection tool for cardiac muscle bundles: A pilot study. *Proceedings of International Society for Magnetic Resonance in Medicine*, Salt Lake City, UT.

Choi, S.I., Kang, J.W., Chun, E.J., Choi, S.H., and Lim, T.H. (2010). High-resolution diffusion tensor MR imaging for evaluating myocardial anisotropy and fiber tracking at 3T: The effect of the number of diffusion-sensitizing gradient directions. *Korean J Radiol* **11**(1): 54–59.

Clayton, R.H., Bernus, O., Cherry, E.M., Dierckx, H., Fenton, F.H., Mirabella, L., Panfilov, A.V., Sachse, F.B., Seemann, G., and Zhang, H. (2011). Models of cardiac tissue electrophysiology: Progress, challenges and open questions. *Prog Biophys Mol Biol* **104**(1–3): 22–48.

Clerc, L. (1976). Directional differences of impulse spread in trabecular muscle from mammalian heart. *J Physiol* **255**(2): 335–346.

Collins, M.J., Ozeki, T., Zhuo, J., Gu, J., Gullapalli, R., Pierson, R.N., Griffith, B.P., Fedak, P.W., and Poston, R.S. (2007). Use of diffusion tensor imaging to predict myocardial viability after warm global ischemia: Possible avenue for use of non-beating donor hearts. *J Heart Lung Transplant* **26**(4): 376–383.

Costa, K.D., Takayama, Y., McCulloch, A.D., and Covell, J.W. (1999). Laminar fiber architecture and three-dimensional systolic mechanics in canine ventricular myocardium. *Am J Physiol* **276**(2 Pt 2): H595–H607.

Criscione, J.C., Rodriguez, F., and Miller, D.C. (2005). The myocardial band: Simplicity can be a weakness. *Eur J Cardiothorac Surg* **28**(2): 363–364; author reply 364–367.

Cui, Z., Zhong, S., Xu, P., He, Y., and Gong, G. (2013). PANDA: A pipeline toolbox for analyzing brain diffusion images. *Front Hum Neurosci* **7**: 42.

de Crespigny, A.J., Marks, M.P., Enzmann, D.R., and Moseley, M.E. (1995). Navigated diffusion imaging of normal and ischemic human brain. *Magn Reson Med* **33**(5): 720–728.

Dierckx, H., Benson, A.P., Gilbert, S.H., Ries, M.E., Holden, A.V., Verschelde, H., and Bernus, O. (2009). Intravoxel fibre structure of the left ventricular free wall and posterior left-right ventricular insertion site in canine myocardium using Q-Ball imaging. *Lect Note Comput Sci* **5528**: 495–504.

Donoho, D. (2006). Compressed sensing. *IEEE Trans Info Theory* **52**: 1289–1306.

Dorri, F., Niederer, P.F., Lunkenheimer, P.P., and Anderson, R.H. (2010). The architecture of the left ventricular myocytes relative to left ventricular systolic function. *Eur J Cardiothorac Surg* **37**(2): 384–392.

Dorri, F., Niederer, P.F., Redmann, K., Lunkenheimer, P.P., Cryer, C.W., and Anderson, R.H. (2007). An analysis of the spatial arrangement of the myocardial aggregates making up the wall of the left ventricle. *Eur J Cardiothorac Surg* **31**(3): 430–437.

Dossel, O., Krueger, M.W., Weber, F.M., Wilhelms, M., and Seemann, G. (2012). Computational modeling of the human atrial anatomy and electrophysiology. *Med Biol Eng Comput* **50**(8): 773–799.

Dou, J., Reese, T.G., Tseng, W.Y., and Wedeen, V.J. (2002). Cardiac diffusion MRI without motion effects. *Magn Reson Med* **48**(1): 105–114.

Dou, J., Tseng, W.Y., Reese, T.G., and Wedeen, V.J. (2003). Combined diffusion and strain MRI reveals structure and function of human myocardial laminar sheets in vivo. *Magn Reson Med* **50**(1): 107–113.

Edelman, R.R., Gaa, J., Wedeen, V.J., Loh, E., Hare, J.M., Prasad, P., and Li, W. (1994). In vivo measurement of water diffusion in the human heart. *Magn Reson Med* **32**(3): 423–428.

Eggen, M.D., Swingen, C.M., and Iaizzo, P.A. (2012). Ex vivo diffusion tensor MRI of human hearts: Relative effects of specimen decomposition. *Magn Reson Med* **67**(6): 1703–1709.

Einstein, A. (1956). *Investigations on the Theory of the Brownian Movement*. Dover Publications, New York.

Ennis, D.B., Nguyen, T.C., Riboh, J.C., Wigstrom, L., Harrington, K.B., Daughters, G.T., Ingels, N.B., and Miller, D.C. (2008). Myofiber angle distributions in the ovine left ventricle do not conform to computationally optimized predictions. *J Biomech* **41**(15): 3219–3224.

Ferreira, P., Kilner, P.J., McGill, L.A., Nielles-Vallespin, S., Scott, A., Spottiswoode, B.S., Zhong, X. et al. (2014a). Aberrant myocardial sheetlet mobility in hypertrophic cardiomyopathy detected using in vivo cardiovascular magnetic resonance diffusion tensor imaging. *J Cardiovasc Magn Reson* **16**(Suppl 1): P338.

Ferreira, P., Nielles-Vallespin, S., Gatehouse, P., de Silva, R., Keegan, J., Speier, P., Feiweier, T. et al. (2013a). Helix angle (HA) healthy statistical average technique for HA quantification in vivo cardiac diffusion tensor imaging. *Proceedings of International Society for Magnetic Resonance in Medicine*, Salt Lake City, UT.

Ferreira, P., Nielles-Vallespin, S., Gatehouse, P., de Silva, R., Keegan, J., Speier, P., Feiweier, T. et al. (2013b). Improved navigator based diffusion tensor MRI of the human heart in vivo. *Proceedings of International Society for Magnetic Resonance in Medicine*, Salt Lake City, UT.

Ferreira, P.F., Kilner, P.J., McGill, L.A., Nielles-Vallespin, S., Scott, A.D., Ho, S.Y., McCarthy, K.P et al. (2014b). In vivo cardiovascular magnetic resonance diffusion tensor imaging shows evidence of abnormal myocardial laminar orientations and mobility in hypertrophic cardiomyopathy. *J Cardiovasc Magn Reson* **16**: 87.

Fick, A. (1855). Ueber diffusion. *Ann Phys* **170**: 59–86.

Fonseca, C.G., Backhaus, M., Bluemke, D.A., Britten, R.D., Chung, J.D., Cowan, B.R., Dinov, I.D. et al. (2011). The Cardiac Atlas Project—An imaging database for computational modeling and statistical atlases of the heart. *Bioinformatics* **27**(16): 2288–2295.

Frank, L.R. (2001). Anisotropy in high angular resolution diffusion-weighted MRI. *Magn Reson Med* **45**(6): 935–939.

Freeman, G.L., LeWinter, M.M., Engler, R.L., and Covell, J.W. (1985). Relationship between myocardial fiber direction and segment shortening in the midwall of the canine left ventricle. *Circ Res* **56**(1): 31–39.

Frindel, C., Robini, M., Croisille, P., and Zhu, Y.M. (2009). Comparison of regularization methods for human cardiac diffusion tensor MRI. *Med Image Anal* **13**(3): 405–418.

Frindel, C., Robini, M., Rapacchi, S., Stephant, E., Zhu, Y.M., and Croisille, P. (2007). Towards in vivo diffusion tensor MRI on human heart using edge-preserving regularization. *Conf Proc IEEE Eng Med Biol Soc* **2007**: 6008–6011.

Frindel, C., Robini, M., Schaerer, J., Croisille, P., and Zhu, Y.M. (2010). A graph-based approach for automatic cardiac tractography. *Magn Reson Med* **64**(4): 1215–1229.

Froeling, M., Mazzoli, V., Nederveen, A.J., Luijten, P.R., and Strijkers, G.J. (2014a). Ex vivo cardiac DTI: On the effects of diffusion time and b-value. *J Cardiovasc Magn Reson* **16**(Suppl 1): P77.

Froeling, M., Strijkers, G.J., Nederveen, A.J., Chamuleau, S.A., and Luijten, P.R. (2014b). Feasibility of in vivo whole heart DTI and IVIM with a 15 minute acquisition protocol. *J Cardiovasc Magn Reson* **16**(Suppl 1): O15.

Fung, Y.C. (2010). *Biomechanics: Mechanical Properties of Living Tissues*. Springer, New York.

Gahm, J.K., Wisniewski, N., Kindlmann, G., Kung, G.L., Klug, W.S., Garfinkel, A., and Ennis, D.B. (2012). Linear invariant tensor interpolation applied to cardiac diffusion tensor MRI. *Med Image Comput Comput Assist Interv* **15**(Pt 2): 494–501.

Gamper, U., Boesiger, P., and Kozerke, S. (2007). Diffusion imaging of the in vivo heart using spin echoes—Considerations on bulk motion sensitivity. *Magn Reson Med* **57**(2): 331–337.

Gao, C., Ye, W., Li, L., Zhang, T., Ren, C., Cheng, L., and Yan, J. (2009). Investigation on the structure of ventricular mass using magnetic resonance diffusion tensor imaging. *Heart Surg Forum* **12**(2): E85–E89.

Garrido, L., Wedeen, V.J., Kwong, K.K., Spencer, U.M., and Kantor, H.L. (1994). Anisotropy of water diffusion in the myocardium of the rat. *Circ Res* **74**(5): 789–793.

Geerts, L., Bovendeerd, P., Nicolay, K., and Arts, T. (2002). Characterization of the normal cardiac myofiber field in goat measured with MR-diffusion tensor imaging. *Am J Physiol Heart Circ Physiol* **283**(1): H139–H145.

Giannakidis, A., Ferreira, P., Scott, A., Nielles-Vallespin, S., Babu-Narayan, S.V., Kilner, P.J., Pennell, D.J., and Firmin, D. (2014). Scanner-efficient diffusion tensor imaging of human cardiac microstructure using the fast composite splitting reconstruction algorithm. *J Cardiovasc Magn Reson* **16**(Suppl 1): W5.

Giannakidis, A., Melkus, G., Liu, J., Saloner, D.A., Majumdar, S., and Gullberg, G.T. (2013). Fast-track cardiac diffusion tensor imaging with compressed sensing based on a novel circular cartesian undersampling. *Proceedings of International Society for Magnetic Resonance in Medicine*, Salt Lake City, UT.

Giannakidis, A., Rohmer, D., Veress, A.I., and Gullberg, G.T. (2012). Diffusion tensor MRI-derived myocardial fiber disarray in hypertensive left ventricular hypertrophy: Visualization, quantification and the effect on mechanical function. In

Cardiac Mapping. M. Shenasa, G. Hindricks, M. Borggrefe, G. Breithardt, and M.E. Josephson (eds.). Wiley-Blackwell, Chichester, U.K.

Gilbert, S.H., Benoist, D., Benson, A.P., White, E., Tanner, S.F., Holden, A.V., Dobrzynski, H., Bernus, O., and Radjenovic, A. (2012a). Visualization and quantification of whole rat heart laminar structure using high-spatial resolution contrast-enhanced MRI. *Am J Physiol Heart Circ Physiol* **302**(1): H287–H298.

Gilbert, S.H., Benson, A.P., Li, P., and Holden, A.V. (2007). Regional localisation of left ventricular sheet structure: Integration with current models of cardiac fibre, sheet and band structure. *Eur J Cardiothorac Surg* **32**(2): 231–249.

Gilbert, S.H., Sands, G.B., LeGrice, I.J., Smaill, B.H., Bernus, O., and Trew, M.L. (2012b). A framework for myoarchitecture analysis of high resolution cardiac MRI and comparison with diffusion tensor MRI. *Conf Proc IEEE Eng Med Biol Soc* **2012**: 4063–4066.

Greenbaum, R.A., Ho, S.Y., Gibson, D.G., Becker, A.E., and Anderson, R.H. (1981). Left ventricular fibre architecture in man. *Br Heart J* **45**(3): 248–263.

Griswold, M.A., Jakob, P.M., Heidemann, R.M., Nittka, M., Jellus, V., Wang, J., Kiefer, B., and Haase, A. (2002). Generalized auto-calibrating partially parallel acquisitions (GRAPPA). *Magn Reson Med* **47**(6): 1202–1210.

Guccione, J.M., Kassab, G., and Ratcliffe, M.B. (2010). *Computational Cardiovascular Mechanics: Modeling and Applications in Heart Failure.* Springer, New York.

Guccione, J.M. and McCulloch, A.D. (1993). Mechanics of active contraction in cardiac muscle: Part I—Constitutive relations for fiber stress that describe deactivation. *J Biomech Eng* **115**(1): 72–81.

Guccione, J.M., Waldman, L.K., and McCulloch, A.D. (1993). Mechanics of active contraction in cardiac muscle: Part II—Cylindrical models of the systolic left ventricle. *J Biomech Eng* **115**(1): 82–90.

Gullberg, G.T., Defrise, M., Panin, V.Y., and Zeng, G.L. (2001). Efficient cardiac diffusion tensor MRI by three-dimensional reconstruction of solenoidal tensor fields. *Magn Reson Imaging* **19**(2): 233–256.

Hagmann, P., Jonasson, L., Maeder, P., Thiran, J.P., Wedeen, V.J., and Meuli, R. (2006). Understanding diffusion MR imaging techniques: From scalar diffusion-weighted imaging to diffusion tensor imaging and beyond. *Radiographics* **26**(Suppl 1): S205–S223.

Hales, P.W., Schneider, J.E., Burton, R.A., Wright, B.J., Bollensdorff, C., and Kohl, P. (2012). Histo-anatomical structure of the living isolated rat heart in two contraction states assessed by diffusion tensor MRI. *Prog Biophys Mol Biol* **110**(2–3): 319–330.

Harmer, J., Stoeck, C.T., Chan, R.W., Toussaint, N., Von Deuster, C., Atkinson, D., and Kozerke, S. (2013a). In-vivo high resolution diffusion tensor imaging of the human heart at 3T: Fat suppression in the presence of b0 field inhomogeneities. *Proceedings of International Society for Magnetic Resonance in Medicine*, Salt Lake City, UT.

Harmer, J., Toussaint, N., Pushparajah, K., Stoeck, C.T., Chan, R.W., Razavi, R., Atkinson, D., and Kozerke, S. (2013b). In-vivo diffusion tensor imaging of the systemic right ventricle at 3T. *Proceedings of International Society for Magnetic Resonance in Medicine*, Salt Lake City, UT.

Harrington, K.B., Rodriguez, F., Cheng, A., Langer, F., Ashikaga, H., Daughters, G.T., Criscione, J.C., Ingels, N.B., and Miller, D.C. (2005). Direct measurement of transmural laminar architecture in the anterolateral wall of the ovine left ventricle: New implications for wall thickening mechanics. *Am J Physiol Heart Circ Physiol* **288**(3): H1324–H1330.

Hasan, K.M., Walimuni, I.S., Abid, H., and Hahn, K.R. (2011). A review of diffusion tensor magnetic resonance imaging computational methods and software tools. *Comput Biol Med* **41**(12): 1062–1072.

Haselgrove, J.C. and Moore, J.R. (1996). Correction for distortion of echo-planar images used to calculate the apparent diffusion coefficient. *Magn Reson Med* **36**(6): 960–964.

Healy, L.J., Jiang, Y., and Hsu, E.W. (2011). Quantitative comparison of myocardial fiber structure between mice, rabbit, and sheep using diffusion tensor cardiovascular magnetic resonance. *J Cardiovasc Magn Reson* **13**: 74.

Helm, P., Beg, M.F., Miller, M.I., and Winslow, R.L. (2005a). Measuring and mapping cardiac fiber and laminar architecture using diffusion tensor MR imaging. *Ann N Y Acad Sci* **1047**: 296–307.

Helm, P.A., Tseng, H.J., Younes, L., McVeigh, E.R., and Winslow, R.L. (2005b). Ex vivo 3D diffusion tensor imaging and quantification of cardiac laminar structure. *Magn Reson Med* **54**(4): 850–859.

Helm, P.A., Younes, L., Beg, M.F., Ennis, D.B., Leclercq, C., Faris, O.P., McVeigh, E., Kass, D., Miller, M.I., and Winslow, R.L. (2006). Evidence of structural remodeling in the dyssynchronous failing heart. *Circ Res* **98**(1): 125–132.

Holdsworth, S.J., Skare, S., Newbould, R.D., and Bammer, R. (2009). Robust GRAPPA-accelerated diffusion-weighted readout-segmented (RS)-EPI. *Magn Reson Med* **62**(6): 1629–1640.

Holmes, A.A., Scollan, D.F., and Winslow, R.L. (2000). Direct histological validation of diffusion tensor MRI in formaldehyde-fixed myocardium. *Magn Reson Med* **44**(1): 157–161.

Hort, W. (1960). Macroscopic and micrometric research on the myocardium of the left ventricle filled to varying degrees. *Virchows Arch Pathol Anat Physiol Klin Med* **333**: 523–564.

Hsu, E.W., Buckley, D.L., Bui, J.D., Blackband, S.J., and Forder, J.R. (2001). Two-component diffusion tensor MRI of isolated perfused hearts. *Magn Reson Med* **45**(6): 1039–1045.

Hsu, E.W. and Henriquez, C.S. (2001). Myocardial fiber orientation mapping using reduced encoding diffusion tensor imaging. *J Cardiovasc Magn Reson* **3**(4): 339–347.

Hsu, E.W., Muzikant, A.L., Matulevicius, S.A., Penland, R.C., and Henriquez, C.S. (1998). Magnetic resonance myocardial fiber-orientation mapping with direct histological correlation. *Am J Physiol* **274**(5 Pt 2): H1627–H1634.

Huang, H. (2010). Delineating neural structures of developmental human brains with diffusion tensor imaging. *Scientific World Journal* **10**: 135–144.

Huang, S. and Sosnovik, D.E. (2010). Molecular and microstructural imaging of the myocardium. *Curr Cardiovasc Imaging Rep* **3**(1): 26–33.

Humphrey, J.D. (2002). *Cardiovascular solid mechanics: Cells, tissues, and organs.* Springer, New York.

Hunter, P.J., McCulloch, A.D., and ter Keurs, H.E. (1998). Modelling the mechanical properties of cardiac muscle. *Prog Biophys Mol Biol* **69**(2–3): 289–331.

Hunter, P.J., Nielsen, P.M., Smaill, B.H., LeGrice, I.J., and Hunter, I.W. (1992). An anatomical heart model with applications to myocardial activation and ventricular mechanics. In *High Performance Computing in Biomedical Research.* T.C. Pilkington, B. Loftis, J.F. Thompson et al. (eds.). CRC Press, Boca Raton, FL.

Jensen, J.H., Helpern, J.A., Ramani, A., Lu, H., and Kaczynski, K. (2005). Diffusional kurtosis imaging: The quantification of non-gaussian water diffusion by means of magnetic resonance imaging. *Magn Reson Med* **53**(6): 1432–1440.

Jiang, Y., Guccione, J.M., Ratcliffe, M.B., and Hsu, E.W. (2007). Transmural heterogeneity of diffusion anisotropy in the sheep myocardium characterized by MR diffusion tensor imaging. *Am J Physiol Heart Circ Physiol* **293**(4): H2377–H2384.

Jiang, Y., Pandya, K., Smithies, O., and Hsu, E.W. (2004). Three-dimensional diffusion tensor microscopy of fixed mouse hearts. *Magn Reson Med* **52**(3): 453–460.

Jones, D.K., Horsfield, M.A., and Simmons, A. (1999a). Optimal strategies for measuring diffusion in anisotropic systems by magnetic resonance imaging. *Magn Reson Med* **42**(3): 515–525.

Jones, D.K., Simmons, A., Williams, S.C., and Horsfield, M.A. (1999b). Non-invasive assessment of axonal fiber connectivity in the human brain via diffusion tensor MRI. *Magn Reson Med* **42**(1): 37–41.

Koay, C.G., Chang, L.C., Carew, J.D., Pierpaoli, C., and Basser, P.J. (2006). A unifying theoretical and algorithmic framework for least squares methods of estimation in diffusion tensor imaging. *J Magn Reson* **182**(1): 115–125.

Kocica, M.J., Corno, A.F., Lackovic, V., and Kanjuh, V.I. (2007). The helical ventricular myocardial band of Torrent-Guasp. *Semin Thorac Cardiovasc Surg Pediatr Card Surg Annu*: 52–60.

Kohler, S., Hiller, K.H., Waller, C., Bauer, W.R., Haase, A., and Jakob, P.M. (2003). Investigation of the microstructure of the isolated rat heart: A comparison between T*2- and diffusion-weighted MRI. *Magn Reson Med* **50**(6): 1144–1150.

Kramer, C.M. (2009). Insights into myocardial microstructure during infarct healing and remodeling: Pathologists need not apply. *Circ Cardiovasc Imaging* **2**(1): 4–5.

Kuijpers, N.H., Hermeling, E., Bovendeerd, P.H., Delhaas, T., and Prinzen, F.W. (2012). Modeling cardiac electromechanics and mechanoelectrical coupling in dyssynchronous and failing hearts: Insight from adaptive computer models. *J Cardiovasc Transl Res* **5**(2): 159–169.

Kung, G.L., Nguyen, T.C., Itoh, A., Skare, S., Ingels, N.B., Jr., Miller, D.C., and Ennis, D.B. (2011). The presence of two local myocardial sheet populations confirmed by diffusion tensor MRI and histological validation. *J Magn Reson Imaging* **34**(5): 1080–1091.

Lau, A.Z., Tunnicliffe, E.M., Frost, R., Koopmans, P.J., Tyler, D.J., and Robson, M.D. (2015). Accelerated human cardiac diffusion tensor imaging using simultaneous multislice imaging. *Magn Reson Med* **73**(3): 995–1004.

Le Bihan, D., Breton, E., Lallemand, D., Aubin, M.L., Vignaud, J., and Laval-Jeantet, M. (1988). Separation of diffusion and perfusion in intravoxel incoherent motion MR imaging. *Radiology* **168**(2): 497–505.

Le Bihan, D., Mangin, J.F., Poupon, C., Clark, C.A., Pappata, S., Molko, N., and Chabriat, H. (2001). Diffusion tensor imaging: Concepts and applications. *J Magn Reson Imaging* **13**(4): 534–546.

Le Bihan, D. and Turner, R. (1992). The capillary network: A link between IVIM and classical perfusion. *Magn Reson Med* **27**(1): 171–178.

Le Bihan, D., Turner, R., and MacFall, J.R. (1989). Effects of intravoxel incoherent motions (IVIM) in steady-state free precession (SSFP) imaging: Application to molecular diffusion imaging. *Magn Reson Med* **10**(3): 324–337.

Legrice, I.J., Hunter, P.J., and Smaill, B.H. (1997). Laminar structure of the heart: A mathematical model. *Am J Physiol* **272**(5 Pt 2): H2466–H2476.

LeGrice, I.J., Smaill, B.H., Chai, L.Z., Edgar, S.G., Gavin, J.B., and Hunter, P.J. (1995a). Laminar structure of the heart: Ventricular myocyte arrangement and connective tissue architecture in the dog. *Am J Physiol* **269**(2 Pt 2): H571–H582.

LeGrice, I.J., Takayama, Y., and Covell, J.W. (1995b). Transverse shear along myocardial cleavage planes provides a mechanism for normal systolic wall thickening. *Circ Res* **77**(1): 182–193.

Lekadir, K., Lange, M., Zimmer, V.A., Hoogendoorn, C., and Frangi, A.F. (2016). Statistically-driven 3D fiber reconstruction and denoising from multi-slice cardiac DTI using a Markov random field model. *Med Image Anal* **27**: 105–116.

Li, T.Q., Takahashi, A.M., Hindmarsh, T., and Moseley, M.E. (1999). ADC mapping by means of a single-shot spiral MRI technique with application in acute cerebral ischemia. *Magn Reson Med* **41**(1): 143–147.

Lin, C.P., Tseng, W.Y., Cheng, H.C., and Chen, J.H. (2001). Validation of diffusion tensor magnetic resonance axonal fiber imaging with registered manganese-enhanced optic tracts. *Neuroimage* **14**(5): 1035–1047.

Liu, C., Bammer, R., Kim, D.H., and Moseley, M.E. (2004). Self-navigated interleaved spiral (SNAILS): Application to high-resolution diffusion tensor imaging. *Magn Reson Med* **52**(6): 1388–1396.

Lohezic, M., Teh, I., Bollensdorff, C., Peyronnet, R., Hales, P.W., Grau, V., Kohl, P., and Schneider, J.E. (2014). Interrogation of living myocardium in multiple static deformation states with diffusion tensor and diffusion spectrum imaging. *Prog Biophys Mol Biol* **115**(2–3): 213–225.

Lonyai, A., Dubin, A.M., Feinstein, J.A., Taylor, C.A., and Shadden, S.C. (2010). New insights into pacemaker lead-induced venous occlusion: Simulation-based investigation of alterations in venous biomechanics. *Cardiovasc Eng* **10**(2): 84–90.

Luciani, A., Vignaud, A., Cavet, M., Nhieu, J.T., Mallat, A., Ruel, L., Laurent, A., Deux, J.F., Brugieres, P., and Rahmouni, A. (2008). Liver cirrhosis: Intravoxel incoherent motion MR imaging—Pilot study. *Radiology* **249**(3): 891–899.

Lunkenheimer, P.P., Niederer, P., Sanchez-Quintana, D., Murillo, M., and Smerup, M. (2013). Models of ventricular structure and function reviewed for clinical cardiologists. *J Cardiovasc Transl Res* **6**(2): 176–186.

Lunkenheimer, P.P., Redmann, K., Kling, N., Jiang, X., Rothaus, K., Cryer, C.W., Wubbeling, F. et al. (2006). Three-dimensional architecture of the left ventricular myocardium. *Anat Rec A Discov Mol Cell Evol Biol* **288**(6): 565–578.

Lunkenheimer, P.P., Redmann, K., Niederer, P., Schmid, P., Smerup, M., Stypmann, J., Dabritz, S., Rothaus, K., and Anderson, R.H. (2008). Models versus established knowledge in describing the functional morphology of the ventricular myocardium. *Heart Fail Clin* **4**(3): 273–288.

Lustig, M., Donoho, D., and Pauly, J.M. (2007). Sparse MRI: The application of compressed sensing for rapid MR imaging. *Magn Reson Med* **58**(6): 1182–1195.

Masutani, Y., Aoki, S., Abe, O., Hayashi, N., and Otomo, K. (2003). MR diffusion tensor imaging: Recent advance and new techniques for diffusion tensor visualization. *Eur J Radiol* **46**(1): 53–66.

Mattiello, J., Basser, P.J., and LeBihan, D. (1994). Analytical expressions for the b matrix in NMR diffusion imaging and spectroscopy. *J Magn Reson A* **108**: 131–141.

Mazumder, R., Choi, S., Clymer, B.D., White, R.D., and Kolipaka, A. (2013). Diffusion tensor imaging of fresh and formalin fixed porcine hearts: A comparison study of fiber tracts. *Proceedings of International Society for Magnetic Resonance in Medicine*, Salt Lake City, UT.

Mazumder, R., Clymer, B.D., White, R.D., and Kolipaka, A. (2014). Estimation of helical angle of the left ventricle using diffusion tensor imaging with minimum acquisition time. *J Cardiovasc Magn Reson* **16**(Suppl 1): P359.

McCulloch, A.D. (2000). Cardiac biomechanics. In *The Biomedical Engineering Handbook*. J.D. Bronzino, and D.R. Peterson (eds.). CRC Press, Boca Raton, FL.

McDowell, K.S., Vadakkumpadan, F., Blake, R., Blauer, J., Plank, G., MacLeod, R.S., and Trayanova, N.A. (2012). Methodology for patient-specific modeling of atrial fibrosis as a substrate for atrial fibrillation. *J Electrocardiol* **45**(6): 640–645.

McGill, L., Scott, A., Ferreira, P., Nielles-Vallespin, S., Ismail, T., Kilner, P., Gatehouse, P., Prasad, P., Giannakidis, A., Firmin, D., and Pennell, D.J. (2015). Heterogeneity of diffusion tensor imaging measurements of fractional anisotropy and mean diffusivity in normal human hearts in vivo. *J Cardiovasc Magn Reson* **17**(Suppl 1): O1.

McGill, L.A., Ferreira, P., Scott, A.D., Nielles-Vallespin, S., Ismail, T., Silva, R., Kilner, P.J., Firmin, D., and Pennell, D.J. (2014). Influence of subject characteristics on DTI parameters in the normal heart. *J Cardiovasc Magn Reson* **16**(Suppl 1): P7.

McLean, M. and Prothero, J. (1991). Myofiber orientation in the weanling mouse heart. *Am J Anat* **192**(4): 425–441.

McNab, J.A. and Miller, K.L. (2008). Sensitivity of diffusion weighted steady state free precession to anisotropic diffusion. *Magn Reson Med* **60**(2): 405–413.

Mekkaoui, C., Chen, H.H., Chen, Y., Kostis, W., Jackowski, M., Reese, T., and Sosnovik, D. (2015a). Detection of diffuse myocardial fibrosis in vivo using diffusion tensor imaging with the supertoroidal model. *Proceedings of International Society for Magnetic Resonance in Medicine*, Toronto, Ontario, Canada.

Mekkaoui, C., Chen, I., Chen, H.H., Kostis, W., Pereira, F., Jackowski, M., and Sosnovik, D. (2015b). Differential response of the left and right ventricles to pressure overload revealed with diffusion tensor MRI tractography of the heart in vivo. *J Cardiovasc Magn Reson* **17**(Suppl 1): O3.

Mekkaoui, C., Huang, S., Chen, H.H., Dai, G., Reese, T.G., Kostis, W.J., Thiagalingam, A. et al. (2012). Fiber architecture in remodeled myocardium revealed with a quantitative diffusion CMR tractography framework and histological validation. *J Cardiovasc Magn Reson* **14**: 70.

Mekkaoui, C., Jackowski, M., Reese, T., and Sosnovik, D. (2013a). Sheet tractography provides a multi-dimensional representation of architecture in normal and infarcted hearts. *Proceedings of International Society for Magnetic Resonance in Medicine*, Salt Lake City, UT.

Mekkaoui, C., Jackowski, M.P., Thiagalingam, A., Kostis, W.J., Nielles-Vallespin, S., Firmin, D., Bhat, H., Ruskin, J.N., Reese, T.G., and Sosnovik, D.E. (2014a). Correlation of DTI tractography with electroanatomic mapping in normal and infarcted myocardium. *J Cardiovasc Magn Reson* **16**(Suppl 1): O68.

Mekkaoui, C., Nielles-Vallespin, S., Jackowski, M.P., Reese, T., Gatehouse, P., Firmin, D., and Sosnovik, D. (2013b). Dynamics of the fiber architecture matrix in the human heart in vivo. *Proceedings of International Society for Magnetic Resonance in Medicine*, Salt Lake City, UT.

Mekkaoui, C., Nielles-Vallespin, S., Jackowski, M.P., Reese, T., Gatehouse, P., Firmin, D., and Sosnovik, D. (2013c). Improved tractography of the human heart in vivo by motion correction of multi-breathold diffusion tensor MRI. *Proceedings of International Society for Magnetic Resonance in Medicine*, Salt Lake City, UT.

Mekkaoui, C., Porayette, P., Jackowski, M.P., Kostis, W.J., Dai, G., Sanders, S., and Sosnovik, D. (2013d). Diffusion MRI tractography of the developing human fetal heart. *Proceedings of International Society for Magnetic Resonance in Medicine*, Salt Lake City, UT.

Mekkaoui, C., Porayette, P., Jackowski, M.P., Kostis, W.J., Dai, G., Sanders, S., and Sosnovik, D.E. (2013e). Diffusion MRI tractography of the developing human fetal heart. *PLoS One* **8**(8): e72795.

Mekkaoui, C., Reese, T., Cauley, S., Setsompop, K., Bhat, H., Kostis, W., Jackowski, M., and Sosnovik, D. (2015c). Free-breathing diffusion tensor MRI of the entire human heart in vivo using simultaneous multislice excitation and spatio-temporal registration. *Proceedings of International Society for Magnetic Resonance in Medicine*, Toronto, Ontario, Canada.

Mekkaoui, C., Reese, T.G., Jackowski, M.P., Bhat, H., Kostis, W.J., and Sosnovik, D.E. (2014b). In vivo fiber tractography of the right and left ventricles using diffusion tensor MRI of the entire human heart. *J Cardiovasc Magn Reson* **16**(Suppl 1): P17.

Merboldt, K.D., Hanicke, W., Bruhn, H., Gyngell, M.L., and Frahm, J. (1992). Diffusion imaging of the human brain in vivo using high-speed STEAM MRI. *Magn Reson Med* **23**(1): 179–192.

Mistry, N.N. and Hsu, E.W. (2006). Retrospective distortion correction for 3D MR diffusion tensor microscopy using mutual information and Fourier deformations. *Magn Reson Med* **56**(2): 310–316.

Mori, S., Crain, B.J., Chacko, V.P., and van Zijl, P.C. (1999). Three-dimensional tracking of axonal projections in the brain by magnetic resonance imaging. *Ann Neurol* **45**(2): 265–269.

Moseley, M.E., Cohen, Y., Mintorovitch, J., Chileuitt, L., Shimizu, H., Kucharczyk, J., Wendland, M.F., and Weinstein, P.R. (1990). Early detection of regional cerebral ischemia in cats: Comparison of diffusion- and T2-weighted MRI and spectroscopy. *Magn Reson Med* **14**(2): 330–346.

Moulin, K., Croisille, P., Feiweier, T., Delattre, B.M., Wei, H., Roberts, B., Beuf, O., and Viallon, M. (2015). In-vivo free-breathing DTI & IVIM of the whole human heart using a real-time slice-followed SE-EPI navigator-based sequence: A reproducibility study in healthy volunteers. *Proceedings of International Society for Magnetic Resonance in Medicine*, Toronto, Ontario, Canada.

Mukherjee, P., Berman, J.I., Chung, S.W., Hess, C.P., and Henry, R.G. (2008). Diffusion tensor MR imaging and fiber tractography: Theoretic underpinnings. *Am J Neuroradiol* **29**(4): 632–641.

Munoz-Moreno, E., Cardenes, R., and Frangi, A.F. (2010). Analysis of the helix and transverse angles of the muscle fibers in the myocardium based on Diffusion Tensor Imaging. *Conf Proc IEEE Eng Med Biol Soc* **2010**: 5720–5723.

Muzikant, A.L., Hsu, E.W., Wolf, P.D., and Henriquez, C.S. (2002). Region specific modeling of cardiac muscle: Comparison of simulated and experimental potentials. *Ann Biomed Eng* **30**(7): 867–883.

Nasiraei-Moghaddam, A. and Gharib, M. (2009). Evidence for the existence of a functional helical myocardial band. *Am J Physiol Heart Circ Physiol* **296**(1): H127–H131.

Nguyen, C., Fan, Z., Bi, X., and Li, D. (2015). In vivo cardiac DTI on a widely-available clinical scanner. *Proceedings of International Society for Magnetic Resonance in Medicine*, Toronto, Ontario, Canada.

Nielles-Vallespin, S., Ferreira, P., Gatehouse, P., Keegan, J., de Silva, R., Ismail, T., Scott, A. et al. (2013a). Time-resolved in vivo cardiac diffusion tensor MRI of the human heart. *Proceedings of International Society for Magnetic Resonance in Medicine*, Salt Lake City, UT.

Nielles-Vallespin, S., Mekkaoui, C., Gatehouse, P., Reese, T.G., Keegan, J., Ferreira, P.F., Collins, S. et al. (2013b). In vivo diffusion tensor MRI of the human heart: Reproducibility of breath-hold and navigator-based approaches. *Magn Reson Med* **70**(2): 454–465.

Nielsen, E., Smerup, M., Agger, P., Frandsen, J., Ringgard, S., Pedersen, M., Vestergaard, P. et al. (2009). Normal right ventricular three-dimensional architecture, as assessed with diffusion tensor magnetic resonance imaging, is preserved during experimentally induced right ventricular hypertrophy. *Anat Rec (Hoboken)* **292**(5): 640–651.

Nielsen, P.M., Le Grice, I.J., Smaill, B.H., and Hunter, P.J. (1991). Mathematical model of geometry and fibrous structure of the heart. *Am J Physiol* **260**(4 Pt 2): H1365–H1378.

Nordsletten, D.A., Niederer, S.A., Nash, M.P., Hunter, P.J., and Smith, N.P. (2011). Coupling multi-physics models to cardiac mechanics. *Prog Biophys Mol Biol* **104**(1–3): 77–88.

O'Dell, W.G. and McCulloch, A.D. (2000). Imaging three-dimensional cardiac function. *Annu Rev Biomed Eng* **2**: 431–456.

Omens, J.H., Rockman, H.A., and Covell, J.W. (1994). Passive ventricular mechanics in tight-skin mice. *Am J Physiol* **266**(3 Pt 2): H1169–H1176.

Ozarslan, E. and Mareci, T.H. (2003). Generalized diffusion tensor imaging and analytical relationships between diffusion tensor imaging and high angular resolution diffusion imaging. *Magn Reson Med* **50**(5): 955–965.

Pashakhanloo, F., Schar, M., Beinart, R., Zviman, M.M., Halperin, H., Mori, S., Gai, N.D., Bluemke, D.A., McVeigh, E.R., and Herzka, D.A. (2013). 3D high-resolution diffusion tensor imaging of heart ex-vivo after myocardial infarction in porcine model. *Proceedings of International Society for Magnetic Resonance in Medicine*, Salt Lake City, UT.

Pearlman, E.S., Weber, K.T., and Janicki, J.S. (1981). Quantitative histology of the hypertrophied human heart. *Fed Proc* **40**(7): 2042–2047.

Pearlman, E.S., Weber, K.T., Janicki, J.S., Pietra, G.G., and Fishman, A.P. (1982). Muscle fiber orientation and connective tissue content in the hypertrophied human heart. *Lab Invest* **46**(2): 158–164.

Peeters, T.H., Vilanova, A., Strijkers, G.J., and ter Haar Romeny, B.M. (2006). Visualization of the fibrous structure of the heart. *Vision, Modeling and Visualization*, Aachen, Germany.

Pervolaraki, E., Reynolds, S., Bucur, A., Frangi, A., Anderson, R., Paley, M., and Holden, A. (2013). High resolution 3D imaging of post-mortem human fetal hearts. *Proceedings of International Society for Magnetic Resonance in Medicine*, Salt Lake City, UT.

Pipe, J.G., Farthing, V.G., and Forbes, K.P. (2002). Multishot diffusion-weighted FSE using PROPELLER MRI. *Magn Reson Med* **47**(1): 42–52.

Plank, G., Burton, R.A., Hales, P., Bishop, M., Mansoori, T., Bernabeu, M.O., Garny, A. et al. (2009). Generation of histo-anatomically representative models of the individual heart: Tools and application. *Philos Trans A Math Phys Eng Sci* **367**(1896): 2257–2292.

Poveda, F., Gil, D., Marti, E., Andaluz, A., Ballester, M., and Carreras, F. (2013). Helical structure of the cardiac ventricular anatomy assessed by diffusion tensor magnetic resonance imaging with multiresolution tractography. *Rev Esp Cardiol* **66**(10): 782–790.

Poveda, F., Marti, E., Gil, D., Carreras, F., and Ballester, M. (2012). Helical structure of ventricular anatomy by diffusion tensor cardiac MR tractography. *JACC Cardiovasc Imaging* **5**(7): 754–755.

Pravdin, S.F., Berdyshev, V.I., Panfilov, A.V., Katsnelson, L.B., Solovyova, O., and Markhasin, V.S. (2013). Mathematical model of the anatomy and fibre orientation field of the left ventricle of the heart. *Biomed Eng Online* **12**: 54.

Pruessmann, K.P., Weiger, M., Scheidegger, M.B., and Boesiger, P. (1999). SENSE: Sensitivity encoding for fast MRI. *Magn Reson Med* **42**(5): 952–962.

Rapacchi, S., Wen, H., Viallon, M., Grenier, D., Kellman, P., Croisille, P., and Pai, V.M. (2011). Low b-value diffusion-weighted cardiac magnetic resonance imaging: Initial results in humans using an optimal time-window imaging approach. *Invest Radiol* **46**(12): 751–758.

Reese, T.G., Heid, O., Weisskoff, R.M., and Wedeen, V.J. (2003). Reduction of eddy-current-induced distortion in diffusion MRI using a twice-refocused spin echo. *Magn Reson Med* **49**(1): 177–182.

Reese, T.G., Wedeen, V.J., and Weisskoff, R.M. (1996). Measuring diffusion in the presence of material strain. *J Magn Reson B* **112**(3): 253–258.

Reese, T.G., Weisskoff, R.M., Smith, R.N., Rosen, B.R., Dinsmore, R.E., and Wedeen, V.J. (1995). Imaging myocardial fiber architecture in vivo with magnetic resonance. *Magn Reson Med* **34**(6): 786–791.

Rijcken, J., Arts, T., Bovendeerd, P., Schoofs, B., and van Campen, D. (1996). Optimization of left ventricular fibre orientation of the normal heart for homogeneous sarcomere length during ejection. *Eur J Morphol* **34**(1): 39–46.

Rijcken, J., Bovendeerd, P.H., Schoofs, A.J., van Campen, D.H., and Arts, T. (1999). Optimization of cardiac fiber orientation for homogeneous fiber strain during ejection. *Ann Biomed Eng* **27**(3): 289–297.

Ripplinger, C.M., Li, W., Hadley, J., Chen, J., Rothenberg, F., Lombardi, R., Wickline, S.A., Marian, A.J., and Efimov, I.R. (2007). Enhanced transmural fiber rotation and connexin 43 heterogeneity are associated with an increased upper limit of vulnerability in a transgenic rabbit model of human hypertrophic cardiomyopathy. *Circ Res* **101**(10): 1049–1057.

Robb, J.S. and Robb, R.D. (1942). The normal heart: Anatomy and physiology of the structural units. *Am Heart J* **23**: 455–467.

Roberts, D.E., Hersh, L.T., and Scher, A.M. (1979). Influence of cardiac fiber orientation on wavefront voltage, conduction velocity, and tissue resistivity in the dog. *Circ Res* **44**(5): 701–712.

Roberts, T.P. and Schwartz, E.S. (2007). Principles and implementation of diffusion-weighted and diffusion tensor imaging. *Pediatr Radiol* **37**(8): 739–748.

Rohmer, D., Sitek, A., and Gullberg, G.T. (2007). Reconstruction and visualization of fiber and laminar structure in the normal human heart from ex vivo diffusion tensor magnetic resonance imaging (DTMRI) data. *Invest Radiol* **42**(11): 777–789.

Ross, M.A. and Streeter, D.D., Jr. (1975). Nonuniform subendocardial fiber orientation in the normal macaque left ventricle. *Eur J Cardiol* **3**(3): 229–247.

Rushmer, R.F., Crystal, D.K., and Wagner, C. (1953). The functional anatomy of ventricular contraction. *Circ Res* **1**(2): 162–170.

Sachse, F.B. (2004). *Computational Cardiology: Modeling of Anatomy, Electrophysiology, and Mechanics*. Springer, New York.

Sachse, F.B., Werner, C.D., Meyer-Waarden, K., and Dossel, O. (2000). Development of a human body model for numerical calculation of electrical fields. *Comput Med Imaging Graph* **24**(3): 165–171.

Schmid, P., Jaermann, T., Boesiger, P., Niederer, P.F., Lunkenheimer, P.P., Cryer, C.W., and Anderson, R.H. (2005). Ventricular myocardial architecture as visualised in postmortem swine hearts using magnetic resonance diffusion tensor imaging. *Eur J Cardiothorac Surg* **27**(3): 468–472.

Schmid, P., Lunkenheimer, P.P., Redmann, K., Rothaus, K., Jiang, X., Cryer, C.W., Jaermann, T., Niederer, P., Boesiger, P., and Anderson, R.H. (2007). Statistical analysis of the angle of intrusion of porcine ventricular myocytes from epicardium to endocardium using diffusion tensor magnetic resonance imaging. *Anat Rec (Hoboken)* **290**(11): 1413–1423.

Schmitt, B., Fedarava, K., Falkenberg, J., Rothaus, K., Bodhey, N.K., Reischauer, C., Kozerke, S. et al. (2009). Three-dimensional alignment of the aggregated myocytes in the normal and hypertrophic murine heart. *J Appl Physiol* (1985) **107**(3): 921–927.

Scollan, D.F., Holmes, A., Winslow, R., and Forder, J. (1998). Histological validation of myocardial microstructure obtained from diffusion tensor magnetic resonance imaging. *Am J Physiol* **275**(6 Pt 2): H2308–H2318.

Scollan, D.F., Holmes, A., Zhang, J., and Winslow, R.L. (2000). Reconstruction of cardiac ventricular geometry and fiber orientation using magnetic resonance imaging. *Ann Biomed Eng* **28**(8): 934–944.

Scott, A., Ferreira, P., Nielles-Vallespin, S., McGill, L., Pennell, D.J., and Firmin, D. (2015a). Directions vs. averages: An in-vivo comparison for cardiac DTI. *J Cardiovasc Magn Reson* **17**(Suppl 1): P25.

Scott, A., Nielles-Vallespin, S., Ferreira, P., McGill, L., Pennell, D.J., and Firmin, D. (2015b). Improving the accuracy of cardiac DTI by averaging the complex data. *J Cardiovasc Magn Reson* **17**(Suppl 1): O38.

Scott, A., Nielles-Vallespin, S., Ferreira, P., McGill, L., Pennell, D.J., and Firmin, D. (2015c). "Squashing the Peanut": What it means for in-vivo cardiac DTI. *Proceedings of International Society for Magnetic Resonance in Medicine*, Toronto, Ontario, Canada.

Scott, A.D., Ferreira, P., Nielles-Vallespin, S., McGill, L.A., Kilner, P.J., Pennell, D.J., and Firmin, D. (2014). Improved in-vivo cardiac DTI using optimal b-values. *J Cardiovasc Magn Reson* **16**(Suppl 1): O27.

Scott, A.D., Ferreira, P.F., Nielles-Vallespin, S., Gatehouse, P., McGill, L.A., Kilner, P., Pennell, D.J., and Firmin, D.N. (2015). Optimal diffusion weighting for in vivo cardiac diffusion tensor imaging. *Magn Reson Med* **74**(2): 420–430.

Seemann, G., Hoper, C., Sachse, F.B., Dossel, O., Holden, A.V., and Zhang, H. (2006). Heterogeneous three-dimensional anatomical and electrophysiological model of human atria. *Philos Trans A Math Phys Eng Sci* **364**(1843): 1465–1481.

Sengupta, P.P., Khandheria, B.K., and Narula, J. (2008a). Twist and untwist mechanics of the left ventricle. *Heart Fail Clin* **4**(3): 315–324.

Sengupta, P.P., Tajik, A.J., Chandrasekaran, K., and Khandheria, B.K. (2008b). Twist mechanics of the left ventricle: Principles and application. *JACC Cardiovasc Imaging* **1**(3): 366–376.

Shi, Y., Jiang, Y., and Hsu, E.W. (2007). Comparison of diffusion tensor and Q-Ball imaging of the canine myocardium. *Proceedings of International Society for Magnetic Resonance in Medicine*, Berlin, Germany.

Skare, S., Newbould, R.D., Clayton, D.B., and Bammer, R. (2006). Propeller EPI in the other direction. *Magn Reson Med* **55**(6): 1298–1307.

Smerup, M., Agger, P., Nielsen, E.A., Ringgaard, S., Pedersen, M., Niederer, P., Anderson, R.H., and Lunkenheimer, P.P. (2013a). Regional and epi- to endocardial differences in transmural angles of left ventricular cardiomyocytes measured in ex vivo pig hearts: Functional implications. *Anat Rec (Hoboken)* **296**(11): 1724–1734.

Smerup, M., Nielsen, E., Agger, P., Frandsen, J., Vestergaard-Poulsen, P., Andersen, J., Nyengaard, J. et al. (2009). The three-dimensional arrangement of the myocytes aggregated together within the mammalian ventricular myocardium. *Anat Rec (Hoboken)* **292**(1): 1–11.

Smerup, M., Partridge, J., Agger, P., Ringgaard, S., Pedersen, M., Petersen, S., Hasenkam, J.M., Niederer, P., Lunkenheimer, P.P., and Anderson, R.H. (2013b). A mathematical model of the mechanical link between shortening of the cardiomyocytes and systolic deformation of the left ventricular myocardium. *Technol Health Care* **21**(1): 63–79.

Song, X., Zhu, Y.M., Yang, F., and Luo, J.H. (2010). Quantitative study of fiber tracking results in human cardiac DTI. *IEEE International Conference on Digital Signal Processing (ICSP)*, Beijing, China.

Sosnovik, D.E., Mekkaoui, C., Huang, S., Chen, H.H., Dai, G., Stoeck, C.T., Ngoy, S. et al. (2014). Microstructural impact of ischemia and bone marrow-derived cell therapy revealed with diffusion tensor magnetic resonance imaging tractography of the heart in vivo. *Circulation* **129**(17): 1731–1741.

Sosnovik, D.E., Wang, R., Dai, G., Reese, T.G., and Wedeen, V.J. (2009a). Diffusion MR tractography of the heart. *J Cardiovasc Magn Reson* **11**: 47.

Sosnovik, D.E., Wang, R., Dai, G., Wang, T., Aikawa, E., Novikov, M., Rosenzweig, A., Gilbert, R.J., and Wedeen, V.J. (2009b). Diffusion spectrum MRI tractography reveals the presence of a complex network of residual myofibers in infarcted myocardium. *Circ Cardiovasc Imaging* **2**(3): 206–212.

Sowerby, A.J., Harries, J., Diakun, G.P., Towns-Andrews, E., Bordas, J., and Stier, A. (1994). X-ray diffraction studies of whole rat heart during anoxic perfusion. *Biochem Biophys Res Commun* **202**(3): 1244–1251.

Spotnitz, H.M. (2000). Macro design, structure, and mechanics of the left ventricle. *J Thorac Cardiovasc Surg* **119**(5): 1053–1077.

Stejskal, E.O. and Tanner, J.E. (1965). Spin diffusion measurements: Spin echoes in the presence of a time-dependent field gradient. *J Chem Phys* **42**: 288–292.

Stieltjes, B., Kaufmann, W.E., van Zijl, P.C., Fredericksen, K., Pearlson, G.D., Solaiyappan, M., and Mori, S. (2001). Diffusion tensor imaging and axonal tracking in the human brainstem. *Neuroimage* **14**(3): 723–735.

Stoeck, C.T., Kalinowska, A., von Deuster, C., Harmer, J., Chan, R.W., Niemann, M., Manka, R. et al. (2014). Dual-phase cardiac diffusion tensor imaging with strain correction. *PLoS One* **9**(9): e107159.

Stoeck, C.T., von Deuster, C., Cesarovic, N., Genet, M., Emmert, M., and Kozerke, S. (2015a). Direct comparison of in-vivo and post-mortem spin-echo based diffusion tensor imaging in the porcine heart. *J Cardiovasc Magn Reson* **17**(Suppl 1): P76.

Stoeck, C.T., von Deuster, C., Genet, M., Atkinson, D., and Kozerke, S. (2015b). First and second order motion compensated spin-echo diffusion tensor imaging of the human heart. *Proceedings of International Society for Magnetic Resonance in Medicine*, Toronto, Ontario, Canada.

Stoeck, C.T., von Deuster, C., Genet, M., Atkinson, D., and Kozerke, S. (2015c). Second order motion compensated spin-echo diffusion tensor imaging of the human heart. *J Cardiovasc Magn Reson* **17**(Suppl 1): P81.

Stoeck, C.T., von Deuster, C., Toussaint, N., and Kozerke, S. (2013). High-resolution single-shot DTI of the in-vivo human heart using asymmetric diffusion encoding. *Proceedings of International Society for Magnetic Resonance in Medicine*, Salt Lake City, UT.

Streeter, D.D., Gross morphology and fiber geometry of the heart. Berne R, Sperelakis N; *Handbook of Physiology*. Section 2. The Cardiovascular System, Vol. 1, 1979, Williams & Wilkins, Baltimore, MD, pp. 61–112.

Streeter, D.D., Jr. and Hanna, W.T. (1973a). Engineering mechanics for successive states in canine left ventricular myocardium. I. Cavity and wall geometry. *Circ Res* **33**(6): 639–655.

Streeter, D.D., Jr. and Hanna, W.T. (1973b). Engineering mechanics for successive states in canine left ventricular myocardium. II. Fiber angle and sarcomere length. *Circ Res* **33**(6): 656–664.

Streeter, D.D., Jr., Spotnitz, H.M., Patel, D.P., Ross, J., Jr., and Sonnenblick, E.H. (1969). Fiber orientation in the canine left ventricle during diastole and systole. *Circ Res* **24**(3): 339–347.

Strijkers, G.J., Bouts, A., Blankesteijn, W.M., Peeters, T.H., Vilanova, A., van Prooijen, M.C., Sanders, H.M., Heijman, E., and Nicolay, K. (2009). Diffusion tensor imaging of left ventricular remodeling in response to myocardial infarction in the mouse. *NMR Biomed* **22**(2): 182–190.

Takayama, Y., Costa, K.D., and Covell, J.W. (2002). Contribution of laminar myofiber architecture to load-dependent changes in mechanics of LV myocardium. *Am J Physiol Heart Circ Physiol* **282**(4): H1510–H1520.

Tang, D., Yang, C., Geva, T., Gaudette, G., and Del Nido, P.J. (2010). Effect of patch mechanical properties on right ventricle function using MRI-based two-layer anisotropic models of human right and left ventricles. *Comput Model Eng Sci* **56**(2): 113–130.

Tezuka, F., Hort, W., Lange, P.E., and Nurnberg, J.H. (1990). Muscle fiber orientation in the development and regression of right ventricular hypertrophy in pigs. *Acta Pathol Jpn* **40**(6): 402–407.

Torrent-Guasp, F. (1957). *Anatomia Funciónal del Corazón*. La actividad ventricular diastólica y sistólica. Paz Montalvo, Madrid, Spain.

Torrent-Guasp, F. (1980). Macroscopic structure of the ventricular myocardium. *Rev Esp Cardiol* **33**: 265–287.

Torrent-Guasp, F., Buckberg, G.D., Clemente, C., Cox, J.L., Coghlan, H.C., and Gharib, M. (2001). The structure and function of the helical heart and its buttress wrapping. I. The normal macroscopic structure of the heart. *Semin Thorac Cardiovasc Surg* **13**(4): 301–319.

Torrey, H.C. (1956). Bloch equations with diffusion terms. *Phys Rev* **104**: 563–565.

Tournier, J.D., Mori, S., and Leemans, A. (2011). Diffusion tensor imaging and beyond. *Magn Reson Med* **65**(6): 1532–1556.

Toussaint, N., Sermesant, M., Stoeck, C.T., Kozerke, S., and Batchelor, P.G. (2010). In vivo human 3D cardiac fibre architecture: Reconstruction using curvilinear interpolation of diffusion tensor images. *Med Image Comput Comput Assist Interv* **13**(Pt 1): 418–425.

Toussaint, N., Stoeck, C.T., Schaeffter, T., Kozerke, S., Sermesant, M., and Batchelor, P.G. (2013a). In vivo human cardiac fibre architecture estimation using shape-based diffusion tensor processing. *Med Image Anal* **17**(8): 1243–1255.

Toussaint, N., Stoeck, C.T., Schaeffter, T., Sermesant, M., and Kozerke, S. (2013b). Cardiac laminae structure dynamics from in-vivo diffusion tensor imaging. *Proceedings of International Society for Magnetic Resonance in Medicine*, Salt Lake City, UT.

Trayanova, N.A., O'Hara, T., Bayer, J.D., Boyle, P.M., McDowell, K.S., Constantino, J., Arevalo, H.J., Hu, Y., and Vadakkumpadan, F. (2012). Computational cardiology: How computer simulations could be used to develop new therapies and advance existing ones. *Europace* **14**(Suppl 5): v82–v89.

Tseng, W.Y., Dou, J., Reese, T.G., and Wedeen, V.J. (2006). Imaging myocardial fiber disarray and intramural strain hypokinesis in hypertrophic cardiomyopathy with MRI. *J Magn Reson Imaging* **23**(1): 1–8.

Tseng, W.Y., Reese, T.G., Weisskoff, R.M., Brady, T.J., Dinsmore, R.E., and Wedeen, V.J. (1997). Mapping myocardial fiber and sheet function in humans by magnetic resonance imaging (MRI). *Circulation* **96**: 1096.

Tseng, W.Y., Reese, T.G., Weisskoff, R.M., Brady, T.J., and Wedeen, V.J. (2000). Myocardial fiber shortening in humans: Initial results of MR imaging. *Radiology* **216**(1): 128–139.

Tseng, W.Y., Reese, T.G., Weisskoff, R.M., and Wedeen, V.J. (1999). Cardiac diffusion tensor MRI in vivo without strain correction. *Magn Reson Med* **42**(2): 393–403.

Tseng, W.Y., Wedeen, V.J., Reese, T.G., Smith, R.N., and Halpern, E.F. (2003). Diffusion tensor MRI of myocardial fibers and sheets: Correspondence with visible cut-face texture. *J Magn Reson Imaging* **17**(1): 31–42.

Tu, J.V., Brien, S.E., Kennedy, C.C., Pilote, L., Ghali, W.A., and Canadian Cardiovascular Outcomes Research, T. (2003). Introduction to the canadian cardiovascular outcomes research team's (CCORT) Canadian cardiovascular atlas project. *Can J Cardiol* **19**(3): 225–229.

Tubbs, R.S., Gianaris, N., Shoja, M.M., Loukas, M., and Cohen Gadol, A.A. (2012). "The heart is simply a muscle" and first description of the tetralogy of "Fallot". Early contributions to cardiac anatomy and pathology by bishop and anatomist Niels Stensen (1638–1686). *Int J Cardiol* **154**(3): 312–315.

Tuch, D.S. (2004). Q-ball imaging. *Magn Reson Med* **52**(6): 1358–1372.

Tuch, D.S., Reese, T.G., Wiegell, M.R., Makris, N., Belliveau, J.W., and Wedeen, V.J. (2002). High angular resolution diffusion imaging reveals intravoxel white matter fiber heterogeneity. *Magn Reson Med* **48**(4): 577–582.

Vadakkumpadan, F., Arevalo, H., Ceritoglu, C., Miller, M., and Trayanova, N. (2012). Image-based estimation of ventricular fiber orientations for personalized modeling of cardiac electrophysiology. *IEEE Trans Med Imaging* **31**(5): 1051–1060.

Vadakkumpadan, F., Arevalo, H., Prassl, A.J., Chen, J., Kickinger, F., Kohl, P., Plank, G., and Trayanova, N. (2010). Image-based models of cardiac structure in health and disease. *Wiley Interdiscip Rev Syst Biol Med* **2**(4): 489–506.

Vendelin, M., Bovendeerd, P.H., Engelbrecht, J., and Arts, T. (2002). Optimizing ventricular fibers: Uniform strain or stress, but not ATP consumption, leads to high efficiency. *Am J Physiol Heart Circ Physiol* **283**(3): H1072–H1081.

Vetter, F.J. and McCulloch, A.D. (1998). Three-dimensional analysis of regional cardiac function: A model of rabbit ventricular anatomy. *Prog Biophys Mol Biol* **69**(2–3): 157–183.

Vignaud, A., Rodriguez, I., Ennis, D.B., DeSilva, R., Kellman, P., Taylor, J., Bennett, E., and Wen, H. (2006). Detection of myocardial capillary orientation with intravascular iron-oxide nanoparticles in spin-echo MRI. *Magn Reson Med* **55**(4): 725–730.

Vilanova, A., Zhang, S., Kindlmann, G., and Laidlaw, D. (2005). An introduction to visualization of diffusion tensor imaging and its applications. In *Visualization and Image Processing of Tensor Fields*, J. Weickert and H. Hagen (eds.). Springer-Verlag, New York.

von Deuster, C., Stoeck, C.T., Giese, D., Harmer, J., Chan, R.W., Atkinson, D., and Kozerke, S. (2013). Concurrent dual-slice cardiac DTI of the in-vivo human heart. *Proceedings of International Society for Magnetic Resonance in Medicine*, Salt Lake City, UT.

Waldman, L.K., Nosan, D., Villarreal, F., and Covell, J.W. (1988). Relation between transmural deformation and local myofiber direction in canine left ventricle. *Circ Res* **63**(3): 550–562.

Walker, J.C., Guccione, J.M., Jiang, Y., Zhang, P., Wallace, A.W., Hsu, E.W., and Ratcliffe, M.B. (2005a). Helical myofiber orientation after myocardial infarction and left ventricular surgical restoration in sheep. *J Thorac Cardiovasc Surg* **129**(2): 382–390.

Walker, J.C., Ratcliffe, M.B., Zhang, P., Wallace, A.W., Fata, B., Hsu, E.W., Saloner, D., and Guccione, J.M. (2005b). MRI-based finite-element analysis of left ventricular aneurysm. *Am J Physiol Heart Circ Physiol* **289**(2): H692–H700.

Walker, J.C., Ratcliffe, M.B., Zhang, P., Wallace, A.W., Hsu, E.W., Saloner, D.A., and Guccione, J.M. (2008). Magnetic resonance imaging-based finite element stress analysis after linear repair of left ventricular aneurysm. *J Thorac Cardiovasc Surg* **135**(5): 1094–1102, e1091–e1092.

Wang, T.T., Kwon, H.S., Dai, G., Wang, R., Mijailovich, S.M., Moss, R.L., So, P.T., Wedeen, V.J., and Gilbert, R.J. (2010). Resolving myoarchitectural disarray in the mouse ventricular wall with diffusion spectrum magnetic resonance imaging. *Ann Biomed Eng* **38**(9): 2841–2850.

Wedeen, V.J., Hagmann, P., Tseng, W.Y., Reese, T.G., and Weisskoff, R.M. (2005). Mapping complex tissue architecture with diffusion spectrum magnetic resonance imaging. *Magn Reson Med* **54**(6): 1377–1386.

Wei, H., Viallon, M., Delattre, B.M., Moulin, K., Yang, F., Croisille, P., and Zhu, Y. (2015). Free-breathing diffusion tensor imaging and tractography of the human heart in healthy volunteers using wavelet-based image fusion. *IEEE Trans Med Imaging* **34**(1): 306–316.

Wei, H., Viallon, M., Delattre, B.M., Pai, V.M., Wen, H., Xue, H., Guetter, C., Jolly, M.P., Croisille, P., and Zhu, Y. (2013a). In vivo diffusion tensor imaging of the human heart with free-breathing in healthy volunteers. *Proceedings of International Society for Magnetic Resonance in Medicine*, Salt Lake City, UT.

Wei, H., Viallon, M., Delattre, B.M., Wang, L., Pai, V.M., Wen, H., Croisille, P., and Zhu, Y. (2013b). Quantitative analysis of cardiac motion effects on in vivo diffusion tensor parameters. *Proceedings of International Society for Magnetic Resonance in Medicine*, Salt Lake City, UT.

Wei, H., Viallon, M., Delattre, B.M., Wang, L., Pai, V.M., Wen, H., Xue, H., Guetter, C., Croisille, P., and Zhu, Y. (2013c). Assessment of cardiac motion effects on the fiber architecture of the human heart in vivo. *IEEE Trans Med Imaging* **32**(10): 1928–1938.

Weiss, D.L., Keller, D.U., Seemann, G., and Dossel, O. (2007). The influence of fibre orientation, extracted from different segments of the human left ventricle, on the activation and repolarization sequence: A simulation study. *Europace* **9**(Suppl 6): vi96–104.

Welsh, C., Di Bella, E., and Hsu, E. (2015). Higher-order motion-compensation for in vivo cardiac diffusion tensor imaging in rats. *IEEE Trans Med Imaging* **34**(9): 1843–1853.

Welsh, C.L., Dibella, E.V., Adluru, G., and Hsu, E.W. (2013). Model-based reconstruction of undersampled diffusion tensor k-space data. *Magn Reson Med* **70**(2): 429–440.

Wenk, J.F., Sun, K., Zhang, Z., Soleimani, M., Ge, L., Saloner, D., Wallace, A.W., Ratcliffe, M.B., and Guccione, J.M. (2011). Regional left ventricular myocardial contractility and stress in a finite element model of posterobasal myocardial infarction. *J Biomech Eng* **133**(4): 044501.

Westin, C.F., Maier, S.E., Mamata, H., Nabavi, A., Jolesz, F.A., and Kikinis, R. (2002). Processing and visualization for diffusion tensor MRI. *Med Image Anal* **6**(2): 93–108.

Winklhofer, S., Stoeck, C.T., Berger, N., Thali, M., Manka, R., Kozerke, S., Alkadhi, H., and Stolzmann, P. (2014). Post-mortem cardiac diffusion tensor imaging: Detection of myocardial infarction and remodeling of myofiber architecture. *Eur Radiol* **24**(11): 2810–2818.

Winslow, R.L., Scollan, D.F., Holmes, A., Yung, C.K., Zhang, J., and Jafri, M.S. (2000). Electrophysiological modeling of cardiac ventricular function: From cell to organ. *Annu Rev Biomed Eng* **2**: 119–155.

Wu, E.X., Wu, Y., Nicholls, J.M., Wang, J., Liao, S., Zhu, S., Lau, C.P., and Tse, H.F. (2007a). MR diffusion tensor imaging study of postinfarct myocardium structural remodeling in a porcine model. *Magn Reson Med* **58**(4): 687–695.

Wu, E.X., Wu, Y., Tang, H., Wang, J., Yang, J., Ng, M.C., Yang, E.S. et al. (2007b). Study of myocardial fiber pathway using magnetic resonance diffusion tensor imaging. *Magn Reson Imaging* **25**(7): 1048–1057.

Wu, M.T., Su, M.Y., Huang, Y.L., Chiou, K.R., Yang, P., Pan, H.B., Reese, T.G., Wedeen, V.J., and Tseng, W.Y. (2009). Sequential changes of myocardial microstructure in patients postmyocardial infarction by diffusion-tensor cardiac MR: Correlation with left ventricular structure and function. *Circ Cardiovasc Imaging* **2**(1): 32–40, 36 p. following 40.

Wu, M.T., Tseng, W.Y., Su, M.Y., Liu, C.P., Chiou, K.R., Wedeen, V.J., Reese, T.G., and Yang, C.F. (2006). Diffusion tensor magnetic resonance imaging mapping the fiber architecture remodeling in human myocardium after infarction: Correlation with viability and wall motion. *Circulation* **114**(10): 1036–1045.

Wu, Y., Chen, Y., Liu, X., Yeh, F., Hitchens, T., Gabriel, G., and Lo, C. (2015). Diffusion-tensor imaging study of myocardial architecture of Situs Inversus and Situs Solitus mutant mouse hearts. *Proceedings of International Society for Magnetic Resonance in Medicine*, Toronto, Ontario, Canada.

Wu, Y. and Wu, E.X. (2009). MR investigation of the coupling between myocardial fiber architecture and cardiac contraction. *Conf Proc IEEE Eng Med Biol Soc* **2009**: 4395–4398.

Wu, Y., Zou, C., Liu, W., Liao, W., Yang, W., Porter, D.A., Liu, X., and Wu, E.X. (2013). Effect of B-value in revealing postinfarct myocardial microstructural remodeling using MR diffusion tensor imaging. *Magn Reson Imaging* **31**(6): 847–856.

Xing, D., Papadakis, N.G., Huang, C.L., Lee, V.M., Carpenter, T.A., and Hall, L.D. (1997). Optimised diffusion-weighting for measurement of apparent diffusion coefficient (ADC) in human brain. *Magn Reson Imaging* **15**(7): 771–784.

Yagi, N., Shimizu, J., Mohri, S., Araki, J., Nakamura, K., Okuyama, H., Toyota, H. et al. (2004). X-ray diffraction from a left ventricular wall of rat heart. *Biophys J* **86**(4): 2286–2294.

Yang, F., Zhu, Y.M., Magnin, I.E., Luo, J.H., Croisille, P., and Kingsley, P.B. (2012). Feature-based interpolation of diffusion tensor fields and application to human cardiac DT-MRI. *Med Image Anal* **16**(2): 459–481.

Young, A.A., Legrice, I.J., Young, M.A., and Smaill, B.H. (1998). Extended confocal microscopy of myocardial laminae and collagen network. *J Microsc* **192**(Pt 2): 139–150.

Zhang, L., Allen, J., Hu, L., Caruthers, S.D., Wickline, S.A., and Chen, J. (2013). Cardiomyocyte architectural plasticity in fetal, neonatal, and adult pig hearts delineated with diffusion tensor MRI. *Am J Physiol Heart Circ Physiol* **304**(2): H246–H252.

Zhang, S., Crow, J.A., Yang, X., Chen, J., Borazjani, A., Mullins, K.B., Chen, W., Cooper, R.C., McLaughlin, R.M., and Liao, J. (2010). The correlation of 3D DT-MRI fiber disruption with structural and mechanical degeneration in porcine myocardium. *Ann Biomed Eng* **38**(10): 3084–3095.

Zhang, Y., Liang, X., Ma, J., Jing, Y., Gonzales, M.J., Villongco, C., Krishnamurthy, A. et al. (2012). An atlas-based geometry pipeline for cardiac Hermite model construction and diffusion tensor reorientation. *Med Image Anal* **16**(6): 1130–1141.

Zhukov, L. and Barr, A.H. (2003). Heart-muscle fiber reconstruction from diffusion tensor MRI. *IEEE Visualization (VIS)*, Seattle, WA.

6 Continuum Mechanics and Mechanical Cardiac Models

El-Sayed H. Ibrahim, PhD and Ahmed S. Fahmy, PhD

CONTENTS

LIST OF ABBREVIATIONS

Abbreviation	Meaning
1D	One-dimensional
2D	Two-dimensional
3D	Three-dimensional
ADC	Apparent diffusion coefficient
ED	End diastole
ES	End systole
FA	Fractional anisotropy
FEM	Finite element method
HARP	Harmonic phase
LV	Left ventricle
MAP	Maximum a posteriori
MRF	Markov random field
MTR	Magnetization transfer rate
PCA	Principal component analysis
RV	Right ventricle
RVH	RV hypertrophy
SAX	Short-axis
SNR	Signal-to-noise ratio

6.1 INTRODUCTION

6.1.1 MECHANICAL CARDIAC MODELS AND CARDIAC FUNCTIONAL ANALYSIS

Cardiac models that depend only on geometrical representation of the heart face the possibility of producing unreasonable results of the heart function and deformation, especially in the case of low signal-to-noise ratio (SNR), imaging artifacts, or lack of sufficient texture or contrast in the image. The incorporation of realistic mechanical modeling in cardiac image analysis ensures that the generated deformation maps represent realistic heart function. Computational models of the heart have been developed based on geometry (Nielsen et al. 1991, Hooks et al. 2002), microstructure (Legrice et al. 1997), material properties (Hunter et al. 1998, Dokos et al. 2002), and electrophysiology (Pollard and Barr 1991, ten Tusscher et al. 2004, Trayanova 2006).

Theories of continuum mechanics are fundamental in modeling the behavior of the myocardium in response to different forces and stresses. In continuum mechanics, the spatial distribution of forces and deformations is described, and the appropriate relationships among them are established. Such relationships involve a representation of the tissue properties at each spatial location. In addition, continuum mechanics provide a theoretical framework for representing other physical processes and factors attributing to the cardiac contraction-relaxation mechanism, cycle such as distribution of electrical potential, oxygen consumption, temperature, and metabolite concentrations within the myocardium.

6.1.2 CHAPTER OUTLINE

In this chapter, we introduce the basic continuum mechanics definitions and concepts necessary for understanding the results of the different techniques presented throughout the book, and discuss the basic biomechanical models used in myocardial deformation analysis. The chapter starts by reviewing basic mathematical preliminaries, including vectors, scalar and vector products, tensors, vector and tensor calculus, and the eigensystem. The chapter then reviews the basics of continuum mechanics, including tissue definition as a continuum material, reference and deformed configurations, as well as Lagrangian and Eulerian descriptions of deformation. Different types of deformation are then reviewed, including homogeneous deformation and rigid-body motion. Deformation gradient and stress tensor are also reviewed, including infinitesimal stress and rotation tensors as well as normal and shear strains. Volume change under deformation is also discussed. The next section reviews constitutive equations and elasticity. Hooke's law is presented along with the properties of monoclinic, orthotropic, isotropic, and transverse-isotropic materials. The concepts of conservation of mass and momentum are then reviewed, followed by a description of the equilibrium condition and equations of motion. The chapter then reviews the finite element method, including shape approximation, mesh construction, global and natural coordinate systems, shape functions, element strains and stresses, and dynamic equations. After reviewing the continuum mechanics basics, the chapter reviews famous biomechanical models used for estimating myocardial deformation, including models for estimating 3D deformation from planar myocardial contours, sparse 2D measurements, and fused magnitude and phase-contrast MRI images. Finally, hyperelastic warping models and incompressible models are reviewed, along with methods for estimating in vivo material mechanical properties of the myocardium.

6.2 MATHEMATICAL PRELIMINARIES

Before getting into the mechanical behavior of tissues, we first review fundamental mathematical and geometric definitions and properties that will be extensively used in this chapter.

6.2.1 VECTORS

The vector entity is used to describe a geometric or physical quantity that has a magnitude and a direction. Usually, it is formed by stacking a number of scalar elements in a vertical arrangement. In this chapter, **boldface italic**

(small and capital) letters are used as the notation for vectors. For example, the vector representing the position of a tissue particle can be written as x or X. The elements (or coordinates) of such vectors take the same form but in nonbold font, that is, $x = \begin{bmatrix} x_1 & x_2 & x_3 \end{bmatrix}^T$ and $X = \begin{bmatrix} X_1 & X_2 & X_3 \end{bmatrix}^T$.

The magnitude of vector x is denoted by $|x|$ or $\|x\|$, which is a scalar value representing the vector's length. A vector can be represented as a multiplication of its magnitude and direction, that is,

$$x = |x| n_x, \tag{6.1}$$

where n_x is a unit vector in the direction of the vector x; that is, $|n_x| = 1$. In three-dimensional (3D) space, the principal coordinate axes are usually represented by perpendicular unit vectors denoted by e_1, e_2, and e_3. That is, any vector in space can be written in terms of its different components:

$$x = x_1 e_1 + x_2 e_2 + x_3 e_3. \tag{6.2}$$

6.2.2 SCALAR AND VECTOR PRODUCTS

Multiplying a vector by a scalar is equivalent to multiplying each element in the vector by this scalar, that is,

$$\beta x = \begin{bmatrix} \beta x_1 \\ \beta x_2 \\ \beta x_3 \end{bmatrix}, \tag{6.3}$$

where β is any scalar value.

The *inner product*, a.k.a. *dot product*, of two vectors results in a scalar value given by

$$x \cdot y = x_1 y_1 + x_2 y_2 + x_3 y_3. \tag{6.4}$$

The inner product can be also represented by the magnitude and angle between the vectors as follows:

$$x \cdot y = |x|\,|y|\cos(\theta), \tag{6.5}$$

where θ is the angle between the vectors x and y. In matrix notation, the dot product is represented by

$$x \cdot y = x^T y, \tag{6.6}$$

where x^T is a row vector representing the transpose of the (column) vector x.

The *cross product*, a.k.a. *vector product*, is defined as

$$x \times y = |x|\,|y|\sin(\theta) n_\perp, \tag{6.7}$$

where $n_\perp$ is a unit vector perpendicular to the plane containing the vectors x and y.

6.2.3 TENSORS

Tensors are geometric objects that describe a linear mapping from one space to another. They can be represented by a multi-dimensional array of numerical values. Therefore, scalars and vectors are special cases of tensors. In fact, second-order tensors are simply represented by two-dimensional (2D) arrays, that is, matrices, and thus all matrix algebra operations can be applied to such tensors. In this chapter, matrices and tensors are denoted by **boldface nonitalic** (capital or small) letters with their scalar elements denoted by nonbold letters. For example, a tensor that rotates vectors in the 3D space around the z-axis with angle θ is represented by

$$\mathbf{R} = \begin{bmatrix} R_{11} & R_{12} & R_{13} \\ R_{21} & R_{22} & R_{23} \\ R_{31} & R_{32} & R_{33} \end{bmatrix} = \begin{bmatrix} \cos(\theta) & \sin(\theta) & 0 \\ -\sin(\theta) & \cos(\theta) & 0 \\ 0 & 0 & 1 \end{bmatrix}. \quad (6.8)$$

Similarly, the Eulerian strain tensor is represented by

$$\mathbf{e} = \begin{bmatrix} e_{11} & e_{12} & e_{13} \\ e_{21} & e_{22} & e_{23} \\ e_{31} & e_{32} & e_{33} \end{bmatrix}. \quad (6.9)$$

6.2.4 VECTOR AND TENSOR CALCULUS

6.2.4.1 Partial Derivative

Given a first-order tensor, that is, vector, x, the partial derivative of the vector x with respect to t is given by

$$\frac{\partial}{\partial t} x = \begin{bmatrix} \dfrac{\partial x_1}{\partial t} \\ \dfrac{\partial x_2}{\partial t} \\ \dfrac{\partial x_3}{\partial t} \end{bmatrix}. \quad (6.10)$$

For higher-order tensors, for example, matrices, similar equations can be derived where all elements are differentiated with respect to t.

6.2.4.2 Gradient Operator

Let us consider a surface in 3D space that is represented by a function of three variables, $f(x_1, x_2, x_3)$. The gradient of this surface calculates the slope of the surface along each of the three coordinate directions, that is,

$$\nabla f(x_1, x_2, x_3) = \begin{bmatrix} \dfrac{\partial}{\partial x_1} \\ \dfrac{\partial}{\partial x_2} \\ \dfrac{\partial}{\partial x_3} \end{bmatrix} f(x_1, x_2, x_3) = \begin{bmatrix} \dfrac{\partial f}{\partial x_1} \\ \dfrac{\partial f}{\partial x_2} \\ \dfrac{\partial f}{\partial x_3} \end{bmatrix}. \quad (6.11)$$

It is worth noting that the slope of the surface in an arbitrary direction defined by a unit vector, n, can be calculated as

$$\frac{df(x_1, x_2, x_3)}{ds} = n \cdot \nabla f, \quad (6.12)$$

where ds is a differential step along the direction n.

Now, let us consider a vector, f, whose elements represent three surfaces, then, its *gradient* results in a tensor given by

$$\mathbf{grad}\, f \equiv \nabla f = \nabla \begin{bmatrix} f_1(x_1,x_2,x_3) \\ f_2(x_1,x_2,x_3) \\ f_3(x_1,x_2,x_3) \end{bmatrix}^{\mathrm{T}} = \begin{bmatrix} \dfrac{\partial f_1}{\partial x_1} & \dfrac{\partial f_1}{\partial x_2} & \dfrac{\partial f_1}{\partial x_3} \\ \dfrac{\partial f_2}{\partial x_1} & \dfrac{\partial f_2}{\partial x_2} & \dfrac{\partial f_2}{\partial x_3} \\ \dfrac{\partial f_3}{\partial x_1} & \dfrac{\partial f_3}{\partial x_2} & \dfrac{\partial f_3}{\partial x_3} \end{bmatrix}. \quad (6.13)$$

The *divergence* of a vector is given by

$$\mathbf{div}\, f \equiv \nabla \cdot f = \frac{\partial f_1}{\partial x_1} + \frac{\partial f_2}{\partial x_2} + \frac{\partial f_3}{\partial x_3}. \quad (6.14)$$

If we take the divergence of the gradient vector in Equation 6.11, we obtain the *Laplacian* of the surface $f(x_1, x_2, x_3)$:

$$\mathbf{div}(\nabla f) \equiv \nabla \cdot \nabla f = \nabla^2 f = \frac{\partial^2 f}{\partial x_1^2} + \frac{\partial^2 f}{\partial x_2^2} + \frac{\partial^2 f}{\partial x_3^2}. \quad (6.15)$$

Given a second-order tensor **F**, its divergence is a vector defined by

$$\mathbf{div}\, \mathbf{F} \equiv \nabla \cdot \mathbf{F} = \begin{bmatrix} \dfrac{\partial f_{11}}{\partial x_1} + \dfrac{\partial f_{12}}{\partial x_2} + \dfrac{\partial f_{13}}{\partial x_3} \\ \dfrac{\partial f_{21}}{\partial x_1} + \dfrac{\partial f_{22}}{\partial x_2} + \dfrac{\partial f_{23}}{\partial x_3} \\ \dfrac{\partial f_{31}}{\partial x_1} + \dfrac{\partial f_{32}}{\partial x_2} + \dfrac{\partial f_{33}}{\partial x_3} \end{bmatrix}. \quad (6.16)$$

The *curl* of a vector is defined by

$$\mathbf{curl}\, f \equiv \nabla \times f = \begin{vmatrix} \hat{x}_1 & \hat{x}_2 & \hat{x}_3 \\ \dfrac{\partial}{\partial x} & \dfrac{\partial}{\partial y} & \dfrac{\partial}{\partial z} \\ f_1 & f_2 & f_3 \end{vmatrix}, \quad (6.17)$$

where

$\hat{x}_i$ is a unit vector in the x_i direction

|**M**| represents the determinant of matrix **M**

6.2.5 EIGENVECTORS AND EIGENVALUES

Let us now consider tensors as operators that change a vector into another vector. In this regard, the *eigenvectors* of a given tensor are vectors that do not change their direction under this tensor operation. That is, only the magnitude of the eigenvectors is changed with a value referred to as the *eigenvalue*. An eigenvector v of a tensor $\mathbf{A}$ must satisfy the following equation:

$$\mathbf{A}v = \lambda v, \tag{6.18}$$

where λ is the corresponding eigenvalue of v. An important characteristic of symmetric tensors is that the eigenvectors associated with distinct eigenvalues are orthogonal. That is, if three eigenvalues of a third-order tensor are all distinct, then the three corresponding eigenvectors are mutually orthogonal.

6.3 TISSUE AS A CONTINUUM MATTER

One fundamental assumption in mechanical heart modeling is that the heart tissue is spatially continuous (Chadwick 1982). That is, regardless of spatial resolution, the tissue properties and behavior can be represented by a continuous function. Let us consider a piece of the myocardium occupying a region $\mathbf{B}_t$ in space with volume V_t at time t. According to the continuum assumption, each particle of this piece of tissue has a position $x = (x_1, x_2, x_3)$, where x_i is a continuous variable defined over the region occupied by the tissue, that is, $x \in \mathbf{B}_t$. For example, the continuity assumption implies that the volume of the considered piece of tissue is given by the following integral equation:

$$V_t = \iiint_{x_1, x_2, x_3 \in \mathbf{B}_t} dx_1 \cdot dx_2 \cdot dx_3. \tag{6.19}$$

6.3.1 REFERENCE CONFIGURATION

The positions of all the particles representing the tissue at time $t = t_o$ are referred to as the *reference configuration* or the *undeformed configuration*, as shown in Figure 6.1. The particles of this configuration are called the *material points*. The mathematical convention is to write the coordinates of the reference configuration with capital letters; that is, $x = X$ at $t = t_o$, where $X = (X_1, X_2, X_3)$.

Similar to the coordinate variables x_i, the variables X_i are also continuous but defined over the region occupied by the tissue at t_o. To emphasize the convention that there are two different coordinate systems, we rewrite the volume equation in the undeformed configuration as

$$V_o = \iiint_{X_1, X_2, X_3 \in \mathbf{B}_o} dX_1 \cdot dX_2 \cdot dX_3. \tag{6.20}$$

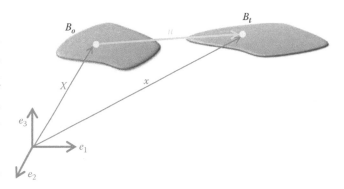

FIGURE 6.1 Reference and deformed configurations. Tissue deformation is represented by the displacement, u, of each particle from the reference configuration, B_o, to the deformed configuration, B_t.

As will be discussed later, if a tissue is incompressible, then its volume will be the same at every configuration, for example, $V_o = V_t$ for all t.

It is worth noting that in cardiac functional analysis, the end-diastolic (ED) phase is usually considered the reference configuration. The reason is that most electrocardiogram (ECG)-gated imaging techniques start data acquisition immediately after the QRS wave of the ECG, that is, at ED. Nevertheless, from a mathematical point of view, the reference configuration can be taken at any point in the cardiac cycle.

6.3.2 DEFORMED CONFIGURATION

A deforming (e.g., contracting or stretching) tissue has its particles moved from their reference position, X, at time t_o to a new position, x, at time t. The new arrangement of particles' positions are referred to as the *deformed configuration*, as shown in Figure 6.1. Because the tissue particles cannot vanish or be duplicated (assuming that the tissue is incompressible and cannot be ruptured), then there is a one-to-one mapping between the reference and deformed configurations. That is, the position of a tissue particle in the deformed configuration can be written as a function of the particle's position in the reference configuration and vice versa.

6.3.3 LAGRANGIAN DESCRIPTION OF DEFORMATION

If the particle's position in the reference configuration X is chosen as the independent variable, then, at time t, the particle's position in the deformed configuration can be written as a continuous function as follows:

$$x = x(X, t). \tag{6.21}$$

To study tissue deformation, one needs to determine the displacement of each particle as shown in Figure 6.1. The displacement of a particle which moved from position X to position x is a vector, u, given by

$$u(X, t) = x - X. \tag{6.22}$$

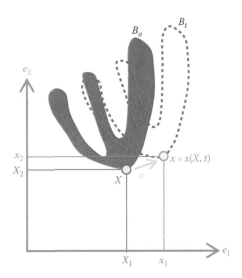

FIGURE 6.2 Lagrangian description of deformation. Each material point (e.g., myocardium tissue particle) is studied while tracking it from the reference (B_o; red) to the deformed (B_t; dotted) configuration. The example here illustrates the apex movement.

Equations 6.21 and 6.22 represent a *Lagrangian* description of deformation where, at any time point, one is concerned only with the deformation of each particle with respect to the reference configuration, that is, the material points. For example, in cardiac image analysis of a sequence of timeframes throughout the cardiac cycle, one might be interested in estimating some mechanical property, for example, stiffness, of the apex at each timeframe. In this case, the apex is considered a material point, and thus at each timeframe we need to locate its new position, $x(X, t)$, and calculate the stiffness at this location (see Figure 6.2).

6.3.4 EULERIAN DESCRIPTION OF DEFORMATION

If, on the other hand, the particle's position in the deformed configuration is chosen as the independent variable, then the reference position of this particle can be represented as

$$X = X(x,t). \tag{6.23}$$

In this case, the displacement of this particle is given by

$$u(x,t) = X - x. \tag{6.24}$$

Equations 6.23 and 6.24 represent the *Eulerian* description of deformation where, at any time point, one observes the deformation at a fixed location in the deformed configuration (see Figure 6.3). For example, given a sequence of images of the aorta, it is sometimes required to estimate the speed of blood flow at certain location inside the vessel lumen. In this case, we do the calculations at a specific location in the lumen, x, ignoring the fact that the blood particles at this location at time t are not the same as those at time t_o.

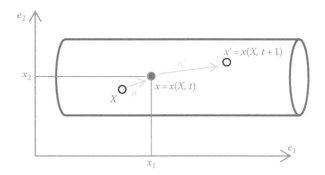

FIGURE 6.3 Eulerian description of deformation. It is more suitable to study fluid dynamics using the Eulerian description, where the speed (or flow) of the material points is studied at fixed points in space, for example, the point (x_1, x_2).

6.4 DEFORMATION

When the myocardium deforms, the analysis of the displacement distribution of its particles, or material points, is important to reveal the underlying heart mechanics. In this perspective, Equation 6.22 is usually rewritten as

$$x = X + u(X,t). \tag{6.25}$$

Depending on the functional form of $u(X, t)$, there are different types of deformation that can be experienced by the tissue.

6.4.1 HOMOGENEOUS DEFORMATION

The main feature of homogeneous deformation is that the deformation parameters are independent of the particle's location. That is, in this type of motion, the particle's position in the deformed configuration is given by

$$x(t) = \mathbf{A}(t)X + d(t), \tag{6.26}$$

where $\mathbf{A}(t)$ is a second-order tensor with constant entries (independent of the elements of X) that applies deformation to the tissue particles from certain time point to another and $d(t)$ is a constant global translation vector.

6.4.2 RIGID-BODY MOTION

Rigid-body motion is a special case of homogeneous deformation, which is usually used to describe global motion of the studied object. The global displacement of the heart caused by respiratory motion or patient movements is just one example of rigid-body motion. A main feature distinguishing rigid-body motion is that the distance between any two material points is preserved in all deformed configurations. In general, there are two types of rigid-body motions: translation and rotation. The general equation for a particle's position at time t when the tissue undergoes both translation and rotation is given by

$$x = \mathbf{R}(t)(X - c) + d(t), \tag{6.27}$$

where

$\mathbf{R}(t)$ is a rotation matrix about the origin

$\boldsymbol{c}$ is a constant vector representing the center of rotation

$\boldsymbol{d}(t)$ is a translation vector

Initially, $\mathbf{R}(0) = \mathbf{I}$, where $\mathbf{I}$ is the identity matrix, and $\boldsymbol{d}(0) = \boldsymbol{c}$. As can be seen from Equation 6.27, the parameters of motion, namely, $\mathbf{R}(t)$, $\boldsymbol{d}(t)$, and $\boldsymbol{c}$, are independent of $\boldsymbol{X}$. It is worth noting that the general case of motion is nonrigid, where the distances between the material points change with time.

6.4.3 DEFORMATION GRADIENT

Usually, it is more interesting to examine the behavior of two adjacent material points. For example, the local function of the myocardium can be evaluated by calculating the change in tissue length that takes place between end-diastole (ED) and end-systole (ES). Consider a myocardium point that has the coordinates $\boldsymbol{X}$ in the reference configuration and undergoes a displacement $\boldsymbol{u}(\boldsymbol{X}, t)$ to move to point $\boldsymbol{x}$ in the deformed configuration, where

$$\boldsymbol{x} = \boldsymbol{X} + \boldsymbol{u}(\boldsymbol{X}, t). \tag{6.28}$$

Similarly, a material point located at $\boldsymbol{X} + d\boldsymbol{X}$, where $d\boldsymbol{X} = (dX_1, dX_2, dX_3)$, would have a displacement $\boldsymbol{u}(\boldsymbol{X} + d\boldsymbol{X}, t)$ and move to point $\boldsymbol{x} + d\boldsymbol{x}$. Substituting in Equation 6.25, then

$$\boldsymbol{x} + d\boldsymbol{x} = (\boldsymbol{X} + d\boldsymbol{X}) + \boldsymbol{u}(\boldsymbol{X} + d\boldsymbol{X}, t). \tag{6.29}$$

Subtracting Equation 6.28 from Equation 6.29 results in

$$d\boldsymbol{x} = (\mathbf{I} + \nabla \boldsymbol{u}) d\boldsymbol{X}, \tag{6.30}$$

where $(\nabla \boldsymbol{u}) d\boldsymbol{X}$ is the displacement gradient along the direction of $d\boldsymbol{X}$. The displacement gradient, $\nabla \boldsymbol{u}$, is a 2D matrix defined by

$$\nabla \boldsymbol{u} = \begin{bmatrix} \dfrac{\partial u_1}{\partial X_1} & \dfrac{\partial u_1}{\partial X_2} & \dfrac{\partial u_1}{\partial X_3} \\ \dfrac{\partial u_2}{\partial X_1} & \dfrac{\partial u_2}{\partial X_2} & \dfrac{\partial u_2}{\partial X_3} \\ \dfrac{\partial u_3}{\partial X_1} & \dfrac{\partial u_3}{\partial X_2} & \dfrac{\partial u_3}{\partial X_3} \end{bmatrix}. \tag{6.31}$$

The *deformation gradient* is defined as

$$\mathbf{F} = \mathbf{I} + \nabla \boldsymbol{u}, \tag{6.32}$$

then, Equation 6.30 can be written as

$$d\boldsymbol{x} = \mathbf{F} d\boldsymbol{X}. \tag{6.33}$$

Since the mapping from the reference to the deformed configurations is one-to-one, then the deformation gradient is invertible, and thus

$$d\boldsymbol{X} = \mathbf{F}^{-1} d\boldsymbol{x}. \tag{6.34}$$

It can be noticed that if the deformation gradient, $\mathbf{F}$, is given by a constant matrix everywhere in the tissue, then we have a homogeneous deformation. In addition, if $\mathbf{F}$ is equal to the identity matrix everywhere in the tissue, then the tissue is at most undergoing translation; that is, there is no deformation or rotation.

As a second-order tensor, the deformation gradient, $\mathbf{F}$, can be decomposed (using *polar decomposition*) into the product of two tensors, that is,

$$\mathbf{F} = \mathbf{RU}, \tag{6.35}$$

where

$\mathbf{R}$ is an orthogonal tensor representing rotation

$\mathbf{U}$ is a positive definite symmetric tensor representing stretch

6.4.4 DEFORMATION AND STRAIN TENSORS

Now, let us consider the question of how the distance, dS, between two material points in the reference configuration is related to that, ds, in the deformed configuration. First, notice that, using the Euclidian distance, the length ds can be calculated by the dot product between the differential vector, $d\boldsymbol{x}$, and itself, that is,

$$ds^2 = \|d\boldsymbol{x}\|^2 = d\boldsymbol{x} \cdot d\boldsymbol{x}. \tag{6.36}$$

Using Equation 6.33, the distance in the deformed configuration can be written as

$$ds^2 = \mathbf{F} d\boldsymbol{X} \cdot \mathbf{F} d\boldsymbol{X} = d\boldsymbol{X} \cdot (\mathbf{F}^\mathrm{T}\mathbf{F}) d\boldsymbol{X}, \tag{6.37}$$

That is,

$$ds^2 = d\boldsymbol{X} \cdot \mathbf{C} d\boldsymbol{X}, \tag{6.38}$$

where the matrix $\mathbf{C}$ is known as the *right Cauchy–Green deformation tensor*, given by

$$\mathbf{C} = \mathbf{F}^\mathrm{T}\mathbf{F}. \tag{6.39}$$

It is worth noting that for rigid-body motions, that is, when $ds = dS$, the tensor $\mathbf{C} = \mathbf{I}$. From Equation 6.32, we have

$$\mathbf{C} = \mathbf{F}^\mathrm{T}\mathbf{F} = (\mathbf{I} + \nabla \boldsymbol{u})^\mathrm{T} (\mathbf{I} + \nabla \boldsymbol{u}). \tag{6.40}$$

That is,

$$\mathbf{C} = \mathbf{I} + \nabla \boldsymbol{u} + (\nabla \boldsymbol{u})^\mathrm{T} + (\nabla \boldsymbol{u})^\mathrm{T} (\nabla \boldsymbol{u}). \tag{6.41}$$

From Equations 6.35 and 6.39, and noticing that $\mathbf{R}^\mathrm{T}\mathbf{R} = \mathbf{I}$, the right Cauchy–Green deformation tensor can be represented by

$$\mathbf{C} = \mathbf{U}^2. \tag{6.42}$$

6.4.4.1 Lagrangian Strain Tensor

Let

$$\mathbf{E}^* = \frac{1}{2}\left[\nabla u + \left(\nabla u\right)^T + \left(\nabla u\right)^T\left(\nabla u\right)\right], \qquad (6.43)$$

then Equation 6.43 becomes

$$\mathbf{E}^* = \frac{1}{2}\left(\mathbf{C} - \mathbf{I}\right) = \frac{1}{2}\left(\mathbf{F}^T\mathbf{F} - \mathbf{I}\right). \qquad (6.44)$$

The tensor $\mathbf{E}^*$ is known as the *Lagrangian strain tensor*, which characterizes the *change* in length between the reference and deformed configurations.

6.4.4.2 Eulerian Strain Tensor

To describe strain in terms of spatial coordinates in the deformed configuration, let us define the *Eulerian strain tensor* as

$$\mathbf{e}^* = \frac{1}{2}\left(\mathbf{I} - \left(\mathbf{F}\mathbf{F}^T\right)^{-1}\right) = \frac{1}{2}\left(\mathbf{I} - \mathbf{B}^{-1}\right), \qquad (6.45)$$

where $\mathbf{B} = \mathbf{F}\mathbf{F}^T$ is the *left Cauchy–Green deformation tensor*. To illustrate the geometric meaning of the components of $\mathbf{e}^*$, let us consider two vectors in the deformed configuration, $dx = ds n_1$ and $dx' = ds' n_2$. Using Equation 6.34, and denoting the corresponding differential vectors in the reference configuration by $dX = dS m_1$ and $dX' = dS' m_2$, then

$$dX \cdot dX' = \mathbf{F}^{-1}dx \cdot \mathbf{F}^{-1}dx' = dx \cdot \left(\mathbf{F}\mathbf{F}^T\right)^{-1}dx' = dx \cdot \mathbf{B}^{-1}dx'. \qquad (6.46)$$

That is, if $dS^2 = dX \cdot dX$, then

$$\frac{dS^2}{ds^2} = [\mathbf{B}^{-1}]_{11}, \qquad (6.47)$$

where the right-hand side of Equation 6.47 represents the first diagonal element in the tensor $\mathbf{B}^{-1}$. It can also be shown that

$$\frac{ds^2 - dS^2}{2ds^2} = \mathbf{e}^*_{11}. \qquad (6.48)$$

Similar relations can be derived for the other diagonal elements of $\mathbf{B}^{-1}$ and $\mathbf{e}^*$. It can be also shown that

$$\frac{dSdS'}{dsds'}\cos(\theta) = [\mathbf{B}^{-1}]_{11}, \qquad (6.49)$$

where θ is the angle between the vectors m_1 and m_2. In terms of the spatial displacement in the deformed configuration, the Eulerian strain tensor can be written as

$$\mathbf{e}^* = \frac{1}{2}\left[\nabla_t u + \left(\nabla_t u\right)^T - \left(\nabla_t u\right)\left(\nabla_t u\right)^T\right], \qquad (6.50)$$

where the gradient operator, ∇_t, is applied with respect to the coordinates of the deformed configuration, that is,

$$\nabla_t u = \begin{bmatrix} \dfrac{\partial u_1}{\partial x_1} & \dfrac{\partial u_1}{\partial x_2} & \dfrac{\partial u_1}{\partial x_3} \\[2mm] \dfrac{\partial u_2}{\partial x_1} & \dfrac{\partial u_2}{\partial x_2} & \dfrac{\partial u_2}{\partial x_3} \\[2mm] \dfrac{\partial u_3}{\partial x_1} & \dfrac{\partial u_3}{\partial x_2} & \dfrac{\partial u_3}{\partial x_3} \end{bmatrix}. \qquad (6.51)$$

6.4.4.3 Infinitesimal Strain Tensor

When the displacement gradient is very small, the second-order terms in Equation 6.41 can be ignored; that is,

$$\mathbf{C} \approx \mathbf{I} + 2\mathbf{E}, \qquad (6.52)$$

where $\mathbf{E}$ is called the *infinitesimal strain tensor*, given by

$$\mathbf{E} = \frac{1}{2}\left(\nabla u + \left(\nabla u\right)^T\right). \qquad (6.53)$$

From Equation 6.31, recall that

$$\nabla u = \begin{bmatrix} \dfrac{\partial u_1}{\partial X_1} & \dfrac{\partial u_1}{\partial X_2} & \dfrac{\partial u_1}{\partial X_3} \\[2mm] \dfrac{\partial u_2}{\partial X_1} & \dfrac{\partial u_2}{\partial X_2} & \dfrac{\partial u_2}{\partial X_3} \\[2mm] \dfrac{\partial u_3}{\partial X_1} & \dfrac{\partial u_3}{\partial X_2} & \dfrac{\partial u_3}{\partial X_3} \end{bmatrix}, \qquad (6.54)$$

and thus, the infinitesimal strain tensor $\mathbf{E}$ can be written as

$$\mathbf{E} = \begin{bmatrix} \dfrac{\partial u_1}{\partial X_1} & \dfrac{1}{2}\left(\dfrac{\partial u_1}{\partial X_2} + \dfrac{\partial u_2}{\partial X_1}\right) & \dfrac{1}{2}\left(\dfrac{\partial u_1}{\partial X_3} + \dfrac{\partial u_3}{\partial X_1}\right) \\[3mm] \dfrac{1}{2}\left(\dfrac{\partial u_1}{\partial X_2} + \dfrac{\partial u_2}{\partial X_1}\right) & \dfrac{\partial u_2}{\partial X_2} & \dfrac{1}{2}\left(\dfrac{\partial u_2}{\partial X_3} + \dfrac{\partial u_3}{\partial X_2}\right) \\[3mm] \dfrac{1}{2}\left(\dfrac{\partial u_1}{\partial X_3} + \dfrac{\partial u_3}{\partial X_1}\right) & \dfrac{1}{2}\left(\dfrac{\partial u_2}{\partial X_3} + \dfrac{\partial u_3}{\partial X_2}\right) & \dfrac{\partial u_3}{\partial X_3} \end{bmatrix}. \qquad (6.55)$$

Similar formulas for tensor $\mathbf{E}$ can be written in the cylindrical and spherical coordinate systems (Slaughter 2002).

6.4.4.3.1 Normal and Shear Strains

To understand the meaning of the strain tensor, let us consider a differential vector, $dX = dS n$, that represents a line segment connecting two closely-located material points, where dS is its length and n is a unit vector indicating its direction. In the deformed configuration, let the vector dX be deformed to a vector dx whose length is ds. Substituting Equation 6.52 into Equation 6.38 yields

$$ds^2 = dX \cdot \mathbf{C}dX = dX \cdot \left(dX + 2\mathbf{E}dX\right), \qquad (6.56)$$

or

$$ds^2 = dS^2 + 2dS^2 \left(\boldsymbol{n} \cdot \mathbf{E}\boldsymbol{n} \right), \qquad (6.57)$$

which can be written as

$$\boldsymbol{n} \cdot \mathbf{E}\boldsymbol{n} = \frac{ds^2 - dS^2}{2dS^2} = \frac{(ds - dS)(ds + dS)}{2dS^2} \approx \frac{ds - dS}{dS}. \qquad (6.58)$$

The last approximation in this equation is directly deduced from the infinitesimal deformation assumption, where the length ds is very similar to dS, and thus the term $(ds + dS) \approx 2dS$. Equation 6.58 shows that the relative change in the tissue's length along any direction, $\boldsymbol{n}$, can be calculated by simple matrix–vector multiplication given by $\boldsymbol{n} \cdot \mathbf{E}\boldsymbol{n}$. One case that is of a special interest to us is when the direction of the vector $d\boldsymbol{X}$ is aligned with any of the principal coordinate axes. For example, when $\boldsymbol{n} = \begin{bmatrix} 1 & 0 & 0 \end{bmatrix}^T$, then

$$\boldsymbol{n} \cdot \mathbf{E}\boldsymbol{n} = E_{11} = \frac{\partial u_1}{\partial X_1} = \frac{ds - dS}{dS}, \qquad (6.59)$$

where E_{ii} is the ith element in the diagonal of the tensor $\mathbf{E}$. Similarly, the other diagonal elements are given by $E_{22} = (\partial u_2 / \partial X_2) = (ds - dS)/dS$ and $E_{33} = (\partial u_3 / \partial X_3) = (ds - dS)/dS$. The diagonal elements of the tensor $\mathbf{E}$ are known as *normal strains*.

It is also interesting to consider the geometric meaning of the off-diagonal elements of the tensor $\mathbf{E}$. First, let us consider two perpendicular tissue line segments $d\boldsymbol{X} = dS\boldsymbol{n}$ and $d\boldsymbol{X}' = dS'\boldsymbol{n}'$. In the deformed configuration, let the two segments deform to $d\boldsymbol{x}$ and $d\boldsymbol{x}'$ with lengths ds and ds', respectively. Let the angle between the two vectors $d\boldsymbol{x}$ and $d\boldsymbol{x}'$ be denoted by θ. Then,

$$d\boldsymbol{x} \cdot d\boldsymbol{x}' = \mathbf{F}d\boldsymbol{X} \cdot \mathbf{F}d\boldsymbol{X}' = d\boldsymbol{X} \cdot \mathbf{C}d\boldsymbol{X}'. \qquad (6.60)$$

Substitution from Equation 6.52 yields

$$d\boldsymbol{x} \cdot d\boldsymbol{x}' = d\boldsymbol{X} \cdot d\boldsymbol{X}' + 2d\boldsymbol{X} \cdot \mathbf{E}d\boldsymbol{X}'. \qquad (6.61)$$

From the orthogonality of $d\boldsymbol{X}$ and $d\boldsymbol{X}'$, the first term in the right-hand side vanishes; then using the definition of inner product between two vectors, we have

$$ds \, ds' \cos(\theta) = \left(2dS \, dS'\right)\mathbf{n} \cdot \mathbf{E}\boldsymbol{n}'. \qquad (6.62)$$

Now, let $\varphi = \pi/2 - \theta$, where φ is the change in the angle between the two vectors that takes place during tissue deformation from the reference configuration to the deformed configuration (at time t). The angular change, φ, is referred to as the *shear strain*. Using the assumption of very small deformation, which implies that $\sin(\varphi) \approx \varphi$, $ds \approx dS$, and $ds' \approx dS'$, we get the following useful formula for calculating the shear strain:

$$\varphi = 2\boldsymbol{n} \cdot \mathbf{E}\boldsymbol{n}'. \qquad (6.63)$$

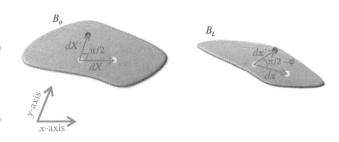

FIGURE 6.4 General body deformation inducing a shear strain that represents the angular change between two vectors.

The special case when the two vectors are aligned with the coordinate axes (as shown in Figure 6.4) can be useful to understand the meaning of off-diagonal elements of the tensor $\mathbf{E}$ as follows. First, let $\mathbf{n}$ and $\mathbf{n}'$ be aligned with the x- and y-axes, then it can be shown that

$$\varphi = 2E_{12} = \frac{\partial u_1}{\partial X_2} + \frac{\partial u_2}{\partial X_1}. \qquad (6.64)$$

Similarly, if $\mathbf{n}$ and $\mathbf{n}'$ are aligned with the x- and z-axes, then

$$\varphi = 2E_{13} = \frac{\partial u_1}{\partial X_3} + \frac{\partial u_3}{\partial X_1}, \qquad (6.65)$$

and if $\mathbf{n}$ and $\mathbf{n}'$ are aligned with the y- and z-axes, then

$$\varphi = 2E_{23} = \frac{\partial u_2}{\partial X_3} + \frac{\partial u_3}{\partial X_2}. \qquad (6.66)$$

6.4.4.4 Infinitesimal Rotation Tensor

When expressing the displacement gradient, $\nabla\boldsymbol{u}$, as a sum of symmetric and antisymmetric components, we get

$$\nabla\boldsymbol{u} = \frac{1}{2}\left(\nabla\boldsymbol{u} + \left(\nabla\boldsymbol{u}\right)^{\mathrm{T}}\right) + \frac{1}{2}\left(\nabla\boldsymbol{u} - \left(\nabla\boldsymbol{u}\right)^{\mathrm{T}}\right). \qquad (6.67)$$

Assuming infinitesimal deformation, then the symmetric term in this equation is the infinitesimal strain tensor, $\mathbf{E}$, defined by Equation 6.53. The antisymmetric (a.k.a. skew-symmetric) term is referred to as the *infinitesimal rotation tensor*

$$\boldsymbol{\Omega} = \frac{1}{2}\left(\nabla\boldsymbol{u} - \left(\nabla\boldsymbol{u}\right)^{\mathrm{T}}\right). \qquad (6.68)$$

One important characteristic of an antisymmetric tensor is that it contains only three independent components. This is because the diagonal elements are canceled out, $\Omega_{ii} = 0$, and the upper off-diagonal elements are the negatives of the lower off-diagonal elements, that is, $\Omega_{ij} = -\Omega_{ji}$. Let the three independent components of the rotation tensor $\boldsymbol{\Omega}$ form a vector $\boldsymbol{\omega}$; then given a vector, $\boldsymbol{x}$, it can be shown that (Lai et al. 2009)

$$\boldsymbol{u} = \boldsymbol{\Omega}\boldsymbol{x} = \boldsymbol{\omega} \times \boldsymbol{x}. \qquad (6.69)$$

That is, the antisymmetric part of the displacement gradient has indeed an effect of uniform rotation about the origin.

6.4.4.5 Principal Strains

The eigenvectors of a symmetric tensor, $\mathbf{E}$, are mutually orthogonal, and can therefore be used to diagonalize the tensor. That is, if the eigenvectors of $\mathbf{E}$ are given by $\boldsymbol{n}_1$, $\boldsymbol{n}_2$, and $\boldsymbol{n}_3$, then

$$\mathbf{N}^{\mathrm{T}}\mathbf{E}\mathbf{N} = \begin{bmatrix} \lambda_1 & 0 & 0 \\ 0 & \lambda_2 & 0 \\ 0 & 0 & \lambda_3 \end{bmatrix}, \quad (6.70)$$

where $\mathbf{N}$ is a matrix whose columns are $\boldsymbol{n}_1$, $\boldsymbol{n}_2$, and $\boldsymbol{n}_3$. The directions of these eigenvectors are known as the *principal directions*, and the corresponding eigenvalues, λ_1, λ_2, and λ_3, are known as the *principal strains*. Now, in Equation 6.63, let $\boldsymbol{n} = \boldsymbol{n}_i$ and $\boldsymbol{n}' = \boldsymbol{n}_j$ with $i \neq j$; then

$$\varphi = 2\boldsymbol{n}_i \cdot \mathbf{E}\boldsymbol{n}_j = 2\mathrm{E}_{ij} = 0. \quad (6.71)$$

That is, any pair of perpendicular line segments aligned in the directions of $\boldsymbol{n}_1$, $\boldsymbol{n}_2$, and $\boldsymbol{n}_3$ will remain perpendicular in the deformed configuration. Moreover, the change in the length of a line segment, that is, $(ds - dS)$, originally oriented along the $\boldsymbol{n}_i$ direction is given by $\lambda_i dS$. It is worth noting that, in the general case, the line segment in the deformed configuration, $d\boldsymbol{x}$, does not remain in its original direction; that is, $d\boldsymbol{x} \neq \lambda_i dS\boldsymbol{n}_i$.

6.4.5 Volume Change under Deformation

Consider a rectangular parallelepiped in a given reference configuration whose sides are aligned with the principal directions and have lengths dS_1, dS_2, and dS_3. The volume of this parallelepiped in the reference configuration is thus given by

$$dV_0 = dS_1 dS_2 dS_3. \quad (6.72)$$

From the previous section, the volume of the parallelepiped in the deformed configuration is given by

$$dV = ds_1 ds_2 ds_3 = (1+\lambda_1)dS_1(1+\lambda_2)dS_2(1+\lambda_3)dS_3. \quad (6.73)$$

Ignoring higher-order terms of λ_i, the change in the volume per unit reference volume is referred to as the *dilation*, D_v, and is given by

$$D_v = \frac{dV - dV_0}{dV_0} \approx \lambda_1 + \lambda_2 + \lambda_3. \quad (6.74)$$

Recalling the definition of the tensor $\mathbf{E}$, the dilation is also given by

$$D_v = \frac{\partial u_1}{\partial X_1} + \frac{\partial u_2}{\partial X_2} + \frac{\partial u_3}{\partial X_3} = \mathrm{div}\,\boldsymbol{u}. \quad (6.75)$$

When the tissue does not change in volume during deformation, that is, $dV = dV_0$, the tissue is said to be *incompressible* and the deformation is said to be *isochoric*. In this case,

$$D_v = \mathrm{div}\,\boldsymbol{u} = 0. \quad (6.76)$$

It should be noticed that the incompressibility property given by Equation 6.76 is practically valid in almost all soft tissues, and hence it is widely used for mechanical modeling of the heart tissue.

6.4.6 Applied Forces and Stress Tensor

Stress represents the amount of force per unit area exerted on any point of a given body. While force is represented by a vector whose elements vary from one location to another, stress is represented by a second-order tensor, that is, a matrix. That is, stress not only depends on the location of the point within the body, but also on the direction of the plane passing through this point. For example, let us consider a plane (out of possibly infinite number of planes) passing through a given point $\boldsymbol{x} = [x_1, x_2, x_3]^{\mathrm{T}}$ and forming a tetrahedron by its intersections with the coordinate planes as shown in Figure 6.5. Let this plane be represented by its normal vector, $\boldsymbol{n}$. Then, the force per unit area, $\boldsymbol{\sigma}$, exerted on this plane at point $\boldsymbol{x}$ has three components along the three principal axes, that is, $\boldsymbol{\sigma} = [\sigma_1, \sigma_2, \sigma_3]^{\mathrm{T}}$. If the plane is rotated in any direction, then the three stress components will change accordingly. Representing these stress components as a linear function of the components of vector $\boldsymbol{n}$ yields

$$\boldsymbol{\sigma} = \mathbf{t}\,\boldsymbol{n}, \quad (6.77)$$

where

  $\mathbf{t}$ is a (second-order) stress tensor whose elements can be given as functions of x_1, x_2, and x_3
  $\boldsymbol{\sigma}$ is the stress for a specific plane orientation $\boldsymbol{n}$

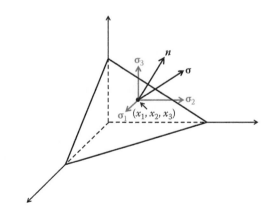

FIGURE 6.5 Traction vectors on the surface of a tetrahedron. The main force, $\boldsymbol{\sigma}$, is shown decomposed into its components in the direction of the three main axes. Vector $\boldsymbol{n}$ is normal to the plane.

Although the tensor **t** contains nine elements, it can be shown that it is a symmetric tensor containing only six independent components (Slaughter 2002, Lai et al. 2009), that is,

$$\mathbf{t} = \begin{bmatrix} t_{11} & t_{12} & t_{13} \\ t_{12} & t_{22} & t_{23} \\ t_{13} & t_{23} & t_{33} \end{bmatrix}. \qquad (6.78)$$

It is worth noting that **t** is referred to as *Cauchy Stress Tensor*, which is the stress measured in the deformed configuration. On the other hand, stress tensors can be defined in the undeformed configuration, which are known as *Piola–Kirchhoff stress tensors*.

To understand the meaning of the different components of the stress tensor, consider a patch of area ΔA on a plane passing through *x* with *n* parallel to the *x*-axis. Then, an arbitrary force, $\Delta f = [\Delta f_1, \Delta f_2, \Delta f_3]^T$ passing through *x*, would result in stresses in the three main directions given by $\sigma = [t_{11}, t_{12}, t_{13}]^T = [\Delta f_1/\Delta A, \Delta f_2/\Delta A, \Delta f_3/\Delta A]^T$. That is, t_{11} represents the stress normal to the plane (along *x*-direction), while t_{12} and t_{13} represent the *shear stress* components. Similar interpretation can be made for the other components of the stress tensor.

Similar to those of the strain tensors, the eigenvectors of the stress tensors are of special importance. They represent the directions of three orthogonal planes that experience only normal stress, that is, no shear stress. These planes are referred to as the *principal planes* and the corresponding stresses (eigenvalues) are known as the *principal stresses*.

6.5 CONSTITUTIVE EQUATIONS

In the previous sections, the strain and stress tensors were defined and discussed independently. In this section, we introduce the relationship between both quantities, which is defined by the constitutive equations. Constitutive equations are mathematical models that are used to describe the response (e.g., in terms of strain) of a given material when it experiences some activity (e.g., external stress). That is, the mathematical form and parameters of the constitutive equations are determined solely based on the assumptions made about the material. In the following sections, we will introduce some frequently used constitutive equations that allow *theoretical* modeling and prediction of the material mechanical properties. It is worth noting that thermal conditions play an important role in continuum mechanics; for example, heating a piece of tissue induces strain and stress distribution depending on the tissue type. Nevertheless, in the following sections, we assume isothermal conditions, unless explicitly mentioned otherwise.

6.5.1 Elastic Materials

An elastic material tends to completely return to its original shape upon removal of the forces that cause the deformation.

6.5.1.1 Cauchy Elastic Materials

A *Cauchy elastic material* (also referred to as simple, or ideal, elastic material) is a material whose stress at any given point is determined only by the current state of deformation, and vice versa; that is, there is one-to-one mapping between stress and deformation. At a given point, the constitutive equation of a Cauchy elastic material is given by

$$\mathbf{t} = \mathbf{t}(\mathbf{F}), \qquad (6.79)$$

where

t is the Cauchy stress tensor
F is the deformation gradient with respect to an arbitrary reference configuration
$\mathbf{t}(\cdot)$ is a function that maps 2D matrices into second-order tensors

The material coefficients that specify the constitutive relationship between the stress and strain components are assumed to be constant during the deformation, for example, independent of deformation, gravity, or inertia. It follows from the above definition that the stress in a Cauchy elastic material does not depend on the deformation history that induced the state of current deformation, for example, the time-deformation curve. It also implies that the stress at a given point depends only on the deformation within an infinitesimal neighborhood of that point regardless of the deformation of the rest of the body.

6.5.1.2 Hyperelastic Materials

A *hyperelastic* (or *Green elastic*) material is a special case of Cauchy's elasticity, where the stress–strain relation is derived from the strain energy density function $W(\mathbf{E})$, such that the stress component, t_{ij}, in Equation 6.78 is given by

$$t_{ij} = \frac{\partial W}{\partial E_{ij}}, \qquad (6.80)$$

where E_{ij} is the corresponding element of the infinitesimal strain tensor defined in Equation 6.53. The strain energy density function W is usually given in the form of a polynomial function (using Taylor's series expansion) of the strain elements. For example, the strain energy density function of the Venant–Kirchhoff model is given by

$$W(\mathbf{E}) = \frac{\lambda}{2}\left[tr(\mathbf{E})\right]^2 + \mu\, tr(\mathbf{E}^2), \qquad (6.81)$$

where

λ and μ are Lame coefficients
$tr(\cdot)$ is the trace of a matrix given by the summation of all diagonal elements

The second Lame coefficient, μ, is also known as the shear modulus, while the first Lame coefficient is related to the bulk modulus, K, through the relation $K = \lambda + 2\mu/3$.

6.5.2 Hooke's Law

The constitutive equation of linear elastic (or Hookean) materials is given by $\mathbf{t} = \mathbf{CE}$, where $\mathbf{C}$ is a fourth-order tensor that maps the strain tensor $\mathbf{E}$ to the stress tensor $\mathbf{t}$. Such linear relationship is referred to as Hooke's law and is only a first-order approximation of the actual material response to the applied force. For simplicity, it is common to use the engineering notation to represent this equation, where the elements of the stress and strain tensors are stacked to form stress and strain vectors, respectively. In this case, the mapping can be written in terms of the *stiffness tensor*, $\mathbf{C}$; that is,

$$\begin{bmatrix} t_{11} \\ t_{22} \\ t_{33} \\ t_{12} \\ t_{13} \\ t_{23} \end{bmatrix} = \begin{bmatrix} C_{11} & C_{12} & C_{13} & C_{14} & C_{15} & C_{16} \\ C_{21} & C_{22} & C_{23} & C_{24} & C_{25} & C_{26} \\ C_{31} & C_{32} & C_{33} & C_{34} & C_{35} & C_{36} \\ C_{41} & C_{42} & C_{43} & C_{44} & C_{45} & C_{46} \\ C_{51} & C_{52} & C_{53} & C_{54} & C_{55} & C_{56} \\ C_{61} & C_{62} & C_{63} & C_{64} & C_{65} & C_{66} \end{bmatrix} \begin{bmatrix} E_{11} \\ E_{22} \\ E_{33} \\ 2E_{12} \\ 2E_{13} \\ 2E_{23} \end{bmatrix}. \tag{6.82}$$

The multiplication by a factor of 2 is used to explicitly represent the *engineering* shear strain variables. As mentioned earlier, the stress–strain relation for elastic materials is a one-to-one mapping, which means that the matrix $\mathbf{C}$ has an inverse $\mathbf{G} = \mathbf{C}^{-1}$ (referred to as the *compliance matrix*), which can be used to estimate the strain tensor given the stress tensor. The elements of the compliance matrix, and thus stiffness, are usually determined by engineering quantities such as Young's modulus, Poisson's ratio, shear modulus, etc. *Young's modulus* is a mechanical property of linear elastic solid materials that provides a measure of the force (per unit area) required to stretch a material sample; *Poisson's ratio* is the negative ratio of transverse to axial strain; and *shear modulus* is the ratio of shear stress to shear strain. It is worth noting that the structure of the stiffness matrix depends on the material type. The following are some examples of common materials.

6.5.2.1 Monoclinic Materials

A monoclinic material has a plane of symmetry; therefore, its stiffness matrix can be represented as

$$\mathbf{C} = \begin{bmatrix} C_{11} & C_{12} & C_{13} & 0 & 0 & C_{16} \\ C_{21} & C_{22} & C_{23} & 0 & 0 & C_{26} \\ C_{31} & C_{32} & C_{33} & 0 & 0 & C_{36} \\ 0 & 0 & 0 & C_{44} & C_{45} & 0 \\ 0 & 0 & 0 & C_{45} & C_{55} & 0 \\ C_{16} & C_{26} & C_{36} & 0 & 0 & C_{66} \end{bmatrix}. \tag{6.83}$$

6.5.2.2 Orthotropic Materials

An orthotropic material has two or three mutually orthogonal twofold axes of *rotational symmetry*; therefore, its mechanical properties are different along each axis. Its stiffness matrix is represented as

$$\mathbf{C} = \begin{bmatrix} C_{11} & C_{12} & C_{13} & 0 & 0 & 0 \\ C_{12} & C_{22} & C_{23} & 0 & 0 & 0 \\ C_{13} & C_{23} & C_{33} & 0 & 0 & 0 \\ 0 & 0 & 0 & C_{44} & 0 & 0 \\ 0 & 0 & 0 & 0 & C_{55} & 0 \\ 0 & 0 & 0 & 0 & 0 & C_{66} \end{bmatrix}. \tag{6.84}$$

In terms of engineering material quantities, its compliance matrix is given by

$$\mathbf{G} = \mathbf{C}^{-1} = \begin{bmatrix} \dfrac{1}{\varepsilon_1} & -\dfrac{\nu_{21}}{\varepsilon_2} & -\dfrac{\nu_{31}}{\varepsilon_3} & 0 & 0 & 0 \\ -\dfrac{\nu_{12}}{\varepsilon_1} & \dfrac{1}{\varepsilon_2} & -\dfrac{\nu_{32}}{\varepsilon_3} & 0 & 0 & 0 \\ -\dfrac{\nu_{13}}{\varepsilon_1} & -\dfrac{\nu_{23}}{\varepsilon_2} & \dfrac{1}{\varepsilon_3} & 0 & 0 & 0 \\ 0 & 0 & 0 & \dfrac{1}{\mu_{23}} & 0 & 0 \\ 0 & 0 & 0 & 0 & \dfrac{1}{\mu_{13}} & 0 \\ 0 & 0 & 0 & 0 & 0 & \dfrac{1}{\mu_{12}} \end{bmatrix}, \tag{6.85}$$

where
  ε_i is Young's modulus of the material in the i-direction
  ν_{ij} is Poisson's ratio (strain in the j-direction relative to that in the i-direction when the material is stressed in the i-direction)
  μ_{ij} is the shear modulus in the i–j plane

6.5.2.3 Isotropic Materials

The properties of an isotropic material do not change from direction to another, and it can be shown that the compliance matrix is given by

$$\mathbf{G} = \begin{bmatrix} \dfrac{1}{\varepsilon} & -\dfrac{\nu}{\varepsilon} & -\dfrac{\nu}{\varepsilon} & 0 & 0 & 0 \\ -\dfrac{\nu}{\varepsilon} & \dfrac{1}{\varepsilon} & -\dfrac{\nu}{\varepsilon} & 0 & 0 & 0 \\ -\dfrac{\nu}{\varepsilon} & -\dfrac{\nu}{\varepsilon} & \dfrac{1}{\varepsilon} & 0 & 0 & 0 \\ 0 & 0 & 0 & \dfrac{2(1+\nu)}{\varepsilon} & 0 & 0 \\ 0 & 0 & 0 & 0 & \dfrac{2(1+\nu)}{\varepsilon} & 0 \\ 0 & 0 & 0 & 0 & 0 & \dfrac{2(1+\nu)}{\varepsilon} \end{bmatrix}. \tag{6.86}$$

6.5.2.4 Transverse-Isotropic Materials

In some cases, the material might have stiffness that is symmetric about a certain axis. That is, the material properties are indifferent in a plane perpendicular to the axis of symmetry (Hadjicharalambous et al. 2015). Examples include a bundle of fibers with circular cross sections positioned parallel to the z-axis. In this case, the compliance matrix takes the following form:

$$
\mathbf{G} = \begin{bmatrix}
\dfrac{1}{\varepsilon_p} & -\dfrac{\nu_p}{\varepsilon_p} & -\dfrac{\nu_{fp}}{\varepsilon_f} & 0 & 0 & 0 \\[2mm]
-\dfrac{\nu_p}{\varepsilon_p} & \dfrac{1}{\varepsilon_p} & -\dfrac{\nu_{fp}}{\varepsilon_f} & 0 & 0 & 0 \\[2mm]
-\dfrac{\nu_{pf}}{\varepsilon_p} & -\dfrac{\nu_{pf}}{\varepsilon_p} & \dfrac{1}{\varepsilon_f} & 0 & 0 & 0 \\[2mm]
0 & 0 & 0 & \dfrac{2(1+\nu_p)}{\varepsilon_p} & 0 & 0 \\[2mm]
0 & 0 & 0 & 0 & \dfrac{1}{\mu_f} & 0 \\[2mm]
0 & 0 & 0 & 0 & 0 & \dfrac{1}{\mu_f}
\end{bmatrix},
$$

$$(6.87)$$

where

ε_p and ε_f are Young's modulus values in the plane and the axial directions, respectively

ν_p is Poisson's ratio (when stress is applied in any of the planar directions)

ν_{fp} is Poisson's ratio (when stress is applied along the axial direction)

μ_f is the shear modulus across the axis of symmetry

6.6 CONSERVATION OF MASS AND MOMENTUM

6.6.1 Conservation of Mass

Let ρ be the mass density of a given body $\mathbf{B}_t$. The conservation of mass principle states that the total mass of any part $\tilde{\mathbf{B}}_t \subset \mathbf{B}_t$ is equal to the amount of mass flowing into the volume (v) occupied by this body through its surface. That is,

$$
\frac{d}{dt}\int_{\tilde{\mathbf{B}}_t} \rho\, dv = -\int_{\partial \tilde{\mathbf{B}}_t} \left(\rho \dot{x}\right) \mathbf{n}\, da, \qquad (6.88)
$$

where

$\mathbf{n}\, da$ is a surface patch on the *closed* body surface $\partial \mathbf{B}_t$

da is the area of the patch

$\mathbf{n}$ is a vector normal to the patch

The negative sign is due to the convention that $\mathbf{n}$ is pointing outward the body (indicating the direction of "leaving" the body). From the divergence theory, we can show that, for an infinitesimal volume of the body at location $\mathbf{x}$, the conservation of mass can be represented by

$$
\frac{\partial \rho}{\partial t} + \nabla \cdot (\rho \dot{x}) = 0, \qquad (6.89)
$$

where ∇ is the divergence operator.

6.6.2 Forces and Momenta

Linear momentum and angular momentum (with respect to a point $\mathbf{x}_o$) of a body $\mathbf{B}_t$ are defined by

$$
\text{Lin. momentum} \overset{def}{=} \int_{\mathbf{B}_t} \rho \dot{x}\, dv,
$$

$$(6.90)$$

$$
\text{Ang. momentum} \overset{def}{=} \int_{\mathbf{B}_t} \rho \left(\mathbf{x} - \mathbf{x}_o\right) \times \dot{x}\, dv,
$$

where

ρ is density (mass per unit volume) of the body, which is a function of position $\mathbf{x}$

$\dot{x}$ is the speed of point $\mathbf{x}$

Forces acting on the body cause a change of its momentum. In general, there are two types of forces: body (or internal) forces and surface tractions. Examples of body forces include gravitational, thermal, and electromagnetic forces. The total internal force of a given body $\mathbf{B}_t$ is represented by the integration (over the body volume) of the internal force per unit volume, f. That is,

$$
\text{Total body force} = \int_{\mathbf{B}_t} f\, dv. \qquad (6.91)
$$

Surface tractions are direct stresses applied to the body surface by another body, for example, the force applied to the vessels' surface caused by pulsatile blood flow. The total traction applied to the surface $\partial \mathbf{B}_t$ of a given body is represented by the integration (over the body surface area) of the stress per unit area. That is,

$$
\text{Total traction} = \int_{\partial \mathbf{B}_t} \mathbf{t}\, \mathbf{n}\, da, \qquad (6.92)
$$

where

$\mathbf{t}$ is the stress tensor at the differential patch $\mathbf{n}\, da$ of the *closed* body surface $\partial \mathbf{B}_t$

da is the area of the patch

$\mathbf{n}$ is a vector normal to the patch

6.6.3 Conservation of Momentum

From Newton's second law of motion, the net force acting on an object is equal to the rate of change of linear momentum.

That is, force can be thought of as the time derivative of linear momentum. Mathematically, this is represented by

$$\int_{\mathbf{B}_t} f dv + \int_{\partial \mathbf{B}_t} \mathbf{t}\, n da = \frac{d}{dt} \int_{\mathbf{B}_t} \rho \dot{x} dv. \tag{6.93}$$

Similarly, the following equation represents the conservation of angular momentum:

$$\int_{\mathbf{B}_t} x \times f dv + \int_{\partial \mathbf{B}_t} x \times \mathbf{t}\, n da = \frac{d}{dt} \int_{\mathbf{B}_t} \rho (x - x_o) \times \dot{x} dv. \tag{6.94}$$

6.6.4 Equilibrium Condition and Equations of Motion

From the conservation of momentum principle, the net force acting on a given body $\mathbf{B}_t$ (or even any arbitrary part of the body, $\tilde{\mathbf{B}}_t$) is zero at equilibrium conditions, that is,

$$\int_{\bar{\mathbf{B}}_t} f dv + \int_{\partial \bar{\mathbf{B}}_t} \mathbf{t}\, n da = 0. \tag{6.95}$$

From the divergence theorem in calculus, the second integral in Equation 6.95 can be replaced by an integration over the entire volume instead of the surface. Therefore, Equation 6.95 can be represented as

$$\int_{\bar{\mathbf{B}}_t} (f + \nabla \cdot \mathbf{t}) dv = 0, \tag{6.96}$$

where $\nabla \cdot \mathbf{t}$ is the divergence of the stress tensor $\mathbf{t}$. Since the above integral vanishes for any arbitrary body region $\tilde{\mathbf{B}}_t$, the term inside the integration should be identical to zero, that is,

$$f + \nabla \cdot \mathbf{t} = 0. \tag{6.97}$$

A similar formula for the conservation of angular momentum can be written as

$$\int_{\mathbf{B}_t} x \times f dv + \int_{\partial \mathbf{B}_t} x \times \mathbf{t}\, n da = 0, \tag{6.98}$$

where x is the position vector. Using the divergence theorem, we can arrive at the important property of the stress tensor symmetry, that is,

$$\mathbf{t} = \mathbf{t}^{\mathrm{T}}. \tag{6.99}$$

While deformation is taking place, the *equation of motion* is a differential equation that describes how the material points move in response to the applied forces. From Equation 6.93,

the equation of motion can be deduced using the divergence theorem and is given by

$$f + \nabla \cdot \mathbf{t} = \rho \frac{d}{dt} \dot{x}$$
$$= \rho \ddot{x}. \tag{6.100}$$

6.7 FINITE ELEMENT METHOD

6.7.1 Basic Concept

Analytical (closed-form) solutions of complex mechanical problems are usually not possible. Instead, numerical methods are used to obtain an approximate, yet acceptable, solution. One of the most powerful numerical techniques is the finite element method (FEM). The method is widely used in practice to find numerical solutions to boundary value problems governed by partial differential equations, for example, estimating tissue elasticity, motion, or deformation (Zhang et al. 2012). The FEM method typically includes few major steps:

1. Approximate the geometry of the tissue being studied using a number of small building blocks, the finite elements.
2. Determine the elements' specifications, for example, type, number of nodes, and shape function.
3. Develop the differential equation for each element.
4. Formulate the global problem as an integration of the developed subproblems (each is at the level of the finite elements).
5. Solve the problem to estimate the solution at the nodes of the elements, for example, the displacement of each node.
6. Use the estimated nodal solution to calculate (by interpolation) the solution at any given point within the element.

In the following sections, we will provide a brief overview of some basic concepts of FEM. The objective here is to provide the reader with the background needed in later sections of the chapter as well as in other chapters in the book. For complete discussion of FEM analysis, the reader is recommended to review textbooks on FEM (Reddy 2005, Zienkiewicz et al. 2013).

6.7.2 Shape Approximation

6.7.2.1 Basic Elements

The elements of the FEM model are defined by their dimensionality (one-dimensional (1D), 2D, or 3D), shapes (e.g., triangles or rectangles), and number of nodes. Figure 6.6 shows different elements that are usually used in FEM formulation.

It is worth noting that decomposition of a given structure into a set of smaller elements is not a trivial task and is application-specific. For example, while it is simpler to use the same type of elements to build the model, different element

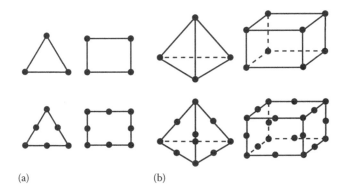

(a)   (b)

FIGURE 6.6 Typical (a) 2D and (b) 3D FEM elements for surface and volume tessellation, respectively. The small black circles represent the nodes for each element. The lower row shows the same elements as in the upper row, but with more number of nodes.

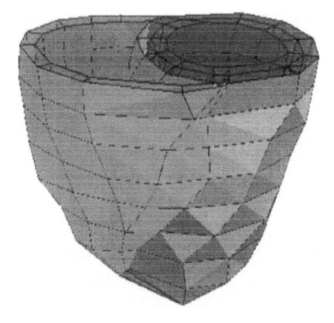

FIGURE 6.7 Finite element model of the left and right ventricles built with different 3D elements. (Reproduced from Haber, I. et al., *Med. Image Anal.*, 4(4), 335, 2000. With permission.)

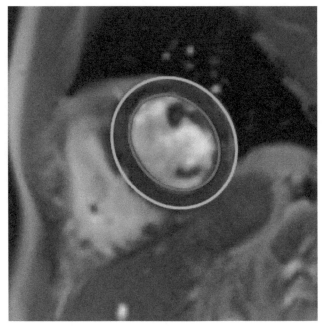

FIGURE 6.8 Cine short-axis image of the heart with the endo- (red) and epicardium (green) segmented.

2D contours can be obtained by manual or automatic segmentation. Figure 6.8 shows endo- and epicardial contours of the LV in a short-axis (SAX) cine MRI image. In other applications, the anatomical structures are determined from the tagged images. Figure 6.9 shows reconstructed taglines superimposed on a SAX tagged image. After obtaining the set of taglines, they are resampled to obtain a set of nodes that will be used later to create the FEM elements. The sampling density is usually increased at the regions of high curvature or with fine details. A 3D mesh is then constructed by connecting the nodes of multiple 2D contours. It is worth noting that the regularity of the elemental shapes shown in Figure 6.6 is usually disrupted due to nonrigid deformation of the object. For example, the straight edges of the elements can take curved shapes of unequal lengths.

6.7.3 GLOBAL AND NATURAL COORDINATE SYSTEMS

Two types of coordinate systems are encountered in FEM. The first type is the *global coordinate system*, which is used to identify the location of a given point relative to the structure, for example, the entire heart. The second type of coordinate system is the *natural coordinate system*, which is used to define a point within an element in terms of its nodes. To illustrate these two types of coordinate system, consider a four-noded 2D rectangular element that is used to tile the surface of the myocardium. Let the four corners of this element be P_1, P_2, P_3, and P_4; that is, $P_i = (x_i, y_i, z_i)$ with $i = 1, 2, 3,$ or 4. For simplicity, let these points be located on the same plane, say, the x–y plane at all deformed configurations; that is, $z_i = 0$. From simple geometric properties, any point within this rectangular

types can be combined to adopt the local shapes of complicated geometries. For example, Haber et al. (2000) used six-noded 3D element to model the apical part of the heart while used eight-noded 3D elements to model the remaining parts, as shown in Figure 6.7. In a more recent study, Zhang et al. (2012) presented a novel atlas-based geometry pipeline for constructing 3D cubic Hermite FEM meshes of the whole human heart from tomographic cardiac images.

6.7.2.2 Mesh Construction

In cardiac analysis, approximating the ventricle's shape using the selected type(s) of elements is done through a number of steps. The first step is to delineate some cardiac anatomical structures to obtain a set of contours. In some applications, the structures of interest are the inner and outer surfaces of the left ventricle (LV). In this case,

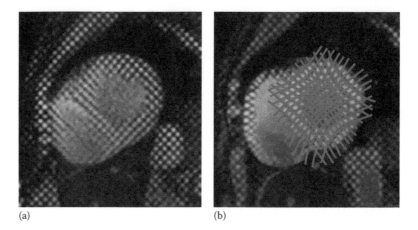

(a) (b)

FIGURE 6.9 Short-axis tagged image of the heart at (a) end-diastole and (b) end-systole. Curves passing through the deformed taglines are shown imposed on the image at end-systole.

element, $P = (x_p, y_p)$, can be represented by a linear combination, or weightings, of the corner points. That is,

$$x_p = \sum_{i=1}^{4} N_i x_i,$$

$$y_p = \sum_{i=1}^{4} N_i y_i,$$

(6.101)

where N_i are weights that can be written in terms of the normalized areas, A_i, of the subrectangles shown in Figure 6.10b; that is, $N_i = A_i/A$, where A is the total area of the element.

A more convenient, and simpler, way of writing these weights is achieved by considering the natural coordinates

of the element. To illustrate the meaning of the natural coordinates, let us isolate the element from the entire mesh and transform it into a standard shape: a square centered in the origin with corner nodes located at (−1, −1), (1, −1), (1, 1), and (−1, 1), as shown in Figure 6.10c. The point P on the new coordinate system is located at (r, s) such that the relative areas of the subrectangles are similar to those on the global coordinates.

Now, if the heart deforms, the rectangular element might deform to an arbitrary quadrilateral shape (orange quadrilateral shape in Figure 6.11a), that is, each node has its own value of displacement. In the natural coordinates, however,

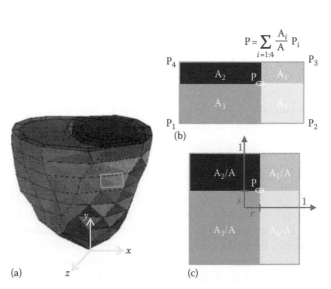

(a) (b) (c)

FIGURE 6.10 Global and natural coordinate systems for a FEM element representation before deformation. (a) Geometrical model of the heart at end-diastole, showing the undeformed element (orange rectangle). (b) Element representation in the global coordinate system. (c) Element representation in the natural coordinate system. (Reproduced from Haber, I. et al., *Med. Image Anal.*, 4(4), 335, 2000. With permission.)

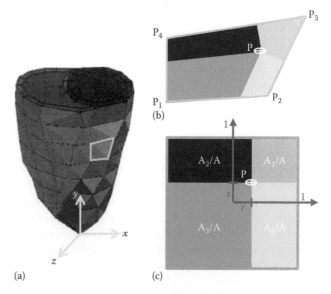

(a) (b) (c)

FIGURE 6.11 Global and natural coordinate systems for a FEM element representation after deformation. (a) Geometrical model of the heart at end-diastole, showing the deformed element (orange quadrilateral shape). (b) Element representation in the global coordinate system. (c) Element representation in the natural coordinate system. (Reproduced from Haber, I. et al., *Med. Image Anal.*, 4(4), 335, 2000. With permission.)

the coordinates of any given element point, (r, s), do not change. We can think of it as if all the points move while maintaining their positions relative to the element nodes governed by the condition that the areas of the subrectangles are kept constant. That is, in the deformed configuration, the new positions are still related to each other by Equation 6.101:

$$x'_p = \sum_{i=1}^{4} N_i x'_i,$$
$$y'_p = \sum_{i=1}^{4} N_i y'_i,$$
(6.102)

where the prime mark indicates the point's location in the deformed configuration. Subtracting Equation 6.101 from Equation 6.102 results in the relation between the nodal displacements (u_i, v_i) and the displacement at an interior element point (u_p, v_p), that is,

$$u_p = \sum_{i=1}^{4} N_i u_i,$$
$$v_p = \sum_{i=1}^{4} N_i v_i.$$
(6.103)

This property has been used in FEM to solve the displacement problems only at the element nodes and estimate the displacement of the interior points using their natural coordinates.

As will be shown later, the same approach can be used to solve the strain and stress problems.

6.7.4 SHAPE FUNCTIONS

In FEM literature, shape functions are the functions that are used to interpolate the nodal values to estimate the values at any point within the element. In other words, they are just the weights, N_i, given as functions of the natural coordinates (r, s). For example, referring to Figure 6.11c, N_i can be calculated as follows:

$$N_1 = \frac{(1-r)(1-s)}{4},$$
$$N_2 = \frac{(1+r)(1-s)}{4},$$
$$N_3 = \frac{(1+r)(1+s)}{4},$$
$$N_4 = \frac{(1-r)(1+s)}{4}.$$
(6.104)

Figure 6.12 shows a plot of these functions. Clearly, they are represented by the common planar (bilinear) interpolation functions.

If higher-order interpolation is required, then the number of nodes on the element should be increased, and hence the number of shape functions. For example, the nine-noded quadrilateral

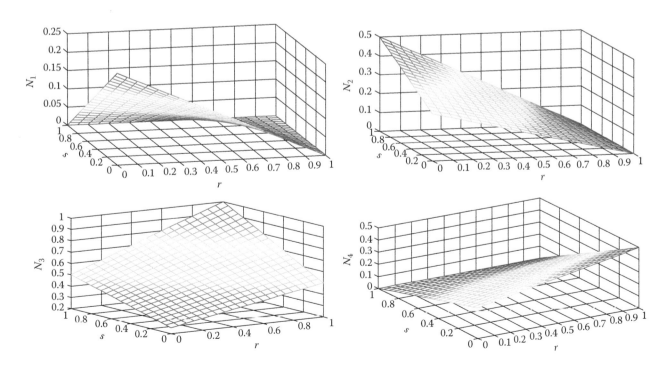

FIGURE 6.12 Shape functions for a 4-noded rectangular element, calculated based on the formulas in Equation 6.104.

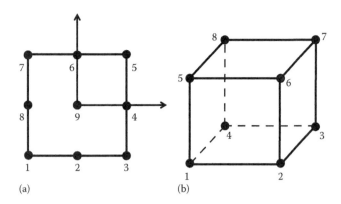

FIGURE 6.13 (a) Nine-noded 2D quadrilateral element; and (b) eight-noded 3D cubic element.

element shown in Figure 6.13a has nine shape functions, given by (note that node 9 lies at the element's center, where $r = s = 0$)

$$N_1 = \frac{1}{4}(r-1)(s-1)rs,$$

$$N_2 = \frac{1}{4}(r+1)(s-1)rs,$$

$$N_3 = \frac{1}{4}(r+1)(s+1)rs,$$

$$N_4 = \frac{1}{4}(r-1)(s+1)rs,$$

$$N_5 = -\frac{1}{2}(1-r^2)(1-s)s, \qquad (6.105)$$

$$N_6 = -\frac{1}{2}(1+r)(s^2-1)r,$$

$$N_7 = -\frac{1}{2}(r^2-1)(1+s)s,$$

$$N_8 = -\frac{1}{2}(r-1)(s^2-1)r,$$

$$N_9 = (1-r^2)(1-s^2).$$

Generalization of the above quadrilateral elements to 3D is straightforward. For example, the eight-noded 3D element in Figure 6.13b has shape functions given by (Zienkiewicz et al. 2013)

$$
\begin{aligned}
N_1 &= (1+r)(1+s)(1+t)/8, \\
N_2 &= (1+r)(1+s)(1-t)/8, \\
N_3 &= (1-r)(1+s)(1-t)/8, \\
N_4 &= (1-r)(1+s)(1+t)/8, \\
N_5 &= (1+r)(1-s)(1+t)/8, \\
N_6 &= (1+r)(1-s)(1-t)/8, \\
N_7 &= (1-r)(1-s)(1-t)/8, \\
N_8 &= (1-r)(1-s)(1+t)/8.
\end{aligned}
\qquad (6.106)
$$

where r, s, and t are the three dimensions in the natural coordinates of the element (the point $r = s = t = 0$ lies in the center of the element, whose sides have equal lengths = 2).

In FEM analysis, matrix representation is preferred to describe the relation between the displacement, or position, of the element points in terms of the nodal displacements. For example, Equation 6.103 for a 4-noded element can be written as

$$d_p = \mathbf{N} \cdot d, \qquad (6.107)$$

where

$$d_p = \begin{bmatrix} u_p \\ v_p \end{bmatrix}$$

$$N = \begin{bmatrix} N_1 & 0 & N_2 & 0 & N_3 & 0 & N_4 & 0 \\ 0 & N_1 & 0 & N_2 & 0 & N_3 & 0 & N_4 \end{bmatrix}$$

$$d = [u_1\, v_1\, u_2\, v_2\, u_3\, v_3\, u_4\, v_4]^{\mathrm{T}}$$

6.7.5 Element Strains and Stresses

In the previous sections, we showed that the displacement of any point within the element can be calculated from the nodal displacements using the shape functions. In many applications, it is required to calculate strain and stress at the interior points given the displacements at the nodes. It can be shown that strain, ε_p, and stress, σ_p, at an interior point, p, are related to the nodal displacements, d, by the following equation (Slaughter 2002):

$$
\begin{aligned}
\varepsilon_p &= \mathbf{B}\, d, \\
\sigma_p &= \mathbf{C}\,\mathbf{B}\, d.
\end{aligned}
\qquad (6.108)
$$

where

   B is the *strain–displacement matrix* whose entries are functions of the derivatives of the shape functions

   C is the *stiffness tensor* that depends on the constitutive model of the material

It is worth noting that the term "*stiffness tensor*," also referred to as the "*constitutive matrix*" in FEM literature, is used to represent the material stiffness in general. In FEM analysis, however, the global problem is formulated in terms of the stiffness of the element nodes. That is, a "*stiffness matrix*," $\mathbf{k}_e$, that summarizes the material constitutive properties within each element, is needed. The latter is obtained by the following integration applied over all points constituting this element:

$$\mathbf{k}_e = \int_{\forall(x,y,z)\in element} \mathbf{B}^{\mathrm{T}}\mathbf{C}\mathbf{B}\, dx\, dy\, dz. \qquad (6.109)$$

As expected, the analytical solution of this integration is difficult, and thus numerical calculation methods are used to approximate the value of the stiffness matrix at each element.

6.7.6 Matrix Formulation of the Dynamic Equation

The matrix formulation of the equation of motion is more suitable for numerical solutions and is thus more convenient in FEM analysis. The general form of the dynamic equation of motion for an element, or an entire structure, is given by (Kojic et al. 2008)

$$\mathbf{M}\ddot{X} + \mathbf{D}\dot{X} + \mathbf{K}X = \mathbf{F}, \tag{6.110}$$

where

  M, **D**, and **K** are the mass, damping, and stiffness matrices of the structure, respectively
  F is the external load acting on the nodes
  X, $\dot{X}$, and $\ddot{X}$ are the displacement, velocity, and acceleration vectors of the nodes

If the equation refers to the entire 3D structure, then the length of the vector X is $3N_e$, where N_e is the total number of elements in the structure. Subsequently, the coefficient matrices of Equation 6.110 are of size $3N_e \times 3N_e$. For an individual element, the stiffness matrix, $\mathbf{K}_e$, is also of the same size ($3N_e \times 3N_e$), but with nonzero entries only corresponding to the nodes of this element. It can be shown that, under equilibrium conditions, the stiffness matrix of the entire structure, **K**, is given by the summation of the stiffness matrices of the individual elements, that is,

$$\mathbf{K} = \sum_{\forall elements} \mathbf{K}_e. \tag{6.111}$$

It is worth noting that the three terms on the left-hand side of Equation 6.110 are referred to as the inertia, damping, and elastic forces, respectively. Different mechanical models can ignore one or more terms from these forces, depending on the model. For example, Haber et al. (2000) used a reduced form of Equation 6.110, where the inertia term was omitted and the damping matrix was set to the identity matrix, that is,

$$\dot{X} + \mathbf{K}X = \mathbf{F}. \tag{6.112}$$

In another formulation, Hu et al. (2003) also ignored the inertia force and formulated the problem as

$$\dot{X} + \mathbf{K}(X - X_0) = \mathbf{F}, \tag{6.113}$$

where X_0 is the displacement generated by the residual strain, which was used to represent the summation of the blood pressure in the LV cavity and the active force generated by the myocardium fibers. A further simplification, which maintains only the damping term, was used by Park et al. (1996a) to control the motion of a global model representing the LV, as follows:

$$\mathbf{D}\dot{X} = \mathbf{F}. \tag{6.114}$$

6.8 BIOMECHANICAL MODELS FOR ESTIMATING 3D HEART DEFORMATION

A number of MRI imaging techniques, for example, myocardial tagging, are available that allow for estimating the displacement of a grid of myocardium points. Usually, these points

are 2D, sparse in space, and the estimated displacement values are vulnerable to image artifacts. Estimating the myocardium deformation is even less accurate because it involves taking the derivatives of these inaccurate displacement values. In this regard, mechanical models could be implemented to enforce constraints on the heart displacement, and thus ensure a smooth and dense 3D deformation field. Usually, the problem can be formulated as follows: given the 2D displacement (or, possibly velocity) at *some* myocardium points, it is required to estimate the 3D deformation or material properties at *all* myocardium points. Figure 6.14 shows a typical problem that will be discussed later. Given a set of images from which the 2D displacement (d_x and d_y) can be measured at the myocardium border points (blue dots) and midwall points (red dots), it is required to estimate the 3D deformation (e.g., strain) at all points lying between the endocardium and epicardium surfaces.

A number of mechanical models have been implemented for cardiac functional analysis from MRI images. In this section and the following sections, we provide a brief description of some of these models (for detailed discussion of tagged image analysis, the reader is referred to Chapter 7 of this book and Chapters 2 and 3 of *Heart Mechanics: Magnetic Resonance Imaging—Advanced Techniques, Clinical Applications, and Future Trends*, respectively). In 1995, Benayoun and Ayache (1995) used modal analysis (Nastar 1994) for instantaneous analysis and smoothing of the computed displacement field. Modal analysis changes the standard canonical basis to the vibration basis of a deformable model defined by its elastic and mass properties:

$$\mathbf{K}\varnothing = \omega^2 \mathbf{M}\varnothing, \tag{6.115}$$

where

  $\varnothing$ contains the system eigenvectors
  K is the stiffness matrix
  M is the mass matrix
  ω is the mode frequency

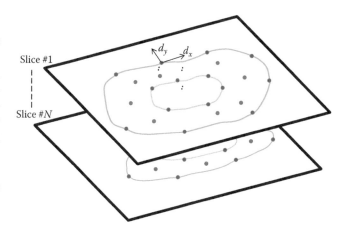

FIGURE 6.14 Estimating myocardium deformation from a set of 2D images. Given a set of sparse 2D displacement measurements (d_x and d_y) at the myocardium borders and midwall points (blue and red dots, respectively), it is required to estimate the 3D deformation at all myocardium points.

In 1999, Papademetris et al. (1999) proposed a deformation model based by continuum mechanics, where regularization is accomplished by measuring the internal energy of the myocardial tissue, assuming a linear elastic body model. It should be noted that one limitation of the linear elasticity model is that it does not capture the progressive hardening of any material when it is stretched (Papademetris et al. 2002).

Pham et al. (2001) presented a 3D active region model, which consists of a geometric template of the heart and a constitutive equation defining its dynamical behavior. The developed model was immersed into the image data and submitted to a force field that pulls the model interfaces toward the image's edges. The equilibrium of the model is achieved by minimizing the following energy function:

$$E = E_{Elastic} + E_{Data},\qquad(6.116)$$

where

$E_{Elastic}$ represents the deformation energy of the model
E_{Data} is the energy due to the external forces

The elastic energy is given by

$$E_{Elastic} = \frac{1}{2}\int_{\Omega}\sigma^T\varepsilon\,d\Omega,\qquad(6.117)$$

where

σ and ε are the stress and strain vectors, respectively
Ω is the space occupied by the object

The image data energy is given by

$$E_{Data}(u) = -\int_{\Gamma}t\,u\,d\Gamma,\qquad(6.118)$$

where

Γ is the object's border
t is the surface field
u is the displacement

In another study, Zhuang et al. (2005) presented a biomechanically constrained technique for simultaneously performing segmentation and deformation recovery of the myocardium from MRI images. The model was solved by minimizing an energy function that integrated both external image-based and prior model-based forces. Recently, Chapelle et al. (2012) proposed an approach for sequential data assimilation adapted to a biomechanical heart model (Sainte-Marie et al. 2006) with image data obtained from cine MRI images. The developed approach adjusted the biomechanical model to individual subjects and showed to be capable of localizing and quantifying myocardial infarction using regional contractility parameters. In another study, multiparametric MRI has been used for quantitative evaluation of mechanical cardiac tissue properties (Perie et al. 2013). Specifically, the authors used T_1, T_2, and T_2^* relaxation ratios, magnetization transfer ratio (MTR), apparent diffusion coefficient (ADC), and fractional anisotropy (FA) for estimating Young's modulus. Regression analysis showed that only 45% of Young's modulus can be explained by the derived MRI parameters. Principal component analysis (PCA) helped reduce the number of independent variables to two or three principal components with total of 63% or 80% variabilities, respectively. In another study, the authors presented a method for modeling and estimating global cardiac stress and strain of a dynamically controlled cardiac phantom using MRI and computational fluid dynamics (Charalambous et al. 2013). The results have been validated using the solutions of the Navier–Stokes equations along with bench experimentation and data from phase-contrast MRI images. More recently, 3D MRI tagging has been used for parameter estimation and analysis of passive cardiac constitutive laws (Hadjicharalambous et al. 2015). The fidelity of the developed model has been tested by comparing the derived laws with the transversely isotropic Guccione law (Guccione and McCulloch 1993) by characterizing the passive ED pressure–volume relation behavior as well as in an in vivo case.

6.9 3D CARDIAC DEFORMATION FROM PLANAR MYOCARDIAL CONTOURS

6.9.1 METHOD DESCRIPTION

Papademetris et al. (2002) proposed a biomechanical model that can be used to refine image-derived information, aiming to accurately estimating the cardiac deformation. The method begins with an interactive segmentation of the myocardium contours, which are used to reconstruct the 3D myocardium surfaces in the acquired images. Then, given two images at consecutive timeframes, a shape-tracking approach is used to establish the correspondence between the myocardium surfaces in the two images. The obtained correspondence between the surfaces provides a 3D displacement field that is sparse and not smooth, and thus a mechanical model is used to interpolate and smooth the displacement field and thus accurately calculate myocardium deformation (or strain). Figure 6.15 shows an outline of the basic steps of this method, and the following sections describe the method in details.

6.9.2 ASSUMPTIONS REGARDING DEFORMATION

The biomechanical model assumes infinitesimal deformation, that is,

$$\mathbf{F} = \mathbf{I} + \nabla u = \mathbf{I} + \mathbf{E} + \mathbf{\Omega},\qquad(6.119)$$

where

$\mathbf{F}$ is the deformation gradient (as defined in (6.32))
$\mathbf{E}$ and $\mathbf{\Omega}$ are the infinitesimal strain (symmetric) and rotation (antisymmetric) tensors, respectively

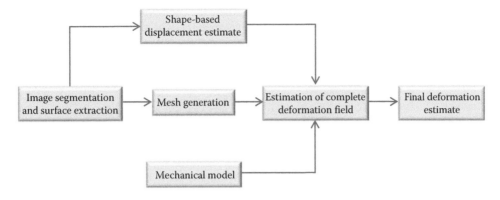

FIGURE 6.15 Outline of the algorithm implemented for accurate estimation of the myocardium strain using mechanical modeling.

Due to the symmetry and antisymmetry properties of these two tensors, they can be represented by the following two vectors:

$$e = [E_{11} E_{22} E_{33} E_{12} E_{13} E_{23}]^{\mathrm{T}},$$
$$\omega = [0\ 0\ 0\ \Omega_{12}\ \Omega_{13}\ \Omega_{23}]^{\mathrm{T}}. \tag{6.120}$$

From Equations 6.53 and 6.68, it can be easily shown that

$$E_{ij} = \frac{1}{2}\left(\frac{\partial u_i}{\partial X_j} + \frac{\partial u_j}{\partial X_i}\right),$$
$$\Omega_{ij} = \frac{1}{2}\left(\frac{\partial u_i}{\partial X_j} - \frac{\partial u_j}{\partial X_i}\right). \tag{6.121}$$

It is also worth noting that under the assumption of infinitesimal deformation, we have $\partial u / \partial X = \partial u / \partial x$, which can be used to simplify a lot of mathematical expressions within the model.

6.9.3 Assumptions Regarding the Material Properties

When a piece of tissue undergoes deformation, its internal energy increases as a function of this deformation. Nevertheless, because the material properties are invariant under rigid transformation, its internal energy can be represented by the *strain energy function* that depends only on the strain tensor. A linear elastic strain function, W, is assumed, that is,

$$W = \frac{1}{2} e^{\mathrm{T}} \mathbf{C} e, \tag{6.122}$$

where
e is given by Equation 6.120
$\mathbf{C}$ is a 6×6 matrix that defines the material properties of the deforming body

The simplest model would assume isotropic tissue material, that is, its mechanical properties are the same in all directions. In this case, the matrix $\mathbf{C}$ takes the following form:

$$\mathbf{C}^{-1} = \frac{1}{\varepsilon}\begin{bmatrix} 1 & -\nu & -\nu & & & \\ -\nu & 1 & -\nu & & \mathbf{0} & \\ -\nu & -\nu & 1 & & & \\ & & & 2(1+\nu) & 0 & 0 \\ & \mathbf{0} & & 0 & 2(1+\nu) & 0 \\ & & & 0 & 0 & 2(1+\nu) \end{bmatrix}, \tag{6.123}$$

where
ε is Young's modulus that represents the stiffness of the tissue
ν is Poisson's ratio that represents a measure of incompressibility

A more realistic, yet simple, model of the LV assumes a transversely isotropic material, that is, a material whose stiffness in the longitudinal direction is different from that in the radial and circumferential directions. The reason for differentiating the longitudinal direction was an attempt to account for different stiffness values of the myocardium fibers. In this case, the matrix takes the form of that in Equation 6.87:

$$\mathbf{C}^{-1} = \begin{bmatrix} \dfrac{1}{\varepsilon_p} & \dfrac{-\nu_p}{\varepsilon_p} & \dfrac{-\nu_{fp}}{\varepsilon_f} & & & \\ \dfrac{-\nu_p}{\varepsilon_p} & \dfrac{1}{\varepsilon_p} & \dfrac{-\nu_{fp}}{\varepsilon_f} & & \mathbf{0} & \\ \dfrac{-\nu_{pf}}{\varepsilon_p} & \dfrac{-\nu_{pf}}{\varepsilon_p} & \dfrac{1}{\varepsilon_f} & & & \\ & & & \dfrac{2(1+\nu_p)}{\varepsilon_p} & 0 & 0 \\ & \mathbf{0} & & 0 & \dfrac{1}{\mu_f} & 0 \\ & & & 0 & 0 & \dfrac{1}{\mu_f} \end{bmatrix}, \tag{6.124}$$

where

ε_f and ε_p are the Young's modulus values in the fiber and cross-fiber directions, respectively

ν_{fp} and ν_p are the corresponding Poisson's ratios

μ_f is the shear modulus across the fibers

6.9.4 PROBABILISTIC FORMULATION OF THE MECHANICAL MODEL

The mechanical model described earlier defines the relationship between myocardium deformation and its material properties. Given an initial estimate of the deformation values that needs to be refined, a probabilistic formulation can be used to model the uncertainty (or randomness) of the measurements. The probabilistic formulation is based on Markov random fields (MRF) and Gibbs probability density function (Geman and Geman 1984). In this formulation, the tissue displacements, u, are assumed to have a Gibbs (exponential) probability density distribution, that is,

$$p(u) = k_1 e^{(-W)}, \qquad (6.125)$$

where k_1 is a normalization factor that guarantees a total probability not exceeding one. It is worth noting that using MRF and Gibbs distribution is a widely common approach in medical image analysis problems (Christensen et al. 1994, Gee et al. 1997). The basic assumption here is that the displacement or strain (or, from a wider perspective, the tissue properties) at certain location depends on the displacements of its immediate neighboring locations. Having a probabilistic relation between the displacements of different myocardium points, smoothing the initial displacement measurements can be achieved using standard probabilistic estimation techniques such as the Bayesian framework (Komo 1987).

6.9.5 DEFORMATION ESTIMATION USING BAYESIAN FRAMEWORK

In a number of studies (Papademetris et al. 1999, 2001, 2002), techniques based on Bayesian estimation have been used to identify myocardial deformation. Given the set of initially estimated displacements, $u^m = u + n$, where n is a zero-mean white Gaussian noise and u is the true (unknown) displacement field, it is required to estimate a refined smooth version, $\hat{u}$, that better approximates the true displacement. For this purpose, the Bayesian framework is used to find a set of optimal displacements that maximizes the posterior probability density function $p(u|u^m)$. That is to say, given a set of measurements, u^m, what is the most probable u that have generated these measurements? The solution to this problem is obtained by finding the optimal set represented by the following equation:

$$\hat{u} = \arg\max_u \left(\log\left(p(u)\right) + \log\left(p(u^m \mid u)\right) \right), \quad (6.126)$$

where the conditional probability $p(u^m|u)$ is obtained from the (assumed) Gaussian probability of the noise, that is,

$$p(u^m \mid u) = k_2 e^{((-1/2)(u^m - u)^{\mathrm{T}} \Sigma^{-1} (u^m - u))}, \qquad (6.127)$$

where

k_2 is a normalization factor

Σ is the covariance matrix, which is a diagonal matrix for white Gaussian noise

In order to solve the optimization problem of Equation 6.126 for the whole set of myocardium points, we need first to stack the individual displacements in a long vector U^m with the corresponding true displacement vector U. By substituting from Equations 6.125 and 6.127, using $\mathbf{K}$ as global stiffness matrix, and converting the optimality condition from maximization to minimization by multiplying the exponent in Equation 6.127 by a negative sign, we get

$$\hat{U} = \arg\min_U \left(\frac{1}{2} \left(e^{\mathrm{T}} \mathbf{K} e + \left(U^m - U\right)^{\mathrm{T}} \Sigma^{-1} \left(U^m - U\right) \right) \right). \quad (6.128)$$

Differentiating the term to be minimized with respect to U and equating to zero yields the final solution:

$$\hat{U} = \left(\Sigma^{-1} + \mathbf{K} \right)^{-1} \Sigma^{-1} U^m. \qquad (6.129)$$

The optimization problem can be solved using the finite element formulation (Bathe 1982). In this formulation, the segmented myocardium volume in each timeframe is divided into a large number of hexahedral elements. Then, Equation 6.129 is solved to estimate the true displacement of this set of elements, whose initial positions are then adjusted to lie on the endo- and epicardial surfaces at the next frame using the nearest-neighbor method, and solving the equation once more using this added constraint. This ensures that there is a reduction of the bias in deformation estimation. The developed shape-based tracking algorithm has been extended to segment 3D cine MRI images, where the strain measurements were derived from the resulting displacements and compared to results from implanted markers (Papademetris et al. 2001). The results from the developed technique showed strong correlations with radial and circumferential strains, and lower correlation with longitudinal strains (Papademetris et al. 2002).

6.9.6 CLINICAL APPLICATION

The method described in the previous sections has been applied to segmented MRI images of four canine heart (Papademetris et al. 2002). For validation purpose, physical copper markers were implanted inside the myocardium of the imaged hearts. These markers can be reliably tracked in the images; therefore, the ground truth of the displacement field at the locations of these markers can be determined. Table 6.1 shows the mean and standard deviation strain values measured by tracking the implanted markers (column 1) and the

TABLE 6.1

Mean ± Standard Deviation Strain Values for Both the Implanted Markers and Biomechanical Model Techniques

	Markers	Isotropic Model			Transversely Isotropic Model		
		$\nu = 0.325$	0.4	0.475	0.325	0.4	0.475
P_1	27 ± 12.4	34.4 ± 15.1	35.8 ± 15.1	38.8 ± 14.9	36.0 ± 15.1	36.2 ± 14.2	39.8 ± 14.8
P_2	−10.4 ± 4.4	−6.2 ± 1.3	−6.5 ± 1.7	−7.3 ± 2.3	−6.6 ± 1.7	−7.4 ± 1.5	−8.3 ± 2.3
P_3	−30.8 ± 6.2	−27.8 ± 3.9	−27.2 ± 3.7	−29.8 ± 5.1	−25.8 ± 3.9	−26.1 ± 3.5	−30.0 ± 4.0

strain values estimated by the proposed biomechanical model (columns 2–7). The table shows the results of the mechanical model under the assumption of isotropic tissue (columns 2–4) and transversely isotropic tissue (columns 5–7) with different Poisson's ratio, ν, as indicated in the table.

The Bayesian approach has been also used for recursively estimating the LV boundaries using nonlinear dynamics, where the LV was represented by level sets (Sun et al. 2005). The model dynamics were built from a training dataset by finding a nonparametric density estimate of the current boundary based on previous boundaries. During implementation, a maximum a posteriori (MAP) estimate of the LV boundary was estimated using curve evolution.

6.10 3D CARDIAC DEFORMATION FROM SPARSE 2D DISPLACEMENT MEASUREMENTS

6.10.1 BACKGROUND

A number of MRI acquisition techniques, for example, myocardial tagging (Ibrahim 2011), provide information to track different myocardium points throughout the cardiac cycle. Due to the planar nature of the acquired tagged images, deformation and motion across the plane in which the images were acquired (through-plane motion) cannot be captured. Several model-based methods have been proposed to estimate the 3D motion field from multiple 2D views of the heart acquired using MRI myocardial tagging. This includes using sparse displacements measured from the tagged images to estimate the parameters of a 3D model representing the displacement field (O'Dell et al. 1995). The method can be thought of as solving a simple interpolation problem where the displacement field is expressed as an analytical series. The interpolation is performed using the prolate spheroidal coordinate system (more details about different geometrical coordinate systems are covered in Chapter 2 of *Heart Mechanics: Magnetic Resonance Imaging—Advanced Techniques, Clinical Applications, and Future Trends*), which efficiently describes the curvilinear deformations of the heart. In fact, the prolate spheroidal coordinate system allows for incorporating the boundary conditions of the approximately elliptical LV shape. A quantitative comparison among some other methods proposed by the same group can be found in Declerck et al. (2000).

Physics-based deformable models, whose parameters are functions of the spatial coordinates of the myocardium, can be used for analyzing cardiac motion (Park et al. 1996b). In this case, the model allows for accurate representation of the local shape variations using only few parameters. Simplified Lagrange equations of motion can be used to describe the model dynamics. In this simplified version, the inertia term is set to zero, that is,

$$\mathbf{D}\dot{q} = f_q, \tag{6.130}$$

where

q is a vector containing the model parameters
$\mathbf{D}$ is a diagonal damping matrix
f_q is a vector containing the external forces (as a function of time and spatial position)

The vector q includes parameters that control the myocardial shape variation under different types of radial, longitudinal, and twisting deformations (Young and Cowan 2012). This model showed the capability of analyzing the motion and shape of the LV midwall in normal subjects as well as patients.

6.10.2 NON-CARTESIAN COORDINATE SYSTEMS-BASED HEART MODELS

Studies of tagged images have revealed three important properties of the LV twist (Azhari et al. 1992). First, the twist angle is higher at the endocardium than epicardium. Second, twist increases toward the apex. Third, radial taglines (in a SAX view) are slightly curved at ES. Many LV models have been proposed approximating the LV geometry by a cylindrical shape. Nevertheless, the cylindrical shape does not account for longitudinal torsional shear variation, which results in that the epicardial twist is higher than, or equal to, the endocardial twist, which is in contrary to actual measurements. Therefore, Azhari et al. (1992) suggested using a conical-based model for describing the LV deformation pattern, as shown in Figure 6.16. In this case, the model deformation is calculated assuming that the torsion moments are represented by external moments applied to a hollow cone with a constant shear modulus. In the developed model, the epicardial and endocardial surfaces are represented by cones

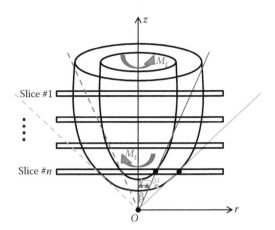

FIGURE 6.16 A schematic depiction of the hollow conical geometry used to approximate the LV. α and β are the epicardial and endocardial cone angles, respectively, M_t is the applied moment, and Slice # n is the measured tomographic slice number n. Note that the common origin, O, lies below the actual anatomical apex.

of angles α and β, respectively, with a common origin, O. The angle of twist $\psi(r,z)$ is thus given by

$$\psi(r,z) = -M_t \Big/ 6\pi G \Big[\big(\cos\alpha - \cos\beta\big) + 1/3\big(\cos^3\beta - \cos^3\alpha\big)\Big]$$

$$\times \big(r^2 + z^2\big)^{3/2}, \qquad (6.131)$$

where
    M_t is the applied moment
    G is the shear modulus of elasticity

In another work by Waks et al. (1996), the authors developed an LV motion simulator that incorporates a 13-parameter model of LV motion based on the work by Arts et al. (1992). The basis of the developed geometric model is the prolate sphere, as shown in Figure 6.17. A prolate sphere is defined by a constant radius λ, which determines its size, and a fixed parameter δ, known

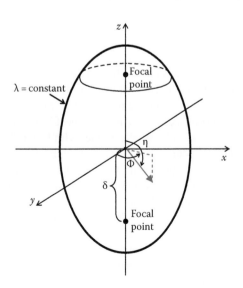

FIGURE 6.17   Prolate spheroidal coordinate system.

as the focal radius. A point (λ, η, ϕ) in the prolate spheroidal coordinates has the following Cartesian coordinates:

$$x = \delta \sinh\lambda \sin\eta \cos\phi, \qquad (6.132)$$

$$y = \delta \sinh\lambda \sin\eta \sin\phi, \qquad (6.133)$$

$$z = \delta \cosh\lambda \cos\eta. \qquad (6.134)$$

On the other hand, a point (x, y, z) in the Cartesian coordinates has the following prolate spheroidal coordinates:

$$r_1 = \sqrt{x^2 + y^2 + (z + \delta)^2}, \qquad (6.135)$$

$$r_2 = \sqrt{x^2 + y^2 + (z - \delta)^2}, \qquad (6.136)$$

$$\lambda = \cosh^{-1}\frac{r_1 + r_2}{2\delta}, \quad \lambda > 0, \qquad (6.137)$$

$$\eta = \cos^{-1}\frac{r_1 - r_2}{2\delta}, \quad 0 \le \eta \le 180, \qquad (6.138)$$

$$\phi = \tan^{-1}\frac{y}{x}, \quad 0 \le \phi \le 360, \qquad (6.139)$$

where r_1 and r_2 are the distances between (x, y, z) and the focus point. The LV can thus be modeled by defining it to lie between a pair of confocal prolate spheres with radii λ_i and λ_o, such that $\lambda_i < \lambda_o$, as shown in Figure 6.18. Complex motion in this model is achieved by applying a series of 13 3D transformations controlled by 13 motion parameters, c_1 through c_{13}, as shown in Table 6.2 (Waks et al. 1996).

Motion in the LV is described by a transformation that maps a material point (a specific location defined on the model LV) to a corresponding spatial point (the material point's location in space at a certain time point) at time t. As the LV deforms, the spatial coordinates of each material point change. This can be expressed mathematically as $\mathbf{r} = r(\mathbf{p}, t)$, where the material point $\mathbf{p}$ moves to the spatial point $\mathbf{r}$ at time t. The inverse transformation is thus given by $\mathbf{p} = p(\mathbf{r}, t)$. The overall

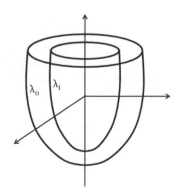

FIGURE 6.18   LV model as the difference between two prolate spheroidal shapes.

TABLE 6.2

Description of the 13c Parameters

Parameters	Meaning
c_1	Radially dependent compression
c_2	Left ventricular torsion
c_3	Ellipticallization in long-axis planes
c_4	Ellipticallization in short-axis planes
c_5	Shear in x-direction
c_6	Shear in y-direction
c_7	Shear in z-direction
c_8	Rotation about x-axis
c_9	Rotation about y-axis
c_{10}	Rotation about z-axis
c_{11}	Translation in x-direction
c_{12}	Translation in y-direction
c_{13}	Translation in z-direction

matrix equation that transforms point $\mathbf{p} = (p_x, p_y, p_z, 1)$ inside the model LV into spatial point $\mathbf{r} = (r_x, r_y, r_z, 1)$ is given by

$$\mathbf{r} = G_a G_6 G_5 G_4 G_3 G_2 G_1 G_0 \mathbf{p}, \qquad (6.140)$$

where

$$G_0 = \begin{bmatrix} d^{1/3} & 0 & 0 & 0 \\ 0 & d^{1/3} & 0 & 0 \\ 0 & 0 & d^{-2/3} & 0 \\ 0 & 0 & 0 & 1 \end{bmatrix}, \qquad (6.141)$$

$$G_1 = \begin{bmatrix} \varepsilon & 0 & 0 & 0 \\ 0 & \varepsilon & 0 & 0 \\ 0 & 0 & \varepsilon & 0 \\ 0 & 0 & 0 & 1 \end{bmatrix}, \qquad (6.142)$$

$$\varepsilon = \sqrt[3]{1 + \frac{3c_1 V_w}{4\pi |G_0 \mathbf{p}|^3}}, \qquad (6.143)$$

(d is a correctional parameter and V_w is the wall volume)

$$G_2 = \begin{bmatrix} \cos dc_2 z / |\mathbf{r}_1| & -\sin dc_2 z / |\mathbf{r}_1| & 0 & 0 \\ \sin dc_2 z / |\mathbf{r}_1| & \cos dc_2 z / |\mathbf{r}_1| & 0 & 0 \\ 0 & 0 & 1 & 0 \\ 0 & 0 & 0 & 1 \end{bmatrix}, \qquad (6.144)$$

$$\mathbf{r}_1 = G_1 G_0 \mathbf{p} = \begin{bmatrix} x \\ y \\ z \\ 1 \end{bmatrix}, \qquad (6.145)$$

$$G_3 = \begin{bmatrix} d^{-1/3} e^{c_4 - (c_3/2)} & 0 & 0 & 0 \\ 0 & d^{-1/3} e^{c_4 - (c_3/2)} & 0 & 0 \\ 0 & 0 & d^{2/3} e^{c_3} & 0 \\ 0 & 0 & 0 & 1 \end{bmatrix}, \qquad (6.146)$$

$$G_4 = \begin{bmatrix} 1 & c_5 & 0 & 0 \\ c_5 & 1 + c_5^2 & 0 & 0 \\ 0 & 0 & 1 & 0 \\ 0 & 0 & 0 & 1 \end{bmatrix}, \qquad (6.147)$$

$$G_5 = \begin{bmatrix} 1 & 0 & c_6 & 0 \\ 0 & 1 & 0 & 0 \\ c_6 & 0 & 1 + c_6^2 & 0 \\ 0 & 0 & 0 & 1 \end{bmatrix}, \qquad (6.148)$$

$$G_6 = \begin{bmatrix} 1 & 0 & 0 & 0 \\ 0 & 1 & c_7 & 0 \\ 0 & c_7 & 1 + c_7^2 & 0 \\ 0 & 0 & 0 & 1 \end{bmatrix}, \qquad (6.149)$$

$$G_a = B_4 B_3 B_2 B_1, \qquad (6.150)$$

$$B_1 = \begin{bmatrix} 1 & 0 & 0 & 0 \\ 0 & \cos c_8 & -\sin c_8 & 0 \\ 0 & \sin c_8 & \cos c_8 & 0 \\ 0 & 0 & 0 & 1 \end{bmatrix}, \qquad (6.151)$$

$$B_2 = \begin{bmatrix} \cos c_9 & 0 & \sin c_9 & 0 \\ 0 & 1 & 0 & 0 \\ -\sin c_9 & 0 & \cos c_9 & 0 \\ 0 & 0 & 0 & 1 \end{bmatrix}, \qquad (6.152)$$

$$B_3 = \begin{bmatrix} \cos c_{10} & -\sin c_{10} & 0 & 0 \\ \sin c_{10} & \cos c_{10} & 0 & 0 \\ 0 & 0 & 1 & 0 \\ 0 & 0 & 0 & 1 \end{bmatrix}, \qquad (6.153)$$

$$B_4 = \begin{bmatrix} 1 & 0 & 0 & c_{11} \\ 0 & 1 & 0 & c_{12} \\ 0 & 0 & 1 & c_{13} \\ 0 & 0 & 0 & 1 \end{bmatrix}. \qquad (6.154)$$

6.10.3 RV MYOCARDIAL DEFORMATION ANALYSIS

While the aforementioned methods can be successfully applied for analyzing the LV motion, they cannot be directly used for analyzing the right ventricle (RV). This is mainly due to the many challenges attributed to the complex shape and motion pattern of the RV. For example, simple geometric shapes (with few parameters) cannot accurately represent the RV surfaces. Also, the RV wall motion varies temporally and spatially with significant amount, which makes it difficult to describe concisely. In addition, typical resolution of the tag-lines is about 6 mm, while the free wall thickness of the RV is approximately 8 mm in normal subjects. That is, a limited number of tags lie on the RV wall, and thus the estimated motion field is of a very limited resolution (Harper and Tello 2003). A method has been proposed to overcome the challenges posed by the RV shape (Haber et al. 2000). The main modification in this method is that the model parameters are no more global functions of position because it is difficult to find a global frame of reference that can describe the complex geometry and motion of the RV. Instead, the method uses a set of large number of parameters to represent the displacement vector at each node of the model. In other words, an FEM model is used to represent and solve the problem of estimating the 3D wall motion of the RV. The equation of motion that governs the displacement of the model nodes is given by

$$\dot{q} + \mathbf{K}q = f_q, \qquad (6.155)$$

where

q is a vector containing the displacements of the different nodes
f_q is a vector of the image-derived forces
$\mathbf{K}$ is a finite element stiffness matrix

Then, for each node, i, the equation of motion can be written as

$$\dot{q}_i = f_{i,int} + f_{i,ext}, \qquad (6.156)$$

where

$f_{i,int} = [\mathbf{K}q]_i$ is an internal stiffness force that resists the node displacement
$f_{i,ext}$ is an external image-derived force (e.g., the displacement estimated from the tagged image)

In this method, the model elements are assumed isotropic, linear, and compressible with Poisson's ratio of 0.4 (nearly incompressible material) and Young's modulus of 0.02 (chosen empirically) (Haber et al. 2000). The external force has two types depending on the node location within the model. First, the nodes on the midwall are affected (only) by tag forces, $f_{i,tag}$, $i \in$ midwall. The calculation of $f_{i,tag}$ is based on a postprocessing analysis algorithm that tracks the location of the tag surfaces from one timeframe to the next one. Next, the tag force is calculated based on the distance between the model nodes and its projection on the tracked tag surfaces. That is, the tag force tries to pull the model toward the locations estimated from the processed images. Because of the large tag separation relative to the thickness of the RV free wall, few or no tags may fall within the RV free wall. To overcome this problem, and to adequately constrain the motion of the model, another type of external forces, namely, the

contour forces, $f_{i,cntr}$, is used to estimate the forces affecting the boundary nodes. That is, the force at a boundary node, i, is given by

$$f_{i,ext} = w f_{i,cntr} + (1-w) f_{i,tag}, \quad i \in \text{boundary}, \quad (6.157)$$

where w is an appropriate weight (set to 0.25 in this work).

Similar to the concept of the tag forces, the contour forces are calculated to pull the boundary points toward the estimated locations of the myocardium surfaces, which are determined by semiautomatic segmentation of the myocardium boundaries using active contour (Kass et al. 1988). After calculating all the forces, the differential equation (6.156) is solved using Euler's method with an appropriate time step, h (initially = 0.01), to calculate the displacement of each node at time t as follows:

$$q_{i,t+1} = q_{i,t} + h\left(f_{i,int} + f_{i,ext}\right). \qquad (6.158)$$

Figure 6.19 shows the estimated trajectories of the myocardium surface calculated at the centers of the model elements. The color of the element's face represents the displacement of the endocardial wall. As can be seen, the displacement is nonuniform with maximum value occurring in the basal slice. In addition, the magnitude and range of displacements are smaller in the septum. The results reported in this study were in agreement with earlier studies of the RV motion in normal subjects and patients with hypertrophy.

6.11 3D CARDIAC DEFORMATION USING MECHANICS-BASED DATA FUSION

6.11.1 MAGNITUDE AND PHASE-CONTRAST MRI IMAGES

Because of the advanced capabilities of MRI scanners, a number of functional and anatomical images can be captured in one imaging session. Fusion of such data can be useful in many applications, including the estimation of myocardium deformation. For example, phase-contrast MRI imaging can simultaneously produce four types of images of the same cross-section (Meyer et al. 1996). The first type includes the "magnitude" images (Figure 6.20a), which depict the changes of the shapes of different anatomical structures. The other three types include "phase" images that contain information about the velocity in the three principal coordinate directions (Figure 6.20b through d). While the latter is sufficient to estimate a dense 3D displacement field, technical challenges limit its ability to accurately estimate the displacement at the myocardium borders (Shi et al. 1998). For complete coverage of analyzing heart mechanics using phase-contrast MRI, the reader is referred to Chapter 7 of *Heart Mechanics: Magnetic Resonance Imaging—Advanced Techniques, Clinical Applications, and Future Trends.*

As tracking the endo- and epicardial contours provides information only about wall motion development, a hybrid analysis technique has been developed to integrate information about the myocardial velocity within the midwall region

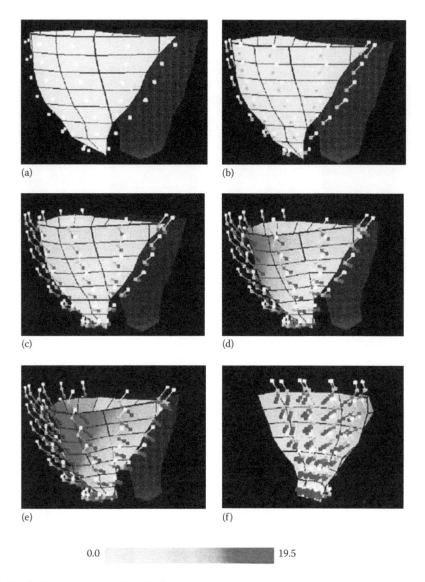

(a)

(b)

(c)

(d)

(e)

(f)

0.0 ▭ 19.5

FIGURE 6.19 Normal RV displacement. (a–e) The RV free wall is shown through four phases of systole. The LV wall is drawn shaded for reference. (f) Septal wall at end-systole from the vantage point of the LV. (Reproduced from Haber, I. et al., *Med. Image Anal.*, 4(4), 335, 2000. With permission.)

from the phase-contrast images with information about the boundary displacement from the endo- and epicardial contours (Shi et al. 1995a,b, 1998). In this respect, the information about boundary displacement is used to generate velocity estimates at the interface between structures, where the phase-contrast images are noisy and generate unreliable measurements. The information from boundary tracking and phase velocity maps is integrated in a continuum mechanical model of the LV to generate complete information about myocardial deformation, as explained in the following sections. In fact, this framework can be also extended to integrate data from other sources of measurements, such as MRI tagging and echocardiographic Doppler.

6.11.2 MECHANICAL MODELING

The adopted mechanical model considers the myocardium as a Hookean material (Shi et al. 1995a,b, 1998). The equation of

motion used in this method includes terms representing stiffness, mass, damping, and loads, that is,

$$\mathbf{M}\ddot{X} + \mathbf{D}\dot{X} + \mathbf{K}X = \mathbf{F}, \qquad (6.159)$$

where

  M, **D**, and **K** are the mass, damping, and stiffness matrices of the tissue, respectively
  F is the external load acting on the nodes
  X, $\dot{X}$, and $\ddot{X}$ are the displacement, velocity, and acceleration vectors, respectively, of the nodes

To integrate the boundary conditions (e.g., the displacements measured at the nodes lying on the myocardium borders) into the model while maintaining the same mathematical representation of the model, the motion equations at the boundary points are changed as follows. Given that the displacement X_i

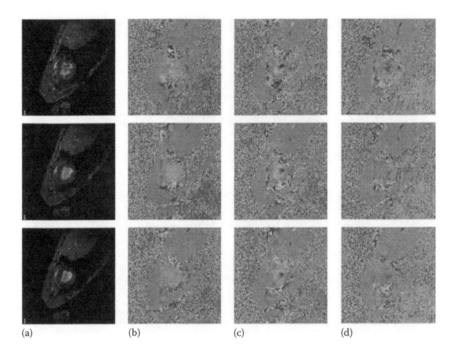

(a)   (b)   (c)   (d)

FIGURE 6.20   (a) Magnitude, (b) *x*-velocity, (c) *y*-velocity, and (d) *z*-velocity images of basal (top), mid-ventricular (middle), and apical (bottom) short-axis images. (Reproduced from Duncan, J. et al., *Prog. Biophys. Mol. Biol.*, 69(2–3), 333, 1998. With permission.)

of node *i* is calculated from the image and found to be equal to *b*, then the *i*th equation (thus the *i*th row in Equation 6.159) is changed to the following form:

$$\sum_{j=1}^{3N} \mathbf{M}_{ij}\ddot{X}_j + \sum_{j=1}^{3N} \mathbf{D}_{ij}\dot{X}_j + \sum_{j=1}^{3N} \mathbf{K}_{ij}X_j + kX_i = \mathbf{F}_i + kb, \quad (6.160)$$

where

N is the number of nodes in the model (with 3 degrees of freedom per each node)

k is an arbitrary multiplying factor that is larger than $\mathbf{K}_{ij}$ for all values of *j*

Consequently, it can be easily shown that the solution of this modified equation results in a displacement $X_i \cong b$ at the boundary node.

In this formulation, the simplest constitutive equation of a linear and isotropic elastic material under infinitesimal deformation is assumed. The model's parameters are Young's modulus = 75 kPa, Poisson's ratio ≈ 0.5 (incompressible material), myocardium density = 1.5 g/mm³, and damping parameter = 0.1. The velocity values at the midwall points are used as the initial velocity conditions, and the surface displacements are used as the displacement boundary conditions. A time step of 0.003125 is used while iteratively solving the differential motion equation. The model has been applied to estimate myocardial deformation in canine hearts.

6.11.3   3D Deformation

The hybrid myocardial deformation technique explained in the previous section has been extended for estimating

volumetric deformation from intrinsic velocity data and geometrical displacement information (Shi et al. 1998). The problem is solved for the unknown displacement vectors, although velocity and acceleration information could be also derived. Figure 6.21 shows a dense endocardial

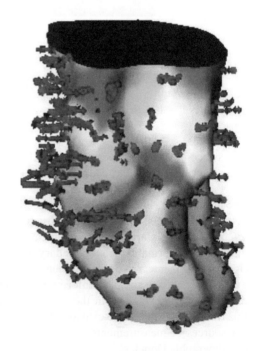

FIGURE 6.21   Shape-tracked dense endocardial displacement vector field of an MRI dataset from end-diastole to end-systole, subsampled for visualization purpose. The trajectories are shown against the rendered endocardial Gaussian curvature map at end-systole. (Reproduced from Shi, P. et al., *Int. J. Comput. Vision*, 35, 65, 1998. With permission.)

displacement vector field (from ED to ES) of a real MRI dataset. The trajectories of some endocardial points are shown against the rendered endocardial surface at ES. Because the process of estimating the displacement from the myocardium contours can fail, a measure of confidence is estimated and only those points that are tracked with high confidence are used to constrain the model. The other measurements included in Shi's model are the velocity measurements at the midwall points, that is, points that are located at more than one pixel distance from the myocardium boundaries. Figure 6.22 shows a complete shape-tracked trajectory of an endocardial point through the cardiac cycle. Figure 6.23 shows different (normal and shear) components of the strain tensor for the deformation between ED and ES. While these results show the potential of the developed method, it cannot be used to infer clinical observations without further validation on a larger dataset.

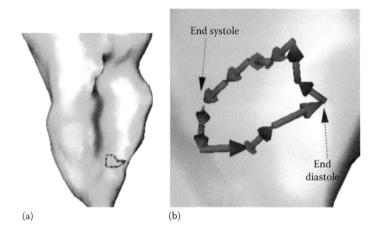

(a) (b)

FIGURE 6.22 Shape-tracked complete trajectory of an endocardial point over the cardiac cycle, superimposed onto the endocardial surface at end-systole. (a) Overview image. (b) Detailed image. (Reproduced from Shi, P. et al., *Int. J. Comput. Vision*, 35, 65, 1998. With permission.)

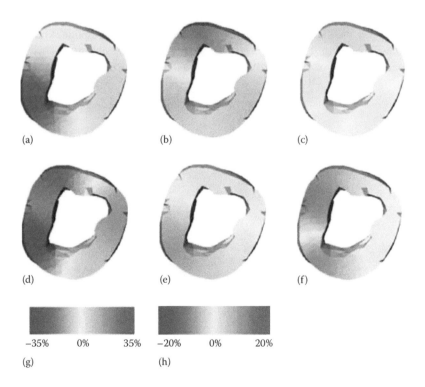

FIGURE 6.23 3D strain maps (end-diastole to end-systole) at mid-ventricle. (a) *x*-direction normal strain; (b) *y*-direction normal strain; (c) *z*-direction normal strain; (d) *xy*-direction shear strain; (e) *yz*-direction shear strain; (f) *zx*-direction shear strain; (g) color scale for *x*-direction normal strain; (h) color scale for all other strains. (Reproduced from Shi, P. et al., *Int. J. Comput. Vision*, 35, 65, 1998. With permission.)

6.11.4 MYOCARDIUM AS A TRANSVERSELY ISOTROPIC ELASTIC MATERIAL

A comprehensive 3D shape-based technique has been developed for measuring regional myocardial deformation from cine MRI images (Sinusas et al. 2001). In the developed technique, the endo- and epicardial surfaces were tracked through the entire cardiac cycle and were used to deform a mesh that represents the LV myocardial volume. The myocardium was modeled as a transversely isotropic elastic solid continuum with preferential stiffness along the fiber directions (Chadwick 1982, Guccione and McCulloch 1991, Hadjicharalambous et al. 2015), and the generated set of partial differential equations were solved using the FEM method. Using the developed technique on dog cine MRI images, it has been shown that the radial and circumferential ES strains are fairly uniform; however, there was a significant apex-to-base gradient in the longitudinal strain and radial-longitudinal shear. Further, transmural epi- to endocardial strain gradients have been observed (Sinusas et al. 2001).

6.12 OTHER CARDIAC MODELS

6.12.1 HYPERELASTIC WARPING MODELS

A hyperelastic warping technique has been developed and validated for myocardial strain measurement from cine MRI images (Veress et al. 2005). The technique is based on an FEM model that is deformed using both image-based and material-based forces. Deformable registration was implemented by minimizing an energy function that includes two components: one component depends on image intensity, and the other provides regularization on the deformation map. The hyperelastic warping technique has the advantages of ensuring diffeomorphic (one-to-one, onto, differentiable, and

invertible) deformation (Christensen et al. 1996, Miller et al. 2002), objectivity to large strains and rotations, relative insensitivity to changes in material coefficients, and high spatial resolution (Veress et al. 2001, Phatak et al. 2007), although at the expense of large computational cost. Veress et al. (2001) showed that hierarchical implementation of the warping technique using sequential spatial filtering avoids the technique's susceptibility to converging to local minima.

Recently, Phatak et al. (2009) validated and implemented a hyperelastic warping technique to provide comprehensive description of myocardial contraction (Figure 6.24). The developed technique included constraints from both image data and active fiber contraction, combined with the hyperelastic constitutive model (Guccione and McCulloch 1993). In regions of the model where the image has large signal intensity or recognized texture, the image data governs the computational process, while in other regions, material-based forces are implemented (Rabbitt et al. 1995, Weiss et al. 1998). The resulting circumferential and radial strain measurements from the developed technique were strongly correlated with those obtained from tagged images analyzed with the harmonic phase (HARP) technique (Phatak et al. 2009). Further, the results for fiber stretch, LV twist, and transmural strain distribution were in good agreement with experimental values in the literature.

6.12.2 INCOMPRESSIBLE MODELS

One problem with nonrigid registration is its tendency to underestimate the ventricular volume size (Rohlfing and Maurer 2001). One solution to this problem is to impose the incompressibility constraint on myocardial deformation. This is a reasonable assumption, knowing that the myocardium is nearly incompressible (total myocardium volume change is less than 4% during the cardiac cycle (Bistoquet et al. 2007)).

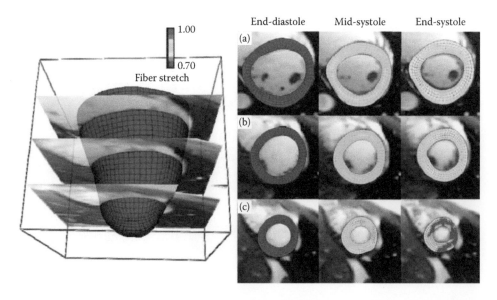

FIGURE 6.24 LV fiber stretch at end-diastole (left column), mid-systole (middle column), and end-systole (right column) with hyperelastic warping, shown at (a) basal (b) mid-cavity, and (c) apical slices. (Reproduced from Phatak, N.S. et al., *Med. Image Anal.*, 13(2), 354, 2009. With permission.)

Therefore, continuity and incompressibility constraints can be imposed in cardiac mechanical modeling (Song and Leahy 1991, Song et al. 1994), where the resulting Euler–Lagrange equations include a set of coupled partial differential equations that can be easily solved, for example, using the conjugate gradient method. The continuity equation is based on the conservation of mass principle: for a certain region V, let f be the density distribution, m be the volume integral over f, and s be the velocity in Lagrangian description; then the continuity constraint states that the rate of m leaving V is canceled by the flux of m across the surface enclosing V, represented mathematically as

$$f_t + \nabla \cdot \left(fs \right) = 0, \tag{6.161}$$

where $f_t = \partial f / \partial t$. For an incompressible material, the density f does not change with time during the particle's movement, which yields the incompressibility constraint

$$f_t \cdot \nabla f \cdot s = 0. \tag{6.162}$$

Therefore, the continuity equation for incompressible material becomes

$$f \nabla \cdot s = 0, \tag{6.163}$$

that is, for an incompressible material, the divergence of the velocity field is zero for regions where f is nonzero, that is,

$$\nabla \cdot s = 0, \tag{6.164}$$

which is the divergence-free constraint.

In one study that used nearly incompressible transformation on point r, the transformation Jacobian J, which represents the relative change of the local volume, was represented as (Bistoquet et al. 2008)

$$J \approx 1 + tr \frac{\partial U}{\partial r}, \tag{6.165}$$

where

U represents the displacement field
r is a point in the domain
tr represents the matrix trace

Therefore, for an incompressible material where

$$\nabla \cdot U = tr \frac{\partial U}{\partial r} = 0, \tag{6.166}$$

the following condition is met:

$$J \approx 1 \tag{6.167}$$

In another study (Rohlfing and Maurer 2001), the incompressibility constraint was also implemented based on the Jacobian determinant of the deformation. A Jacobian-based penalty term can therefore be added to the energy function, which showed to be an efficient and effective way for ensuring incompressible deformation.

6.13 ESTIMATION OF IN VIVO MYOCARDIAL MATERIAL PROPERTIES

Using tissue deformation, or strain, to evaluate the cardiac function proved to be successful in a large number of studies, as illustrated in the previous sections. Nevertheless, it should be noted that strain alone cannot be used to characterize the mechanical tissue properties. For example, the same strain value can be obtained from two different materials by changing the applied stress. This has motivated researchers to take one step further and try to estimate the material properties of the myocardium based on measurements of the myocardium displacement and blood pressure. It is worth noting that the early trials for studying the material properties of the myocardium were based on data measured from ex vivo tissues. Examples include the work of Pinto and Fung (1973) and Pao et al. (1980) who used uniaxial mechanical tests to estimate the myocardium mechanical properties and Demer and Yin (1983) and Yin et al. (1987) who used biaxial mechanical tests to show that the myocardium is an anisotropic material and provided the corresponding constitutive relationships (Humphrey and Yin 1987, 1989).

6.13.1 Early Studies

One of the earliest attempts to estimate in vivo mechanical properties of the heart from MRI was presented by Moulton et al. (1996). In this method, a simple mechanical model of the myocardium is assumed and finite element formulation is used to solve for the model parameters. In the adopted model, the myocardium strain is estimated from tagged MRI images while the blood pressure in the LV and RV is measured using a pair of catheters placed in both ventricles. Given the boundary conditions of the pressure (or stress), a nonlinear optimization problem is formulated and iteratively solved to find the material properties that minimize the difference between the strain values estimated by the model, ε_{est}, and those measured from the images, ε_{meas}. That is, the target is to find a set of parameters that minimizes the objective function, S, given by

$$S = \sum_i \sum_j \left(\varepsilon_{meas;i,j} - \varepsilon_{est;i,j} \right)^2. \tag{6.168}$$

A mechanical model of a simple isotropic Hookean material is used to approximate the pressure–volume relationship during *passive* myocardium expansion. An exponential strain energy function, W, is used to describe the relationship between strain and stress as follows:

$$W = W_L e^{2cW_L}, \tag{6.169}$$

$$W_L = \frac{1}{2}\varepsilon^T D\,\varepsilon,$$

$$= \frac{1}{2}\begin{bmatrix} \varepsilon_{11} & \varepsilon_{22} & \varepsilon_{12} \end{bmatrix}\begin{bmatrix} D_1 & D_2 & D_4 \\ 0 & D_3 & D_5 \\ 0 & 0 & D_6 \end{bmatrix}\begin{bmatrix} \varepsilon_{11} \\ \varepsilon_{22} \\ \varepsilon_{12} \end{bmatrix}, \quad (6.170)$$

where

W_L is a linear isotropic strain energy

c is a constant

D_i is a material property that is function of the elastic modulus and Poisson's ratio

The stress components in this model are obtained by differentiating Equation 6.169 with respect to ε, which yields the stress components

$$\sigma_{ij} = \frac{\partial W}{\partial \varepsilon_{ij}}, \quad (6.171)$$

$$\sigma = (1 + 2cW_L)e^{2cW_L}D\,\varepsilon, \quad (6.172)$$

where $\sigma = \begin{bmatrix} \sigma_{11} & \sigma_{22} & \sigma_{12} \end{bmatrix}^T$, and Poisson's ratio is set equal to 0.45 (nearly incompressible material). It is worth noting that this formulation describes only the ventricles' free relaxation during the diastolic phase with no active force exerted by the muscles. The initial mesh of the model is constructed by selecting few points on the LV and RV contours to create 16 quadratic elements at early diastole, as shown in Figure 6.25. The model is then loaded with the blood

pressure measured in the LV and RV during scanning. To model the pericardial effects on the myocardial deformation, linear spring constraints were applied on the epicardial boundaries. These springs have an additional function that prevents rigid-body motion (ensuring that the model is not moving in space).

One interesting issue in this model is the initial stress-free state. The problem is that to compare the estimated material properties of different hearts, one needs to start from the same initial conditions, that is, the same frame of reference. Nevertheless, each studied subject has a different early-diastolic pressure, and thus different initial states of stress and strain. Usually, the unloaded (stress-free) state is preferred as an initial reference state, but truly stress-free state is difficult to obtain during in vivo experiments. Alternatively, the initial state can be accounted for by first estimating the material properties and using them to solve a forward FEM problem to estimate the initial stress and strain (Moulton et al. 1996).

It should be noted that the method described in this section has a number of limitations, including the simplified assumptions of homogeneous material properties, considering only 2D strain (in-plane motion), and inability to account for the active stress exerted by the heart muscle. These effects have impacted the ability of the method to accurately estimate the material properties of the myocardium.

6.13.2 Fiber-Reinforced Composite Material Modeling

A method has been developed to avoid the limitations of the model described in the previous section (Hu et al. 2003). The method includes a fiber-reinforced composite material model for in vivo stress estimation in the LV and RV. The composite material used in this model consists of two constituents, as shown in Figure 6.26. The first constituent is the muscle fibers (or the reinforcing phase) that is embedded in the other constituent, the collagen (or the matrix).

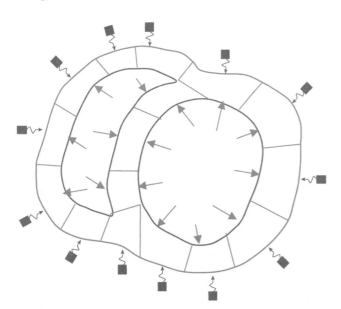

FIGURE 6.25 Two-dimensional model of the heart constructed from MRI images. The model has 16 quadratic elements. Early-late trans-diastolic pressure is measured in the LV and RV during scanning (blue arrowheads). Linear spring constraints (red spring symbols) model the effects of the pericardial pressure on the myocardium and prevent rigid-body motion.

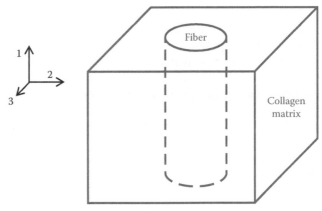

FIGURE 6.26 The model's material is composed of muscle fibers immersed in a matrix of collagen. In the material coordinate system, the first coordinate direction is aligned with the fiber direction.

According to Kaw (1997), for such composite material, Young's moduli along the fiber orientation (ε_1) and across the fibers (ε_2), that is, in the material local coordinate system, are

$$\varepsilon_1 = \varepsilon_f V_f + \varepsilon_c V_c, \qquad (6.173)$$

$$\varepsilon_2 = \frac{1}{V_f/\varepsilon_f + V_c/\varepsilon_c}, \qquad (6.174)$$

where

V_f and V_c are the fiber and matrix volume fractions, respectively

ε_f and ε_c are Young's moduli of the fiber and matrix, respectively

Similarly, Poisson's ratio (ν_{12}) and in-plane shear modulus (G_{12}) are (Hyer 1998)

$$\nu_{12} = \nu_f V_f + \nu_c V_c, \qquad (6.175)$$

$$\mu_{12} = \frac{1}{V_f/\mu_f + V_c/\mu_c}, \qquad (6.176)$$

where

ν_f and ν_c are Poisson's ratios of the fiber and matrix, respectively

μ_f and μ_c are the in-plane shear moduli of the fiber and matrix, respectively

Assuming a Hookean isotropic material, then the stress–strain relationship is given by

$$\varepsilon = \begin{bmatrix} 1/\varepsilon_1 & -\nu_{12}/\varepsilon_1 & -\nu_{12}/\varepsilon_1 & & & \\ -\nu_{12}/\varepsilon_1 & 1/\varepsilon_2 & -\nu_{23}/\varepsilon_2 & & \mathbf{0} & \\ -\nu_{12}/\varepsilon_1 & -\nu_{23}/\varepsilon_2 & 1/\varepsilon_2 & & & \\ & & & 2(1+\nu_{23})/\varepsilon_2 & 0 & 0 \\ & \mathbf{0} & & 0 & 1/\mu_{12} & 0 \\ & & & 0 & 0 & 1/\mu_{12} \end{bmatrix} \sigma,$$

$$= \mathbf{G}\sigma \qquad (6.177)$$

where

ν_{12} and ν_{23} are Poisson's ratios (set to 0.4) corresponding to ε_1 and ε_2

μ_{12} is the shear modulus

Since the stress–strain relation of the myocardium is nonlinear, both Young's moduli are assumed piecewise linear. That is, four linear elasticity intervals are used to approximate the stress–strain relation in the myocardium. The parameter μ_{12} is assumed to be equal to $\varepsilon_2/(1+\nu_{23})$, and $\mathbf{G}$ is called the compliance matrix.

Because the fibers change their orientation (in-plane rotation by angle θ) from the base to apex and from endo- to epicardium, the stress in the local fiber coordinates (1, 2, 3) can

be transformed into global element coordinates (x, y, z) (Hyer 1998) by

$$\sigma_{123} = \begin{bmatrix} \sigma_1 \\ \sigma_2 \\ \sigma_3 \\ \sigma_{23} \\ \sigma_{31} \\ \sigma_{12} \end{bmatrix}$$

$$= \begin{bmatrix} \cos^2\theta & \sin^2\theta & 0 & 0 & 0 & 2\sin\theta\cos\theta \\ \sin^2\theta & \cos^2\theta & 0 & 0 & 0 & -2\sin\theta\cos\theta \\ 0 & 0 & 1 & 0 & 0 & 0 \\ 0 & 0 & 0 & \cos\theta & -\sin\theta & 0 \\ 0 & 0 & 0 & \sin\theta & \cos\theta & 0 \\ -\sin\theta\cos\theta & \sin\theta\cos\theta & 0 & 0 & \cos^2\theta & -\sin^2\theta \end{bmatrix} \begin{bmatrix} \sigma_x \\ \sigma_y \\ \sigma_z \\ \sigma_{yz} \\ \sigma_{zx} \\ \sigma_{xy} \end{bmatrix}$$

$$= \mathbf{T}\sigma_{xyz}. \qquad (6.178)$$

The strain transformation can be also expressed in tensor form as

$$\varepsilon_{123} = \mathbf{T}\varepsilon_{xyz}. \qquad (6.179)$$

From these two equations, a relationship between stress and strain in the global coordinate system can be obtained.

The equation of motion is formulated as follows:

$$\dot{\mathbf{X}} + \mathbf{K}\left(\mathbf{X} - \mathbf{X}_o\right) = \mathbf{F}_p + \mathbf{F}_a, \qquad (6.180)$$

where

$\mathbf{X}$ is the displacement

$\mathbf{F}_p$ is the boundary force (generated by blood pressure in the ventricular cavity)

$\mathbf{F}_a$ is the active force exerted by the cardiac muscle fibers

$\mathbf{K}$ is the stiffness matrix

In this formulation, the boundary condition is a function of time representing the blood pressure within the ventricular cavities, which can be simplified using a piecewise function.

To account for residual strain, both the circumferential and residual strains are assumed to vary linearly from the epicardium to the endocardium. Using the experimental data presented by Costa (1996), the exact values of the circumferential/radial strains are set to 0.05/−0.05 and −0.05/0.05 at the epi- and endocardium, respectively. The developed geometric model here (Hu et al. 2003) is similar to that previously proposed by Haber et al. (2000). The FEM mesh of the model contained 264 eight-noded elements and 327 nodes for the LV, and 80 eight-noded elements and 146 nodes for the RV. To model the variation of the fiber orientation, a higher precision is needed, and thus each element is interpolated to create 27 subelements. Figure 6.27 shows the orientation of the fibers after interpolation. Figures 6.28 and 6.29 show the biventricular stress distributions of a normal volunteer and an RV

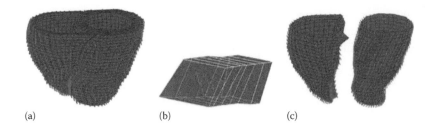

(a)   (b)   (c)

FIGURE 6.27 Fibers of the normal heart shown in (a) epicardium, (b) zoomed-in region covering volume from the epicardium (left side of the volume) to the endocardium (right side of the volume), and in (c) endocardium. (Reproduced from Hu, Z. et al., *Med. Image Anal.*, 7(4), 435, 2003. With permission.)

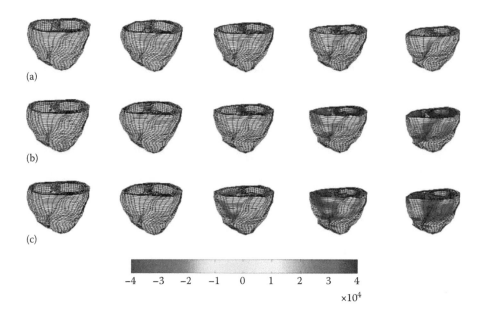

FIGURE 6.28 Stress distribution in a normal heart. (a) Radial, (b) circumferential, and (c) longitudinal components from end-diastole (left) to end-systole (right). (Reproduced from Hu, Z. et al., *Med. Image Anal.*, 7(4), 435, 2003. With permission.)

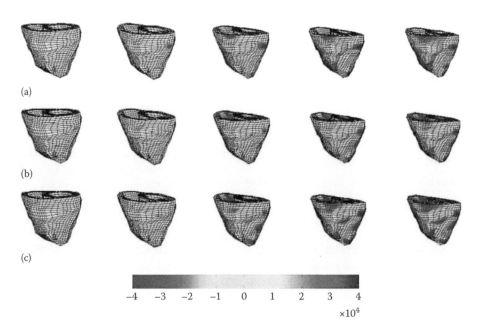

FIGURE 6.29 Stress distribution in a heart with RV hypertrophy (RVH). (a) Radial, (b) circumferential, and (c) longitudinal components from end-diastole (left) to end-systole (right). (Reproduced from Hu, Z. et al., *Med. Image Anal.*, 7(4), 435, 2003. With permission.)

hypertrophy (RVH) patient during one contraction cycle. As can be shown in the figures, radial stresses are generally positive (in contrast to circumferential and longitudinal stresses that are negative).

While the fiber orientation in this model has been estimated based on data reported by Nielsen et al. (1991) and Vetter and McCulloch (1998), a more recent study (Augenstein et al. 2006) showed that it can be measured using diffusion tensor MRI, as explained in Chapter 5. In this case, an FEM of a transverse-isotropic hyperelastic material can be used to estimate in vivo elasticity of the myocardium. The constitutive material parameters are determined such that the difference between the predicted and imaged deformation fields is minimized, similar to the work of Moulton et al. (1996). However, unlike the latter, in this case a 3D displacement field (rather than in-plan 2D deformation) is estimated from the tagged MRI images and used to solve for the model parameters. Unlike the work of Hu et al. (2003), Augenstein et al. (2006) generated different levels of pressure inside the ventricular cavity and measured it using special hardware.

6.14 SUMMARY AND KEY POINTS

6.14.1 SUMMARY

Understanding the basics of continuum mechanics is essential for proper understanding of the myocardial tissue properties, assumption and concepts of operation of different analysis techniques, and the meaning of the derived measurements. The adoption of biomechanical models in heart functional analysis has the advantage of providing smooth and realistic results. It should be noted, though, that the derived measurements could change under different assumptions and based on the implemented mechanical model. The basic concepts covered in this chapter will allow in better understanding of the techniques covered in the rest of the book.

6.14.2 KEY POINTS

- Mechanical models of the heart are used to understand, study, and evaluate the heart function.
- Theories of continuum mechanics are fundamental in modeling the behavior of the myocardium in response to different forces and stresses.
- Tensors are geometric objects that describe linear mapping from one space to another. They can be represented by a multidimensional array of numerical values.
- One fundamental assumption in mechanical modeling of the heart is that the heart tissue is spatially continuous.
- In the Lagrangian description of deformation, one is concerned only with the deformation of each particle with respect to the reference configuration.
- In the Eulerian description of deformation, one observes the deformation at a fixed location in the deformed configuration.

- The main feature of homogeneous deformation is that the deformation parameters are independent of the particle's location.
- Rigid-body motion is a special case of homogeneous deformation, which is usually used to describe global motion of the studied object.
- Stress represents the amount of force per unit area exerted on any point of a given body.
- In Cauchy stress tensors, stress is measured in the deformed configuration.
- In Piola–Kirchhoff stress tensors, stress is measured in the undeformed configuration.
- When the tissue does not change in volume during deformation, the tissue is said to be incompressible and the deformation is said to be isochoric.
- The constitutive equations describe the relationship between stress and strain under certain conditions.
- A Cauchy elastic material is a material whose stress at any given point is determined only by the current state of deformation, that is, there is one-to-one mapping between stress and deformation.
- A hyperelastic material is a special case of Cauchy's elasticity, where the stress–strain relation is derived from the strain energy density function.
- The constitutive equation of linear elastic materials is given by the Hooke's law, which relates stress to strain through the stiffness tensor.
- A monoclinic material has a plane of symmetry.
- An orthotropic material has two or three mutually orthogonal twofold axes of rotational symmetry, so that its mechanical properties are different along each axis.
- An isotropic material has properties that do not change from direction to another.
- A transverse-isotropic material has properties that are indifferent in a plane perpendicular to the axis of symmetry.
- The conservation of mass principle states that the total mass of any part of the body is equal to the amount of mass flowing into the volume occupied by this body through its surface.
- According to the conservation of momentum principle, the net force acting on a given body is zero at equilibrium conditions.
- The equation of motion is a differential equation that describes how the material points move in response to the applied forces.
- The FEM method is a powerful numerical analysis technique that has been successfully implemented in myocardial deformation analysis.
- The FEM method relies on approximating the geometry of the tissue under study using a number of small building blocks called the finite elements.
- In FEM, shape functions are the functions that are used to interpolate the nodal values to estimate the values at any point within the element.

REFERENCES

Arts, T., Hunter, W. C., Douglas, A., Muijtjens, A. M., and Reneman, R. S. (1992). Description of the deformation of the left ventricle by a kinematic model. *J Biomech* **25**(10): 1119–1127.

Augenstein, K. F., Cowan, B. R., LeGrice, I. J., and Young, A. A. (2006). Estimation of cardiac hyperelastic material properties from MRI tissue tagging and diffusion tensor imaging. *Med Image Comput Comput Assist Interv* **9**(Pt 1): 628–635.

Azhari, H., Buchalter, M., Sideman, S., Shapiro, E., and Beyar, R. (1992). A conical model to describe the nonuniformity of the left ventricular twisting motion. *Ann Biomed Eng* **20**: 149–165.

Bathe, K. J. (1982). *Finite Element Procedures in Engineering Analysis.* Upper Saddle River, NJ: Prentice Hall.

Benayoun, S. and Ayache, N. (1995). Dense non-rigid motion estimation in sequences of medical images using differential constraints. *Lect Notes Comput Sci* **970**: 254–261

Bistoquet, A., Oshinski, J., and Skrinjar, O. (2007). Left ventricular deformation recovery from cine MRI using an incompressible model. *IEEE Trans Med Imaging* **26**(9): 1136–1153.

Bistoquet, A., Oshinski, J., and Skrinjar, O. (2008). Myocardial deformation recovery from cine MRI using a nearly incompressible biventricular model. *Med Image Anal* **12**(1): 69–85.

Chadwick, R. S. (1982). Mechanics of the left ventricle. *Biophys J* **39**(3): 279–288.

Chapelle, D., Le Tallec, P., Moireau, P., and Sorine, M. (2012). An energy-preserving muscle tissue model: Formulation and compatible discretizations. *J Multiscale Comput Eng* **10**: 189–211.

Charalambous, N., Michaelides, K., Psimolofitis, E., Tzangarakis, V., Michaelides, D., Angeli, S., and Constantinides, C. (2013). Stress-strain characterization of a dynamically-controlled cardiac phantom with fluid and structural dynamics. *Proceedings of the International Society of Magnetic Resonance in Medicine*, Salt Lake City, UT, p. 4449.

Christensen, G. E., Rabbitt, R. D., and Miller, M. I. (1994). 3D brain mapping using a deformable neuroanatomy. *Phys Med Biol* **39**(3): 609–618.

Christensen, G. E., Rabbitt, R. D., and Miller, M. I. (1996). Deformable templates using large deformation kinematics. *IEEE Trans Image Process* **5**(10): 1435–1447.

Costa, K. (1996). The structural basis of three-dimensional ventricular mechanics. PhD dissertation, University of California, San Diego, CA.

Declerck, J., Denney, T. S., Ozturk, C., O'Dell, W., and McVeigh, E. R. (2000). Left ventricular motion reconstruction from planar tagged MR images: A comparison. *Phys Med Biol* **45**(6): 1611–1632.

Demer, L. L. and Yin, F. C. (1983). Passive biaxial mechanical properties of isolated canine myocardium. *J Physiol* **339**: 615–630.

Dokos, S., Smaill, B. H., Young, A. A., and LeGrice, I. J. (2002). Shear properties of passive ventricular myocardium. *Am J Physiol Heart Circ Physiol* **283**(6): H2650–H2659.

Duncan, J., Shi, P., Constable, T., and Sinusas, A. (1998). Physical and geometrical modeling for image-based recovery of left ventricular deformation. *Prog Biophys Mol Biol* **69**(2–3): 333–351.

Gee, J. C., Haynor, D. R., Le Briquer, L., and Bajcsy, R. K. (1997). Advances in elastic matching theory and its implementation. *Lect Notes Comput Sci* **1205**: 63–72.

Geman, D. and Geman, S. (1984). Stochastic relaxation, Gibbs distribution and Bayesian restoration of images. *IEEE Trans Pattern Anal Machine Intell* **6**: 721–741.

Guccione, J. and McCulloch, A. (1991). Finite element modeling of ventricular mechanics. In *Theory of Heart*, P. Hunter, A. McCulloch, and P. Nielsen (eds.). Berlin, Germany: Springer-Verlag, pp. 122–144.

Guccione, J. M. and McCulloch, A. D. (1993). Mechanics of active contraction in cardiac muscle: Part I—Constitutive relations for fiber stress that describe deactivation. *J Biomech Eng* **115**(1): 72–81.

Haber, I., Metaxas, D. N., and Axel, L. (2000). Three-dimensional motion reconstruction and analysis of the right ventricle using tagged MRI. *Med Image Anal* **4**(4): 335–355.

Hadjicharalambous, M., Chabiniok, R., Asner, L., Sammut, E., Wong, J., Carr-White, G., Lee, J., Razavi, R., Smith, N., and Nordsletten, D. (2015). Analysis of passive cardiac constitutive laws for parameter estimation using 3D tagged MRI. *Biomech Model Mechanobiol* **14**(4): 807–828.

Harper, K. W. and Tello, R. (2003). Prediction rule for diagnosis of arrhythmogenic right ventricular dysplasia based on wall thickness measured on MR imaging. *Comput Med Imaging Graph* **27**(5): 363–371.

Hooks, D. A., Tomlinson, K. A., Marsden, S. G., LeGrice, I. J., Smaill, B. H., Pullan, A. J., and Hunter, P. J. (2002). Cardiac microstructure: Implications for electrical propagation and defibrillation in the heart. *Circ Res* **91**(4): 331–338.

Hu, Z., Metaxas, D., and Axel, L. (2003). In vivo strain and stress estimation of the heart left and right ventricles from MRI images. *Med Image Anal* **7**(4): 435–444.

Humphrey, J. D. and Yin, F. C. (1987). On constitutive relations and finite deformations of passive cardiac tissue: I. A pseudostrain-energy function. *J Biomech Eng* **109**(4): 298–304.

Humphrey, J. D. and Yin, F. C. (1989). Biomechanical experiments on excised myocardium: Theoretical considerations. *J Biomech* **22**(4): 377–383.

Hunter, P. J., McCulloch, A. D., and ter Keurs, H. E. (1998). Modelling the mechanical properties of cardiac muscle. *Prog Biophys Mol Biol* **69**(2–3): 289–331.

Hyer, M. W. (1998). *Stress Analysis of Fiber-Reinforced Composite Materials.* New York: McGraw-Hill.

Ibrahim, El-S. H. (2011). Myocardial tagging by cardiovascular magnetic resonance: Evolution of techniques—Pulse sequences, analysis algorithms, and applications. *J Cardiovasc Magn Reson* **13**: 36.

Kass, M., Witkin, A., and Terzopoulos, D. (1988). Snakes: Active contour models. *Int J Comput Vision* **1**: 321–331.

Kaw, A. K. (1997). *Mechanics of Composite Materials.* Boca Raton, FL: CRC Press.

Kojic, M., Filipovic, N., Stojanovic, B., and Kojic, N. (2008). *Computer Modeling in Bioengineering: Theoretical Background, Examples and Software.* West Sussex, U.K.: John Wiley & Sons.

Komo, J. J. (1987). *Random Signal Analysis in Engineering Systems.* Waltham, MA: Academic Press.

Lai, W. M., Rubin, D., and Krempl, E. (2009). *Introduction to Continuum Mechanics.* Burlington, MA: Elsevier.

Legrice, I. J., Hunter, P. J., and Smaill, B. H. (1997). Laminar structure of the heart: A mathematical model. *Am J Physiol* **272**(5 Pt 2): H2466–H2476.

Meyer, F. G., Constable, R. T., Sinusas, A. J., and Duncan, J. S. (1996). Tracking myocardial deformation using phase contrast MR velocity fields: A stochastic approach. *IEEE Trans Med Imaging* **15**(4): 453–465.

Miller, M. I., Trouve, A., and Younes, L. (2002). On the metrics and Euler-Lagrange equations of computational anatomy. *Annu Rev Biomed Eng* **4**: 375–405.

Moulton, M. J., Creswell, L. L., Downing, S. W., Actis, R. L., Szabo, B. A., and Pasque, M. K. (1996). Myocardial material property determination in the in vivo heart using magnetic resonance imaging. *Int J Card Imaging* **12**(3): 153–167.

Nastar, C. (1994). Vibration modes for nonrigid motion analysis in 3D images. *Proceedings of the Third European Conference on Computer Vision (ECCV)*, Stockholm, Sweden, pp. 231–236.

Nielsen, P. M., Le Grice, I. J., Smaill, B. H., and Hunter, P. J. (1991). Mathematical model of geometry and fibrous structure of the heart. *Am J Physiol* **260**(4 Pt 2): H1365–H1378.

O'Dell, W. G., Moore, C. C., Hunter, W. C., Zerhouni, E. A., and McVeigh, E. R. (1995). Three-dimensional myocardial deformations: Calculation with displacement field fitting to tagged MR images. *Radiology* **195**(3): 829–835.

Pao, Y. C., Nagendra, G. K., Padiyar, R., and Ritman, E. L. (1980). Derivation of myocardial fiber stiffness equation based on theory of laminated composite. *J Biomech Eng* **102**(3): 252.

Papademetris, X., Shi, P., Dione, D. P., Sinusas, A. J., Constable, R. T., and Duncan, J. S. (1999). Recovery of soft tissue object deformation from 3D image sequences using biomechanical models. *Lect Notes Comput Sci* **1613**: 352–357.

Papademetris, X., Sinusas, A. J., Dione, D. P., Constable, R. T., and Duncan, J. S. (2002). Estimation of 3-D left ventricular deformation from medical images using biomechanical models. *IEEE Trans Med Imaging* **21**(7): 786–800.

Papademetris, X., Sinusas, A. J., Dione, D. P., and Duncan, J. S. (2001). Estimation of 3D left ventricular deformation from echocardiography. *Med Image Anal* **5**: 17–28.

Park, J., Metaxas, D., and Axel, L. (1996a). Analysis of left ventricular wall motion based on volumetric deformable models and MRI-SPAMM. *Med Image Anal* **1**(1): 53–71.

Park, J., Metaxas, D., Young, A. A., and Axel, L. (1996b). Deformable models with parameter functions for cardiac motion analysis from tagged MRI data. *IEEE Trans Med Imaging* **15**(3): 278–289.

Perie, D., Dahdah, N., Foudis, A., and Curnier, D. (2013). Multiparametric MRI as an indirect evaluation tool of the mechanical properties of in-vitro cardiac tissues. *BMC Cardiovasc Disord* **13**: 24.

Pham, Q. C., Vincent, F., Clarysse, P., Croisille, P., and Magnin, I. E. (2001). A FEM-based deformable model for the 3D segmentation and tracking of the heart in cardiac MRI. *Proceedings of the Second International Symposium on Image and Signal Processing and Analysis*, Pula, Croatia, pp. 250–254.

Phatak, N. S., Maas, S. A., Veress, A. I., Pack, N. A., Di Bella, E. V., and Weiss, J. A. (2009). Strain measurement in the left ventricle during systole with deformable image registration. *Med Image Anal* **13**(2): 354–361.

Phatak, N. S., Sun, Q., Kim, S. E., Parker, D. L., Sanders, R. K., Veress, A. I., Ellis, B. J., and Weiss, J. A. (2007). Noninvasive determination of ligament strain with deformable image registration. *Ann Biomed Eng* **35**(7): 1175–1187.

Pinto, J. G. and Fung, Y. C. (1973). Mechanical properties of the heart muscle in the passive state. *J Biomech* **6**(6): 597–616.

Pollard, A. E. and Barr, R. C. (1991). Computer simulations of activation in an anatomically based model of the human ventricular conduction system. *IEEE Trans Biomed Eng* **38**(10): 982–996.

Rabbitt, R. D., Weiss, J. A., Christensen, G. E., and Miller, M. I. (1995). Mapping of hyperelastic deformable templates using the finite element method. *Proc SPIE* **2573**: 252–265.

Reddy, J. (2005). *An Introduction to the Finite Element Method*. New York: McGraw-Hill.

Rohlfing, T. and Maurer, C. R. (2001). Intensity-based non-rigid registration using adaptive multilevel free-form deformation with an incompressibility constraint. *Lect Notes Comput Sci* **2208**: 111–119.

Sainte-Marie, J., Chapelle, D., Cimrman, R., and Sorine, M. (2006). Modeling and estimation of the cardiac electromechanical activity. *Comput Struct* **84**: 1743–1759.

Shi, P., Robinson, G., Chakraborty, A., Staib, L., Constable, R., Sinusas, A., and Duncan, J. (1995a). A unified framework to assess myocardial function from 4D images. *Proceedings of the First International Conference on Computer Vision, Virtual Reality and Robotics in Medicine*, Nice, France, pp. 1–11.

Shi, P., Robinson, G., Constable, R. T., and Sinusas, A. (1995b). A model-based integrated approach to track myocardial deformation using displacement and velocity constraints. *Proceedings of the Fifth International Conference on Computer Vision*, Cambridge, MA, pp. 687–692.

Shi, P., Sinusas, A. J., Constable, R. T., and Duncan, J. S. (1998). Volumetric deformation analysis using mechanics-based data fusion: Applications in cardiac motion recovery. *Int J Comput Vision* **35**: 65–85.

Sinusas, A. J., Papademetris, X., Constable, R. T., Dione, D. P., Slade, M. D., Shi, P., and Duncan, J. S. (2001). Quantification of 3-D regional myocardial deformation: Shape-based analysis of magnetic resonance images. *Am J Physiol Heart Circ Physiol* **281**(2): H698–H714.

Slaughter, W. S. (2002). *The Linearized Theory of Elasticity*. Boston, MA: Birkhauser.

Song, S. M. and Leahy, R. M. (1991). Computation of 3-D velocity fields from 3-D cine CT images of a human heart. *IEEE Trans Med Imaging* **10**(3): 295–306.

Song, S. M., Leahy, R. M., Boyd, D. P., Brundage, B. H., and Napel, S. (1994). Determining cardiac velocity fields and intraventricular pressure distribution from a sequence of ultrafast CT cardiac images. *IEEE Trans Med Imaging* **13**(2): 386–397.

Sun, W., Qetin, M., Chan, R., Reddy, V., Holmvang, G., Chandar, V., and Willsky, A. (2005). Segmenting and tracking the left ventricle by learning the dynamics in cardiac images. *Inf Process Med Imaging* **19**: 553–565.

ten Tusscher, K. H., Noble, D., Noble, P. J., and Panfilov, A. V. (2004). A model for human ventricular tissue. *Am J Physiol Heart Circ Physiol* **286**(4): H1573–H1589.

Trayanova, N. (2006). Defibrillation of the heart: Insights into mechanisms from modelling studies. *Exp Physiol* **91**(2): 323–337.

Veress, A. I., Gullberg, G. T., and Weiss, J. A. (2005). Measurement of strain in the left ventricle during diastole with cine-MRI and deformable image registration. *J Biomech Eng* **127**(7): 1195–1207.

Veress, A. I., Weiss, J. A., Rabbitt, R. D., Lee, J. N., and Gullberg, G. T. (2001). Measurement of 3D left ventricular strains during diastole using image warping and untagged MRI images. *Comput Cardiol* **28**:165–168.

Vetter, F. J. and McCulloch, A. D. (1998). Three-dimensional analysis of regional cardiac function: A model of rabbit ventricular anatomy. *Prog Biophys Mol Biol* **69**(2–3): 157–183.

Waks, E., Prince, J. L., and Douglas, A. S. (1996). Cardiac motion simulator for tagged MRI. *Proceedings of the IEEE Workshop Mathematical Methods in Biomedical Image Analysis*, San Francisco, CA, pp. 182–191.

Weiss, J. A., Rabbitt, R. D., Bowden, A. E., and Maker, B. N. (1998). Incorporation of medical image data in finite element models to track strain in soft tissues. *Proc SPIE* **3254**: 477–484.

Yin, F. C., Strumpf, R. K., Chew, P. H., and Zeger, S. L. (1987). Quantification of the mechanical properties of noncontracting canine myocardium under simultaneous biaxial loading. *J Biomech* **20**(6): 577–589.

Young, A. A. and Cowan, B. R. (2012). Evaluation of left ventricular torsion by cardiovascular magnetic resonance. *J Cardiovasc Magn Reson* **14**: 49.

Zhang, Y., Liang, X., Ma, J., Jing, Y., Gonzales, M. J., Villongco, C., Krishnamurthy, A. et al. (2012). An atlas-based geometry pipeline for cardiac Hermite model construction and diffusion tensor reorientation. *Med Image Anal* **16**(6): 1130–1141.

Zhuang, L., Liu, H., Liang, X., Bao, H., Hu, H., and Shi, P. (2005). A simultaneous framework for recovering three dimensional shape and nonrigid motion from cardiac image sequences. *Conf Proc IEEE Eng Med Biol Soc* **6**: 5731–5734.

Zienkiewicz, O. C., Taylor, R. L., and Zhu, J. Z. (2013). *The Finite Element Method: Its Basis and Fundamentals*. Waltham, MA: Butterworth-Heinemann.

7 Cardiac Magnetic Resonance Cine Image Analysis

El-Sayed H. Ibrahim, PhD

CONTENTS

LIST OF ABBREVIATIONS

Abbreviation	Meaning
2D	Two-dimensional
3D	Three-dimensional
4D	Four-dimensional
AAM	Active appearance model
ASM	Active shape model
CRT	Cardiac resynchronization therapy
DENSE	Displacement-encoding with stimulated echo
ECG	Electrocardiogram
EF	Ejection fraction
EM	Expectation-maximization
FEM	Finite-element method
GMI	Geometric moment invariant
HARP	Harmonic phase
HT	Hough transform
ICA	Independent component analysis
ILM	Interlandmark motion
IMM	Interacting multiple model
ISITOAA	Iterative salient isolated threshold optimization ant algorithm
IVD	Interventricular dyssynchrony
LAX	Long-axis
LBBB	Left bundle branch block
LDA	Linear discriminant analysis
LSVM	Linear support vector machine
LV	Left ventricle
LVD	LV dyssynchrony
MI	Myocardial infarction
ML	Maximum likelihood
MMSE	Minimum mean squared error
MRF	Markov random field
NMI	Normalized mutual information
NURBS	Nonuniform rational B-splines
NWT	Normalized wall thickness
OF	Optical flow
PCA	Principal component analysis
PDM	Point distribution modeling
PGC	Periodic generalized cylinder
RV	Right ventricle
SAX	Short-axis
SDE	Shannon's differential entropy
SNR	Signal-to-noise ratio
UKF	Unscented Kalman filter
UKS	Unscented Kalman smoother
WVD	Wigner–Ville distribution

7.1 INTRODUCTION

7.1.1 CARDIAC CINE MAGNETIC RESONANCE IMAGING

Cine MRI imaging is a main component of almost every cardiovascular magnetic resonance (CMR) exam. Typically, a stack of parallel short-axis (SAX) images covering the heart is acquired along with four-chamber, two-chamber, and sometimes three-chamber views. Ventricular contours drawn on the cine images during postprocessing are used to generate measures of global heart function, for example, volumes, mass, and ejection fraction (EF). However, recent efforts have been made to exploit cine images for evaluating regional heart function, for example, measuring myocardial strain and detecting wall motion abnormalities. It should be noted that while the cine images lack the tagging pattern that is used for tracking myocardial deformation in the MRI tagged images, useful information can still be obtained from tracking wall motion during the cardiac cycle. Furthermore, myocardial radial thickening is easier to measure from the cine nontagged images because the tagging pattern sparsely samples the myocardium in the radial direction. Therefore, many image processing and analysis techniques have been developed for evaluating myocardial deformation during the cardiac cycle based on processing the cine images, which is the topic of this chapter. It should be noted that in this chapter we do not address methods for analyzing the cine images using the recently developed feature-tracking techniques. These techniques are covered in detail in the next chapter.

7.1.2 CINE IMAGING COMPARED TO OTHER IMAGING MODALITIES

Since the mid-1980s, findings from cine CMR images have been compared to other more established techniques for evaluating the heart function (Underwood et al. 1986, Sechtem et al. 1987, Lotan et al. 1989, Peshock et al. 1989, Haag et al. 1991, Herbots et al. 2004). In 1986, Underwood et al. (1986) compared CMR to x-ray ventriculography, where the results showed good agreement between the two modalities for assessing ventricular wall motion. In the following year, Sechtem et al. (1987) used electrocardiogram (ECG)-gated cine CMR to quantify systolic left ventricular (LV) wall thickening in patients with different heart diseases and showed that the CMR results are in agreement with two-dimensional (2D) echo for differentiating infarcted regions. Later in 1989, Lotan et al. (1989) showed that the results from cine long-axis (LAX) CMR images are comparable to LV cineangiography for evaluating regional wall motion. In the same year, these conclusions were confirmed in an experimental study on dogs (Peshock et al. 1989), where the CMR results showed good agreement not only with cineangiography, but also with histochemical evidence of infarction with wall thickening being an accurate parameter for identifying myocardial infarction. In other studies (Haag et al. 1991, Herbots et al. 2004), CMR has been compared to M-mode echocardiography. For example, Haag et al. (1991) showed that LV wall thickness and chamber diameter measured from CMR images are precise, but satisfactory accurate, markers for evaluating the heart function in volunteers and patients with coronary artery disease (CAD). In another study (Herbots et al. 2004), M-mode MRI images were constructed by sampling the cine CMR images along a line drawn across the inferolateral wall, from which radial strain was measured, which was well correlated with results from M-mode echocardiography throughout the whole cardiac cycle.

7.1.3 CHAPTER OUTLINE

This chapter covers different techniques that have been implemented for evaluating regional heart function from cine CMR images. The chapter starts by covering simple techniques for quantifying ventricular wall motion, including wall motion thickening, centerline and centersurface methods, wall motion patterns, and still-frame parametric maps. Atlas-based techniques are then covered, starting by a brief review of cardiac segmentation and registration techniques, and followed by discussing probabilistic and statistical atlases. Geometrical modeling is then discussed, including basic LV models and simple geometrical fitting techniques. The chapter then covers nonrigid deformation techniques, including active contours, thin plates, B-splines, nonuniform rational B-splines (NURBS), active shape models (ASM) and active appearance models (AAM), nonrigid registration, and differential geometrical properties. The next section covers intensity-based analysis techniques, including optical flow (OF), Wigner–Ville distribution (WVD), harmonic analysis, level sets, and other intensity distribution techniques. Spatiotemporal registration and recursive filters are then covered, followed by Kalman filters and smoothers, where the last section includes continuous, discrete, and hybrid Kalman filters, information theoretic measures, and interacting multiple models. It should be noted that some of the techniques covered in this chapter apply also to tagged image analysis (Chapters 2 and 3 of *Heart Mechanics: Magnetic Resonance Imaging—Advanced Techniques, Clinical Applications, and Future Trends*); however, they are described in each chapter based on the application at hand.

7.2 WALL MOTION ANALYSIS: SIMPLE TECHNIQUES

7.2.1 VENTRICULAR WALL THICKENING

7.2.1.1 2D Implementation

Different techniques have been presented for quantitative assessment of regional heart function from cine CMR images

(Tseng 2000). Specifically, ventricular wall thickening (Figure 7.1), defined as the percentage change in wall thickness between end-diastole and end-systole, showed to be a sensitive marker for detecting dysfunctional myocardium (Tseng 2000, van der Geest et al. 2000).

7.2.1.2 3D Implementation

Different studies (Buller et al. 1995, Holman et al. 1997) focused on correcting for errors in wall thickness measurements due to inaccurate positioning of the heart's LAX direction, which is exaggerated with heart motion (Figure 7.2). An algorithm has been developed for three-dimensional (3D) wall thickness calculation based on planar 2D wall thickness measurements (Buller et al. 1995). The developed technique is based on calculating the oblique angle between the imaging slice and ventricular wall from a set of 2D SAX images in order to reverse the overestimation effect in wall thickness measurement (Figure 7.3).

In the 3D wall thickness measurement technique, a 3D surface (dashed midwall surface in Figure 7.3) is generated through all midpoints of the centerline chords in a set of parallel SAX slices, from which the vectors normal to the myocardium are constructed at all points (Holman et al. 1997). The oblique angle α between the myocardial normal vector (tilted dashed line) and the vector normal to the imaging slice (vertical dashed line) is then measured, and the 3D "true" wall thickness (WT_{3D}) is obtained from the apparent "exaggerated" measured 2D wall thickness (WT_{2D}) as follows:

$$WT_{3D} = WT_{2D} \times \sin\alpha. \tag{7.1}$$

Numerical simulations showed that the proposed technique has errors of only 1.6% and 10.6% in wall thickness measurement at the basal/mid and apical slices, respectively, compared to errors of 8.1% and 28.6%, respectively, with 2D measurements (Buller et al. 1995).

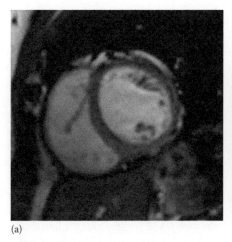 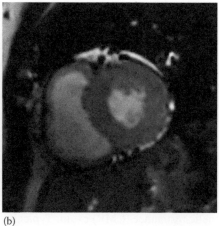

(a)   (b)

FIGURE 7.1 Change in myocardial wall thickness during the cardiac cycle. Short-axis slice at (a) end-diastole and (b) end-systole, showing significant change in wall thickness.

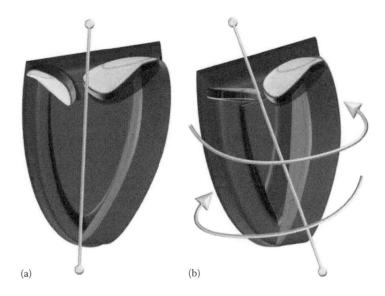

FIGURE 7.2 Error in long-axis (LAX) orientation with respect to the heart position. (a) LAX orientation is correctly determined. (b) LAX orientation is tilted with respect to the heart position, which affects wall thickness measurement, especially with heart motion during the cardiac cycle (the curved arrows show heart twisting during systole). (Courtesy of Dr. Shehab Anwar, Aswan Heart Institute, Aswan, Egypt.)

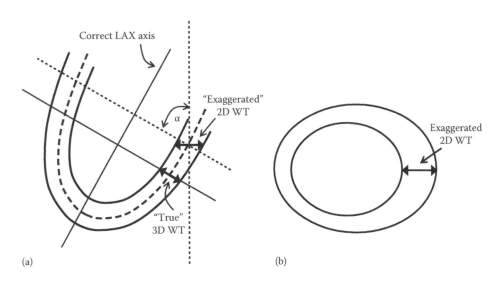

FIGURE 7.3 3D wall thickness measurement. (a) "Exaggerated" 2D wall thickness due to incorrect long-axis (LAX) orientation with respect to the heart position. Angle α is determined to calculate the "true" 3D wall thickness. (b) Tilted short-axis view of the heart showing the "exaggerated" 2D slice thickness. Note that incorrect LAX orientation is exaggerated for illustration purpose in this example.

7.2.1.3 Wall Thickness Measurement Using Laplace Equation

Recently, an improved 3D technique for measuring ventricular wall thickness using Laplace equation has been developed, and the results have been validated against visual scoring by experts (Prasad et al. 2009, 2010). The developed technique is based on modeling the myocardial wall as a series of nested sublayers bounded by the endo- and epicardial surfaces (Figure 7.4). Therefore, the wall thickness is not measured based on a straight-line principle; it is rather measured by integrating along the direction perpendicular to each sublayer between the two surfaces, which provides more accurate results (Prasad et al. 2010).

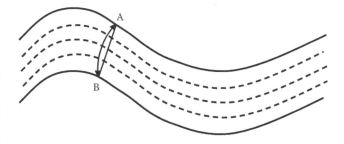

FIGURE 7.4 Wall thickness measurement using Laplace equation. Wall thickness is measured from a curved path drawn normal to the different sublayers between points A and B on the endo- and epicardium. The resulting wall thickness is different from that measured from a straight line drawn between the two points.

7.2.2 Centerline Method

7.2.2.1 2D Implementation

The LV wall thickness could be obtained from a SAX slice by drawing radial lines emanating from a point located at the center of mass of the LV blood pool and measuring the lengths of the line segment between the endocardial and epicardial borders. However, the validity of this straightforward approach has been challenged by reports showing that ventricular motion proceeds toward many points rather than a single center point (Goodyer and Langou 1982), which would result in measurement error due to wall thickness overestimation if the SAX slice is not exactly perpendicular to the local ventricular LAX orientation. The centerline method was developed to eliminate this error in wall thickness measurement (Sheehan et al. 1986). Rather than assuming an LV cross-sectional shape, the centerline method is based on generating a path (centerline) between the endo- and epicardial contours, from which different chords are drawn perpendicular to it at evenly spaced distances (Figure 7.5). Then, the length of the line segment of each cord in-between the endo- and epicardium determines regional ventricular wall thickness, from which wall thickening is measured by conducting the measurement at both end-systole and end-diastole and calculating the percentage increase in the length of the wall segment.

The centerline method has the advantage that it does not require a centroid or a reference coordinate system to correct for in-plane translational motion (Goodyer and Langou 1982). Sheehan et al. (1986) explored the advantages of the centerline method for quantitatively assessing regional heart function by measuring the change in wall thickness between end-systole and end-diastole along 100 chords constructed perpendicular to the centerline drawn midway between the endo- and epicardium. The measurements were represented in units of standard deviation from the mean results in a normal population, which has the advantage of expressing the severity of wall motion abnormality rather than just identifying abnormally contracting regions. Since its introduction, the centerline method has been used in a number of studies for measuring wall motion thickening. For example, Holman et al. (1995) used the centerline method for investigating the accuracy of ventricular wall thickening for identifying wall motion abnormality in eight pigs with induced myocardial infarction (MI) as compared to results from gadolinium delayed-enhancement CMR.

7.2.2.2 Centersurface Method

The centersurface method (Hubka et al. 2002, Beohar et al. 2007) has been developed as a 3D extension of the centerline method. The centersurface method constructs a triangulated surface midway between the endo- and epicardial surfaces, from which lines are constructed at every vertex perpendicular to the centersurface (Beohar et al. 2007). The myocardial wall thickness is then determined by measuring the length of the line segments between the intersection points of the generated lines with the endo- and epicardial surfaces. Therefore, the centersurface method is not affected by the obliquity of the direction of the ventricular wall with respect to the imaging plane, especially that the degree of obliquity changes between end-systole and end-diastole, which introduces an additional error in measuring wall thickening (Beyar et al. 1990). Furthermore, the centersurface method has the advantage that it does not depend on any geometrical assumptions that may introduce errors in wall thickness computation, especially in advanced stages of heart diseases when the heart assumes distorted shapes in response to increased loads. The accuracy of the centersurface method for measuring ventricular thickness has been validated in vitro (Hubka et al. 2002) and for accurately quantifying the infarct size and degree of myocardial contractility impairment in the LV (Beohar et al. 2007).

7.2.3 Wall Motion Patterns

As an extension of measuring wall thickening from end-diastole to end-systole, wall thickness can be measured at various timeframes through the cardiac cycle in order to generate a curve showing the pattern of wall thickness change across the cardiac cycle. This way, accurate assessments of the ventricular function and wall motion abnormality can be obtained.

7.2.3.1 Wall Motion Detection Using Pattern Recognition

Pattern recognition techniques have been implemented for analyzing ventricular wall motion. Recently, a correlation-based classification technique has been presented for identifying regions of abnormal regional wall motion in the LV (Lu et al. 2009). For the classifier to work successfully, a normalization scheme needs to be conducted, which is simplified by working in the polar coordinates system, as shown in Figure 7.6. Briefly, the

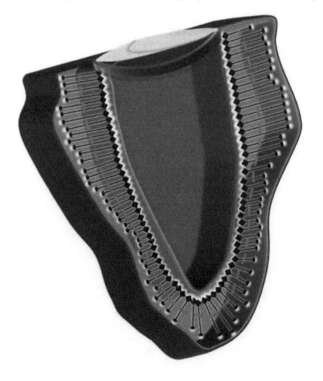

FIGURE 7.5 Centerline method. A centerline is drawn midway between the endo- and epicardium (dashed red line). Wall thickness is calculated from line segments (short black line segments) drawn perpendicular to the generated centerline. (Courtesy of Dr. Shehab Anwar, Aswan Heart Institute, Aswan, Egypt.)

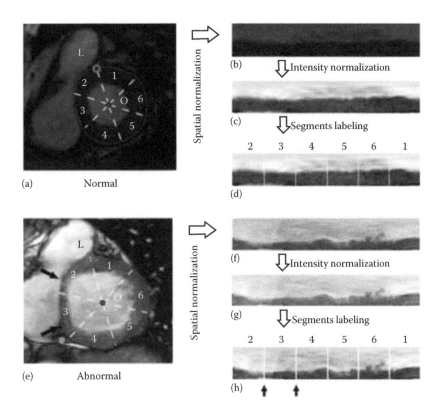

FIGURE 7.6 Examples of the normalization procedure for (a–d) a normal subject and (e–h) a patient with abnormal wall motion. In (a) and (e), "L" is the reference point and "O" is the centroid of the LV. In (e) and (h), the two black arrows point to the abnormal segment. (Reproduced from Lu, Y. et al., *Med. Image Comput. Comput. Assist. Interv.*, 12(Pt 2), 750, 2009. With permission.)

normalization scheme starts by identifying a reference point (usually the anterior end of the interventricular septum) to localize the heart position. The size of the heart is then normalized by the length of the LV radius measured from a SAX slice. Shape normalization is followed by signal intensity normalization, where the intensity of each pixel is set to $(x - \mu)/\sigma$, where x is the original signal intensity and μ and σ are the mean and standard deviation, respectively, of the signal intensity in the myocardium. Following the normalization stage, an intrasegment classifier is used to identify segments with wall motion abnormality.

As shown in Figure 7.7, normalized myocardial segments from all heart phases are concatenated vertically to construct a spatiotemporal image, from which the signal intensity profile is measured by averaging the vertical signal intensity across different angles in the segment (Lu et al. 2009). Finally, correlation coefficients are calculated between the signal intensity profiles of the segment at different cardiac phases and the signal intensity profile at end-diastole in order to measure the segmental motion pattern during the cardiac cycle and identify segments with wall motion abnormality.

7.2.3.2 Normalized Wall Thickening Patterns

Recently, Wael et al. (2015) developed a technique that can detect regional wall motion abnormality based on capturing the variation in the myocardial thickness during the cardiac cycle. In the developed technique, the myocardial wall thickness is normalized by dividing the calculated distances by the mean radius of the epicardium at end-diastole. The normalized wall thickness

(NWT) values of all contour points within each segment in a SAX slice are averaged to one NWT value (Figure 7.8). Principal component analysis (PCA) is then applied to find the directions of data variations. The feature vector that represents the contraction pattern of each segment is created as the projection of its NWT pattern (through the cardiac cycle) on the eigenvectors corresponding to the largest eigenvalues. Feature classification is conducted using the maximum likelihood (ML) criterion with leave-one-out method over each segment (Elisseeff 2002). The results showed the capability of the developed method for identifying regions with abnormal wall motion.

7.2.3.3 Cardiac Dyssynchrony

Myocardial wall motion, assessed by CMR, has recently been used for detecting cardiac dyssynchrony (Foley et al. 2009). In this technique, a stack of cine SAX slices covering the LV is acquired, and a set of 100 radial chords was constructed in each slice to measure radial wall motion at all phases in the cardiac cycle. Each slice was then divided into six segments, in which radial wall motion was quantified by fitting the data to an empirical sine wave function of the form

$$y(t) = a + b \times \sin\left(\frac{t}{RR} + c\right), \tag{7.2}$$

where

RR is the length of the cardiac cycle
a, b, and c are constants

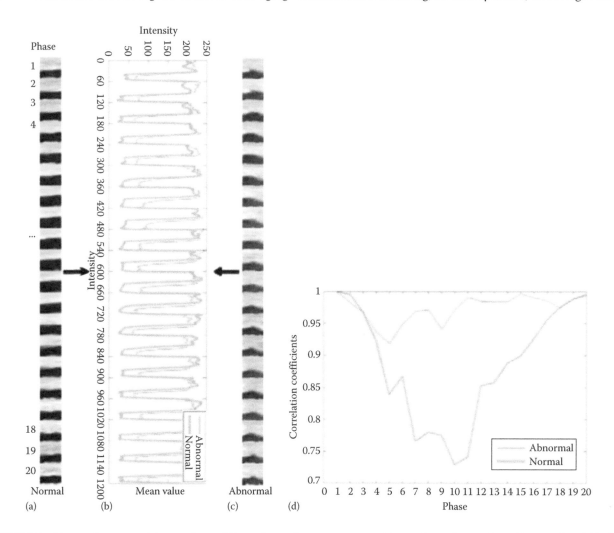

FIGURE 7.7   Temporal segmental images from different heart phases concatenated in a column format from (a) normal and (c) abnormal subjects. (b) Intensity profiles of the column image averaged across segments of the normal (green) and abnormal (red) segment. (d) Intrasegment correlation coefficients of the normal and abnormal segment. (Reproduced from Lu, Y. et al., *Med. Image Comput. Comput. Assist. Interv.*, 12(Pt 2), 750, 2009. With permission.)

The delay between the septal and lateral wall motion is measured as the time difference between the time-to-peak inward wall motion of the septal and lateral segments. Figure 7.9 shows the resulting dyssynchrony map, which shows the existence of cardiac dyssynchrony in patients with heart failure (Foley et al. 2009). In a more recent study, Suever et al. (2014) applied cross-correlation analysis on endocardial boundary radial displacement curves, generated from cine CMR images, to determine the delay time between each generated curve and a patient-specific reference. The measured delay times were projected onto the American Heart Association 17-segment model to create regional dyssynchrony maps.

7.2.3.4   Factors Affecting Wall Motion Measurements

The wall thickness curves (during the cardiac cycle) derived from the cine images are subject to a measurement error, which is represented by large differences in the results from neighboring regions (in the absence of regional wall abnormality). In this respect, low-pass filtering (LPF) of the wall thickness curves is expected to minimize the errors in the

cardiac functional parameters generated from these curves. In their study, Lamb et al. (1995) showed that LPF has the effect of reducing the differences in peak wall thinning rate and time-to-peak wall thinning rate between neighboring segments from 0.31% to 0.15% mean wall thickness/ms and from 35 to 19 ms, respectively, which results in better representation and more accurate estimation of the myocardial wall motion.

The capability of deriving clinically useful measures of the heart wall motion and myocardial thickening from real-time cine CMR imaging is appealing; however, the compromise in image quality due to real-time imaging may affect the measurements accuracy. Using a turbo field echo–echo planar imaging sequence, Plein et al. (2001) found differences between the measurements obtained from conventional and real-time cine images, with the largest disagreement in the anterior and lateral segments. The measurement differences could be attributed to chemical shift artifacts, susceptibility artifacts, and lower spatial resolution with real-time imaging, which limit the technique's capability of accurately quantifying measures of regional

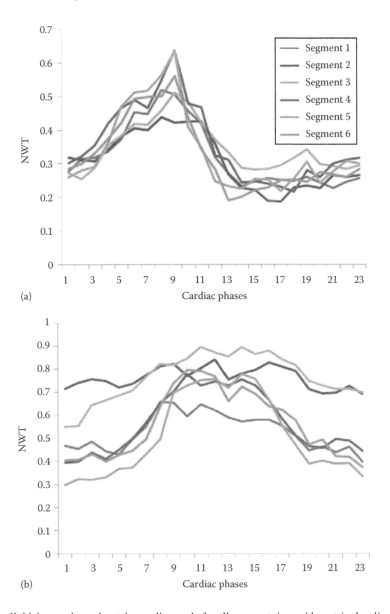

FIGURE 7.8 Normalized wall thickness throughout the cardiac cycle for all segments in a mid-ventricular slice from (a) normal (volunteer) and (b) patient with hypertrophic cardiomyopathy.

heart function. In a recent study (Contijoch et al. 2014), global LV elastance was dynamically measured using real-time cine CMR images to obtain regional LV elastance. LV motion was evaluated from wall thickness measurements in a large number of real-time image frames. The authors assessed different motion tracking algorithms and described their performance with respect to true motion labeled by experts. The results showed that symmetric diffeomorphic image registration with moderate spatial scale allows for accurate tracking of myocardial motion from a large number of real-time image frames.

7.2.3.5 Longitudinal Strain from Long-Axis Images

A number of studies have recently discussed the capability of measuring global longitudinal strain from LAX cine images (Kawakubo et al. 2013, Dusch et al. 2014, Gjesdal et al. 2014). Gjesdal et al. (2014) used LAX strain, measured from cine CMR images, as an index of global LV function, and compared it to that

measured from echocardiography in a post-infarct patient population. The results showed that the measurement of LAX strain was fast and reproducible by both CMR and echocardiography with good agreement between the two measurements. In another study, LAX strain has been used for the evaluation of cardiac dyssynchrony based on LV dyssynchrony (LVD) and interventricular dyssynchrony (IVD) indices, as shown in Figure 7.10 (Kawakubo et al. 2013). The results showed that LVD is significantly longer in patients with indication for CRT compared to those without indication for CRT. Further, both LVD and IVD are significantly longer in CRT responders than in CRT nonresponders. In a similar study, longitudinal LV fractional shortening has been used for assessing diastolic dysfunction confirmed by transthoracic echocardiography (Dusch et al. 2014). Finally, Riffel et al. (2015) proposed a standardized cardiac deformation approach based on the assessment of global longitudinal and circumferential strains from CMR and echocardiography images.

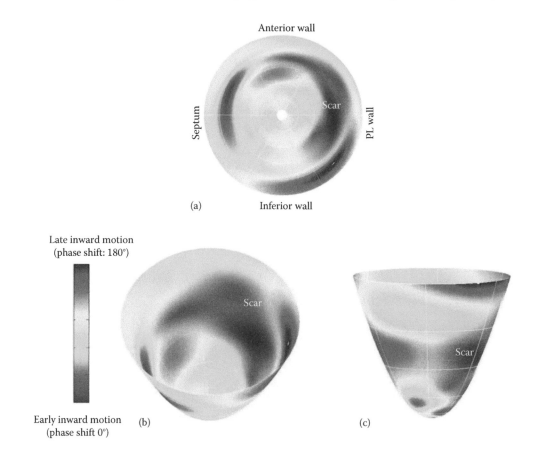

FIGURE 7.9   Spatial distribution of endocardial wall motion in heart failure. The color-encoded regional delay of radial inward motion is mapped onto (a) a bull's-eye map and three-dimensional surfaces of the left ventricular pictured (b) from above and (c) from the side. Timing of the radial inward motion is expressed as a phase delay ranging from 0° to 180°. A phase delay of 0° (blue color) represents early ventricular motion concordant with initial ventricular electrical activation, while a phase delay of 180° (red color) represents diastolic inward motion. (Reproduced from Foley, P.W. et al., *J. Cardiovasc. Magn. Reson.*, 11, 50, 2009.)

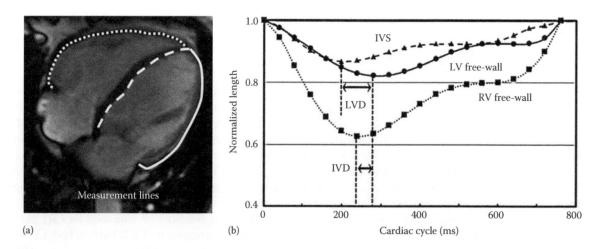

FIGURE 7.10   Definition of longitudinal left ventricular dyssynchrony (LVD) and interventricular dyssynchrony (IVD) indices for assessing cardiac dyssynchrony. (a) Longitudinal lengths of the LV free wall (solid line), the interventricular septum (IVS, dashed line), and the right ventricular (RV) free wall (dotted line) are measured at 20 timepoints throughout the cardiac cycle on a 4-chamber cine MRI image. (b) The longitudinal strain curves are obtained from normalized lengths of LV and RV free walls, and IVS based on timing of the onset of myocardial contraction. The index of LVD is defined as the difference between the times of minimum LV free-wall length and IVS length. The index of IVD is defined as the difference between the times of minimum LV and RV free-wall lengths. (Reproduced from Kawakubo, M. et al., *Eur. J. Radiol.*, 82(12), 2212, 2013. With permission.)

7.2.4 STILL-FRAME PARAMETRIC MAPS

7.2.4.1 Cyclic Wall Motion Variation

Besides measuring wall thickening, cine CMR images have been used for generating still-frame parametric images of wall motion (Caiani et al. 2004, Kachenoura et al. 2007). One idea is to generate an image in which each pixel is assigned a gray value representing the cyclic variation of local signal intensity at different timepoints in the cardiac cycle (Caiani et al. 2004). The resulting image shows bright bands of signal intensity at the endo- and epicardial borders, with the band's width reflecting the degree of wall motion. This is especially evident in the endocardial region and in steady-state free precession (SSFP) images, which have high contrast between the myocardium and blood pool. The parametric map is generated by fitting the pixel signal intensity change through the cardiac cycle as a sinusoidal function in the form of (Figure 7.11)

$$y(t) = A_1 \times \sin(\omega t + \varphi_1) + A_2 \times \sin(2\omega t + \varphi_2), \quad (7.3)$$

where the period of this function, $T = (2\pi\omega)^{-1}$, is determined from the ECG RR interval. The sum of the amplitudes of the first and second harmonics of the sinusoidal function, as shown in Equation 7.3, is then used to determine the intensity value for each pixel. In the resulting parametric image, hypokinetic myocardium shows thinner band and darker signal intensity than healthy regions, as shown in Figure 7.12 (Caiani et al. 2004). It should be noted that the incorporation of the amplitude of the second higher harmonic component in calculation helps reduce the intensity dropout, which could be misinterpreted as hypokinesis. Despite its capability of providing accurate information about wall motion abnormality, the developed technique is sensitive to motion caused by tissue translation. Further, the papillary muscle and myocardial trabeculations may affect the generated parametric image.

7.2.4.2 Pixel Signal Intensity Transition Mode

The cine CMR images can be used for generating parametric maps of wall motion for fast and robust evaluation of regional

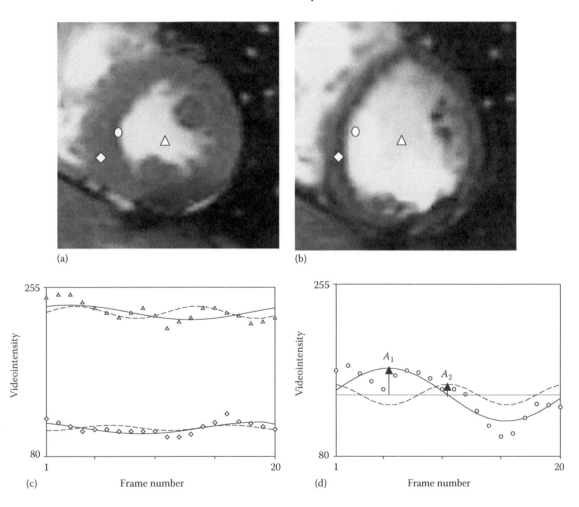

FIGURE 7.11 Parametric imaging of left ventricular wall motion. Three pixels at fixed positions are marked on the (a) end-systolic and (b) end-diastolic cardiovascular magnetic resonance images with three different symbols: a triangle, a diamond, and a circle. (c) Signal intensity of the pixels that remain in the myocardium or in the ventricular cavity throughout the cardiac cycle (diamond and triangle, respectively) is not expected to change beyond image noise. (d) In contrast, the intensity in the pixel represented by the circle changes considerably as the endocardium moves in and out. The sum of the amplitudes of the first two harmonics (A_1 and A_2) of the best-fit function, which is the parameter displayed in the parametric images in Figure 7.12, can thus differentiate between these classes of pixels and therefore depict the extent of endocardial motion. (Reproduced from Caiani, E.G. et al., *J. Cardiovasc. Magn. Reson.*, 6(3), 619, 2004.)

End-diastole   Parametric map   End-systole

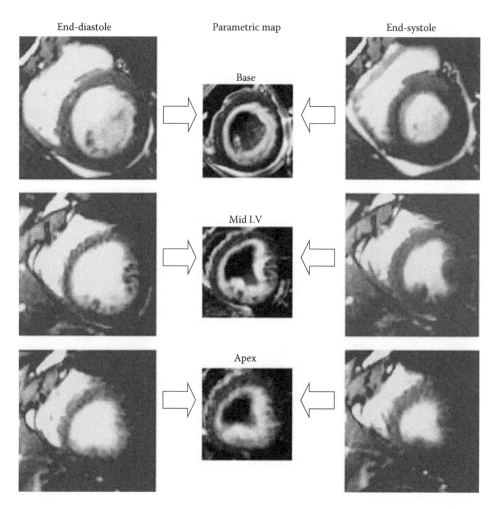

FIGURE 7.12 Parametric maps generated based on the first and second harmonic components of the sinusoidally modeled wall motion, as explained in Figure 7.11, in a patient with septal wall motion abnormality. End-diastolic (left column) and end-systolic (right column) short-axis cardiovascular magnetic resonance images obtained at three different levels of the left ventricle. Note the reduced myocardial thickening (left and right columns) concomitant with the thinning of the bright band (middle column) in the septal area at all ventricular levels. (Reproduced from Caiani, E.G. et al., *J. Cardiovasc. Magn. Reson.*, 6(3), 619, 2004.)

heart function (Kachenoura et al. 2007). This technique is similar to the analysis criteria used in echocardiography, where a nonlinear transition model is used to generate parametric maps based on changes in the pixels' signal intensity during the cardiac cycle (Ruiz Dominguez et al. 2005). In this regard, three groups of pixels could be identified in the image based on the pattern of signal intensity change during the cardiac cycle: (1) pixels that remain within the myocardium, (2) pixels that remain inside the blood pool, and (3) pixels that are inside the blood pool during diastole and become part of the myocardium during systole. Actually, it is this last group of pixels that is of particular importance as it represents ventricular wall motion during the cardiac cycle, which could be used to identify the regions of abnormal wall motion based on a number of derived parameters.

Two transition times (T_{ON} and T_{OFF}) could be determined from the signal intensity variation of the third group of pixels, with the generated T_{ON} and T_{OFF} images showing bands of increasing and decreasing signal intensity, respectively, from the endocardial end-diastolic boundary toward the center of the blood pool. The mean contraction time image, T_M (defined as the

average of T_{ON} and T_{OFF}), shows information about inward and outward wall motion, which is important for identifying contraction delays between different ventricular segments. Further, the mean radial velocity, V_m (defined as the slope of the transition time), and the time-to-first contraction of the endocardium, T_{fc} (defined as the shortest transition time), could be obtained as additional means for wall motion characterization. Kachenoura et al. (2007) showed a promising role of the developed technique for identifying wall motion abnormality, where the technique showed that T_{fc} and T_M increased, and V_m decreased in MI, while large time delays were observed in left bundle branch block (LBBB) (Figure 7.13). Nevertheless, it should be noted that this technique is sensitive to global heart motion.

7.2.5 INTERLANDMARK MOTION ANALYSIS

Besides the importance of studying wall motion thickening during the cardiac cycle for analyzing regional heart motion, the inclusion of multiple reference points (or landmarks) in the analysis allows for more accurate results. In this respect,

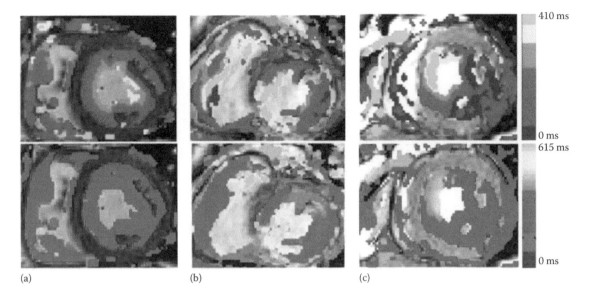

(a) (b) (c)

FIGURE 7.13 Parametric T_{ON} (top) and T_{M} (bottom) maps for three subjects: (a) control subject, (b) subject with inferior myocardial infarction, (c) subject with left ventricular bundle branch block. (Reproduced from Kachenoura, N. et al., *J. Magn. Reson. Imaging*, 26(4), 1127, 2007. With permission.)

the interlandmark motion (ILM) analysis technique has been developed for identifying myocardial abnormality (Lekadir et al. 2007, 2011). The technique is based on analyzing the relationship between landmarks at two regions in the LV during the whole cardiac cycle. The ILM vectors could include information about the LV shape, size, and wall thickness and displacement, which when combined result in an efficient approach for localizing abnormal myocardial regions. Specifically, a generalization form of the barycentric coordinates is used for modeling the probability distribution of a certain point ($\boldsymbol{x}$) based on known positions of non-coplanar landmarks ($\mathbf{x}_1$, $\mathbf{x}_2$, and $\mathbf{x}_3$) (Lekadir et al. 2011):

$$\boldsymbol{x} = u_1 x_1 + u_2 x_2 + u_3 x_3, \qquad (7.4)$$

where the coefficients u_1, u_2, and u_3 sum up to 1 to ensure invariance of the shape orientation, and their absolute values do not exceed 1 to avoid large displacements (Figure 7.14). As a large number of samples are used during the training phase of the method, the coefficient vectors can be calculated by forming the system of equations as a linear optimization problem, which can be solved using a number of available techniques, for example, Lagrange multipliers.

The analysis of the relationship between two landmarks (Figure 7.15) starts by forming an invariant multivariate vector $\mathbf{v}(p_i, p_j)$ that describes the coupled geometry between two landmarks p_i and p_j:

$$\mathbf{v}(p_i, p_j) = (a_{ij1}, \ldots, a_{ijF})^T, \qquad (7.5)$$

where

    F is the number of temporal frames

    a_{ijt} is a univariate ILM descriptor at frame # t

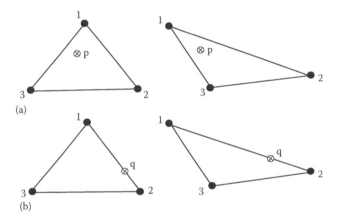

(a)

(b)

FIGURE 7.14 Barycentric coordinates. (a) Point p has the same barycentric coordinates (relative positioning within the triangle) with respect to vertices 1, 2, and 3 despite the difference in the shape of the two triangles (on the top). (b) Another example for point q shown on two triangles on the bottom.

A set of ILM vectors describing normal spatiotemporal properties is used in the training phase to define the normal range of motion variation (tolerance region, R_v). The variability in a normal population is represented by a multivariate normal distribution, where R_v is estimated as follows (Lekadir et al. 2011):

$$R_v = \left\{ \mathbf{v} \mid (\mathbf{v} - \bar{\mathbf{v}})^T \mathbf{S}_v^{-1} (\mathbf{v} - \bar{\mathbf{v}}) < L \right\} \qquad (7.6)$$

where

    $\bar{\mathbf{v}}$ and $\mathbf{S}_v$ represent the mean vector and covariance matrix, respectively, of $\mathbf{v}$

    L is a certain threshold value

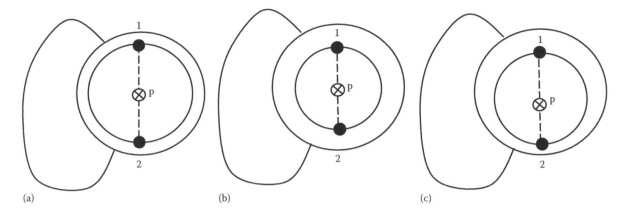

(a)   (b)   (c)

FIGURE 7.15   Interlandmark motion (ILM). Difference in ILM of point p at end-systole in (b) normal and (c) inferior wall motion abnormality cases with respect to reference end-diastole in (a).

A new vector can be then identified as representing a normal or abnormal ILM observation based on whether it belongs or does not belong to the tolerance region:

$$f_d(\mathbf{v}) = \begin{cases} 1, & \text{if } \mathbf{v} \in R_v \\ 0, & \text{if } \mathbf{v} \notin R_v \end{cases}. \qquad (7.7)$$

The ILM technique has a number of advantages: (1) it is invariant to similarity transformations, which waives the necessity for a preparatory shape alignment stage; (2) it decomposes the global shape pattern into local constraints, which facilitates image analysis; and (3) it provides an uncertainty matrix based on geometrical and statistical properties.

7.3   ATLAS-BASED TECHNIQUES

Model-based cardiac image analysis is an active area of research. Model-based analysis techniques provide a powerful approach for fast and accurate evaluation of the heart images. By customizing anatomical and functional cardiac models to images from an individual subject, information about the heart's shape and function can be obtained, which is helpful for studying normal ranges of variation in the population and differences in pathological cases. Compared to model-free approaches, the model-based techniques have the advantage that they provide information about the expected shapes of the structures of interest, which makes it easier to identify these structures in images with low signal-to-noise ratio (SNR) or in the presence of imaging artifacts. Further, the structures of interest can be described with a small number of parameters, and all image analysis and shape modeling steps can be conducted in a common framework. Model-based analysis techniques have been implemented for evaluating global (Matheny and Goldgof 1995, Staib and Duncan 1996) and regional (Huang and Goldgof 1993, Benayoun and Ayache 1998, Papademetris et al. 1999, Shi et al. 2000) heart function, and for investigating new descriptors of cardiac function (Friboulet et al. 1992, 1993, Nastar and Ayache 1996, Clarysse et al. 1997).

Future research trends in model-based analysis include evaluating current models' reliability and performance, examining new functional descriptors of the heart, and developing multidisciplinary models (Frangi et al. 2001).

Building cardiac atlases is an active area of research that is useful for both heart segmentation and identifying abnormal cases. In this respect, the cardiac atlas could be simply thought of as an average labeled image representation of the heart based on a training dataset. Given a new dataset, image registration is used to map the new dataset to the atlas, based on which the heart could be segmented and abnormal cases could be identified. Despite their advantages, it should be noted that the implementation of medical atlases in clinical practice is limited by the need for extensive manual segmentation during the training process and the possibility of missing important cases during the training phase that could limit the atlas's capability of identifying similar cases during implementation.

Although this chapter is not intended to cover all segmentation and registration techniques available in the image processing literature, a succinct overview of different techniques that have been implemented for studying myocardial deformation is presented in the first part of this section.

7.3.1   INTRODUCTION TO HEART SEGMENTATION AND REGISTRATION

7.3.1.1   Myocardial Segmentation

Heart segmentation techniques can be broadly divided into two categories (Sun et al. 2005, 2010) based on whether they depend on prior information (e.g., from previous timeframes (Geiger et al. 1995, Jolly et al. 2001, Zhou et al. 2005), active shape models (ASMs) (Mitchell et al. 2001, 2002, Zambal et al. 2006, van Assen et al. 2008, Zhang et al. 2010), or atlases (Lorenzo-Valdes et al. 2004, Zhuang et al. 2008)) or depend on intensive user intervention (Hautvast et al. 2006, Ben Ayed et al. 2009b, 2012). While the first category is characterized by automatic heart segmentation, it depends on time-consuming preprocessing steps. Nevertheless, cardiac segmentation based on finding a region in the segmented image that matches certain model or shape features usually provides excellent results (Adam et al. 2009, Ben Ayed et al. 2009b, 2010, 2012, Hochbaum and Singh 2009, Mukherjee et al. 2009, Ni et al. 2009, Pham et al. 2011, Nambakhsh et al. 2013, Suinesiaputra et al. 2014).

7.3.1.1.1 Gradient-Based Segmentation

A number of cardiac segmentation techniques use gradient-based methods to identify the object's boundary (Goshtasby and Turner 1995, Chakraborty et al. 1996, Weng et al. 1997, Jolly et al. 2001, Paragios 2002, Tsai et al. 2003), which results in optimal segmentation when the statistics inside and outside the object are different from each other. Gradient-based segmentation is implemented to determine a threshold that approximately localizes the boundaries of the ventricles, which correspond to a sharp rising or falling of the intensity profile (Weng et al. 1997), as shown in Figure 7.16. The detected boundaries are used to segment the image based on an attention map that approximates the region of interest in SAX images of the heart. A likelihood function is usually used to fine-tune the results.

7.3.1.1.2 Region-Based Segmentation

Region-based segmentation is used to divide the CMR images into separate clusters and determine the cluster that best represents the LV based on a voting procedure (Jolly et al. 2001). Specifically, multiple iterations of the Dijkstra's algorithm are usually run with increasing size of the search area (Duncan and Ayache 2000). The inclusion of the same pixels in the resulting contours in consecutive iterations is used as an indicator that these pixels represent a stable edge and should be included in the final segmentation. The developed algorithm determines the final contour based on best fit in the image by enforcing two constraining conditions: (1) the endocardium stays inside the epicardium and (2) the myocardial thickness stays about the same in all segments.

7.3.1.1.3 Artificial Intelligence Techniques

Artificial intelligence techniques have been implemented for segmenting CMR images. Besides the techniques based on artificial neural networks (Zurada 2012), fuzzy clustering (Miyamoto et al. 2008), and genetic algorithms (Simon 2013), new techniques have been developed based on deep

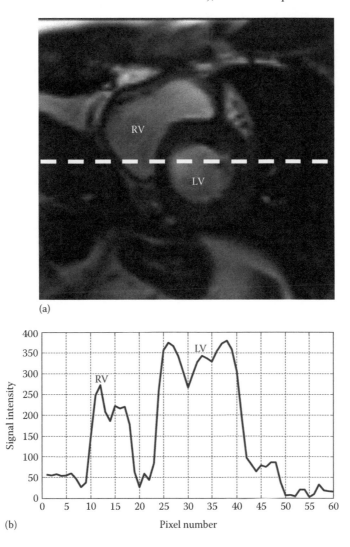

(a)

(b)

FIGURE 7.16 Gradient-based segmentation. (a) Short-axis image showing the location (dotted line) where signal intensity profile is calculated. (b) Signal intensity profile showing large gradients marking the ventricular boundaries. LV, left ventricle; RV, right ventricle.

learning and ant colony optimization. One example of the latter group is the iterative salient isolated threshold optimization ant algorithm (ISITOAA) technique that has been developed for segmenting the LV and RV from SAX images (Ibrahim et al. 2012). The ISITOAA algorithm is composed of two stages that are iteratively implemented: (1) adaptive segmentation (using salient thresholding) and (2) boundary detection (using the trapped ant algorithm [TAA]), as shown in Figure 7.17. The technique works by simulating the adaptive process by which ants find food and transfer it to their nest, where they communicate by dispersing pheromone on the path they have traveled. When ants encounter pheromone, they move accordingly with stochastic rules. Ants are considered to be in the same salient region if they cross each other's path in the same region (share one or more boundary points). The resulting set of boundary

points is associated with the number of ants belonging to it, which provides a measure of solution stability. An ant dies if it is found to be in a nonsalient region or if it encounters a pixel greater than a certain threshold in a specified number of movements. When an ant encounters a pixel greater than that threshold, it adds its location to the set of pixels it predicts to be in the boundary. Ants continue to process until a specified time limit is reached, where they are removed from the image. The ISITOAA technique is significantly faster (parallel processing with different intelligent agents (ants)) and more consistent than manual segmentations. The technique showed the capability of successfully detecting the endocardial borders in the case of severe trabeculations, which is a challenging task for automatic segmentation (Figure 7.18).

7.3.1.2 Heart Registration Techniques

Several review papers have been published in the field of medical image registration (Lucas and Kanade 1981, Maurer and Fizpatrick 1993, van den Elsen et al. 1993, Maintz and Viergever 1998, Hill et al. 2001). A thorough review of cardiac image registration is provided in Makela et al. (2002), where the registration techniques are divided into two main categories based on using either geometric image features or voxel similarity measures. The first category is divided into two subgroups based on the registration of a set of points or edges/surfaces. The second category is divided into three subgroups based on measuring moments and principal axes, intensity differences and correlation, or mutual information. We hereby provide a brief description of each of these groups. For more details, the reader is referred to the article by Makela et al. (2002).

The point-based registration techniques use anatomical landmarks, which are registered with the corresponding

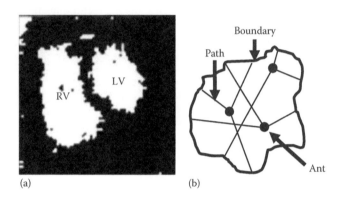

(a)   (b)

FIGURE 7.17 Ant colony optimization technique. (a) A threshold image. (b) Boundary detection based on ants' movement along various paths.

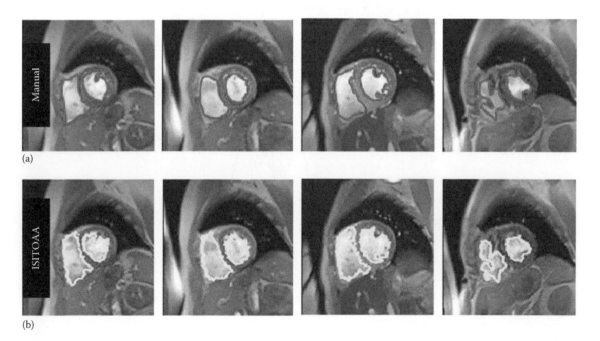

FIGURE 7.18   (a) Manual– and (b) iterative salient isolated threshold optimization ant algorithm (ISITOAA)–segmented short-axis images at different positions in the left ventricle.

points on the reference image, usually using the noniterative least-squares method (Arun et al. 1987). Although this group of techniques can be applied to any imaging modality, they have limited implementation in cardiac image registration because only few landmark points can be defined on non-tagged cine images, for example, the papillary muscles and insertion points of the RV into the interventricular septum. The edge- and surface-based registration techniques depend on minimizing a distance map defined on the segmented surfaces, usually using the chamfer method (Borgefors 1986, 1988). The surface-based cardiac registration techniques usually result in good registration of the areas of interest, although the results are affected by the choice of the surface to be registered, for example, epicardium versus endocardium.

The intensity-based registration techniques have the advantage that they do not require a priori extraction of registration features as in the geometry-based techniques. The moments- and principal-axes-based registration techniques measure statistical factors extracted from the images: the distribution of the image's intensity (moments) or the principal axes of the object of interest. The intensity difference- and correlation-based registration techniques maximize the similarity between two images based on the assumption that the pixel values in the registered images are strongly correlated. The mutual information-based registration techniques measure the statistical dependence of one image on the other, that is, the amount of information in one image that can be inferred from the other one (Wells et al. 1996, Maes et al. 1997).

Data interpolation may be required before conducting image registration to ensure that the two images have the same spatial resolution and to compensate for nonisotropic resolution in case of 3D imaging, where slice thickness is usually larger than in-plane pixel size. Nevertheless, one approach to reduce the computational time is to implement multiresolution registration techniques. In this case, the solution is obtained by an iterative implementation of the registration process at successively increasing resolution levels. However, it should be noted that successful registration depends on providing a compromise between accuracy, robustness, and speed.

7.3.2 Probabilistic Atlases

A probabilistic atlas provides information about the probability that a certain structure appears at a certain location in the image. The general steps for constructing a probabilistic atlas (Figure 7.19) include (Lotjonen et al. 2004) (1) segmenting and registering the heart images in a training dataset of a reference subject, (2) blurring the registered images with a Gaussian filter, and (3) averaging the blurred images. A similarity measure, for example, normalized mutual information (NMI), is usually used to assess the similarity between the source and destination data. NMI is given by

$$NMI = \frac{H(S) + H(D)}{H(S, D)}, \qquad (7.8)$$

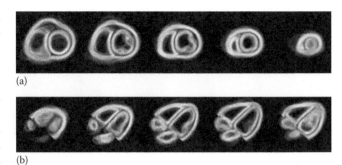

(a)

(b)

FIGURE 7.19   (a) Short-axis and (b) long-axis slices from a probabilistic atlas. (Reproduced from Lotjonen, J. et al., *Med. Image Anal.*, 8(3), 371, 2004. With permission.)

where
H(S) and H(D) are marginal entropies
H(S, D) is a joint entropy of the source data S and destination data D

Basically, entropy is a measure of uncertainty in a random variable based on probability P, given by

$$H(x) = -\sum_i P(x_i) \log P(x_i). \qquad (7.9)$$

A probability cardiac atlas has been developed to generate spatiotemporal probability maps of the LV and RV based on four-dimensional (4D) CMR data from 14 healthy volunteers (Lorenzo-Valdes et al. 2004). The developed atlas was used for developing a segmentation technique using the expectation-maximization (EM) technique (Dempster et al. 1977) and Markov random field (MRF) algorithm (Van Leemput et al. 1999), where the probabilistic atlas helped in estimating the initial model parameters and incorporating prior information for structure classification. The developed technique includes five steps that are repeated until convergence or until a maximum number of iterations is reached (Lorenzo-Valdes et al. 2004):

1. Classification of the voxels using the initial model parameters
2. Estimation of the Gaussian parameters of the model
3. Estimation of the MRF parameters
4. Classification using all parameters
5. Computation of the largest connected component for each structure

Figure 7.20 shows an example of the segmentation results of applying this technique in a healthy volunteer and a patient. In the developed classifier, the generated probabilistic maps serve the purpose of automating the estimation of the initial parameters for each structure and providing a priori information about the likelihood of spatial and temporal variation of different anatomical structures.

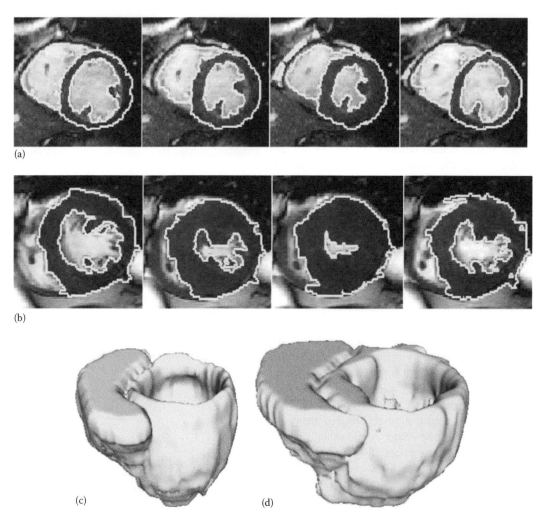

FIGURE 7.20 (a, b) 2D heart segmentation and (c, d) 3D reconstruction in (a and c) healthy volunteer and (b and d) patient based on a probabilistic atlas. (Reproduced from Lorenzo-Valdes, M. et al., *Med. Image Anal.*, 8(3), 255, 2004. With permission.)

7.3.3 STATISTICAL ATLASES

7.3.3.1 Basic Idea

Statistical atlases are used to identify changes in the cardiac anatomy due to shape variation in a certain population. They have the advantage of combining the concepts of population-based atlases and model-based image analysis. Similar to the probability atlases, the statistical atlases provide information about data variability in the heart structure. Furthermore, the statistical atlases provide information about the exact type of variability, which could be used for adapting the average atlas to the images from a certain subject. Statistical atlases can be therefore used in different cardiac image analysis applications, including identification of heart functional abnormalities. Frangi et al. (2002), Mitchell et al. (2002), and Lotjonen et al. (2004) were the first to develop ventricular statistical atlases of the human heart. Ordas et al. (2007) then developed a statistical atlas of the entire heart using registration-based techniques. Beg et al. (2004) constructed a statistical cardiac atlas based on large-deformation diffeomorphic mapping. Later, Perperidis et al. (2005b) and Lorenzo-Valdés et al. (2002) developed 4D spatiotemporal statistical cardiac atlases. In the latter study, the

constructed statistical atlas has been used to provide a priori information about intensity and spatial variation in the heart, where the technique showed to be capable of tracking the LV and RV with accuracies of 99% and 96%, respectively.

The construction of a statistical atlas requires at least three steps (Perperidis et al. 2012): (1) segmenting the CMR images and extracting the structures' surfaces, (2) propagating the landmarks from the reference model to the images of a certain subject, and (3) statistically analyzing the changes in the structures' shape using modal analysis.

7.3.3.2 Modal Analysis

Modal analysis is a mathematical technique for reducing the number of degrees of freedom in a certain model, which results in constructing an overdetermined problem that can be solved for shape recovery. Point distribution modeling (PDM) is one of the well-established techniques for shape representation (Cootes et al. 1995). In PDM, the mean shape model and shape variation are defined using PCA, which is applied on a training dataset to determine the major trends of variation in the model by decomposing the variability into a set of orthogonal modes along with their associated variances (Cootes et al. 1994). PDM has been implemented for detecting cardiac shape abnormalities (Mitchell et al. 2003). Cardiac shape deformation could be also determined using statistical deformation models (SDM) (Rueckert et al. 2001), as will be explained later in the chapter. Despite its many advantages, a limitation of PDM is its tendency to overconstrain the space of valid shapes, which could be addressed by adopting a hierarchical shape representation approach (Davatzikos et al. 2003), combining statistical and synthetic modes (Wang and Staib 2000), or using nonorthogonal subspace projection (Comaniciu et al. 2004).

7.3.3.2.1 Principal Component Analysis

In PCA, the distribution of the landmarks (represented by a landmark vector $\mathbf{x}$) is approximated by a linear model of the form (Lotjonen et al. 2004, Perperidis et al. 2005a)

$$\mathbf{x} = \bar{\mathbf{x}} + \Phi\mathbf{b}, \qquad (7.10)$$

where

$\bar{\mathbf{x}} = (1/n)\sum_{i=1}^{n}\mathbf{x}_i$ is the average landmark vector

$\mathbf{b}$ is the model's shape parameter vector

Φ is a matrix whose columns are obtained by performing PCA on the covariance matrix $\mathbf{C} = (1/(n-1))\sum_{i=1}^{n}(\mathbf{x}_i - \bar{\mathbf{x}})(\mathbf{x}_i - \bar{\mathbf{x}})^T$.

PCA determines the eigenvalues and eigenvectors of the covariance matrix using singular value decomposition:

$$\mathbf{C} = \mathbf{Q}\mathbf{D}\mathbf{Q}^T, \qquad (7.11)$$

where

$\mathbf{D}$ is a diagonal matrix of eigenvalues

$\mathbf{Q}$ is an orthogonal matrix of eigenvectors

As the eigenvectors represent the modes of variation in the system and the eigenvalues represent the variances in these directions, only the eigenvectors corresponding to the largest eigenvalues are considered when forming the statistical model because they represent the major modes of variation in the training dataset. For normal distributions, the shape variance in a certain mode is represented by the corresponding eigenvalue λ_i. Therefore, by considering normal shape variation within three standard deviations (SD) from the mean shape (from $-3\sqrt{\lambda_i}$ to $3\sqrt{\lambda_i}$), we ensure that 99.7% of the shape variations are encompassed in the model, as shown in Figure 7.21 (Lotjonen et al. 2003). A new shape, $\mathbf{y}$, that is not part of the training dataset can then be represented as

$$\hat{\mathbf{y}} = \bar{\mathbf{x}} + \Phi\mathbf{b}_y, \qquad (7.12)$$

where $\mathbf{b}_y$ is obtained by the least-squares solution of the equation

$$\mathbf{b}_y = \Phi^T(\mathbf{y} - \bar{\mathbf{x}}). \qquad (7.13)$$

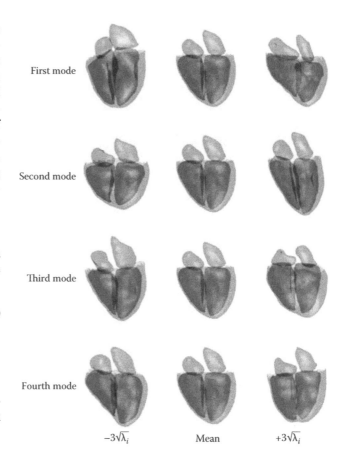

First mode

Second mode

Third mode

Fourth mode

$-3\sqrt{\lambda_i}$ Mean $+3\sqrt{\lambda_i}$

FIGURE 7.21 Four principal component analysis modes showing mean and mean ± 3SD models. (Reproduced from Lotjonen, J. et al., *Med. Image Anal.*, 8(3), 371, 2004. With permission.)

If $\mathbf{y}$ is similar to one of the examples in the training dataset, then $\mathbf{b}_y$ resembles one of the $\mathbf{b}$ vectors (normal or healthy heart shape). Otherwise (pathological case), $\mathbf{b}_y$ lies outside the distribution of the set of $\mathbf{b}$ vectors. It should be noted that a shape alignment step, for example, using Procrustes alignment (Dryden and Mardia 1998), is usually implemented before conducting PCA to eliminate variations in location, size, and shape orientation.

7.3.3.2.2 Independent Component Analysis

Suinesiaputra et al. (2004a,b, 2005, 2009) took statistical cardiac modeling one step further by implementing independent component analysis (ICA) in the statistical modeling instead of using PCA. Similar to PCA, ICA is a linear generative model; however, ICA poses the additional constraint of statistical independency of the vectors of the Ψ matrix in the following equation:

$$\mathbf{b} = \Psi(\mathbf{x} - \bar{\mathbf{x}}). \qquad (7.14)$$

Therefore, the independent components of the system are given by

$$\Phi = \Psi^{-1}, \qquad (7.15)$$

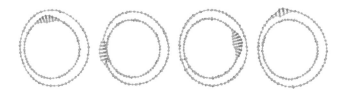

FIGURE 7.22 Four independent components of wall motion variation. (Reproduced from Suinesiaputra, A. et al., *Inf. Process Med. Imaging*, 19, 321, 2005. With permission.)

where the matrix Ψ is estimated using mathematical optimization. Replacing PCA by ICA has the advantages of allowing for simple joint probability density function estimation from different components (Figure 7.22) and of being more suitable for local feature extraction compared to global feature extraction with PCA (Uzumcu et al. 2003). It should be noted that as the number of computed independent components increases, the accuracy of detecting shape variation increases. ICA modeling has been implemented for identifying improvement in myocardial contractility, as shown in Figure 7.23 (Suinesiaputra et al. 2005).

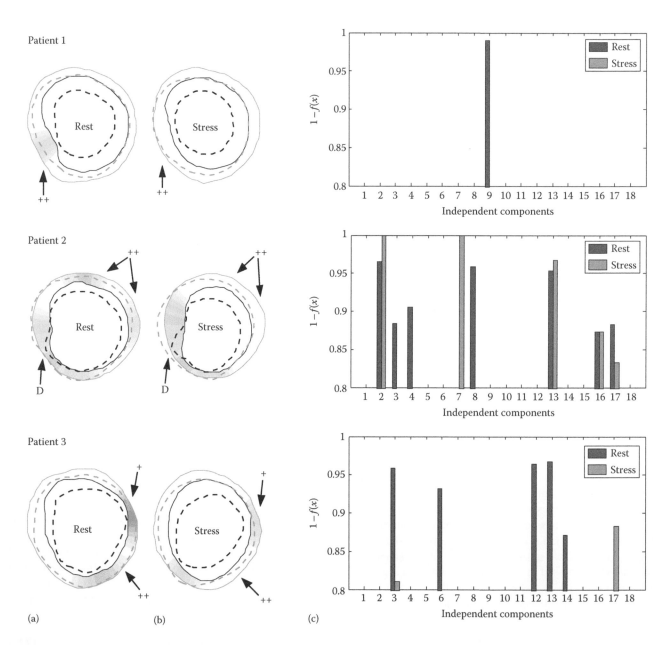

FIGURE 7.23 Prediction of myocardial contractility improvement from three patients based on independent component analysis. Quantification of abnormal regions from (a) rest and (b) stress states. The end-diastolic and end-systolic contours are drawn in solid and dashed lines, respectively. (c) Abnormal independent components. "+" and "++" point to regions that showed contractility improvement and a lot of contractility improvement, respectively. "D" points to abnormal regions that that has small contraction at rest and improved contraction, but abnormal motion, at stress. $f(x)$ is the probability density function for each independent component. (Reproduced from Suinesiaputra, A. et al., *Inf. Process Med. Imaging*, 19, 321, 2005. With permission.)

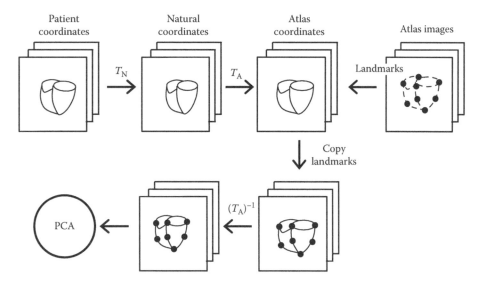

FIGURE 7.24 Atlas-based automatic landmarking. The datasets are matched to the atlas through quasi-affine (T_N) and nonrigid (T_A) transformations before landmarking. The T_A transformation is then reversed and principal component analysis (PCA) is implemented. Because of the applied transformations, the PCA modes of variation represent nonrigid deformations, but not differences in the heart pose or size.

An automated tool has been developed to detect and localize regional wall motion abnormality based on ICA modeling (Suinesiaputra et al. 2009). In this respect, CMR images from normal volunteers are used to train the system, based on which the classification algorithm detects abnormally contracting regions of the myocardium. The performance of the ICA modeling technique for identifying regional wall motion abnormality has been compared to myocardial infarction determined by delayed enhancement CMR, as well as for detecting wall motion improvement from rest to stress (Suinesiaputra et al. 2004b, 2011).

7.3.3.3 3D Statistical Models

Three-dimensional statistical shape models of the heart have been constructed based on automatic landmark generation (Frangi et al. 2002). The developed models have the advantages that they can process multiple-part structures and require less restrictive assumptions on the structure's topology. Once the atlas is built, the landmarks are propagated to data from individual subjects by warping each labeled volume into the atlas with a transformation that is composed of both global and local components, as shown in Figure 7.24. Specifically, for each location in the reference shape, the corresponding locations in the individual shapes are obtained by maximizing a voxel similarity measure between the corresponding labels.

A 3D statistical model of the heart consisting of the ventricles, atria, and epicardium has also been developed (Lotjonen et al. 2003, 2004). The model is constructed by combining images from SAX and LAX images using both PCA and ICA techniques in addition to non-parametric landmark probability distributions (Figure 7.25). Another 3D statistical atlas has been constructed using the PDM method trained from a population of 90 cases including common pathologies (Cootes et al. 1995, van Assen et al. 2003). The developed atlas was

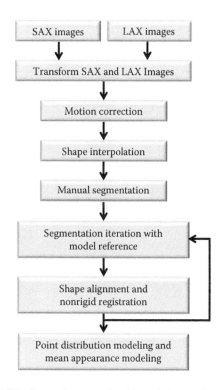

FIGURE 7.25 Steps of constructing 3D statistical model of the heart.

implemented for evaluating regional cardiac function parameters using cardiac ASM.

Four-dimensional statistical atlases of the heart have been also developed (Perperidis et al. 2005a). The technique divides the distribution space of the heart shapes into two subspaces that account for intersubject and intrasubject (changes in the shape during the cardiac cycle) shape variations, as shown in Figures 7.26 and 7.27. The developed technique has been implemented for differentiating between images

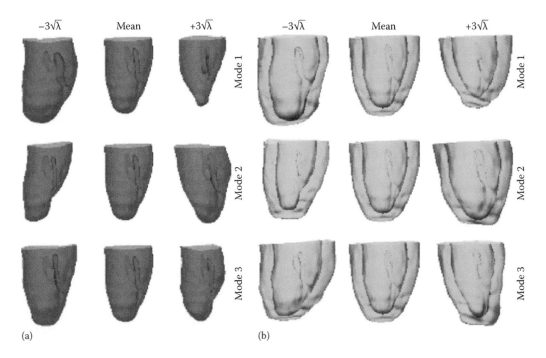

FIGURE 7.26   The significant modes of variation across subjects of the (a) left ventricle and (b) myocardium. (Reproduced from Perperidis, D. et al., *Med. Image Comput. Comput. Assist. Interv.*, 8(Pt 2), 402, 2005a. With permission.)

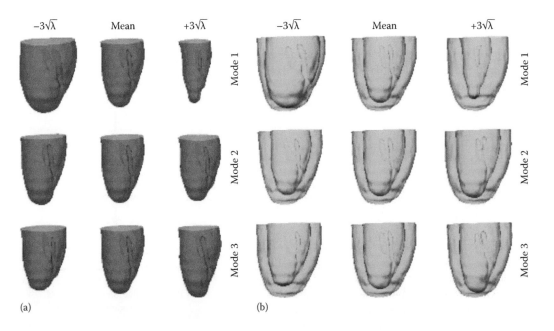

FIGURE 7.27   The significant modes of variation across the cardiac cycle of the (a) left ventricle and (b) myocardium. (Reproduced from Perperidis, D. et al., *Med. Image Comput. Comput. Assist. Interv.*, 8(Pt 2), 402, 2005a. With permission.)

from normal volunteers and patients with hypertrophic cardiomyopathy using a k-weighted nearest neighbor classifier. Statistical cardiac atlases have been also developed for analyzing the anatomical phenotype of different normal mouse strains (Perperidis et al. 2012).

In a recent study, Roohi and Zoroofi (2013) developed a 4D statistical LV model from cine SAX CMR images. In the developed technique, kernel PCA is used to explore the nonlinear variation in a population, where the distribution of the landmarks is divided into inter- and intrasubject subspaces. The developed technique has been applied for segmenting all phases of a cardiac cycle, and the results were compared to those from conventional ASM analysis. The extended registration approach implemented in the developed technique allowed for better temporal and spatial alignment of the cardiac dataset, showing that nonlinear PCA is more appropriate to approximate the LV 4D statistical model than conventional techniques.

7.4 GEOMETRICAL MODELING

7.4.1 HISTORICAL BACKGROUND

Geometrical modeling of the heart has the advantage of providing a simple and computationally inexpensive way for overall assessment of the cardiac function. It provides simple parametric representation of the heart shape that usually results in satisfactory results with acceptable accuracy, especially in cases without severe deviations from the model assumptions. When adopted, this approach replaces finite-element modeling (usually implemented on tagged CMR images) with its associated expensive computational cost. Despite the simple analytical approach with geometrical modeling, it has been implemented for deriving many cardiac functional parameters including LV volume, EF, wall motion, and myocardial twist (Bardinet et al. 1996). In their review article, Frangi et al. (2001) provided an overview of various geometrical models of the LV that have been used in cardiac analysis, including the truncated bullet (combination of an ellipsoid and cylinder) model (Cauvin et al. 1993), superquadrics (Metaxas and Terzopoulos 1993, Chen et al. 1995), sinusoidal basis functions (Staib and Duncan 1996), harmonic functions (Matheny and Goldgof 1995), deformable cylinders (Goshtasby 1993, Goshtasby and Turner

1995), and planispheric-based representation (Declerck et al. 1998). Notwithstanding, ellipsoids have been widely used for LV modeling (Janz et al. 1980, Chadwick 1982, Dulce et al. 1993). Other studies investigated geometric modeling of the RV using the ellipsoidal shell (difference between two ellipsoids) model (Denslow 1994) and biquadric surface patches (Sacks et al. 1993). Recently, Zhang et al. (2012) developed an atlas-based geometry pipeline for cardiac Hermite model reconstruction. The authors also developed an optical flow-based technique for deforming the constructed atlas to align with images from individual patients.

7.4.2 BASIC LV MODELS

Thiele et al. (2002) presented a nice comparison between different geometrical models for evaluating the LV volume. The studied models included those that use only SAX slices (Group A: modified Simpson, hemisphere cylinder, and Teichholz models), LAX slices (Group B: biplane ellipsoid and single-phase ellipsoid models), and both LAX and SAX slices (Group C: combined triplane model), as shown in Figure 7.28.

One of the problems when using only SAX slices is the through-plane motion effect, especially for the basal slices,

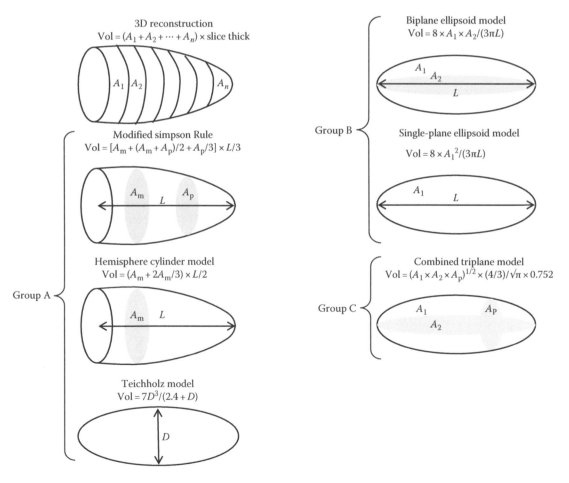

FIGURE 7.28 3D geometric models of the left ventricle (LV) and formula for volume measurement. A_m, short-axis (SAX) area of the LV at the mitral valve level; A_p, SAX area of left ventricle at the papillary muscle level; L, length of the LV; D, SAX diameter of the LV at the mitral valve level. (Reproduced from Thiele, H. et al., *J. Cardiovasc. Magn. Reson.*, 4(3), 327, 2002.)

which results in incomplete coverage of the LV during the whole cardiac cycle and introduces measurements errors. This difficulty could be addressed by combining SAX and LAX slices in the model, which improves the measurements accuracy and reduces inter- and intra-observer variability (Thiele et al. 2002). This observation was discussed in a study by Kuwahara and Eiho (1991), who found that 3D reconstruction of the heart is better achieved by combining slices from different orientations than by stacking a set of parallel slices from one orientation.

The geometrical models shown in Figure 7.28 have been tested on 25 subjects in order to compare the accuracy of ventricular function measurements from SSFP and gradient echo (GRE) images (Thiele et al. 2002). The results showed that with SSFP, most models yield good correlations with volumetric data, although the LV volume and EF were higher and lower, respectively, with SSFP than with GRE images. The combined triplane model showed the highest measurements accuracy, while the biplane and single-plane ellipsoid models resulted in low correlations between the measurements from the two image sequences.

In a recent study, a method has been developed for estimating LV functional parameters from a small number of cine SAX images and one LAX image (El-Rewaidy et al. 2014). Specifically, the developed method is based on using the LAX contour to swipe the SAX contours and fill in the missed LV surface between the SAX slices. The proposed geometrical modeling method showed to be superior to other standard modeling techniques.

7.4.3 SIMPLE GEOMETRICAL FITTING TECHNIQUES

7.4.3.1 Parametric Fitting

Simple parametric LV models have been tested for determining changes in the ventricular function between normal and diseased hearts (Wise et al. 1999). Specifically, 3D rotationally symmetric analytical functions (paraboloid, Equation 7.16; quadratic function, Equation 7.17; and ellipsoid, Equation 7.18) have been implemented to model the LV shape:

Paraboid

$$z = z_0 + a((x - x_0)^2 + (y - y_0)^2), \qquad (7.16)$$

Quadratic function

$$z = z_0 + a((x - x_0)^2 + (y - y_0)^2)^2, \qquad (7.17)$$

Ellipsoid

$$R^2 = (x - x_0)^2 + (y - y_0)^2 + a^2(z - z_0)^2, \qquad (7.18)$$

where

(x_0, y_0, z_0) represents the center of the geometrical shape
R is the radius of the shape
a is a constant

The constraint of finite extent of the heart is imposed on the developed models. For the sampled LV endo- and epicardial borders (obtained from SAX slices) to fit the geometric models, the actual LV contour in the SAX image are replaced with a best-fit circle. In their study, Wise et al. (1999) showed the capability of the geometrical model-based analysis of identifying the differences in LV dynamics in normal and hypertensive rats, especially with the ellipsoidal model, which successfully predicted the endo- and epicardial borders and LV volumes during the whole cardiac cycle.

7.4.3.2 Superquadric Fitting

Superquadrics represent a family of surfaces obtained by extending conventional quadrics (Barr 1981). Geometrical cardiac models based on a superquadric geometrical fitting have been developed for analyzing LV deformation during the cardiac cycle (Bardinet et al. 1995, 1996), where the 3D LV model is represented as

$$\left(\left(\left(\frac{x}{a_1} \right)^{2/\epsilon_2} + \left(\frac{y}{a_2} \right)^{2/\epsilon_2} \right)^{\epsilon_2/\epsilon_1} + \left(\frac{z}{a_3} \right)^{2/\epsilon_1} \right)^{\epsilon_1/2} = 1, \qquad (7.19)$$

where ϵ_1 and ϵ_2 are constants, and the geometrical fitting is achieved by minimizing the energy function

$$E = \sum \left(1 - F\left(x, y, z, a_1, a_2, a_3, \epsilon_1, \epsilon_2 \right) \right)^2, \qquad (7.20)$$

where F is the function defined in Equation 7.19.

7.4.3.3 Polynomial Fitting

The LV shape could be analytically represented using global polynomials. For example, ellipsoids, expressed as a polynomial series in the prolate spheroidal coordinates, have been used to represent the LV shape (O'Dell and McCulloch 2000). In this case, the radial coordinate λ can be represented as a function of the circumferential, θ, and longitudinal angles, φ, as

$$\lambda = \sum_{l=0}^{L} \sum_{m=-l}^{l} a_j P_l^m \left(\cos\theta \right) e^{im\varphi}, \qquad (7.21)$$

where

P_l^m are Legendre polynomials
The coefficients a_j are fit to the endo- and epicardial contours obtained from SAX images

The planispheric coordinate system has been adopted for LV representation as it is an efficient approach for representing myocardial deformation (Declerck et al. 1997, 1998).

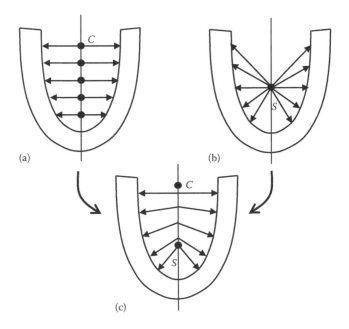

(a)

(b)

(c)

FIGURE 7.29 (a) Cylindrical, (b) spherical, and (c) planispheric models of the left ventricle. The 3D planispheric model is a combination of the cylindrical and spherical geometries. *C* and *S* are contraction centers.

The planispheric coordinate system combines cylindrical and spherical representations, such that points near the base and apex are roughly described by cylindrical and spherical coordinates, respectively (Figure 7.29). The shape is differentiable in space and time and can represent the heart motion by a small number of parameters that have simple relationships with canonical directions of the myocardial deformation (radial, circumferential, and longitudinal). In the Cartesian space, a 3D planispheric system is defined by points *S* and *C* in the centers of the LV cavity and base, respectively, and by orthogonal vectors in the longitudinal and radial directions, respectively, as shown in Figure 7.29.

7.4.3.4 Deformable Parameterized Primitives

A family of deformable parameterized primitives has been introduced for presenting cardiac structures (Park et al. 1994). The unique feature about these physics-based deformable models is that the value of their parameter functions can vary across the primitive shape, as opposed to being constant as in other primitives such as superquadrics, which allows for creating complex shapes that represent deformed cardiac structures with high accuracy. Figure 7.30 shows an example of a superquadric ellipsoid with fixed shape and a generalized primitive with varying radius across the main axis.

7.4.3.5 Deformable Periodic Generalized Cylinder

A deformable model representing closed contours with periodic motion has been implemented for cardiac modeling (O'Donnell et al. 1994). The developed model is called

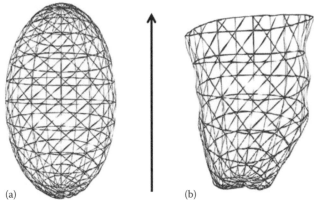

(a)

(b)

FIGURE 7.30 (a) A superquadric ellipsoid with fixed shape and (b) a generalized primitive with varying radius across the main axis (arrow).

deformable periodic generalized cylinder, and it combines global and local motion components based on Lagrangian dynamics (Terzopoulos and Metaxas 1991). In this type of modeling, the central axis represents time, through which the model's cross-sectional changes periodically, as shown in Figure 7.31. In this regard, the equation of the model's

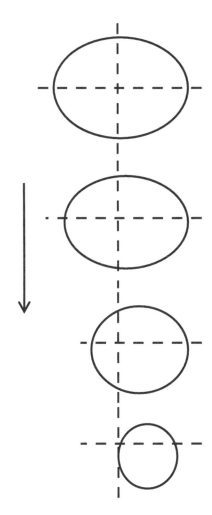

FIGURE 7.31 Change in the cross-sectional shape of a deformable periodic generalized model with time (arrow).

cross-section (ellipse in our case) can be represented by its x- and y-coordinates (A and B here) as

$$A(t,\theta) = r_1(t)\cos\theta + a(t), \quad 0 < \theta < 2\pi, \quad (7.22)$$

$$B(t,\theta) = r_2(t)\sin\theta + b(t), \quad 0 < \theta < 2\pi, \quad (7.23)$$

where

t represents time

θ is the sweeping angle

a and b represent translation

r_1 and r_2 are scaling factors

7.5 NONRIGID DEFORMATION

7.5.1 GENERAL OVERVIEW

In contrast to rigid motion that includes gross object motion, for example, translation and rotation, nonrigid motion describes the object's change in shape (deformation) over time. Therefore, object-centered deformation parameters, such as strain, are used to describe this regional motion instead of the frame-oriented parameters, for example, displacement and rotation. Nevertheless, nonrigid motion detection techniques are limited by image quality and the accumulation of tracking error in the case of nonrigid image registration.

Deformable heart models can be classified into two main categories: parametric and geometrical. The parametric models are based on active contours, a.k.a. snakes, introduced by Kass et al. (1988). McInerney and Terzopoulos (1996) provided a review of different active contours along with their characteristics, implementations, and limitations. The geometrical models implement curve and surface propagation techniques for detecting myocardial wall motion through the minimization of an energy function to ensure that the deformation results match the image data and satisfy the smoothness condition. Various deformable templates (Terzopoulos 1986, Terzopoulos et al. 1987, Yuille et al. 1989, Lipson et al. 1990, Gilchrist et al. 2004) and active shapes (Clarysse et al. 1995, McInerney and Terzopoulos 1995b, Ranganath 1995, Blake and Isard 1997) have been developed based on the original snake concept to improve motion detection performance, especially in images with low SNR (Paragios 2002). Further, 3D models constructed from a set of 2D snakes (Ranganath 1995) or polyhedral meshes (Friboulet et al. 1992, Costa et al. 1996, Nastar and Ayache 1996, Benayoun and Ayache 1998) have been developed.

Recently, deformable models have been implemented for myocardial segmentation (Sliman et al. 2013) and strain estimation (Elnakib et al. 2015) from cine CMR images. In one study (Sliman et al. 2013), first-order visual appearance inside and outside the deformable model is modeled using an adaptive linear combination of discrete Gaussian functions. Further, second-order visual appearance of the LV wall is modeled with a translational and rotation-invariant second-order Markov-Gibbs random field. The incorporation of these appearance features along with the boundary information allowed for accurate heart segmentation, as evidenced by both the Dice similarity coefficient and a distance metric on a dataset from 15 subjects. In another study (Elnakib et al. 2015), the LV wall borders are segmented using a level set–based deformable model guided by a stochastic force derived from a second-order Markov-Gibbs random field model that incorporates information about the object's shape and appearance features. A geometrical Laplace-based method is then used to measure myocardial strain by tracking corresponding points on successive myocardial contours throughout the cardiac cycle.

7.5.2 PARAMETRIC TECHNIQUES

7.5.2.1 Active Contours and Surfaces

7.5.2.1.1 Snakes

Active contour models, or snakes, were introduced by Kass et al. (1988) to model deformable contours under internal constraints (that ensure their smoothness) and external constraints from the image features or prior knowledge (Ranganath 1995). The name "snake" comes from the nature of operation of these contours when they change their shape to achieve the minimum energy that satisfies both internal and external constraints. The snake is defined parametrically by the curve $\mathbf{x}(s) = [x(s), y(s)]$, $s \in [0, 1]$, which minimizes the following energy function (Yeo et al. 2007):

$$E = \int_0^1 \left(\alpha\,|\mathbf{x}'(s)|^2 + \beta\,|\mathbf{x}''(s)|^2 + \gamma E_{\text{ext}}(\mathbf{x}(s)) \right) ds, \quad (7.24)$$

where α and β are weighting parameters. The first and second derivatives of $\mathbf{x}(s)$ control the curve's tension and rigidity, respectively, which together represent internal energy. The external energy E_{ext} is usually defined as the negative value of the magnitude of the image's gradient, weighed by a third parameter, γ (Jolly et al. 2001). Another model for describing flexible shape templates has been developed based on a training set that describes the important points to be varied and associated with statistical behaviors (Cootes et al. 1994). The model is similar to the snake concept, except that it incorporates global shape constraints based on the examples provided in the training set. Snakes have been implemented for extracting contours from cine CMR images with minimal user interaction (Ranganath 1995, Jolly et al. 2001). The method showed to be reliable for extracting the contours despite image noise, artifacts, and low temporal resolution.

7.5.2.1.2 Balloons

Deformable surfaces, or balloons, are 3D extensions of snakes. They are capable of representing the shape of the deformed cardiac surface under different internal and external energy components, similar to the idea of snakes (Duncan et al. 1991a, Cohen and Cohen 1993, O'Dell and McCulloch 2000). In their paper, McInerney and Terzopoulos (1995a) used a thin plate-based dynamic balloon model to fit the elastically deforming cardiac surface under internal surface smoothness constraints and external forces generated using Lagrangian equations of motion.

7.5.2.2 Thin Plates

The elastic deformation energy of a thin plate is given by (McInerney and Terzopoulos 1995a):

$$E(\mathbf{x}) = \iint \left(\alpha_{10} \left| \frac{\partial \mathbf{x}}{\partial u} \right|^2 + \alpha_{01} \left| \frac{\partial \mathbf{x}}{\partial v} \right|^2 + \beta_{20} \left| \frac{\partial^2 \mathbf{x}}{\partial u^2} \right|^2 \right.$$

$$\left. + \beta_{11} \left| \frac{\partial^2 \mathbf{x}}{\partial u \partial v} \right|^2 + \beta_{02} \left| \frac{\partial^2 \mathbf{x}}{\partial v^2} \right|^2 \right) du\, dv, \quad (7.25)$$

where $\mathbf{x}(u, v) = [x(u, v), y(u, v), z(u, v)]^T$ represents the position of material point (u, v) relative to a reference frame in the 3D Euclidean space. The constants α_{10} and α_{01} control the tensions in the u and v directions, respectively, while β_{20} and β_{02} control the corresponding bending rigidities, and β_{11} controls the twisting rigidity. In Lagrangian dynamics, the behavior of a balloon model during the fitting process is governed by the total energy function:

$$\mu \frac{\partial^2 \mathbf{x}}{\partial t^2} + \gamma \frac{\partial \mathbf{x}}{\partial t} + \delta_{\mathbf{x}} E = f, \quad (7.26)$$

where the first term represents the inertial forces due to the mass density $\mu(u, v)$, the second term represents the damping forces due to the damping density $\gamma(u, v)$, and the third term represents the elastic forces $\delta_{\mathbf{x}}$ and E. Finally, $f(u, v, t)$ represents the forces derived from the image data. In a recent study, using thin plate-based active deformation, Yeo et al. (2007) elucidated the LV wall motion during isovolumetric contraction.

7.5.2.3 B-Splines and NURBS

7.5.2.3.1 B-Splines

Most surface reconstruction techniques use piecewise polynomial surfaces, for example, B-splines or bicubic Hermite surface patches (Frangi et al. 2001). Nonrigid registration has been used to estimate myocardial motion from cine CMR images with B-splines implemented as the basis functions for parametric transformation (Ledesma-Carbayo et al. 2006). The developed technique computes the displacement field, $\mathbf{g}(t, \mathbf{x})$, as a series of transformations between consecutive pairs of images, $\mathbf{g}'_t(\mathbf{x})$:

$$\mathbf{g}(t, \mathbf{x}) = \mathbf{g}_t(\mathbf{x}), \quad (7.27)$$

where

$t \in \{0, \ldots, T-1\}$
$\mathbf{x} = (x_1, x_2)$

and

$$\mathbf{g}_t(\mathbf{x}) = \mathbf{g}'_t(\mathbf{x}_{t-1}), \quad (7.28)$$

where

$\mathbf{x}_{t-1} = \mathbf{g}_{t-1}(\mathbf{x})$
$\mathbf{g}_0(\mathbf{x}) = \mathbf{x}$

The transformation between consecutive frames $\mathbf{g}'_t$ is defined as a linear combination of B-splines (Kybic and Unser 2003, Sorzano et al. 2005):

$$\mathbf{g}'_t(\mathbf{x}) = \sum c_j B_r(\mathbf{x}/h - j), \quad (7.29)$$

where

h determines the knot spacing
The coefficients c_j control the solution smoothness

The implemented B-spline cubic basis function is defined as follows:

$$B_0(u) = \frac{(1-u)^3}{6},$$

$$B_1(u) = \frac{(3u^3 - 6u^2 + 4)}{6},$$

$$B_2(u) = \frac{(-3u^3 + 3u^2 + 3u + 1)}{6},$$

$$B_3(u) = \frac{u^3}{6}. \quad (7.30)$$

In another study, myocardial deformation was computed using B-splines-based nonrigid registration, and the results were compared to those obtained from tagged images (Bajo et al. 2007). The study showed that the strain values measured from the cine images are overestimated, with strain in the septum providing the least overestimation. In a similar study, the end-diastolic and end-systolic contours were used to measure myocardial strain using nonrigid registration (Feng et al. 2008). In this case, the inter-frame deformation was modeled with low-resolution B-splines, and the gradient information around the myocardial wall, blood pool, and papillary muscles was used to derive the registration in the adjacent areas that have low gradients (Kybic and Unser 2003). The cost function was formulated as the difference between the template and source images, which was solved using the Levenberg algorithm (Aster et al. 2012). The results of this study showed good correlation between the strain values measured from the cine and tagged images. However, in contrast to the results from Bajo et al. (2007), the authors here found that the cine-derived circumferential strain during diastole and radial strain during the whole cardiac cycle are more accurate than those measured from the tagged images. In a different study, a technique was developed for tracking myocardial deformation based on parametric modeling of the LV using free-form deformation; this time defined by Bernstein polynomials rather than B-splines (Bardinet et al. 1996).

7.5.2.3.2 NURBS

Third-order nonuniform rational B-splines (NURBS) have been used to model deformable surfaces. A surface S is represented by NURBS as

$$S(s,t) = (x(s,t), y(s,t), z(s,t)) \frac{\sum_{i=1}^{n}\sum_{j=1}^{m} B_{ik}(s)B_{jl}(t)h_{ij}P_{ij}}{\sum_{i=1}^{n}\sum_{j=1}^{m} B_{ik}(s)B_{jl}(t)h_{ij}},$$

(7.31)

where
  P_{ij} is a control point
  $B_{ij}(s)$ is the ith basis polynomial of order j
  h_{ij} are weighting parameters

NURBS surfaces allow for an efficient geometrical representation from a relatively few data points. NURBS have been used to generate an accurate and complete representation of the heart's biventricular geometry to any desired level of details (Creswell et al. 1992). In this case, a finite-element model is built using solid models that represent the epicardium, LV cavity, and RV cavity. In a similar study, a 3D biventricular solid model has been created using geometric data extracted from ex vivo canine heart, where the individual profiles were created by fitting the NURBS to contour points from the extracted data (Pirolo et al. 1993). Recently, Moyer et al. (2013) presented a method for assessing global and regional mechanical atrial function using finite-element surface fitting, where the fitted surface was used to measure the left atrial volume, regional motion, and spatial motion heterogeneity in healthy subjects and atrial fibrillation patients.

7.5.2.4 Active Shape Models/Active Appearance Models

7.5.2.4.1 Methods Description

ASMs and AAMs are popular parametric models. Cardiac ASMs were developed by Cootes et al. (1994, 1995) to statistically model the shape and associated shape variation of a certain object based on a set of training examples (Zhang et al. 2010). ASMs have been used for detecting cardiac deformation by minimizing an energy function that measures the difference between the model and image data. In subsequent studies, cardiac AAMs have been developed as extension of ASMs (Cootes et al. 1998, 1999). In contrast to ASMs that provide local appearance information in the vicinity of each landmark using separate appearance models, AAMs represent the object's average shape and shape variation along with the appearance of a complete image dataset in an integral statistical model (Mitchell et al. 2001). AAMs showed to be robust for detecting the heart deformation because they include prior information about the heart shape and image appearance based on the training examples. On the other side, it should be noted that because of the strict optimization constraints, ASMs and AAMs can be easily trapped at local minima, which generates tracking errors that propagate through various timeframes. Therefore, these techniques require a good initialization and a carefully selected training dataset so that the algorithms are not disturbed by nontarget objects in the image.

Recently, automatic training and reliability estimation have been studied for a 3D ASM model applied for cardiac segmentation from cine CMR images (Tobon-Gomez et al. 2012). Specifically, the technique's performance was evaluated with point-to-surface and volume errors. The results showed that the inclusion of the reliability measures reduced volume errors in hypertrophic and heart failure patients. In another study, ASM has been combined with inter-profile modeling paradigm for right ventricular (RV) segmentation (ElBaz and Fahmy 2012). The proposed technique includes two modifications to the standard ASM algorithm. The first modification is implementing PCA to capture inter-profile relations among the shape's neighboring landmarks, which are used to model the inter-profile variations in the training set. The second modification is using a multistage searching algorithm to find the best profile match (best shape fitting) iteratively. The results showed that the developed technique can reduce the segmentation error by about 0.4 mm and increase the contour overlap by about 4% compared to the standard ASM technique.

7.5.2.4.2 Combined ASM/AAM

Two studies investigated the implementation of combined ASM/AAM techniques for detecting cardiac deformation (Mitchell et al. 2001, Zhang et al. 2010). In 2001, Mitchell et al. (2001) developed a multistage ASM/AAM hybrid technique for segmenting the LV and RV while avoiding local minima during the search for a solution. In the following year, the same group developed a 3D AAM technique that has been successfully implemented on SAX CMR slices (Mitchell et al. 2002). Recently, Zhang et al. (2010) developed a combined ASM/AAM technique for segmenting 4D CMR images of the LV and RV in normal and Tetralogy of Fallot conditions. The developed technique starts by building a PDM that describes the cardiac shape variation based on a training dataset. During segmentation, the shape landmarks are iteratively updated and the intensity pattern is modeled by a texture model. The shape and texture parameters are then combined into a single appearance vector that is statistically modeled. Model matching is achieved by searching for the optimal parameters that minimize the difference between the model and target vectors. After the segmentation process is completed, different motion features are extracted and used to differentiate between normal volunteers and patients. The technique showed to be capable of differentiating between normal subjects and Tetralogy of Fallot patients with sensitivity and specificity of 90%–100%.

7.5.2.5 Nonrigid Registration

7.5.2.5.1 Method Description

Nonrigid registration is used to map feature points in one timeframe to the corresponding points in another timeframe. This concept has been used to model myocardial deformation during the cardiac cycle (Lorenzo-Valdés et al. 2002). Specifically, a combined transformation model that includes both global and local components is implemented:

$$T(x,y,z) = T_{\text{global}}(x,y,z) + T_{\text{local}}(x,y,z), \quad (7.32)$$

where the global transformation component describes an affine transformation that represents translation, rotation, and scaling

$$T_{\text{global}}(x,y,z) = \begin{pmatrix} \theta_{11} & \theta_{12} & \theta_{13} \\ \theta_{21} & \theta_{22} & \theta_{23} \\ \theta_{31} & \theta_{32} & \theta_{33} \end{pmatrix} \times \begin{pmatrix} x \\ y \\ z \end{pmatrix} + \begin{pmatrix} \theta_{14} \\ \theta_{24} \\ \theta_{34} \end{pmatrix} \quad (7.33)$$

and the local transformation component describes a free-form deformation based on B-splines

$$T_{\text{local}}(x,y,z) = \sum_{l=0}^{3}\sum_{m=0}^{3}\sum_{n=0}^{3} B_l(u)B_m(v)B_n(w)P_{i+l,j+m,k+n}, \quad (7.34)$$

where

P denotes the control points that parameterize the transformation

u, v, and w denote the lattice coordinates of x, y, and z

B_i is the ith B-spline cubic basis function

Based on the previously defined transformation T, the deformation between the reference end-diastolic timeframe ($n = 1$) and any other timeframe, N, can be defined as the sum of local transformations (Figure 7.32):

$$T_{N,1}(x,y,z) = \sum_{n=1}^{N-1} T_{n+1,n}(x,y,z). \quad (7.35)$$

7.5.2.5.2 Implementation

A nonrigid registration technique has been recently developed for cardiac motion estimation using the sum of squared pixel intensity differences between the reference and deformed images as a similarity measure (Li et al. 2008). Levenberg-Marquardt non-linear least squares algorithm was used for optimization, and finite-element registration was implemented to track the points in both the forward and backward directions. A flexible global-to-local parameter map was used to link the global lattice P to the local lattices P^e:

$$x = u(X) = \sum \Psi^e(X)P^e, \quad (7.36)$$

where

x is the current coordinates

u is the displacement field

X is the reference coordinates

Ψ represents bi-cubic Bezier basis functions (Biswas and Lovell 2010)

A graphics processing unit was dedicated for image processing, which resulted in a high processing rate of 0.5 s/frame.

Nonrigid registration algorithms have been also implemented on the MRI scanner computer during image reconstruction for automatic tracking of the image features (Figure 7.33; Li et al. 2010). The inline implementation of the algorithm resulted in a 10 s delay in image display on the scanner console; however, this capability allowed for faster evaluation of the ventricular function than using off-line postprocessing.

Recently, nonrigid registration has been applied to standard cine CMR images to measure myocardial strain, and the results were compared to strain values measured using the

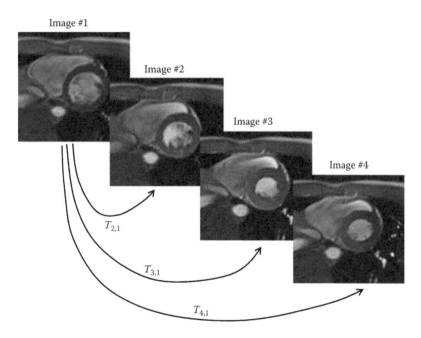

FIGURE 7.32 Tracking of a cardiac motion based on nonrigid registration. $T_{m,n}$ is a transformation that maps a point in the heart at timeframe n into the corresponding point at timeframe m.

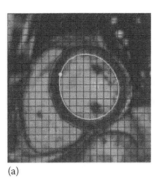 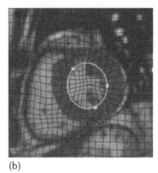 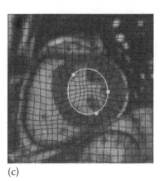

(a)   (b)   (c)

FIGURE 7.33 Deformation maps based on nonrigid registration. (a) Short-axis slice at end-diastole, with undeformed tracking grid and manual contours. The dots show the location of manually placed guide points. (b) The same slice at end-systole with validated off-line tracking. (c) The same slice at end-systole with in-line tracking. (Reproduced from Li, B. et al., *JACC Cardiovasc. Imaging*, 3(8), 860, 2010. With permission.)

displacement-encoding with stimulated echo (DENSE) pulse sequence (Allan et al. 2011). The results showed less than 3% error between strain measurements obtained by the two techniques. This capability of nonrigid registration for measuring myocardial strain from cine images has been also confirmed in more recent study by Tsai et al. (2015). In another study, a hierarchical transformation model, including both global and local LV deformations, has been developed to analyze LV strain and strain rate from cine CMR images using nonrigid registration (Gan et al. 2015). In the developed technique, an additional term was added to the cost function to constrain the transformation based on expert hints. The hints are represented by a set of landmarks that are used to adjust the registration algorithm toward the correct solution. Specifically, the landmark information are used to tie each pair of corresponding points together. Further, the endocardial/epicardial contour information is used to tie each pair of corresponding contours together. Therefore, the developed technique has the advantage of using information from the whole myocardium instead of only using wall motion information. In a similar study, Hu et al. (2014) developed an automatic cardiac segmentation method using local binary fitting and dynamic programming. The developed method combines deformable modeling with image-based information to improve the segmentation performance. Dynamic programming is used to obtain the epicardial boundary, where prior information about spatial relationships between the acquired images is incorporated in the analysis.

7.5.2.5.3 Myocardial Incompressibility

The condition of myocardial incompressibility has been added to nonrigid registration for more realistic results (Bistoquet et al. 2007, 2008). A curvilinear coordinate system was used, based on which the myocardial midsurface was defined from the endo- and epicardial boundaries. With this presentation, any point, **r**, on the LV myocardium could be represented as

$$\mathbf{r}(\hat{\mathbf{u}}, \gamma) = \mathbf{m}(\hat{\mathbf{u}}) + \gamma\hat{\mathbf{n}}(\hat{\mathbf{u}}),\qquad(7.37)$$

where
γ is the distance of the point from the midsurface
$\hat{\mathbf{n}}(\hat{\mathbf{u}})$ is the surface normal at point $\mathbf{m}(\hat{\mathbf{u}})$

Besides including the incompressibility condition, a nontransmural bending assumption was implemented to ensure that any point on the myocardium remains at the normal direction to the same point on the midsurface during deformation. LV deformation was obtained by searching for the nodes that maximize the similarity between the reference frame and the current frame. The developed technique has been successfully implemented for differentiating between healthy volunteers and patients with ventricular dyssynchrony (Bistoquet et al. 2007). The technique showed to behave uniformly in all regions and was capable of generating realistic cardiac deformation patterns. Furthermore, the technique provided a compromise between computational complexity and information comprehensiveness. Incompressible nonrigid deformation has been also implemented to develop a method for biventricular myocardial deformation recovery (Figure 7.34; Bistoquet et al. 2008). The developed technique was successfully validated against results from tagged CMR images.

7.5.2.5.4 RV Deformation

Compared to the LV, the RV deformation is hard to detect due to the ventricle's thin wall, ill-defined shape, and complex nature of deformation. Nonrigid registration has been used to define RV deformation between a reference timeframe and any other timeframe in the cardiac cycle (Punithakumar et al. 2013b). In another study (Satriano et al. 2015), a novel 4D strain analysis tool has been used for measuring RV strain from cine CMR images. The authors measured peak principal strain amplitude and normalized time-to-peak strain for each model node and calculated a new metric as the ratio between these two measurements. This new metric showed to be capable of differentiating between patients with severe versus nonsevere pulmonary hypertension.

7.5.3 DIFFERENTIAL GEOMETRICAL PROPERTIES

7.5.3.1 Curvature Measurements

Various techniques for tracking the heart motion depend on measuring the changes in differential geometric properties of the curves, for example, curvature and torsion, from one image to another (Millman and Parker 1977). In 1991,

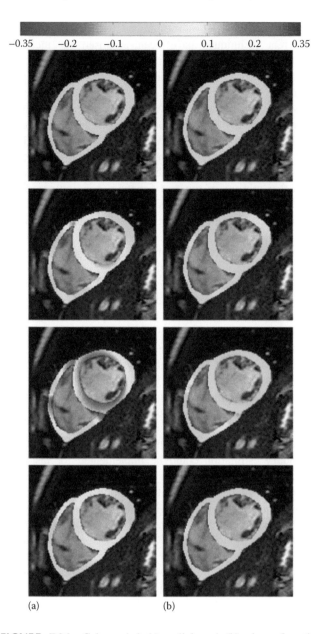

(a)   (b)

FIGURE 7.34 Color-coded (a) radial and (b) circumferential Lagrangian strains in a normal subject over the cardiac cycle. The first and third rows represent end-diastole and end-systole, respectively. (Reproduced from Bistoquet, A. et al., *Med. Image Anal.*, 12(1), 69, 2008. With permission.)

Amini et al. (1991) presented a nice description of these parameters and their implementation for analyzing cine CMR images. There are two fundamental forms that describe different surface properties. The first form represents intrinsic (stretching-related) properties of the surface $\mathbf{r}(u,v)$, which is given by the quadratic form

$$I(du,dv) = (d\mathbf{r}, d\mathbf{r}) = \begin{bmatrix} du & dv \end{bmatrix} \begin{bmatrix} E & F \\ F & G \end{bmatrix} \begin{bmatrix} du \\ dv \end{bmatrix}, \quad (7.38)$$

where the surface position $d\mathbf{r} = \mathbf{r}_u du + \mathbf{r}_v dv$ (subscripts represent derivatives), $E = (\mathbf{r}_u, \mathbf{r}_u)$, $F = (\mathbf{r}_u, \mathbf{r}_v)$, and $G = (\mathbf{r}_v, \mathbf{r}_v)$.

The second fundamental form represents extrinsic (bending-related) surface properties, which measures the correlation between change in the normal vector $d\mathbf{n}$ and change in the surface position $d\mathbf{r}$ at (u, v):

$$II(du,dv) = \begin{bmatrix} du & dv \end{bmatrix} \begin{bmatrix} L & M \\ M & N \end{bmatrix} \begin{bmatrix} du \\ dv \end{bmatrix} = -(d\mathbf{r}, d\mathbf{n}), \quad (7.39)$$

where

$L = (\mathbf{r}_{uu}, \mathbf{n})$

$M = (\mathbf{r}_{uv}, \mathbf{n})$

$N = (\mathbf{r}_{vv}, \mathbf{n})$

By combining the two fundamental forms, we obtain β:

$$\beta = \begin{bmatrix} E & F \\ F & G \end{bmatrix}^{-1} \begin{bmatrix} L & M \\ M & N \end{bmatrix}, \quad (7.40)$$

from which the Gaussian curvature (K) and mean curvature (H), which represent the intrinsic and extrinsic surface properties, respectively, could be obtained

$$K(u,v) = \det(\beta) = \frac{LN - M^2}{EG - F^2}, \quad (7.41)$$

$$H(u,v) = \frac{1}{2}\operatorname{tr}(\beta) = \frac{EN + GL - 2FM}{2(EG - F^2)}. \quad (7.42)$$

Other curvature properties of interest are obtained from the normal curvature k_n at a point on the surface, which could be parameterized as a function of the angle θ at that point:

$$k_n(\theta) = k_1 \cos^2(\theta) + k_2 \sin^2(\theta), \quad (7.43)$$

where k_1 and k_2 are the principal curvatures that represent the minimum and maximum normal curvatures at that point, which are related to the Gaussian and mean curvatures by

$$\frac{k_1^2 + k_2^2}{2} = 2H^2(u,v) - K(u,v). \quad (7.44)$$

7.5.3.2 LV Deformation

The curvature properties have been used to analyze 3D LV motion (Friboulet et al. 1993). By iteratively computing the Gaussian curvature over the LV surface, it has been shown that the curvature remains stable throughout the cardiac cycle. In another study, regional curvature properties have been used to analyze the LV deformation from 3D CMR images acquired throughout the cardiac cycle (Clarysse et al. 1997). The curvature description of the surface provides two indices that decouple the curvature's shape and magnitude of curviness. By tracking the endocardial motion, the curvature-based technique showed to be capable of differentiating between normal and abnormal LVs. Recently, Wan et al. (2014) developed a technique for analyzing regional LV shape dynamics from 3D cine CMR images. In the developed technique, 3D LV models were reconstructed and restored for possible motion distortion. The curvedness values were computed on a segmental basis throughout the cardiac cycle and were fitted using a second-order Fourier series. Unsupervised learning was then applied on the extracted Fourier coefficients to differentiate between data from normal subjects and patients.

7.5.3.3 RV Deformation

Surface curvature has been used to analyze RV deformation (Sacks et al. 1993). The RV free wall surface is approximated by biquadratic patches of the form

$$S(u,v) = au^2 + 2buv + cv^2, \tag{7.45}$$

where a, b, and c are determined for each surface node. The minor (k_1) and major (k_2) principal curvatures are then computed as follows:

$$k_1 = a + c + \sqrt{(a-c)^2 + 4b^2}, \tag{7.46}$$

$$k_2 = a + c - \sqrt{(a-c)^2 + 4b^2}, \tag{7.47}$$

which enable representing the biquadric surface patch $S(x_1, x_2)$ as

$$S(u,v) = k_1 u^2 + k_2 v^2. \tag{7.48}$$

The developed method has been evaluated on CMR images from a dog, where the results showed that while the RV free wall undergoes small changes during systole, its overall curvature remains constant (Sacks et al. 1993).

7.5.3.4 Wall Motion Tracking Based on Differential Geometrical Properties

7.5.3.4.1 Method Description

A number of ventricular wall motion tracking techniques search for similarities between differential geometric shape properties of corresponding points in consecutive timeframes using mathematical optimization and smoothness constraints (Shi et al. 2000). The ventricular surface is usually represented by local surface patches modeled as flexible thin plates. Using curvature parameters, the bending energy required to bend a surface patch from an initial state to a deformed state is given by

$$\epsilon_{bc} = A \left(\frac{\left(k_1 - \bar{k}_1\right)^2 + \left(k_2 - \bar{k}_2\right)^2}{2} \right), \tag{7.49}$$

where

- k_1 and k_2 are the minor and major principal curvatures, respectively, of the initial surface patch
- $\bar{k}_1$ and $\bar{k}_2$ are the corresponding parameters after deformation

7.5.3.4.2 Implementation

Different techniques have been proposed for measuring myocardial deformation by tracking the evolution of differential geometric landmark features of the studied objects, for example, local extreme curvature points or curvature zero-crossing points, under the assumption that these features change smoothly between consecutive timeframes (Duncan et al. 1994, Shi et al. 1994, 2000). For each landmark in the first timeframe, a small search area centered at this location is constructed in the second timeframe. The point in this search area that minimizes the cost function (bending area in the case of curvature) is used as the corresponding point. The deformation trajectory during the cardiac cycle is then built by concatenating the motion vectors between corresponding points in consecutive timeframes. Regional ventricular measures, for example, strain and strain rate, can then be derived from these trajectories.

The shape characteristics of the endocardial border could be studied and used to guide the development of myocardial deformation (Duncan et al. 1991a,b). In this respect, the 2D endocardial boundary is modeled as a flexible rod, whose local segments are tracked through successive timeframes. Motion computation involves minimizing the bending energy between the segments in successive timeframes (Duncan et al. 1991b), where the contour determined in one timeframe is used as the initial estimate of the contour in the next timeframe (Staib and Duncan 1992). In this respect, multiscale boundary estimation could be implemented for faster and efficient computation (Shi et al. 1994). A feedback mechanism could be also implemented to minimize the differences between actual and predicted boundary movements.

A hybrid method has been presented for measuring myocardial wall motion between two timeframes in the cardiac cycle (Benayoun and Ayache 1995). For each feature point in the first image, the method searches for the corresponding point in the second image by minimizing a mechanically based energy function that includes two terms: a curvature-based term that matches differential singularities in the two images and a gradient-based term that constrains the field's regularity. To reduce the computational time, an adaptive mesh is used whose resolution depends on the presence of high gradient, and modal analysis is implemented for compact representation of the analyzed parameters.

7.6 INTENSITY-BASED TECHNIQUES

Many techniques have been presented for extracting cardiac motion fields from cine CMR images using both 2D and 3D approaches (Shi et al. 1999, McEachen et al. 2000, Wang et al. 2001, Perperidis et al. 2005b). These techniques can be categorized into two groups: intensity-based and boundary-based techniques. The first group is based on detecting changes in the pixels' signal intensity in a sequence of images using OF or other intensity-based techniques (Tistarelli and Marcenaro 1994, Makela et al. 2002, Perperidis et al. 2005b). The second group of techniques is based on extracting the boundary of the cardiac wall and tracking its displacement from one timeframe to another, as described in the previous section (Amini et al. 1991, Shi et al. 2000, Papademetris et al. 2001, Wang et al. 2001). In this section, we cover the first group of techniques.

7.6.1 Optical Flow

7.6.1.1 Basic Concepts

Optical flow (OF) is an image processing technique that uses image brightness variation between consecutive time-frames to compute motion of object points in the image. The OF technique was introduced in the late 1950s and adopted in the early 1980s for image analysis applications (Horn and Schunck 1981, Meyering et al. 2000a). The OF techniques have been generalized in 3D using the divergence-free constraint (Gorce et al. 1997). Methods for obtaining OF can be divided into differential, matching, frequency-based, and phase-based techniques (Carranza et al. 2007). It should be noted that OF techniques are discussed again in Chapter 3 of *Heart Mechanics: Magnetic Resonance Imaging—Advanced Techniques, Clinical Applications, and Future Trends*, but for analyzing tagged CMR images.

7.6.1.2 Differential OF

7.6.1.2.1 First-Order Differential OF

OF is estimated from the derivatives of the image intensity over space and time. The differential techniques are based on the assumption of minimal change in signal intensity (brightness) inside a local region in the image between consecutive timeframes, which is mathematically represented as

$$I(\mathbf{x},t) = I(\mathbf{x}+\delta\mathbf{x}, t+\delta t), \qquad (7.50)$$

where

$I(\mathbf{x}, t)$ is the signal intensity at position $\mathbf{x}$ and time t
δ represents a minimal change

This assumption leads to setting the derivative of the image signal intensity (with respect to time) to zero. Expanding the left-hand side of Equation 7.50 with a Taylor series leads to the OF constraint equation, which is solved for the image velocity $\mathbf{v}$ (assumed to be uniform):

$$\nabla I \mathbf{v} + I_t = 0, \qquad (7.51)$$

where

$\nabla I = (\partial I/\partial x, \partial I/\partial y)$
$I_t = \partial I / \partial t$
$\mathbf{v} = (v_x, v_y)$

Using OF, Denney and McVeigh (1997) presented a model-free motion tracking technique that depends on energy minimization by penalizing large deformation gradients.

7.6.1.2.2 Second-Order Differential OF

A second-order differential approach has been adopted to constrain 2D velocity (Uras et al. 1988, Barron et al. 1994):

$$I_{xx}(\mathbf{x},t)v_x + I_{yx}(\mathbf{x},t)v_y + I_{tx}(\mathbf{x},t) = 0, \qquad (7.52)$$

$$I_{xy}(\mathbf{x},t)v_x + I_{yy}(\mathbf{x},t)v_y + I_{ty}(\mathbf{x},t) = 0. \qquad (7.53)$$

Equations 7.52 and 7.53 could be used by themselves or in combination with Equation 7.51 to obtain motion velocity. It should be noted that the second-order approach provides less accurate results than the first-order approach in case of data sparsity (Barron et al. 1994). Generally, the differential OF techniques are challenging in the cases of noisy images, aliasing, or small temporal support, which may be addressed by incorporating regularization terms or switching to other approaches (Barron et al. 1992, 1994).

7.6.1.3 Horn–Schunck OF

Horn and Schunck (1981) combined the gradient constraints with a smoothness term to constrain the velocity field by minimizing the following energy function

$$\int_D \left((I_x v_x + I_y v_y + I_t)^2 + \gamma^2 (\|\nabla v_x\|^2 + \|\nabla v_y\|^2) \right) dx, \quad (7.54)$$

which is defined over a domain of interest D, where γ is a weighting factor (usually set to 100).

7.6.1.4 Lucas–Kanade OF

Lucas and Kanade (1981) set the OF problem as a weighted least-squares fitting of the measurements in Equation 7.51 to a constant velocity in each local region R by minimizing the following energy function:

$$\sum_{\mathbf{x}\in R} W^2(\mathbf{x})\left((\nabla I(\mathbf{x},t))^T \mathbf{v} + I_t(\mathbf{x},t)\right)^2, \qquad (7.55)$$

where $W(\mathbf{x})$ is a window function. The solution of the Lucas–Kanade equation is given by

$$A^T W^2 A\mathbf{v} = A^T W^2 \mathbf{b}, \qquad (7.56)$$

where

$A = [\nabla I(x_1), ..., \nabla I(x_n)]^T$
$W = \text{diag}(W(x_1), ..., W(x_n))$
$\mathbf{b} = -[I_t(x_1), ..., I_t(x_n)]^T$

Equation 7.55, therefore, represents a weighted least-squares estimate of $\mathbf{v}$ from estimates of normal velocities $v_n \mathbf{n}$:

$$\sum_{\mathbf{x}\in R} W^2(\mathbf{x})c^2(\mathbf{x})(\mathbf{v}^T\mathbf{n}(\mathbf{x}) + v_n(\mathbf{x}))^2, \qquad (7.57)$$

where the coefficients $c^2(\mathbf{x})$ reflect the confidence in the normal velocity estimates, given by $c(\mathbf{x}) = \|\nabla I(\mathbf{x}, t)\|$.

7.6.1.5 Matching Techniques

In the matching (or region-based) techniques, motion velocity is computed by matching certain features in the image between consecutive timeframes based on least-squares or correlation criteria. In this respect, velocity is obtained by calculating the shift, s, that results in the best fit between a small region around $\mathbf{x}_0$ in a certain timeframe and the corresponding region around $\mathbf{x}_0 + s$ in the next timeframe (Burt et al. 1983, Little and Verri 1989).

7.6.1.6 Frequency-Based Techniques

The frequency (energy)-based techniques are based on the output of velocity-tuned filters in the frequency domain (Adelson and Bergen 1986, Barman et al. 1991, Fleet 1992). The Fourier transform of the translating pattern in Equation 7.51 is represented as

$$\hat{I}(\mathbf{k},\omega) = \hat{I}_0(\mathbf{k})\delta(\omega + \mathbf{v}^T\mathbf{k}), \qquad (7.58)$$

where

$\hat{I}(\mathbf{k})$ is the Fourier transform of $I(\mathbf{x}_0)$
$\delta(\cdot)$ is a Dirac delta function
ω is frequency

This shows that all nonzero power lies on a plane in the Fourier space. The frequency-based techniques showed to be more robust than the gradient-based (Meyering et al. 2000b) or matching (Beauchemin and Barron 1995) techniques.

7.6.1.7 Phase-Based Techniques

In the phase-based techniques, the motion fields are obtained by analyzing the phase behavior of the output of selectively oriented band-pass filters applied to the image (Waxman and Bergholm 1988, Fleet 1992). Recently, Xavier et al. (2012) developed a method for local myocardial motion estimation from cine CMR images using a modified phase-based OF technique. The estimated phase-based OF measurements showed good agreement with those measured using a reference standard OF method as well as with results in the literature. The advantage of the developed method is its robustness with respect to Rician noise and to brightness changes usually observed in the cine images, especially in basal SAX slices due to cardiac through-plane motion.

7.6.2 WIGNER–VILLE DISTRIBUTION (WVD)

7.6.2.1 Basic Technique

Spatiotemporal analysis of the cardiac motion using OF based on WVD has been presented in a number of studies (Meyering et al. 2000a, Carranza et al. 2006, 2007). The WVD is defined as follows (Carranza et al. 2006):

$$W_I(x,y,t,w_x,w_y,w_t)$$

$$= \iiint R_I(x,y,t,\alpha,\beta,\tau)e^{-j(\alpha w_x + \beta w_y + \tau w_t)}d\alpha\,d\beta\,d\tau, \qquad (7.59)$$

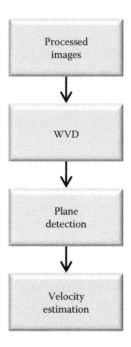

FIGURE 7.35 Schematic diagram of Wigner–Ville distribution implementation for measuring cardiac motion.

where (* denotes complex conjugation)

$$R_I(x,y,t,\alpha,\beta,\tau) = I(x+\alpha,y+\beta,t+\tau)$$

$$\times I^*(x-\alpha,y-\beta,t-\tau) \qquad (7.60)$$

and an image sequence can be represented by a function $I_0(x, y)$, for example,

$$I(x,y,t) = I_0(x - v_x t, y - v_y t), \qquad (7.61)$$

under the assumption that the moving objects have uniform velocity and constant signal intensity. The WVD of the time-varying image $I(x, y, t)$ can then be given by

$$W_I(x,y,t,w_x,w_y,w_t) = \delta(v_x w_x + v_y w_y + w_t)$$

$$\times W_I(x - v_x t, y - v_y t, w_x, w_y). \qquad (7.62)$$

Therefore, the WVD of a linearly translating image with velocity (v_x, v_y) is zero everywhere, except in the plane defined by

$$\{(x,y,t,w_x,w_y,w_t): v_x w_x + v_y w_y + w_t = 0\}. \qquad (7.63)$$

Figure 7.35 shows a schematic diagram of WVD implementation (Carranza et al. 2006).

7.6.2.2 WVD with Hough Transform

The Hough transform has been added to WVD in order to provide a value of the displacement field from the spatiotemporal representation (Carranza et al. 2007). Further, a Gaussian-based probabilistic approach was adopted to improve the accuracy of motion detection. This motion detection technique showed

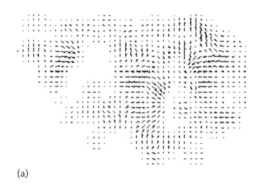

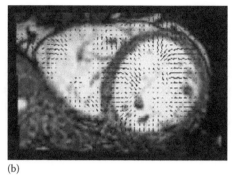

(a)   (b)

FIGURE 7.36 Wigner–Ville distribution based on Hough transform for measuring cardiac motion. (a) Optical flow (OF) results obtained during systole. (b) OF measurements superimposed on the end-diastolic frame. (Reproduced from Carranza, N. et al., *Opt. Spectrosc.*, 103, 877, 2007. With permission.)

to be robust to noise and have the ability to discard features from other structures (Figure 7.36). The developed technique could be implemented in a hierarchical fashion to accurately and efficiently capture both large and detailed motion components (Beauchemin and Barron 1995). Nevertheless, it should be noted that nonrigid heart motion introduces cross-terms in the resulting spectrum, which can affect the technique's performance for plane detection.

7.6.3 HARMONIC ANALYSIS

7.6.3.1 Harmonic Functions

Due to the heart's periodic motion, its motion can be represented by harmonic functions of a spatiotemporal nature. Four-dimensional spherical harmonics can be used to efficiently model the LV motion (Chen et al. 1994), especially that the heart can be mapped into a sphere after properly selecting its center, toward which about 90% of wall motion is directed (Potel et al. 1984). Time-dependent harmonic functions, Ψ, form the solution of the equation (Matheny and Goldgof 1995)

$$\frac{\partial^2 \Psi}{\partial x^2} + \frac{\partial^2 \Psi}{\partial y^2} + \frac{\partial^2 \Psi}{\partial z^2} + \frac{1}{c^2}\frac{\partial^2 \Psi}{\partial t^2} = 0, \qquad (7.64)$$

where c is a constant. Spherical harmonics are parameterized by two numbers, m and n, forming a set of functions that are continuous, orthogonal, and complete on the sphere (MacRobert 1967). The basic functions $U_{nm}(\phi, \theta)$ and $V_{nm}(\phi, \theta)$ are defined in the spherical coordinate system as

$$U_{nm}(\phi,\theta) = \cos m\phi \, P_{n,m}(\cos\theta), \qquad (7.65)$$

$$V_{nm}(\phi,\theta) = \sin m\phi \, P_{n,m}(\cos\theta), \qquad (7.66)$$

where $P_{n,m}(.)$ is the general Legendre function, given by

$$P_{n,m}(x) = (1-x^2)^{m/2}\frac{d^m}{dx^m}P_n(x), \qquad (7.67)$$

and $P_n(.)$ is the Legendre polynomial of degree n. Therefore, to represent an arbitrary shape, its radius $r(\phi, \theta)$ is calculated as a linear sum of spherical harmonic base functions:

$$r(\phi,\theta) \approx \sum_{n=1}^{N}\sum_{m=0}^{n}\left(A_{nm}U_{nm}(\phi,\theta) + B_{nm}V_{nm}(\phi,\theta)\right). \qquad (7.68)$$

Chen et al. (1994) adopted a hierarchical coarse-to-fine approach to represent the LV motion with spherical harmonic, where the chamber's translation and rotation are described by the heart's global rigid motion, its twisting and scaling are described by its global nonrigid motion, and finally local deformation (the residue of the global motion) is represented by spherical harmonics.

The LV's nonrigid motion has been also efficiently described by hyperspherical harmonics (Matheny and Goldgof 1995), defined as

$$x = s\sin(\eta)\sin(\theta)\cos(\phi),$$

$$y = s\sin(\eta)\sin(\theta)\sin(\phi),$$

$$z = s\sin(\eta)\cos(\theta),$$

$$t = \frac{s}{c}\cos\eta, \qquad (7.69)$$

where

c is a scaling constant
θ and ϕ are the latitude and longitude angles
η is the hyperlatitude angle
s is the radial displacement, given by

$$s = \sqrt{x^2 + y^2 + z^2 + c^2 t^2}. \qquad (7.70)$$

7.6.3.2 Frequency Analysis

Frequency analysis of the periodic heart motion provides a means for identifying its different excitation modes. Temporal smoothing of the heart motion can be implemented by retaining only the main Fourier harmonics based on modal analysis (Nastar and Ayache 1996). Fourier analysis has been combined with contour detection for fast localization of the heart without user intervention (Lin et al. 2006). In this respect, the average (DC (direct current) term) and first-harmonic images of the heart are obtained by Fourier analysis, and are used, in addition to a priori shape information, to determine a region of interest and a threshold for precisely delineating the LV.

7.6.4 LEVEL SETS

7.6.4.1 Method Description
The level set method (Sethian 1999) is based on representing an n-dimensional boundary by a zero level set of an $n + 1$ dimension (the level set function, φ), such that

$$\varphi(x(t),t) = 0. \tag{7.71}$$

Therefore, instead of tracking each point on the boundary, the boundary deformation is tracked by measuring the evolution of φ:

$$\varphi_t + F.|\nabla\varphi|, \tag{7.72}$$

where the subscript represents derivative, ∇ represents gradient, and F is the normal component of the boundary velocity, defined as

$$F = -g(v_0 + \varepsilon k) - \nabla g \cdot \frac{\nabla\varphi}{|\nabla\varphi|}, \tag{7.73}$$

where

  v_0 is a constant velocity
  k is the local curvature acting as a regularization term weighted by ε
  g is a contour indicator function (Randrianarisolo et al. 2008)

7.6.4.2 Implementation
Using the level set method, a technique has been developed for segmenting CMR images by propagating the epi- and endocardial contours and representing the visual information by vector gradients based on estimating the signal intensity characteristics of different objects (Paragios 2002). In another study, a level set-based segmentation technique has been implemented for detecting the endocardial contours from a set of 2D images acquired during consecutive timeframes in the cardiac cycle (Figure 7.37; Chenoune et al. 2005). The set of successively segmented contours are matched using global alignment and a level set-based morphing technique is used to measure myocardial deformation.

In a similar study, the level set method has been implemented for myocardial segmentation from a set of 2D+t images (Randrianarisolo et al. 2008). In this method, the initial interface is represented by a simple polyhedral surface centered at the ventricular cavity. An interpolation technique is then used to detect myocardial velocity, from which relevant information about the heart function can be obtained.

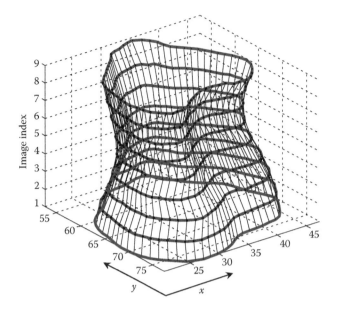

FIGURE 7.37   Segmentation and matching of the endocardial borders in a cine MRI sequence using the level set method. (Reproduced from Chenoune, Y. et al., *Comput. Med. Imaging Graph.*, 29(8), 607, 2005. With permission.)

The results have been validated against strain measurements from tagged images analyzed with the harmonic phase (HARP) technique. Recently, Ben Ayed et al. (2009b) developed a technique for automatic myocardial tracking using a level set-based global distribution matching.

7.6.4.3 Graph Cuts
The graph cut method has been implemented for segmenting the LV using a discrete kernel matching energy (Ben Ayed et al. 2009c). The method is based on the Bhattacharyya measure (described later in the chapter), which provides nearly real-time results. The region of interest in each frame is obtained by optimizing geometric and photometric priors that measure the distribution similarity between that region and the model in the first frame. The developed technique has the advantage that it does not require complex training or optimization. In general, compared to active contours, the graph cuts techniques provide significant improvement with respect to computational speed and complexity (Ben Ayed et al. 2010, 2011, Pham et al. 2011, Punithakumar et al. 2012b).

7.6.5 INTENSITY DISTRIBUTION TECHNIQUES

7.6.5.1 General Overview
Identifying different heart structures, for example, through image segmentation, is necessary for tracking their deformation during the cardiac cycle. In this respect, prior information from training examples or a manually segmented reference timeframe could be used to improve the segmentation process. The prior information could be related to the intensity distribution or shape variation in the CMR images, which can be embedded in the system via variational level sets (Zhang and Freedman 2005, Cremers et al. 2007) or

ASMs/AAMs (Cootes et al. 2001). In the level sets approach, the ML method has been used for minimizing a cost function that includes shape and intensity constraints (Lynch et al. 2006, 2008). Alternatively, ASMs and AAMs depend on maximizing the similarities between certain points in the image and the corresponding points in the model (Freedman et al. 2005). However, neither the level sets nor the ASMs/AAMs embed global information about the overlap between the intensity distributions within different regions in the image (e.g., myocardium, blood pool, and background), which could help eliminate the need for obtaining shape priors or making assumptions about the intensity/shape distributions in the image (Ben Ayed et al. 2008).

In a series of studies, Ben Ayed et al. (2008, 2009a,b) addressed this issue by embedding information about the intensity overlap in the images for improved segmentation and efficient motion tracking of different cardiac structures. Starting from a manually segmented reference timeframe (usually the first timeframe at end-diastole), two curves are identified to represent the endo- and epicardial contours. The evolution of these contours is followed through all the timeframes (Hautvast et al. 2006, Zhu et al. 2010) by maximizing a function that includes two components (Ben Ayed et al. 2009b): (1) the Bhattacharyya coefficient (Ben Ayed et al. 2010, Pham et al. 2011), which is a similarity measure between the intensity distribution in the regions inside and outside the identified boundaries, and (2) a gradient term that ensures the smoothness of the contours (Adam et al. 2009, Mitiche and Ben Ayed 2010).

7.6.5.2 Bhattacharyya Coefficient

The Bhattacharyya coefficient has been studied in information theory (Aherne et al. 1998), which showed to have the following advantages: (1) simple geometric interpretation, and (2) normalized range, which provides a convenient way to measure shape similarity (Ben Ayed et al. 2012). The Bhattacharyya coefficient aims to find a region $R \subset \Omega$ whose distribution most closely matches a given reference distribution M by Bhattacharyya measure (Nambakhsh et al. 2011):

$$B(P, M) = \sum_{z \in Z} \sqrt{P(z) M(z)}, \qquad (7.74)$$

where $P(z)$ is a nonparametric estimate of the distribution within R, given by

$$P(z) = \frac{\int_R K_z(x) dx}{|R|}, \quad \forall z \in Z, \qquad (7.75)$$

where
$|R|$ is the area of region R
$K_z(\cdot)$ is a kernel (typically Gaussian) function

$$K_z(x) = \frac{1}{(2\pi\sigma^2)^{n/2}} e^{-\left(\frac{\|z - I(x)\|^2}{2\sigma^2}\right)}, \qquad (7.76)$$

where I represents the image.

7.6.5.3 Convex Segmentation

Recently, the convex relaxation condition has been added to the distribution matching technique for fast and robust detection of the LV epi- and endocardial surfaces, as shown in Figure 7.38 (Nambakhsh et al. 2013). The developed technique eliminates the need for large training sets and can detect different cardiac structures regardless of changes in their shapes due to tissue deformation. The developed technique requires only a simple user input (single mouse clicks in the myocardium and blood pool) to start the segmentation process. The resulting system is solved by optimizing two energy functions that include the following priors: (1) distance distribution, (2) intensity distribution, and (3) surface smoothness.

7.6.5.4 Max-Flow Segmentation

Max-flow segmentation has been implemented for developing a method for fast detection of the LV boundaries through the optimization of two cost functions (Ben Ayed et al. 2012). The developed method showed to provide excellent real-time results based on the information from the first timeframe, which relaxes the need for a large training dataset and makes the segmentation process insensitive to biases from geometrical shape deformations.

The LV segmentation problem can be formulated as an iterative convex max-flow relaxation approach, which is solved by optimizing two discrete cost functions of global intensity and geometric constraints based on the Bhattacharyya similarity (Aherne et al. 1998). Specifically, the solution is obtained by finding the optimal regions of blood cavity (R_c) and myocardium (R_m) that match given distributions (M_c and M_m, respectively), subject to a tight region boundaries constraint. The problem is formulated as follows (Nambakhsh et al. 2011):

$$\min_{R_c, R_m} \left(-D_c(R_c) - D_m(R_m) + \gamma \left(|\partial R_c| + |\partial R_m| \right) \right), \qquad (7.77)$$

subject to the geometrical prior

$$R_c \subset R_m, \qquad (7.78)$$

where $|\partial R|$ measures the perimeter of region R and $D(R)$ is given by

$$D_c(R_c) = \alpha_c B(P_c^I, M_c^I) + (1 - \alpha_c) B(P_c^D, M_c^D),$$

$$D_m(R_m) = \alpha_m B(P_m^I, M_m^I) + (1 - \alpha_m) B(P_m^D, M_m^D), \qquad (7.79)$$

where the first terms in Equation 7.78 are the Bhattacharyya coefficients (defined in Equation 7.74) of intensity distribution (superscript I) and the second terms are the Bhattacharyya coefficients of radial distance distribution (superscript D).

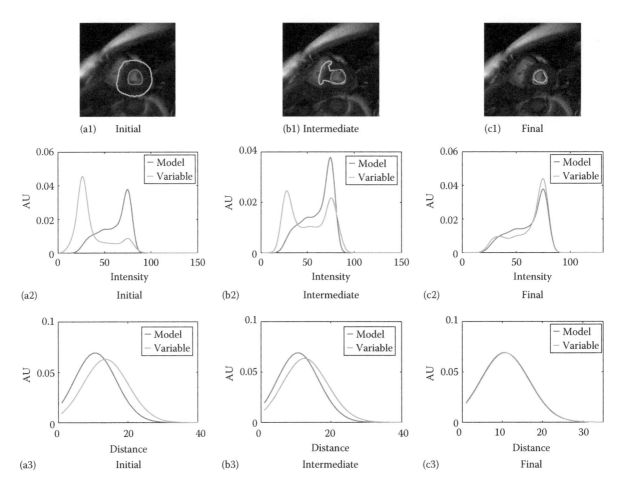

FIGURE 7.38   Three examples showing the evolution of segmentation and the corresponding intensity distributions during an iterative distribution matching process. (Reproduced from Nambakhsh, C.M. et al., *Med. Image Anal.*, 17(8), 1010, 2013. With permission.)

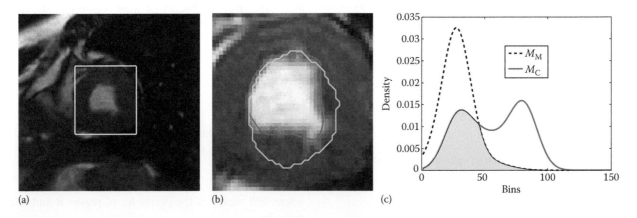

FIGURE 7.39   Max-flow segmentation. (a) Segmentation is limited to a region of interest around the left ventricle. (b) The green curve shows the expert (ground truth) delineation and the red curve shows the segmentation obtained by implementing the max-flow method. (c) M_C and M_M show the distribution of image data within the ground truth cavity (inside the green curve) and the myocardium (outside the green curve), respectively. (Reproduced from Ben Ayed, I. et al., *Med. Image Anal.*, 16(1), 87, 2012. With permission.)

α_c and α_m are weighting constants. The developed technique results in fast segmentation of the CMR images and provides accurate results that correlate well with manual segmentation. Further, the technique is shape-invariant and intrinsically handles ventricular shape variation, as shown in Figure 7.39 (Nambakhsh et al. 2011).

7.6.5.5 Segmental Contraction

A technique has been recently developed for characterizing segmental cardiac function based on Bhattacharyya coefficients to measure the similarity between the image distribution within each cardiac segment and the distribution of the corresponding user-provided segment (Afshin et al.

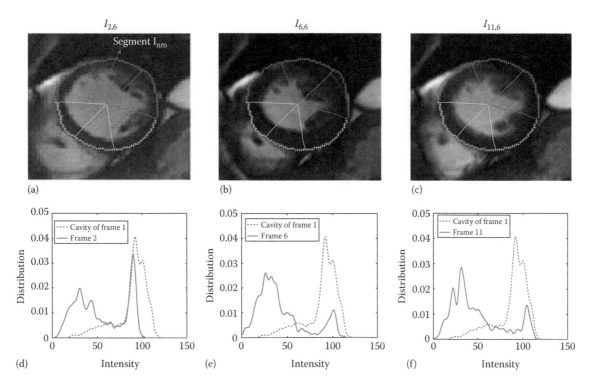

FIGURE 7.40 Left ventricle detection using segmental contraction. (a–c) Regional myocardial segments based on Bhattacharyya coefficients and (d–f) the corresponding image statistics. (Reproduced from Afshin, M. et al., *Med. Image Comput. Comput. Assist. Interv.*, 14(Pt 3), 107, 2011. With permission.)

2011, 2014). The developed technique requires only minimal user interface in the first timeframe, after which, it automatically builds the regional segments in all subsequent timeframes. The statistical features are generated as the proportion of blood within each segment (Figure 7.40), which is related to segmental contraction. The direction in which the generated image features are most significant is then determined using linear discriminant analysis (LDA), the results of which are fed to a linear support vector machine (LSVM) classifier for real-time identification of abnormal myocardial contraction.

7.7 SPATIOTEMPORAL REGISTRATION AND RECURSIVE FILTERS

Myocardial analysis techniques that work on static images are limited by the data available in that specific timeframe; they do not benefit from the information in the previous and following timeframes. Nevertheless, temporal characteristics of the heart motion can be incorporated in dynamic modeling for more accurate results (Jacob et al. 2001, Liu and Shi 2007, Punithakumar et al. 2010b).

7.7.1 Spatiotemporal Registration

7.7.1.1 Accounting for Global and Local Transformations

Spatiotemporal registration has been implemented for identifying different heart structures and distinguishing normal volunteers from patients with hypertrophic cardiomyopathy

(Perperidis et al. 2005a,b). The technique is based on a 4D deformable transformation model that includes both spatial and temporal components. The spatial transformation consists of both global and local parts, where the global part is represented by an affine transformation to address differences in size, orientation, and translation of the heart; and the local part is represented by a B-splines-based free-form deformation model to address differences in the heart's shape. Similar to spatial transformation, the temporal transformation consists of both global and local parts. Conducting the temporal and spatial optimization simultaneously results in better registration results than performing them separately, albeit at the cost of increased computational complexity (Perperidis et al. 2005b). Importantly, performing the temporal transformation using the cross-correlation method provides results similar to those obtained from the combined spatial and temporal approach.

7.7.1.2 Implementing Geometric Moment Invariants

Spatiotemporal registration can be implemented based on geometric moment invariants (GMIs) (Shen et al. 2005). Three-dimensional images acquired at different timepoints in the cardiac cycle are registered simultaneously, and the estimated motion is forced to follow spatiotemporal smooth constraints (Figure 7.41). The technique starts by assigning an attribute vector to each point in the dataset. The attribute vector includes information about the image intensity, boundary, and GMIs. The GMIs are calculated at different scales and are concatenated in the attribute vector. The registration technique can be applied

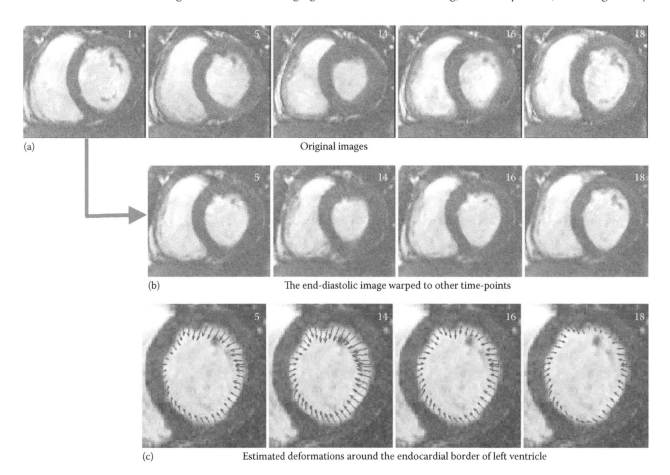

(a)   Original images

(b)   The end-diastolic image warped to other time-points

(c)   Estimated deformations around the endocardial border of left ventricle

FIGURE 7.41   Deformation estimation based on spatiotemporal registration. (a) Five selected cardiac images at different timeframes. (b) The results of warping end-diastole to other timepoints in the cardiac cycle. (c) Deformations around the left ventricle, estimated from the end-diastolic image. (Reproduced from Shen, D. et al., *Med. Image Comput. Comput. Assist. Interv.*, 8(Pt 2), 902, 2005. With permission.)

hierarchically for faster image processing and reduced chances of being trapped at local minima. The technique could also work in a multiresolution framework, where each resolution provides a certain level of transformation based on the total transformations estimated from the previous resolutions. The results of this technique have compared favorably with those obtained from tagged CMR images (Sundar et al. 2009).

7.7.1.3   Diffeomorphic Temporal Registration

Diffeomorphic temporal registration has been implemented to measure strain from a sequence of 3D cardiac images (De Craene et al. 2010). In this technique, the displacement field is computed by forward Eulerian integration of the velocity field, and temporal consistency is ensured by representing the velocity field as a summation of spatiotemporal B-splines. The temporal consistency of the developed technique allows for computing myocardial displacement/velocity at any timepoint in the cardiac cycle, which is particularly useful in the presence of image noise or artifacts. The developed technique has been implemented for detecting improvements in strain measurements after cardiac resynchronization therapy (CRT) (De Craene et al. 2010).

7.7.2   Recursive Filters

Recursive estimation-based myocardial segmentation depends on using the ventricular boundaries to construct a dynamic system for estimating myocardial deformation (Sun et al. 2005). Therefore, displacement estimation at a certain timepoint does not only depend on the observed data at that timepoint, but also on the results from past segmentations (Figure 7.42).

In a series of studies, McEachen et al. (1994, 1995, 2000, McEachen and Duncan 1997) used recursive filter–based temporal analysis for measuring myocardial deformation. The developed technique uses 2D harmonic estimation to model the periodic nature of the heart motion, which showed the capability of providing smoothly varying mapping functions. Recursive tracking can be improved by including information from phase-contrast cine CMR images in addition to the shape information obtained from the cine images (McEachen et al. 1995). Such improvement results in better trajectory estimates, especially in the regions where the shape information is not reliable. The resulting trajectory estimates are usually fed into a recursive least-squares filter to ensure the temporal periodicity and spatial smoothness of the final trajectories. The combined shape/phase recursive technique provided

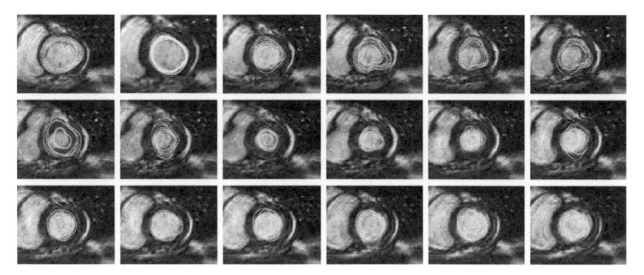

FIGURE 7.42 Curves representing predictions of the left ventricle segmentation in different frames in the cardiac cycle (from top left to bottom right) using recursive estimation. (Reproduced from Sun, W. et al., *Inf. Process. Med. Imaging*, 19, 553, 2005. With permission.)

results in good agreement with those from implanted markers (McEachen et al. 1995).

Recursive filtering has been also implemented for quantifying nonrigid motion of the LV wall by conducting three steps (McEachen and Duncan 1997): (1) initial estimation of local contour displacement by matching shape features between consecutive images, (2) smoothing the results, and (3) mapping the results to their closest points on the target contour. These three steps are repeated for all contours, and the resulting vectors are assembled into complete paths. The developed recursive filtering techniques are unique in that they are capable of modeling motion trajectories across multiple frames based on adaptive filtering (McEachen et al. 2000). Adaptive filtering makes it possible for the filter to work in cases where complete information about the image's signal characteristics is not available. Nevertheless, it should be noted that in the case of stationary environments, the recursive filter converges to the optimal Wiener solution after a number of iterations (Haykin 1986).

7.8 KALMAN FILTERS

7.8.1 Continuous Kalman Filter

As early as 1993, Metaxas and Terzopoulos (1993) used continuous nonlinear Kalman filter (Kalman 1960) to reconstruct a cardiac recursive shape and motion estimator. Here, Lagrange equations are used as a system model to continuously synthesize nonrigid heart motion based on the differences between data observations and estimated model state. The developed technique showed the capability of providing 3D nonrigid cardiac shape estimation for real-time applications. In a more recent study, the heart spatiotemporal motion in the whole image sequence has been measured by estimating the coefficients of harmonic series based on Lagrangian representation of motion (Delhay et al. 2007). In this technique, the parameters are considered as stochastic signals and

stored in a state vector, which is not directly measurable, but can be recursively estimated based on a set of successive measurements using Kalman filter.

7.8.2 Extended Kalman Filter

A stochastic finite-element model has been presented for simultaneous estimation of both heart kinematics and material properties from periodic cardiac images (Figures 7.43 and 7.44; Shi and Liu 2003). This joint probabilistic estimation approach is of particular interest to achieve robust and accurate motion estimates in the case of uncertain material properties or noisy images. The developed technique combines differential equations of myocardial dynamics with FEM modeling, where the material parameters and imaging data are treated as random variables. The extended Kalman filter is implemented to linearize the equations and provide joint estimates. The technique's implementation showed that the material parameters have better sensitivity for deriving transmural properties than do the motion parameters, an observation that has been validated by histology (Shi and Liu 2003).

The state-space representation of the continuous linear stochastic system is as follows (Shi and Liu 2003):

$$\dot{x}(t) = A_c x(t) + B_c w(t), \qquad (7.80)$$

where $x(t)$ is the kinematic state vector, represented as

$$x(t) = \begin{bmatrix} U(t) \\ \dot{U}(t) \end{bmatrix}, \qquad (7.81)$$

where U is the displacement vector. The system matrices, A_c and B_c, and the control term w are derived as follows:

$$A_c = \begin{bmatrix} 0 & I \\ -M^{-1}K & -M^{-1}C \end{bmatrix}, \qquad (7.82)$$

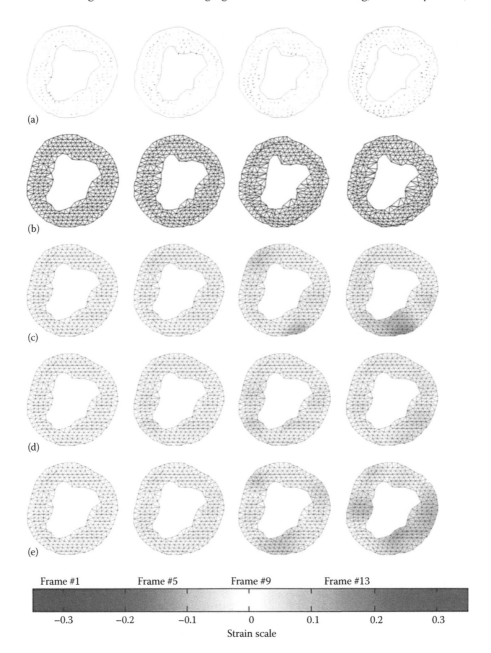

FIGURE 7.43 Myocardial deformation results based on a stochastic finite-element method model using extended Kalman filter. (a) Frame-to-frame displacement maps. (b) Deforming myocardial meshes. (c) Radial, (d) circumferential, and (e) radial–circumferential shear strains. (Reproduced from Shi, P. and Liu, H., *Med. Image Anal.*, 7(4), 445, 2003. With permission.)

$$B_c = \begin{bmatrix} 0 & 0 \\ 0 & M^{-1} \end{bmatrix}, \quad (7.83)$$

$$w(t) = \begin{bmatrix} 0 \\ R(t) \end{bmatrix}, \quad (7.84)$$

where
  M, C, and K are the mass, damping, and stiffness matrices, respectively
  R is the load vector

The associated measurement equation, which describes the observations $y(t)$ provided by the images, is expressed as

$$y(t) = Dx(t) + e(t), \quad (7.85)$$

where
  $e(t)$ is the measurement noise
  D is the measurement matrix

$$D = \begin{bmatrix} D_U \\ D_{\dot{U}} \end{bmatrix}. \quad (7.86)$$

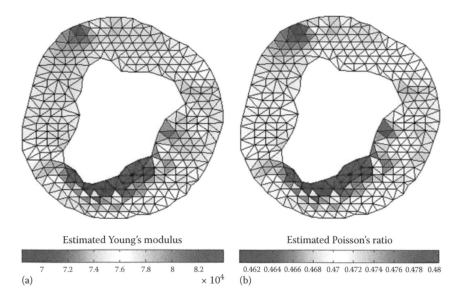

FIGURE 7.44 Estimated (a) Young's modulus and (b) Poisson's ratio based on a stochastic finite-element method model using extended Kalman filter. (Reproduced from Shi, P. and Liu, H., *Med. Image Anal.*, 7(4), 445, 2003. With permission.)

Assuming hidden Markov model for the state equations, Equation 7.80 can be discretized and written as

$$x\big((k+1)T\big) = Ax(kT) + Bw(kT),$$ (7.87)

where

$$A = e^{A_c T},$$ (7.88)

$$B = A_c^{-1}(e^{A_c T} - I)B_c.$$ (7.89)

7.8.3 DISCRETE STATE-SPACE MODEL

A discrete state-space model that describes the cyclic motion of a point is given by (Punithakumar et al. 2010c)

$$\xi_{k+1} = F_{cy}(k)\xi_k + w_k,$$ (7.90)

where

$$F_{cy}(k) = \begin{bmatrix} 1 & 0 & 0 \\ 1 - \cos(\omega T) & \cos(\omega T) & \frac{1}{\omega}\sin(\omega T) \\ \omega\sin(\omega T) & -\omega\sin(\omega T) & \cos(\omega T) \end{bmatrix},$$ (7.91)

where
- (x, y) is a Cartesian point on the endocardial boundary $k(s)$
- $\xi = \begin{bmatrix} \bar{x} \ x \ \dot{x} \end{bmatrix}^T$ is a state vector that describes the dynamics of the point in the x-direction ($\dot{x}$ and $\bar{x}$ denote velocity and mean position over a cardiac cycle, respectively)
- ω is angular frequency
- $w(t)$ is a white noise

Let $s = [\bar{x}\, x\, \dot{x}\, \bar{y}\, y\, \dot{y}]^T$ be the state vector that describes the dynamics in the x–y plane. The discrete state-space model in the x–y plane can be then given by

$$s_{k+1} = \begin{bmatrix} F_{cy}(k) & \mathbf{0}_{3\times 3} \\ \mathbf{0}_{3\times 3} & F_{cy}(k) \end{bmatrix} s_k + v_k,$$ (7.92)

where v_k is noise. The Kalman filter is applied for state estimation. Let $z_k = [z_{k,x}\ z_{k,y}]^T$ be the measurement at timepoint $k \in [1, ..., K]$. Then, the measurement equation is given by

$$z_k = H_k s_k + \eta_k,$$ (7.93)

where

$$H_k = \begin{bmatrix} 0 & 1 & 0 & 0 & 1 & 0 \\ 0 & 0 & 0 & 0 & 0 & 0 \end{bmatrix},$$ (7.94)

and η_k is a zero-mean Gaussian noise.

7.8.4 CONTINUOUS-DISCRETE KALMAN FILTER

A hybrid continuous-discrete Kalman filter has been developed for recovering cardiac motion from periodic cine CMR images (Figure 7.45; Tong and Shi 2006). In this technique, the state estimates are predicted according to the original continuous state equation and then updated with new measurements at discrete observation timepoints. Both minimum-mean-squared-error and min–max $H\infty$ optimization techniques are implemented to couple the continuous dynamics with the discrete observations. The spatiotemporal

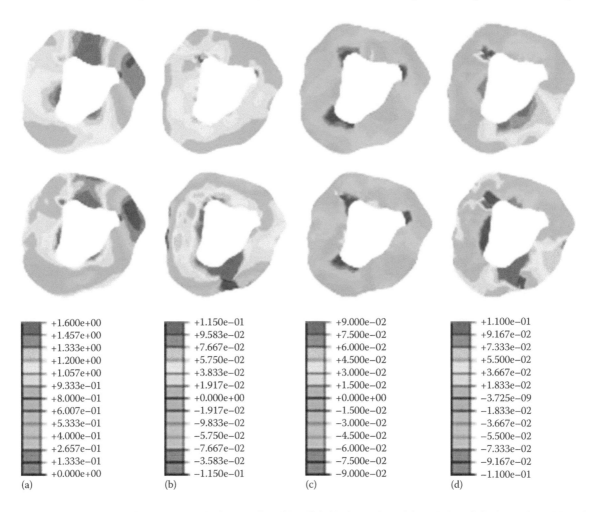

+1.600e+00	+1.150e−01	+9.000e−02	+1.100e−01
+1.457e+00	+9.583e−02	+7.500e−02	+9.167e−02
+1.333e+00	+7.667e−02	+6.000e−02	+7.333e−02
+1.200e+00	+5.750e−02	+4.500e−02	+5.500e−02
+1.057e+00	+3.833e−02	+3.000e−02	+3.667e−02
+9.333e−01	+1.917e−02	+1.500e−02	+1.833e−02
+8.000e−01	+0.000e+00	+0.000e+00	−3.725e−09
+6.007e−01	−1.917e−02	−1.500e−02	−1.833e−02
+5.333e−01	−9.833e−02	−3.000e−02	−3.667e−02
+4.000e−01	−5.750e−02	−4.500e−02	−5.500e−02
+2.657e−01	−7.667e−02	−6.000e−02	−7.333e−02
+1.333e−01	−3.583e−02	−7.500e−02	−9.167e−02
+0.000e+00	−1.150e−01	−9.000e−02	−1.100e−01
(a)	(b)	(c)	(d)

FIGURE 7.45 Estimated (a) displacement magnitude as well as (b) radial, (c) circumferential, and (d) radial–circumferential strain maps. Top: continuous-discrete Kalman filter results. Middle: $H\infty$ results. Bottom: color scales. (Reproduced from Tong, S. and Shi, P., *Med. Image Comput. Comput. Assist. Interv.*, 9(Pt 1), 744, 2006. With permission.)

biomechanical constraints are adopted using the following dynamic equation (Shi and Liu 2003):

$$M\ddot{U} + C\dot{U} + KU = R, \qquad (7.95)$$

where

M, C, and K are the mass, damping, and stiffness matrices, respectively
R is the load vector
U is the displacement vector

The first analysis step involves transforming Equation 7.95 into a state-space equation, as previously described in Equations 7.80 through 7.86. The continuous-discrete Kalman filter is a recursive filter consisting of prediction and update stages. In the prediction stage (between observation time instants), the state estimate $\hat{x}(t)$ and its covariance $P(t)$ propagate as follows (Bar-Sharlom et al. 2001):

$$\dot{\hat{x}}(t) = A(t)\hat{x}(t) + B(t)w(t), \qquad (7.96)$$

$$\dot{P}(t) = A(t)P(t) + P(t)A(t)' + \tilde{Q}(t), \qquad (7.97)$$

where $\tilde{Q}$ is the covariance of noise $v(t)$, while in the update stage, the state estimate and its covariance are updated using the standard discrete Kalman filter

$$\hat{x}(kT) = \hat{x}(kT^-) + W(k)(y(k) - D\hat{x}(kT^-)), \qquad (7.98)$$

$$P(kT) = P(kT^-) - W(k)S(k)W^T(k), \qquad (7.99)$$

where

$$S(k) = DP(kT^-)D^T + V(k) \qquad (7.100)$$

and the Kalman gain $W(k)$ is given by

$$W(k) = P(kT^-)D^T S(k) - 1, \qquad (7.101)$$

7.8.5 Kalman Filters and Information-Theoretic Measures

In a series of studies, Punithakumar et al. (2009, 2010c) presented the use of information measures and Bayesian filtering for detecting LV motion abnormality. Briefly, a cyclic model is constructed

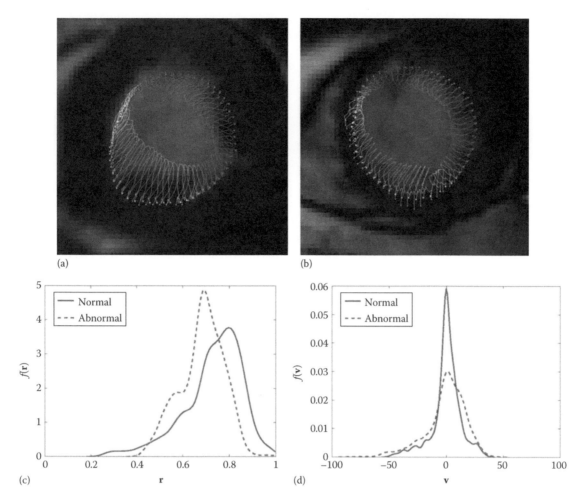

(a)

(b)

(c)

(d)

FIGURE 7.46 Potential of the Shannon's differential entropy measure for detecting motion abnormality. (a) Normal motion. (b) Abnormal motion. (c, d) show radial distance and radial velocity distributions, respectively, for both the normal and abnormal cases. Despite significant overlap between normal and abnormal motion distributions, the Shannon's differential entropy results are relatively different. f is the kernel density estimate. (Reproduced from Punithakumar, K. et al., *Med. Image Comput. Comput. Assist. Interv.*, 12(Pt 2), 373, 2009. With permission.)

to characterize the dynamics of the myocardial points' motion during the cardiac cycle, and Kalman filter is implemented for state estimation, which is subsequently analyzed using Shannon's differential entropy (SDE) to study distributions of the normalized radial motion estimates. Figure 7.46 shows the technique's capability of differentiating between normal and abnormal myocardial motion distributions (Punithakumar et al. 2010c).

7.8.5.1 Shannon's Differential Entropy

The SDE is given by (Punithakumar et al. 2010c)

$$S_f = -\int_{\mathbf{r} \in R} \frac{\sum_{i,k} K_\sigma\left(r_k^i - \mathbf{r}\right)}{NK} \times \left(\ln \sum_{i,k} K_\sigma\left(r_k^i - \mathbf{r}\right) - \ln NK \right) d\mathbf{r}, \tag{7.102}$$

where
- N is the number of samples
- K is the number of frames
- K_σ is the kernal function, given by

$$K_\sigma(y) = \frac{1}{\sqrt{2\pi\sigma^2}} e^{-\frac{y^2}{2\sigma^2}}, \tag{7.103}$$

and r_k^i is the normalized radial distance, given by

$$r_k^i = \frac{\sqrt{\left(\hat{x}_k^i - \frac{1}{N}\sum_i \hat{x}_k^i\right)^2 + \left(\hat{y}_k^i - \frac{1}{N}\sum_i \hat{y}_k^i\right)^2}}{\max_i \sqrt{\left(\hat{x}_k^i - \frac{1}{N}\sum_i \hat{x}_k^i\right)^2 + \left(\hat{y}_k^i - \frac{1}{N}\sum_i \hat{y}_k^i\right)^2}}, \tag{7.104}$$

where $\hat{x}_k^i$ and $\hat{y}_k^i$ are the estimates of x_k^i and y_k^i.

7.8.5.2 Unscented Kalman Filters and Smoothers

A Kalman filter-based method has been developed for detecting the heart wall motion abnormality from a multi-view fusion of cine CMR images (Figures 7.47 and 7.48; Punithakumar et al. 2012a). The method first obtains a

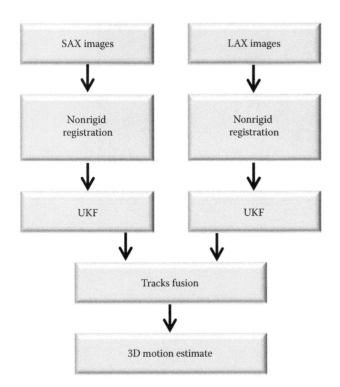

FIGURE 7.47 Algorithm steps for 3D motion estimation using unscented Kalman filters (UKF).

sequence of corresponding points using nonrigid registration. The selected points are then mapped to a 3D space and tracked using unscented Kalman filter (UKF) (Julier and Uhlmann 2004), which showed to provide high accuracy for nonlinear filtering applications (Punithakumar et al. 2012a).

An ML fusion approach is adopted to track the points from different views, and an SDE classifier is used to detect regions of abnormal myocardial structure.

In more details, the likelihood function is given by (Punithakumar et al. 2012a)

$$L(\mathbf{s}) = -\ln p(\mathbf{s}^s, \mathbf{s}^l | \mathbf{s}) \propto \left(\begin{bmatrix} \mathbf{s}^s \\ \mathbf{s}^l \end{bmatrix} - \begin{bmatrix} I \\ I \end{bmatrix} \mathbf{s} \right)^T P^{-1} \left(\begin{bmatrix} \mathbf{s}^s \\ \mathbf{s}^l \end{bmatrix} - \begin{bmatrix} I \\ I \end{bmatrix} \mathbf{s} \right), \tag{7.105}$$

where $\mathbf{s}^s$ and $\mathbf{s}^l$ are the motion estimates obtained from the SAX and LAX images, respectively, using unscented Kalman smoother (UKS). The state vectors $\mathbf{s}^s, \mathbf{s}^l \in ([\bar{x}\ \dot{x}\ \bar{y}\ y\ \dot{y}\ \bar{z}\ z\ \dot{z}\ \omega]^T)$, where (x, y, z) is a myocardial point in the 3D reference coordinate system corresponding to a pixel (i, j) in the image coordinate system, $[\dot{x}\ \dot{y}\ \dot{z}]$ is the velocity vector, $[\bar{x}\ \bar{y}\ \bar{z}]$ is the mean position of (x, y, z) over the cardiac cycle, and ω angular frequency. In the previous equation,

$$P = \begin{bmatrix} P^s & P^{sl} \\ P^{ls} & P^l \end{bmatrix}, \tag{7.106}$$

where
P^s and P^l are the covariance matrices of $\mathbf{s}^s$ and $\mathbf{s}^l$, respectively
P^{sl} is the cross-covariance matrix between $\mathbf{s}^s$ and $\mathbf{s}^l$
I is the identity matrix

The ML solution is given by

$$\mathbf{s}^{ML} = \max_{\mathbf{s}} L(\mathbf{s}) = P^l (P^s + P^l)^{-1} \mathbf{s}^s + P^s (P^s + P^l)^{-1} \mathbf{s}^l, \tag{7.107}$$

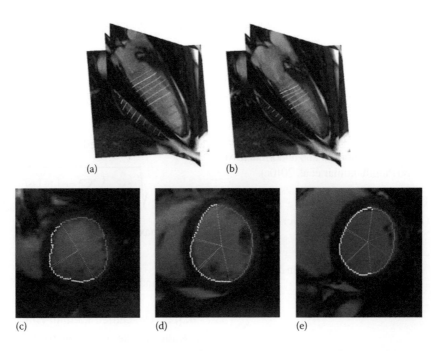

FIGURE 7.48 Cardiac segmentation results using unscented Kalman filters. The segmentation results fused on (a) end-diastolic and (b) end-systolic long-axis images, as well as (c) apical, (d) midcavity, and (e) basal short-axis images. (Reproduced from Punithakumar, K. et al., *Med. Image Comput. Comput. Assist. Interv.*, 15(Pt 2), 527, 2012a. With permission.)

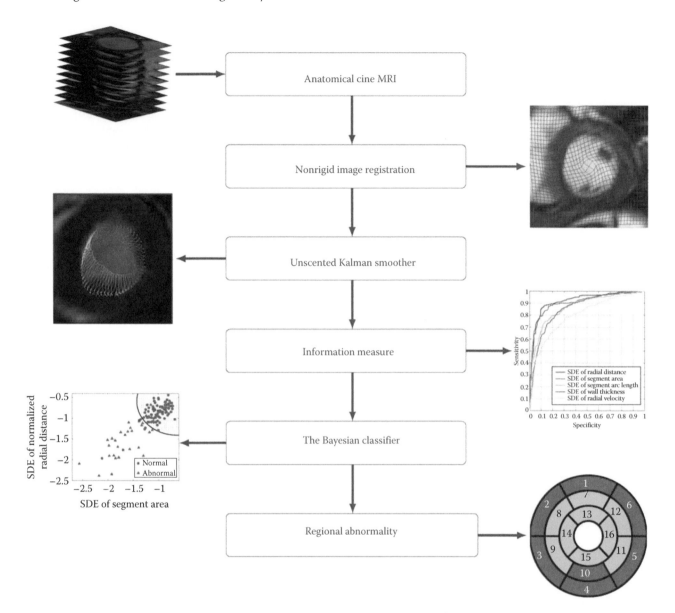

FIGURE 7.49 Algorithm for detecting wall motion abnormality based on unscented Kalman smoother. (Reproduced from Punithakumar, K. et al., *Med. Image Anal.*, 17(3), 311, 2013a. With permission.)

where the cross-covariances P^{sl} and P^{ls} between SAX and LAX observations are assumed to be zeroes.

A cyclic dynamic model that includes a time-varying angular frequency component can be implemented to generate accurate description of different heart phases (Figure 7.49; Punithakumar et al. 2010a, 2013a). The method is based on obtaining point correspondences between two images T_1 and T_k by optimizing a similarity measure ϕ (Chen et al. 2010):

$$\phi = \underset{\phi}{\text{opt}}\, E_s(T_1, T_k, \phi(\xi)) \tag{7.108}$$

for each location $\xi \in \Omega$, where $\phi: \Omega \to \Omega$ is a transformation function, and $E_s(\cdot)$ is a similarity measure. UKS (Sarkka 2008) is then implemented to generate the state estimates, which are used to measure regional LV function using SDE.

Finally, a naive Bayesian classifier (Seber 1984) is constructed from the SDEs of classifier features to detect heart regions with abnormal wall motion.

7.8.6 Interacting Multiple Models

Cardiac motion tracking can be conducted based on multiple models that represent different phases of the cardiac cycle (Punithakumar et al. 2010b). In this case, an interacting multiple model (IMM) estimation algorithm is implemented to switch between different Markovian models. The IMM provides a model probability, which is used to identify the model that best matches the heart motion. Each cycle of the IMM filter is composed of four steps: interaction, model-specific filtering, model probability update, and model combination.

During the interaction step, the individual filter estimates are mixed with respect to the predicted model probabilities. The mixing probability $\mu_k^{i|j}$ for models M_i and M_j are calculated as follows:

$$\mu_k^{i|j} = \frac{p_{ij}\mu_{k-1}^i}{\bar{c}_j}, \tag{7.109}$$

where

$$\bar{c}_j = \sum_{i=1}^{n} p_{ij}\mu_{k-1}^i; \tag{7.110}$$

the system M consists of n models $M = (M_1, \ldots, M_n)$; $\mu_k^j = p(M_j)$ is the probability of model M_j at time step k; p_{ij} is the model's transition probability; and μ_{k-1}^i is the model probability at time step $k-1$. The mean (m) and covariance (P) inputs to each filter j are calculated as follows:

$$m_{k-1}^{0j} = \sum_{i=1}^{n} \mu_k^{i|j} m_{k-1}^i, \tag{7.111}$$

$$P_{k-1}^{0j} = \sum_{i=1}^{n} \mu_k^{i|j} \left[P_{k-1}^i + \left(m_{k-1}^i - m_{k-1}^{0j}\right)\left(m_{k-1}^i - m_{k-1}^{0j}\right)^T \right]. \tag{7.112}$$

During the model-specific filtering step, each filter predicts and updates its state estimates using its dynamic model assumption. Kalman filter is used to calculate the mode-conditioned state estimates for each model. The prediction and update equations are given by

$$\left[m_k^{-i}, P_k^{-i} \right] = \mathrm{KF}_p\left(m_{k-1}^{0j}, P_{k-1}^{0j}, F\left(\omega^i\right), Q_k^i\right), \tag{7.113}$$

$$\left[m_k^i, P_k^i \right] = \mathrm{KF}_u\left(m_k^{-i}, P_k^{-i}, z_k, H_k^i, R_k^i\right), \tag{7.114}$$

where

Q and R are covariances of the noises
F and H are defined in Equations 7.91 and 7.94, respectively
KF_p and KF_u are the prediction and update equations, respectively, of the Kalman filter

During the model's probability update step, the probability of the model is updated with respect to the difference (residual) between the actual and predicted measurements. The probability μ_k^i of mode M_k^j is given by

$$\mu_k^i = \frac{\Lambda_k^i \bar{c}_i}{\sum_{i=1}^{n} \Lambda_k^i \bar{c}_i}, \tag{7.115}$$

where Λ_k^i is the likelihood of model M_i at time step k, given by

$$\Lambda_k^i = N(v_k^i; 0, S_k^i), \tag{7.116}$$

where

v_k^i is the measurement residual
S_k^i is the innovation covariance for model M_i in the Kalman filter update step

Finally, during the combination step, the estimate of the IMM algorithm is calculated by combining individual mode-conditioned filter estimates using mode probabilities

$$m_k = \sum_{i=1}^{n} \mu_k^i m_k^i, \tag{7.117}$$

$$P_k = \sum_{i=1}^{n} \mu_k^i \left[P_k^i + \left(m_k^i - m_k\right)\left(m_k^i - m_k\right)^T \right]. \tag{7.118}$$

7.9 SUMMARY AND KEY POINTS

7.9.1 SUMMARY

Despite the development of advanced and complicated MRI sequences for measuring cardiac function (that will be covered in the rest of the book), cine MRI images remain the basic building block in almost every cardiac MRI scan. Therefore, different analysis techniques have been developed throughout the years for estimating myocardial deformation parameters and identifying cardiac motion abnormalities from the cine images. Besides the advantage of these techniques for evaluating regional heart function in case the tagging images are not acquired, they also allow for retrospective cardiac functional analysis from existing datasets. Although the accuracy and level of details from such techniques are suboptimal to those from advanced tagging and phase-contrast based techniques, they provide a valuable means for general evaluation of the cardiac function and identification of abnormal wall motion without additional scan time or processing steps as required for advanced tagging techniques. Further, with advanced and complicated mathematical and statistical models, the results from cine-based analysis techniques are expected to improve.

7.9.2 KEY POINTS

- Cine imaging is the main component of almost every cardiac MRI scan.
- Ventricular wall thickening is a sensitive marker for detecting dysfunctional myocardium.
- Wall thickness measurement could be exaggerated if the imaging plane is not perpendicular to the heart's LAX direction.
- The centerline and centersurface methods reduce the errors in wall thickness measurements by correcting for LAX misalignment.
- Still-frame parametric images could be generated from the cine images to represent cardiac function.

- Compared to model-free approaches, the model-based techniques have the advantage that they provide information about the expected shapes of the structures of interest, which makes it easier to identify these structures in images with low SNR or in the presence of imaging artifacts.
- Artificial intelligence techniques provide a powerful tool for analyzing myocardial deformation.
- Probabilistic atlases provide information about the probability that a certain cardiac structure appears at a certain location in the image.
- Statistical atlases are used to identify changes in the cardiac anatomy due to shape variation in a certain population.
- The construction of a statistical atlas requires at least three steps: (1) segmenting the CMR images and extracting the structures' surfaces, (2) propagating the landmarks from the reference model to the images of a certain subject, and (3) statistically analyzing the changes in the structures' shape using modal analysis.
- Modal analysis (e.g., PCA or ICA) is a mathematical technique for reducing the number of degrees of freedom in a model, which results in constructing an overdetermined problem that can be easily solved for shape recovery.
- PCA and ICA allow for identifying the basic models of variation in cardiac motion.
- Similar to PCA, ICA is a linear generative model; however, ICA poses the additional constraint of statistical independency of the individual components.
- Geometrical modeling of the heart has the advantage of providing a simple and computationally inexpensive way for overall assessment of the cardiac function, albeit at the cost of measurements' accuracy.
- Nonrigid registration is used to map feature points in one timeframe to the corresponding points in another timeframe. This concept has been used to model myocardial deformation during the cardiac cycle.
- Most surface reconstruction techniques use piecewise polynomial surfaces, for example, B-splines or bicubic Hermite surface patches.
- Active contour models, or snakes, model deformable contours under internal constraints that ensure their smoothness and external constraints from the image features or prior knowledge.
- Snakes have been implemented for extracting contours from the cine images with minimal user interaction.
- ASMs and ASMs are popular parametric models for nonrigid registration.
- Various techniques for tracking the heart motion depend on measuring changes in differential geometric properties of the curves, for example, curvature and torsion, from one image to another.

- OF is an image processing technique that uses the image brightness variation between consecutive timeframes to compute motion of the object points in the image. OF techniques have been extensively implemented for quantifying myocardial deformation.
- Due to the heart's periodic motion, its motion can be represented by harmonic functions that describe a spatiotemporal relationship.
- The level set and graph cut techniques have been implemented for heart segmentation. Compared to active contours, these techniques provide significant improvement with respect to computational speed and complexity.
- Intensity distribution–based techniques have been developed for identifying different heart structures.
- Myocardial analysis techniques that work on static images do not benefit from the information in the previous and following timeframes. Spatiotemporal analysis addresses this limitation by simultaneously analyzing the data in both the space and time domains.
- Recursive estimation-based segmentation techniques depend on using the ventricular boundaries to construct a dynamic system for estimating myocardial deformation.
- Kalman filters provide an efficient and accurate means for evaluating the heart motion based on spatiotemporal analysis.
- Information theoretic measures have been combined with stochastic techniques for improving the accuracy of regional functional analysis.

REFERENCES

Adam, A., Kimmel, R., and Rivlin, E. (2009). On scene segmentation and histograms-based curve evolution. *IEEE Trans Pattern Anal Mach Intell* **31**(9): 1708–1714.

Adelson, E. and Bergen, J. (1986). The extraction of spatiotemporal energy in human and machine vision. *IEEE Motion Workshop*, Charleston, SC, pp. 151–156.

Afshin, M., Ben Ayed, I., Punithakumar, K., Law, M., Islam, A., Goela, A., Peters, T., and Li, S. (2014). Regional assessment of cardiac left ventricular myocardial function via MRI statistical features. *IEEE Trans Med Imaging* **33**: 481–494.

Afshin, M., Ben Ayed, I., Punithakumar, K., Law, M. W., Islam, A., Goela, A., Ross, I., Peters, T., and Li, S. (2011). Assessment of regional myocardial function via statistical features in MR images. *Med Image Comput Comput Assist Interv* **14**(Pt 3): 107–114.

Aherne, F. J., Thacker, N. A., and Rockett, P. (1998). The Bhattacharyya metric as an absolute similarity measure for frequency coded data. *Kybernetika* **34**: 363–368.

Allan, A., Gao, H., McComb, C., and Berry, C. (2011). Myocardial strain estimated from standard cine MRI closely represents strain estimated from dedicated strain-encoded MRI. *Conf Proc IEEE Eng Med Biol Soc* **2011**: 2650–2653.

Amini, A. A., Owen, R. L., Anandan, A., and Duncan, J. S. (1991). Non-rigid motion models for tracking the left-ventricular wall. *Lect Notes Comput Sci* **511**: 343–357.

Arun, K. S., Huang, T. S., and Blostein, S. D. (1987). Least-squares fitting of two 3-d point sets. *IEEE Trans Pattern Anal Mach Intell* **9**(5): 698–700.

Aster, R. C., Borchers, B., and Thurber, C. H. (2012). *Parameter Estimation and Inverse Problems*. Waltham, MA: Academic Press.

Bajo, A., Ledesma-Carbayo, M. J., Marta, C. S., David, E. P., Garcia-Fernandez, M. A., Desco, M., and Santos, A. (2007). Cardiac motion analysis from magnetic resonance imaging: Cine magnetic resonance versus tagged magnetic resonance. *Computers in Cardiology*, Durham, NC, pp. 81–84.

Bar-Sharlom, Y., Li, X., and Kirubarajan, T. (2001). *Estimation with Applications to Tracking and Navigation*. Hoboken, NJ: Wiley.

Bardinet, E., Cohen, L. D., and Ayache, N. (1995). Tracking medical 3D data with a parametric deformable model. *Proceedings of the International Symposium on Computer Vision*, Coral Gables, FL, pp. 299–304.

Bardinet, E., Cohen, L. D., and Ayache, N. (1996). Tracking and motion analysis of the left ventricle with deformable super-quadrics. *Med Image Anal* **1**(2): 129–149.

Barman, H., Haglund, L., Knutsson, H. and Granlund, G. (1991). Estimation of velocity, acceleration and disparity in time sequences. *Proceedings of the IEEE Motion Workshop*, Princeton, NJ, pp. 44–51.

Barr, A. H. (1981). Superquadrics and angle-preserving deformations. *IEEE Comput Graph Appl* **1**: 11–23.

Barron, J. L., Fleet, D. J., and Beauchemin, S. S. (1994). Performance of optical flow techniques. *Int J Comput Vision* **12**: 43–77.

Barron, J. L., Fleet, D. J., Beauchemin, S. S. and Burkitt, T. A. (1992). Performance of optical flow techniques. *Proceedings of the IEEE Computer Vision and Pattern Recognition (CVPR)*, Champaign, IL, pp. 236–242.

Beauchemin, S. S. and Barron, J. L. (1995). The computation of optical flow. *ACM Comput Surveys* **27**: 433–467.

Beg, M. F., Helm, P. A., McVeigh, E., Miller, M. I., and Winslow, R. L. (2004). Computational cardiac anatomy using MRI. *Magn Reson Med* **52**(5): 1167–1174.

Ben Ayed, I., Chen, H., Punithakumar, K., Ross, I., and Li, S. (2010). Graph cut segmentation with a global constraint: Recovering region distribution via a bound of the Bhattacharyya measure. *Proceedings of the IEEE Conference on Computer Vision and Pattern Recognition (CVPR)*, San Francisco, CA, pp. 3288–3295.

Ben Ayed, I., Chen, H. M., Punithakumar, K., Ross, I., and Li, S. (2012). Max-flow segmentation of the left ventricle by recovering subject-specific distributions via a bound of the Bhattacharyya measure. *Med Image Anal* **16**(1): 87–100.

Ben Ayed, I., Li, S., and Ross, I. (2009a). Embedding overlap priors in variational left ventricle tracking. *IEEE Trans Med Imaging* **28**(12): 1902–1913.

Ben Ayed, I., Li, S., Ross, I., and Islam, A. (2009b). Myocardium tracking via matching distributions. *Int J Comput Assist Radiol Surg* **4**(1): 37–44.

Ben Ayed, I., Lu, Y., Li, S., and Ross, I. (2008). Left ventricle tracking using overlap priors. *Med Image Comput Comput Assist Interv* **11**(Pt 1): 1025–1033.

Ben Ayed, I., Punithakumar, K., Garvin, G., Romano, W., and Li, S. (2011). Graph cuts with invariant object-interaction priors: application to intervertebral disc segmentation. *Inf Process Med Imaging* **22**: 221–232.

Ben Ayed, I., Punithakumar, K., Li, S., Islam, A., and Chong, J. (2009c). Left ventricle segmentation via graph cut distribution matching. *Med Image Comput Comput Assist Interv* **12**(Pt 2): 901–909.

Benayoun, S. and Ayache, N. (1995). Dense non-rigid motion estimation in sequences of medical images using differential constraints. *Lect Notes Comput Sci* **970**: 254–261

Benayoun, S. and Ayache, N. (1998). Dense and nonrigid motion estimation in sequences of medical images using differential constraints. *Int J Comput Vision* **26**: 25–40.

Beohar, N., Flaherty, J. D., Davidson, C. J., Vidovich, M. I., Brodsky, A., Lee, D. C., Wu, E., Bolson, E. L., Bonow, R. O., and Sheehan, F. H. (2007). Quantitative assessment of regional left ventricular function with cardiac MRI: Three-dimensional centersurface method. *Catheter Cardiovas Interven* **69**: 721–728.

Beyar, R., Shapiro, E. P., Graves, W. L., Rogers, W. J., Guier, W. H., Carey, G. A., Soulen, R. L., Zerhouni, E. A., Weisfeldt, M. L., and Weiss, J. L. (1990). Quantification and validation of left ventricular wall thickening by a three-dimensional volume element magnetic resonance imaging approach. *Circulation* **81**(1): 297–307.

Bistoquet, A., Oshinski, J., and Skrinjar, O. (2007). Left ventricular deformation recovery from cine MRI using an incompressible model. *IEEE Trans Med Imaging* **26**(9): 1136–1153.

Bistoquet, A., Oshinski, J., and Skrinjar, O. (2008). Myocardial deformation recovery from cine MRI using a nearly incompressible biventricular model. *Med Image Anal* **12**(1): 69–85.

Biswas, S. and Lovell, B. C. (2010). *Bezier and Splines in Image Processing and Machine Vision*. London, U.K.: Springer-Verlag.

Blake, A. and Isard, M. (1997). *Active Contours*. Berlin, Germany: Springer-Verlag.

Borgefors, G. (1986). Distance transformations in digital images. *Comput Vision Graph Image Process* **34**: 344–371.

Borgefors, G. (1988). Hierarchical chamfer matching: A parametric edge matching algorithm. *IEEE Trans Pattern Anal Mach Intell* **10**: 849–865.

Buller, V. G., van der Geest, R. J., Kool, M. D., and Reiber, J. H. (1995). Accurate three-dimensional wall thickness measurement from multi-slice short-axis MR imaging. *Computers in Cardiology*, Vienna, Austria, pp. 245–248.

Burt, P., Yen, C., and Xu, X. (1983). Multi resolution flow-through motion analysis. *Proceedings of the IEEE CVPR*, Washington, DC, pp. 246–252.

Caiani, E. G., Toledo, E., MacEneaney, P., Collins, K. A., Lang, R. M., and Mor-Avi, V. (2004). The role of still-frame parametric imaging in magnetic resonance assessment of left ventricular wall motion by non-cardiologists. *J Cardiovasc Magn Reson* **6**(3): 619–625.

Carranza, N., Cristobal, G., Bayerl, P., and Neumann, H. (2007). Motion estimation of magnetic resonance cardiac images using the Wigner–Ville and Hough Transforms. *Opt Spectrosc* **103**: 877–885.

Carranza, N., Cristobal, G., Ledesma-Carbayo, M. J., and Santos, A. (2006). A new cardiac motion estimation method based on a spatio-temporal frequency approach and Hough transform. *Computers in Cardiology*, Valencia, Spain, pp. 805–808.

Cauvin, J. C., Boire, J. Y., Zanca, M., Bonny, J. M., Maublant, J., and Veyre, A. (1993). 3D modeling in myocardial 201TL SPECT. *Comput Med Imaging Graph* **17**(4–5): 345–350.

Chadwick, R. S. (1982). Mechanics of the left ventricle. *Biophys J* **39**(3): 279–288.

Chakraborty, A., Staib, L. H., and Duncan, J. S. (1996). Deformable boundary finding in medical images by integrating gradient and region information. *IEEE Trans Med Imaging* **15**(6): 859–870.

Chen, C. W., Huang, T. S., and Arrott, M. (1994). Modeling, analysis, and visualization of left ventricle shape and motion by hierarchical decomposition. *IEEE Trans Pattern Anal Mach Intell* **16**: 342–356.

Chen, C. W., Luo, J., Parker, K. J., and Huang, T. S. (1995). CT volumetric data-based left ventricle motion estimation: An integrated approach. *Comput Med Imaging Graph* **19**(1): 85–100.

Chen, H. M., Goela, A., Garvin, G. J., and Li, S. (2010). A parameterization of deformation fields for diffeomorphic image registration and its application to myocardial delineation. *Med Image Comput Comput Assist Interv* **13**(Pt 1): 340–348.

Chenoune, Y., Delechelle, E., Petit, E., Goissen, T., Garot, J., and Rahmouni, A. (2005). Segmentation of cardiac cine-MR images and myocardial deformation assessment using level set methods. *Comput Med Imaging Graph* **29**(8): 607–616.

Clarysse, P., Friboulet, D., and Magnin, I. E. (1997). Tracking geometrical descriptors on 3-D deformable surfaces: Application to the left-ventricular surface of the heart. *IEEE Trans Med Imaging* **16**(4): 392–404.

Clarysse, P., Poupon, F., Barbier, B., and Magnin, I. E. (1995). 3D boundary extraction of the left ventricle by a deformable model with a priori information. *Proceedings of the International Conference on Image Processing*, Washington, DC, pp. 492–495.

Cohen, L. D. and Cohen, I. (1993). Finite-element methods for active contour models and balloons for 2-D and 3-D images. *IEEE Trans Pattern Anal Mach Intell* **15**: 1131–1147.

Comaniciu, D., Zhou, X. S., and Krishnan, S. (2004). Robust real-time myocardial border tracking for echocardiography: An information fusion approach. *IEEE Trans Med Imaging* **23**(7): 849–860.

Contijoch, F., Rogers, K., Avants, A., Yushkevich, P., Hoshmand, V., Gorman, R. C., Han, Y., and Witschey, W. R. (2014). Quantification of left ventricular deformation fields from undersampled radial, real-time cardiac MRI. *J Cardiovasc Magn Reson* **16**(Suppl. 1): P366.

Cootes, T. F., Beeston, C., Edwards, G. J., and Taylor, C. J. (1999). A unified framework for atlas matching using active appearance models. *Lect Notes Comput Sci* **1613**: 322–333.

Cootes, T. F., Edwards, G. J., and Taylor, C. J. (1998). Active appearance models. *Lect Notes Comput Sci* **1407**: 484–498.

Cootes, T. F., Edwards, G. J., and Taylor, C. J. (2001). Active appearance models. *IEEE Trans Pattern Anal Mach Intell* **23**: 681–685.

Cootes, T. F., Hill, A., Taylor, C. J., and Haslam, J. (1994). The use of active shape models for locating structures in medical images. *Image and Vision Comput* **12**: 355–366.

Cootes, T. F., Taylor, C. J., Cooper, D. H., and Graham, J. (1995). Active shape models-their training and application. *Comput Vision Image Understand* **61**: 38–59.

Costa, K. D., Hunter, P. J., Wayne, J. S., Waldman, L. K., Guccione, J. M., and McCulloch, A. D. (1996). A three-dimensional finite element method for large elastic deformations of ventricular myocardium: II—Prolate spheroidal coordinates. *J Biomech Eng* **118**(4): 464–472.

Cremers, D., Rousson, M., and Deriche, R. (2007). A review of statistical approaches to level set segmentation: Integrating color, texture, motion and shape. *Int J Comput Vision* **72**: 195–215.

Creswell, L. L., Wyers, S. G., Pirolo, J. S., Perman, W. H., Vannier, M. W., and Pasque, M. K. (1992). Mathematical modeling of the heart using magnetic resonance imaging. *IEEE Trans Med Imaging* **11**(4): 581–589.

Davatzikos, C., Tao, X., and Shen, D. (2003). Hierarchical active shape models, using the wavelet transform. *IEEE Trans Med Imaging* **22**(3): 414–423.

De Craene, M., Piella, G., Duchateau, N., Silva, E., Doltra, A., Gao, H., D'Hooge, J. et al. (2010). Temporal diffeomorphic free-form deformation for strain quantification in 3D-US images. *Med Image Comput Comput Assist Interv* **13**(Pt 2): 1–8.

Declerck, J., Feldmar, J., and Ayache, N. (1997). Definition of a 4D continuous polar transformation for the tracking and the analysis of LV motion. *Lect Notes Comput Sci* **1205**: 33–42.

Declerck, J., Feldmar, J., and Ayache, N. (1998). Definition of a four-dimensional continuous planispheric transformation for the tracking and the analysis of left-ventricle motion. *Med Image Anal* **2**(2): 197–213.

Delhay, B., Clarysse, P., and Magnin, I. E. (2007). Locally adapted spatio-temporal deformation model for dense motion estimation in periodic cardiac image sequences. *Lect Notes Comput Sci* **4466**: 393–402.

Dempster, A. P., Laird, N. M., and Rubin, D. B. (1977). Maximum likelihood from incomplete data via the EM algorithm. *J R Statist Soc Ser B* **39**: 1–38.

Denney, T. S., Jr. and McVeigh, E. R. (1997). Model-free reconstruction of three-dimensional myocardial strain from planar tagged MR images. *J Magn Reson Imaging* **7**(5): 799–810.

Denslow, S. (1994). An ellipsoidal shell model for volume estimation of the right ventricle from magnetic resonance images. *Acad Radiol* **1**(4): 345–351.

Dryden, I. L. and Mardia, K. V. (1998). *Statistical Shape Analysis*. New York: Wiley.

Dulce, M. C., Mostbeck, G. H., Friese, K. K., Caputo, G. R., and Higgins, C. B. (1993). Quantification of the left ventricular volumes and function with cine MR imaging: Comparison of geometric models with three-dimensional data. *Radiology* **188**(2): 371–376.

Duncan, J. S. and Ayache, N. (2000). Medical image analysis: Progress over two decades and the challenges ahead. *IEEE Trans Pattern Anal Mach Intell* **22**: 85–106.

Duncan, J. S., Lee, F. A., Smeulders, A. M., and Zaret, B. L. (1991a). A bending energy model for measurement of cardiac shape deformity. *IEEE Trans Med Imaging* **10**(3): 307–320.

Duncan, J. S., Owen, R. L., Staib, L. H., and Anandan, P. (1991b). Measurement of non-rigid motion using contour shape descriptors. *Proceedings of the IEEE Computer Vision and Pattern Recognition (CVPR)*, Maui, HI, pp. 318–324.

Duncan, J. S., Shi, P., Amini, A. A., Constable, R. T., Staib, L. H., Dione, D. P., Shi, Q. et al. (1994). Toward reliable, noninvasive measurement of myocardial function from 4D images. *Proc SPIE* **2168**: 149–161.

Dusch, M. N., Thadani, S. R., Dhillon, G. S. and Hope, M. D. (2014). Diastolic function assessed by cardiac MRI using longitudinal left ventricular fractional shortening. *Clin Imaging* **38**(5): 666–668.

El-Rewaidy, H., Khalifa, A., and Fahmy, A. S. (2014). Accurate estimation of the myocardium global function from reduced magnetic resonance image acquisitions. *Conf Proc IEEE Eng Med Biol Soc* **2014**: 6728–6731.

ElBaz, M. S. and Fahmy, A. S. (2012). Active shape model with inter-profile modeling paradigm for cardiac right ventricle segmentation. *Med Image Comput Comput Assist Interv* **15**(Pt 1): 691–698.

Elisseeff, A. (2002). *Leave-One-Out Error and Stability of Learning Algorithms with Applications*. Amsterdam, the Netherlands: IOS Press.

Elnakib, A., Beache, G. M., Gimel'farb, G., and El-Baz, A. (2015). Intramyocardial strain estimation from cardiac cine MRI. *Int J Comput Assist Radiol Surg* **10**(8):1299–1312.

Feng, W., Denney, T. S., Lloyd, S., Dell'Italia, L., and Gupta, H. (2008). Contour regularized left ventricular strain analysis from cine MRI. *Proceedings of the Fifth IEEE International Symposium on Biomedicine Imaging (ISBI)*, Paris, France, pp. 520–523.

Fleet, D. (1992). *Measurement of Image Velocity*. Norwell, MA: Kluwer Academic Publication.

Foley, P. W., Khadjooi, K., Ward, J. A., Smith, R. E., Stegemann, B., Frenneaux, M. P., and Leyva, F. (2009). Radial dyssynchrony assessed by cardiovascular magnetic resonance in relation to left ventricular function, myocardial scarring and QRS duration in patients with heart failure. *J Cardiovasc Magn Reson* **11**: 50.

Frangi, A. F., Niessen, W. J., and Viergever, M. A. (2001). Three-dimensional modeling for functional analysis of cardiac images: A review. *IEEE Trans Med Imaging* **20**(1): 2–25.

Frangi, A. F., Rueckert, D., Schnabel, J. A., and Niessen, W. J. (2002). Automatic construction of multiple-object three-dimensional statistical shape models: Application to cardiac modeling. *IEEE Trans Med Imaging* **21**(9): 1151–1166.

Freedman, D., Radke, R. J., Zhang, T., Jeong, Y., Lovelock, D. M., and Chen, G. T. (2005). Model-based segmentation of medical imagery by matching distributions. *IEEE Trans Med Imaging* **24**(3): 281–292.

Friboulet, D., Magnin, I. E., Mathieu, C., Pommert, A., and Hoehne, K. H. (1993). Assessment and visualization of the curvature of the left ventricle from 3D medical images. *Comput Med Imaging Graph* **17**(4–5): 257–262.

Friboulet, D., Magnin, I. E., and Revel, D. (1992). Assessment of a model for overall left ventricular three-dimensional motion from MRI data. *Int J Card Imaging* **8**(3): 175–190.

Gan, Y., Chen, Q., Zhang, S., Ju, S., and Li, Z. Y. (2015). MRI-based strain and strain rate analysis of left ventricle: A modified hierarchical transformation model. *Biomed Eng Online* **14**(Suppl. 1): S9.

Geiger, D., Gupta, A., Costa, L. A., and Vlontzos, J. (1995). Dynamic programming for detecting, tracking, and matching deformable contours. *IEEE Trans Pattern Anal Mach Intell* **17**: 294–302.

Gilchrist, C. L., Xia, J. Q., Setton, L. A., and Hsu, E. W. (2004). High-resolution determination of soft tissue deformations using MRI and first-order texture correlation. *IEEE Trans Med Imaging* **23**(5): 546–553.

Gjesdal, O., Almeida, A. L., Hopp, E., Beitnes, J. O., Lunde, K., Smith, H. J., Lima, J. A., and Edvardsen, T. (2014). Long axis strain by MRI and echocardiography in a postmyocardial infarct population. *J Magn Reson Imaging* **40**(5): 1247–1251.

Goodyer, A. V. and Langou, R. A. (1982). The multicentric character of normal left ventricular wall motion. Implications for the evaluation of regional wall motion abnormalities by contrast angiography. *Cathet Cardiovasc Diagn* **8**(3): 225–232.

Gorce, J. M., Friboulet, D., and Magnin, I. E. (1997). Estimation of three-dimensional cardiac velocity fields: Assessment of a differential method and application to three-dimensional CT data. *Med Image Anal* **1**(3): 245–261.

Goshtasby, A. (1993). Design and recovery of 2-D and 3-D shapes using rational Gaussian curves and surfaces. *Int J Comput Vis* **10**: 233–256.

Goshtasby, A. and Turner, D. A. (1995). Segmentation of cardiac cine MR images for extraction of right and left ventricular chambers. *IEEE Trans Med Imaging* **14**(1): 56–64.

Haag, U. J., Hess, O. M., Maier, S. E., Jakob, M., Liu, K., Meier, D., Jenni, R., Boesiger, P., Anliker, M., and Krayenbuehl, H. P. (1991). Left ventricular wall thickness measurements by magnetic resonance: A validation study. *Int J Card Imaging* **7**(1): 31–41.

Hautvast, G., Lobregt, S., Breeuwer, M., and Gerritsen, F. (2006). Automatic contour propagation in cine cardiac magnetic resonance images. *IEEE Trans Med Imaging* **25**(11): 1472–1482.

Haykin, S. S. (1986). *Adaptive Filter Theory*. Englewood Cliffs, NJ: Prentice-Hall.

Herbots, L., Maes, F., D'Hooge, J., Claus, P., Dymarkowski, S., Mertens, P., Mortelmans, L. et al. (2004). Quantifying myocardial deformation throughout the cardiac cycle: A comparison of ultrasound strain rate, grey-scale M-mode and magnetic resonance imaging. *Ultrasound Med Biol* **30**(5): 591–598.

Hill, D. L., Batchelor, P. G., Holden, M., and Hawkes, D. J. (2001). Medical image registration. *Phys Med Biol* **46**(3): R1–R45.

Hochbaum, D. S. and Singh, V. (2009). An efficient algorithm for co-segmentation. *Proceedings of the IEEE 12th International Conference on Computer Vision (ICCV)*, Kyoto, Japan, pp. 269–276.

Holman, E. R., Buller, V. G., de Roos, A., van der Geest, R. J., Baur, L. H., van der Laarse, A., Bruschke, A. V., Reiber, J. H., and van der Wall, E. E. (1997). Detection and quantification of dysfunctional myocardium by magnetic resonance imaging. A new three-dimensional method for quantitative wall-thickening analysis. *Circulation* **95**(4): 924–931.

Holman, E. R., Vliegen, H. W., van der Geest, R. J., Reiber, J. H., van Dijkman, P. R., van der Laarse, A., de Roos, A., and van der Wall, E. E. (1995). Quantitative analysis of regional left ventricular function after myocardial infarction in the pig assessed with cine magnetic resonance imaging. *Magn Reson Med* **34**(2): 161–169.

Horn, B. K. and Schunck, B. G. (1981). Determining optical flow. *Artif Intell* **17**: 185–203.

Hu, H., Gao, Z., Liu, L., Liu, H., Gao, J., Xu, S., Li, W., and Huang, L. (2014). Automatic segmentation of the left ventricle in cardiac MRI using local binary fitting model and dynamic programming techniques. *PLoS One* **9**(12): e114760.

Huang, W. C. and Goldgof, D. (1993). Adaptive-size meshes for rigid and nonrigid analysis and synthesis. *IEEE Trans Pattern Anal Mach Intell* **15**: 611–616.

Hubka, M., Lipiecki, J., Bolson, E. L., Martin, R. W., Munt, B., Maza, S. R., and Sheehan, F. H. (2002). Three-dimensional echocardiographic measurement of left ventricular wall thickness: In vitro and in vivo validation. *J Am Soc Echocardiogr* **15**(2): 129–135.

Ibrahim, El-S. H., Birchell, S., and Elfayoumy, S. (2012). Artificial intelligent technique for measuring heart volume from MRI images using iterative salient isolated threshold optimization ant algorithm (ISITOAA). *Proceedings of the International Society for Magnetic Resonance in Medicine*, Melbourne, Victoria, Australia, p. 1248.

Jacob, G., Noble, J. A., Kelion, A. D., and Banning, A. P. (2001). Quantitative regional analysis of myocardial wall motion. *Ultrasound Med Biol* **27**(6): 773–784.

Janz, R. F., Kubert, B. R., Pate, E. F., and Moriarty, T. F. (1980). Effect of shape on pressure-volume relationships of ellipsoidal shells. *Am J Physiol* **238**(6): H917–H926.

Jolly, M., Duta, N., and Funka-Lea, G. (2001). Segmentation of the left ventricle in cardiac MR images. *Proceedings of the Eighth IEEE Conference on Computer Vision*, Vancouver, British Columbia, Canada, pp. 501–508.

Julier, S. J. and Uhlmann, J. K. (2004). Unscented filtering and non-linear estimation. *Proc IEEE* **92**: 401–422.

Kachenoura, N., Redheuil, A., Balvay, D., Ruiz-Dominguez, C., Herment, A., Mousseaux, E., and Frouin, F. (2007). Evaluation of regional myocardial function using automated wall motion analysis of cine MR images: Contribution of parametric images, contraction times, and radial velocities. *J Magn Reson Imaging* **26**(4): 1127–1132.

Kalman, R. E. (1960). A new approach to linear filtering and prediction problems. *J Basic Eng* **82**: 35–45.

Kass, M., Witkin, A., and Terzopoulos, D. (1988). Snakes: Active contour models. *Int J Comput Vision* 1: 321–331.

Kawakubo, M., Nagao, M., Kumazawa, S., Chishaki, A. S., Mukai, Y., Nakamura, Y., Honda, H., and Morishita, J. (2013). Evaluation of cardiac dyssynchrony with longitudinal strain analysis in 4-chamber cine MR imaging. *Eur J Radiol* **82**(12): 2212–2216.

Kuwahara, M. and Eiho, S. (1991). 3-D heart image reconstructed from MRI data. *Comput Med Imaging Graph* **15**(4): 241–246.

Kybic, J. and Unser, M. (2003). Fast parametric elastic image registration. *IEEE Trans Image Process* **12**(11): 1427–1442.

Lamb, H. J., Singleton, R. R., van der Geest, R. J., Pohost, G. M., and de Roos, A. (1995). MR imaging of regional cardiac function: Low-pass filtering of wall thickness curves. *Magn Reson Med* **34**(3): 498–502.

Ledesma-Carbayo, M. J., Bajo, A., Santa Marta, C., Perez-David, E., Caso, I., Garcia-Fernandez, M. A., Santos, A., and Desco, M. (2006). Cardiac motion analysis from cine MR sequences using non-rigid registration techniques. *Computers in Cardiology*, Valencia, Spain, pp. 65–68.

Lekadir, K., Keenan, N., Pennell, D., and Yang, G. Z. (2007). Shape-based myocardial contractility analysis using multivariate outlier detection. *Med Image Comput Comput Assist Interv* **10**(Pt 2): 834–841.

Lekadir, K., Keenan, N. G., Pennell, D. J., and Yang, G. Z. (2011). An inter-landmark approach to 4-D shape extraction and interpretation: Application to myocardial motion assessment in MRI. *IEEE Trans Med Imaging* **30**(1): 52–68.

Li, B., Liu, Y., Occleshaw, C. J., Cowan, B. R., and Young, A. A. (2010). In-line automated tracking for ventricular function with magnetic resonance imaging. *JACC Cardiovasc Imaging* **3**(8): 860–866.

Li, B., Young, A. A., and Cowan, B. R. (2008). GPU accelerated non-rigid registration for the evaluation of cardiac function. *Med Image Comput Comput Assist Interv* **11**(Pt 2): 880–887.

Lin, X., Cowan, B. R., and Young, A. A. (2006). Automated detection of left ventricle in 4D MR images: Experience from a large study. *Med Image Comput Comput Assist Interv* **9**(Pt 1): 728–735.

Lipson, P., Yuille, A. L., O'Keeffe, D., Cavanaugh, J., Taaffe, J., and Rosenthal, D. (1990). Deformable templates for feature extraction from medical images. *Lect Notes Comput Sci* **427**: 413–417.

Little, J. and Verri, A. (1989). Analysis of differential and matching methods for optical flow. *IEEE Motion Workshop*, Irvine, CA, pp. 173–180.

Liu, H. and Shi, P. (2007). State-space analysis of cardiac motion with biomechanical constraints. *IEEE Trans Image Process* **16**(4): 901–917.

Lorenzo-Valdes, M., Sanchez-Ortiz, G. I., Elkington, A. G., Mohiaddin, R. H., and Rueckert, D. (2004). Segmentation of 4D cardiac MR images using a probabilistic atlas and the EM algorithm. *Med Image Anal* **8**(3): 255–265.

Lorenzo-Valdés, M., Sanchez-Ortiz, G. I., Mohiaddin, R., and Rueckert, D. (2002). Atlas-based segmentation and tracking of 3D cardiac MR images using non-rigid registration. *Lect Notes Comput Sci* **2488**: 642–650.

Lotan, C. S., Cranney, G. B., Bouchard, A., Bittner, V., and Pohost, G. M. (1989). The value of cine nuclear magnetic resonance imaging for assessing regional ventricular function. *J Am Coll Cardiol* **14**(7): 1721–1729.

Lotjonen, J., Kivisto, S., Koikkalainen, J., Smutek, D., and Lauerma, K. (2004). Statistical shape model of atria, ventricles and epicardium from short- and long-axis MR images. *Med Image Anal* **8**(3): 371–386.

Lotjonen, J., Koikkalainen, J., Smutek, D., Kivisto, S., and Lauerma, K. (2003). Four-chamber 3-D statistical shape model from cardiac short-axis and long-axis MR images. *Lect Notes Comput Sci* **2878**: 459–466.

Lu, Y., Radau, P., Connelly, K., Dick, A., and Wright, G. (2009). Pattern recognition of abnormal left ventricle wall motion in cardiac MR. *Med Image Comput Comput Assist Interv* **12**(Pt 2): 750–758.

Lucas, B. D. and Kanade, T. (1981). An iterative image registration technique with an application to stereo vision. *Proceedings of the Seventh International Joint Conference on Artificial Intelligence (IJCAI)*, Vancouver, British Columbia, Canada, pp. 674–679.

Lynch, M., Ghita, O., and Whelan, P. F. (2006). Left-ventricle myocardium segmentation using a coupled level-set with a priori knowledge. *Comput Med Imaging Graph* **30**(4): 255–262.

Lynch, M., Ghita, O., and Whelan, P. F. (2008). Segmentation of the left ventricle of the heart in 3-D+t MRI data using an optimized nonrigid temporal model. *IEEE Trans Med Imaging* **27**(2): 195–203.

MacRobert, T. M. (1967). *Spherical Harmonics*. New York: Pergamon Press.

Maes, F., Collignon, A., Vandermeulen, D., Marchal, G., and Suetens, P. (1997). Multimodality image registration by maximization of mutual information. *IEEE Trans Med Imaging* **16**(2): 187–198.

Maintz, J. B. and Viergever, M. A. (1998). A survey of medical image registration. *Med Image Anal* **2**(1): 1–36.

Makela, T., Clarysse, P., Sipila, O., Pauna, N., Pham, Q. C., Katila, T., and Magnin, I. E. (2002). A review of cardiac image registration methods. *IEEE Trans Med Imaging* **21**(9): 1011–1021.

Matheny, A. and Goldgof, D. B. (1995). The use of three- and four-dimensional surface harmonics for rigid and nonrigid shape recovery and representation. *IEEE Trans Pattern Anal Mach Intell* **17**: 967–981.

Maurer, C. R. and Fitzpatrick, J. M. (1993). A review of medical image registration. *Interactive Image-guided Neurosurgery*. In: R.J. Maciunas (Ed.), American Association of Neurological Surgeons, Parkridge, IL, pp. 17–44.

McEachen, J. C., 2nd and Duncan, J. S. (1997). Shape-based tracking of left ventricular wall motion. *IEEE Trans Med Imaging* **16**(3): 270–283.

McEachen, J. C., Meyer, F. G., Constable, R. T., Nehorai, A., and Duncan, J. S. (1995). A recursive filter for phase velocity assisted shape-based tracking of cardiac non-rigid motion *Proceedings of the Fifth International Conference on Computer Vision*, Cambridge, MA, pp. 653–658.

McEachen, J. C., Nehorai, A., and Duncan, J. S. (1994). A recursive filter for temporal analysis of cardiac motion. *Proceedings of the IEEE Workshop on Biomedical Image Analysis*, Seattle, WA, pp. 124–133.

McEachen, J. C., Nehorai, A., and Duncan, J. S. (2000). Multiframe temporal estimation of cardiac nonrigid motion. *IEEE Trans Image Process* **9**(4): 651–665.

McInerney, T. and Terzopoulos, D. (1995a). A dynamic finite element surface model for segmentation and tracking in multidimensional medical images with application to cardiac 4D image analysis. *Comput Med Imaging Graph* **19**(1): 69–83.

McInerney, T. and Terzopoulos, D. (1995b). Topologically adaptable snakes. *Proceedings of the Fifth International Conference on Computer Vision*, Cambridge, MA, pp. 840–845.

McInerney, T. and Terzopoulos, D. (1996). Deformable models in medical image analysis: A survey. *Med Image Anal* 1(2): 91–108.

Metaxas, D. and Terzopoulos, D. (1993). Shape and nonrigid motion estimation through physics-based synthesis. *IEEE Trans Pattern Anal Mach Intell* 15: 580–591.

Meyering, W. I., Gutierrez, M. A., Furuie, S. S., Rebelo, M. S., and Melo, C. P. (2000a). Spatiotemporal-frequency analysis applied to motion detection. *Proceedings of the 22nd IEEE Annual International Conference on EMBS*, Chicago, IL, pp. 1720–1723.

Meyering, W. I., Gutierrez, M. A., Furuie, S. S., Rebelo, M. S., and Melo, C. P. (2000b). Wigner-Ville distribution applied to cardiac motion estimation. *Computers in Cardiology*, Cambridge, MA, pp. 619–622.

Millman, R. and Parker, G. (1977). *Elements of Differential Geometry*. Englewood Cliffs, NJ: Prentice-Hall.

Mitchell, S. C., Bosch, J. G., Lelieveldt, B. P., van der Geest, R. J., Reiber, J. H., and Sonka, M. (2002). 3-D active appearance models: Segmentation of cardiac MR and ultrasound images. *IEEE Trans Med Imaging* 21(9): 1167–1178.

Mitchell, S. C., Lelieveldt, B. P., Bosch, H. G., Reiber, J. H., and Sonka, M. (2003). Disease characterization of active appearance model coefficients. *Proc SPIE* 5032: 38–49.

Mitchell, S. C., Lelieveldt, B. P., van der Geest, R. J., Bosch, H. G., Reiber, J. H., and Sonka, M. (2001). Multistage hybrid active appearance model matching: Segmentation of left and right ventricles in cardiac MR images. *IEEE Trans Med Imaging* 20(5): 415–423.

Mitiche, A. and Ben Ayed, I. (2010). *Variational and Level Set Methods in Image Segmentation*. Berlin, Germany: Springer-Verlag.

Miyamoto, S., Ichihashi, H., and Honda, K. (2008). *Algorithms for Fuzzy Clustering: Methods in c-Means Clustering with Applications*. Berlin, Germany: Springer.

Moyer, C. B., Helm, P. A., Clarke, C. J., Budge, L. P., Kramer, C. M., Ferguson, J. D., Norton, P. T., and Holmes, J. W. (2013). Wall-motion based analysis of global and regional left atrial mechanics. *IEEE Trans Med Imaging* 32(10): 1765–1776.

Mukherjee, L., Singh, V., and Dyer, C. R. (2009). Half-Integrality based algorithms for cosegmentation of images. *Proceedings of the IEEE Computer Society Conference on Computer Vision and Pattern Recognition*, Miami, FL, pp. 2028–2035.

Nambakhsh, C. M., Yuan, J., Punithakumar, K., Goela, A., Rajchl, M., Peters, T. M., and Ayed, I. B. (2013). Left ventricle segmentation in MRI via convex relaxed distribution matching. *Med Image Anal* 17(8): 1010–1024.

Nambakhsh, M. S., Yuan, J., Ben Ayed, I., Punithakumar, K., Goela, A., Islam, A., Peters, T., and Li, S. (2011). A convex max-flow segmentation of LV using subject-specific distributions on cardiac MRI. *Inf Process Med Imaging* 22: 171–183.

Nastar, C. and Ayache, N. (1996). Frequency-based nonrigid motion analysis: Application to four dimensional medical images. *IEEE Trans Pattern Anal Mach Intell* 18: 1067–1079.

Ni, K., Bresson, X., Chan, T., and Esedoglu, S. (2009). Local histogram based segmentation using the Wasserstein distance. *Int J Compt Vision* 84: 97–111.

O'Dell, W. G. and McCulloch, A. D. (2000). Imaging three-dimensional cardiac function. *Annu Rev Biomed Eng* 2: 431–456.

O'Donnell, T., Gupta, A., and Boult, T. E. (1994). A periodic generalized cylinder model with local deformations for tracking closed contours exhibiting repeating motion. *Proceedings of the 12th IAPR International Conference on Pattern Recognition*, Jerusalem, Israel, pp. 397–402.

Ordas, S., Oubel, E., Sebastian, R., and Frangi, A. F. (2007). Computational anatomy atlas of the heart. *Proceedings of the Fifth International Symposium Image and Signal Processing Analysis*, Istanbul, Turkey, pp. 338–342.

Papademetris, X., Shi, P., Dione, D. P., Sinusas, A. J., Constable, R. T., and Duncan, J. S. (1999). Recovery of soft tissue object deformation from 3D image sequences using biomechanical models. *Lect Notes Comput Sci* 1613,: 352–357.

Papademetris, X., Sinusas, A. J., Dione, D. P., and Duncan, J. S. (2001). Estimation of 3D left ventricular deformation from echocardiography. *Med Image Anal* 5: 17–28.

Paragios, N. (2002). A variational approach for the segmentation of the left ventricle in cardiac image analysis. *Int J Comput Vision* 50: 345–362.

Park, J., Metaxas, D., and Young, A. (1994). Deformable models with parameter functions: Application to heart-wall modeling. *Proceedings of the IEEE Computer Vision Pattern Recognition (CVPR)*, Seattle, WA, pp. 437–442.

Perperidis, D., Bucholz, E., Johnson, G. A., and Constantinides, C. (2012). Morphological studies of the murine heart based on probabilistic and statistical atlases. *Comput Med Imaging Graph* 36(2): 119–129.

Perperidis, D., Mohiaddin, R., and Rueckert, D. (2005a). Construction of a 4D statistical atlas of the cardiac anatomy and its use in classification. *Med Image Comput Comput Assist Interv* 8(Pt 2): 402–410.

Perperidis, D., Mohiaddin, R. H., and Rueckert, D. (2005b). Spatio-temporal free-form registration of cardiac MR image sequences. *Med Image Anal* 9(5): 441–456.

Peshock, R. M., Rokey, R., Malloy, G. M., McNamee, P., Buja, L. M., Parkey, R. W., and Willerson, J. T. (1989). Assessment of myocardial systolic wall thickening using nuclear magnetic resonance imaging. *J Am Coll Cardiol* 14(3): 653–659.

Pham, V., Takahashi, K., and Naemura, T. (2011). Foreground-background segmentation using iterated distribution matching. *Proceedings of the IEEE Conference on Computer Vision and Pattern Recognition (CVPR)*, Providence, RI, pp. 2113–2120.

Pirolo, J. S., Bresina, S. J., Creswell, L. L., Myers, K. W., Szabo, B. A., MW, V. A., and Pasque, M. K. (1993). Mathematical three-dimensional solid modeling of biventricular geometry. *Ann Biomed Eng* 21(3): 199–219.

Plein, S., Smith, W. H., Ridgway, J. P., Kassner, A., Beacock, D. J., Bloomer, T. N., and Sivananthan, M. U. (2001). Qualitative and quantitative analysis of regional left ventricular wall dynamics using real-time magnetic resonance imaging: Comparison with conventional breath-hold gradient echo acquisition in volunteers and patients. *J Magn Reson Imaging* 14(1): 23–30.

Potel, M. J., MacKay, S. A., Rubin, J. M., Aisen, A. M., and Sayre, R. E. (1984). Three-dimensional left ventricular wall motion in man. Coordinate systems for representing wall movement direction. *Invest Radiol* 19(6): 499–509.

Prasad, M., Ramesh, A., Kavanagh, P., Gerlach, J., Germano, G., Berman, D., and Slomka, P. (2009). Myocardial wall thickening from gated magnetic resonance images using Laplace's equation. *Proc SPIE Int Soc Opt Eng.* 2009 Feb 10; 7260: 72602I.

Prasad, M., Ramesh, A., Kavanagh, P., Tamarappoo, B. K., Nakazato, R., Gerlach, J., Cheng, V. et al. (2010). Quantification of 3D regional myocardial wall thickening from gated magnetic resonance images. *J Magn Reson Imaging* 31(2): 317–327.

Punithakumar, K., Ben Ayed, I., Islam, A., Goela, A., and Lil, S. (2012a). Regional heart motion abnormality detection via multiview fusion. *Med Image Comput Comput Assist Interv* 15(Pt 2): 527–534.

Punithakumar, K., Ben Ayed, I., Islam, A., Goela, A., Ross, I. G., Chong, J., and Li, S. (2013a). Regional heart motion abnormality detection: An information theoretic approach. *Med Image Anal* **17**(3): 311–324.

Punithakumar, K., Ben Ayed, I., Islam, A., Ross, I. G., and Li, S. (2010a). Regional heart motion abnormality detection via information measures and unscented Kalman filtering. *Med Image Comput Comput Assist Interv* **13**(Pt 1): 409–417.

Punithakumar, K., Ben Ayed, I., Islam, A., Ross, I. G., and Li, S. (2010b). Tracking endocardial motion via multiple model filtering. *IEEE Trans Biomed Eng* **57**(8): 2001–2010.

Punithakumar, K., Ben Ayed, I., Ross, I. G., Islam, A., Chong, J., and Li, S. (2010c). Detection of left ventricular motion abnormality via information measures and Bayesian filtering. *IEEE Trans Inf Technol Biomed* **14**(4): 1106–1113.

Punithakumar, K., Li, S., Ben Ayed, I., Ross, I., Islam, A., and Chong, J. (2009). Heart motion abnormality detection via an information measure and Bayesian filtering. *Med Image Comput Comput Assist Interv* **12**(Pt 2): 373–380.

Punithakumar, K., Noga, M., and Boulanger, P. (2013b). Cardiac right ventricular segmentation via point correspondence. *Conf Proc IEEE Eng Med Biol Soc* **2013**: 4010–4013.

Punithakumar, K., Yuan, J., Ben Ayed, I., Li, S., and Boykov, Y. (2012b). A convex max-flow approach to distribution-based figure-ground separation. *SIAM J Imaging Sci* **5**: 1333–1354.

Randrianarisolo, S., Delechelle, E., Petit, E., Rahmouni, A., and Garot, J. (2008). Assessment of myocardial deformations from untagged cardiac cine MRI. *Conf Proc IEEE Eng Med Biol Soc* **2008**: 3401–3404.

Ranganath, S. (1995). Contour extraction from cardiac MRI studies using snakes. *IEEE Trans Med Imaging* **14**(2): 328–338.

Riffel, J., Keller, M. G., Aurich, M., Sander, Y., Andre, F., Giusca, S., aus dem Siepen, F. et al. (2015). Standardized assessment of global longitudinal and circumferential strain—A modality independent software approach. *J Cardiovasc Magn Reson* **17**(Suppl. 1): Q9.

Roohi, S. F. and Zoroofi, R. A. (2013). 4D statistical shape modeling of the left ventricle in cardiac MR images. *Int J Comput Assist Radiol Surg* **8**(3): 335–351.

Rueckert, D., Frangi, A. F., and Schnabel, J. A. (2001). Automatic construction of 3D statistical deformation models using non-rigid registration. *Lect Notes Comput Sci* **2208**: 77–84.

Ruiz Dominguez, C., Kachenoura, N., De Cesare, A., Delouche, A., Lim, P., Gerard, O., Herment, A., Diebold, B., and Frouin, F. (2005). Assessment of left ventricular contraction by parametric analysis of main motion (PAMM): Theory and application for echocardiography. *Phys Med Biol* **50**(14): 3277–3296.

Sacks, M. S., Chuong, C. J., Templeton, G. H., and Peshock, R. (1993). In vivo 3-D reconstruction and geometric characterization of the right ventricular free wall. *Ann Biomed Eng* **21**(3): 263–275.

Sarkka, S. (2008). Unscented Rauch-Tung-Striebel smoother. *IEEE Trans Automat Control* **53**: 845–849.

Satriano, A., Kandalam, V., Jivraj, K., Mikami, Y., Medwid, H., Lydell, C., Merchant, N., Howarth, A. G., Elliot, T. L., and White, J. A. (2015). 4-Dimensional strain imaging of the right ventricle: Application in patients with severe pulmonary hypertension. *J Cardiovasc Magn Reson* **17**(Suppl 1): Q56.

Seber, G. A. (1984). *Multivariate Observations*. Hoboken, NJ: John Wiley & Sons Inc.

Sechtem, U., Sommerhoff, B. A., Markiewicz, W., White, R. D., Cheitlin, M. D., and Higgins, C. B. (1987). Regional left ventricular wall thickening by magnetic resonance imaging: Evaluation in normal persons and patients with global and regional dysfunction. *Am J Cardiol* **59**(1): 145–151.

Sethian, J. A. (1999). *Level Set Methods and Fast Marching Methods*. Cambridge, U.K.: Cambridge University Press.

Sheehan, F. H., Bolson, E. L., Dodge, H. T., Mathey, D. G., Schofer, J., and Woo, H. W. (1986). Advantages and applications of the centerline method for characterizing regional ventricular function. *Circulation* **74**(2): 293–305.

Shen, D., Sundar, H., Xue, Z., Fan, Y., and Litt, H. (2005). Consistent estimation of cardiac motions by 4D image registration. *Med Image Comput Comput Assist Interv* **8**(Pt 2): 902–910.

Shi, P., Amini, A., Robinson, G. and Sinusas, A. (1994). Shape-based 4D left ventricular myocardial function analysis. *Proceedings of the IEEE Workshop on Biomedical Image Analysis*, Seattle, WA, pp. 88–97.

Shi, P. and Liu, H. (2003). Stochastic finite element framework for simultaneous estimation of cardiac kinematic functions and material parameters. *Med Image Anal* **7**(4): 445–464.

Shi, P., Sinusas, A. J., Constable, R. T., and Duncan, J. (1999). Volumetric deformation analysis using mechanics-based data fusion: Applications in cardiac motion recovery. *Int J Compt Vision* **35**: 65–85.

Shi, P., Sinusas, A. J., Constable, R. T., Ritman, E., and Duncan, J. S. (2000). Point-tracked quantitative analysis of left ventricular surface motion from 3-D image sequences. *IEEE Trans Med Imaging* **19**(1): 36–50.

Simon, D. (2013). *Evolutionary Optimization Algorithms*. Hoboken, NJ: John Wiley & Sons.

Sliman, H., Khalifa, F., Elnakib, A., Soliman, A., El-Baz, A., Beache, G. M., Elmaghraby, A., and Gimel'farb, G. (2013). Myocardial borders segmentation from cine MR images using bidirectional coupled parametric deformable models. *Med Phys* **40**(9): 092302.

Sorzano, C. O., Thevenaz, P., and Unser, M. (2005). Elastic registration of biological images using vector-spline regularization. *IEEE Trans Biomed Eng* **52**(4): 652–663.

Staib, L. H. and Duncan, J. S. (1992). Boundary finding with parametrically deformable models. *IEEE Trans Pattern Anal Mach Intell* **14**: 1061–1075.

Staib, L. H. and Duncan, J. S. (1996). Model-based deformable surface finding for medical images. *IEEE Trans Med Imaging* **15**(5): 720–731.

Suever, J. D., Fornwalt, B. K., Neuman, L. R., Delfino, J. G., Lloyd, M. S., and Oshinski, J. N. (2014). Method to create regional mechanical dyssynchrony maps from short-axis cine steady-state free-precession images. *J Magn Reson Imaging* **39**(4): 958–965.

Suinesiaputra, A., Cowan, B. R., Al-Agamy, A. O., Elattar, M. A., Ayache, N., Fahmy, A. S., Khalifa, A. M. et al. (2014). A collaborative resource to build consensus for automated left ventricular segmentation of cardiac MR images. *Med Image Anal* **18**(1): 50–62.

Suinesiaputra, A., Frangi, A. F., Kaandorp, T. A., Lamb, H. J., Bax, J. J., Reiber, J. H., and Lelieveldt, B. P. (2009). Automated detection of regional wall motion abnormalities based on a statistical model applied to multislice short-axis cardiac MR images. *IEEE Trans Med Imaging* **28**(4): 595–607.

Suinesiaputra, A., Frangi, A. F., Kaandorp, T. A., Lamb, H. J., Bax, J. J., Reiber, J. H., and Lelieveldt, B. P. (2011). Automated regional wall motion abnormality detection by combining rest and stress cardiac MRI: Correlation with contrast-enhanced MRI. *J Magn Reson Imaging* **34**(2): 270–278.

Suinesiaputra, A., Frangi, A. F., Lamb, H. J., Reiber, J. H., and Lelieveldt, B. P. (2005). Automatic prediction of myocardial contractility improvement in stress MRI using shape morphometrics with independent component analysis. *Inf Process Med Imaging* **19**: 321–332.

Suinesiaputra, A., Frangi, A. F., Uzumcu, M., Reiber, J. H., and Lelieveldt, B. P. (2004a). Extraction of myocardial contractility patterns from short-axes MR images using independent component analysis. *Lect Notes Comput Sci* **3117**: 75–86.

Suinesiaputra, A., Uzumcu, M., Frangi, A. F., Kaandorp, T. A., Reiber, J. H., and Lelieveldt, B. P. (2004b). Detecting regional abnormal cardiac contraction in short-axis MR images using independent component analysis. *Lect Notes Comput Sci* **3216**: 737–744

Sun, H., Frangi, A. F., Wang, H., Sukno, F. M., Tobon-Gomez, C., and Yushkevich, P. A. (2010). Automatic cardiac MRI segmentation using a biventricular deformable medial model. *Med Image Comput Comput Assist Interv* **13**(Pt 1): 468–475.

Sun, W., Qetin, M., Chan, R., Reddy, V., Holmvang, G., Chandar, V., and Willsky, A. (2005). Segmenting and tracking the left ventricle by learning the dynamics in cardiac images. *Inf Process Med Imaging* **19**: 553–565.

Sundar, H., Litt, H., and Shen, D. (2009). Estimating myocardial motion by 4D image warping. *Pattern Recogn* **42**(11): 2514–2526.

Terzopoulos, D. (1986). Regularization of inverse visual problems involving discontinuities. *IEEE Trans Pattern Analysis Machine Intell* **8**: 413–424.

Terzopoulos, D. and Metaxas, D. (1991). Dynamic 3D models with local and global deformations: Deformable superquadrics. *Proceedings of the Third International Conference on Computer Vision*, Osaka, Japan, pp. 606–615.

Terzopoulos, D., Platt, J., Barr, A., and Fleischer, K. (1987). Elastically deformable models. *Comput Graph* **21**: 205–214.

Thiele, H., Paetsch, I., Schnackenburg, B., Bornstedt, A., Grebe, O., Wellnhofer, E., Schuler, G., Fleck, E., and Nagel, E. (2002). Improved accuracy of quantitative assessment of left ventricular volume and ejection fraction by geometric models with steady-state free precession. *J Cardiovasc Magn Reson* **4**(3): 327–339.

Tistarelli, M. and Marcenaro, G. (1994). Using optical flow to analyze the motion of human body organs from bioimages. *Proceedings of the IEEE Workshop on Biomedical Image Analysis*, Seattle, WA, pp. 100–109.

Tobon-Gomez, C., Sukno, F. M., Butakoff, C., Huguet, M., and Frangi, A. F. (2012). Automatic training and reliability estimation for 3D ASM applied to cardiac MRI segmentation. *Phys Med Biol* **57**(13): 4155–4174.

Tong, S. and Shi, P. (2006). Cardiac motion recovery: Continuous dynamics, discrete measurements, and optimal estimation. *Med Image Comput Comput Assist Interv* **9**(Pt 1): 744–751.

Tsai, A., Yezzi, A., Jr., Wells, W., Tempany, C., Tucker, D., Fan, A., Grimson, W. E., and Willsky, A. (2003). A shape-based approach to the segmentation of medical imagery using level sets. *IEEE Trans Med Imaging* **22**(2): 137–154.

Tsai, Y. J., Liu, Y., Greiser, A., Hayes, C., Lam, H., Occleshaw, C., Young, A., and Cowan, B. (2015). Fully automated strain analysis from SSFP cines of the heart using non-rigid registration techniques. *Proceedings of the International Society of Magnetic Resonance in Medicine*, Toronto, Ontario, Canada, p. 4529.

Tseng, W. Y. (2000). Magnetic resonance imaging assessment of left ventricular function and wall motion. *J Formosan Med Assoc = Taiwan yi zhi* **99**(8): 593–602.

Underwood, S. R., Rees, R. S., Savage, P. E., Klipstein, R. H., Firmin, D. N., Fox, K. M., Poole-Wilson, P. A., and Longmore, D. B. (1986). Assessment of regional left ventricular function by magnetic resonance. *Br Heart J* **56**(4): 334–340.

Uras, S., Girosi, F., Verri, A., and Torre, V. (1988). A computational approach to motion perception. *Biol Cyber* **60**: 79–97.

Uzumcu, M., Frangi, A. F., Reiber, J. H., and Lelieveldt, B. P. (2003). Independent component analysis in statistical shape models. *Proc SPIE* **5032**: 375–383.

van Assen, H. C., Danilouchkine, M. G., Behloul, F., Lamb, H. J., van der Geest, R. J., Reiber, J. H., and Lelieveldt, B. P. (2003). Cardiac LV segmentation using a 3D active shape model driven by fuzzy inference. *Lect Notes Comput Sci* **2878**: 533–540.

van Assen, H. C., Danilouchkine, M. G., Dirksen, M. S., Reiber, J. H., and Lelieveldt, B. P. (2008). A 3-D active shape model driven by fuzzy inference: Application to cardiac CT and MR. *IEEE Trans Inf Technol Biomed* **12**(5): 595–605.

van den Elsen, P. A., Pol, E. J., and Viergever, M. A. (1993). Medical image matching—A review with classification. *IEEE Eng Med Biol Mag* **12**: 26–39.

van der Geest, R. J., Lelieveldt, B. P., and Reiber, J. H. (2000). Quantification of global and regional ventricular function in cardiac magnetic resonance imaging. *Top Magn Reson Imaging* **11**(6): 348–358.

Van Leemput, K., Maes, F., Vandermeulen, D., and Suetens, P. (1999). Automated model-based tissue classification of MR images of the brain. *IEEE Trans Med Imaging* **18**(10): 897–908.

Wael, M., Ibrahim, El-S. H., and Fahmy, A. S. (2015). Normalized wall thickening patterns for detecting cardiac functional abnormality from cine MRI images. *Proceedings of the International Society of Magnetic Resonance in Medicine*, Toronto, Ontario, Canada, p. 4477.

Wan, M., Kng, T. S., Yang, X., Zhang, J., Zhao, X., Thai, W. S., Wan, C. L., Zhong, L., Tan, R. S., and Su, Y. (2014). Left ventricular regional shape dynamics analysis by three-dimensional cardiac magnetic resonance imaging associated with left ventricular function in first-time myocardial infarction patients. *Conf Proc IEEE Eng Med Biol Soc* **2014**: 5113–5116.

Wang, Y. and Staib, L. H. (2000). Boundary finding with prior shape and smoothness models. *IEEE Trans Pattern Anal Mach Intell* **22**: 738–743.

Wang, Y. P., Chen, Y., and Amini, A. A. (2001). Fast LV motion estimation using subspace approximation techniques. *IEEE Trans Med Imaging* **20**(6): 499–513.

Waxman, A., Wu, J., and Bergholm, F. (1988). Convicted activation profiles: Receptive fields for real-time measurement of short-range visual motion. *Proceedings of the IEEE CVPR*, Ann Arbor, MI, pp. 717–723.

Wells, W. M., 3rd, Viola, P., Atsumi, H., Nakajima, S., and Kikinis, R. (1996). Multi-modal volume registration by maximization of mutual information. *Med Image Anal* **1**(1): 35–51.

Weng, J., Singh, A., and Chiu, M. Y. (1997). Learning-based ventricle detection from cardiac MR and CT images. *IEEE Trans Med Imaging* **16**(4): 378–391.

Wise, R. G., Huang, C. L., Al-Shafei, A. I., Carpenter, T. A., and Hall, L. D. (1999). Geometrical models of left ventricular contraction from MRI of the normal and spontaneously hypertensive rat heart. *Phys Med Biol* **44**(10): 2657–2676.

Xavier, M., Lalande, A., Walker, P. M., Brunotte, F., and Legrand, L. (2012). An adapted optical flow algorithm for robust quantification of cardiac wall motion from standard cine-MR examinations. *IEEE Trans Inf Technol Biomed* **16**(5): 859–868.

Yeo, S. Y., Zhong, L., Su, Y., Tan, R. S., and Ghista, D. N. (2007). Analysis of left ventricular surface deformation during isovolumic contraction. *Conf Proc IEEE Eng Med Biol Soc* **2007**: 787–790.

Yuille, A. L., Cohen, D. S. and Hallinan, P. W. (1989). Feature extraction from faces using deformable templates. *Proceedings of the IEEE CVPR*, San Diego, CA, pp. 104–109.

Zambal, S., Hladuvka, J., and Buhler, K. (2006). Improving segmentation of the left ventricle using a two-component statistical model. *Med Image Comput Comput Assist Interv* **9**(Pt 1): 151–158.

Zhang, H., Wahle, A., Johnson, R. K., Scholz, T. D., and Sonka, M. (2010). 4-D cardiac MR image analysis: Left and right ventricular morphology and function. *IEEE Trans Med Imaging* **29**(2): 350–364.

Zhang, T. and Freedman, D. (2005). Improving performance of distribution tracking through background mismatch. *IEEE Trans Pattern Anal Mach Intell* **27**(2): 282–287.

Zhang, Y., Liang, X., Ma, J., Jing, Y., Gonzales, M. J., Villongco, C., Krishnamurthy, A. et al. (2012). An atlas-based geometry pipeline for cardiac Hermite model construction and diffusion tensor reorientation. *Med Image Anal* **16**(6): 1130–1141.

Zhou, X. S., Comaniciu, D., and Gupta, A. (2005). An information fusion framework for robust shape tracking. *IEEE Trans Pattern Anal Mach Intell* **27**(1): 115–129.

Zhu, Y., Papademetris, X., Sinusas, A. J., and Duncan, J. S. (2010). Segmentation of the left ventricle from cardiac MR images using a subject-specific dynamical model. *IEEE Trans Med Imaging* **29**(3): 669–687.

Zhuang, X., Rhode, K., Arridge, S., Razavi, R., Hill, D., Hawkes, D., and Ourselin, S. (2008). An atlas-based segmentation propagation framework locally affine registration—Application to automatic whole heart segmentation. *Med Image Comput Comput Assist Interv* **11**(Pt 2): 425–433.

Zurada, J. M. (2012). *Introduction to Artificial Neural Systems*. Jaico Publishing House, Mumbai, India.

8 Cardiovascular Magnetic Resonance Feature Tracking

El-Sayed H. Ibrahim, PhD and Rolf Baumann, MSc

CONTENTS

ABBREVIATIONS

Abbreviation	Meaning
1D	One-dimensional
2D	Two-dimensional
AF	Atrial fibrillation
ARVC	Arrhythmogenic right ventricular cardiomyopathy
CMR-FT	CMR feature tracking
CRT	Cardiac resynchronization therapy
CSPAMM	Complementary spatial modulation of magnetization
CSS	Churg–Strauss syndrome
DCM	Dilated cardiomyopathy
Ecc	Circumferential strain
ECG	Electrocardiogram
EF	Ejection fraction
Ell	Longitudinal strain
Err	Radial strain
FT	Feature tracking
HARP	Harmonic phase
HCM	Hypertrophic cardiomyopathy
HFpEF	Heart failure with preserved ejection fraction
ICC	Intraclass correlation
LA	Left atrium
LAD	Left anterior descending
LAX	Long-axis
LBBB	Left bundle branch block
LGE	Late gadolinium enhancement
LV	Left ventricle
MI	Myocardial infarction
NYHA	New York Heart Association
PH	Pulmonary hypertension
RA	Right atrium
RV	Right ventricle
RVOTO	Right ventricular outflow tract obstruction
SAX	Short-axis
SCS	Systolic circumferential strain
SD	Standard deviation
SENC	Strain encoding
SNR	Signal-to-noise ratio
SR	Strain rate
SRcc	Circumferential strain rate
SRll	Longitudinal strain rate
SRrr	Radial strain rate
SSFP	Steady-state free precession
STE	Speckle tracking echocardiography
STEMI	ST-segment elevation myocardial infarction
SV	Single ventricle
TA	Trans-apical
TAPSE	Tricuspid annular plane systolic excursion
TAVI	Transcatheter aortic valve implantation
TF	Trans-femoral
TOF	Tetralogy of Fallot
VVI	Velocity vector imaging

8.1 INTRODUCTION

8.1.1 Feature Tracking in CMR

Cardiovascular magnetic resonance (CMR) applications are evolving very rapidly. For the assessment of heart function, the interest has gone from pure volumetric analysis, where the only interest is tracking the inner surface of the heart chambers, to actual assessment of myocardium contractility, studying the deformation patterns of this complex muscular structure. A number of different CMR techniques have been developed for pursuing the goal of assessing the heart mechanics. All of these techniques, however, require specific acquisition procedures that add time to the overall CMR exam. This added exam time may limit the implementation of these techniques to specific cases where standard nontagged cine images cannot provide sufficient diagnostic information about myocardial contractility.

Visual assessment is typically used for evaluating heart function based on cine CMR images, which provide more details besides volumes and mass measurements. However, visual assessment is limited by interobserver variability and lack of quantitation. CMR feature tracking (CMR-FT) is a new image analysis technique that has been recently developed for measuring myocardial contractility patterns from nontagged cine CMR images. CMR-FT stemmed from the more established speckle tracking echocardiography (STE) imaging. Therefore, it is natural to start this chapter by introducing STE and explaining how it was adopted to develop CMR-FT.

8.1.2 Chapter Outline

This chapter starts by introducing STE, the technique based on which the idea of CMR-FT is developed. Along with STE, the topics of STE validation, velocity vector imaging (VVI), and echo feature tracking (Echo-FT) are addressed to lay the foundation for introducing CMR-FT in the rest of the chapter. The chapter then describes the anatomical features in CMR images that are tracked through the cardiac cycle and addresses the adaptation of the feature tracking technique to the heart physiology and CMR imaging. The next sections in the chapter describe in details the different steps in the CMR-FT algorithm, as well as the derived cardiac functional parameters and the relationships among them.

The reproducibility of the CMR-FT technique and its validation against STE and CMR tagging are then addressed. The next sections in the chapter address the limitations and practical implementation of CMR-FT. Finally, the chapter reviews different clinical applications of CMR-FT, which have been extensively increased in the past four years. It should be noted that almost all CMR-FT clinical applications are discussed in its chapter; not in the clinical application chapters in the end of the book. This is related to the novelty of the technique and its implementation constraints, as described later in the chapter, which make it more appropriate to group the technique's applications in this chapter rather than merging them with more established techniques in Chapters 9 and 10 of *Heart Mechanics: Magnetic Resonance Imaging—Advanced Techniques, Clinical Applications, and Future Trends*.

8.2 FEATURE TRACKING IN ECHOCARDIOGRAPHY

8.2.1 SPECKLE TRACKING ECHOCARDIOGRAPHY

As it is the case with several medical imaging techniques that have been developed by taking advantage of some kind of imaging artifact and turning it into a new imaging technique, STE is based on tracking ultrasound speckles, which are randomly generated due to reflection, refraction, and scattering of the echo beams and considered as artifacts in echocardiography (Figure 8.1). Nevertheless, as the resulting interference pattern remains relatively stable within a small region of interest, then instead of being sources of signal noise in the image, the speckles can be considered as intrinsic tissue markers, which can then be tracked through the cardiac cycle to measure regional myocardial deformation; the concept behind STE. In 2001, Kaluzynski et al. (2001) demonstrated the STE concept by measuring strain in a deformable phantom model. Shortly after, STE has been used for measuring global strain in patients with myocardial infarction (MI) (Reisner et al. 2004). A couple of years later, in a key study by Amundsen et al. (2006), the authors validated STE against gold standard sonomicrometry (see Chapter 9) as well as CMR tagging (see Chapters 10 and 11).

In STE, a cluster of pixels (kernel) is defined and tracked from timeframe to another using a search algorithm based on optical flow (Horn and Schunk 1981) (optical flow techniques are described in more detail in Chapter 3 of *Heart Mechanics: Magnetic Resonance Imaging—Advanced Techniques, Clinical Applications, and Future Trends*) and other image processing techniques to identify the kernel displacement (Bohs and Trahey 1991) with the goal of minimizing the difference between similar clusters in consecutive timeframes (Figure 8.2) (Pavlopoulos and Nihoyannopoulos 2008, Blessberger and Binder 2010a, Mondillo et al. 2011). In this respect, two parameters are defined in the processing algorithm: the size of the search region and size of the kernel, which determine the velocity range and velocity resolution, respectively (Bohs et al. 2000, Malpica et al. 2004).

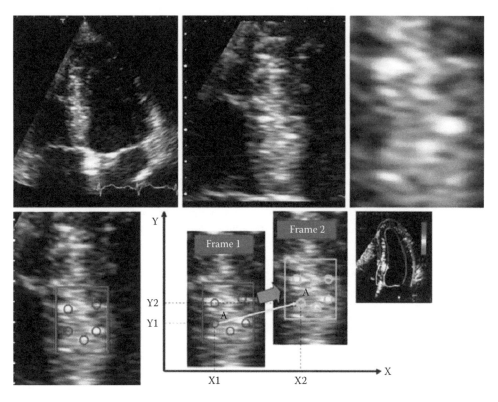

FIGURE 8.1 An echocardiography image (successively magnified from left to right) showing the speckle pattern on the myocardial wall and the searching algorithm for the kernel inside the red/green squares in two subsequent frames. (Reproduced from Pavlopoulos, H. and Nihoyannopoulos, P., *Int. J. Cardiovasc. Imaging*, 24(5), 479, 2008. With permission.)

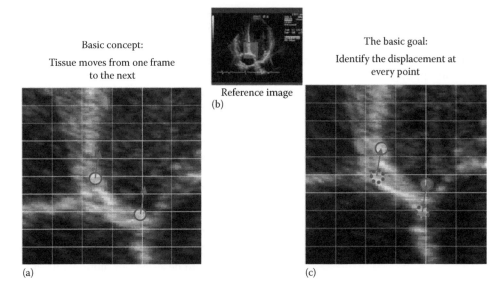

Basic concept:

Tissue moves from one frame
to the next

Reference image
(b)

The basic goal:

Identify the displacement at
every point

(a)

(c)

FIGURE 8.2   The concept of tracking the displacement of certain features inside the search window (square box in image (b)) from (a) the reference frame to (c) the next frame.

STE has been implemented in various studies (Blessberger and Binder 2010b) for examining wall motion abnormality (Anwar et al. 2012), ischemic heart disease (Gjesdal et al. 2007, Roes et al. 2009, Bansal et al. 2010), MI (Takeuchi et al. 2007, Amundsen et al. 2009, Sjoli et al. 2009), cardiac dyssynchrony (Tops et al. 2009), Duchenne muscular dystrophy (Ryan et al. 2013), hemodialysis (Mendes et al. 2008), and right ventricular (RV) mechanics (Gustafsson et al. 2008, Lemarie et al. 2015), as well as in pediatrics (Lorch et al. 2008, Koopman et al. 2011) and young athletes (Stefani et al. 2009a,b).

8.2.2   STE Validation

STE has been validated against other more established techniques for measuring myocardial deformation. As early as 2003, Konofagou et al. (2003) showed that tissue displacement and strain measured from STE have good agreement with measurements from one-dimensional (1D) CMR tagging. A couple of years later, an important study by Helle-Valle et al. (2005) showed that STE-derived myocardial rotation measurements in healthy volunteers are consistent with measurements from CMR tagging. In the same year, Notomi et al. (2005) drew the same conclusion in a study for measuring ventricular torsion. Lee et al. (2007) conducted a similar study for validating in-plane displacement and strain measurements from STE against CMR tagging. Another important study came in 2006 from Amundsen et al. (2006), who, using sonomicrometry and CMR tagging as the gold standards, validated STE as an angle-independent technique (e.g., as opposed to Doppler imaging) for measuring regional myocardial deformation. Subsequently, two different STE techniques have been compared to harmonic-phase (HARP) tagging analysis, where the results showed good agreement between STE and HARP for measuring myocardial contractility (Bansal et al. 2008). The same conclusion was also reached by Lee et al. (2008), who compared STE to HARP,

and illustrated the STE capability of differentiating between abnormal and normal myocardium (Figure 8.3). In another study, the accuracy and speed of STE for evaluating the left ventricular (LV) volume and ejection fraction (EF) have been compared to volume measurements from cine MRI using Simpson's approximation (Di Bella et al. 2010). Finally, two-dimensional (2D) STE has been validated against hemodynamics, tissue Doppler, MRI tagging, and sonomicrometry for evaluating cardiac systolic and diastolic functions and identifying subclinical markers of cardiac myopathies (Biswas et al. 2013).

8.2.3   Velocity Vector Imaging

VVI is another new echocardiographic image analysis technique that is similar to, and based on, STE. In VVI, vectors emanating from the endocardial border and showing tissue deformation from the first timeframe to the last one are displayed overlaid on the echo image, where each vector's direction and magnitude represent the direction and magnitude, respectively, of the velocity component at that particular tissue point (Vannan et al. 2005, Cannesson et al. 2006, Masuda et al. 2008, Biswas et al. 2013), as shown in the example in Figure 8.4. VVI uses an algorithm that implements STE using features of the myocardial structure (e.g., mitral annulus and border of the heart chamber) for tracking the endocardial wall motion (Chen et al. 2007b, Biswas et al. 2013), which makes it faster and more precise than STE. This advantage could be attributed to the lack of the signal intensity averaging process (across the myocardial thickness) that is implemented in STE (Burns et al. 2008). VVI assumes coherent tracked kernel, where tracking is performed by following the reference points to guide the tracking algorithm, and implementing snakes (see Chapter 7) to track the whole length of the endocardial border (Bansal et al. 2008). To improve the tracking results, VVI applies a sequence of intermediate steps to track motion of the

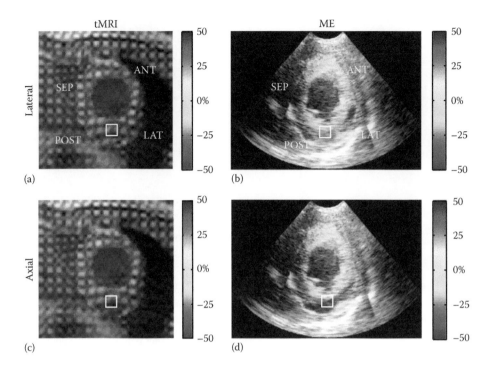

FIGURE 8.3 Two-dimensional end-systolic strain from cardiovascular magnetic resonance (CMR) tagging and echo images of myocardial elastography. (a) and (c) show the lateral and axial strains (see echo images on the right for strain directions) from tagged CMR images, respectively; (b) and (d) show the lateral and axial strains from echo images, respectively. The figure shows close agreement between results from CMR tagging and echocardiography. ANT, anterior; LAT, lateral; POST, posterior; SEP, septal. (Reproduced from Lee, W.N. et al., *Ultrasound Med. Biol.*, 34(12), 1980, 2008. With permission.)

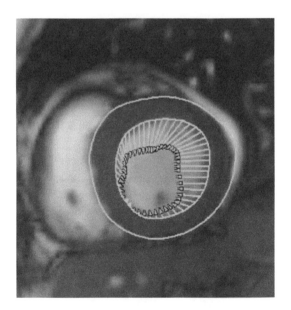

FIGURE 8.4 Velocity imaging in a short-axis cardiovascular magnetic resonance image showing inferoseptal wall motion abnormality.

tissue material points. Two-dimensional tracking is usually conducted as a sequence of two 1D operations (pixels from cuts perpendicular and parallel to the border) (Masuda et al. 2008). Cross-correlation and Fourier techniques are implemented to enhance the measurements' accuracy and ensure periodicity of the cardiac cycle (Pirat et al. 2008).

Recently, Kim et al. (2009) performed a head-to-head comparison between VVI and STE for measuring myocardial rotation, where the authors concluded that caution should be taken when interpreting the results due to the possible measurement differences between the two techniques as a result of implementing different tracking algorithms. VVI has been successfully implemented in various studies for examining ischemic heart disease (Yang et al. 2012), MI (Jurcut et al. 2008, Masuda et al. 2008), LV hypertrophy (Chen et al. 2007a), RV contractility (Pirat et al. 2006, Kutty et al. 2008, Tugcu et al. 2010), as well as in fetuses (Ishii et al. 2012) and normal subjects (Carasso et al. 2012).

8.2.4 ECHOCARDIOGRAPHY FEATURE TRACKING

Echo-FT is a recently developed technique that gained a lot of interest because it combines the advantages of both STE and VVI. Echo-FT operation can be summarized in a few steps (Figures 8.5 through 8.11), which will lay the foundation for introducing CMR-FT in the following sections:

Step 0: A preprocessing step, including manual tracing of the endocardium by the operator (Figure 8.5)
Step 1: Tracking the up- and down-motion of the mitral annulus (Figure 8.6)
Step 2: Motion rescaling and application to other points on the endocardium (Figure 8.7)

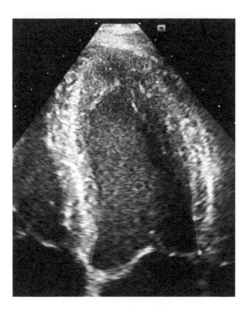

FIGURE 8.5 Preprocessing step in feature tracking: manual tracing of the endocardium.

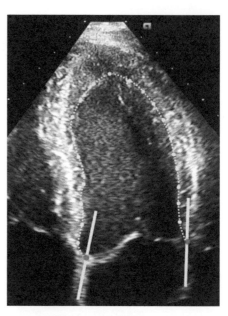

FIGURE 8.7 Step 2 in feature tracking: rescaling the motion and application to other points on the endocardium (small yellow dots).

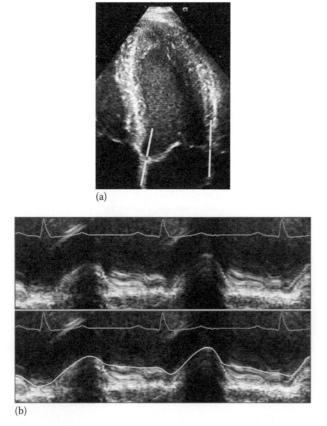

(a)

(b)

FIGURE 8.6 Step 1 in feature tracking: tracking the up- and down-motion of the mitral annulus. (a) Echo image showing the location of the tracked points on the mitral annulus. (b) Reconstructed M-mode image showing the movement of the tracked pints with time.

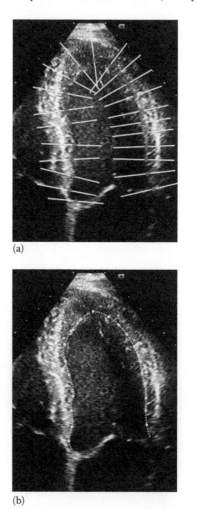

(a)

(b)

FIGURE 8.8 Step 3 in feature tracking: motion tracking across the wall. (a) Line segments aligned in the directions orthogonal to the ventricle boundary. (b) The intersection points (small dots) of the ventricle boundary and orthogonal line segments in (a).

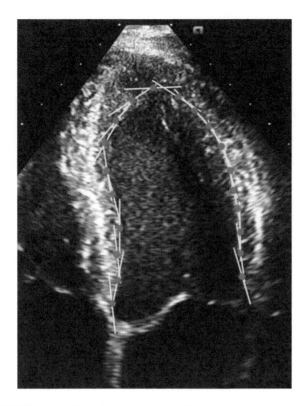

FIGURE 8.9 Step 4 in feature tracking: evaluation of tissue displacement along the heart wall relative to the moving border.

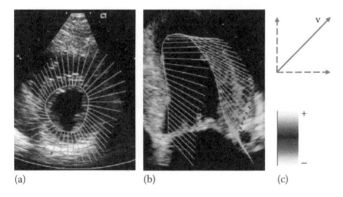

(a)   (b)   (c)

FIGURE 8.10 Calculation of tissue displacement and velocity. Velocity is shown on (a) short-axis and (b) long-axis images. (c) A velocity vector (solid line) can be split into two orthogonal components (dashed lines); positive and negative velocities are represented by red and blue colors, respectively, for parametric display.

Step 3: Motion tracking in the direction orthogonal to the identified boundary (Figure 8.8)

Step 4: Evaluation of tissue displacement along the heart wall relative to the moving border (Figure 8.9)

Step 5: Calculation of tissue displacement and velocity (Figures 8.10 and 8.11)

Figures 8.12 through 8.14 show examples of using Echo-FT for deriving different functional measures of the heart mechanics.

8.3 CMR-FT: TECHNIQUE DESCRIPTION

8.3.1 CONCEPT OF WORK

Inspired by the STE and VVI techniques, CMR-FT has been recently introduced for measuring regional myocardial deformation from cine CMR images based on intrinsic anatomical features, for example, mitral annulus, valves, papillary muscles, tissue/cavity border, myocardial septum, and distinct trabecular structures of the endocardial surface (Remme et al. 2005; Figures 8.15 and 8.16), and periodicity of the heart motion (Hor et al. 2010, 2011, Schuster et al. 2011, Schuster and Nagel 2011).

Feature tracking proceeds in a way broadly comparable to particle image velocimetry (Adrian 1991, Willert and Gharib 1991) and other pattern tracking approaches (Singh 1992, Barron et al. 1994), which have been developed over a number of years for fluid dynamic and other engineering or image processing applications. Feature tracking has been applied in different fields, and although the basic concept of work is the same, it needs adaptation to the specific application in hand. Specifically, the heart muscle has distinct characteristics that are not found in other applications. Therefore, optimizing the feature tracking technology for cardiac imaging is necessary. Feature tracking needs also to be adapted to the specific imaging modality. CMR cine imaging, particularly using steady-state free precession (SSFP) sequences, provides high image quality as well as moderate spatial and temporal resolutions, with the notion that temporal resolution can be improved at the expense of spatial resolution and/or image quality. It should be also noted that the cine images are not acquired in real time; they are rather reconstructed from data acquired over a number of cardiac cycles (segmented data acquisition, described in more details in Chapter 4). While CMR temporal resolution rarely approaches that of echocardiography, its achieved image quality is superior.

8.3.2 ADAPTATION TO CMR

Feature tracking is based on defining a relatively small window centered at a certain anatomical pattern (feature) in one image at a certain timeframe and searching for the as-much-as-possible similar local pattern in a window, of the same size and in the vicinity of the original window, in the image at the next timeframe. The displacement found between the two patterns represents local tissue displacement.

Information about the complex heart motion pattern is used to optimize the feature tracking algorithm. For example, knowing that the absolute heart motion decreases along the cardiac border in the longitudinal direction from base to apex, then the heart base is expected to have a significantly larger motion during the cardiac cycle compared to the apex. Additional guiding information is based on the facts that the apical myocardium has radial or circumferential displacement components rather than longitudinal ones and that circumferential motion decreases toward the mid-ventricle and

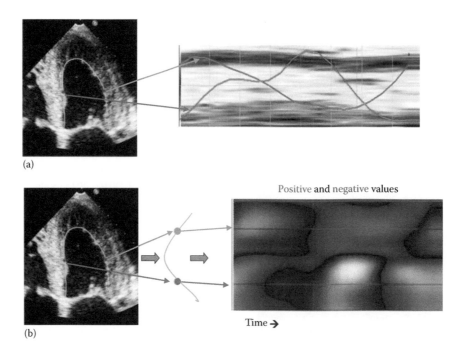

FIGURE 8.11   Velocity change through the cardiac cycle. (a) Two curves showing velocity change through the cardiac cycle at two points on the endocardium. (b) Parametric display of velocity change along the entire endocardial border through the cardiac cycle. Red and blue represent positive and negative velocities, respectively.

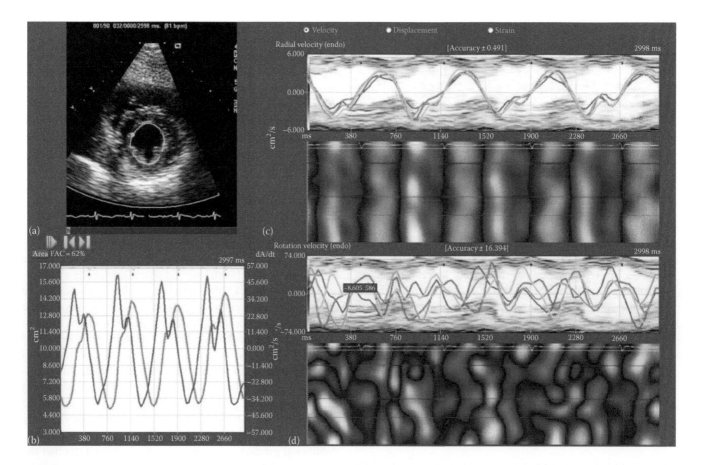

FIGURE 8.12   Velocity analysis with echo feature tracking. (a) Echo image showing the points at which velocity is measured. (b) Curves showing ventricular area change (red curve) and area rate of change (blue curve) with time. (c) Radial velocity curves and parametric map. (d) Rotational velocity curves and parametric map.

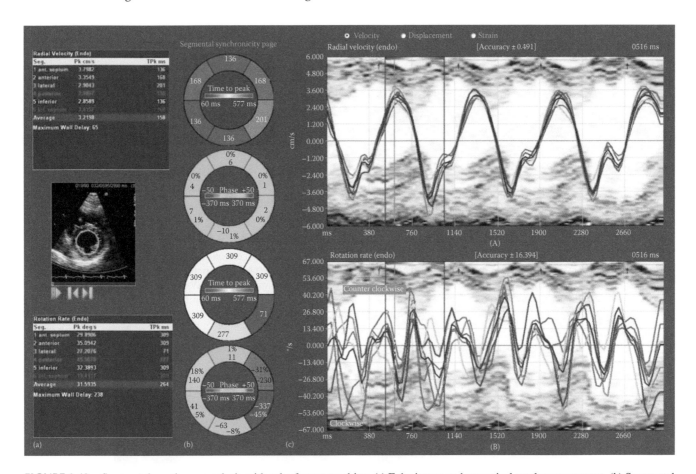

FIGURE 8.13 Segmental synchrony analysis with echo feature tracking. (a) Echo image and numerical results per segment. (b) Segmental time-to-peak and synchrony phase. (c) Segmental (A) radial velocity and (B) rotation rate.

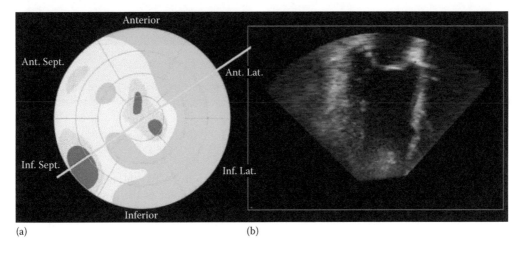

FIGURE 8.14 Echo feature tracking results showing dyskinetic basal septum and akinetic apex. (a) Color-coded 17-segment AHA model showing dyskinetic inferior septum (red) and akinetic apex (light brown). (b) The echo image showing the tracked points (small red dots).

it is in opposite directions at the basal and apical myocardium. Motion periodicity is another characteristic of the heart motion that is used for feature tracking optimization such that any unrealistic movements that might have been caused by artifacts can be detected and excluded. It should be noted that the last feature may inadvertently lead to missing subtle wall motion abnormality in the case of arrhythmia.

It is evident that a large interrogation window is necessary to detect large tissue displacements, although this comes at the expense of reduced accuracy because displacement would

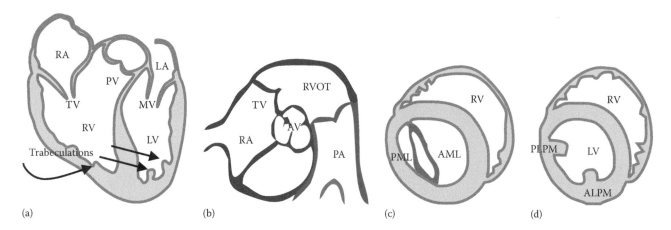

FIGURE 8.15   Cardiac features that can be tracked in cardiovascular magnetic resonance feature tracking. (a) Four-chamber long-axis view. (b) Aortic, tricuspid, and pulmonic valve level. (c) Mitral valve short-axis level. (d) Mid-ventricular short-axis level. The features and abbreviations are as follows: ALPM, anterior lateral plate mesoderm; AML, anterior mitral leaflet; AV, aortic valve; LV, left ventricle; PA, pulmonary artery; PLPM, posterior lateral plate mesoderm; PML, posterior mitral leaflet; RA, right atrium; RV, right ventricle; RVOT, RV outflow tract; TV, tricuspid valve. (Courtesy of Dr. Tamer Basha, Harvard University, Cambridge, MA.)

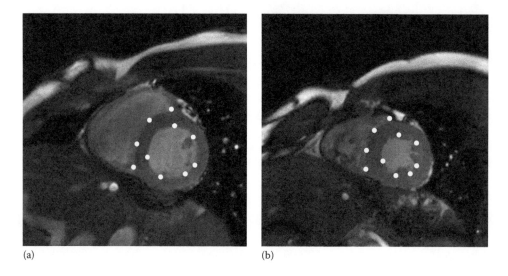

FIGURE 8.16   Cardiac features that can be tracked with the cardiovascular magnetic resonance feature tracking technique. The tracked points are shown at (a) diastole and (b) systole.

be averaged over a large area. On the other hand, although a small interrogation window improves accuracy, the window cannot be too small, or otherwise the motion pattern would not be detectable. Experience from different applications suggests that the length of the window side to be at least 8 pixels. Based on these concerns, a complete tracking method must employ a hierarchical sequence of tracking steps that starts with a large search window to detect large displacements and progressively proceeds to smaller windows to improve accuracy. The low temporal resolution in CMR can be problematic for fast movements. Therefore, when a cardiac structure experiences a large displacement from one frame to another, for example, movement of the mitral valve leaflets during diastole, the interrogation window has to be large enough to catch this displacement at the expense of lower accuracy. For reliable feature tracking, a minimum temporal resolution of around 25 frames/s should be maintained.

8.3.3   Method Description

8.3.3.1   Basic Idea

Similar to Echo-FT, the basic concept of CMR-FT is that the displacement of the gray-scale patterns during the cardiac cycle corresponds to the displacement of the actual muscle tissue being represented by this gray-scale pattern (Figure 8.17).

8.3.3.2   Motion Tracking

Feature tracking follows ("tracks") the gray-scale pattern by searching for a certain anatomical feature identified in the reference timeframe inside the surrounding neighborhood in the next frame (Figure 8.18).

As the location of the gray-scale pattern in the subsequent imaging frame is identified, a displacement vector, and associated tissue velocity, can be determined (Figure 8.19). This procedure is

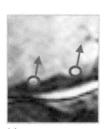

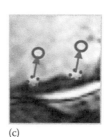

FIGURE 8.17 Feature tracking concept and analysis goal. The reference image (b) shows the region of interest (orange square) within which the anatomical features are tracked. The cardiovascular magnetic resonance image (a) shows the features to be tracked in the first timeframe. The image (c) shows the the new locations of the tracked features in the second timeframe, which is used to determine tissue displacement at every pixel.

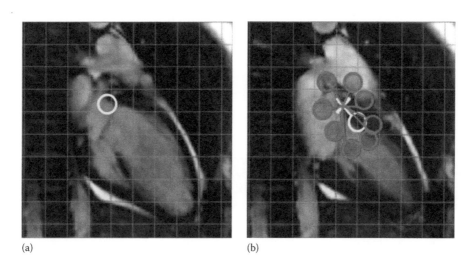

FIGURE 8.18 The basic concept of feature tracking is that the tissue displacement corresponds to the displacement of its gray-scale pattern from one timepoint ((a) frame one) to the next one ((b) frame two). The region of interest in frame one (yellow circle) is tracked in frame two (the red circles represent possible new locations of the region of interest).

performed on a certain number of myocardial regions throughout the complete cardiac cycle, resulting in displacement information about different heart regions at any timepoint in the cardiac cycle. Maximum displacement of a certain myocardial region, or displacement at a specific cardiac event, can then be derived.

8.3.3.3 Steps of the Feature Tracking Processing Algorithm

Figure 8.20 shows an example of the basic workflow for CMR-FT implementation. The detailed steps of CMR-FT are illustrated in Figures 8.20 and 8.21 (Hor et al. 2011).

Step 0: Initial Processing Step

The initial processing step consists of manually selecting a number of N points (markers) (x_i, y_i) on the endo-, mid-, or epicardial border in one image (timeframe). The border can be open, as in long-axis (LAX) views, or it can be closed, where the last point connects to the first one, as in short-axis (SAX) views. The importance of this initial step should be emphasized, as the measurements' accuracy and processing time depend on the number and distribution of these points. Based on this initial processing step, three successive tracking steps are conducted:

Step 1: Detection and compensation for large motion components

First, the large inward–outward motion of the cavity–tissue interface is detected. Tracking along a specified direction is performed using the method of transmural cuts (Figure 8.22), where a line segment perpendicular to the myocardial border and cutting through the myocardial thickness is generated at each marker point. Feature tracking is conducted by generating the signal pattern in the vicinity of each preselected point

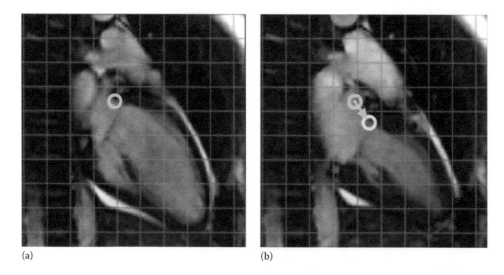

(a)   (b)

FIGURE 8.19   A displacement vector (arrow) representing the displacement from a certain position in frame 1 (green circle in (a)) to the corresponding position in frame 2 (yellow circle in (b)).

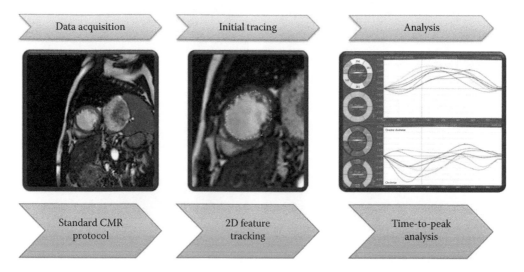

Data acquisition   Initial tracing   Analysis

Standard CMR   2D feature   Time-to-peak
protocol   tracking   analysis

FIGURE 8.20   The basic workflow in cardiovascular magnetic resonance feature tracking, starting with data acquisition using a standard cardiovascular magnetic resonance protocol, followed by ventricle boundary tracing using feature extraction, and finally data analysis (segmental radial displacements and rotation angles in this case).

in the first frame, usually at end-diastole, and shifting it in the surrounding neighborhood until the most closely matching pattern is found in the following frame. In LAX views only, a preliminarily step is conducted to detect the large motion of the mitral annulus, searching for apparent displacement of relatively large-scale image patterns ("features") in the vicinity of the atrioventricular junction. Subsequently, the processing algorithm proportionally adjusts the tracking process along the entire myocardial border for such large motion from the base to apex. These tracking procedures are performed on a thin interrogation windows (4 pixels wide) elongated along the dominant sought displacement direction with window length progressively reduced from 48 to 8 pixels (hierarchical search). Two-dimensional spatiotemporal images are then formed for each marker point such that the transmural cuts

(at that point) from consecutive timeframes form the lines of the image (the columns of the matrix representing the image) from left to right, as shown in Figure 8.22. Therefore, the resulting image shows displacement of the marker point through the cardiac cycle, where border tracking is conducted on the resulting image. In that sense, the resulting image is similar to an M-mode echo image.

Assuming that a marker point needs to be tracked through M timeframes, then the constructed image would have M columns, x_i, where i ranges from 1 to M. The algorithm then determines a sequence of real numbers y_i that represent the vertical positions of points x_i. Staring from a known position y_k of point x_k, the vertical displacement from y_k to y_{k+1} is determined as the shift that maximizes the cross-correlation between the columns x_k and x_{k+1}. This process is repeated for estimating y_{k+2},

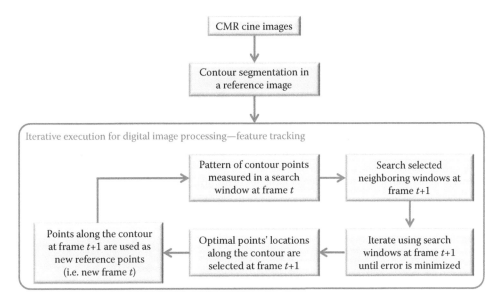

FIGURE 8.21 Overview of the feature tracking algorithm. The technique starts with the selected contour to be traced and is iteratively solved by minimizing the errors in subsequent image frames.

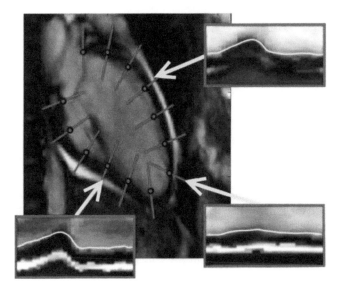

FIGURE 8.22 Motion tracking along transmural cuts at different points on the ventricular boundary. The insets show the constructed "M-mode" images that show wall motion through the cardiac cycle.

y_{k+3}, and so on. The vertical displacements are then iteratively refined to improve the tracking process using a smaller image (image with reduced vertical dimension) around the first estimates. Finally, the active snake algorithm (see Chapter 7) is applied to smooth the point displacement between consecutive frames (Bohs et al. 2000). To improve tracking accuracy, another round of border tracking is conducted with thick cuts parallel to the border line. Finally, a three-point low-pass filter is applied to the results to ensure spatial coherence.

Step 2: Local motion refinement

The moving-window technique is used for matching the feature points between consecutive frames (Figure 8.23).

A relatively large $M \times M$ (typically 16×16) window is firstly selected in the reference timeframe to provide a rough estimation of the feature's new position in the following timeframe. A smaller window (one-fourth of the size of the first one; i.e., 8×8) is then centered at that first estimation for another tracking round to fine-tune the results.

The tracking algorithm involves implementing the optical flow method for tracking the 2D movement of the feature points between consecutive timeframes. The optical flow method is based on the assumption that the image intensity pattern changes slightly with time in a small searching window, that is,

$$\frac{dI(x,t)}{dt} = 0, \qquad (8.1)$$

where $I(x, t)$ is the image intensity pattern at location x and time t. By applying the same concept in the spatial domain, the resulting equations can be written in the form of a gradient constraint equation:

$$\nabla I(x,t).m + I_t(x,t), \qquad (8.2)$$

where

    ∇I is the spatial image gradient
    I_t is the temporal derivative of the image
    $m = (u(x), v(x))$ is the motion field
    u and v are the two velocity components

Step 3: Motion refinement along the tracked border

Tissue tracking is finalized by tracking along an M-mode representation of the extracted border (one spatial dimension along the length of the curved border, unwrapped against time). The search is centered at each of the estimated border points. Again, the search zones start large and are progressively reduced in size. It should be noted that the shape (geometry) of

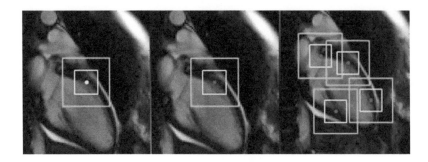

FIGURE 8.23 Refinement of the search region for different locations in the myocardium. The search starts with the large (green) windows, and then it is fine-tuned using the smaller (yellow) windows, as shown in the right panel.

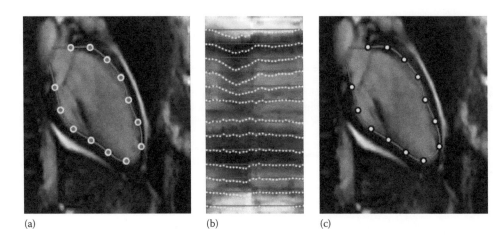

(a) (b) (c)

FIGURE 8.24 Tracking along the left ventricular (LV) border. The geometry is not changed between the panels (a) and (c); only the points' distribution along the border is changed. Panel (b) shows the temporal evolution of the points along the endocardial border of the LV (horizontal axis represents time).

the border is not changed; only the redistribution of the marker points along it (Figure 8.24).

Comments

When epicardial tracking is also required, the epicardial motion is initially estimated as a percentage of the endocardial motion; then, the same previously mentioned steps are performed with the additional constraint that the epicardium cannot cross the endocardium. All the steps described earlier are performed enforcing the periodicity constraint, implicating that the last frame in the cardiac cycle is followed by the first one, which improves the tracking accuracy by avoiding drifts due to error accumulation. Therefore, drift is not corrected for; it is rather implicitly excluded in the calculation itself.

8.3.4 Measured Parameters

8.3.4.1 Global and Regional Analysis

Applying feature tracking to regular gray-scale cine images leads to quantitative information about tissue motion in the first place. This information is only the starting point for quantification of tissue mechanics. The tracked points are assumed as representing material tissue regions; therefore, the tracking results immediately report the displacements of such regions, which can be subdivided into radial and longitudinal displacements in LAX images, or radial and circumferential displacements in SAX images. From tissue motion information, further parameters like velocity, strain, and strain rate (SR) can be derived and analyzed. Global analysis can be performed to generate representative values, for example, global strain, which describe the deformation of the whole ventricle in certain directions. Regional analysis, on the other hand, investigates local regions by subdividing the myocardium into segments that are reasonably sized for a clinically relevant diagnosis. Figure 8.25 shows an example of different display schemes of the generated measurements, and Figure 8.26 shows global and regional assessment of myocardial mechanics.

8.3.4.2 Integral and Differential Quantities

Once the border geometry and displacement velocities are obtained, dynamics-related measures can be derived (Figures 8.27 and 8.28). It is advisable to focus on integral quantities, for example, displacement and strain, which report cumulative values, especially in datasets where the temporal resolution is limited. These parameters

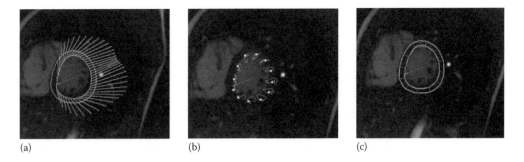

FIGURE 8.25 Different display methods for feature tracking. (a) Velocity vectors. (b) Tracking paths. (c) Segmental analysis.

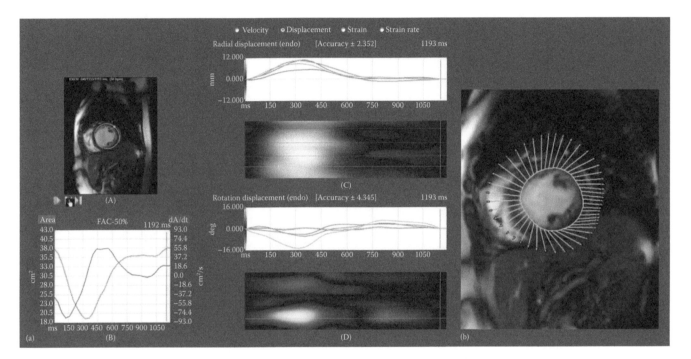

FIGURE 8.26 Global and regional analysis of myocardial mechanics. (a) (A) Cine image; (B) area change (red curve) and area rate of change (blue curve); (C) radial displacement; and (D) rotation displacement. (b) Velocity vectors across the left ventricular boundary.

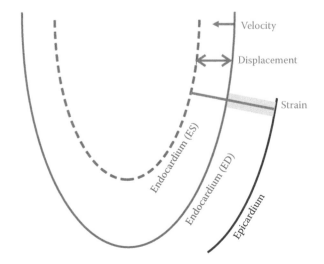

FIGURE 8.27 Heart mechanics parameters measured from 2D long-axis images. Strain is measured as the relative change in tissue length (between the thin red and thick pink lines). ED, end-diastole; ES, end-systole.

characterize global heart motion during a certain time period, for example, systole. Differential quantities (computed by the differentiation of other measures), for example, SR, require sufficient signal-to-noise ratio (SNR) and high temporal resolution to ensure appropriate measurement accuracy (in echo, it is assumed that at least 60 frames/s or more are required).

8.3.4.3 Displacement

Displacement is a cumulative parameter that represents the distance a piece of tissue moves during a period of time, for example, during systole, represented by the maximum displacement in the distance–time curve (Figure 8.29). The later part of the curve corresponds to the diastolic heart phase where the displacement returns back to zero.

8.3.4.4 Velocity

The velocity vector is computed as the rate of change of displacement with time (difference in tissue displacement between two timeframes divided by the time interval

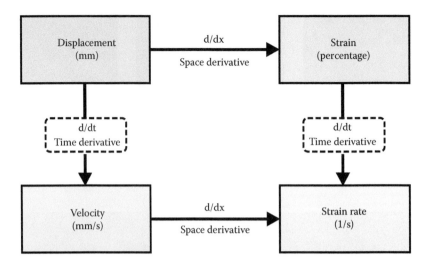

FIGURE 8.28   Parameters measured using cardiovascular magnetic resonance feature tracking and the mathematical relationships among them.

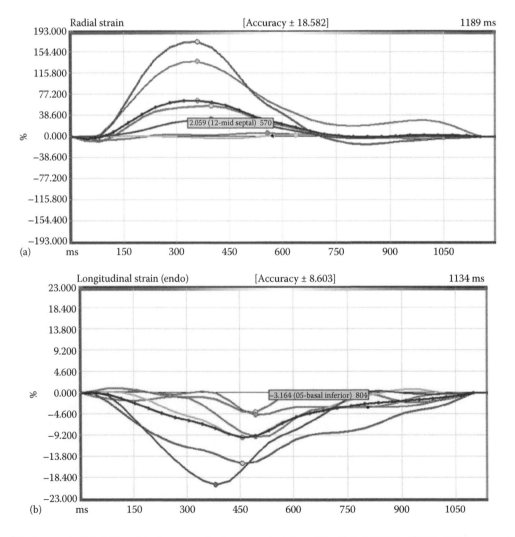

FIGURE 8.29   Displacement of six left ventricular segments, shown as percentage (a) radial and (b) longitudinal displacement change (strain).

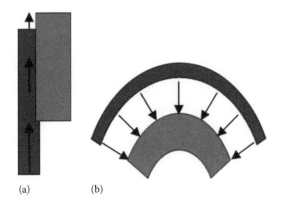

(a)   (b)

FIGURE 8.30 (a) Longitudinal compression and (b) radial stretching during systole. Brown and red represent the initial and modified states, respectively.

in-between). Velocity is a differential quantity that bears the risks described earlier.

8.3.4.5 Strain

Strain is an integral property that represents deformation, for example, effective local tissue shortening during systole. Strain is calculated as

$$S(t) = \frac{L(t) - L_0}{L_0}, \tag{8.3}$$

where L and L_0 are the new and original lengths of the tissue segment, respectively. Therefore, strain shows whether the length of the tissue segment gets smaller (contracting tissue; negative strain) or larger (elongating tissue; positive strain) with respect to the initial length (usually measured at end-diastole). Strain occurs due to velocity difference, where the two ends of the tissue segment move with different velocities. For example, during systole, the myocardium is shortened in the longitudinal direction and lengthened in the radial direction (Figure 8.30); the opposite occurs during diastole.

8.3.4.6 Strain Rate

SR is defined as the time derivative of strain. However, as mentioned for velocity, this is a differential measure with associated precautions. Moreover, as strain is computed after conducting spatial differentiation, the accuracy of measuring SR is low, especially that the frame rate of cine CMR imaging is usually insufficient for reliable measurements, that is, suboptimal to that of echo imaging.

8.3.4.7 Torsion

In a SAX view, the absolute rotation during systole can be measured. This rotation varies in the SAX slices from apical to basal levels. In healthy subjects, a counterclockwise rotation is observed in the apical slices (as seen from the apex), while the basal slices show a clockwise rotation (Figure 8.31). In the slices around the papillary muscle level, rotation is very little. Torsion represents the differential rotation from base to apex, divided by the ventricle length (the distance from base to apex).

8.4 VALIDATION

8.4.1 CMR-FT VERSUS STE

8.4.1.1 Pros and Cons

STE is more established than CMR-FT. However, compared to STE, CMR-FT is more reliable due to the inherently high image quality with CMR compared to echo, which allows for accurate myocardial border detection. Further, CMR imaging is not affected by the acoustic window, geometric assumptions, or operator dependency as in echo (echo's image quality largely depends on the sonographer's experience). On the other hand, CMR is not as good as echo in terms of temporal and spatial resolutions as well as the exam's cost. Further, CMR-FT lacks intrinsic speckles, which are nature in echocardiography. Therefore, the intramyocardial features that can be tracked in CMR-FT are limited compared to STE. Other limitations of CMR-FT include the measurements' dependency on image quality, initial myocardial boundary determined in the first timeframe, and selected landmarks, as well as the technique's incapability for detecting through-plane motion. It should be noted that the lower limit of the tracked velocity depends on the images' spatial and temporal resolutions. For example, improving the temporal resolution allows for capturing larger velocities; nevertheless, a corresponding improvement of spatial resolution is required to ensure the measurements' accuracy.

8.4.1.2 Validation against STE

8.4.1.2.1 Congenital Heart Disease

A number of studies have been conducted to compare CMR-FT to STE. Kempny et al. (2012) compared CMR-FT to STE and simple endocardial border delineation for evaluating biventricular myocardial function in tetralogy of Fallot (TOF) patients and healthy volunteers. The results showed similar interobserver variability between CMR-FT and STE for measuring global LV longitudinal strain (Ell); however, CMR-FT was more reproducible than STE for measuring global circumferential and LV radial strain (Err). The reproducibility of measuring regional strain was, however, poor by CMR-FT. In the RV, CMR-FT showed higher interobserver reproducibility for measuring global Ell; besides,

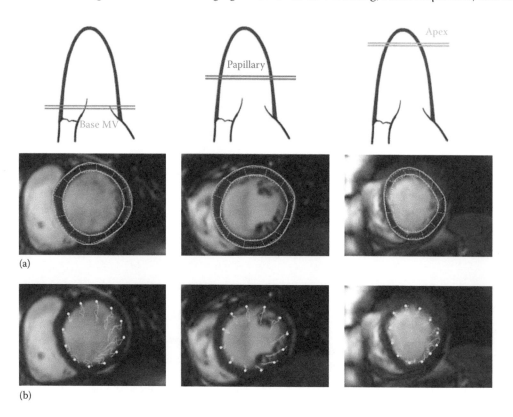

FIGURE 8.31   Rotation in three different short-axis slices (base, mid, and apex). The (a) and (b) images display segmental rotation and tracking paths of the myocardium.

global circumferential strain (Ecc) and Err were measurable only by CMR-FT. Finally, endocardial border delineation gave similar results to CMR-FT for measuring global strain. In another study on TOF (Padiyath et al. 2013), CMR-FT and STE showed similar qualitative results for myocardial tracking from SAX images; however, CMR-FT showed suboptimal results from 4-chamber images (Figure 8.32).

The best intermodality agreement occurred for measuring Ecc, while Err showed poor intermodality agreement.

8.4.1.2.2   Cardiomyopathies

In a study on normal subjects and patients with cardiomyopathy, using CMR tagging as the common gold standard, the performance of CMR-FT showed to be similar to STE

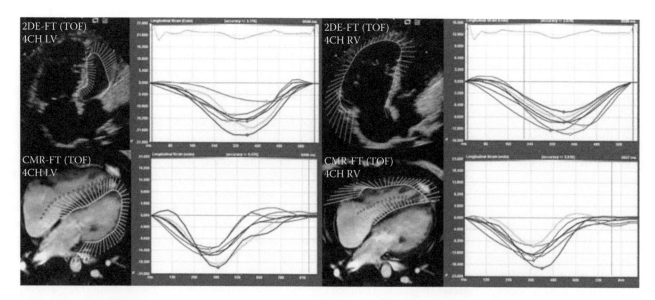

FIGURE 8.32   Two-dimensional echo feature tracking (top panels) and cardiovascular magnetic resonance feature tracking (bottom panels) images and longitudinal strains of the left ventricle (left panels) and right ventricle (right panels) in tetralogy of Fallot on four-chamber images. (Reproduced from Padiyath, A. et al., *Echocardiography*, 30(2), 203, 2013. With permission.)

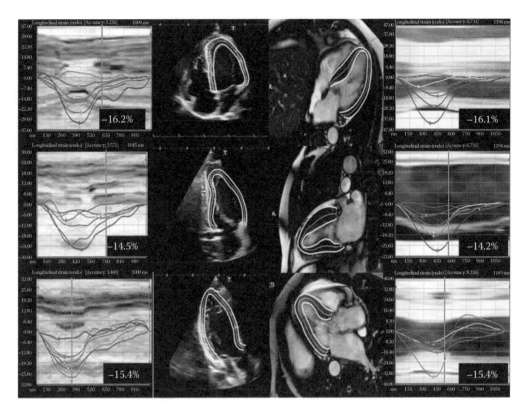

FIGURE 8.33 Representative endocardial longitudinal strain curves and average strain values from echocardiography (left) and cardiovascular magnetic resonance (right) images, demonstrating assessments in the 4-chamber view (top), 2-chamber view (middle), and 3-chamber/left ventricular outflow tract view (bottom). The figure shows similar global values (demonstrated in the bottom right of each figure) and strain curves obtained by both techniques. (Reproduced from Williams, L.K. et al., *J. Am. Soc. Echocardiogr.*, 26(10), 1153, 2013. With permission.)

for measuring LV rotational mechanics and related principal strains (Li et al. 2012). CMR-FT has been validated for measuring LV strain and rotation in hypertrophic cardiomyopathy (HCM), using echocardiographic strain assessment by VVI as a reference (Figures 8.33 and 8.34) (Williams et al. 2013). Although both global Ell and Ecc from CMR-FT and echo VVI demonstrated excellent agreements, there was a stronger correlation between the two techniques for measuring Ell. In another study (Orwat et al. 2014), LV Ell, Ecc, and longitudinal and circumferential strain rates (SRll and SRcc) were measured in normal volunteers and HCM patients using CMR-FT and STE. A good agreement was found between global LV Ell measured with CMR-FT (normals, 20.8%; HCM, 17.6%) and STE (normals, 19.4%; HCM, 16.6%), while the agreement was worse for Ecc and all SR measurements. In both LV and RV, the interobserver reproducibility was higher for the strain measurements compared to SR, while the coefficients of variation were lowest for LV Ell by CMR-FT. The results of this study support the observation that CMR-FT benefits from the RV trabeculations, which results in reproducible measurements that compare well with those from STE.

8.4.1.2.3 Other Heart Diseases

In a study on 50 consecutive patients with a wide range of electrocardiogram (ECG) QRS width and EF value, an agreement was reported between CMR-FT and STE for showing that radial dyssynchrony is significantly higher in patients with wide QRS than in patients with narrow QRS (Figures 8.35 and 8.36) (Onishi et al. 2011, 2013). Specifically, the CMR-FT dyssynchrony measurements were significantly higher in patients with wide QRS (>120 ms) and low EF (<35%), and showed good correlation with those from STE (R = 0.89). These results suggest that CMR-FT holds promise for evaluating patients for cardiac resynchronization therapy (CRT).

In patients with ischemic cardiomyopathy who underwent both CMR and echocardiography, RV Ell by VVI and STE showed relatively good correlations with RVEF and Ell by CMR-FT, despite underestimated STE measurements (compared to CMR-FT) of septal and global RV Ell (Park et al. 2015). Further, strain measurements by STE showed significantly lower intraobserver variability compared to VVI and CMR-FT measurements. Recently, CMR-FT has been compared to STE for evaluating LV function in 73 patients with clinically suspected heart failure symptoms, who underwent both echocardiography and CMR exams within 3–5 days (Onishi et al. 2015). The results showed that global Ell (averaged from three standard longitudinal views) and global Ecc (measured from a mid-LV SAX plane) were closely correlated with STE measurements. Further, the strain measurements from CMR-FT and STE were inversely correlated with EF measured from the CMR images.

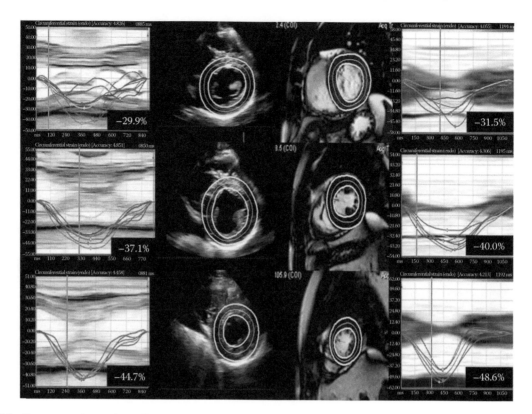

FIGURE 8.34   Representative endocardial circumferential strain curves and average strain values from echocardiography (left) and cardiovascular magnetic resonance (right) images, demonstrating assessment at the basal (top), mid-ventricle (middle), and apical (bottom) levels. (Reproduced from Williams, L.K. et al., *J. Am. Soc. Echocardiogr.*, 26(10), 1153, 2013. With permission.)

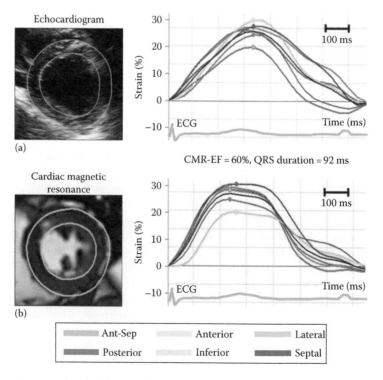

FIGURE 8.35   Example of radial time–strain curves by (a) speckle tracking echocardiography and (b) cardiovascular magnetic resonance feature tracking in a patient with normal left ventricular function and without dyssynchrony, demonstrating synchronous time-to-peak-strain curves. (Reproduced from Onishi, T. et al., *Proc. Am. Coll. Cardiol.*, 1086, 2011; Onishi, T. et al., *J. Cardiovasc. Magn. Reson.*, 15, 95, 2013.)

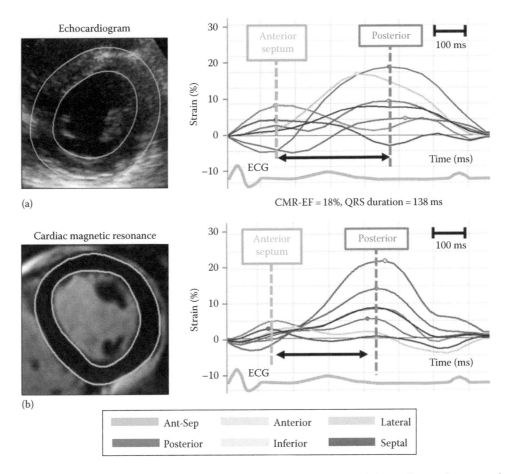

FIGURE 8.36 Radial time–strain curves by (a) speckle tracking echocardiography and (b) cardiovascular magnetic resonance feature tracking in left ventricular dyssynchrony, demonstrating dyssynchronous time-to-peak strain with early peak strain in the anterior septum (green line) and delayed peak strain in the posterior lateral wall (blue line). (Reproduced from Onishi, T. et al., *J. Cardiovasc. Magn. Reson.*, 15, 95, 2013.)

8.4.1.2.4 Techniques' Disagreement

Despite the techniques' agreement reported earlier in this section, some studies illustrated techniques' disagreement. Schmidt et al. (2014) implemented CMR-FT and STE in Fontan patients. While at least one myocardial segment could not be adequately quantified with STE in 63% of the patients, CMR-FT allowed for complete visualization of all wall segments. The results from this study showed poor agreement between the two techniques, despite a good or moderate interobserver variability in CMR-FT. The parameters derived from CMR-FT correlated significantly with age at Fontan completion, New York Heart Association (NYHA) class, and peak oxygen uptake in cardiopulmonary exercise testing. In another study on 45 phenylketonuria patients and 24 arterial hypertension patients, no agreement was observed between STE and either CMR-FT or tagging for measuring Ecc on both global and segmental levels (Schneeweis et al. 2015). Recently, CMR-FT analysis has been performed on 29 hypertensive patients using the TomTec and cvi42 analysis packages (Almutairi et al. 2015). The results showed significant differences between Ecc measurements from the two software packages,

whereas the radial and Ell values showed no clear trends. Such results emphasize the need for a gold standard validation to assess the accuracy of cardiac motion analysis software packages.

8.4.2 CMR-FT versus Tagging

8.4.2.1 Pros and Cons

Compared to CMR tagging, CMR-FT is simpler and faster as it does not require additional tagging sequences and the accompanying complicated, and sometimes time-consuming, tag analysis. Further, CMR-FT provides both global (e.g., EF) and regional (e.g., strain) cardiac functional measures from the same set of cine images, it can be applied retrospectively on previously acquired datasets that do not include tagged images, and it has short processing time (few minutes), which allows for its application on a large number of existing datasets. Nevertheless, the accuracy of CMR-FT is suboptimal to CMR tagging as the intrinsic tissue markers used in CMR-FT are much less than, and not as uniformly distributed as, the taglines in the CMR tagged images.

8.4.2.2 Validation against Tagging

8.4.2.2.1 Normal Subjects

A number of studies have been conducted for validating CMR-FT against more established techniques, especially CMR tagging, for measuring regional heart function. In a study by Augustine et al. (2013), the authors used the TomTec software to compare CMR-FT to CMR tagging in a group of healthy volunteers. The processing time of CMR-FT was shorter than that of CMR tagging (mean ± SD of 8.8 ± 4.7 minutes versus 15.4 ± 4.9 minutes for CMR-FT and CMR tagging, respectively). The results showed that the circumferential, but not longitudinal or radial, global strain measurements had reasonable agreement between the two techniques. Further, the CMR-FT measurements were overestimated compared to those from CMR tagging. In another study (Alshammari et al. 2014), the Circle cvi42 tissue tracking prototype software has been implemented for measuring Ecc and Err in 15 healthy volunteers, and the results have been compared to tagging and STE (Figure 8.37). The analysis time for CMR-FT was less than 1 minute (excluding the time required to identify the LV contours) compared to 10 minutes for tag analysis using HARP. The resulting global Err and Ecc from CMR-FT showed favorable agreement with those from tagging (R = 0.91, p < 0.01) and STE (R = 0.83, p < 0.01). Specifically, the peak global systolic Err/Ecc (mean ± SD) from CMR-FT, tagging, and STE were 22% ± 8%/−16% ± 3%, 16% ± 5%/−16% ± 5%, and 17% ± 6%/−17% ± 2%, respectively.

8.4.2.2.2 Myocardial Infarction

In postacute ST-segment elevation myocardial infarction (STEMI), global LV Ecc and Ell measured by CMR-FT showed to be higher than those measured with tagging (Khan et al. 2015b,c). Global strain showed high intra- and interobserver agreements, while segmental strain showed good intra- and interobserver agreements (intraclass correlation [ICC] > 0.7), except for segmental Ell measured by tagging, which showed poor agreement. Further, Ecc measured by CMR-FT correlated significantly with total infarct size and segmental infarct extent, which allowed for successfully distinguishing infarcted, adjacent, and remote segments.

8.4.2.2.3 Diastolic Dysfunction and Heart Failure

In a study on diastolic dysfunction patients (Kuetting et al. 2015), global and regional early-diastolic SR, peak-diastolic SR, twist, untwist, and torsion measurements were calculated using both CMR tagging and CMR-FT. Global early diastolic SR by CMR-FT showed good agreement with tagging, as well as low intra- and interobserver variabilities. However, compared to CMR-FT, tagging showed higher accuracy and reproducibility of both global and regional diastolic strain, and provided reliable information about diastolic myocardial rotation and untwisting. Recently, CMR-FT has been compared to complementary spatial modulation of magnetization (CSPAMM) tagging for measuring strain in 43 subjects (15 healthy, 19 with systolic heart failure, and 9 with diastolic heart failure) (Raman et al. 2014). The cine and tagged images were analyzed using multimodality tissue tracking (MTT; Toshiba, v.6.0, Tokyo, Japan) and HARP software packages, respectively. The results showed good agreement between the two techniques for measuring strain and SR. However, the feature tracking technique resulted in larger inter- and intraobserver agreements for measuring Err compared to HARP.

8.4.2.2.4 Cardiomyopathies

The VVI software (VVI v. 2.0, Siemens Medical Solutions USA Inc., Malvern, PA) has been used for comparing CMR-FT to CMR tagging in patients with HCM and normal volunteers (Figure 8.38; Harrild et al. 2012). The results showed close agreement between the measurements from the two techniques, although peak segmental strain showed less agreement. The measurements' agreement was better in the volunteers than in the patients group, and the degree of disagreement became larger with increasing measurement values. The authors noticed that the CMR-FT technique performed better at the endocardial surface despite the large difference in the processing time between the two techniques (1–2 minutes versus 12–15 minutes for CMR-FT and CMR tagging, respectively).

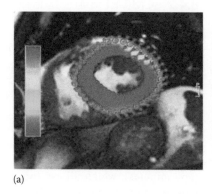 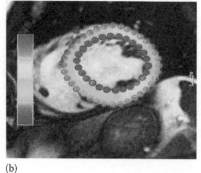

(a) (b)

FIGURE 8.37 Left ventricular short-axis image at (a) end-systole and (b) end-diastole with tissue tracking overlays. Analysis was conducted using the Circle cvi42 tissue tracking prototype software. (Reproduced from Alshammari, Q.T. et al., Cardiovascular magnetic resonance radial and circumferential strain: Comparison between SSFP feature tracking, MRI tagging, and speckle tracking echocardiography, *Proceedings of the International Society for Magnetic Resonance in Medicine*, Milan, Italy, 2014, p. 3977. With permission.)

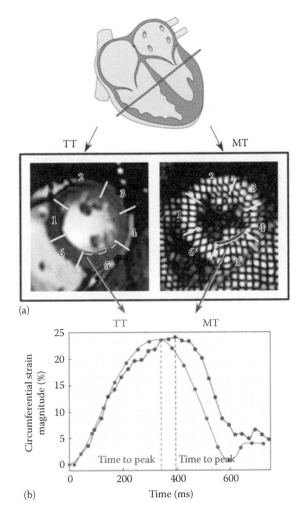

(a)

(b)

FIGURE 8.38 Representative myocardial strain analysis of cardiovascular magnetic resonance tagging and cine steady-state free precession (SSFP) short-axis images at the mid-papillary level from a normal subject. (a) The myocardium is divided into six matching segments on the tagged and SSFP images. (b) Myocardial tagging and tissue tracking analysis techniques were performed to calculate the average endocardial circumferential strain within each segment throughout the cardiac cycle. (Reproduced from Harrild, D.M. et al., *Int. J. Cardiovasc. Imaging*, 28(8), 2009, 2012. With permission.)

A recent study on cardiomyopathic patients and normal subjects showed good agreement between CMR-FT and tagging for measuring peak-systolic global Ecc and SRcc as well as early-diastolic global SRcc at the subendocardium (Moody et al. 2015). The study also showed good agreement for measuring peak-systolic global Ell and SRll. However, the weakest agreement between the two techniques was observed for measuring early-diastolic global SRll.

8.4.2.2.5 Other Heart Diseases

The initial validation of CMR-FT has been conducted using mathematical models (Hor et al. 2011), where the ground truth was known. In the clinical setting, Hor et al. (2010) used the TomTec image analysis package (TomTec Imaging

Systems, Munich, Germany) to compare CMR-FT to HARP tag analysis for measuring myocardial strain in 191 boys with Duchenne muscular dystrophy. Ecc was measured at a mid-ventricular SAX slice, where the measurements from CMR-FT showed excellent correlation with those from HARP (R = 0.899) and appropriately classified the patients into four groups of different disease stages. In a recent study (Wu et al. 2014), segmental peak-systolic Ecc and time-to-peak Ecc were measured in patients with left bundle branch block (LBBB) and patients with hypertrophic obstructive cardiomyopathy using CMR-FT at endocardial and mid-wall regions (CMR-FT-endo and CMR-FT-mid, respectively), and the measurements were compared to those obtained using CMR tagging. The results showed that peak Ecc was higher with CMR-FT-endo compared to tissue tagging and CMR-FT-mid. Differences in time-to-peak Ecc were present between the three analysis methods. The intra- and interobserver agreements of segmental peak Ecc and time-to-peak Ecc were substantially lower with CMR-FT-mid compared to tissue tagging. All three analysis methods showed high intraobserver agreement of time-to-peak Ecc. Nevertheless, the intraobserver agreement of mean time-to-peak Ecc measured with CMR-FT-endo was higher than that measured with CMR-FT-mid.

Feature tracking showed moderate agreement with grid-tagged HARP analysis for measuring Ecc in Fontan patients, with a trend toward lower strain values with CMR-FT (Anwar et al. 2014b). In another study on pediatric cancer survivors, Lu et al. (2014a,b) compared LV strain measurements obtained using CMR-FT and HARP tagging from patient who underwent a CMR scan more than 5 years after completing anthracycline chemotherapy. While mid-ventricular Ecc by CMR-FT showed good agreement with that measured by HARP (−20.8 ± 3.4 and 19.5 ± 2.5, respectively), Err showed poor agreement between the two techniques. CMR-FT intra- and interobserver reproducibilities were excellent for Ecc; however, reproducibility was poor for Err.

Recently, CMR-FT has been compared to HARP and strain-encoding (SENC) in pulmonary hypertension (PH) patients and normal subjects (Ohyama et al. 2015). CMR-FT-derived RV Ell correlated closely with SENC measurements. LV Ell, quantified by CMR-FT, showed moderate correlation with SENC, and LV Ecc by CMR-FT showed moderate correlation with HARP. In the PH patients, RV Ell negatively correlated with RVEF and positively correlated with mean pulmonary arterial pressure.

8.5 REPRODUCIBILITY, LIMITATIONS, AND PRACTICAL IMPLEMENTATION OF CMR-FT

8.5.1 MEASUREMENTS REPRODUCIBILITY

Measuring reproducibility of newly developed techniques is important as high reproducibility means that less subjects are needed for clinical studies, which is translated into higher cost efficiency (Bellenger et al. 2000). Besides reproducibility results from different studies shown in the previous sections, the reproducibility of the CMR-FT technique has been specifically investigated in a couple of studies from Eike Nagel's group (Morton et al. 2012, Schuster et al. 2013a). In both studies, Ell and Err were calculated from LAX images, while Ecc was calculated from midventricular SAX images. The RV upper septal insertion point was manually defined to ensure accurate segmentation. The first study investigated the feature tracking technique's intraobserver reproducibility and whether it is affected by the magnetic field strength (Schuster et al. 2013a). In that study, the authors conducted CMR-FT on two groups, each consisting of 10 healthy subjects, imaged on 1.5 T or 3 T scanners. The analysis was conducted twice with 4 weeks in-between, and intraobserver reproducibility was determined by comparing the results from the first and the second analyses in both groups. The results showed no difference in strain, LV volume, or EF at different field strengths. However, there existed a considerable variability in segmental measurements. Ecc in the LV was the most reproducible parameter, while Ell in the RV was the least reproducible parameter. In the second study, interstudy reproducibility of CMR-FT was investigated (Morton et al. 2012). In that study, 16 healthy volunteers were imaged three times within a single day. The first and second scans were fasting, while the third scan was nonfasting. The results showed that the interstudy reproducibility varied among different measured parameters. It was better for global than for segmental analysis. Similar to the previous study (Schuster et al. 2013a), LV Ecc and RV Ell were the most and least reproducible parameters, respectively. Err was the least reproducible global measure, while the reproducibility of the LV volume and EF was excellent.

Recently, the feasibility and reproducibility of CMR-FT for measuring LV torsion and diastolic recoil has been evaluated in ten healthy volunteers scanned during rest and dobutamine stress (Figures 8.39 and 8.40; Kowallick et al. 2014b). Torsion was defined as the difference between apical and basal rotations, divided by the distance between the two slices. Depending on the distance between the most apical (defined as 0% LV distance) and most basal (defined as 100% LV distance) slices, four different models were examined for calculating torsion: model 1 (25%–75%), model 2 (0%–100%), model 3 (25%–100%), and model 4 (0%–75%). Reproducibility was good to excellent for all torsion and recoil rate parameters, but was especially high when using an apical level at 25% distance instead of the most apical slice. There was no significant difference between the different models at rest. Nevertheless, only model 1 (25%–75%) discriminated between the rest and stress measurements (global torsion 2.7 ± 1.5°/cm, 3.6 ± 2.0°/cm, 5.1 ± 2.2°/cm and global recoil rate −30.1 ± 11.1°/cm/s, −46.9 ± 15.0°/cm/s, −68.9 ± 32.3°/cm/s, for rest, 10, and 20 µg/kg/min of dobutamine stimulation, respectively). In another study (Ainslie et al. 2015), an in-house developed software has been used to validate torsion measured from CMR images. The results showed strong and weak correlations for twist (difference (in degrees) between basal and apical rotations) and torsion, respectively, with increasing dobutamine dose.

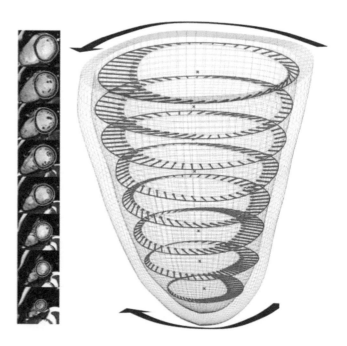

FIGURE 8.39 Three-dimensional model of left ventricular rotational displacement by cardiovascular magnetic resonance feature tracking. Rotation between timepoints (angular difference between red (epicardium) and green (endocardium) contours) is computed in each slice, and it is then linearly interpolated between slices. The 3D ventricular model is automatically fitted to the contours and is used here for illustration. (Reproduced from Kowallick, J.T. et al., *PLoS One*, 9(10), e109164, 2014b.)

8.5.2 TECHNIQUE'S LIMITATIONS

CMR-FT is capable of detecting displacement of the features that move 1 or more pixels between two successive timeframes. If a feature is displaced by less than 1 pixel, it apparently does not move. It follows that the displacement measurements could be associated with an unavoidable error depending on image resolution. The velocity's maximum accuracy is equal to 1 pixel size divided by the time interval between two consecutive timeframes (that turns out to be about 2 or 3 cm/s). For strain measurement, the intrinsic error is approximately given by the square root of the number of timeframes divided by the number of pixels along the border line, which in the clinical imaging settings gives an error of about 2%–4%.

Tracking the displacement of local features among consecutive timeframes is based on the search for maximum agreement between two regions. This requires detection of the displacement (shift) value that maximizes the correlation function (or, equivalently, the value that minimizes the error function in the smooth surface representing the boundary). Searching for the maximum value of a smooth surface is a difficult task, and, further, the actual position of such maximum can vary significantly when the surface is slightly modified. Therefore, small differences in the tracking process can lead to different results. The presence of this potential variability requires the inclusion of a relevant smoothing step in the end-user software to avoid unrealistic changes in the local

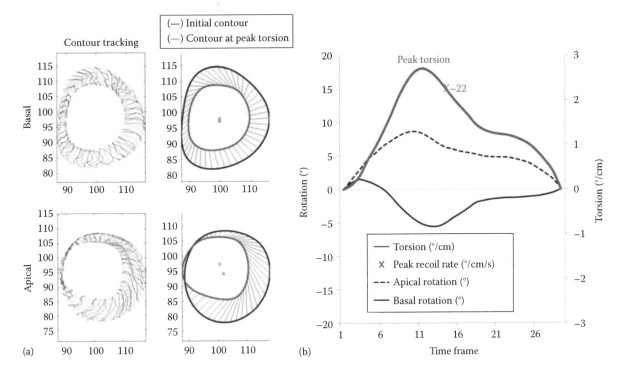

FIGURE 8.40 Evaluation of myocardial rotation using cardiovascular magnetic resonance feature tracking. (a) Rotational displacement of 48 voxels tracked throughout the cardiac cycle. (b) Left ventricular torsion calculated as the difference in counterclockwise (positive) apical rotation and clockwise (negative) basal rotation, divided by the interslice distance. (From Kowallick, J.T. et al., *PLoS One*, 9(10), e109164, 2014b.)

behavior of tissue motion. Nevertheless, this additional step results in smoothing out fine regional deformations that may be masked and hardly detected. This difficulty can somehow be resolved by using a multiscale tracking procedure that conducts multiple steps and performs redundant calculations capable of smoothing the variability out. The user can then visually check the myocardial border motion to avoid evident erroneous estimates and may sometimes need to repeat the calculations to verify the repeatability of the sought measurements.

8.5.3 Practical Implementation

CMR-FT provides rapidly and easily attainable quantitative results of heart mechanics. However, following the previous discussion on the technique's limitations, it must be stressed that CMR-FT should be used to look at global parameters or parameters in reasonably sized regions. We hereby discuss some practical implementation guidelines. First of all, the feature tracking analysis must be performed in properly controlled slices of the LV where the tissue is well visible and out-of-plane motion is presumably small. Further, the analysis should be conducted on high-quality images with high spatial resolution (<1 mm) and temporal resolution (<50 ms between successive timeframes). It should be noted that even with high-quality images, the results may present with large variability. Therefore, multiple tracings, with the aid of visual assessment, are necessary to reduce the risk of erroneous results. In particular, in LAX views, tracking the mitral

annulus must be visually checked as this factor alone may substantially influence the result.

Secondly, it must be understood that different parameters of mechanical function are associated with different degrees of reliability. As a general rule, integral variables, for example, displacement and strain, are more reliable than differential ones, for example, velocity and SR. Therefore, the measurements from differential variables should be interpreted with caution. Moreover, given the relative large time interval between consecutive timeframes in CMR imaging, velocity and SR measurements cannot reproduce mechanical variations that last for one or few of timeframes (like the spikes at isovolumic phases); on the contrary, the measurements can be corrupted by these rapid variations. Among different measurements, myocardial rotation values are smaller and theoretically hold a larger intrinsic error. At the same time, in many cases, myocardial thickness and radial strain could be very small, which leads to partial overlap between neighboring interrogation windows and results in substantial measurement errors.

Thirdly, the measurement variability between adjacent regions and the necessarily applied smoothing process influence regional or rapidly varying motion. Therefore, quantitative assessment by CMR-FT should be largely considered for global measures or measures in reasonably sized regions (e.g., global strain, average inward wall motion, and mean rotation). Regional measures can still be evidenced in terms of standard deviation (SD) or other whole measures that are based on appropriate combination of all values. Similarly, differences in timing are better measured for cardiac phases (e.g., systole or diastole) rather than at instantaneous events (e.g., time-to-peak strain). In summary, CMR-FT must be performed on representative datasets with sufficient image quality. The measurements' reliability can be improved by repeating the analysis. Overall, the CMR-FT results can be used as an initial and fast step of interpreting the images. Quantitative analysis must then be considered in terms of global parameters (or measurements on reasonably sized region) calculated from reliable measurements, for example, displacement and global strain.

8.6 CLINICAL APPLICATIONS

Although it has been developed only a few years ago, CMR-FT has already been implemented in different clinical studies, as outlined in this section.

8.6.1 AGE- AND GENDER-SPECIFIC DIFFERENCES

CMR-FT has been used for studying strain variation based on gender and age. In one study (Kadiyala et al. 2011), CMR-FT has been used to determine normal gender-specific strain values in three LAX views and three SAX views at different levels (base, mid-ventricle, and apex) in 60 healthy subjects. The results revealed significant variation in global and regional strains among men and women. Another study (Augustine et al. 2013) confirmed these findings and showed that radial deformation has significant variation, especially in females, a finding that has been confirmed by CMR tagging in the same study.

In a recent study (Andre et al. 2015) on 150 healthy volunteers (75 male and 75 female) of three age tertiles, global peak-systolic Err, endocardial Ecc, mid-myocardial Ecc, endocardial Ell, and mid-myocardial Ell were (mean ± SD) 36.3% ± 8.7%, −27.2% ± 4.0%, −21.3 ± 3.3%, −23.4% ± 3.4%, and −21.6% ± 3.2%, respectively. Global peak early-diastolic radial, endocardial circumferential, mid-myocardial circumferential, endocardial longitudinal, and mid-myocardial longitudinal SR values were −2.1 ± 0.5 s⁻¹, 2.1 ± 0.6 s⁻¹, 1.7 ± 0.5 s⁻¹, 1.8 (1.5–2.2) s⁻¹, and 1.6 (1.4 – 2.0) s⁻¹, respectively. Compared to women, men showed higher Err and lower Ecc and Ell. Further, SRcc and SRll in men were significantly lower than in women. Err increased significantly with age, whereas all SR measurements showed a decreasing trend with age. In a similar study (Taylor et al. 2015), CMR-FT has been used for evaluating LV strain and SR in 100 healthy patients (10 men and 10 women in each of five age deciles from 20 to 70 years). Peak-systolic Ell, Ecc, and Err were −21.3% ± 4.8%, −26.1% ± 3.8%, and 39.8% ± 8.3%, respectively. Peak-systolic Ecc and Err showed the highest and lowest interobserver agreements, respectively. The magnitude of peak-systolic Ecc showed increasing trend with age, and there was a significant gender difference in peak-systolic Ell, with larger deformation magnitude in women (−22.7%) than in men (−19.3%).

Recently, a study has been conducted to record reference atrial and ventricular Ell values in 115 subjects during childhood and adolescence using CMR-FT (Shang et al. 2015). The study explored correlations between Ell and age, body surface area, gender, end-diastolic volume, and EF. Ell measurements in the RA, RV, LA, and LV were 26.6% ± 10%, 18% ± 5%, 26.5% ± 10.6%, and 17.5% ± 5%, respectively. There were significant positive correlations between Ell measurements in the LA, LV, RA, and RV and corresponding EF increase. However, the correlations with age and body surface area were generally weak, and gender-wise differences were not significant for atrial and ventricular Ell.

8.6.2 MYOCARDIAL CONTRACTILITY AT REST AND STRESS

In 2011, Schuster et al. (2011) conducted a study to investigate the ability of CMR-FT for quantifying myocardial wall motion at rest and during dobutamine stress in healthy volunteers. The results showed the capability of CMR-FT for differentiating between wall motion at rest and stress, despite a considerable inter- and intraobserver variability for all parameters. In another study (Cheng et al. 2014), CMR-FT showed an improvement in myocardial mechanical performance after an in-scanner exercise using a supine ergometer. Normal subjects showed more favorable myocardial mechanical reserve than patients with cardiomyopathy. Most recently, CMR-FT analysis has been conducted using the Circle cvi42 tissue tracking software for measuring Err and Ecc during exercise ergometry using an MRI bicycle combined with multislice cine imaging and compressed-sensing image reconstruction (Figure 8.41; Hamilton-Craig et al. 2014).

8.6.3 RV FUNCTION

CMR-FT has been implemented for semiautomatic quantification of tricuspid annular plane systolic excursion (CMR-TAPSE), analogous to echocardiography TAPSE, in order to predict normal RV systolic function (Botelho et al. 2014). The results showed that CMR-TAPSE is promising for efficient prediction of normal RV systolic function with similar performance to echo-TAPSE and good correlation with CMR-derived RVEF. In another study on 50 patients who underwent right heart catheterization, reduced RV longitudinal and radial displacements as well as septal Ecc and Err were associated with reduced RVEF (Muthukumar et al. 2015). Further, regional wall motion, including Ell as well as septal Ecc and Err, significantly correlated with pulmonary wedge pressure and mean pulmonary arterial pressure.

8.6.4 ATRIAL IMAGING

A number of studies have been recently conducted to investigate the feasibility of using CMR-FT for evaluating atrial function (Habibi et al. 2014). In a study on 10 young and 10 elderly healthy subjects as well as 20 patients with severe aortic stenosis, CMR-FT has been used to measure regional and global Ell and SRll, radial motion fraction, and relative velocity for the three LA motion phases: reservoir, conduit, and contraction (Figures 8.42 and 8.43; Evin et al. 2015).

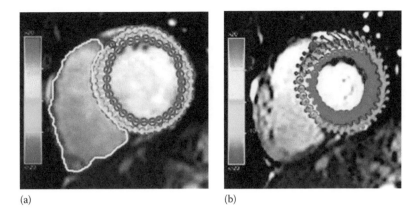

(a) (b)

FIGURE 8.41 Left ventricular short-axis image at (a) end-diastole and (b) end-systole with feature tracking overlays. Analysis was conducted using the Circle cvi42 tissue tracking prototype software. (Reproduced from Hamilton-Craig, C. et al., Radial and circumferential strain using feature tracking from cine SSFP imaging with compressed sensing at rest and with MRI exercise ergometry, *Proceedings of the International Society for Magnetic Resonance in Medicine*, Milan, Italy, 2014, p. 3906. With permission.)

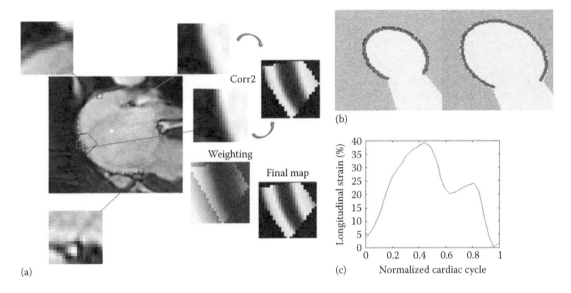

(a) (b) (c)

FIGURE 8.42 Description of the feature tracking algorithm for atrial motion tracking and an example of a synthetic phantom along with the normal longitudinal strain curve used for its generation. (a) Spatial correlation between two regions of interest weighted by the distance map to the left atrium (LA) edge and/or active contour, resulting in a final map. (b) Ellipsoidal phantom with realistic size fitted on real LA data, and the maximum dilatation and minimum contraction obtained from (c) typical normal longitudinal strain curve, derived from literature. The phantom had pixel size of 0.73 mm and 60 frames. (Reproduced from Evin, M. et al., *J. Magn. Reson. Imaging*, 42(2), 379, 2015. With permission.)

The results showed that all LA functional parameters were significantly impaired in aortic stenosis. Further, subclinical age-related variations resulted in a decreasing trend in all LA parameters, which was significant only in the radial conduit function parameters. Finally, the LA functional parameters characterized atrial alteration in aortic stenosis with higher sensitivity than conventional LA volumetric parameters.

CMR-FT has been used for measuring left atrial (LA) Ell and SRll in 10 healthy volunteers, 10 patients with HCM, and 10 patients with heart failure and preserved ejection fraction (HFpEF) (Kowallick et al. 2014a, 2015a). Specifically, the following parameters were measured (Figure 8.44): LA reservoir function (total strain [ε_s], peak positive strain rate [SR_s]), LA

conduit function (passive strain [ε_e], peak-early negative strain rate [SR_e]), and LA booster pump function (active strain [ε_a], peak-late negative SR [SR_a]). The results showed impaired LA reservoir function in HCM and HFpEF compared to healthy controls (ε_s [%], HCM = 22.1 ± 5.5, HFpEF = 16.3 ± 5.8, controls = 29.1 ± 5.3; SR_s [s^{-1}], HCM = 0.9 ± 0.2, HFpEF = 0.8 ± 0.3, controls = 1.1 ± 0.2) and impaired LA conduit function (ε_e [%], HCM = 10.4 ± 3.9, HFpEF = 11.9 ± 4.0, controls = 21.3 ± 5.1; SR_e [s^{-1}], HCM = −0.5 ± 0.2, HFpEF = −0.6 ± 0.1, controls = −1.0 ± 0.3). Further, the LA booster pump function was increased in HCM while decreased in HFpEF (ε_a [%], HCM = 11.7 ± 4.0, HFpEF = 4.5 ± 2.9, controls = 7.8 ± 2.5; SR_a [s^{-1}], HCM = −1.2 ± 0.4, HFpEF = −0.5 ± 0.2,

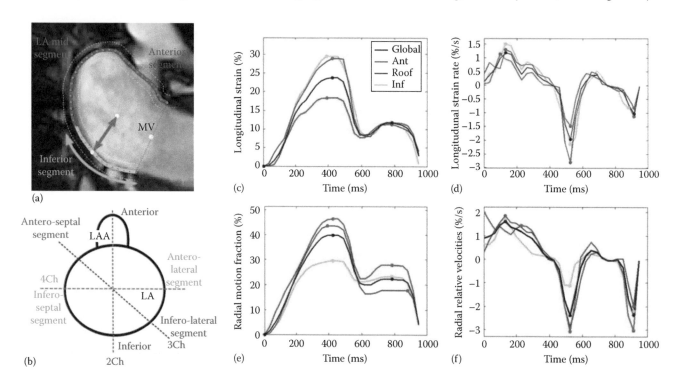

FIGURE 8.43 Global and regional left atrium (LA) functional parameters based on cardiovascular magnetic resonance feature tracking analysis. (a) Two-chamber view restricted to the LA. (b) Schematic view of the LA orientation and segments. (c) Longitudinal strain curves. (d) Longitudinal strain rate curves. (e) Radial motion fraction. (f) Radial relative velocities for a control subject. Ant, anterior segment; Inf, inferior segment; Long, longitudinal; LAA, left atrium appendage; MV, mitral valve; Roof, LA roof segment. (Reproduced from Evin, M. et al., *J. Magn. Reson. Imaging*, 42(2), 379, 2015. With permission.)

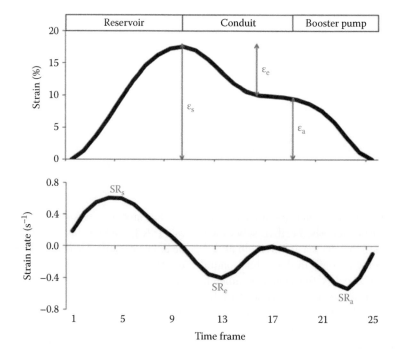

FIGURE 8.44 Left atrial strain and strain rate profiles. The left atrial function compromises reservoir, conduit, and contractile booster pump functions. Total strain (ε_s) and peak positive strain rate (SR_s) correspond to reservoir function. Passive strain (ε_e) and peak-early negative strain rate (SR_e) correspond to conduit function. Active strain (ε_a) and peak-late negative strain rate (SR_a) correspond to contractile booster pump function. (Reproduced from Kowallick, J.T. et al., *J. Cardiovasc. Magn. Reson.*, 16, 60, 2014a.)

controls = −0.9 ± 0.3). In another study from the same group (Kowallick et al. 2015b), the authors investigated the interstudy reproducibility of the developed technique for quantifying atrial dynamics. The results showed that interstudy reproducibility was better for volumetric indexes and strain than for SR parameters, and it was better for LA than for right atrial (RA) dynamics. Among the different functional components, the reservoir function was the most reproducibly assessed by either technique, followed by the conduit and booster pump functions.

A recent study investigated the capability of CMR-FT for quantifying LA deformation in patients with atrial fibrillation (AF) (Inoue et al. 2015). The LA volume, emptying fraction (EF), strain, and SR were assessed in 169 patients with a history of AF in sinus rhythm at the time of preablation (Figures 8.45 and 8.46). The patients with a history of stroke or transient ischemic attack had greater LA volumes, lower LA total EF, lower LA maximum and preatrial contraction strains, and lower absolute SR values during LV systole and early-diastole than the patients without stroke or transient ischemic attack. Further, the LA reservoir function was associated with stroke or transient ischemic attack.

A recent study from the multiethnic study of atherosclerosis (MESA) trial showed an association between LA function using CMR-FT and myocardial fibrosis (Imai et al. 2014). Compared to controls, patients with scar had significantly higher minimum LA volume; lower LA EF, maximum LA strain (E_{max}), maximum LA strain rate (SR_{max}), absolute LA strain rate at early-diastolic peak (SRE), and LA strain rate at atrial contraction peak (SRA). Tissue T1 time-constant measured 12 minutes after contrast injection was significantly associated with E_{max}, SR_{max}, SRE, and SRA, while T1 time-constant measured 25 minutes after contrast injection was significantly associated with SR_{max} and SRA. In another study, Peters et al. (2015) showed that LA strain, measured by CMR-FT, is correlated with atrial fibrosis, measured by late gadolinium enhancement (LGE) CMR, in AF patients (Figure 8.47).

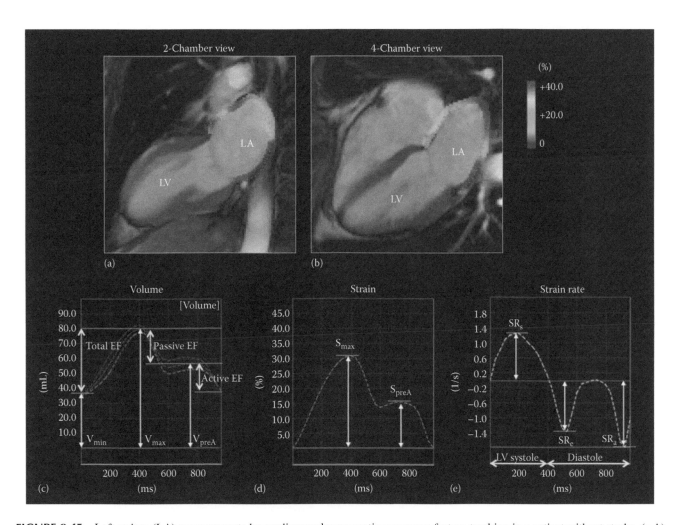

FIGURE 8.45 Left atrium (LA) measurements by cardiovascular magnetic resonance feature tracking in a patient without stroke. (a, b) LA longitudinal strain in the 2- and 4-chamber views at the end of left ventricular (LV) systole. (c) LA volume curve. The pink dotted line is the average of the values of volume in the 2- and 4-chamber views. The LA maximum volume (V_{max}), preatrial contraction volume (V_{preA}), and minimum volume (V_{min}) are identified. The LA emptying fractions are calculated using V_{max}, V_{preA}, and V_{min}. (d, e) The LA strain and strain rate curves. The LA maximum strain (S_{max}) and preatrial contraction strain (S_{preA}) are identified from the strain curve. The strain rates during LV systole (SR_s), LV early-diastole (SR_e), and atrial contraction (SR_a) are analyzed from the strain rate curve. (Reproduced from Inoue, Y.Y. et al., *J. Am. Heart Assoc.*, 4(4), 2015.)

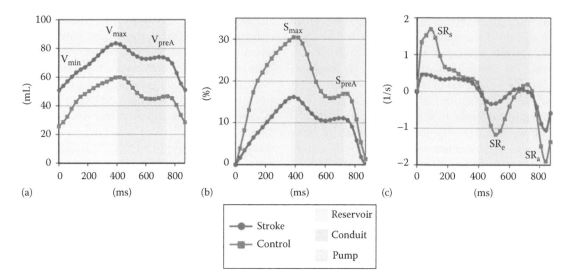

FIGURE 8.46 Left atrium (LA) measurements by cardiovascular magnetic resonance feature tracking in patients with and without stroke. (a) LA volume. (b) LA global longitudinal strain. (c) LA strain rate in a patient with stroke (red lines) and without stroke (blue lines). The patient with stroke has larger LA volume and smaller strain and strain rate. The LA serves as a reservoir during left ventricular (LV) systole, as a conduit during LV early diastole, and as an active pump during late diastole. S_{max}, maximum strain; S_{preA}, preatrial contraction strain; SR_a, strain rate at atrial contraction; SR_e, strain rate at LV early diastole; SR_s, maximum strain rate; V_{max}, maximum indexed volume; V_{min}, minimum indexed volume; V_{preA}, preatrial contraction indexed volume. (Reproduced from Inoue, Y.Y. et al., *J. Am. Heart Assoc.*, 4(4), 2015.)

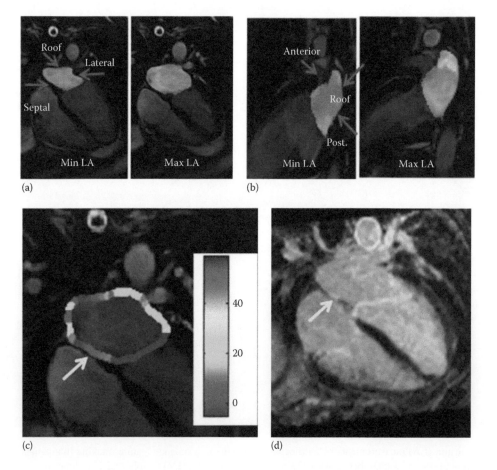

FIGURE 8.47 Strain correlation with fibrosis in the left atrium. Begin- and end-systole (a) 4-chamber and (b) 2-chamber images are contoured, excluding veins, and regions are identified. (c) Color-coded strain map (%) displayed on a cine image. (d) Reformatted late gadolinium enhancement image showing fibrosis in a corresponding region of low strain. Strains in the valvular regions and at ostial locations are excluded. (Reproduced from Peters, D.C. et al., Left atrial strain is correlated to atrial fibrosis by late gadolinium enhancement, in an AF population, *Proceedings of the International Society for Magnetic Resonance in Medicine*, Toronto, Ontario, Canada, 2015, p. 4469. With permission.)

Recently, CMR-FT has been implemented for studying atrial function in MI and in Cushing's syndrome. In a study on 101 patients who underwent CMR 3–5 days and 6 months after first STEMI treated with primary percutaneous coronary intervention, CMR-FT showed that average LA strain is an independent predictor of LV remodeling observed in the 6 months follow-up scan (Karwat et al. 2015). Finally, CMR-FT showed that the reservoir, conduit, and contraction phases of LA function are impaired in Cushing's syndrome, and that both the reservoir and contraction functions improve after treatment, while the conduit function does not, emphasizing the effect of LV filling pressures in Cushing's syndrome (Charles et al. 2015).

8.6.5 ISCHEMIC HEART DISEASE AND MYOCARDIAL INFARCTION

In a study by Schuster et al. (2013b), the authors investigated the capability of CMR-FT for evaluating viability in patients with ischemic cardiomyopathy. CMR-FT showed to be capable of quantifying wall motion changes between the rest and stress conditions (Figure 8.48), with parameter variability that was largest and smallest for measuring Err and Ecc, respectively. Further, the CMR-FT results correlated well with scar transmurality, which makes CMR-FT a simple and fast tool for assessing myocardial viability, especially by nonexperienced observers (Schuster et al. 2015). Similar results have been shown by Schneeweis et al. (2014), where strain analysis with CMR-FT during adenosine stress showed significant differences between normal and ischemic myocardium.

In an important study by Maret et al. (2009), CMR-FT was capable of identifying scar defined by LGE CMR (Figures 8.49 and 8.50). The infarcted regions showed lower functional measures than those in the healthy segments. Specifically, Err was the most significant parameter for differentiating between scarred and nonscarred myocardium. A cutoff value of 38.8% for Err identified >50% transmural scars in the left anterior descending (LAD) artery-supplied region with sensitivity and specificity of 80% and 86%, respectively. The radial deformation measurements showed good reproducibility, and the global measures agreed with other global measures of the heart function. In another study from the same group (Maret et al. 2015), CMR-FT has been used for measuring longitudinal and radial phase delays of velocity, displacement, and strain in 30 patients 4–8 weeks after STEMI treated with percutaneous coronary intervention. The results showed that standard deviation of phase in the radial measurements could differentiate patients with scar from those without scar. Further, SD of time-to-peak velocity, displacement, and strain in the radial measurements performed better than the longitudinal measurements.

CMR-FT showed to be capable of characterizing global and regional strain in patients with prior MI, as well as determining the relationship between strain, infarct size (based on computer-assisted planimetry of LGE images) and EF

(Shafi et al. 2011). Specifically, global Ecc was reduced in all MI patients, while Ell was preserved in the majority of the infarcts. Further, global Ecc at the endocardium was superior to infarct size for predicting EF reduction. In a similar study (Buss et al. 2015), CMR-FT performed on 74 consecutive patients 2–4 days after successfully reperfused STEMI showed that a cutoff value of −19.3% for global Ecc could identify patients with preserved EF (≥50%) at 6 months follow-up with sensitivity and specificity of 76% and 85%, respectively. These results were superior to those obtained from Ell and noninferior to those provided by LGE imaging (Giusca et al. 2015), a finding that has been confirmed in another study (Khan et al. 2015a). Finally, CMR-FT has been used for detecting subtle changes in myocardial Ecc 3 months after intracoronary stem cell infusion in patients with MI (Bhatti et al. 2013).

8.6.6 NONISCHEMIC CARDIOMYOPATHIES

In dilated cardiomyopathy (DCM), myocardial strain measured by CMR-FT showed to be related to survival, which may aid in risk stratification of such patients independent of age, clinical parameters, and established cardiac risk markers (Buss et al. 2014). In a study that compared myocardial mechanical properties in DCM (Choudhary et al. 2014), CMR-FT showed that LV Ecc, Ell, SRcc, and SRll are highly dependent on LVEF reduction. Despite significant differences in the degrees of strain and SR reduction between DCM patients with and without acute heart failure, the reduction of the relaxation rate at early diastole was similarly high in both groups. In another study about nonischemic DCM (Taylor et al. 2014a), CMR-FT showed that mid-wall fibrosis (MWF) is associated with impaired myocardial contraction in the circumferential direction (Figure 8.51), which may account for the negative effects of MWF on patients undergoing CRT. In a recent study conducted on 82 patients diagnosed with DCM and 30 healthy volunteers, CMR-FT showed that the DCM patients had significantly lower apical and basal rotations, resulting in significantly lower LV twist and LV torsion (Ochs et al. 2015). Further, an inversed rotational pattern was observed in many of the DCM patients.

Recently, CMR-FT showed that the strain-to-stress ratio is a promising noninvasive myocardial contractile index, which can depict the contribution of contractile depression to reduced myocardial function in cardiomyopathy (Merchant et al. 2014). Another study showed similar results about the importance of CMR-FT-derived strain for identifying nonischemic cardiomyopathies with preserved EF (Collins et al. 2015). Recently, Taylor et al. (2014b) showed that dyssynchrony measures derived from CMR-FT, such as circumferential (CURE) and radial uniformity ratio estimates (RURE) based on myocardial strain (both CURE and RURE range from 0 to 1, where 0 and 1 represent complete dyssynchrony and perfect synchrony, respectively), can efficiently differentiate cardiomyopathic patients from healthy subjects. The CURE and RURE measures are ratios of the spatial uniformity of strain,

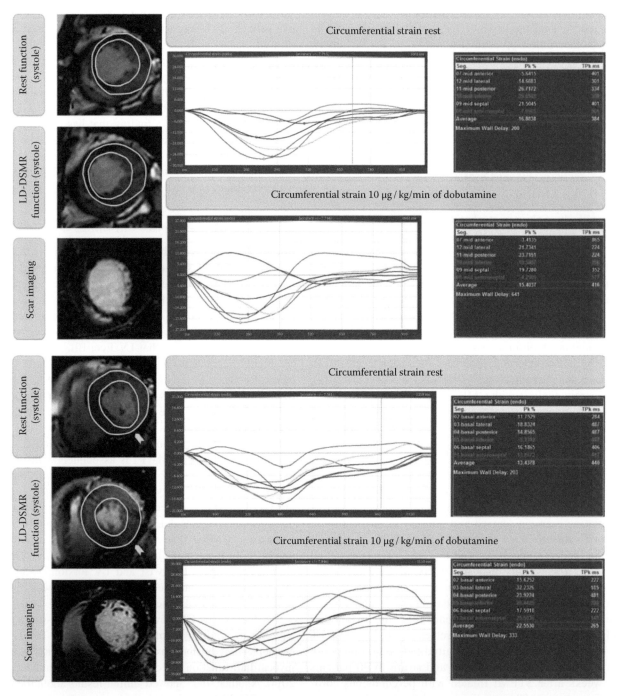

FIGURE 8.48 Two examples of end-systolic cine images at rest and with dobutamine stress, late gadolinium enhanced images, and segmental circumferential subendocardial strain curves at rest and with dobutamine stress. The example in the upper panel shows transmural anteroseptal myocardial scarring and corresponding akinesia that is not reversible with low-dose dobutamine. There is no improvement in circumferential strain. The example in the lower panel shows wall motion abnormality at rest that is reversible with low-dose dobutamine (arrowheads) in the basal inferior segment. There is nontransmural late gadolinium enhancement. LD-DSMR, low-dose dobutamine stress magnetic resonance. (Reproduced from Schuster, A. et al., *Int. J. Cardiol.*, 166(2), 413, 2013b. With permission.)

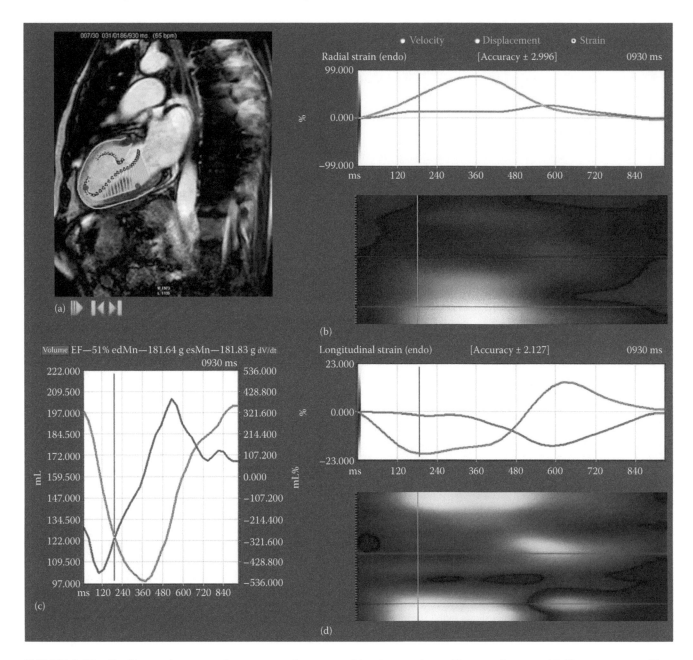

FIGURE 8.49 Cardiovascular magnetic resonance feature tracking in a patient with extensive scar. (a) Vector arrows of late systolic velocity tracing, 190 ms after QRS. (b) Radial strain tracing of the entire cardiac cycle. Blue represents the apex showing very low strain values, and red represents normal posterior wall. (c) Volume curve (red) and emptying velocity (dV/dt; blue). (d) Longitudinal traces from the same locations, showing postsystolic strain in the apex. (Reproduced from Maret, E. et al., *Cardiovasc. Ultrasound*, 7, 53, 2009.)

averaged over time and over all slices. Mathematically, they are represented as

$$\text{CURE or RURE} = \sqrt{\sum_{\text{slices}\,(s)} \sum_{\text{time}\,(t)} \frac{a_0^s(t)}{a_0^s(t) + 2a_1^s(t)}}, \quad (8.4)$$

where a_0 and a_1 are the zeroth and first-order terms from Fourier analysis of the time–strain graphs. Based on studying 108 cardiomyopathic patients and 55 healthy subjects, CURE (0.79 ± 0.14 vs. 0.97 ± 0.02) and RURE (0.71 ± 0.14 vs.

0.91 ± 0.04) were significantly reduced in the patients compared to the healthy controls ($p < 0.0001$).

CMR-FT has been used for evaluating biventricular function in arrhythmogenic right ventricular cardiomyopathy (ARVC) (Heermann et al. 2014). The results showed that the RV global SRll in ARVC (-0.68 ± 0.36 s^{-1}) and borderline ARVC (-0.85 ± 0.36 s^{-1}) was significantly reduced compared to healthy volunteers (-1.38 ± 0.52 s^{-1}). Further, the RV global Ecc and SRcc at the basal level in ARVC (Ecc = -5.1 ± 2.7, SRcc = -0.31 ± 0.13 s^{-1}) were significantly reduced compared to healthy volunteers (Ecc = -9.2% $\pm$

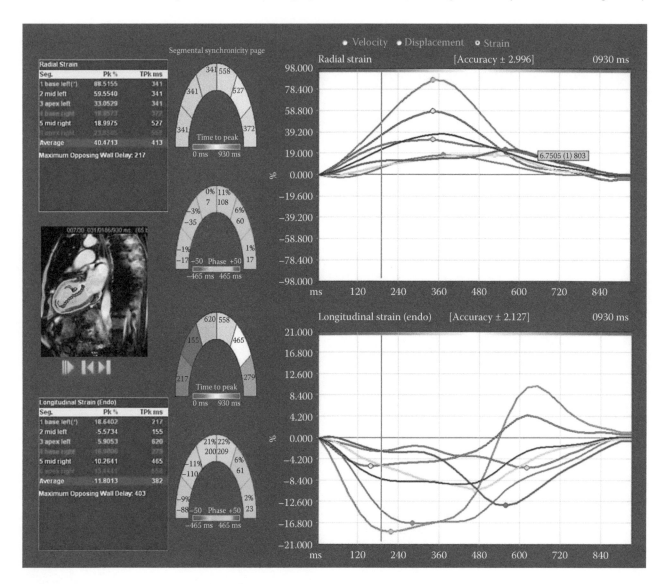

FIGURE 8.50 Measurement window of feature tracking software in ischemic heart disease. The left blue boxes show peak strain values and time-to-peak strain of corresponding segments. The middle column shows graphical displays of six segments, three anterior and three inferoposterior. The upper right panel shows radial strain tracings from the six segments. The lower right panel shows the corresponding longitudinal strain values. (Reproduced from Maret, E. et al., *Cardiovasc. Ultrasound*, 7, 53, 2009.)

3.6%, SRcc = −0.61 ± 0.21 s⁻¹). In patients with ARVC or borderline ARVC and normal RVEF, the global SRll (−0.9 ± 0.3 s⁻¹) was significantly reduced compared to healthy volunteers (−1.4 ± 0.5 s⁻¹). Finally, ARVC patients with Plakophilin-2 mutation showed a clear trend toward having a significantly reduced RV global SRll. In another recent study on cardiomyopathy (Amaki et al. 2014), CMR-FT showed that global Ell was significantly lower in restrictive cardiomyopathy than in constrictive pericarditis, and that the diagnostic value of CMR-FT is similar to that of tissue Doppler echocardiography.

8.6.7 CONGENITAL HEART DISEASE

CMR-FT has been implemented for studying regional heart function in a number of congenital heart diseases. Truong et al. (2010) used CMR-FT for measuring strain and rotational

deformation in patients with single ventricle (SV), where the results showed significantly increased dyssynchrony and decreased Ecc and apical rotation in SV patients compared to normal volunteers (Figure 8.52). In another study on SV Fontan patients (Anwar et al. 2014a), CMR-FT showed moderate correlation between strain and measures of ventricular output (stroke volume and cardiac index) at rest and after exercise, which were not directly related to ventricular size or EF.

CMR-FT has been implemented for studying TOF. Ortega et al. (2011) used CMR-FT to show an association between LV dyssynchrony and adverse outcomes (ventricular tachycardia and death) in patients with repaired TOF. Among different measures of dyssynchrony, the maximum difference (among the six ventricular segments) of time-to-peak Ecc was the best outcome discriminator (Figure 8.53). These results show that CMR-FT could be a useful tool for selecting lead placement sites for cardiac resynchronization.

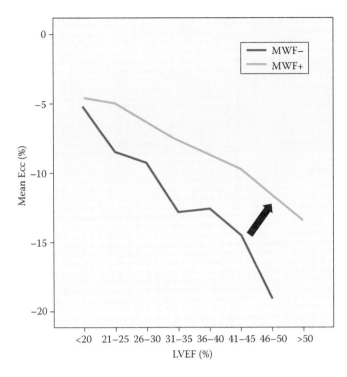

FIGURE 8.51 Mean circumferential strain (Ecc) versus left ventricular ejection fraction in patients with and without mid-wall fibrosis (MWF). (Reproduced from Taylor, R. et al., *J. Cardiovasc. Magn. Reson.*, 16(Suppl 1), P308, 2014.)

Recently, Moon et al. (2015) showed that patients with repaired TOF who experience adverse outcomes (ventricular tachycardia or death) have lower strain measurements than those who do not experience adverse outcomes, and that reduced Ell in both ventricles is strongly associated with adverse clinical outcomes. Specifically, compared to the TOF control group (n = 32), the adverse events group (n = 16) showed significantly reduced median strain in both LV (Ecc = 17% vs. 23%, p = 0.003; Ell = 13% vs. 18%, p < 0.001) and RV (Ecc = 10% vs. 16%, p = 0.001; Ell = 11% vs. 18%, p < 0.001). In another study (Latus et al. 2015), CMR-FT has been used for studying the impact of RV outflow tract obstruction (RVOTO) on biventricular function in patients with repaired TOF. The results showed that patients with RVOTO have significantly higher RV Ecc and Err measurements compared to TOF patients without RVOTO, whereas RV Ell did not differ between the two groups. Further, the degree of RVOTO showed significant correlation with RV Ecc and Err, while RV Ell was unrelated to RVOTO. Finally, interventricular dyssynchrony was significantly higher in the group without RVOTO, while the LV Ell and LV intraventricular synchrony were reduced in the RVOTO group.

In a study on young adults long after aortic coarctation repair, CMR-FT showed reduced global Ell and Err and preserved global Ecc (Figures 8.54 and 8.55; Kutty et al. 2013). The reduction in global Ell was more pronounced in the presence of LV hypertrophy; therefore, it may be a useful indicator of early LV dysfunction. In another study, CMR-FT has been implemented for evaluating RV mechanics in transposition of

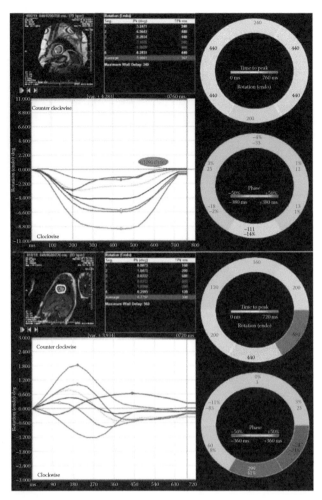

FIGURE 8.52 Cardiovascular magnetic resonance feature tracking in single-ventricle patients. The left ventricular (LV) endocardium of non–single ventricle (non-SV) subjects is traced using velocity vector imaging and depicted in the upper panel. SV endocardium is traced and depicted in the lower panel. Rotational displacement of each of the 6 LV segments, as well as the average value, is recorded. The maximum wall motion delay in the non-SV endocardium is 240 ms, compared to 560 ms in SV, indicating a wider dispersion of time-to-peak curve in the latter. (Reproduced from Truong, U.T. et al., *Am. J. Cardiol.*, 105(10), 1465, 2010. With permission.)

the great arteries after atrial and arterial switch operations (Thattaliyath et al. 2015). The results showed that the atrial switch group had reduced RVEF and increased ventricular volumes compared to the arterial switch group, whereas there was no difference in LVEF and LV volumes between the two groups. Further, the atrial switch group had decreased Ecc, Ell, SRcc, and SRll.

8.6.8 VALVULAR HEART DISEASES

In 43 consecutive patients with symptomatic moderate-to-severe mitral regurgitation patients undergoing percutaneous mitral valve replacement, Zuern et al. (2013) used CMR-FT to show that successful MitraClip procedure can reverse the

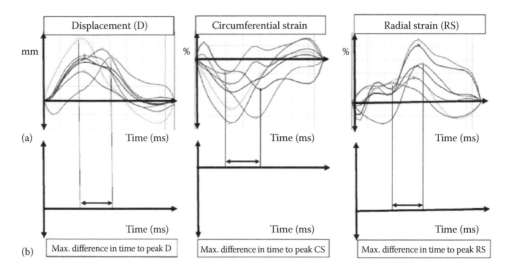

FIGURE 8.53 Dyssynchrony indices in patients with repaired tetralogy of Fallot, calculated using cardiovascular magnetic resonance feature tracking. (a) Radial displacement, circumferential strain, and radial strain curves for six short-axis segments. (b) Maximum differences in segmental times-to-peak displacement and strain. (Reproduced from Ortega, M. et al., *Am. J. Cardiol.*, 107(10), 1535, 2011. With permission.)

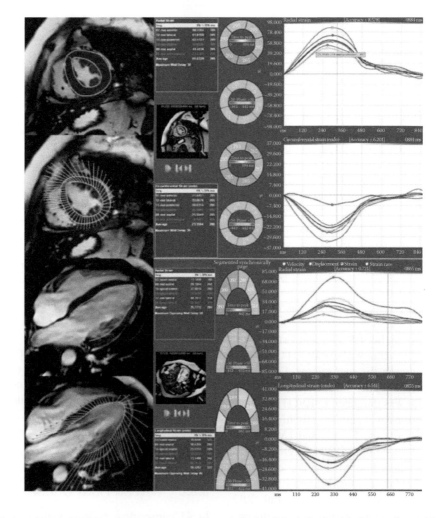

FIGURE 8.54 Cardiovascular magnetic resonance feature tracking analysis of the left ventricle in a patient with repaired coarctation of the aorta. The top panel shows endocardial tracing and tracking in a short-axis image, with the circumferential and radial strain curves displayed. The bottom panel shows endocardial tracing and tracking in a 4-chamber image, with the longitudinal strain curves displayed. (Reproduced from Kutty, S. et al., *Int. J. Cardiovasc. Imaging*, 29(1), 141, 2013. With permission.)

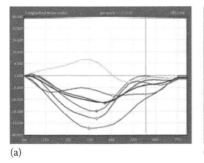 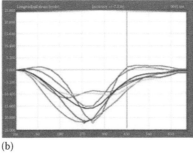 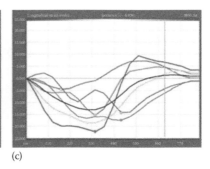

(a)   (b)   (c)

FIGURE 8.55 Representative examples of segmental and global longitudinal strain curves in (a) normal adult control, (b) aortic coarctation with normal left ventricular (LV) mass, and (c) aortic coarctation with LV hypertrophy. (Reproduced from Kutty, S. et al., *Int. J. Cardiovasc. Imaging*, 29(1), 141, 2013. With permission.)

process of LV remodeling within 3 months. In contrast to the improvement of global Ell, there were no significant changes of global Err or Ecc, which may be attributed to the damage from chronic volume overload that primarily affects the subendocardial longitudinally aligned fibers. In a similar study by Lurz et al. (2014), the authors showed that in severely compromised mitral regurgitation patients, marked reduction in mitral regurgitation by MitraClip implantation might not result in improved cardiac output and effective biventricular forward flow.

A couple of recent studies examined LV function in the presence of aortic stenosis. The first study (Cavalcante et al. 2015) showed that global Ell and Ecc correlated well with LVEF regardless of myocardial mass index in aortic stenosis patients with increased LV mass. The second study (Merchant et al. 2015) showed reduced Ecc and Ell in aortic stenosis without significantly increased afterload. Further, contractility, expressed as strain/(end-systolic pressure × volume/mass), was reduced in aortic stenosis, despite that wall stress-based indices and SR were not. Further, there were strong correlations between contractility and EF, although the regression slopes for contractility versus EF and versus strain itself were significantly higher in aortic stenosis patients compared to normals.

In a study on patients with aortic pathology, CMR-FT showed no relationship between aortic stiffness and global measures of LV systolic function following the Ross procedure (Christensen et al. 2014). However, a correlation has been shown between systemic hypertension and preoperative diagnosis of aortic insufficiency with worsened LV Ecc. In another study on patients with RV outflow tract conduit dysfunction, CMR-FT showed that transcatheter pulmonary valve replacement is associated with improved global LV strain, RV strain, and LV synchrony in certain patient groups (Harrild et al. 2013). Recently, CMR-FT has been implemented for evaluating regional LV function after trans-apical (TA) versus trans-femoral (TF) transcatheter aortic valve implantation (TAVI) (Meyer et al. 2014). CMR was performed 3 months after TAVI on 44 patients who had normal EF prior to TAVI. CMR-FT analysis showed no differences in peak-systolic Err and Ell for the basal and mid-ventricular myocardial segments between the TA-TAVI and TF-TAVI groups. However, these measurements were reduced in the apical segments and apical cap in the TA-TAVI group compared to the TF-TAVI group.

8.6.9 Cardiac Electrophysiology

Ceelen et al. (2013) studied 28 consecutive patients with paroxysmal AF who underwent pulmonary vein isolation, where CMR imaging was conducted about 3 days before and 3 months after ablation. CMR-FT was used to measure myocardial velocity, strain, SR, and torsion (Figures 8.56 and 8.57). The results showed that AF patients undergoing ablation appear to have near normal cardiac wall motion, which does not improve following successful ablation.

8.6.10 Other Heart Diseases

CMR-FT has been implemented for studying cardiac involvement in Churg–Strauss syndrome (CSS) (Szczeklik et al. 2011, Miszalski-Jamka et al. 2013). In one study (Szczeklik et al. 2011), CMR-FT showed that CSS patients with impaired LV function have reduced myocardial Ecc compared to subjects with normal LV function. In another study (Miszalski-Jamka et al. 2013), CMR-FT has been implemented for identifying cardiac functional abnormalities in CSS and Wegener's patients with normal ECG and echo. The results showed that despite normal systolic heart function these patients had reduced peak-systolic strain in all directions, which is a sensitive marker of contractile dysfunction. Further, the CSS patients showed less number of segments with reduced peak-systolic Err and Ecc compared to the Wagner's patients. There are two quick notes about that study: (1) the reported reproducibility of segmental strain was better than those previously reported (Schuster et al. 2011, Morton et al. 2012) and (2) the scans were conducted on a 1.5 T scanner that produces less field inhomogeneities than 3.0 T scanners (Morton et al. 2012).

In myocarditis with preserved EF, CMR-FT showed reduced Ell whereas Ecc was not significantly impaired (Andre et al. 2014b). In a similar study, apical peak radial strain rate (SRrr) and peak longitudinal velocity showed significant reduction between baseline and 3 months followup in myocarditis patients with preserved EF (Khanji et al. 2015). Further, the baseline peak longitudinal velocity was

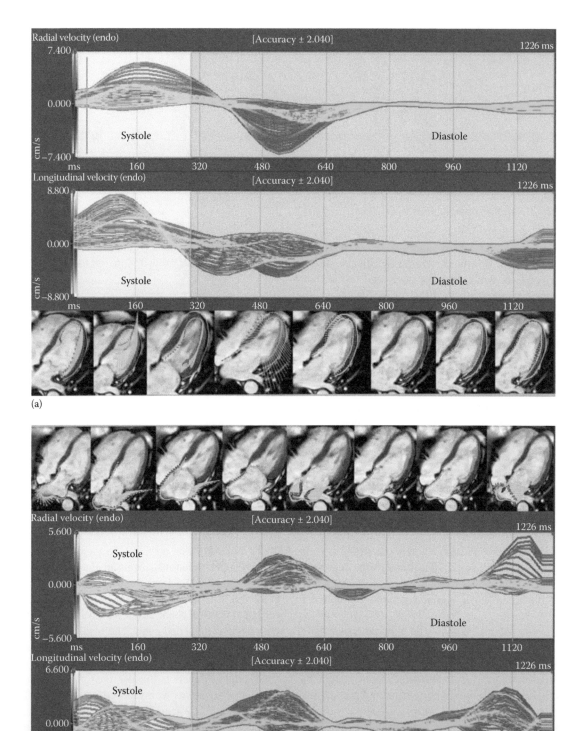

FIGURE 8.56   Feasibility of cardiovascular magnetic resonance feature tracking velocity analysis of the left ventricle (LV) and left atrium (LA) in patients with paroxysmal atrial fibrillation. Feature tracking analysis of the radial and longitudinal velocities in the (a) LV and (b) LA. The blue lines represent tracking of the endocardial borders. The length of the green vectors in the 4-chamber images represents absolute values of velocities. (Reproduced from Ceelen, F. et al., *Int. J. Cardiovasc. Imaging*, 29(8), 1807, 2013. With permission.)

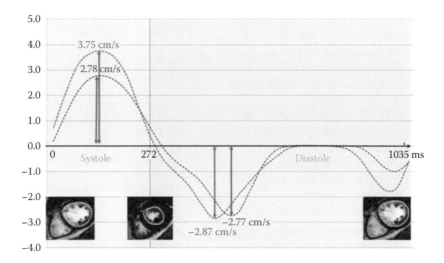

FIGURE 8.57 Radial velocity curves of the endocardium in patients with paroxysmal atrial fibrillation. The figure shows baseline (blue) and 3 months follow-up (red) curves of radial velocity (cm/s) in a mid-ventricular short-axis view. (Reproduced from Ceelen, F. et al., *Int. J. Cardiovasc. Imaging*, 29(8), 1807, 2013. With permission.)

independently associated with EF change, with higher velocities predicting improvement in EF over time. In another study (Weigand et al. 2015), Ell and global Ecc showed good sensitivity and specificity for detecting troponin leak and LGE existence in myocarditis with preserved EF.

In a recent study, CMR-FT showed disturbed contraction in patients with systemic light chain amyloidosis (Andre et al. 2014a). A similar study confirmed reduced myocardial twist and untwist rates in amyloidosis (Hussain et al. 2015). CMR-FT has been also used for studying Kawasaki disease convalescent patients with preserved conventional functional indices (Bratis et al. 2015), where the results showed a trend for lower Ecc and Ell in Kawasaki disease patients, compared to normal controls, irrespective of their coronary artery status.

8.7 SUMMARY AND KEY POINTS

8.7.1 Summary

CMR-FT is a new tool for measuring heart mechanics from standard cine CMR images without the need for running special CMR sequences or conducting complicated image post-processing. Despite being relatively new, the technique has been validated against STE and CMR tagging with satisfactory results. Further, CMR-FT has been implemented in different clinical studies. Nevertheless, the practical implementation of the technique needs to be conducted with caution due to its limitations. The technique is best utilized for measuring global motion parameters, for example, global myocardial strain and displacement. Further, it should be applied on images with good image quality and on reasonably sized regions. The measurements should be repeated to examine reproducibility, and wall motion abnormalities should be interpreted with caution. Although the technique needs further improvements to enhance its reliability and widen its applications, it holds promise to be part of the analysis tools in cardiac imaging labs, at least for fast quantitative assessment of cardiac function.

8.7.2 Key Points

- STE is based on tracking movement of the ultrasound speckles, as intrinsic markers of the myocardium, in the echo images.
- STE has been validated against implanted markers and CMR tagging for measuring regional myocardial deformation.
- VVI is a new echocardiographic image analysis technique that is similar to, and based on, STE.
- Echocardiography feature tracking is a recently developed technique that gained a lot of interest because it combines the advantages of both STE and VVI.
- Inspired by the STE and VVI techniques, CMR-FT has been recently introduced for measuring regional myocardial deformation from cine CMR images based on intrinsic anatomical features and periodicity of the heart motion.
- Feature tracking is based on defining a relatively small window centered at a certain anatomical pattern (feature) in one image and searching for the as-much-as-possible similar local pattern in a window, of the same size and in the vicinity of the original window, in the following image (timeframe).
- CMR-FT employs a hierarchical sequence of tracking steps that starts with a large search window to detect large displacements and progressively proceeds to smaller windows to improve accuracy.
- CMR-FT consists of the following steps: initial preprocessing, feature detection, compensation for large motion components, refinement of local motion, and refinement of motion along the tracked border.
- The following parameters can be measured using CMR-FT: myocardial displacement, velocity, strain, strain rate, rotation, and torsion.

- The measured parameters can be classified as either integral, for example, displacement and strain, or differential, for example, velocity and strain rate.
- The integral parameters are more robust and reproducible, and less affected by low image quality and noise than the differential parameters.
- Compared to STE, CMR-FT is more reliable due to the inherently better image quality with CMR than with echo, which allows for accurate myocardial border detection. Further, CMR imaging is not affected by acoustic window, geometric assumptions, or operator dependency as in echo.
- CMR-FT has been validated against STE in a number of studies on healthy volunteers and patients.
- A number of studies have been conducted to validate CMR-FT against CMR tagging for measuring regional heart function in healthy volunteers and patients.
- Compared to CMR tagging, CMR-FT is simpler and faster as it does not require an additional tagging sequence and the accompanying complicated, and sometimes time-consuming, tag analysis step.
- Generally, the accuracy of CMR-FT is suboptimal to CMR tagging as the intrinsic tissue markers used in CMR-FT are much less than, and not as uniformly distributed as, the taglines in the CMR tagged images.
- CMR-FT has certain limitations with respect to sensitivity to spatial and temporal changes in the tracked pattern, which depend on the acquired images' spatial and temporal resolutions, respectively. Therefore, precautions should be taken into consideration to avoid these limitations.
- Practical implementation of CMR-FT requires proper understanding of the technique and its capabilities, such that the resulting measures become meaningful and useful. In this respect, CMR-FT can be a useful initial and fast technique for evaluating the heart mechanics, although its accuracy for evaluating regional myocardial function is suboptimal to CMR tagging.
- Although being a relatively new technique, CMR-FT has been implemented in a number of clinical applications, including gender- and age-specific strain differences, RV mechanics, atrial imaging, myocardial contractility at rest and stress, ischemic heart disease and MI, nonischemic cardiomyopathies, congenital heart diseases, valvular diseases, and cardiac electrophysiology.

REFERENCES

Adrian, R. J. (1991). Particle-image technique for experimental fluid mechanics. *Ann Rev Fluid Mech* **23**: 261–304.

Ainslie, M. P., Reid, A., Miller, C. A., Clark, D., Francis, L., and Schmitt, M. (2015). Evaluation of left ventricular torsion using cardiac MRI. Validation of feature tracking. *J Cardiovasc Magn Reson* **17**(Suppl 1): O47.

Almutairi, H. M., Zemrak, F., Treibel, T. A., Sado, D., Boubertakh, R., Miquel, M. E., and Petersen, S. E. (2015). A comparison of cardiac motion analysis software packages: Application to left ventricular deformation analysis in hypertensive patients. *J Cardiovasc Magn Reson* **17**(Suppl 1): P57.

Alshammari, Q. T., Strugnell, W. E., Chan, J., Burstow, D. J., and Hamilton-Craig, C. (2014). Cardiovascular magnetic resonance radial and circumferential strain: Comparison between SSFP feature tracking, MRI tagging, and speckle tracking echocardiography. *Proceedings of the International Society for Magnetic Resonance*, Milan, Italy, p. 3977.

Amaki, M., Savino, J., Ain, D. L., Sanz, J., Pedrizzetti, G., Kulkarni, H., Narula, J., and Sengupta, P. P. (2014). Diagnostic concordance of echocardiography and cardiac magnetic resonance-based tissue tracking for differentiating constrictive pericarditis from restrictive cardiomyopathy. *Circ Cardiovasc Imaging* **7**(5): 819–827.

Amundsen, B. H., Crosby, J., Steen, P. A., Torp, H., Slordahl, S. A., and Stoylen, A. (2009). Regional myocardial long-axis strain and strain rate measured by different tissue Doppler and speckle tracking echocardiography methods: A comparison with tagged magnetic resonance imaging. *Eur J Echocardiogr* **10**(2): 229–237.

Amundsen, B. H., Helle-Valle, T., Edvardsen, T., Torp, H., Crosby, J., Lyseggen, E., Stoylen, A. et al. (2006). Noninvasive myocardial strain measurement by speckle tracking echocardiography: Validation against sonomicrometry and tagged magnetic resonance imaging. *J Am Coll Cardiol* **47**(4): 789–793.

Andre, F., Kammerer, R., Breuninger, K., Kristen, A. V., Galuschky, C., Schoenland, S., Hegenbart, U. et al. (2014a). Cardiac magnetic resonance strain imaging in systemic light chain amyloidosis. *J Cardiovasc Magn Reson* **16**(Suppl 1): P321.

Andre, F., Steen, H., Matheis, P., Westkott, M., Breuninger, K., Sander, Y., Kammerer, R. et al. (2015). Age- and gender-related normal left ventricular deformation assessed by cardiovascular magnetic resonance feature tracking. *J Cardiovasc Magn Reson* **17**: 25.

Andre, F., Stock, F. T., Breuninger, K., aus dem Siepen, F., Giannitsis, E., Korosoglou, G., Katus, H. A., and Buss, S. (2014b). Assessment of myocardial strain in patients with myocarditis by cardiac magnetic resonance imaging. *J Cardiovasc Magn Reson* **16**(Suppl 1): P314.

Anwar, A. M. (2012). Global and segmental myocardial deformation by 2D speckle tracking compared to visual assessment. *World J Cardiol* **4**(12): 341–346.

Anwar, S., Doddasomayajula, R., Keller, M. S., Harris, M. A., Yoganathan, A., Fogel, M. A., and Whitehead, K. K. (2014a). Strain to evaluate ventricular function in Fontan patients undergoing exercise cardiac magnetic resonance imaging. *J Cardiovasc Magn Reson* **16**(Suppl 1): P123.

Anwar, S., Fogel, E. J., Doddasomayajula, R., Davidson, A., Keller, M. S., Harris, M. A., Whitehead, K. K., and Fogel, M. A. (2014b). Feature tracking strain is similar to harmonic phase cardiac magnetic resonance in Fontan patients: A validation study. *J Cardiovasc Magn Reson* **16**(Suppl 1): P106.

Augustine, D., Lewandowski, A. J., Lazdam, M., Rai, A., Francis, J., Myerson, S., Noble, A. et al. (2013). Global and regional left ventricular myocardial deformation measures by magnetic resonance feature tracking in healthy volunteers: Comparison with tagging and relevance of gender. *J Cardiovasc Magn Reson* **15**: 8.

Bansal, M., Cho, G. Y., Chan, J., Leano, R., Haluska, B. A., and Marwick, T. H. (2008). Feasibility and accuracy of different techniques of two-dimensional speckle based strain and validation with harmonic phase magnetic resonance imaging. *J Am Soc Echocardiogr* **21**(12): 1318–1325.

Bansal, M., Jeffriess, L., Leano, R., Mundy, J., and Marwick, T. H. (2010). Assessment of myocardial viability at dobutamine echocardiography by deformation analysis using tissue velocity and speckle-tracking. *JACC Cardiovasc Imaging* **3**(2): 121–131.

Barron, J. L., Fleet, D. J., and Beachchemin, S. (1994). Performance of optical flow techniques. *Int J Computer Vision* **12**: 43–77.

Bellenger, N. G., Davies, L. C., Francis, J. M., Coats, A. J., and Pennell, D. J. (2000). Reduction in sample size for studies of remodeling in heart failure by the use of cardiovascular magnetic resonance. *J Cardiovasc Magn Reson* **2**(4): 271–278.

Bhatti, S., Al-Khalidi, H., Hor, K., Hakeem, A., Taylor, M., Quyyumi, A. A., Oshinski, J. et al. (2013). Assessment of myocardial contractile function using global and segmental circumferential strain following intracoronary stem cell infusion after myocardial infarction: MRI feature tracking feasibility study. *ISRN Radiol* 2013: 371028.

Biswas, M., Sudhakar, S., Nanda, N. C., Buckberg, G., Pradhan, M., Roomi, A. U., Gorissen, W., and Houle, H. (2013). Two- and three-dimensional speckle tracking echocardiography: Clinical applications and future directions. *Echocardiography* **30**(1): 88–105.

Blessberger, H. and Binder, T. (2010a). Non-invasive imaging: Two dimensional speckle tracking echocardiography: Basic principles. *Heart* **96**(9): 716–722.

Blessberger, H. and Binder, T. (2010b). Two dimensional speckle tracking echocardiography: Clinical applications. *Heart* **96**(24): 2032–2040.

Bohs, L. N., Geiman, B. J., Anderson, M. E., Gebhart, S. C., and Trahey, G. E. (2000). Speckle tracking for multi-dimensional flow estimation. *Ultrasonics* **38**(1–8): 369–375.

Bohs, L. N. and Trahey, G. E. (1991). A novel method for angle independent ultrasonic imaging of blood flow and tissue motion. *IEEE Trans Biomed Eng* **38**(3): 280–286.

Botelho, M., Bou Ayache, J., Bogachkov, A., Artang, R., Bi, X., Vazquez, M. R., Carr, J. C., and Collins, J. D. (2014). Application of feature tracking at cine cardiac MR for the semiautomated prediction of normal right ventricular systolic function: A feasibility study. *J Cardiovasc Magn Reson* **16**(Suppl 1): P74.

Bratis, K., Hackmann, P., Child, N., Mavrogeni, S., Krasemann, T., Hussain, T., Botnar, R., Razavi, R., and Greil, G. F. (2015). CMR feature tracking in Kawasaki Disease convalescence. *J Cardiovasc Magn Reson* **17**(Suppl 1): P366.

Burns, A. T., McDonald, I. G., Thomas, J. D., Macisaac, A., and Prior, D. (2008). Doin' the twist: New tools for an old concept of myocardial function. *Heart* **94**(8): 978–983.

Buss, S., Andre, F., Breuninger, K., Lehrke, S., Voss, A., Galuschky, C., Lossnitzer, D. et al. (2014). Prognostic value of myocardial strain analysis with cardiac magnetic resonance in patients with dilated cardiomyopathy. *J Cardiovasc Magn Reson* **16**(Suppl 1): O90.

Buss, S. J., Krautz, B., Hofmann, N., Sander, Y., Rust, L., Giusca, S., Galuschky, C. et al. (2015). Prediction of functional recovery by cardiac magnetic resonance feature tracking imaging in first time ST-elevation myocardial infarction. Comparison to infarct size and transmurality by late gadolinium enhancement. *Int J Cardiol* **183**: 162–170.

Cannesson, M., Tanabe, M., Suffoletto, M. S., Schwartzman, D., and Gorcsan, J., 3rd (2006). Velocity vector imaging to quantify ventricular dyssynchrony and predict response to cardiac resynchronization therapy. *Am J Cardiol* **98**(7): 949–953.

Carasso, S., Biaggi, P., Rakowski, H., Mutlak, D., Lessick, J., Aronson, D., Woo, A., and Agmon, Y. (2012). Velocity vector imaging: Standard tissue-tracking results acquired in normals—The VVI-STRAIN study. *J Am Soc Echocardiogr* **25**(5): 543–552.

Cavalcante, J. L., Delgado-Montero, A., Rijal, S., Schelbert, E. B., and Gorcsan, J. (2015). The association of global longitudinal and global circumferential strain with ejection fraction in patients with aortic stenosis and increased left ventricular mass: A feature tracking CMR study. *J Cardiovasc Magn Reson* **17**(Suppl 1): P226.

Ceelen, F., Hunter, R. J., Boubertakh, R., Sommer, W. H., Armbruster, M., Schilling, R. J., and Petersen, S. E. (2013). Effect of atrial fibrillation ablation on myocardial function: Insights from cardiac magnetic resonance feature tracking analysis. *Int J Cardiovasc Imaging* **29**(8): 1807–1817.

Charles, R., Evin, M., Kamenicky, P., Mousseaux, E., Raissuni, Z., Lamy, J., Cluzel, P., Kachenoura, N., and Redheuil, A. (2015). CMR left atrial characterization in Cushing's syndrome: A feature tracking study. *J Cardiovasc Magn Reson* **17**(Suppl 1): P42.

Chen, J., Cao, T., Duan, Y., Yuan, L., and Wang, Z. (2007a). Velocity vector imaging in assessing myocardial systolic function of hypertensive patients with left ventricular hypertrophy. *Can J Cardiol* **23**(12): 957–961.

Chen, J., Cao, T., Duan, Y., Yuan, L., and Yang, Y. (2007b). Velocity vector imaging in assessing the regional systolic function of patients with post myocardial infarction. *Echocardiography* **24**(9): 940–945.

Cheng, J. Y., Cao, J. J., and Halloran, K. (2014). Feasibility of performing in-scanner exercise testing and assessing myocardial mechanical reserve in normal volunteers and in patients with cardiomyopathy. *J Cardiovasc Magn Reson* **16**(Suppl 1): P255.

Choudhary, N., Kabbli, G., Duncanson, L. J., Passick, M., Halloran, K., and Cao, J. J. (2014). Comparison of myocardial mechanical properties in patients with dilated cardiomyopathy with and without acute heart failure. *J Cardiovasc Magn Reson* **16**(Suppl 1): P239.

Christensen, J., Lu, J. C., Yu, S., Donohue, J., Agarwal, P. P., Mahani, M. G., and Dorfman, A. L. (2014). Pulse wave velocity does not predict ventricular strain in Ross patients. *J Cardiovasc Magn Reson* **16**(Suppl 1): P113.

Collins, J. D., Botelho, M., Stark, M., Lee, D. C., Kalisz, K., Smith, P. M., Allen, B. D. et al. (2015). Cardiac MR feature tracking identifies abnormal biventricular global strain values in biopsy-proven non-ischemic cardiomyopathies. *J Cardiovasc Magn Reson* **17**(Suppl 1): Q8.

Di Bella, G., Zito, C., Gaeta, M., Cusma Piccione, M., Minutoli, F., Donato, R., Recupero, A., Madaffari, A., Coglitore, S., and Carerj, S. (2010). Semiautomatic quantification of left ventricular function by two-dimensional feature tracking imaging echocardiography. A comparison study with cardiac magnetic resonance imaging. *Echocardiography* **27**(7): 791–797.

Evin, M., Cluzel, P., Lamy, J., Rosenbaum, D., Kusmia, S., Defrance, C., Soulat, G. et al. (2015). Assessment of left atrial function by MRI myocardial feature tracking. *J Magn Reson Imaging* **42**(2): 379–389.

Giusca, S., Krautz, B., Sander, Y., Rust, L., Galuschky, C., Seitz, S., Giannitsis, E. et al. (2015). Prediction of functional recovery by cardiac magnetic resonance feature tracking imaging in first time ST-elevation myocardial infarction. Comparison to infarct size and transmurality by late gadolinium enhancement. *J Cardiovasc Magn Reson* **17**(Suppl 1): P87.

Gjesdal, O., Hopp, E., Vartdal, T., Lunde, K., Helle-Valle, T., Aakhus, S., Smith, H. J., Ihlen, H., and Edvardsen, T. (2007). Global longitudinal strain measured by two-dimensional speckle tracking echocardiography is closely related to myocardial infarct size in chronic ischaemic heart disease. *Clin Sci (Lond)* **113**(6): 287–296.

Gustafsson, U., Lindqvist, P., and Waldenstrom, A. (2008). Apical circumferential motion of the right and the left ventricles in healthy subjects described with speckle tracking. *J Am Soc Echocardiogr* **21**(12): 1326–1330.

Habibi, M., Venkatesh, B. A., and Lima, J. A. (2014). Feature tracking cardiac magnetic resonance imaging in the assessment of left atrial function. *J Am Coll Cardiol* **63**(22): 2434–2435.

Hamilton-Craig, C., Strugnell, W., Alshammari, Q., Chapman, M., Morris, N., Seale, H., Kermeen, F., Schmitt, B., M., Z., Chan, J., and La Gerche, A. (2014). Radial and circumferential strain using feature tracking from cine SSFP imaging with compressed sensing at rest and with MRI exercise ergometry. *Proceedings of the International Society for Magnetic Resonance*, Milan, Italy, p. 3906.

Harrild, D. M., Han, Y., Geva, T., Zhou, J., Marcus, E., and Powell, A. J. (2012). Comparison of cardiac MRI tissue tracking and myocardial tagging for assessment of regional ventricular strain. *Int J Cardiovasc Imaging* **28**(8): 2009–2018.

Harrild, D. M., Marcus, E., Hasan, B., Alexander, M. E., Powell, A. J., Geva, T., and McElhinney, D. B. (2013). Impact of transcatheter pulmonary valve replacement on biventricular strain and synchrony assessed by cardiac magnetic resonance feature tracking. *Circ Cardiovasc Interv* **6**(6): 680–687.

Heermann, P., Hedderich, D. M., Paul, M., Schulke, C., Kroeger, J. R., Baessler, B., Wichter, T. et al. (2014). Biventricular myocardial strain analysis in patients with arrhythmogenic right ventricular cardiomyopathy (ARVC) using cardiovascular magnetic resonance feature tracking. *J Cardiovasc Magn Reson* **16**: 75.

Helle-Valle, T., Crosby, J., Edvardsen, T., Lyseggen, E., Amundsen, B. H., Smith, H. J., Rosen, B. D. et al. (2005). New noninvasive method for assessment of left ventricular rotation: Speckle tracking echocardiography. *Circulation* **112**(20): 3149–3156.

Hor, K. N., Baumann, R., Pedrizzetti, G., Tonti, G., Gottliebson, W. M., Taylor, M., Benson, W., and Mazur, W. (2011). Magnetic resonance derived myocardial strain assessment using feature tracking. *J Vis Exp* (48).

Hor, K. N., Gottliebson, W. M., Carson, C., Wash, E., Cnota, J., Fleck, R., Wansapura, J. et al. (2010). Comparison of magnetic resonance feature tracking for strain calculation with harmonic phase imaging analysis. *JACC Cardiovasc Imaging* **3**(2): 144–151.

Horn, B. K. and Schunk, B. G. (1981). Determining optical flow. *Artif Intell* **17**: 185–203.

Hussain, S., Buss, S., Kutty, S., Steen, H., Lossnitzer, D., Beerbaum, P., Lamata, P., and Schuster, A. (2015). Quantitative assessment of myocardial mechanics in patients with cardiac amyloid using cardiovascular magnetic resonance myocardial feature tracking. *J Cardiovasc Magn Reson* **17**(Suppl 1): Q28.

Imai, M., Ambale Venkatesh, B., Samiei, S., Donekal, S., Habibi, M., Armstrong, A. C., Heckbert, S. R., Wu, C. O., Bluemke, D. A., and Lima, J. A. (2014). Multi-ethnic study of atherosclerosis: Association between left atrial function using tissue tracking from cine MR imaging and myocardial fibrosis. *Radiology* **273**(3): 703–713.

Inoue, Y. Y., Alissa, A., Khurram, I. M., Fukumoto, K., Habibi, M., Venkatesh, B. A., Zimmerman, S. L. et al. (2015). Quantitative tissue-tracking cardiac magnetic resonance (CMR) of left atrial deformation and the risk of stroke in patients with atrial fibrillation. *J Am Heart Assoc* **4**(4).

Ishii, T., McElhinney, D. B., Harrild, D. M., Marcus, E. N., Sahn, D. J., Truong, U., and Tworetzky, W. (2012). Circumferential and longitudinal ventricular strain in the normal human fetus. *J Am Soc Echocardiogr* **25**(1): 105–111.

Jurcut, R., Pappas, C. J., Masci, P. G., Herbots, L., Szulik, M., Bogaert, J., Van de Werf, F. et al. (2008). Detection of regional myocardial dysfunction in patients with acute myocardial infarction using velocity vector imaging. *J Am Soc Echocardiogr* **21**(8): 879–886.

Kadiyala, M., Toole, R., Bertman, K., Pollack, S., and Reichek, N. (2011). Feature tracking: A novel method to analyze myocardial strain: Results from the CMR strain study in healthy volunteers. *J Cardiovasc Magn Reson* **13**(Suppl 1): P14.

Kaluzynski, K., Chen, X., Emelianov, S. Y., Skovoroda, A. R., and O'Donnell, M. (2001). Strain rate imaging using two-dimensional speckle tracking. *IEEE Trans Ultrason Ferroelectr Freq Control* **48**(4): 1111–1123.

Karwat, K., Tomala, M., Miszalski-Jamka, K., Mazur, W., Kereiakes, D., Nessler, J., Zmudka, K., and Miszalski-Jamka, T. (2015). Left atrial contractile strain is the independent predictor of LV remodeling after ST-segment elevation myocardial infarction. *J Cardiovasc Magn Reson* **17**(Suppl 1): P151.

Kempny, A., Fernandez-Jimenez, R., Orwat, S., Schuler, P., Bunck, A. C., Maintz, D., Baumgartner, H., and Diller, G. P. (2012). Quantification of biventricular myocardial function using cardiac magnetic resonance feature tracking, endocardial border delineation and echocardiographic speckle tracking in patients with repaired tetralogy of Fallot and healthy controls. *J Cardiovasc Magn Reson* **14**: 32.

Khan, J. N., Greenwood, J. P., Nazir, S. A., Dalby, M., Curzen, N., Hetherington, S. et al. (2015a). Predictive value of segmental extent of late gadolinium enhancement and peak circumferential systolic strain in predicting improvement and normalisation of dysfunctional segments post STEMI. *J Cardiovasc Magn Reson* **17**(Suppl 1): O11.

Khan, J. N., Singh, A., Nazir, S. A., Kanagala, P., Gershlick, A. H., and McCann, G. P. (2015b). Comparison of cardiovascular magnetic resonance feature tracking and tagging for the assessment of left ventricular systolic strain in acute myocardial infarction. *Eur J Radiol* **84**(5): 840–848.

Khan, J. N., Singh, A., Nazir, S. A., Kanagala, P., Greenwood, J. P., Gershlick, A., and McCann, G. P. (2015c). Comparison of cardiovascular magnetic resonance feature tracking and tagging for the assessment of left ventricular systolic strain in acute myocardial infarction. *J Cardiovasc Magn Reson* **17**(Suppl 1): P102.

Khanji, M. Y., Javaid, M. R., Mohiddin, S. A., Boubertakh, R., Sekhri, N., and Petersen, S. E. (2015). Cardiovascular magnetic resonance feature tracking in patients with acute myocarditis and normal ejection fraction: Potential for improved diagnosis and prognosis. *J Cardiovasc Magn Reson* **17**(Suppl 1): M7.

Kim, D. H., Kim, H. K., Kim, M. K., Chang, S. A., Kim, Y. J., Kim, M. A., Sohn, D. W., Oh, B. H., and Park, Y. B. (2009). Velocity vector imaging in the measurement of left ventricular twist mechanics: Head-to-head one way comparison between speckle tracking echocardiography and velocity vector imaging. *J Am Soc Echocardiogr* **22**(12): 1344–1352.

Konofagou, E. E., Manning, W., Kissinger, K., and Solomon, S. D. (2003). Myocardial elastography-comparison to results using MR cardiac tagging. *Proceedings of the IEEE Ultrasonics Symposium*, pp. 130–133.

Koopman, L. P., Slorach, C., Manlhiot, C., McCrindle, B. W., Jaeggi, E. T., Mertens, L., and Friedberg, M. K. (2011). Assessment of myocardial deformation in children using Digital Imaging and Communications in Medicine (DICOM) data and vendor independent speckle tracking software. *J Am Soc Echocardiogr* **24**(1): 37–44.

Kowallick, J. T., Kutty, S., Edelmann, F., Chiribiri, A., Villa, A., Steinmetz, M., Sohns, J. M. et al. (2014a). Quantification of left atrial strain and strain rate using cardiovascular magnetic resonance myocardial feature tracking: A feasibility study. *J Cardiovasc Magn Reson* **16**: 60.

Kowallick, J. T., Kutty, S., Edelmann, F., Chiribiri, A., Villa, A., Steinmetz, M., Sohns, J. M. et al. (2015a). Quantification of left atrial strain and strain rate using cardiovascular magnetic resonance myocardial feature tracking. *J Cardiovasc Magn Reson* **17**(Suppl 1): P66.

Kowallick, J. T., Lamata, P., Hussain, S. T., Kutty, S., Steinmetz, M., Sohns, J. M., Fasshauer, M. et al. (2014b). Quantification of left ventricular torsion and diastolic recoil using cardiovascular magnetic resonance myocardial feature tracking. *PLoS One* **9**(10): e109164.

Kowallick, J. T., Morton, G., Lamata, P., Jogiya, R., Kutty, S., Hasenfuss, G., Lotz, J., Nagel, E., Chiribiri, A., and Schuster, A. (2015b). Quantification of atrial dynamics using cardiovascular magnetic resonance: Inter-study reproducibility. *J Cardiovasc Magn Reson* **17**: 36.

Kuetting, D., Sprinkart, A. M., Doerner, J., Schild, H., and Thomas, D. (2015). Comparison of magnetic resonance feature tracking with harmonic phase imaging analysis (CSPAMM) for assessment of global and regional diastolic function. *Eur J Radiol* **84**(1): 100–107.

Kutty, S., Deatsman, S. L., Nugent, M. L., Russell, D., and Frommelt, P. C. (2008). Assessment of regional right ventricular velocities, strain, and displacement in normal children using velocity vector imaging. *Echocardiography* **25**(3): 294–307.

Kutty, S., Rangamani, S., Venkataraman, J., Li, L., Schuster, A., Fletcher, S. E., Danford, D. A., and Beerbaum, P. (2013). Reduced global longitudinal and radial strain with normal left ventricular ejection fraction late after effective repair of aortic coarctation: A CMR feature tracking study. *Int J Cardiovasc Imaging* **29**(1): 141–150.

Latus, H., Hachmann, P., Gummel, K., Khalil, M., Yerebakan, C., Bauer, J., Schranz, D., and Apitz, C. (2015). Impact of residual right ventricular outflow tract obstruction on biventricular strain and synchrony in patients after repair of tetralogy of Fallot: A cardiac magnetic resonance feature tracking study. *Eur J Cardiothorac Surg* **48**(1): 83–90.

Lee, W. N., Ingrassia, C. M., Fung-Kee-Fung, S. D., Costa, K. D., Holmes, J. W., and Konofagou, E. E. (2007). Theoretical quality assessment of myocardial elastography with in vivo validation. *IEEE Trans Ultrason Ferroelectr Freq Control* **54**(11): 2233–2245.

Lee, W. N., Qian, Z., Tosti, C. L., Brown, T. R., Metaxas, D. N., and Konofagou, E. E. (2008). Preliminary validation of angle-independent myocardial elastography using MR tagging in a clinical setting. *Ultrasound Med Biol* **34**(12): 1980–1997.

Lemarie, J., Huttin, O., Girerd, N., Mandry, D., Juilliere, Y., Moulin, F., Lemoine, S., Beaumont, M., Marie, P. Y., and Selton-Suty, C. (2015). Usefulness of speckle-tracking imaging for right ventricular assessment after acute myocardial infarction: A magnetic resonance imaging/echocardiographic comparison within the relation between aldosterone and cardiac remodeling after myocardial infarction study. *J Am Soc Echocardiogr* **28**(7): 818–827 e814.

Li, P., Meng, H., Liu, S. Z., and Vannan, M. A. (2012). Quantification of left ventricular mechanics using vector-velocity imaging, a novel feature tracking algorithm, applied to echocardiography and cardiac magnetic resonance imaging. *Chin Med J (Engl)* **125**(15): 2719–2727.

Lorch, S. M., Ludomirsky, A., and Singh, G. K. (2008). Maturational and growth-related changes in left ventricular longitudinal strain and strain rate measured by two-dimensional speckle tracking echocardiography in healthy pediatric population. *J Am Soc Echocardiogr* **21**(11): 1207–1215.

Lu, J. C., Connelly, J. A., Zhao, L., Agarwal, P. P., and Dorfman, A. L. (2014a). Comparison of feature tracking and harmonic phase imaging for strain measurement on cardiovascular magnetic resonance in pediatric cancer survivors. *J Cardiovasc Magn Reson* **16**(Suppl 1): P334.

Lu, J. C., Connelly, J. A., Zhao, L., Agarwal, P. P., and Dorfman, A. L. (2014b). Strain measurement by cardiovascular magnetic resonance in pediatric cancer survivors: Validation of feature tracking against harmonic phase imaging. *Pediatr Radiol* **44**(9): 1070–1076.

Lurz, P., Serpytis, R., Balzek, S., Seeburger, J., Mangner, N., Eitel, I., Desch, S. et al. (2014). Assessment of acute changes in biventricular volumes, systolic function and strain after MitraClipTM-implantation using magnetic resonance imaging and feature tracking. *J Cardiovasc Magn Reson* **16**(Suppl 1): P317.

Malpica, N., Santos, A., Zuluaga, M. A., Ledesma, M. J., Perez, E., Garcia-Fernandez, M. A., and Desco, M. (2004). Tracking of regions-of-interest in myocardial contrast echocardiography. *Ultrasound Med Biol* **30**(3): 303–309.

Maret, E., Liehl, M., Brudin, L., Todt, T., Edvardsen, T., and Engvall, J. E. (2015). Phase analysis detects heterogeneity of myocardial deformation on cine MRI. *Scand Cardiovasc J* **49**(3): 149–158.

Maret, E., Todt, T., Brudin, L., Nylander, E., Swahn, E., Ohlsson, J. L., and Engvall, J. E. (2009). Functional measurements based on feature tracking of cine magnetic resonance images identify left ventricular segments with myocardial scar. *Cardiovasc Ultrasound* **7**: 53.

Masuda, K., Asanuma, T., Taniguchi, A., Uranishi, A., Ishikura, F., and Beppu, S. (2008). Assessment of dyssynchronous wall motion during acute myocardial ischemia using velocity vector imaging. *JACC Cardiovasc Imaging* **1**(2): 210–220.

Mendes, L., Ribeiras, R., Adragao, T., Lima, S., Horta, E., Reis, C., Amaral, T., Aguiar, C., Gouveia, R., and Silva, A. (2008). Load-independent parameters of diastolic and systolic function by speckle tracking and tissue Doppler in hemodialysis patients. *Rev Port Cardiol* **27**(9): 1011–1025.

Merchant, T., Janosevic, D., Jayam, M., Kadiyala, M., Pollack, S., Cao, J. J., and Reichek, N. (2014). Myocardial contractility indices based on strain imaging. *J Cardiovasc Magn Reson* **16**(Suppl 1): P333.

Merchant, T., Reichek, N., Barasch, E., Kadiyala, M., Jayam, M., Pollack, S., Cao, J. J., and Young, A. A. (2015). Myocardial contractility and afterload in aortic stenosis. *J Cardiovasc Magn Reson* **17**(Suppl 1): P371.

Meyer, C. G., Frick, M., Lotfi, S., Altiok, E., Koos, R., Kirschfink, A., Lehrke, M., Autschbach, R., and Hoffmann, R. (2014). Regional left ventricular function after transapical vs. transfemoral transcatheter aortic valve implantation analysed by cardiac magnetic resonance feature tracking. *Eur Heart J Cardiovasc Imaging* **15**(10): 1168–1176.

Miszalski-Jamka, T., Szczeklik, W., Sokolowska, B., Karwat, K., Belzak, K., Mazur, W., Kereiakes, D. J., and Musial, J. (2013). Standard and feature tracking magnetic resonance evidence of myocardial involvement in Churg-Strauss syndrome and granulomatosis with polyangiitis (Wegener's) in patients with normal electrocardiograms and transthoracic echocardiography. *Int J Cardiovasc Imaging* **29**(4): 843–853.

Mondillo, S., Galderisi, M., Mele, D., Cameli, M., Lomoriello, V. S., Zaca, V., Ballo, P. et al. (2011). Speckle-tracking echocardiography: A new technique for assessing myocardial function. *J Ultrasound Med* **30**(1): 71–83.

Moody, W. E., Taylor, R. J., Edwards, N. C., Chue, C. D., Umar, F., Taylor, T. J., Ferro, C. J. et al. (2015). Comparison of magnetic resonance feature tracking for systolic and diastolic strain and strain rate calculation with spatial modulation of magnetization imaging analysis. *J Magn Reson Imaging* **41**(4): 1000–1012.

Moon, T. J., Choueiter, N., Geva, T., Valente, A. M., Gauvreau, K., and Harrild, D. M. (2015). Relation of biventricular strain and dyssynchrony in repaired tetralogy of fallot measured by cardiac magnetic resonance to death and sustained ventricular tachycardia. *Am J Cardiol* **115**(5): 676–680.

Morton, G., Schuster, A., Jogiya, R., Kutty, S., Beerbaum, P., and Nagel, E. (2012). Inter-study reproducibility of cardiovascular magnetic resonance myocardial feature tracking. *J Cardiovasc Magn Reson* **14**: 43.

Muthukumar, L., Duncanson, L. J., Schapiro, W., McLaughlin, J., Young, A. A., and Cao, J. J. (2015). Association of reduced right ventricular global and regional wall motion with abnormal right heart hemodynamics. *J Cardiovasc Magn Reson* **17**(Suppl 1): P317.

Notomi, Y., Lysyansky, P., Setser, R. M., Shiota, T., Popovic, Z. B., Martin-Miklovic, M. G., Weaver, J. A. et al. (2005). Measurement of ventricular torsion by two-dimensional ultrasound speckle tracking imaging. *J Am Coll Cardiol* **45**(12): 2034–2041.

Ochs, A., Schuster, A., Riffel, J., Duchting, J., Thome, S., Andre, F., Seitz, S. et al. (2015). LV rotational mechanics in patients with dilated cardiomyopathy compared to healthy individuals: Experience from the European CMR Registry. *J Cardiovasc Magn Reson* **17**(Suppl 1): Q69.

Ohyama, Y., Ambale-Venkatesh, B., Chamera, E., Shehata, M. L., Corona-Villalobos, C. P., Zimmerman, S. L., Hassoun, P. M., Bluemke, D. A., and Lima, J. A. (2015). Comparison of strain measurement from multimodality tissue tracking with strain-encoding MRI and harmonic phase MRI in pulmonary hypertension. *Int J Cardiol* **182**: 342–348.

Onishi, T., Saha, S. K., Delgado-Montero, A., Ludwig, D. R., Onishi, T., Schelbert, E. B., Schwartzman, D., and Gorcsan, J., 3rd (2015). Global longitudinal strain and global circumferential strain by speckle-tracking echocardiography and feature-tracking cardiac magnetic resonance imaging: Comparison with left ventricular ejection fraction. *J Am Soc Echocardiogr* **28**(5): 587–596.

Onishi, T., Saha, S. K., Ludwig, D., Onishi, T., Ahmed, M., Marek, J., Schwartzman, D., and Gorcsan, J. (2011). The utility of novel off-line approach to quantify dyssynchrony from routine cardiac magnetic resonance images: Comparison with echocardiographic speckle tracking. *Proc Am Coll Cardiol* 1086.

Onishi, T., Saha, S. K., Ludwig, D. R., Onishi, T., Marek, J. J., Cavalcante, J. L., Schelbert, E. B., Schwartzman, D., and Gorcsan, J., 3rd (2013). Feature tracking measurement of dyssynchrony from cardiovascular magnetic resonance cine acquisitions: Comparison with echocardiographic speckle tracking. *J Cardiovasc Magn Reson* **15**: 95.

Ortega, M., Triedman, J. K., Geva, T., and Harrild, D. M. (2011). Relation of left ventricular dyssynchrony measured by cardiac magnetic resonance tissue tracking in repaired tetralogy of fallot to ventricular tachycardia and death. *Am J Cardiol* **107**(10): 1535–1540.

Orwat, S., Kempny, A., Diller, G. P., Bauerschmitz, P., Bunck, A., Maintz, D., Radke, R. M., and Baumgartner, H. (2014). Cardiac magnetic resonance feature tracking—A novel method to assess myocardial strain: Comparison with echocardiographic speckle tracking in healthy volunteers and in patients with left ventricular hypertrophy. *Kardiol Pol* **72**(4): 363–371.

Padiyath, A., Gribben, P., Abraham, J. R., Li, L., Rangamani, S., Schuster, A., Danford, D. A., Pedrizzetti, G., and Kutty, S. (2013). Echocardiography and cardiac magnetic resonance-based feature tracking in the assessment of myocardial mechanics in tetralogy of Fallot: An intermodality comparison. *Echocardiography* **30**(2): 203–210.

Park, J. H., Kusunose, K., Motoki, H., Kwon, D. H., Grimm, R. A., Griffin, B. P., Marwick, T. H., and Popovic, Z. B. (2015). Assessment of right ventricular longitudinal strain in patients with ischemic cardiomyopathy: Head-to-head comparison between two-dimensional speckle-based strain and velocity vector imaging using volumetric assessment by cardiac magnetic resonance as a "Gold Standard". *Echocardiography* **32**(6): 956–965.

Pavlopoulos, H. and Nihoyannopoulos, P. (2008). Strain and strain rate deformation parameters: From tissue Doppler to 2D speckle tracking. *Int J Cardiovasc Imaging* **24**(5): 479–491.

Peters, D. C., Cornfeld, D., Sinusas, A. J., Duncan, J. S., Papademetris, X., Grunseich, K., and Chelikani, S. (2015). Left atrial strain is correlated to atrial fibrosis by late gadolinium enhancement, in an AF population. *Proceedings of the International Society for Magnetic Resonance*, Toronto, Ontario, Canada, p. 4469.

Pirat, B., Khoury, D. S., Hartley, C. J., Tiller, L., Rao, L., Schulz, D. G., Nagueh, S. F., and Zoghbi, W. A. (2008). A novel feature-tracking echocardiographic method for the quantitation of regional myocardial function: Validation in an animal model of ischemia-reperfusion. *J Am Coll Cardiol* **51**(6): 651–659.

Pirat, B., McCulloch, M. L., and Zoghbi, W. A. (2006). Evaluation of global and regional right ventricular systolic function in patients with pulmonary hypertension using a novel speckle tracking method. *Am J Cardiol* **98**(5): 699–704.

Raman, F. S., Tee, M., Vigneault, D., Liu, S., and Bluemke, D. A. (2014). Multimodality tissue tracking algorithm of myocardial strain: Initial validation with tagged MRI. *Proceedings of the International Society for Magnetic Resonance*, Milan, Italy, p. 3949.

Reisner, S. A., Lysyansky, P., Agmon, Y., Mutlak, D., Lessick, J., and Friedman, Z. (2004). Global longitudinal strain: A novel index of left ventricular systolic function. *J Am Soc Echocardiogr* **17**(6): 630–633.

Remme, E. W., Augenstein, K. F., Young, A. A., and Hunter, P. J. (2005). Parameter distribution models for estimation of population based left ventricular deformation using sparse fiducial markers. *IEEE Trans Med Imaging* **24**(3): 381–388.

Roes, S. D., Mollema, S. A., Lamb, H. J., van der Wall, E. E., de Roos, A., and Bax, J. J. (2009). Validation of echocardiographic two-dimensional speckle tracking longitudinal strain imaging for viability assessment in patients with chronic ischemic left ventricular dysfunction and comparison with contrast-enhanced magnetic resonance imaging. *Am J Cardiol* **104**(3): 312–317.

Ryan, T. D., Taylor, M. D., Mazur, W., Cripe, L. H., Pratt, J., King, E. C., Lao, K. et al. (2013). Abnormal circumferential strain is present in young Duchenne muscular dystrophy patients. *Pediatr Cardiol* **34**(5): 1159–1165.

Schmidt, R., Orwat, S., Kempny, A., Schuler, P., Radke, R., Kahr, P. C., Hellige, A., Baumgartner, H., and Diller, G. P. (2014). Value of speckle-tracking echocardiography and MRI-based feature tracking analysis in adult patients after Fontan-type palliation. *Congenit Heart Dis* **9**(5): 397–406.

Schneeweis, C., Doltra, A., Nasser, S. B., Hassel, J., Grafe, M., Wellnhofer, E., Schnackenburg, B. et al. (2015). Intraindividual comparison of circumferential strain using speckle tracking by echocardiography versus CMR feature tracking and myocardial tagging in patients. *J Cardiovasc Magn Reson* **17**(Suppl 1): P340.

Schneeweis, C., Schnackenburg, B., Berger, A., Kelle, S., Fleck, E., and Gebker, R. (2014). Value of strain analysis with feature tracking in adenosine stress myocardial perfusion magnetic resonance imaging. *J Cardiovasc Magn Reson* **16**(Suppl 1): P193.

Schuster, A., Kutty, S., Padiyath, A., Parish, V., Gribben, P., Danford, D. A., Makowski, M. R., Bigalke, B., Beerbaum, P., and Nagel, E. (2011). Cardiovascular magnetic resonance myocardial feature tracking detects quantitative wall motion during dobutamine stress. *J Cardiovasc Magn Reson* **13**: 58.

Schuster, A., Morton, G., Hussain, S. T., Jogiya, R., Kutty, S., Asrress, K. N., Makowski, M. R. et al. (2013a). The intraobserver reproducibility of cardiovascular magnetic resonance myocardial feature tracking strain assessment is independent of field strength. *Eur J Radiol* **82**(2): 296–301.

Schuster, A. and Nagel, E. (2011). Toward full quantification of wall motion with MRI. *Curr Cardiovasc Imaging Rep* **4**: 85–86.

Schuster, A., Paul, M., Bettencourt, N., Hussain, S. T., Morton, G., Kutty, S., Bigalke, B. et al. (2015). Myocardial feature tracking reduces observer-dependence in low-dose dobutamine stress cardiovascular magnetic resonance. *PLoS One* **10**(4): e0122858.

Schuster, A., Paul, M., Bettencourt, N., Morton, G., Chiribiri, A., Ishida, M., Hussain, S. et al. (2013b). Cardiovascular magnetic resonance myocardial feature tracking for quantitative viability assessment in ischemic cardiomyopathy. *Int J Cardiol* **166**(2): 413–420.

Shafi, N. A., Bertman, K., Yoon, A., Toole, R., Ronin, M., Pollack, S., Reichek, N., and Kadiyala, M. (2011). Quantitative assessment of global and regional strain in relation to infarct size in patients with myocardial infarction. *J Cardiovasc Magn Reson* P131.

Shang, Q., Kutty, S., Danford, D., Steinmetz, M., Schuster, A., Kuehne, T., Beerbaum, P., and Sarikouch, S. (2015). Myocardial deformation assessed by longitudinal strain: Chamber-specific normative data for CMR-feature tracking from the German competence network for congenital heart defects. *J Cardiovasc Magn Reson* **17**(Suppl 1): P202.

Singh, A. (1992). *Optic Flow Computation: A Unified Perspective.* IEEE Computer Society Press, Los Alamitos, CA.

Sjoli, B., Orn, S., Grenne, B., Ihlen, H., Edvardsen, T., and Brunvand, H. (2009). Diagnostic capability and reproducibility of strain by Doppler and by speckle tracking in patients with acute myocardial infarction. *JACC Cardiovasc Imaging* **2**(1): 24–33.

Stefani, L., De Luca, A., Maffulli, N., Mercuri, R., Innocenti, G., Suliman, I., Toncelli, L. et al. (2009a). Speckle tracking for left ventricle performance in young athletes with bicuspid aortic valve and mild aortic regurgitation. *Eur J Echocardiogr* **10**(4): 527–531.

Stefani, L., Pedrizzetti, G., De Luca, A., Mercuri, R., Innocenti, G., and Galanti, G. (2009b). Real-time evaluation of longitudinal peak systolic strain (speckle tracking measurement) in left and right ventricles of athletes. *Cardiovasc Ultrasound* **7**: 17.

Szczeklik, W., Miszalski-Jamka, T., Mastalerz, L., Sokolowska, B., Dropinski, J., Banys, R., Hor, K. N., Mazur, W., and Musial, J. (2011). Multimodality assessment of cardiac involvement in Churg-Strauss syndrome patients in clinical remission. *Circ J* **75**(3): 649–655.

Takeuchi, M., Nishikage, T., Nakai, H., Kokumai, M., Otani, S., and Lang, R. M. (2007). The assessment of left ventricular twist in anterior wall myocardial infarction using two-dimensional speckle tracking imaging. *J Am Soc Echocardiogr* **20**(1): 36–44.

Taylor, R. J., Moody, W. E., Umar, F., Edwards, N. C., Taylor, T. J., Stegemann, B., Townend, J. N. et al. (2015). Myocardial strain measurement with feature-tracking cardiovascular magnetic resonance: Normal values. *Eur Heart J Cardiovasc Imaging* **16**(8): 871–881.

Taylor, R. J., Umar, F., Lin, L. S., Ahmed, A., Moody, W. E., Stegemann, B., Townend, J. N., Steeds, R. P., and Leyva, F. (2014a). Mechanical effects of midwall fibrosis in non-ischemic dilated cardiomyopathy. *J Cardiovasc Magn Reson* **16**(Suppl 1): P308.

Taylor, R. J., Umar, F., Moody, W. E., Meyyappan, C., Stegemann, B., Townend, J. N., Hor, K. N. et al. (2014b). Feature-tracking cardiovascular magnetic resonance as a novel technique for the assessment of mechanical dyssynchrony. *Int J Cardiol* **175**(1): 120–125.

Thattaliyath, B. D., Forsha, D. E., Stewart, C., Barker, P. C., and Campbell, M. J. (2015). Evaluation of right ventricular myocardial mechanics using velocity vector imaging of cardiac MRI cine images in transposition of the great arteries following atrial and arterial switch operations. *Congenit Heart Dis* **10**(4): 371–379.

Tops, L. F., Delgado, V., and Bax, J. J. (2009). The role of speckle tracking strain imaging in cardiac pacing. *Echocardiography* **26**(3): 315–323.

Truong, U. T., Li, X., Broberg, C. S., Houle, H., Schaal, M., Ashraf, M., Kilner, P. et al. (2010). Significance of mechanical alterations in single ventricle patients on twisting and circumferential strain as determined by analysis of strain from gradient cine magnetic resonance imaging sequences. *Am J Cardiol* **105**(10): 1465–1469.

Tugcu, A., Yildirimturk, O., Tayyareci, Y., Demiroglu, C., and Aytekin, S. (2010). Evaluation of subclinical right ventricular dysfunction in obstructive sleep apnea patients using velocity vector imaging. *Circ J* **74**(2): 312–319.

Vannan, M. A., Pedrizzetti, G., Li, P., Gurudevan, S., Houle, H., Main, J., Jackson, J., and Nanda, N. C. (2005). Effect of cardiac resynchronization therapy on longitudinal and circumferential left ventricular mechanics by velocity vector imaging: Description and initial clinical application of a novel method using high-frame rate B-mode echocardiographic images. *Echocardiography* **22**(10): 826–830.

Weigand, J. D., Nielsen, J., Sengupta, P., Sanz, J., Srivastava, S., and Uppu, S. (2015). Feature tracking derived longitudinal and circumferential myocardial strain abnormalities in clinical myocarditis. *J Cardiovasc Magn Reson* **17**(Suppl 1): P321.

Willert, C. E. and Gharib, M. (1991). Digital particle image velocimetry. *Exp Fluids* **10**: 181–193.

Williams, L. K., Urbano-Moral, J. A., Rowin, E. J., Jamorski, M., Bruchal-Garbicz, B., Carasso, S., Pandian, N. G., Maron, M. S., and Rakowski, H. (2013). Velocity vector imaging in the measurement of left ventricular myocardial mechanics on cardiac magnetic resonance imaging: Correlations with echocardiographically derived strain values. *J Am Soc Echocardiogr* **26**(10): 1153–1162.

Wu, L., Germans, T., Guclu, A., Heymans, M. W., Allaart, C. P., and van Rossum, A. C. (2014). Feature tracking compared with tissue tagging measurements of segmental strain by cardiovascular magnetic resonance. *J Cardiovasc Magn Reson* **16**(1): 10.

Yang, Z. R., Zhou, Q. C., Lee, L., Zou, L., Zeng, S., Tan, Y., and Cao, D. M. (2012). Quantitative assessment of left ventricular systolic function in patients with coronary heart disease by velocity vector imaging. *Echocardiography* **29**(3): 340–345.

Zuern, C. S., Krumm, P., Wurster, T., Kramer, U., Schreieck, J., Henning, A., Bauer, A., Gawaz, M., and May, A. E. (2013). Reverse left ventricular remodeling after percutaneous mitral valve repair: Strain analysis by speckle tracking echocardiography and cardiac magnetic resonance imaging. *Int J Cardiol* **168**(5): 4983–4985.

9 Heart Mechanics
From Implanted Markers to Magnetic Resonance Imaging Tagging

El-Sayed H. Ibrahim, PhD, Andreas Sigfridsson, PhD;
and John-Peder E. Kvitting, MD, PhD

CONTENTS

LIST OF ABBREVIATIONS

Abbreviation	Meaning
2D	Two dimensional
3D	Three dimensional
ASD	Atrial septal defect
CABG	Coronary artery bypass grafting
CRT	Cardiac resynchronization therapy
DANTE	Delay alternating with nutation for tailored excitation
ECG	Electrocardiogram
HARP	Harmonic phase
LAD	Left anterior descending
LAX	Long axis
LV	Left ventricle
LVAD	LV assist device
PH	Pulmonary hypertension
RF	Radio frequency
RV	Right ventricle
SAR	Specific absorption rate
SAX	Short axis
SNR	Signal-to-noise ratio
SPAMM	Spatial modulation of magnetization
TD	Tagging-to-imaging delay
TOF	Tetralogy of Fallot

9.1 INTRODUCTION

9.1.1 COMPLEX NATURE OF MYOCARDIAL DEFORMATION: ASSESSMENT BY INVASIVE AND NONINVASIVE TECHNIQUES

A solid understanding of cardiac mechanics is fundamental to comprehend the normal myocardial contractility pattern, alterations caused by different heart diseases, and potential impact of different medical, catheter-based, or surgical treatments (Buckberg et al. 2004). The heterogeneous three-dimensional (3D) nature of the heart motion has always made analysis of the cardiac function an intricate task (Buckberg et al. 2008). The myocardial deformation tensor has three motion components, nine deformation gradients, and six strains (see Chapter 6 for a detailed coverage of mathematical formulations of heart mechanics). This inherent complexity combined with regional myocardial dysfunction, for example, in the setting of ischemic heart disease, leads to daunting cardiac function analysis. Furthermore, any cardiac imaging modality quantifying regional myocardial function should have the ability to track the same tissue material throughout the cardiac cycle.

In current clinical practice, noninvasive imaging modalities such as echocardiography, myocardial perfusion scintigraphy, and magnetic resonance imaging (MRI) dominate the field for assessment of regional heart function. However, prior to their development, surgically implanted markers provided much of the fundamental knowledge we have today about myocardial motion and deformation. Albeit inherently invasive in nature, surgically implanted markers remain a valuable tool in experimental animal models providing the capability for precise tracking of fiducial markers for quantification of myocardial mechanics and heart valve function. Further, these techniques provide the gold standard against which new noninvasive technique can be validated.

9.1.2 CHAPTER OUTLINE

This chapter outlines the early stages of using surgically implanted markers (radiopaque markers and sonomicrometric crystals) for studying myocardial function, leading up to the seminal paper in October 1988 by Elias Zerhouni from Johns Hopkins University, which introduced myocardial tagging as a noninvasive method for assessing myocardial motion (Zerhouni et al. 1988). The chapter starts by providing a historical background about invasive techniques for evaluating myocardial deformation. The radiopaque markers and sonomicrometry techniques are then discussed in details, starting with implantation procedures and practical considerations, and followed by experimental and clinical applications of both techniques. The next sections in the chapter discuss limitations of the marker implantation-based techniques and their roles in the current era. The original tagging technique developed by Zerhouni et al. (1988) is then discussed in detail, starting with the technique's basic principles, and followed by the magnetization behavior in different cases of the technique's implementation. The technique's technical developments, validation, and applications are then discussed. The chapter concludes by discussing the limitations of this original tagging technique and briefly comparing it to two famous tagging techniques that appeared shortly after: spatial modulation of magnetization (SPAMM) and delay alternating with nutation for tailored excitation (DANTE), which are covered in details in Chapter 10.

9.2 HISTORICAL BACKGROUND OF INVASIVE TECHNIQUES FOR ASSESSING MYOCARDIAL FUNCTION

Prior to the introduction of surgically implanted markers, most data about cardiac physiology were obtained from open-chest animals and isolated perfused hearts (Langendorff hearts). The acute nature of these experiments and the need for anesthesia might have blunted normal physiological reaction in the studied animals and limited the translational value of these findings to humans.

In 1967, Carlsson and Milne (1967) were the first to describe permanent tantalum screws implantation into the endocardium for subsequent functional studies of heart mechanics. These screws were implanted through cardiac catheterization without opening the chest of the animals. Prior to this, Hamilton and Rompf (1932) sutured metal markers to the surface of the heart in a canine model and quantified

their movement with fluoroscopy. Rushmer et al. (1953) used a similar approach to study segmental ventricular contractions in a canine experiment in 1953. Most of the data presented in the early literature described individual markers movement at different locations in the heart, where the results showed that the movement is very consistent in any particular animal. Postmortem examination of dogs was performed by Rushmer et al. (1953), who showed a thin layer of connective tissue covering the stainless steel markers, indicating that the markers could be used for long-term follow-up studies. In 1956, Ellis et al. (1956) introduced the use of sonomicrometers for studying the left ventricular (LV) dimensions by measuring the transit time of the sound waves between two crystals sutured to the surface of the LV.

Apart from biplane cineradiography of implanted tantalum screws, other surgically implanted techniques for assessing regional myocardial function include (Table 9.1) sonomicrometry (LeWinter et al. 1975, Rankin et al. 1976, Sasayama et al. 1976a, Sabbah et al. 1981, Gallagher et al. 1982, 1984, 1985a,b, Freeman et al. 1985, Aversano et al. 1986, Fujita et al. 1989a,b), radio-frequency (RF) coils attached to the epicardial surface (Arts et al. 1982), and ultrasonic echo measurements of myocardial sutures (Myers et al. 1986). Epicardial deformation has been also studied using electromagnetic induction coils (Arts and Reneman 1980, Arts et al. 1982), where data models of the LV mechanics can be verified based on the epicardial deformation.

Although the literature about cardiac surgical markers is quite extensive, the following sections outline some of the most important findings in this field and provide a thorough

---

TABLE 9.1
Invasive Techniques for Assessment of Regional Myocardial Function

Biplane cineradiography of radiopaque markers

Pros

An entirely implantable method allowing for long-term follow-up

High spatial and temporal resolutions

Endovascular implantation possible

Cons

Need for ionizing radiation

Difficulty in differentiating close-by individual markers

Makers possibly affecting the response of the myocardium

Sonomicrometry (i.e., ultrasonic crystals)

Pros

Simultaneous volume and regional myocardial function measurements

High spatial and temporal resolutions

Excellent method for validating the accuracy of noninvasive modalities

Cons

Need for invasive surgery to implant the crystals

Need for exteriorizing the leads, thus impeding long-term follow-up

Leads and crystals possibly affecting the response of the myocardium

Miscellaneous techniques

Electromagnetic induction coils

Ultrasonic echo measurements of myocardial sutures

overview of the two most commonly used techniques: radiopaque markers and sonomicrometric crystals.

9.3 RADIOPAQUE MARKERS

9.3.1 GENERAL OVERVIEW

Several groups worked extensively with surgically implanted radiopaque markers to quantify regional myocardial deformation. The radiopaque markers allow for instantaneous determination of the LV size, shape, and volume in the intact heart in both physiological and pathophysiological studies (Harrison et al. 1963, Carlsson 1969, Mitchell et al. 1969, Wildenthal and Mitchell 1969, McDonald 1970, Ingels et al. 1971, Sandler and Alderman 1974, Vine et al. 1976, Shoukas et al. 1981). The radiopaque markers used in different experimental and human studies are in the form of clips, beads, or screws. The early studies provided information about the intact beating heart to confirm the physiological theories associated with the Frank–Starling mechanism and Laplace's law (Sandler and Alderman 1974). In this respect, the surgically implanted markers enabled tracking a well-defined, albeit limited, number of points of interest in the myocardium, which are time resolved in the Lagrangian coordinate system (Fenton et al. 1978, Shoukas et al. 1981, Walley et al. 1982). An important advantage of biplane cinefluroscopic tracking of the surgically implanted markers is the ability to study the intact unanesthetized animal over a prolonged period of time.

9.3.2 IMPLANTATION TECHNIQUE AND TECHNICAL DATA

9.3.2.1 Marker Types

The surgically implanted radiopaque markers used in most experimental animal studies, as well as some of the human studies, are close-winded turns of a metallurgical grade tantalum wire, as shown in Figure 9.1.

The markers are made of tantalum as this material is known to be nonreactive, and a thin capsule of connective tissue usually covers the screws with time after implantation. Specific tails on the markers facilitate their subsequent identification in the fluoroscopic images (Castro et al. 1993). In the studies performed by Ingels et al. (1975), the markers used measured 0.85 mm × 1.5 mm. The tantalum screws are mounted on an insertor tool, allowing for precise insertion of the screws into the myocardium at a depth of approximately 5 mm. In more recent marker investigations, the depth of the myocardium has been assessed with the help of echocardiography to guide the insertion. The insertor is placed perpendicular to the area of interest and the screw is implanted such that when the insertor is retracted, the screw remains in place (Figure 9.2a). An example of the insertor used in the early clinical studies at Stanford University is shown in Figure 9.2b. The coronary arteries are used as landmarks to ensure consistent placement of the markers.

The use of stainless steel balls implanted on the endocardial, midwall, and epicardial surfaces of the heart has been also reported in the literature (Shoukas et al. 1981). Three

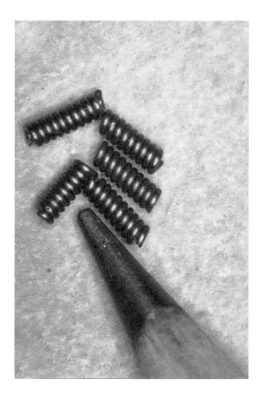

FIGURE 9.1 Tantalum markers. For size relationship, the markers are placed next to a pencil. (Image courtesy of Neil B. Ingels and D. Craig Miller, Department of Thoracic and Cardiovascular Surgery, Stanford University, Stanford, CA.)

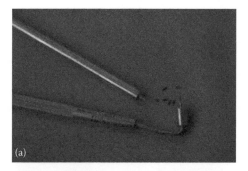

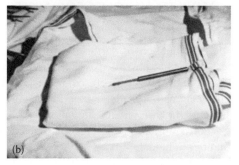

FIGURE 9.2 Marker insertion tool and markers. (a) The marker insertion tool together with a sample of tantalum markers. (b) The insertor used in the early clinical studies conducted at Stanford University. (Images courtesy of Neil B. Ingels and D. Craig Miller, Department of Thoracic and Cardiovascular Surgery, Stanford University, Stanford, CA.)

different sizes of 1.1906, 1.000, and 0.7938 mm have been used for easy identification of the markers on subsequent fluoroscopic images. This particular approach allowed the insertion of a large number of markers (>100 steel balls) into the heart (Garrison et al. 1982). A small capsule, measuring one-tenth of the ball diameter, has been seen 4 months after implantation, where the myocardial fibers seemed to be separated, but not cut or torn (Shoukas et al. 1981).

9.3.2.2 Practical Considerations

The distribution of the radiopaque markers usually outlines the LV, covering the apex and three short-axis (SAX) planes along the anterolateral and inferior margins of the ventricle, as shown in Figure 9.3. Based on the markers' placement, different measurements can be obtained, for example, ventricular dimensions, percentage shortening, and radius of curvature.

The markers outlining the LV provide a cine ventriculogram without the need to administer an intravenous contrast agent. The LV volumes assessed by angiography and implanted markers showed good correlation (Ingels et al. 1977). In both animals and humans, great care should be taken not to implant the markers into any visible branches of the coronary artery system (Figure 9.4).

The accuracy of the surgically implanted marker technique is very high with error of repeated measurements in the range of 1%, error of the measured lengths of about 2.7%, and reproducibility error of the measured lengths in the range of 0.04 cm (Ingels et al. 1975). These excellent numbers make the surgically implanted marker technique unique for detecting subtle changes in the myocardial function, and despite advances in noninvasive imaging modalities, this level of accuracy is difficult to match.

9.3.3 EXPERIMENTAL STUDIES USING RADIOPAQUE MARKERS

9.3.3.1 Animal Preparation

The animal experiments are usually performed in a fully equipped operating room with sterile conditions if the experiment is meant for permanent implantation. Figure 9.5 shows an intraoperative image of the surgeon inserting the markers into a canine cardiac transplant.

For in vivo studies, the implantation of the radiopaque markers is usually performed through a left thoracotomy at the fifth intercostal space, where the heart is suspended in a pericardial cradle (Fann et al. 1991). The depth of the myocardial wall is assessed using either a syringe or epicardial echocardiography. If no additional markers are to be implanted on the mitral or aortic valves, then there is no need for cardiopulmonary bypass to implant the LV markers. The animals usually have a fluid-filled pressure catheter placed via the carotid artery to measure instantaneous aortic or LV pressure, combined with a surface electrocardiogram (ECG). In some studies, the chest is closed with the placement of chest tubes, while in other studies the animal is transported with an open chest to the catheterization laboratory. For transmural bead

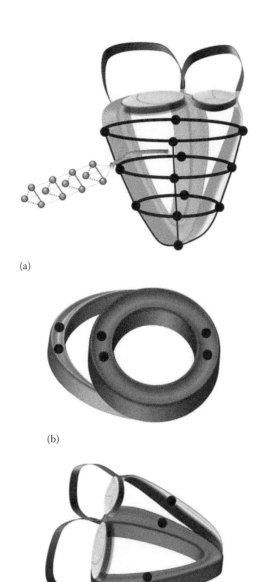

(a)

(b)

(c)

FIGURE 9.3 Markers' placement and measurements derivation. (a) Schematic representation of three short-axis (SAX) planes and an apical point outlining the left ventricle. The figure shows an example of an anterior-septal bead set consisting of four levels of transmural beads. (b) Circumferential and radial displacements as well as the radius of curvature are calculated from the markers in a SAX view. (c) Longitudinal displacement is calculated from the markers in a long-axis view. (Courtesy of Dr. Shehab Anwar, National Heart Institute, Cairo, Egypt.)

implantation, a stabilizing device is used to lock into the surface of the heart and ensure precise insertion of the markers, as shown in Figure 9.6a, b, and c (Cheng et al. 2005).

9.3.3.2 Biplane Imaging

After implantation of the markers, the animals are transported, in a supine position, to the catheterization laboratory for imaging of the markers (or bead columns) using biplane videofluoroscopy, usually at a sampling rate of 60 Hz, giving a

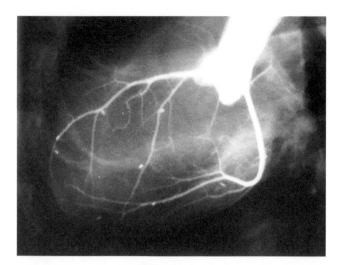

FIGURE 9.4 Fluoroscopic image of the tantalum markers in a human subject. Contrast agent is injected in the aortic root to help visualize the coronary arteries. (Image courtesy of Neil B. Ingels and D. Craig Miller, Department of Thoracic and Cardiovascular Surgery, Stanford University, Stanford, CA.)

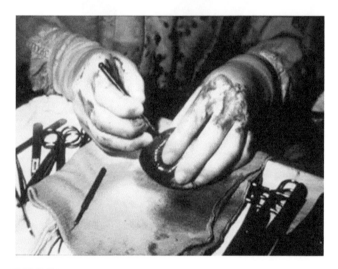

FIGURE 9.5 A surgeon inserting the markers into a canine cardiac transplant. (Image courtesy of Neil B. Ingels and D. Craig Miller, Department of Thoracic and Cardiovascular Surgery, Stanford University, Stanford, CA.)

temporal resolution of 16.7 ms (Figure 9.7a and b). The images are usually acquired at 45° right anterior oblique and 45° left anterior oblique projections to facilitate the separation of the individual implanted markers. The videofluoroscopic images are recorded on a videotape and synchronized with the x-ray pulses (Figure 9.8). In recent marker studies, a complete digital setup replaced this analog interface. In most studies, the experiments end with imaging a radiographic phantom with known markers locations (Daughters et al. 1988). At the end of the animal experiments (acute or chronic), the animal is sacrificed, the heart is explanted, and the positions of the markers are verified.

9.3.3.3 Image Processing and Data Analysis

Most research groups use semiautomated image processing and digitization software to obtain 3D Lagrangian

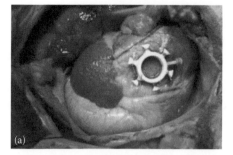

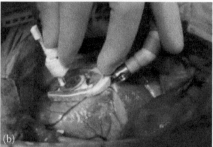

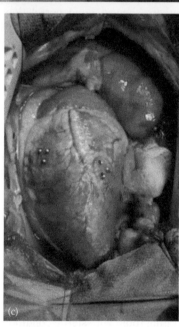

FIGURE 9.6 Markers insertion with a stabilizing device. (a) Prior to insertion of the transmural bead set, a stabilizing device is sewn to the surface of the heart. (b) Using a commercial stabilizing device used in off-pump coronary artery bypass surgery (Octopus Tissue Stabilizer, Medtronic, Minneapolis, MN), the bead set is inserted into the myocardium at predefined levels. (c) An intraoperative view of the locations of the transmural bead set after insertion (in this case in the anterior basal and lateral equatorial parts of the left ventricle). Note that the epicardial bead markers are larger than the markers inserted into the myocardium. (Images courtesy of Neil B. Ingels and D. Craig Miller, Department of Thoracic and Cardiovascular Surgery, Stanford University, Stanford, CA.)

coordinates from the biplane images averaged over several heart beats (Niczyporuk and Miller 1991). Davis et al. (1980) at University of California, San Francisco, described a method for determining the shadows of the markers on the x-ray images, thus facilitating identification of the markers

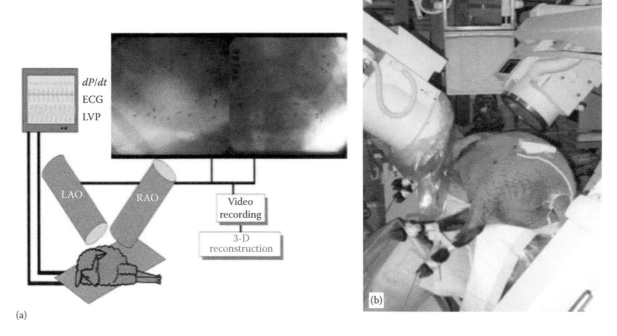

(a)

(b)

FIGURE 9.7 Image acquisition of implanted markers. (a) Schematic drawing of the setup in the catheterization laboratory with simultaneous recording of electrocardiogram and pressure indices during the acquisition of the marker data. Two-dimensional images from each view are digitized from the video recordings and combined to obtain 3D Lagrangian marker coordinates. (b) A sheep in the lateral decubitus position during an acute open-chest experiment on the x-ray table prior to acquisition of the marker data. *dP/dt*, pressure change with time; ECG, electrocardiogram; LAO, left anterior oblique; LVP, LV pressure; RAO, right anterior oblique. (Image courtesy of Tom C. Nguyen, Stanford University, Stanford, CA.)

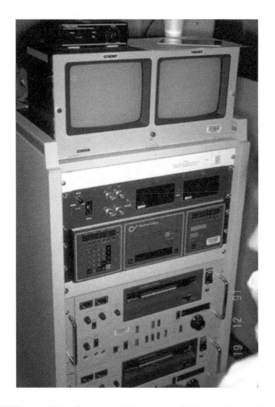

FIGURE 9.8 Videofluoroscopic image acquisition and recording. The analog system of a videotape recorder, on which the videofluoroscopic images are recorded and synchronized with the x-ray pulses. (Image courtesy of Neil B. Ingels and D. Craig Miller, Department of Thoracic and Cardiovascular Surgery, Stanford University, Stanford, CA.)

in the biplane radiographs, and consequently estimating the 3D marker coordinates. The markers are usually placed in front of each film plane to provide a reference to the local XYZ-coordinates system (Davis et al. 1980, Garrison et al. 1982). The data from the Stanford group showed an accuracy of 0.1 ± 0.3 mm for 3D displacement reconstruction (Niczyporuk and Miller 1991), and Garrison et al. (1982) from Johns Hopkins University found a root-mean-square measurement error of 0.07 mm in the X- and Y-directions and 0.05 mm in the Z-direction. In the animal experiments, continuous LV and aortic pressures obtained from micro-manometers allow for relating the data from the markers to the pressure data in different filling states by increasing or decreasing the loading level (often done with balloon occlusion of the inferior vena cava).

9.3.3.4 Myocardial Structure Based on Implanted Markers

Details about the myocardial fiber architecture and its relationship to the heart function became available by studying the transmural myocardial deformation based on multiple layers of surgically implanted beads (Waldman et al. 1985, 1988). The studies by Waldman et al. (1985, 1988) provided unique data reflecting the nonhomogeneous contraction of the myocardium both in normal state and during ischemia. The results described the myocardial fiber orientation that smoothly ranges from a left-handed helix in the epicardial layers to a right-handed helix in the endocardial layers

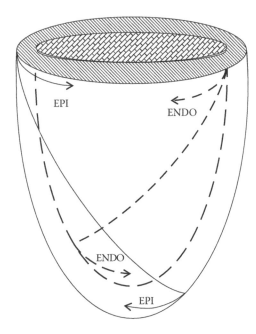

FIGURE 9.9 Schematic of the helical myocardial fiber structure. The figure shows the spiral nature of the myocardial fibers ranging from a left-handed helix (solid line) in the epicardial layers smoothly to a right-handed helix (dashed line) in the endocardial layers. The midwall fibers are circumferentially aligned. ENDO, endocardium; EPI, epicardium.

through circumferentially aligned midwall fibers (Streeter et al. 1969, Greenbaum et al. 1981, Torrent-Guasp et al. 2005), as shown in Figure 9.9. The spiral nature of the myocardial fibers (i.e., their pitch angle) can virtually create any amount of ejection fraction despite an individual fiber shortening of only 15% (Sallin 1969, Ingels 1997). A detailed coverage of the heart microstructure is provided in Chapter 5. The results from marker studies on animal models provided an important insight into how sarcomere shortening translates into the macro level of wall thickening, circumferential shortening, and longitudinal shortening. The dense bead column arrays used in marker studies allow for detailed description and quantification of the fibers' orientation and function (Ashikaga et al. 2004a,c, Harrington et al. 2005). The cine radiography of these bead columns has an excellent spatial resolution of 0.15 mm (Cheng et al. 2006).

9.3.3.5 Applications

The role of LV torsion has been studied in tachycardia-induced cardiomyopathy in an experimental ovine model, showing decreased torsion peak and abolished early-diastolic recoil (Tibayan et al. 2002). These data form the basis for subsequent torsion studies using MRI or echocardiography in patients with cardiomyopathy. The effect of mitral valve replacement on LV torsion has been studied in an experimental animal model, showing that resecting the subvalvular apparatus at the time of valve replacement affects the LV systolic function (DeAnda et al. 1994, 1995).

Meier et al. (1980) implanted radiopaque markers in different regions of the right ventricle (RV): free wall, apex,

midventricle, and outflow tract, where the results showed a contraction sequence beginning at the apex and ending at the conus. A similar contraction pattern has been observed in pigs based on implanted endocardial marker pairs in the LV free wall (Heikkila et al. 1972). The RV function has been studied at the time of LV assist device (LVAD) implantation in closed-chest dogs, showing impaired RV contractility due to a leftward shift of the interventricular septum (Moon et al. 1997a,b). The RV cardiac output can be maintained in the LVAD experiment by reducing the RV afterload, which results in concomitant increase in the RV preload (Moon et al. 1993).

Using tantalum screws implanted in the endocardium in dogs, Raff and Glantz (1981) observed a consistent effect on the LV volume loading after opening the chest or the pericardium. The effect of partial ventriculectomy has been also studied in a passive porcine heart model, with the markers' positions used as input for subsequent simulations (Green et al. 1998).

High-resolution data using transmural bead columns allowed for detecting changes in the epicardial and subendocardial strains, and relating them to the segmental nature of coronary supply both in normal animals and animals with ischemic hearts during intermittent coronary occlusion (Cheng et al. 2005, Rodriguez et al. 2005). For example, the studies by Cheng et al. (2005) and Rodriguez et al. (2005) illustrated alterations in the transmural and fiber-sheet strains adjacent to the area at risk during ischemia, which could reflect a direct mechanical interaction between ischemic and nonischemic myocardium. Two-dimensional strain gradients across the penumbra zone of ischemic myocardium have also been described (Van Leuven et al. 1994). Further, Villarreal et al. (1991) described alterations in 3D cardiac strains. The techniques based on surgically implanted markers can also provide unique data to validate different noninvasive or semi-invasive methods for assessing regional myocardial function. For example, Kong et al. (1971) used a canine model with epicardial radiopaque markers to validate the use of opacified coronary arteries bifurcation as a landmark for quantifying epicardial segmental lengths.

9.3.4 Clinical Studies Using Radiopaque Markers

In the human studies reported in the literature, no intraoperative complications have been described, and during the clinical follow-up, the screws remained in place without signs of migration. Minor tissue reaction in the form of connective tissue fibrosis has been seen around the markers, as observed in postoperative findings in the experimental animal studies.

9.3.4.1 Myocardial Contractility

In the 1960s at the National Institutes of Health (NIH) in the United States, Braunwald et al. (Williams et al. 1965, Glick et al. 1966) surgically implanted markers in five patients undergoing open heart surgery and showed that the RV and

LV dimensions decrease as function of increased heart rate as well as after administration of nitroglycerin. Later, McDonald (1970, 1972) used surgical clips to determine the LV contractility pattern during systole in patients with hypertrophic cardiomyopathy. The hypertrophic cardiomyopathy patients, in whom the markers had been implanted at the time of aortic valve replacement, showed reduced myocardial shortening as measured by the markers after surgery (McDonald 1972).

In one of the early studies using radiopaque markers, the markers have been implanted in a total of 13 cardiac transplants (Stinson et al. 1975), where the results showed correlation between LV function deterioration and signs of graft rejection confirmed by endomyocardial biopsies. In another implanted marker study of the LV function in denervated and innervated cardiac transplants, there was no difference between the two groups in terms of myocardial contractility and cardiac output (Savin et al. 1980). In similar patient groups, the effect of tachycardia, as an inotropic stimulus for improved LV function, as well as the effects of exercise and atrial pacing have been studied in transplanted hearts (McLaughlin et al. 1978, Ricci et al. 1979a,b, Pope et al. 1980, Haskell et al. 1981). Some of these results are in agreement with the experimental atrial pacing and exercise effects in denervated canine hearts, as shown by Mattila et al. (1973). The effects of different drugs have been also tested in the same group of patients with anatomical denervated hearts (Mason et al. 1977, 1978) as well as in patients after coronary artery bypass grafting (CABG) (Kleiman et al. 1978, 1979, McLaughlin et al. 1978, Fowler et al. 1984). In 1978, Brower et al. (1978) used surgically implanted markers in 56 patients after saphenous vein bypass grafting to determine regional epicardial myocardial shortening after revascularization. In that study, the markers allowed for quantifying the improvement in myocardial shortening as seen 6 months postoperative after enhancing the flow to the myocardium distal to the coronary stenosis.

9.3.4.2 Ventricular Twist

In 1975, Ingels et al. (1975) at Stanford University used surgically implanted markers in patients to determine LV function postoperatively. Tantalum markers were implanted in 24 patients who were undergoing coronary revascularization and/or valvular surgery. An example of the setup for the acquisition of early postoperative data in the intensive care unit at Stanford University is shown in Figure 9.10. The markers helped provide a noninvasive ventriculogram of the LV without the need to administer intravenous contrast. An interesting and unique finding from this study was the description of the LV twist–untwist pattern, where the apical segments of the LV rotated in an opposite direction to the basal segments, while the midventricular segments hardly rotated (Ingels et al. 1975), as illustrated in Figure 9.11.

The results showed that the basal segments rotate about 4° counterclockwise while the apical segments rotate 7° in the opposite direction. The opposite rotation of the basal and apical segments during systole is defined as torsion or twist. In fact, this phenomenon has been observed as early

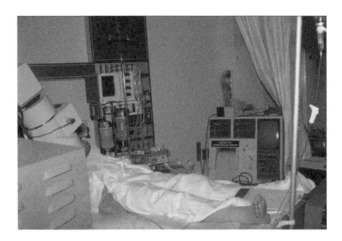

FIGURE 9.10 Image acquisition in a human subject. The acquisition of markers data in a patient during the early hours postoperative in the intensive care unit at Stanford University. (Image courtesy of Neil B. Ingels and D. Craig Miller, Department of Thoracic and Cardiovascular Surgery, Stanford University, Stanford, CA.)

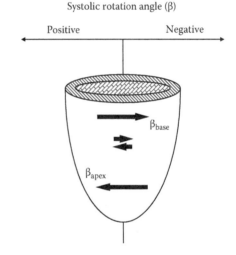

FIGURE 9.11 Schematic illustration of the twisting motion of the left ventricle during systole. Negative rotation is seen for the basal segments, almost no rotation for the midventricular segments, and positive rotation for the apical segments (see the arrows for directions).

as in 1669, when Richard Lower (1968) reported this pattern of myocardial contraction and compared it to "the wringing of a linen to squeeze out the water." This "wringing" motion is accompanied by a parallel base to apex movement of the mitral annulus, where the RV free wall has greater longitudinal movement amplitude than the LV free wall (Lundback 1986, Rogers et al. 1991). These movements are combined with the finding that the apex of the heart is almost stationary throughout the cardiac cycle (Fischer et al. 1994, Rodriguez et al. 2004b).

The LV twist–untwist pattern gained much interest and has been seen as an early marker of myocardial dysfunction. It has been recently described and quantified using different imaging modalities, including echocardiography and MRI (Maier et al. 1992, Lorenz et al. 2000, Helle-Valle et al. 2005).

For example, based on surgically implanted markers, acute cardiac allograft rejection has been associated with altered diastolic untwist mechanism in the absence of any noticeable systolic abnormalities (Yun et al. 1991). Furthermore, the LV twist mechanism during heart failure has gained popularity in recent years, where the effects of surgical management and cardiac resynchronization therapy (CRT) on regional myocardial function remain hard to quantify and predict in the individual patient (Sogaard et al. 2002, Athanasuleas et al. 2004). In this respect, different heart pathologies, such as myocardial hypertrophy, dilatation, ischemia, and fibrosis, may alter normal torsional function of the LV (Yun and Miller 1995, Tibayan et al. 2004). For example, pressure loading in transplanted patients hardly showed any effect on LV systolic twist or early-diastolic untwist, whereas volume loading affected diastolic untwist, and inotropic stimulation increased both systolic twist and diastolic untwist (Moon et al. 1994).

9.3.4.3 Volume and Pressure Loading

The early effects of LV volume loading have been studied in patients immediately after CABG (Daughters et al. 1985, Miller et al. 1985). The effects of closing the pericardium have been studied in the first 10–15 hours postoperatively with the pericardium first closed and then opened. The results showed a clear constraining effect on the LV function, which improved after opening the pericardium (Daughters et al. 1992). The early limitations of LV volume estimation with echocardiography against volume measurement based on implanted markers in patients have been also studied in the same patient group (Schnittger et al. 1982). Vine et al. (1976) implanted epicardial radiopaque markers in 22 subjects undergoing open heart surgery and showed that the time–volume curves based on the markers give similar results to those from angiography.

The effects of intrathoracic pressure changes have been studied by Buda et al. (1979) in eight patients with epicardial markers implanted at the time of CABG or cardiac transplant. The results provided by the markers showed a clear effect of pressure on the LV function, with reciprocal effects on afterload when the intrathoracic pressure was altered with the Valsalva and Muller maneuvers. In transplant patients, RV asynergy has been studied, confirming the complexity of the RV function and the need for multidimensional data to adequately describe its motion (Chin et al. 1989).

9.3.4.4 Valvular Function

Apart from the study of regional myocardial function, the surgically implanted markers have provided fundamental data on aortic and mitral valve function during normal states, in diseased hearts, and after surgical intervention (Glasson et al. 1997, Dagum et al. 1999, Kvitting et al. 2010a). In this respect, several experimental animal studies have been conducted to study alteration in the mitral valve function, such as functional or ischemic mitral regurgitation, along with associated changes in the LV function (Dagum et al. 2000, Tibayan et al. 2003, Rodriguez et al. 2004a).

9.4 SONOMICROMETERS

9.4.1 General Overview

Sonomicrometry is the most common marker implantation technique after tantalum makers, wherein piezoelectric crystals, usually made of ceramic material, are implanted in the myocardium. Each implanted crystal has a dual role: transmitting and receiving signals from other crystals. These crystals operate at frequencies of 1 MHz and higher, and the distance between them is continuously measured with high spatial resolution (~15 μm). Based on the data from the crystals, different indices such as volume, wall thickness, and segmental shortening can be measured (Figure 9.12). An important advantage of the sonomicrometric crystals is that they provide volume measurements simultaneously with regional variables such as wall thickness.

9.4.2 Experimental Studies Using Sonomicrometry

9.4.2.1 Markers Implantation

Sonomicrometric crystals can be used in large as well as small animals such as rats (Matsui et al. 2001) and mice (Feng et al. 2002) to quantify regional myocardial thickening. The crystals are implanted in a similar fashion to the radiopaque markers through a left-sided thoracotomy. An intraoperative photograph of implanted crystals and attached coils in the heart is shown in Figure 9.13. The setup for crystal implantation is similar to that described for the radiopaque marker technique. Villarreal et al. (1988) showed excellent correlation between strain measurements from sonomicrometry and radiopaque markers.

9.4.2.2 Wall Motion and Thickening

Ultrasonic crystals have been used to show linear relationship between regional myocardial blood flow and epicardial wall motion during graded coronary occlusion (Weintraub et al. 1981). In another study, Hattori et al. (1982), using crystals, showed that reduction in segmental shortening in the epicardial and endocardial myocardium followed each other during graded coronary occlusion. The ultrasonic crystals have been also used to measure wall thickening (Heyndrickx et al. 1975, 1978, Ross and Franklin 1976, Sasayama et al. 1976a) and changes in subendocardial segmental shortening (Theroux et al. 1974, 1976, Sasayama et al. 1976b). In another study, the same method showed increased blood flow to nonischemic myocardium during intravenous infusion of a calcium channel blocker, as well as the effects of nitroglycerin on ischemic and nonischemic epicardial segmental lengthening (Weintraub et al. 1982a,b).

An important limitation of individual transducers is that they only measure a single chamber dimension (length, width, or wall thickness) (Sandler and Alderman 1974). Using three piezoelectric crystals arranged in a "crystal triangle," 2D finite strain has been measured in a canine model (Osakada et al. 1980, Villarreal et al. 1988). Using sonomicrometers, Gallagher et al. (1985a) showed that the ratio of inner to outer

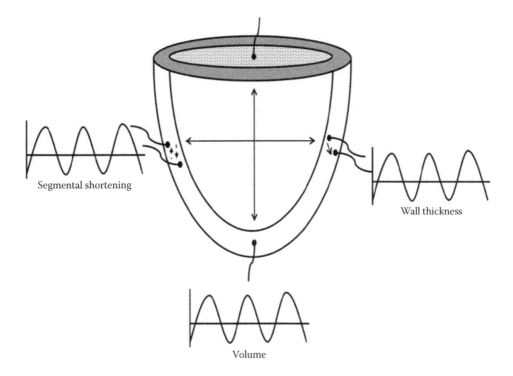

FIGURE 9.12 Schematic representation of the left ventricle and some of the indices that can be measured using sonomicrometric crystals.

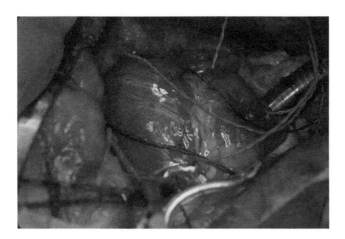

FIGURE 9.13 The piezoelectric sonomicrometric crystals attached to the surface of an ovine left ventricle. (Image courtesy of Neil B. Ingels and D. Craig Miller, Department of Thoracic and Cardiovascular Surgery, Stanford University, Stanford, CA.)

wall thickening is approximately 2.5:1.0 at rest and during moderate exercise in an experimental canine model, which suggests that the wall thickening gradient is affected by the fiber architecture and LV geometry, not by positive chronotropic and inotropic changes. These results confirm the theoretical models predicting fractional shortening of the inner and outer parts of the ventricle to be 67% and 33%, respectively, and assuming a transmural wall thickening gradient (Arts et al. 1979). The transmural gradient has also been verified by epicardial echocardiography (Myers et al. 1986).

Epicardial deformation has been studied using electromagnetic induction coils (Arts and Reneman 1980, Arts et al. 1982), based on which models of the LV mechanics could be

verified. The pericardium effects on LV filling dynamics have been also studied using ultrasonic crystals (Hoit et al. 1993). Further, sonomicrometry has been used to study the physiological effects of LV untwisting rate as a clinical marker of diastolic dysfunction (Opdahl et al. 2012).

9.4.2.3 Advanced Applications

In the field of gene transfer and implantation of mesenchymal stem cells in myocardial infarction models, sonomicrometric crystals have been placed within the ischemic region for measuring wall thickness and contractile function (Shake et al. 2002, Thompson et al. 2003), often in combination with transthoracic echocardiography (Leotta et al. 2002). In cardiac surgery, the order, duration, and frequency of cardioplegia delivery have been studied extensively, where sonomicrometric crystals have been used to determine the effect of the administration regime and type of solution on myocardial function (Jayawant et al. 1999, Kuhn-Regnier et al. 2000, Warner et al. 2001, Klass et al. 2004).

Apart from myocardial mechanics, sonomicrometric crystals have been extensively used to study valvular function in animal models (Hiro et al. 2004, Sacks et al. 2006, Fawzy et al. 2011, Askov et al. 2013, Jensen et al. 2014). A complete overview of the use of sonomicrometric crystals for studying valvular function is outside the scope of this chapter.

9.4.3 CLINICAL STUDIES USING SONOMICROMETER CRYSTALS

Sonomicrometric hemispherical crystals have been used in the setting of open heart surgery, first reported from the Duke Medical Center, in order to obtain objective measurements of global and regional heart function (Hill et al. 1978, Chitwood et al. 1979, 1980, Olsen et al. 1979). The crystals have primarily been implanted in patients undergoing coronary artery bypass grafting (CABG) (Hagl et al. 1978, Tyson et al. 1982), where the implantation was easy with insertion times of only a few minutes.

Despite the inherent invasive nature of the method, no bleeding or major complications have been reported in sonomicrometric studies; further, the crystals showed potential as a monitoring tool (Moores et al. 1984). They are later removed through a midline chest tube in the intensive care unit. Using crystals in the operating room, Brown et al. (1999) studied the effect of off-pump CABG on regional myocardial systolic function before the patients' wounds were closed, as per standard practice. The myocardial damage due to the insertion of the crystals is probably modest (Gelberg et al. 1979) and comparable to the injury caused by temporary ventricular pacing wires. Nevertheless, the trauma associated with the implantation of the crystals has limited its widespread clinical use as well as the rapid development and spread of echocardiography.

9.5 LIMITATIONS OF THE INVASIVE TECHNIQUES

9.5.1 Limitations of Surgically Implanted Marker Studies

One of the main reasons for the limited spread of the surgically implanted marker techniques, particularly in human studies, is the highly invasive nature of these methods. Further, the need for imaging with ionizing radiation makes follow-up studies ethically difficult to justify.

Several problems are associated with the surgically implanted makers. Firstly, the small size of the markers results in poor signal-to-noise ratio (SNR). Secondly, the rapid motion of the markers, combined with the overlap between some of them, makes motion assessment ambiguous in certain regions. Thirdly, since the markers need to be surgically implanted, only diseased human hearts have been studied, and therefore, the data obtained may not reflect normal myocardial function, making generalization based on the obtained results difficult. Another limitation of the marker studies is the time-consuming data analysis, which precludes the technique's widespread clinical use. Also, data from animals must be interpreted with caution since differences between species might occur (Ashikaga et al. 2004a). Finally, the placement of the markers at certain locations in the heart, for example, the interventricular septum, is technically challenging.

The finite number of implanted markers is also an important limitation, and missing or displaced markers are difficult to correct for after implantation. Since the number of markers to be implanted is limited, some *a priori* information is needed to ensure optimal marker placement. Nevertheless, this is not a limitation of noninvasive imaging modalities covering the entire heart (Kvitting et al. 2010b, Zhong et al. 2010). There are, however, some techniques that promise easy implantation of more than 100 markers in the heart (Shoukas et al. 1981).

9.5.2 Markers' Effects on Studied Parameters

An important limitation of the marker studies is that the markers themselves might alter normal myocardial function. For in-depth study of transmural deformation, the metallic bead columns constitute up to one-third of the myocardial wall (McVeigh and Zerhouni 1991). Later studies using deformation data obtained using echocardiography showed that opening of the chest and pericardium affects the intrinsic properties of the myocardium (Wranne et al. 1993, Derumeaux et al. 1998). Stokland et al. (1980) at the University of Oslo showed, by measuring the myocardial chordal lengths with ultrasonic crystals placed in the anterior myocardial wall, that the intact pericardium exerts a moderate restrictive effect on the heart function during volume loading, while the heart function improved after opening the intact pericardium. Walley et al. (1982), however, showed that opening the pleura or performing a sternotomy dislocates the heart within the thoracic cavity, although the magnitude of LV shortening was unaffected in an experimental canine model with implanted radiopaque tantalum markers. For chronic animal studies, pleural and pericardial adhesions because of the markers might alter regional myocardial function (Rushmer 1954), which is not the case with noninvasive imaging.

It has been shown that the markers themselves are quite inert and the tissue reaction is minimal; however, the degree by which the markers might affect the fiber architecture and cardiac function remains unclear. It should be noted that although the clinical studies using surgically implanted markers are invasive at the time of implantation, they do not usually control the main determinants of myocardial function: preload, afterload, heart rate, or contractile state at the time of data acquisition (Brower et al. 1978). For follow-up studies, fibrosis around the markers might have affected the results, particularly for the epicardially placed markers. For the sonomicrometer studies, shear motion of the crystals is an important limitation (Osakada et al. 1980).

9.6 SURGICALLY IMPLANTED MARKERS IN THE CURRENT ERA

9.6.1 Implanted Markers in Experimental Studies

After the introduction of noninvasive imaging modalities, surgically implanted markers still provide important data about different aspects of the heart function, for example, translaminar architecture and myocardial contractility (McCulloch and Omens 1991, LeGrice et al. 1995, Harrington et al. 2005). Ashikaga et al. (2004a,b,c, 2007, 2008, 2009) have extensively studied transmural myocardial mechanics using bead sets in animals. Quantification of transmural strains using bead columns showed that passive ventricular restraint (using the CorCap device) prevents LV remodeling in the setting of myocardial ischemia (Cheng et al. 2006). Such a study, with a sham group, an intervention group that receives passive restraint device, and a control group, would have been impossible to perform in humans. The results provided important information about the mechanism behind the favorable effect of LV remodeling observed in animal and human studies (Chaudhry et al. 2000, Acker 2005).

A 3D array of radiopaque markers has been used to study and quantify residual strain in the anterior midventricular LV in canine, where the results showed epicardial fiber extension and endocardial fiber contraction in the intact unloaded myocardium (Costa et al. 1997). Such a study is infeasible to perform in humans. Finally, the signal void created by the surgically implanted markers have been used to validate 3D motion quantified using phase-contrast MRI (Pelc et al. 1994).

9.6.2 Implanted Markers as the Gold Standard

Sonomicrometry remains the gold standard against which new imaging techniques, for example, speckle tracking echocardiography for measuring myocardial strain (Amundsen et al. 2006, Seo et al. 2011), echocardiographic methods for assessing myocardial work (Russell et al. 2012), optical flow for measuring myocardial strain (Duan et al. 2009), and MRI tagging for evaluating regional myocardial function (Yeon et al. 2001), are validated. The high accuracy of the piezoelectric crystals makes them still attractive in the experimental setting for quantifying subtle changes in systolic segmental shortening and wall thickening in diverse settings, for example, experimental cardiac surgery (Duffy et al. 2009, Abd-Elfattah et al. 2012), and for quantification of LV remodeling after myocardial infarction (Yarbrough et al. 2010) or heart failure (de Souza Vilarinho et al. 2010). Nevertheless, the use of surgically implanted markers, both radiopaque markers and sonomicrometric crystals, in humans has ceased since the introduction of noninvasive imaging modalities such as echocardiography and MRI.

9.7 INFANCY OF MRI TAGGING

9.7.1 Need for Noninvasive Means for Evaluating Cardiac Function

The complex motion of the heart (translation, rotation, twist, tilt, shear, and shortening) in combination with the lack of intrinsic myocardial landmarks poses a fundamental limitation to many cardiac imaging modalities. In the seminal paper by Zerhouni et al. (1988), the authors proposed using MRI for creating virtual tissue tags of saturated magnetization and subsequently tracking the tagged tissue for motion quantification. This idea changed the field altogether.

Before the introduction of MRI tagging, several technical advances have been achieved with imaging modalities such as nuclear imaging and echocardiography to study ventricular wall motion and quantify wall thickening (Feigenbaum 1994). These modalities, however, have inherent limitation in their ability to quantify regional cardiac function. Up to Zerhouni's work, all imaging modalities, including MRI, provided images that show homogeneous signal intensity inside the myocardium, which makes it infeasible to track intramyocardial tissue deformation. The only method available at that time for measuring myocardial deformation depended on surgically implanted markers, as described earlier in the chapter.

9.7.2 Basic Principles of MRI Tagging

The main idea behind the MRI tagging technique presented by Zerhouni et al. is creating a magnetization saturation pattern in the tissue through the implementation of RF saturation pulses to perturb the magnetization in a spatially varying fashion. As the perturbed magnetization follows tissue deformation, the myocardial motion can be detected in the images acquired later in the cardiac cycle after tags preparation.

Motion tracking by MRI tagging involves two main steps: tags preparation and image acquisition, with some time delay in between the two steps. Tags preparation takes place immediately after detection of the R-wave of the ECG; therefore, the MRI tagging sequences are synchronized with the ECG. The time delay usually depends on the information to be acquired, for example, a delay from end-diastole to end-systole is implemented for measuring systolic strain. During the tags preparation step, the magnetization is saturated at selected locations in the myocardium. During the time delay in between tag preparation and image acquisition, the myocardium undergoes deformation, where the saturated magnetization, an intrinsic property of the tissue, follows the deformation. Therefore, in the obtained tagged image, the deformed tag lines identify tissue motion that took place during the time delay.

The selection of the time delay affects the tagging contrast (signal difference between the tagged and nontagged tissues), as the magnetization undergoes relaxation during this period trying to reach equilibrium, which results in reduced tagging contrast. For sufficiently short time delays, the flip angle of the tags preparation RF pulses can be selected to provide optimal tagging contrast such that the signal of the tagged tissue is nulled at the imaging time. This, however, works only for a specific time point after tags preparation, not for multiple timeframe (cine) acquisition. For longer time delays, optimal contrast is not obtained, but the tagging contrast may still be sufficient for tags detection during image analysis.

9.7.3 Original Implementation of MRI Tagging

9.7.3.1 Tagging Patterns

Each tag preparation RF pulse creates one tag line, where the placement of the tag lines can be determined in a number of ways. In the original paper by Zerhouni et al. (1988), three different approaches were implemented:

1. Six parallel tag lines, consisting of two sets of three lines each, were defined on a long-axis (LAX) slice and used for longitudinal motion analysis.
2. Two orthogonal sets of three parallel tag lines each, intersecting in the center of the LV (in a SAX slice), formed a grid-like tagging pattern, which was used for circumferential and radial motion analysis.
3. Three radial tag lines, centered in the LV (in a SAX slice), were created using three tag pulses and used for radial motion analysis.

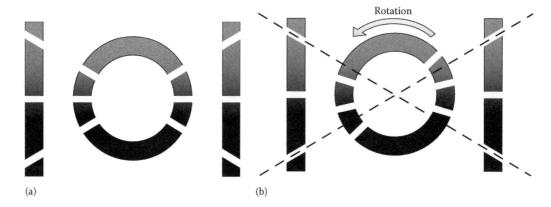

(a)   (b)

FIGURE 9.14   Schematic of the phantom experiment for validating the original tagging technique. (a) Image frame acquired immediately after tags application. Note how the white tag lines are aligned in the both circular and vertical parts of the phantom. (b) Image frame acquired after the circular part of the phantom has rotated. Note that the originally aligned (white) tag lines are not aligned any more (dashed lines).

In its original implementation (Zerhouni et al. 1988), tags preparation used RF pulses of 12 ms each, which produced tag line thickness ≥0.35 cm. It should be noted that by using multiple RF pulses (each for creating a single tag line), the tagging time will be slightly shifted for different tag lines, resulting in different time delays for different tag lines, which may affect their appearance in the acquired image due to magnetization relaxation. Furthermore, each RF pulse contributes to the specific absorption rate (SAR) deposited in the patient, which limits the number of RF pulses that can be used, and thus the number of achievable tag lines.

9.7.3.2   Technique Validation

In order to validate the MRI tagging method, an experiment has been conducted using a 12 cm hollow phantom made out of a gelatin mixture approximating the magnetization T_1 and T_2 relaxation times of the myocardium, which was rotated at different rotation speeds (Zerhouni et al. 1988). First, the phantom was imaged in a stationary position to assess gradient linearity and define reference radial tag lines. The phantom was then rotated, and the displacement of the tags was recorded (Figure 9.14). In the stationary position, the tag lines created in the phantom were straight, as determined by linear regression of the x–y coordinates of 15 points along each tag line, with correlation coefficient of 0.99. A position offset of 4 ± 2 mm (mean ± SD) was, however, found between the prescribed and measured values, which was probably due to inaccuracies in the calibration settings. Because of this fairly large offset, the tag lines in moving tissues needed to be related to the tag lines in nonmoving tissues in the periphery of the image (two poles to the left and right of the rotating phantom in Figure 9.14). Following the phantom experiment, MRI scans have been conducted on eight healthy volunteers from 18 to 36 years old with normal heart rates (54–75 beats per minute). A whole-body 0.38 T MRI scanner (Rx4000, Resonex, Sunnyvale, CA) was used for imaging. The total scan time ranged from 28 to 56 minutes.

These preliminary data showed that MRI tagging holds promise for quantifying motion of different myocardial tissue layers. In two of the volunteers in whom three parallel SAX slices were obtained, translation of the myocardium was higher in the basal (1.7 ± 0.4 cm) compared to the apical (0.2 ± 0.2 cm) planes. Twisting motion of the apex was also demonstrated, with higher degree of rotation in the posterolateral and inferior walls.

As expected, the tag lines were not visible in the ventricular cavity since the rapid blood flow destroys the integrity of the tags. The tags in the myocardium, on the other hand, are not dispersed and can be accurately tracked throughout the contraction phase of the cardiac cycle. By applying the tagging pulses every other heartbeat, the tag persistence could be improved by allowing the magnetization to recover during the even-numbered "dummy" R–R cycles.

9.8   SIGNAL MANIPULATION AND RELAXATION

9.8.1   TAGGING PULSE SEQUENCE

The approach presented by Zerhouni et al. is based on inversion recovery imaging. The tag lines are prepared using slice-selective RF pulses with flip angles in the range from 90° to 180°, where the saturated slices' orientation is orthogonal to the imaging slice. The gradient pulse applied during the RF pulse determines the orientation of the saturated tag plane, which is orthogonal to the direction of the applied gradient. The tags preparation sequence is typically applied right after the detection of the R-wave of the ECG. After tags preparation, the heart undergoes motion, during which the tagged magnetization follows myocardial deformation. Later in the cardiac cycle, data readout takes place to create images of the heart with the tag lines deformed based on the amount of motion that occurred between tags preparation and data acquisition. A schematic diagram of the tagging pulse sequence is shown

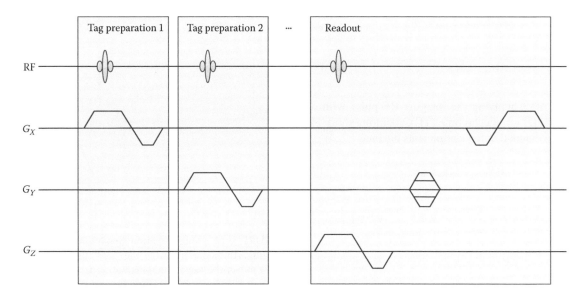

FIGURE 9.15 Schematic pulse sequence diagram of the original tagging technique. The tag lines are created one by one, orthogonal to the imaged slice, using slice-selective saturation radio-frequency (RF) pulses (one vertical line and one horizontal line are shown in the figure). The gradient pulse accompanying the tagging RF pulse determines the tagline orientation. After certain time delay, the readout module is played out, recording an image in which the tag lines have deformed by the motion that occurred during the delay period. Conventional Cartesian data readout is shown in the figure.

in Figure 9.15. The time between the tags preparation pulses and data readout is called the tagging-to-imaging delay (TD). For multiple image acquisition at different points in the cardiac cycle, multiple TDs are required; but for simplicity, only one TD is considered in our analysis in the following section.

9.8.2 Magnetization Manipulation

The tagging RF pulse disturbs the magnetization in the tagged slice based on the applied flip angle. In this section, the magnetization behavior is analyzed based on the tagging and imaging flip angles as well as the magnetization relaxation effects. Three cases are considered here: saturation recovery (tagging flip angle = 90°), inversion recovery (tagging flip angle = 180°), and general case (90° < tagging flip angle < 180°).

9.8.2.1 Saturation Recovery Tagging

Figure 9.16 shows the magnetization behavior for saturation recovery tagging. Immediately after the implementation of the 90° tagging RF pulse (time (t) = 0⁺), the tagged magnetization (red arrow) is completely tipped into the transverse plane, while the untagged magnetization in the surrounding tissues (black arrow) is left intact, described as

$$M_{non\text{-}tag}^{z} = M_0, \tag{9.1}$$

$$M_{non\text{-}tag}^{xy} = 0, \tag{9.2}$$

$$M_{tag}^{z} = 0, \tag{9.3}$$

$$M_{tag}^{xy} = M_0. \tag{9.4}$$

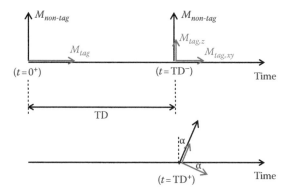

FIGURE 9.16 Magnetization behavior in saturation recovery tagging. Immediately after the 90° tagging radio-frequency (RF) pulse (time (t) = 0⁺), the tagged magnetization is tipped into the transverse plane, while the untagged magnetization is unaffected. The tagged magnetization experiences longitudinal and transverse magnetization relaxation during the tag delay (TD) period. The imaging RF pulse, applied at TD, tips (partially or completely) both the tagged and untagged magnetizations into the transverse plane. An imaging flip angle = α is shown here.

During the tag delay (TD) time duration, the tagged magnetization experiences both transverse (T_2) and longitudinal (T_1) relaxations, while the untagged magnetization is unaffected (assuming full magnetization recovery is achieved before applying the tagging RF pulse). Immediately before applying the imaging RF pulse at t = TD⁻, the magnetization components can be written as

$$M_{non\text{-}tag}^{z} = M_0, \tag{9.5}$$

$$M_{non\text{-}tag}^{xy} = 0, \tag{9.6}$$

$$M_{tag}^z = M_0(1 - e^{-TD/T_1}), \qquad (9.7)$$

$$M_{tag}^{xy} = M_0 e^{-TD/T_2}. \qquad (9.8)$$

Immediately after applying the imaging RF pulse with flip angle α at $t = TD^+$ (or at echo time (TE), assuming short TE), the transverse magnetization components become

$$M_{non\text{-}tag}^{xy} = M_0 \sin \alpha, \qquad (9.9)$$

$$M_{tag}^{xy} = M_0 \left((1 - e^{-TD/T_1}) \sin \alpha + e^{-TD/T_2} \cos \alpha \right). \qquad (9.10)$$

Assuming a 90° imaging flip angle, the transverse magnetization components are

$$M_{non\text{-}tag}^{xy} = M_0, \qquad (9.11)$$

$$M_{tag}^{xy} = M_0 \left(1 - e^{-TD/T_1} \right), \qquad (9.12)$$

which results in tagging contrast (normalized signal difference) between the tagged and nontagged tissues of

$$Tag\_Contrast = e^{-TD/T_1}, \qquad (9.13)$$

which is maximized for TD = 0 (practically using minimum TD).

9.8.2.2 Inversion Recovery Tagging

Figure 9.17 shows the magnetization behavior for inversion recovery tagging. Immediately after the implementation of the 180° tagging RF pulse (time (t) = 0$^+$), the tagged magnetization is inverted in the negative longitudinal direction, while the untagged magnetization in the surrounding tissues is left intact, described as

$$M_{non\text{-}tag}^z = M_0, \qquad (9.14)$$

$$M_{non\text{-}tag}^{xy} = 0, \qquad (9.15)$$

$$M_{tag}^z = -M_0, \qquad (9.16)$$

$$M_{tag}^{xy} = 0. \qquad (9.17)$$

During the TD time duration, the tagged magnetization experiences longitudinal relaxation trying to reach equilibrium, while the untagged magnetization is unaffected. Immediately before applying the imaging RF pulse at $t = TD^-$, the magnetization components can be written as

$$M_{non\text{-}tag}^z = M_0, \qquad (9.18)$$

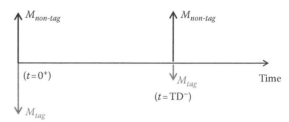

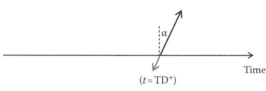

FIGURE 9.17 Magnetization behavior in inversion recovery tagging. Immediately after the 180° tagging radio-frequency (RF) pulse, the tagged magnetization (red arrow) is tipped into the negative longitudinal direction, while the untagged magnetization (black arrow) is unaffected. The tagged magnetization experiences longitudinal magnetization relaxation during the tag delay (TD) period. The imaging RF pulse, applied at TD, tips (partially or completely) both the tagged and untagged magnetizations into the transverse plane. An imaging flip angle = α is shown here.

$$M_{non\text{-}tag}^{xy} = 0, \qquad (9.19)$$

$$M_{tag}^z = -M_0 e^{-TD/T_1} + M_0 \left(1 - e^{-TD/T_1} \right)$$
$$= M_0 \left(1 - 2 e^{-TD/T_1} \right), \qquad (9.20)$$

$$M_{tag}^{xy} = 0, \qquad (9.21)$$

Immediately after applying the imaging RF pulse with flip angle α at $t = TD^+$, the transverse magnetization components become

$$M_{non\text{-}tag}^{xy} = M_0 \sin \alpha, \qquad (9.22)$$

$$M_{tag}^{xy} = M_0 \left(1 - 2 e^{-TD/T_1} \right) \sin\alpha. \qquad (9.23)$$

Assuming a 90° imaging flip angle, the transverse magnetization components are

$$M_{non\text{-}tag}^{xy} = M_0, \qquad (9.24)$$

$$M_{tag}^{xy} = M_0 \left(2 e^{-TD/T_1} - 1 \right), \qquad (9.25)$$

which results in tagging contrast of (magnitude reconstruction is assumed):

$$Tag\_Contrast = 1 - \left| 1 - 2 e^{-TD/T_1} \right|, \qquad (9.26)$$

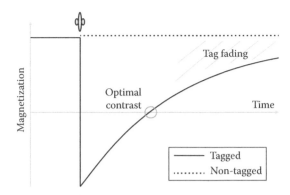

FIGURE 9.18 Illustration of magnetization relaxation after application of the tagging inversion pulse in a simplified case, ignoring readout pulses. Nontagged magnetization (dashed line) is unaffected, while the tagged magnetization (solid line) is inverted (tipped into the negative z-axis) and thus experiences T_1 relaxation. At the zero-crossing time (small gray circle), occurring at TD = ln(2) × T_1 (if a 180° flip angle is used), optimal tagging contrast is obtained. Later in time, the tagged magnetization experiences additional relaxation, approaching the level of nontagged magnetization, leading to reduced tagging contrast (tags fading).

which is maximized when the recovering tagged magnetization crosses the zero line (Figure 9.18), that is, when

$$TD = \ln(2) \times T_1. \tag{9.27}$$

9.8.2.3 General Tagging Case

Figure 9.19 shows the magnetization behavior for a general-case tagging, where the tagging flip angle = 90 + φ°, where 0° < φ < 90°. Immediately after the implementation of the tagging RF pulse (time (t) = 0^+), the tagged magnetization has two components in the longitudinal and transverse directions, while untagged magnetization is left intact, which is described as

$$M_{non\text{-}tag}^z = M_0, \tag{9.28}$$

$$M_{non\text{-}tag}^{xy} = 0, \tag{9.29}$$

$$M_{tag}^z = -M_0 \sin\varphi, \tag{9.30}$$

$$M_{tag}^{xy} = M_0 \cos\varphi. \tag{9.31}$$

During the TD time duration, the tagged magnetization experiences both longitudinal and transverse relaxations, while the untagged magnetization is unaffected. Immediately before applying the imaging RF pulse at t = TD^-, the magnetization components can be written as

$$M_{non\text{-}tag}^z = M_0, \tag{9.32}$$

$$M_{non\text{-}tag}^{xy} = 0, \tag{9.33}$$

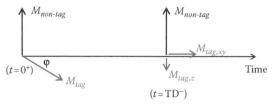

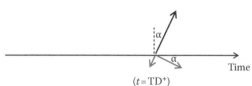

FIGURE 9.19 Magnetization behavior in a general-case tagging. Immediately after the tagging radio-frequency (RF) pulse, the tagged magnetization (red arrow) is tipped (partially or completely) into the transverse plane (tagging angle = 90 + φ° is shown here), while the untagged magnetization (black arrow) is unaffected. The tagged magnetization experiences both longitudinal and transverse magnetization relaxation during the tag delay (TD). The imaging RF pulse, applied at TD period, tips (partially or completely) both the tagged and untagged magnetizations into the transverse plane. An imaging flip angle = α is shown here.

$$M_{tag}^z = -M_0 \sin\varphi\, e^{-TD/T_1} + M_0 \left(1 - e^{-TD/T_1}\right)$$
$$= M_0(1 - (1 + \sin\varphi)e^{-TD/T_1}) = \text{``}v\text{''}, \tag{9.34}$$

$$M_{tag}^{xy} = M_0 \cos\varphi\, e^{-TD/T_2} = \text{``}u\text{''}. \tag{9.35}$$

Immediately after applying the imaging RF pulse with flip angle α at t = TD^+, the transverse magnetization components become

$$M_{non\text{-}tag}^{xy} = M_0 \sin\alpha, \tag{9.36}$$

$$M_{tag}^{xy} = u\cos\alpha + v\sin\alpha = M_0 \cos\varphi\, e^{-TD/T_2} \cos\alpha$$
$$+ M_0(1 - (1 + \sin\varphi)e^{-TD/T_1})\sin\alpha. \tag{9.37}$$

Assuming a 90° imaging flip angle, the transverse magnetization components are

$$M_{non\text{-}tag}^{xy} = M_0, \tag{9.38}$$

$$M_{tag}^{xy} = M_0 \left(1 - (1 + \sin\varphi)e^{-TD/T_1}\right), \tag{9.39}$$

which results in tagging contrast of (magnitude reconstruction is assumed):

$$Tag\_Contrast = 1 - \left|1 - (1 + \sin\varphi)e^{-TD/T_1}\right|, \tag{9.40}$$

which is maximized by nulling the signal from the tagged tissue, that is, when

$$TD = \ln\left(1 + \sin\varphi\right) \times T_1. \qquad (9.41)$$

9.8.2.4 Tagging Contrast Optimization

Figure 9.20 shows the tagging contrast as a function of TD (0 ms ≤ TD ≤ 1000 ms) for different values of the tagging flip angle from 90° (saturation recovery) to 180° (inversion recovery) in steps of 15°, assuming imaging at 1.5 T (T_1 = 850 ms) and heart rate of 60 beats per minute.

From another perspective, the tagging contrast is maximized for a certain TD when the angle φ (in the general-case tagging discussed earlier in Equation 9.41) becomes

$$\varphi = \sin^{-1}\left(e^{TD/T_1} - 1\right). \qquad (9.42)$$

Figure 9.21 shows tagging contrast as a function of the tagging flip angle (= 90 + φ°) for TD ranging from 0 to 1000 ms in steps of 200 ms.

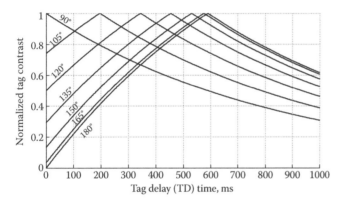

FIGURE 9.20 Normalized tagging contrast for different tag delay times. The figure shows contrast curves for different tagging flip angles from 90° to 180° in steps of 15°.

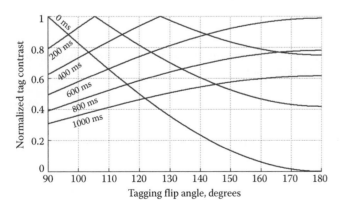

FIGURE 9.21 Normalized tagging contrast for different tagging flip angles. The figure shows contrast curves for different tag delay times from 0 ms to 1000 ms in steps of 200 ms.

9.9 POSTPROCESSING ANALYSIS

The tagged MRI images convey information about the cardiac motion in a visually intuitive way. The tag lines show how the grid or line tagging pattern has deformed due to myocardial motion (Figure 9.22).

If multiple images are acquired during different time points in the cardiac cycle, the sequence of images could be played back in a cine mode to show myocardial deformation during the cardiac cycle. Quantitative analysis of tissue motion requires tracking the tag lines, which can be done either manually, semiautomatically (McVeigh and Zerhouni 1991, Moore et al. 1992), or fully automatically (Bazille et al. 1994). The semiautomatic approaches usually rely on the user identifying seed points at the tag line's intersections with the endocardial and epicardial borders. The processing algorithm then finds the tag line between these points. This way, the tracking process is less subjective and less time consuming. In addition to finding the tag lines, endocardial and epicardial segmentation is also necessary for strain estimation. However, the detection of the tag lines appears to be much more robust than myocardial border segmentation (Bazille et al. 1994). It should be noted that Chapters 2 and 3 of *Heart Mechanics: Magnetic Resonance Imaging—Advanced Techniques, Clinical Applications, and Future Trends* are devoted for tagged image analysis.

Curve-fitting techniques can be implemented to find the tag center with subpixel precision. Using least-squares fitting, which is optimal for linear problems, good results can be achieved for tag center detection, that is, identifying the trough of the signal intensity profile perpendicular to the tag line. While the optimal thickness of the tag lines depends on the application at hand, optimal tag thickness was found in the range of 0.8–1.5 pixels, although it is always better to err on the higher end (Atalar and McVeigh 1994). Additionally, the tags need to be separated by approximately 5 pixels to

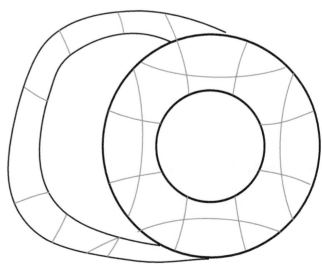

FIGURE 9.22 Illustration of how tag lines are deformed through contraction of the left and right ventricles. Note the tag lines are deformed based on myocardial contraction.

avoid neighboring tag lines from interfering with the estimation of the tag center (Mcveigh and Gao 1993).

9.10 TECHNICAL DEVELOPMENTS

9.10.1 Multispectral Tagging Pulses

The saturation-based tagging techniques has been improved over time. The original work by Zerhouni et al. (1988) allowed for producing the tag lines with minimum width of 0.35 cm, which limited the achievable resolution for myocardial motion detection. Three years after the introduction of Zerhouni's technique, a high-spatial-resolution version of the technique was developed to measure transmural myocardial strain gradient in the normal dog heart (McVeigh and Zerhouni 1991). The pulse sequence included multispectral RF pulses capable of generating high-resolution tagging density (2-mm tag separation). Each RF pulse was designed to have a number of discrete spectral components, and the signal power was adjusted to generate thin tag lines. A tagging grid pattern can be created with the intersection of the two orthogonal sets of parallel tag lines, as shown in Figure 9.23. A tag-detection algorithm was applied on the generated images to measure tag displacement with a precision of 0.1–0.2 mm over the systolic heart phase.

9.10.2 High-Resolution Tagging

Using a modified quadruple gradient set, O'Dell et al. (1994) developed a technique for generating tagging images with very thin tag lines (0.6 mm) for detailed cardiac motion analysis. The gradient coils along the X-, Y-, and Z-directions were capable of generating gradient amplitudes of 113, 47, and 152 mT/cm, respectively, at 100 amps current, with slew rate of 200 mT/cm/ms and ramp time of 150 μs, which are considered advanced characteristics by the standards of that time. The generated field distortions were less than 2% over an 8 cm scanner bore, which allowed for high-resolution tagging with 0.1 mm point tracking precision. Nevertheless, it should be

noted that the axis of the gradient must be aligned perpendicular to the B_0 field, limiting the technique's application to small animals or isolated heart experiments.

9.11 VALIDATION AND CLINICAL APPLICATIONS OF MRI TAGGING

9.11.1 Validation Studies

9.11.1.1 Validation against Sonomicrometry

In order to validate the MRI tagging technique, Lima et al. (1993) implanted sonomicrometers transmurally in a canine model and correlated systolic wall thickening measurements from the surgical markers and MRI tagging. Sonomicrometers were placed transmurally in the left anterior descending (LAD) artery territory in 11 dogs. An MRI-visible imaging marker was sewn to the epicardial crystal. Two adjacent SAX slices were marked with four radial tagging planes, which resulted in segmenting the myocardium into eight volume segments, one of which contained the sonomicrometer (Figure 9.24).

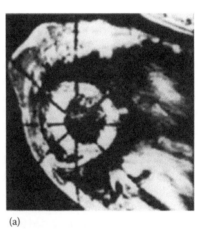

(a)

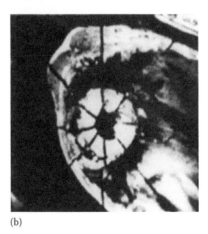

(b)

FIGURE 9.24 Short-axis radially tagged images at (a) end-diastole and (b) end-systole. The small bright epicardial dot adjacent to the upper right tag is an oil-filled marker sewn to the epicardial sonomicrometer crystal. The end-systolic image shows deformation of the tag lines in agreement with the marker displacement. (Reproduced from Lima, J.A., *J. Am. Coll. Cardiol.*, 21(7), 1741, 1993. With permission.)

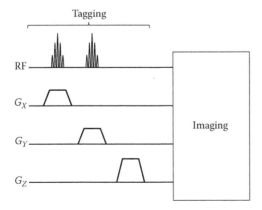

FIGURE 9.23 Multispectral tagging pulse sequence with the tag lines applied in two orthogonal directions to produce a high-resolution tagging grid.

The myocardial thickness was calculated using four methods: (1) "distance" method, the distance between the endo- and epicardial contours in the segment containing the sonomicrometer; (2) "area" method, the segmental SAX area divided by the mean segmental arc length; (3) "biplane" method, the average wall thickness (measured by the "area" method) in the sonomicrometer segment and the adjacent segment in the other SAX slice; and (4) "volume" method, the volume of the sonomicrometer segment divided by the endo- and epicardial surface areas. The results showed excellent correlation between systolic wall thickening (WT) by tagging (WT_MRI) and sonomicrometers (WT_SM), especially using the volume method. The results from regression and correlation analyses were as follows: (1) distance method, WT_MRI = 0.59 + 1.31 WT_SM (R = 0.71, P < 0.0002); (2) area method, WT_MRI = 1.43 + 1.62 WT_SM (R = 0.87, P < 0.0001); (3) biplane method, WT_MRI = 2.09 + 1.46 WT_SM (R = 0.90, P < 0.0001); and (4) volume method, WT_MRI = 0.19 + 1.49 WT_SM (R = 0.95, P < 0.0001). Elaborate in vitro studies have been also conducted to validate MRI tagging for estimating tissue deformation against stroboscopic photographs (Young et al. 1993, Moore et al. 1994).

9.11.1.2 Validation in Normal Subjects

Following Zerhouni's paper, several studies have been conducted to quantify regional inhomogeneity of the human LV motion using the developed MRI tagging technique. Bogaert and Rademakers (2001) implemented MRI tagging to characterize regional LV strain in normal individuals. In this study, five parallel SAX planes and four radially oriented LAX planes were acquired, based on which the LV wall was segmented into 40 small cuboids (Figure 9.25). Regional myocardial strains in the radial, circumferential, and longitudinal directions, as well as shear measurements, were obtained.

The results showed marked morphological nonuniformity in myocardial strain, which in general increased from base to apex

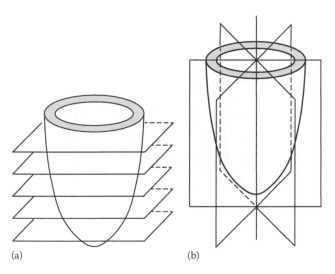

(a)   (b)

FIGURE 9.25 Regional myocardial strain is measured from (a) five parallel short-axis tagged images and (b) four radially oriented long-axis tagged images.

(Figures 9.26 through 9.28). Further, wall thickening showed variable and difficult relation to other functional parameters. For example, the anterior part of the LV was the flattest and thinnest and showed the largest wall thickening (46.6%), while the posterior part wall was thicker, more curved, and showed a lower wall thickening (32.8%). These data correlated well with transmural strain measurements obtained in different LV regions using surgically implanted makers (Cheng et al. 2005). These findings of wall thickening variation have important clinical implication on visual assessment and quantification of wall thickening when comparing different LV regions in an individual patient or interpreting differences between patients.

9.11.2 Applications of MRI Tagging

In this section, we provide a brief coverage of early clinical applications of the originally developed tagging sequence. However, Chapters 9 and 10 of *Heart Mechanics: Magnetic Resonance Imaging—Advanced Techniques, Clinical Applications, and Future Trends* are dedicated for thorough coverage of tagging clinical applications.

9.11.2.1 Transmural Strain Gradients

Using thin tag lines, McVeigh and Zerhouni (1991) were able to measure transmural strain gradients in the myocardium. Strong selection gradients in combination with multifrequency RF pulses allowed for generating thin tag lines. By tracking the tag intersection points, a transmural strain gradient could be found in the dog heart using this high-resolution tagging technique.

9.11.2.2 Through-Plane Motion and 3D Strain Analysis

Moore et al. (1992) used orthogonal tagged slices to recover 3D heart motion. By tracking the tag line intersection points in both SAX and LAX slices, through-plane motion can be accounted for, and using stacks of parallel slices, points covering the whole LV can be tracked in 3D over time. Three-dimensional point tracking enables computation of all nine components of the strain tensor for measuring both normal and shear strains. An additional benefit of tracking through-plane motion is to follow the same tissue material over time, whereas in single-slice (2D) analysis, through-plane motion results in that different material points are tracked at different time points in the cardiac cycle. In a human heart studied with the developed technique, the corrected radial strain values at the LV base were approximately 2.5 times the values measured with a 2D method on a fixed image plane. Another comprehensive study of human LV strain was performed later by Bogaert and Rademakers (2001), who used multiple orthogonal slices to measure 3D strain.

9.11.2.3 Ventricular Torsion Analysis

Several studies used MRI tagging for studying LV torsion, confirming the findings from surgically implanted markers, and providing further information about the role of rapid untwisting during isovolumic relaxation in the early-diastolic filling phase (Buchalter 1990, Rademakers 1992). For example, using

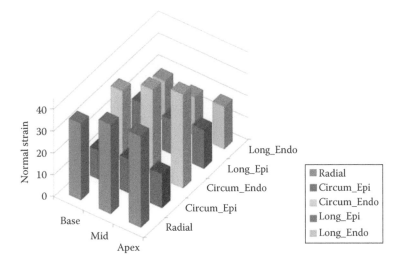

FIGURE 9.26 Normal radial, circumferential (at both endocardial and epicardial positions), and longitudinal (at both endocardial and epicardial slices) strains at basal, midventricular, and apical slices.

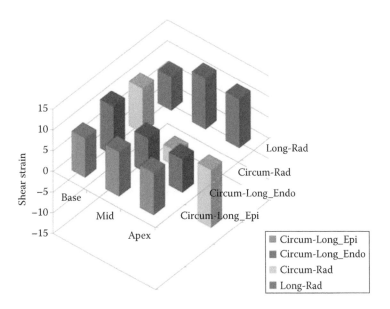

FIGURE 9.27 Shear longitudinal–radial, circumferential–radial, and circumferential–longitudinal (at both endocardial and epicardial positions) strains at basal, midventricular, and apical slices.

MRI tagging, Buchaltar et al. (1990) measured torsion in the LV, where the results showed that torsion in the endocardium was greater than that in the epicardium by approximately two-fold. Less torsion was found in the posterior and posteroseptal regions than in the anterior and anterolateral regions. Further, the torsion difference between the basal and midventricular slice was less than that between the midventricular and apical slices. Looking at torsion variations in the LAX direction, a nonlinear relationship was found, where more torsion variation was reported toward the apex compared to the base of the LV.

In another study, Rademaker et al. (1992) investigated the timing and extent of restoration of the LV systolic torsional deformation with respect to early filling at baseline and with enhanced relaxation. Myocardial untwisting was measured in 10 atrially paced dogs using 8 tag planes intersecting the endo- and epicardium in 3 SAX slices at the basal, midventricular, and apical levels. The results showed that myocardial untwisting occurs mainly during isovolumic relaxation before filling, and it is markedly enhanced in speed and magnitude by catecholamines, offsetting the associated shortening of the filling period. Specifically, apical torsion rapidly changed between its maximum value and the time immediately after mitral valve opening from 12.0° ± 8.5° to 6.9° ± 7.8° at the endocardium and from 7.0° ± 5.8° to 3.2° ± 5.4° at the epicardium. During the same period, there were insignificant changes in the circumferential segment length. After mitral valve opening, however, circumferential segment lengthening was significant, while torsion change was small and insignificant. During dobutamine infusion, there was greater end-systolic torsion with faster and larger changes during isovolumic relaxation.

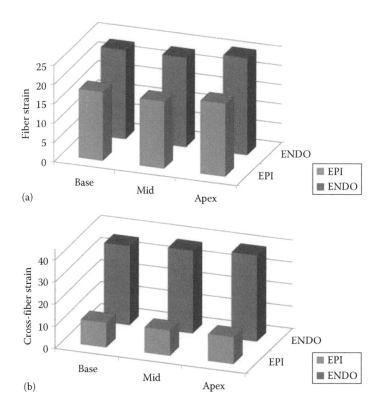

FIGURE 9.28   (a) Fiber and (b) cross-fiber strains at both endocardial and epicardial positions for basal, midventricular, and apical slices.

9.11.2.4 Right Ventricular Deformation

Naito et al. (1995) applied the tagging technique to study myocardial deformation in the RV. Despite the thinner RV free wall, the tag lines could be detected, and fractional shortening could be determined. In another recent study, Chen et al. (2011) implemented MRI tagging on the RV free wall for assessing longitudinal myocardial function in congenital heart disease. The developed method was based on applying a labeling RF pulse prior to image acquisition to generate a tag line across the basal myocardium. RV tag displacement was then measured with automated registration and tracking of the tag line. The developed technique was tested on 84 patients with different diseases (repaired tetralogy of Fallot [rTOF], atrial septal defect [ASD] with pulmonary hypertension [PH], and ASD without PH) and 20 healthy volunteers. The results showed higher RV displacement in the control subjects (26 ± 3 mm) than in rTOF (16 ± 4 mm) and ASD with pulmonary hypertension (18 ± 3 mm) groups, but lower than in the ASD group without pulmonary hypertension (30 ± 4 mm), P < 0.001. The technique was reproducible with interstudy bias ± 95% limits of agreement of 0.7 ± 2.7 mm.

9.12 LIMITATIONS OF THE EARLY MRI TAGGING SEQUENCES

As tissue tagging is based on the principle of magnetization saturation, T_1 relaxation has the effect of reducing the tagging contrast by restoring the magnetization to thermal equilibrium.

This concept is referred to as tag fading, which results in shallow tagging contrast at late cardiac phases, precluding tagging analysis at these phases. This is especially noticed with automatic tag analysis techniques, which are sensitive to tagging contrast variation.

As tagging preparation consists of applying multiple RF pulses (often with 180° flip angles), high SAR may become a problem, limiting the number of tag lines that can be generated. Further, as multiple RF pulses take a certain time to perform, the tag lines are not created simultaneously but are rather slightly shifted in time, which results in different relaxation effects on them, leading to slightly different appearance in the tagged image. Another point is that since the tag lines are created by applying ordinary slice-selective RF pulses, the minimum achievable slice thickness is limited by the duration of the RF pulse and gradient strength, with thinner tag lines and sharper tag profiles requiring long RF pulses and strong gradients.

Zerhouni et al. implemented the initial tagging technique on MRI scanners with very limited hardware capability compared to the MRI systems available today. Further, the capability of controlling data acquisition through pulse sequence programming has been simplified over the years. The MRI systems are now more accurate with respect to timing of the gradients and RF pulses, as well as stable phase clocks. Gradient fidelity and, more importantly, slew rate and maximum gradient strength have been improved considerably. Stronger gradients enable sharper tag lines with less sensitivity to geometric distortions caused by frequency shifts. Zerhouni et al. used a field gradient strength of 0.38 T, whereas the systems of present time are commonly 1.5 or 3 T. Since SNR improves linearly with field strength, this gives more flexibility to SNR-based trade-offs for shorter acquisition time and higher resolution when imaging at high field strength. Since the tag fading is based on T_1 relaxation, and myocardial T_1 is longer at higher field strengths, more tagging contrast is expected with today's MRI systems. This has been reported in several studies comparing tagging at 1.5 and 3 T (Gutberlet et al. 2005, Valeti et al. 2006, Markl et al. 2008, Sigfridsson et al. 2011). Other key improvements in MRI include using receiver coil arrays, which improve local SNR and allow for parallel imaging (Pruessmann et al. 1999) for reduced scan time.

9.13 SPAMM AND DANTE

Although Chapter 10 is devoted to the SPAMM and DANTE tagging techniques, it is worth providing a brief introduction to these two techniques in this section along with their advantages compared to the original tagging technique developed by Zerhouni et al. This is especially important knowing that the SPAMM and DANTE techniques were presented shortly after the introduction of Zerhouni's tagging technique.

9.13.1 SPAMM

In 1989, one year after Zerhouni's original tagging paper was published, Axel and Dougherty (1989a,b) published an alternative approach for MRI tagging: SPAMM, which became the basis of most current-day work on tagging. Figure 9.29 shows the basic pulse sequence of SPAMM tagging, and Figure 9.30 shows magnetization-saturated and SPAMM tagged images.

There are two important differences between magnetization saturation and SPAMM tagging. While in the former the tags are generated with individual RF pulses, in SPAMM all tags can be generated using only two RF pulses.

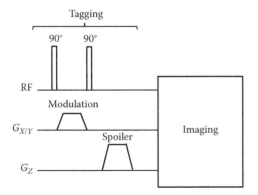

FIGURE 9.29 Pulse sequence diagram of spatial modulation of magnetization (SPAMM) tagging. The tagging part consists of two nonselective 90° radio-frequency pulses, interspersed by a modulation gradient, and followed by a spoiler gradient. Imaging takes place later after tags preparation.

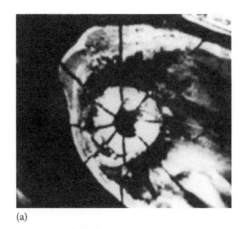

(a)

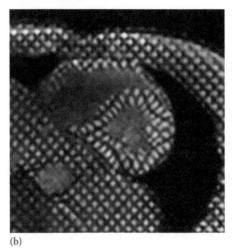

(b)

FIGURE 9.30 Side-by-side MRI tagged images using (a) the original tagging technique and (b) spatial modulation of magnetization (SPAMM) tagging. (a: Reproduced from Lima, J.A., *J. Am. Coll. Cardiol.*, 21(7), 1741, 1993. With permission.)

Although magnetization saturation provides sharper tag lines, high-order binomial SPAMM (Axel and Dougherty 1989a), which uses a binomial number of RF pulses for generating the tag lines, has been proposed for improving the tag profile compared to conventional SPAMM. The other difference between the two tagging techniques is related to tagging analysis. While in magnetization saturation tags tracking takes place in the image space, the harmonic phase (HARP) technique (Osman et al. 1999) can be used for analyzing the SPAMM tagged images based on analyzing the signals in the k-space, which significantly reduces the image processing time.

9.13.2 DANTE

An alternative approach to create tags is to use DANTE tagging, developed by Mosher in 1990. The basic DANTE tagging pulse sequence is shown in Figure 9.31. Compared to the magnetization saturation approach, DANTE tagging has the advantages of encoding many tag lines using one composite RF pulse, depositing less RF energy in the patient, and providing thinner tag lines (Figure 9.32). Additionally, in the DANTE

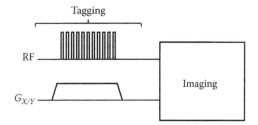

FIGURE 9.31 DANTE tagging pulse sequence. The tagging part consists of multiple nonselective RF pulses applied during continuous application of the tagging gradient. The imaging part follows later after tag preparation.

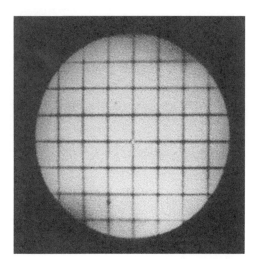

FIGURE 9.32 DANTE tagging in a phantom. The figure shows sharp taglines achieved with DANTE. (Reproduced from Mosher, T.J. and Smith, M.B., *Magn. Reson. Med.*, 15(2), 334, 1990. With permission.)

approach, the RF pulses are applied with a constant gradient, which reduces the eddy currents.

9.14 SUMMARY AND KEY POINTS

9.14.1 SUMMARY

In summary, compared to the early studies using invasive techniques such as surgically implanted radiopaque markers and ultrasonic crystals, MRI tagging opened the door for noninvasive quantification of regional heart function, a field that has been expanding since 1988, as will be detailed in the following chapters. Although advanced noninvasive tagging techniques are currently the gold standard for evaluating regional myocardial function, implanted markers are expected to continue to play a role in such investigations, especially in experimental animal models with the need for detailed information about myocardial deformation in different settings. Further, implanted markers are the gold standard against which new imaging techniques are validated.

9.14.2 KEY POINTS

- Marker implantation experiments allow for instantaneous determination of the LV size, shape, and volume in the intact heart in both physiological and pathophysiological studies.
- Radiopaque markers and sonomicrometer crystals are two famous techniques used in experiments.
- The radiopaque markers are in the form of clips, beads, or screws.
- The distribution of the radiopaque markers usually outlines the LV, covering the apex and three SAX planes along the anterolateral and inferior margins of the ventricle.
- The accuracy of the surgically implanted marker technique is very high with error of repeated measurements in the range of 1%, error of the measured lengths of about 2.7%, and reproducibility errors of the measured lengths in the range of 0.04 cm.
- For in vivo studies, the implantation of the radiopaque markers is usually performed through a left thoracotomy at the fifth intercostal space, where the heart is suspended in a pericardial cradle.
- Images of the implanted markers are acquired using biplane imaging to provide 3D Lagrangian marker coordinates.
- High-resolution data acquired with transmural columns of beads allow for detecting changes in epicardial and subendocardial strains, and relating them to the segmental nature of coronary supply.
- Implanted markers have been used in different studies, including myocardial contractility, ventricular twist, volume and pressure loadings, and valvular function.
- Implanted markers are invasive in nature and are associated with a number of limitations, including their effect on normal myocardial function and the limited number of markers that can be implanted.
- Implanted markers will most probably continue to play a role in studying heart mechanics, especially in animal models of different pathologies.
- The original tagging technique presented by Zerhouni et al. in 1988 opened the door for noninvasive evaluation of regional heart function without the need for markers implantation.
- The original tagging technique developed by Zerhouni et al. is based on saturating the magnetization (using either saturation or inversion recovery techniques) in a plane orthogonal to the imaged slice. The intersection of the saturated plane with the imaged slice creates a tag line that can be tracked during the cardiac cycle for quantifying myocardial deformation.
- The original tagging technique has been validated using a moving phantom and against data from implanted markers.

- The tagging contrast depends on the tagging and imaging flip angles as well as the time delay between tags preparation and data acquisition.
- Technical developments have been added to the original tagging technique to achieve high-resolution tagging.
- The original tagging technique has been implemented for studying transmural strain gradients, 3D myocardial strain, ventricular torsion, and RV deformation.
- The original tagging technique has a number of limitations, including long tag preparation time, high SAR, and nonideal and thick tag profile.
- The SPAMM and DANTE tagging techniques, both developed shortly after Zerhouni's technique appeared, are more advantageous to it. Nevertheless, the original tagging technique by Zerhouni et al. takes the credit for opening the door for noninvasive evaluation of regional heart function with MRI.

REFERENCES

Abd-Elfattah, A. S., Aly, H., Hanan, S., and Wechsler, A. S. (2012). Myocardial protection in beating heart cardiac surgery: I: Pre- or postconditioning with inhibition of es-ENT1 nucleoside transporter and adenosine deaminase attenuates post-MI reperfusion-mediated ventricular fibrillation and regional contractile dysfunction. *J Thorac Cardiovasc Surg* **144**(1): 250–255.

Acker, M. A. (2005). Clinical results with the Acorn cardiac restraint device with and without mitral valve surgery. *Semin Thorac Cardiovasc Surg* **17**(4): 361–363.

Amundsen, B. H., Helle-Valle, T., Edvardsen, T., Torp, H., Crosby, J., Lyseggen, E., Stoylen, A. et al. (2006). Noninvasive myocardial strain measurement by speckle tracking echocardiography: Validation against sonomicrometry and tagged magnetic resonance imaging. *J Am Coll Cardiol* **47**(4): 789–793.

Arts, T. and Reneman, R. S. (1980). Measurement of deformation of canine epicardium in vivo during cardiac cycle. *Am J Physiol* **239**(3): H432–H437.

Arts, T., Reneman, R. S., and Veenstra, P. C. (1979). A model of the mechanics of the left ventricle. *Ann Biomed Eng* **7**(3–4): 299–318.

Arts, T., Veenstra, P. C., and Reneman, R. S. (1982). Epicardial deformation and left ventricular wall mechanisms during ejection in the dog. *Am J Physiol* **243**(3): H379–H390.

Ashikaga, H., Coppola, B. A., Hopenfeld, B., Leifer, E. S., McVeigh, E. R., and Omens, J. H. (2007). Transmural dispersion of myofiber mechanics: Implications for electrical heterogeneity in vivo. *J Am Coll Cardiol* **49**(8): 909–916.

Ashikaga, H., Coppola, B. A., Yamazaki, K. G., Villarreal, F. J., Omens, J. H., and Covell, J. W. (2008). Changes in regional myocardial volume during the cardiac cycle: Implications for transmural blood flow and cardiac structure. *Am J Physiol Heart Circ Physiol* **295**(2): H610–H618.

Ashikaga, H., Criscione, J. C., Omens, J. H., Covell, J. W., and Ingels, N. B., Jr. (2004a). Transmural left ventricular mechanics underlying torsional recoil during relaxation. *Am J Physiol Heart Circ Physiol* **286**(2): H640–H647.

Ashikaga, H., Omens, J. H., and Covell, J. W. (2004b). Time-dependent remodeling of transmural architecture underlying abnormal ventricular geometry in chronic volume overload heart failure. *Am J Physiol Heart Circ Physiol* **287**(5): H1994–H2002.

Ashikaga, H., Omens, J. H., Ingels, N. B., Jr. and Covell, J. W. (2004c). Transmural mechanics at left ventricular epicardial pacing site. *Am J Physiol Heart Circ Physiol* **286**(6): H2401–H2407.

Ashikaga, H., van der Spoel, T. I., Coppola, B. A., and Omens, J. H. (2009). Transmural myocardial mechanics during isovolumic contraction. *JACC Cardiovasc Imaging* **2**(2): 202–211.

Askov, J. B., Honge, J. L., Jensen, M. O., Nygaard, H., Hasenkam, J. M., and Nielsen, S. L. (2013). Significance of force transfer in mitral valve-left ventricular interaction: In vivo assessment. *J Thorac Cardiovasc Surg* **145**(6): 1635–1641, 1641 e1631.

Atalar, E. and McVeigh, E. R. (1994). Optimization of tag thickness for measuring position with magnetic resonance imaging. *IEEE Trans Med Imaging* **13**(1): 152–160.

Athanasuleas, C. L., Buckberg, G. D., Stanley, A. W., Siler, W., Dor, V., Di Donato, M., Menicanti, L. et al. (2004). Surgical ventricular restoration in the treatment of congestive heart failure due to post-infarction ventricular dilation. *J Am Coll Cardiol* **44**(7): 1439–1445.

Aversano, T., Maughan, W. L., Hunter, W. C., Kass, D., and Becker, L. C. (1986). End-systolic measures of regional ventricular performance. *Circulation* **73**(5): 938–950.

Axel, L. and Dougherty, L. (1989a). Heart wall motion: Improved method of spatial modulation of magnetization for MR imaging. *Radiology* **172**(2): 349–350.

Axel, L. and Dougherty, L. (1989b). MR imaging of motion with spatial modulation of magnetization. *Radiology* **171**(3): 841–845.

Bazille, A., Guttman, M. A., McVeigh, E. R., and Zerhouni, E. A. (1994). Impact of semiautomated versus manual image segmentation errors on myocardial strain calculation by magnetic resonance tagging. *Invest Radiol* **29**(4): 427–433.

Bogaert, J. and Rademakers, F. E. (2001). Regional nonuniformity of normal adult human left ventricle. *Am J Physiol Heart Circ Physiol* **280**(2): H610–H620.

Brower, R. W., ten Katen, H. J., and Meester, G. T. (1978). Direct method for determining regional myocardial shortening after bypass surgery from radiopaque markers in man. *Am J Cardiol* **41**(7): 1222–1229.

Brown, P. M., Jr., Kim, V. B., Boyer, B. J., Lust, R. M., Chitwood, W. R., Jr. and Elbeery, J. R. (1999). Regional left ventricular systolic function in humans during off-pump coronary bypass surgery. *Circulation* **100**(19 Suppl): II125–II127.

Buchalter, M. B., Weiss, J. L., Rogers, W. J., Zerhouni, E. A., Weisfeldt, M. L., Beyar, R., and Shapiro, E. P. (1990). Noninvasive quantification of left ventricular rotational deformation in normal humans using magnetic resonance imaging myocardial tagging. *Circulation* **81**(4): 1236–1244.

Buckberg, G., Hoffman, J. I., Mahajan, A., Saleh, S., and Coghlan, C. (2008). Cardiac mechanics revisited: The relationship of cardiac architecture to ventricular function. *Circulation* **118**(24): 2571–2587.

Buckberg, G. D., Weisfeldt, M. L., Ballester, M., Beyar, R., Burkhoff, D., Coghlan, H. C., Doyle, M. et al. (2004). Left ventricular form and function: Scientific priorities and strategic planning for development of new views of disease. *Circulation* **110**(14): e333–e336.

Buda, A. J., Pinsky, M. R., Ingels, N. B., Jr., Daughters, G. T., 2nd, Stinson, E. B., and Alderman, E. L. (1979). Effect of intrathoracic pressure on left ventricular performance. *N Engl J Med* **301**(9): 453–459.

Carlsson, E. (1969). Experimental studies of ventricular mechanics in dogs using the tantalum-labeled heart. *Fed Proc* **28**(4): 1324–1329.

Carlsson, E. and Milne, E. N. (1967). Permanent implantation of endocardial tantalum screws: A new technique for functional studies of the heart in the experimental animal. *J Can Assoc Radiol* **18**(2): 304–309.

Castro, L. J., Moon, M. R., Rayhill, S. C., Niczyporuk, M. A., Ingels, N. B., Jr., Daughters, G. T., 3rd, Derby, G. C., and Miller, D. C. (1993). Annuloplasty with flexible or rigid ring does not alter left ventricular systolic performance, energetics, or ventricular-arterial coupling in conscious, closed-chest dogs. *J Thorac Cardiovasc Surg* **105**(4): 643–658; discussion 658–649.

Chaudhry, P. A., Mishima, T., Sharov, V. G., Hawkins, J., Alferness, C., Paone, G., and Sabbah, H. N. (2000). Passive epicardial containment prevents ventricular remodeling in heart failure. *Ann Thorac Surg* **70**(4): 1275–1280.

Chen, S. S., Keegan, J., Dowsey, A. W., Ismail, T., Wage, R., Li, W., Yang, G. Z., Firmin, D. N., and Kilner, P. J. (2011). Cardiovascular magnetic resonance tagging of the right ventricular free wall for the assessment of long axis myocardial function in congenital heart disease. *J Cardiovasc Magn Reson* **13**: 80.

Cheng, A., Langer, F., Rodriguez, F., Criscione, J. C., Daughters, G. T., Miller, D. C., and Ingels, N. B., Jr. (2005). Transmural cardiac strains in the lateral wall of the ovine left ventricle. *Am J Physiol Heart Circ Physiol* **288**(4): H1546–H1556.

Cheng, A., Nguyen, T. C., Malinowski, M., Langer, F., Liang, D., Daughters, G. T., Ingels, N. B., Jr. and Miller, D. C. (2006). Passive ventricular constraint prevents transmural shear strain progression in left ventricle remodeling. *Circulation* **114**(1 Suppl): I79–I86.

Chin, K. W., Daughters, G. T., Alderman, E. L., and Miller, D. C. (1989). Asynergy of right ventricular wall motion in man. *J Thorac Cardiovasc Surg* **97**(1): 104–109.

Chitwood, W. R., Jr., Hill, R. C., Sink, J. D., Kleinman, L. H., Sabiston, D. C., Jr. and Wechsler, A. S. (1980). Measurement of global ventricular function in patients during cardiac operations using sonomicrometry. *J Thorac Cardiovasc Surg* **80**(5): 724–735.

Chitwood, W. R., Jr., Hill, R. C., Sink, J. D., Sabiston, D. C., Jr. and Wechsler, A. S. (1979). Assessment of ventricular diastolic properties and systolic function in man with sonomicrometry. *Surg Forum* **30**: 266–268.

Costa, K. D., May-Newman, K., Farr, D., O'Dell, W. G., McCulloch, A. D., and Omens, J. H. (1997). Three-dimensional residual strain in midanterior canine left ventricle. *Am J Physiol* **273**(4 Pt 2): H1968–H1976.

Dagum, P., Green, G. R., Nistal, F. J., Daughters, G. T., Timek, T. A., Foppiano, L. E., Bolger, A. F., Ingels, N. B., Jr., and Miller, D. C. (1999). Deformational dynamics of the aortic root: Modes and physiologic determinants. *Circulation* **100**(19 Suppl): II54–II62.

Dagum, P., Timek, T. A., Green, G. R., Lai, D., Daughters, G. T., Liang, D. H., Hayase, M., Ingels, N. B., Jr., and Miller, D. C. (2000). Coordinate-free analysis of mitral valve dynamics in normal and ischemic hearts. *Circulation* **102**(19 Suppl 3): III62–III69.

Daughters, G. T., Derby, G. C., Alderman, E. L., Schwarzkopf, A., Mead, C. W., Ingels, N. B., Jr., and Miller, D. C. (1985). Independence of left ventricular pressure-volume ratio from preload in man early after coronary artery bypass graft surgery. *Circulation* **71**(5): 945–950.

Daughters, G. T., Frist, W. H., Alderman, E. L., Derby, G. C., Ingels, N. B. Jr., and Miller, D. C. (1992). Effects of the pericardium on left ventricular diastolic filling and systolic performance early after cardiac operations. *J Thorac Cardiovasc Surg* **104**(4): 1084–1091.

Daughters, G. T., Sanders, W. J., Miller, D. C., Schwarzkopf, A., Mead, C. W., and Ingels, N. B. (1988). A comparison of two analytical systems for three-dimensional reconstruction for biplane videoradiograms. *Comp Cardiol (IEEE)* **15**: 79–82.

Davis, P. L., Raff, G. L., and Glantz, S. A. (1980). A method to identify implanted radiopaque markers despite rotation of the heart. *Am J Physiol* **239**(4): H573–H580.

de Souza Vilarinho, K. A., Petrucci, O., Baker, R. S., Vassallo, J., Schenka, A. A., Duffy, J. Y., de Oliveira, P. P., and Vieira, R. W. (2010). Early changes in contractility indices and fibrosis in two minimally invasive congestive heart failure models. *Eur J Cardiothorac Surg* **37**(2): 368–375.

DeAnda, A., Jr., Komeda, M., Nikolic, S. D., Daughters, G. T., 2nd, Ingels, N. B., and Miller, D. C. (1995). Left ventricular function, twist, and recoil after mitral valve replacement. *Circulation* **92**(9 Suppl): II458–II466.

DeAnda, A., Jr., Moon, M. R., Yun, K. L., Daughters, G. T., 2nd, Ingels, N. B., Jr., and Miller, D. C. (1994). Left ventricular torsional dynamics immediately after mitral valve replacement. *Circulation* **90**(5 Pt 2): II339–II346.

Derumeaux, G., Ovize, M., Loufoua, J., Andre-Fouet, X., Minaire, Y., Cribier, A., and Letac, B. (1998). Doppler tissue imaging quantitates regional wall motion during myocardial ischemia and reperfusion. *Circulation* **97**(19): 1970–1977.

Duan, Q., Parker, K. M., Lorsakul, A., Angelini, E. D., Hyodo, E., Homma, S., Holmes, J. W., and Laine, A. F. (2009). Quantitative Validation of Optical Flow Based Myocardial Strain Measures Using Sonomicrometry. *Proc IEEE Int Symp Biomed Imaging* **2009**: 454–457.

Duffy, J. Y., McLean, K. M., Lyons, J. M., Czaikowski, A. J., Wagner, C. J., and Pearl, J. M. (2009). Modulation of nuclear factor-kappaB improves cardiac dysfunction associated with cardiopulmonary bypass and deep hypothermic circulatory arrest. *Crit Care Med* **37**(2): 577–583.

Ellis, R. M., Franklin, D. L., and Rushmer, R. F. (1956). Left ventricular dimensions recorded by sonocardiometry. *Circ Res* **4**(6): 684–688.

Fann, J. I., Sarris, G. E., Ingels, N. B., Jr., Niczyporuk, M. A., Yun, K. L., Daughters, G. T., 2nd, Derby, G. C., and Miller, D. C. (1991). Regional epicardial and endocardial two-dimensional finite deformations in canine left ventricle. *Am J Physiol* **261**(5 Pt 2): H1402–H1410.

Fawzy, H., Fukamachi, K., Mazer, C. D., Harrington, A., Latter, D., Bonneau, D., and Errett, L. (2011). Complete mapping of the tricuspid valve apparatus using three-dimensional sonomicrometry. *J Thorac Cardiovasc Surg* **141**(4): 1037–1043.

Feigenbaum, H. (1994). *Echocardiography*. Philadelphia, PA, Lea & Fabier.

Feng, Q., Song, W., Lu, X., Hamilton, J. A., Lei, M., Peng, T., and Yee, S. P. (2002). Development of heart failure and congenital septal defects in mice lacking endothelial nitric oxide synthase. *Circulation* **106**(7): 873–879.

Fenton, T. R., Cherry, J. M., and Klassen, G. A. (1978). Transmural myocardial deformation in the canine left ventricular wall. *Am J Physiol* **235**(5): H523–H530.

Fischer, S. E., McKinnon, G. C., Scheidegger, M. B., Prins, W., Meier, D., and Boesiger, P. (1994). True myocardial motion tracking. *Magn Reson Med* **31**(4): 401–413.

Fowler, M. B., Alderman, E. L., Oesterle, S. N., Derby, G., Daughters, G. T., Stinson, E. B., Ingels, N. B., Mitchell, R. S., and Miller, D. C. (1984). Dobutamine and dopamine after cardiac surgery: Greater augmentation of myocardial blood flow with dobutamine. *Circulation* **70**(3 Pt 2): I103–I111.

Freeman, G. L., LeWinter, M. M., Engler, R. L., and Covell, J. W. (1985). Relationship between myocardial fiber direction and segment shortening in the midwall of the canine left ventricle. *Circ Res* **56**(1): 31–39.

Fujita, M., Mikuniya, A., McKown, D. P., McKown, M. D., and Franklin, D. (1989a). Changes in regional myocardial cross-sectional area during brief coronary occlusion and reperfusion in conscious dogs. *Int J Cardiol* **22**(1): 21–28.

Fujita, M., Sasayama, S., Araie, E., Yamanishi, K., Ohno, A., McKown, D. P., and Franklin, D. (1989b). Changes in isovolumic segment shortening following acute coronary occlusion: Disproportionate effects of anterior versus posterior ischemia. *Int J Cardiol* **22**(1): 29–35.

Gallagher, K. P., Matsuzaki, M., Koziol, J. A., Kemper, W. S., and Ross, J., Jr. (1984). Regional myocardial perfusion and wall thickening during ischemia in conscious dogs. *Am J Physiol* **247**(5 Pt 2): H727–H738.

Gallagher, K. P., Osakada, G., Hess, O. M., Koziol, J. A., Kemper, W. S., and Ross, J., Jr. (1982). Subepicardial segmental function during coronary stenosis and the role of myocardial fiber orientation. *Circ Res* **50**(3): 352–359.

Gallagher, K. P., Osakada, G., Matsuzaki, M., Miller, M., Kemper, W. S., and Ross, J., Jr. (1985a). Nonuniformity of inner and outer systolic wall thickening in conscious dogs. *Am J Physiol* **249**(2 Pt 2): H241–H248.

Gallagher, K. P., Stirling, M. C., Choy, M., Szpunar, C. A., Gerren, R. A., Botham, M. J., and Lemmer, J. H. (1985b). Dissociation between epicardial and transmural function during acute myocardial ischemia. *Circulation* **71**(6): 1279–1291.

Garrison, J. B., Ebert, W. L., Jenkins, R. E., Yionoulis, S. M., Malcom, H., Heyler, G. A., Shoukas, A. A., Maughan, W. L., and Sagawa, K. (1982). Measurement of three-dimensional positions and motions of large numbers of spherical radiopaque markers from biplane cineradiograms. *Comput Biomed Res* **15**(1): 76–96.

Gelberg, H. J., Brundage, B. H., Glantz, S., and Parmley, W. W. (1979). Quantitative left ventricular wall motion analysis: A comparison of area, chord and radial methods. *Circulation* **59**(5): 991–1000.

Glasson, J. R., Komeda, M., Daughters, G. T., Foppiano, L. E., Bolger, A. F., Tye, T. L., Ingels, N. B., Jr., and Miller, D. C. (1997). Most ovine mitral annular three-dimensional size reduction occurs before ventricular systole and is abolished with ventricular pacing. *Circulation* **96**(9 Suppl): II-115–II-122; discussion II-123.

Glick, G., Williams, J. F., Jr., Harrison, D. C., Morrow, A. G., and Braunwald, E. (1966). Cardiac dimensions in intact unanesthetized man. VI. Effects of changes in heart rate. *J Appl Physiol* **21**(3): 947–952.

Green, G. R., Moon, M. R., DeAnda, A., Jr., Daughters, G. T., 2nd, Glasson, J. R., and Miller, D. C. (1998). Effects of partial left ventriculectomy on left ventricular geometry and wall stress in excised porcine hearts. *J Heart Valve Dis* **7**(5): 474–483.

Greenbaum, R. A., Ho, S. Y., Gibson, D. G., Becker, A. E., and Anderson, R. H. (1981). Left ventricular fibre architecture in man. *Br Heart J* **45**(3): 248–263.

Gutberlet, M., Schwinge, K., Freyhardt, P., Spors, B., Grothoff, M., Denecke, T., Ludemann, L., Noeske, R., Niendorf, T., and Felix, R. (2005). Influence of high magnetic field strengths

and parallel acquisition strategies on image quality in cardiac 2D CINE magnetic resonance imaging: Comparison of 1.5 T vs. 3.0 T. *Eur Radiol* **15**(8): 1586–1597.

Hagl, S., Meisner, H., Heimisch, W., and Sebening, F. (1978). Acute effects of aortocoronary bypass surgery on left ventricular function and regional myocardial mechanics: A clinical study. *Ann Thorac Surg* **26**(6): 548–558.

Hamilton, W. F. and Rompf, J. H. (1932). Movements of the base of the ventricle and the relative constancy of the cardiac volume. *Am J Physiol* **102**: 559–565.

Harrington, K. B., Rodriguez, F., Cheng, A., Langer, F., Ashikaga, H., Daughters, G. T., Criscione, J. C., Ingels, N. B., and Miller, D. C. (2005). Direct measurement of transmural laminar architecture in the anterolateral wall of the ovine left ventricle: New implications for wall thickening mechanics. *Am J Physiol Heart Circ Physiol* **288**(3): H1324–H1330.

Harrison, D. C., Goldblatt, A., Braunwald, E., Glick, G., and Mason, D. T. (1963). Studies on cardiac dimensions in intact, unanesthetized man. I. Description of techniques and their validation. II. Effects of respiration. III. Effects of muscular exercise. *Circ Res* **13**: 448–467.

Haskell, W. L., Savin, W. M., Schroeder, J. S., Alderman, E. A., Ingles, N. B., Jr., Daughters, G. T., 2nd, and Stinson, E. B. (1981). Cardiovascular responses to handgrip isometric exercise in patients following cardiac transplantation. *Circ Res* **48**(6 Pt 2): I156–I161.

Hattori, S., Weintraub, W. S., Agarwal, J. B., Bodenheimer, M. M., Banka, V. S., and Helfant, R. H. (1982). Contrasting ischemic contraction patterns by zone and layer in canine myocardium. *Am J Physiol* **243**(6): H852–H855.

Heikkila, J., Tabakin, B. S., and Hugenholtz, P. G. (1972). Quantification of function in normal and infarcted regions of the left ventricle. *Cardiovasc Res* **6**(5): 516–531.

Helle-Valle, T., Crosby, J., Edvardsen, T., Lyseggen, E., Amundsen, B. H., Smith, H. J., Rosen, B. D. et al. (2005). New noninvasive method for assessment of left ventricular rotation: Speckle tracking echocardiography. *Circulation* **112**(20): 3149–3156.

Heyndrickx, G. R., Baig, H., Nellens, P., Leusen, I., Fishbein, M. C., and Vatner, S. F. (1978). Depression of regional blood flow and wall thickening after brief coronary occlusions. *Am J Physiol* **234**(6): H653–H659.

Heyndrickx, G. R., Millard, R. W., McRitchie, R. J., Maroko, P. R., and Vatner, S. F. (1975). Regional myocardial functional and electrophysiological alterations after brief coronary artery occlusion in conscious dogs. *J Clin Invest* **56**(4): 978–985.

Hill, R. C., Kleinman, L. H., Chitwood, W. R., Jr., and Wechsler, A. S. (1978). Segmental mid-wall myocardial dimensions in man recorded by sonomicrometry. *J Thorac Cardiovasc Surg* **76**(2): 235–243.

Hiro, M. E., Jouan, J., Pagel, M. R., Lansac, E., Lim, K. H., Lim, H. S., and Duran, C. M. (2004). Sonometric study of the normal tricuspid valve annulus in sheep. *J Heart Valve Dis* **13**(3): 452–460.

Hoit, B. D., Shao, Y., Gabel, M., and Walsh, R. A. (1993). Influence of pericardium on left atrial compliance and pulmonary venous flow. *Am J Physiol* **264**(6 Pt 2): H1781–H1787.

Ingels, N. B., Jr. (1997). Myocardial fiber architecture and left ventricular function. *Technol Health Care* **5**(1–2): 45–52.

Ingels, N. B., Jr., Daughters, G. T., 2nd, Davies, S. R., and Macdonald, I. B. (1971). Stereo photogrammetric studies on the dynamic geometry of the canine left ventricular epicardium. *J Biomech* **4**(6): 541–550.

Ingels, N. B., Jr., Daughters, G. T., 2nd, Stinson, E. B., and Alderman, E. L. (1975). Measurement of midwall myocardial dynamics in intact man by radiography of surgically implanted markers. *Circulation* **52**(5): 859–867.

Ingels, N. B., Jr., Ricci, D. R., Daughters, G. T., 2nd, Aldersman, E. L., and Stinson, E. B. (1977). Effects of heart rate augmentation on left ventricular volumes and cardiac output of the transplanted human heart. *Circulation* **56**(3 Suppl): II32–II37.

Jayawant, A. M., Stephenson, E. R., Jr., Matte, G. S., Prophet, G. A., LaNoue, K. F., Griffith, J. W., and Damiano, R. J., Jr. (1999). Potassium-channel opener cardioplegia is superior to St. Thomas' solution in the intact animal. *Ann Thorac Surg* **68**(1): 67–74.

Jensen, M. O., Honge, J. L., Benediktsson, J. A., Siefert, A. W., Jensen, H., Yoganathan, A. P., Snow, T. K., Hasenkam, J. M., Nygaard, H., and Nielsen, S. L. (2014). Mitral valve annular downsizing forces: Implications for annuloplasty device development. *J Thorac Cardiovasc Surg* **148**(1): 83–89.

Klass, O., Fischer, U. M., Perez, E., Easo, J., Bosse, M., Fischer, J. H., Tossios, P., and Mehlhorn, U. (2004). Effect of the Na+/H+ exchange inhibitor eniporide on cardiac performance and myocardial high energy phosphates in pigs subjected to cardioplegic arrest. *Ann Thorac Surg* **77**(2): 658–663.

Kleiman, J. H., Alderman, E. L., Goldman, R. H., Ingels, N. B., Daughters, G. T., 2nd, and Stinson, E. B. (1979). Effects of digitalis on normal and abnormal left ventricular segmental dynamics. *Am J Cardiol* **43**(5): 1001–1008.

Kleiman, J. H., Ingels, N. B., Daughters, G., 2nd, Stinson, E. B., Alderman, E. L., and Goldman, R. H. (1978). Left ventricular dynamics during long-term digoxin treatment in patients with stable coronary artery disease. *Am J Cardiol* **41**(5): 937–942.

Kong, Y., Morris, J. J., Jr., and McIntosh, H. D. (1971). Assessment of regional myocardial performance from biplane coronary cineangiograms. *Am J Cardiol* **27**(5): 529–537.

Kuhn-Regnier, F., Fischer, J. H., Jeschkeit, S., Switkowski, R., Bardakcioglu, O., Sobottke, R., and de Vivie, E. R. (2000). Coronary oxygen persufflation combined with HTK cardioplegia prolongs the preservation time in heart transplantation. *Eur J Cardiothorac Surg* **17**(1): 71–76.

Kvitting, J. P., Bothe, W., Goktepe, S., Rausch, M. K., Swanson, J. C., Kuhl, E., Ingels, N. B., Jr., and Miller, D. C. (2010a). Anterior mitral leaflet curvature during the cardiac cycle in the normal ovine heart. *Circulation* **122**(17): 1683–1689.

Kvitting, J. P., Sigfridsson, A., Wigstrom, L., Bolger, A. F., and Karlsson, M. (2010b). Analysis of human myocardial dynamics using virtual markers based on magnetic resonance imaging. *Clin Physiol Funct Imaging* **30**(1): 23–29.

LeGrice, I. J., Takayama, Y., and Covell, J. W. (1995). Transverse shear along myocardial cleavage planes provides a mechanism for normal systolic wall thickening. *Circ Res* **77**(1): 182–193.

Leotta, E., Patejunas, G., Murphy, G., Szokol, J., McGregor, L., Carbray, J., Hamawy, A. et al. (2002). Gene therapy with adenovirus-mediated myocardial transfer of vascular endothelial growth factor 121 improves cardiac performance in a pacing model of congestive heart failure. *J Thorac Cardiovasc Surg* **123**(6): 1101–1113.

LeWinter, M. M., Kent, R. S., Kroener, J. M., Carew, T. E., and Covell, J. W. (1975). Regional differences in myocardial performance in the left ventricle of the dog. *Circ Res* **37**(2): 191–199.

Lima, J. A., Jeremy, R., Guier, W., Bouton, S., Zerhouni, E. A., McVeigh, E., Buchalter, M. B., Weisfeldt, M. L., Shapiro, E. P., and Weiss, J. L. (1993). Accurate systolic wall thickening by nuclear magnetic resonance imaging with tissue tagging: Correlation with sonomicrometers in normal and ischemic myocardium. *J Am Coll Cardiol* **21**(7): 1741–1751.

Lorenz, C. H., Pastorek, J. S., and Bundy, J. M. (2000). Delineation of normal human left ventricular twist throughout systole by tagged cine magnetic resonance imaging. *J Cardiovasc Magn Reson* **2**(2): 97–108.

Lower, R. (1968). *Tractatus de Corde: Item de motu et colore sanguinis*. Early Science in Oxford. R. T. Gunther. Swanson, Pall Mall, Oxford, U.K.

Lundback, S. (1986). Cardiac pumping and function of the ventricular septum. *Acta Physiol Scand Suppl* **550**: 1–101.

Maier, S. E., Fischer, S. E., McKinnon, G. C., Hess, O. M., Krayenbuehl, H. P., and Boesiger, P. (1992). Evaluation of left ventricular segmental wall motion in hypertrophic cardiomyopathy with myocardial tagging. *Circulation* **86**(6): 1919–1928.

Markl, M., Scherer, S., Frydrychowicz, A., Burger, D., Geibel, A., and Hennig, J. (2008). Balanced left ventricular myocardial SSFP-tagging at 1.5T and 3T. *Magn Reson Med* **60**(3): 631–639.

Mason, J. W., Specter, M. J., Ingels, N. B., Daughters, G. T., Ferris, A. C., and Alderman, E. L. (1978). Haemodynamic effects of acebutolol. *Br Heart J* **40**(1): 29–34.

Mason, J. W., Winkle, R. A., Ingels, N. B., Daughters, G. T., Harrison, D. C., and Stinson, E. B. (1977). Hemodynamic effects of intravenously administered quinidine on the transplanted human heart. *Am J Cardiol* **40**(1): 99–104.

Matsui, T., Tao, J., del Monte, F., Lee, K. H., Li, L., Picard, M., Force, T. L., Franke, T. F., Hajjar, R. J., and Rosenzweig, A. (2001). Akt activation preserves cardiac function and prevents injury after transient cardiac ischemia in vivo. *Circulation* **104**(3): 330–335.

Mattila, S., Ingels, N. B., Jr., Daughters, G. T., 2nd, Adler, S. C., Wexler, L., and Dong, E., Jr. (1973). The effects of atrial pacing on the synergy and hemodynamics of the orthotopically transplanted canine heart. *Circulation* **48**(2): 386–391.

McCulloch, A. D. and Omens, J. H. (1991). Non-homogeneous analysis of three-dimensional transmural finite deformation in canine ventricular myocardium. *J Biomech* **24**(7): 539–548.

McDonald, I. G. (1970). The shape and movements of the human left ventricle during systole. A study by cineangiography and by cineradiography of epicardial markers. *Am J Cardiol* **26**(3): 221–230.

McDonald, I. G. (1972). Contraction of the hypertrophied left ventricle in man studied by cineradiography of epicardial markers. *Am J Cardiol* **30**(6): 587–594.

McLaughlin, P. R., Kleiman, J. H., Martin, R. P., Doherty, P. W., Reitz, B., Stinson, E. B., Daughters, G. T., Ingels, N. B., and Alderman, E. L. (1978). The effect of exercise and atrial pacing on left ventricular volume and contractility in patients with innervated and denervated hearts. *Circulation* **58**(3 Pt 1): 476–483.

McVeigh, E. R. and Gao, L. (1993). Precision of tag position estimation in breathhold CINE MRI: The effect of tag spacing. *12th Annual Meeting, Society of Magnetic Resonance in Medicine*, New York.

McVeigh, E. R. and Zerhouni, E. A. (1991). Noninvasive measurement of transmural gradients in myocardial strain with MR imaging. *Radiology* **180**(3): 677–683.

Meier, G. D., Bove, A. A., Santamore, W. P., and Lynch, P. R. (1980). Contractile function in canine right ventricle. *Am J Physiol* **239**(6): H794–H804.

Miller, D. C., Daughters, G. T., Derby, G. C., Mitchell, R. S., Ingels, N. B., Jr., Stinson, E. B., and Alderman, E. L. (1985). Effect of early postoperative volume loading on left ventricular systolic function (including left ventricular ejection fraction determined by myocardial marker) after myocardial revascularization. *Circulation* **72**(3 Pt 2): II207–II215.

Mitchell, J. H., Wildenthal, K., and Mullins, C. B. (1969). Geometrical studies of the left ventricle utilizing biplane cinefluorography. *Fed Proc* **28**(4): 1334–1343.

Moon, M. R., Bolger, A. F., DeAnda, A., Komeda, M., Daughters, G. T., 2nd, Nikolic, S. D., Miller, D. C., and Ingels, N. B., Jr. (1997a). Septal function during left ventricular unloading. *Circulation* **95**(5): 1320–1327.

Moon, M. R., Castro, L. J., DeAnda, A., Tomizawa, Y., Daughters, G. T., 2nd, Ingels, N. B., Jr., and Miller, D. C. (1993). Right ventricular dynamics during left ventricular assistance in closed-chest dogs. *Ann Thorac Surg* **56**(1): 54–66; discussion 66–57.

Moon, M. R., DeAnda, A., Castro, L. J., Daughters, G. T., 2nd, Ingels, N. B., Jr., and Miller, D. C. (1997b). Effects of mechanical left ventricular support on right ventricular diastolic function. *J Heart Lung Transplant* **16**(4): 398–407.

Moon, M. R., Ingels, N. B., Jr., Daughters, G. T., 2nd, Stinson, E. B., Hansen, D. E., and Miller, D. C. (1994). Alterations in left ventricular twist mechanics with inotropic stimulation and volume loading in human subjects. *Circulation* **89**(1): 142–150.

Moore, C. C., O'Dell, W. G., McVeigh, E. R., and Zerhouni, E. A. (1992). Calculation of three-dimensional left ventricular strains from biplanar tagged MR images. *J Magn Reson Imaging* **2**(2): 165–175.

Moore, C. C., Reeder, S. B., and McVeigh, E. R. (1994). Tagged MR imaging in a deforming phantom: Photographic validation. *Radiology* **190**(3): 765–769.

Moores, W. Y., LeWinter, M. M., Long, W. B., Grover, M., Mack, R., and Daily, P. O. (1984). Sonomicrometry: Its application as a routine monitoring technique in cardiac surgery. *Ann Thorac Surg* **38**(2): 117–123.

Mosher, T. J. and Smith, M. B. (1990). A DANTE tagging sequence for the evaluation of translational sample motion. *Magn Reson Med* **15**(2): 334–339.

Myers, J. H., Stirling, M. C., Choy, M., Buda, A. J., and Gallagher, K. P. (1986). Direct measurement of inner and outer wall thickening dynamics with epicardial echocardiography. *Circulation* **74**(1): 164–172.

Naito, H., Arisawa, J., Harada, K., Yamagami, H., Kozuka, T., and Tamura, S. (1995). Assessment of right ventricular regional contraction and comparison with the left ventricle in normal humans: A cine magnetic resonance study with presaturation myocardial tagging. *Br Heart J* **74**(2): 186–191.

Niczyporuk, M. A. and Miller, D. C. (1991). Automatic tracking and digitization of multiple radiopaque myocardial markers. *Comput Biomed Res* **24**(2): 129–142.

O'Dell, W. G., Schoeniger, J. S., Blackband, S. J., and McVeigh, E. R. (1994). A modified quadrupole gradient set for use in high resolution MRI tagging. *Magn Reson Med* **32**(2): 246–250.

Olsen, C. O., Jones, R. N., Attarian, D. E., Hill, R. C., Sink, J. D., Chitwood, W. R., Jr., and Wechsler, A. S. (1979). Relationship of LV compliance to coronary artery perfusion pressure in potassium-arrested canine heart during cardiopulmonary bypass. *Surg Forum* **30**: 246–247.

Opdahl, A., Remme, E. W., Helle-Valle, T., Edvardsen, T., and Smiseth, O. A. (2012). Myocardial relaxation, restoring forces, and early-diastolic load are independent determinants of left ventricular untwisting rate. *Circulation* **126**(12): 1441–1451.

Osakada, G., Sasayama, S., Kawai, C., Hirakawa, A., Kemper, W. S., Franklin, D., and Ross, J., Jr. (1980). The analysis of left ventricular wall thickness and shear by an ultrasonic triangulation technique in the dog. *Circ Res* **47**(2): 173–181.

Osman, N. F., Kerwin, W. S., McVeigh, E. R., and Prince, J. L. (1999). Cardiac motion tracking using CINE harmonic phase (HARP) magnetic resonance imaging. *Magn Reson Med* **42**(6): 1048–1060.

Pelc, L. R., Sayre, J., Yun, K., Castro, L. J., Herfkens, R. J., Miller, D. C., and Pelc, N. J. (1994). Evaluation of myocardial motion tracking with cine-phase contrast magnetic resonance imaging. *Invest Radiol* **29**(12): 1038–1042.

Pope, S. E., Stinson, E. B., Daughters, G. T., 2nd, Schroeder, J. S., Ingels, N. B., Jr., and Alderman, E. L. (1980). Exercise response of the denervated heart in long-term cardiac transplant recipients. *Am J Cardiol* **46**(2): 213–218.

Pruessmann, K. P., Weiger, M., Scheidegger, M. B., and Boesiger, P. (1999). SENSE: Sensitivity encoding for fast MRI. *Magn Reson Med* **42**(5): 952–962.

Rademakers, F. E., Buchalter, M. B., Rogers, W. J., Zerhouni, E. A., Weisfeldt, M. L., Weiss, J. L., and Shapiro, E. P. (1992). Dissociation between left ventricular untwisting and filling. Accentuation by catecholamines. *Circulation* **85**(4): 1572–1581.

Raff, G. L. and Glantz, S. A. (1981). Volume loading slows left ventricular isovolumic relaxation rate. Evidence of load-dependent relaxation in the intact dog heart. *Circ Res* **48**(6 Pt 1): 813–824.

Rankin, J. S., McHale, P. A., Arentzen, C. E., Ling, D., Greenfield, J. C., Jr., and Anderson, R. W. (1976). The three-dimensional dynamic geometry of the left ventricle in the conscious dog. *Circ Res* **39**(3): 304–313.

Ricci, D. R., Orlick, A. E., Alderman, E. L., Ingels, N. B., Jr., Daughters, G. T., 2nd, Kusnick, C. A., Reitz, B. A., and Stinson, E. B. (1979a). Role of tachycardia as an inotropic stimulus in man. *J Clin Invest* **63**(4): 695–703.

Ricci, D. R., Orlick, A. E., Alderman, E. L., Ingels, N. B., Jr., Daughters, G. T., 2nd, and Stinson, E. B. (1979b). Influence of heart rate on left ventricular ejection fraction in human beings. *Am J Cardiol* **44**(3): 447–451.

Rodriguez, F., Langer, F., Harrington, K. B., Cheng, A., Daughters, G. T., Criscione, J. C., Ingels, N. B., and Miller, D. C. (2005). Alterations in transmural strains adjacent to ischemic myocardium during acute midcircumflex occlusion. *J Thorac Cardiovasc Surg* **129**(4): 791–803.

Rodriguez, F., Langer, F., Harrington, K. B., Tibayan, F. A., Zasio, M. K., Liang, D., Daughters, G. T., Ingels, N. B., and Miller, D. C. (2004a). Cutting second-order chords does not prevent acute ischemic mitral regurgitation. *Circulation* **110**(11 Suppl 1): II91–II97.

Rodriguez, F., Tibayan, F. A., Glasson, J. R., Liang, D., Daughters, G. T., Ingels, N. B., Jr., and Miller, D. C. (2004b). Fixed-apex mitral annular descent correlates better with left ventricular systolic function than does free-apex left ventricular long-axis shortening. *J Am Soc Echocardiogr* **17**(2): 101–107.

Rogers, W. J., Jr., Shapiro, E. P., Weiss, J. L., Buchalter, M. B., Rademakers, F. E., Weisfeldt, M. L., and Zerhouni, E. A. (1991). Quantification of and correction for left ventricular systolic long-axis shortening by magnetic resonance tissue tagging and slice isolation. *Circulation* **84**(2): 721–731.

Ross, J., Jr. and Franklin, D. (1976). Analysis of regional myocardial function, dimensions, and wall thickness in the characterization of myocardial ischemia and infarction. *Circulation* **53**(3 Suppl): I88–I92.

Rushmer, R. F. (1954). Continuous measurements of left ventricular dimensions in intact, unanesthetized dogs. *Circ Res* **2**(1): 14–21.

Rushmer, R. F., Crystal, D. K., and Wagner, C. (1953). The functional anatomy of ventricular contraction. *Circ Res* **1**(2): 162–170.

Russell, K., Eriksen, M., Aaberge, L., Wilhelmsen, N., Skulstad, H., Remme, E. W., Haugaa, K. H. et al. (2012). A novel clinical method for quantification of regional left ventricular pressure-strain loop area: A non-invasive index of myocardial work. *Eur Heart J* **33**(6): 724–733.

Sabbah, H. N., Marzilli, M., and Stein, P. D. (1981). The relative role of subendocardium and subepicardium in left ventricular mechanics. *Am J Physiol* **240**(6): H920–H926.

Sacks, M. S., Enomoto, Y., Graybill, J. R., Merryman, W. D., Zeeshan, A., Yoganathan, A. P., Levy, R. J., Gorman, R. C., and Gorman, J. H., 3rd (2006). In-vivo dynamic deformation of the mitral valve anterior leaflet. *Ann Thorac Surg* **82**(4): 1369–1377.

Sallin, E. A. (1969). Fiber orientation and ejection fraction in the human left ventricle. *Biophys J* **9**(7): 954–964.

Sandler, H. and Alderman, E. (1974). Determination of left ventricular size and shape. *Circ Res* **40**(4): 1–8.

Sasayama, S., Franklin, D., Ross, J., Jr., Kemper, W. S., and McKown, D. (1976a). Dynamic changes in left ventricular wall thickness and their use in analyzing cardiac function in the conscious dog. *Am J Cardiol* **38**(7): 870–879.

Sasayama, S., Ross, J., Jr., Franklin, D., Bloor, C. M., Bishop, S., and Dilley, R. B. (1976b). Adaptations of the left ventricle to chronic pressure overload. *Circ Res* **38**(3): 172–178.

Savin, W. M., Alderman, E. L., Haskell, W. L., Schroeder, J. S., Ingels, N. B., Jr., Daughters, G. T., 2nd, and Stinson, E. B. (1980). Left ventricular response to isometric exercise in patients with denervated and innervated hearts. *Circulation* **61**(5): 897–901.

Schnittger, I., Fitzgerald, P. J., Daughters, G. T., Ingels, N. B., Kantrowitz, N. E., Schwarzkopf, A., Mead, C. W., and Popp, R. L. (1982). Limitations of comparing left ventricular volumes by two dimensional echocardiography, myocardial markers and cineangiography. *Am J Cardiol* **50**(3): 512–519.

Seo, Y., Ishizu, T., Enomoto, Y., Sugimori, H., and Aonuma, K. (2011). Endocardial surface area tracking for assessment of regional LV wall deformation with 3D speckle tracking imaging. *JACC Cardiovasc Imaging* **4**(4): 358–365.

Shake, J. G., Gruber, P. J., Baumgartner, W. A., Senechal, G., Meyers, J., Redmond, J. M., Pittenger, M. F., and Martin, B. J. (2002). Mesenchymal stem cell implantation in a swine myocardial infarct model: Engraftment and functional effects. *Ann Thorac Surg* **73**(6): 1919–1925; discussion 1926.

Shoukas, A. A., Sagawa, K., and Maughan, W. L. (1981). Chronic implantation of radiopaque beads on endocardium, midwall, and epicardium. *Am J Physiol* **241**(1): H104–H107.

Sigfridsson, A., Haraldsson, H., Ebbers, T., Knutsson, H., and Sakuma, H. (2011). In vivo SNR in DENSE MRI; temporal and regional effects of field strength, receiver coil sensitivity and flip angle strategies. *Magn Reson Imaging* **29**(2): 202–208.

Sogaard, P., Egeblad, H., Kim, W. Y., Jensen, H. K., Pedersen, A. K., Kristensen, B. O., and Mortensen, P. T. (2002). Tissue Doppler imaging predicts improved systolic performance and reversed left ventricular remodeling during long-term cardiac resynchronization therapy. *J Am Coll Cardiol* **40**(4): 723–730.

Stinson, E. B., Ingels, N. B., Jr., Daughters, G., Alderman, E. L., Griepp, R. B., Oyer, P. R., Copeland, J. G., and Shumway, N. E. (1975). New technique for serial noninvasive measurement of left ventricular dynamics in man: Application to cardiac transplantation. *Surg Forum* **26**: 230–232.

Stokland, O., Miller, M. M., Lekven, J., and Ilebekk, A. (1980). The significance of the intact pericardium for cardiac performance in the dog. *Circ Res* **47**(1): 27–32.

Streeter, D. D., Jr., Spotnitz, H. M., Patel, D. P., Ross, J., Jr., and Sonnenblick, E. H. (1969). Fiber orientation in the canine left ventricle during diastole and systole. *Circ Res* **24**(3): 339–347.

Theroux, P., Franklin, D., Ross, J., Jr., and Kemper, W. S. (1974). Regional myocardial function during acute coronary artery occlusion and its modification by pharmacologic agents in the dog. *Circ Res* **35**(6): 896–908.

Theroux, P., Ross, J., Jr., Franklin, D., Kemper, W. S., and Sasyama, S. (1976). Regional Myocardial function in the conscious dog during acute coronary occlusion and responses to morphine, propranolol, nitroglycerin, and lidocaine. *Circulation* **53**(2): 302–314.

Thompson, R. B., Emani, S. M., Davis, B. H., van den Bos, E. J., Morimoto, Y., Craig, D., Glower, D., and Taylor, D. A. (2003). Comparison of intracardiac cell transplantation: Autologous skeletal myoblasts versus bone marrow cells. *Circulation* **108**(Suppl 1): II264–II271.

Tibayan, F. A., Lai, D. T., Timek, T. A., Dagum, P., Liang, D., Daughters, G. T., Ingels, N. B., and Miller, D. C. (2002). Alterations in left ventricular torsion in tachycardia-induced dilated cardiomyopathy. *J Thorac Cardiovasc Surg* **124**(1): 43–49.

Tibayan, F. A., Lai, D. T., Timek, T. A., Dagum, P., Liang, D., Zasio, M. K., Daughters, G. T., Miller, D. C., and Ingels, N. B., Jr. (2003). Alterations in left ventricular curvature and principal strains in dilated cardiomyopathy with functional mitral regurgitation. *J Heart Valve Dis* **12**(3): 292–299.

Tibayan, F. A., Rodriguez, F., Langer, F., Zasio, M. K., Bailey, L., Liang, D., Daughters, G. T., Ingels, N. B., Jr., and Miller, D. C. (2004). Alterations in left ventricular torsion and diastolic recoil after myocardial infarction with and without chronic ischemic mitral regurgitation. *Circulation* **110**(11 Suppl 1): II109–II114.

Torrent-Guasp, F., Kocica, M. J., Corno, A. F., Komeda, M., Carreras-Costa, F., Flotats, A., Cosin-Aguillar, J., and Wen, H. (2005). Towards new understanding of the heart structure and function. *Eur J Cardiothorac Surg* **27**(2): 191–201.

Tyson, G. S., Jr., Olsen, C. O., Maier, G. W., Davis, J. W., Sethi, G. K., Scott, S. M., Sabiston, D. C., Jr., and Rankin, J. S. (1982). Dimensional characteristics of left ventricular function after coronary artery bypass grafting. *Circulation* **66**(2 Pt 2): I16–I25.

Valeti, V. U., Chun, W., Potter, D. D., Araoz, P. A., McGee, K. P., Glockner, J. F., and Christian, T. F. (2006). Myocardial tagging and strain analysis at 3 Tesla: Comparison with 1.5 Tesla imaging. *J Magn Reson Imaging* **23**(4): 477–480.

Van Leuven, S. L., Waldman, L. K., McCulloch, A. D., and Covell, J. W. (1994). Gradients of epicardial strain across the perfusion boundary during acute myocardial ischemia. *Am J Physiol* **267**(6 Pt 2): H2348–H2362.

Villarreal, F. J., Lew, W. Y., Waldman, L. K., and Covell, J. W. (1991). Transmural myocardial deformation in the ischemic canine left ventricle. *Circ Res* **68**(2): 368–381.

Villarreal, F. J., Waldman, L. K., and Lew, W. Y. (1988). Technique for measuring regional two-dimensional finite strains in canine left ventricle. *Circ Res* **62**(4): 711–721.

Vine, D. L., Dodge, H. T., Frimer, M., Stewart, D. K., and Caldwell, J. (1976). Quantitative measurement of left ventricular volumes in man from radiopaque epicardial markers. *Circulation* **54**(3): 391–398.

Waldman, L. K., Fung, Y. C., and Covell, J. W. (1985). Transmural myocardial deformation in the canine left ventricle. Normal in vivo three-dimensional finite strains. *Circ Res* **57**(1): 152–163.

Waldman, L. K., Nosan, D., Villarreal, F., and Covell, J. W. (1988). Relation between transmural deformation and local myofiber direction in canine left ventricle. *Circ Res* **63**(3): 550–562.

Walley, K. R., Grover, M., Raff, G. L., Benge, J. W., Hannaford, B., and Glantz, S. A. (1982). Left ventricular dynamic geometry in the intact and open chest dog. *Circ Res* **50**(4): 573–589.

Warner, K. G., Sheahan, M. G., Arebi, S. M., Banerjee, A., Deiss-Shrem, J. M., and Khabbaz, K. R. (2001). Proper timing of blood cardioplegia in infant lambs: Superiority of a multiple-dose regimen. *Ann Thorac Surg* **71**(3): 872–876.

Weintraub, W. S., Akizuki, S., Agarwal, J. B., Bodenheimer, M. M., Banka, V. S., and Helfant, R. H. (1982a). Comparative effects of nitroglycerin and nifedipine on myocardial blood flow and contraction during flow-limiting coronary stenosis in the dog. *Am J Cardiol* **50**(2): 281–288.

Weintraub, W. S., Hattori, S., Agarwal, J. B., Bodenheimer, M. M., Banka, V. S., and Helfant, R. H. (1981). The relationship between myocardial blood flow and contraction by myocardial layer in the canine left ventricle during ischemia. *Circ Res* **48**(3): 430–438.

Weintraub, W. S., Hattori, S., Agarwal, J. B., Bodenheimer, M. M., Banka, V. S., and Helfant, R. H. (1982b). The effects of nifedipine on myocardial blood flow and contraction during ischemia in the dog. *Circulation* **65**(1): 49–53.

Wildenthal, K. and Mitchell, J. H. (1969). Dimensional analysis of the left ventricle in unanesthetized dogs. *J Appl Physiol* **27**(1): 115–119.

Williams, J. F., Jr., Glick, G., and Braunwald, E. (1965). Studies on cardiac dimensions in intact unanesthetized man. V. Effects of nitroglycerin. *Circulation* **32**(5): 767–771.

Wranne, B., Pinto, F. J., Siegel, L. C., Miller, D. C., and Schnittger, I. (1993). Abnormal postoperative interventricular motion: New intraoperative transesophageal echocardiographic evidence supports a novel hypothesis. *Am Heart J* **126**(1): 161–167.

Yarbrough, W. M., Mukherjee, R., Stroud, R. E., Meyer, E. C., Escobar, G. P., Sample, J. A., Hendrick, J. W., Mingoia, J. T., and Spinale, F. G. (2010). Caspase inhibition modulates left ventricular remodeling following myocardial infarction through cellular and extracellular mechanisms. *J Cardiovasc Pharmacol* **55**(4): 408–416.

Yeon, S. B., Reichek, N., Tallant, B. A., Lima, J. A., Calhoun, L. P., Clark, N. R., Hoffman, E. A., Ho, K. K., and Axel, L. (2001). Validation of in vivo myocardial strain measurement by magnetic resonance tagging with sonomicrometry. *J Am Coll Cardiol* **38**(2): 555–561.

Young, A. A., Axel, L., Dougherty, L., Bogen, D. K., and Parenteau, C. S. (1993). Validation of tagging with MR imaging to estimate material deformation. *Radiology* **188**(1): 101–108.

Yun, K. L. and Miller, D. C. (1995). Torsional deformation of the left ventricle. *J Heart Valve Dis* **4**(Suppl 2): S214–S220; discussion S220–S212.

Yun, K. L., Niczyporuk, M. A., Daughters, G. T., 2nd, Ingels, N. B., Jr., Stinson, E. B., Alderman, E. L., Hansen, D. E., and Miller, D. C. (1991). Alterations in left ventricular diastolic twist mechanics during acute human cardiac allograft rejection. *Circulation* **83**(3): 962–973.

Zerhouni, E. A., Parish, D. M., Rogers, W. J., Yang, A., and Shapiro, E. P. (1988). Human heart: Tagging with MR imaging—A method for noninvasive assessment of myocardial motion. *Radiology* **169**(1): 59–63.

Zhong, X., Spottiswoode, B. S., Meyer, C. H., Kramer, C. M., and Epstein, F. H. (2010). Imaging three-dimensional myocardial mechanics using navigator-gated volumetric spiral cine DENSE MRI. *Magn Reson Med* **64**(4): 1089–1097.

10 SPAMM and DANTE Tagging

El-Sayed H. Ibrahim, PhD

CONTENTS

LIST OF ABBREVIATIONS

Abbreviation	Meaning
1D	One dimensional
2D	Two dimensional
3D	Three dimensional
AIR-SPAMM	Alternate inversion recovery SPAMM
CABG	Coronary artery bypass grafting
CSI	Chemical shift imaging
CSPAMM	Complementary SPAMM
DANTE	Delays alternating with nutations for tailored excitations
ECG	Electrocardiogram
HARP	Harmonic phase
IR	Inversion recovery
LV	Left ventricle
PC	Phase contrast
RF	Radio frequency
SAR	Specific absorption rate
SNR	Signal-to-noise ratio
SPAMM	Spatial modulation of magnetization
SPAMM n' EGGS	SPAMM with encoded gradients for gauging speed
SPAMM-PAV	SPAMM with polarity alternating velocity-encoding
SR	Saturation recovery

10.1 INTRODUCTION

10.1.1 SPAMM AND DANTE: ROBUST TAGGING METHODS AND THE FOUNDATION OF ADVANCED TECHNIQUES

Different MRI tagging techniques have been proposed for measuring myocardial deformation using MRI (Ibrahim 2011). Generally, these techniques can be divided into magnitude-based and phase-based techniques depending on how the magnetization is manipulated during the MRI scan to reflect tissue motion. The spatial modulation of magnetization (SPAMM) technique covered in this chapter belongs to the first group. Nevertheless, it stands out as the most widely used tagging technique since its introduction by Axel and Dougherty in 1989 until our current day.

Despite being the first MRI tagging technique that allowed for noninvasive evaluation of regional myocardial deformation, the magnetization saturation tagging technique developed by Zerhouni et al. (1988) (see Chapter 9) has limitations that hinder its use in clinical applications. These limitations include the limited number of tag lines that can be created, low tags density, long tags preparation time, and high specific absorption rate (SAR). One year after the introduction of Zerhouni's technique, Axel and Dougherty developed the SPAMM technique (Axel and Dougherty 1989b), which alleviates the aforementioned limitations of the magnetization saturation tagging technique. The SPAMM technique's efficiency and short tags preparation time lead to its adoption in many clinical studies of different heart diseases. Further, SPAMM is the basis for advanced tagging techniques that have been developed later, for example, complementary SPAMM (CSPAMM) by Fischer et al. (1993) and harmonic phase (HARP) by Osman et al. (1999). In this chapter, the SPAMM technique is reviewed in details along with its different development stages. This chapter also covers the delays alternating with nutations for tailored excitations (DANTE) tagging technique. DANTE is one of the early tagging techniques that was developed in 1990 by Mosher and Smith (1990), and despite its limited applications, it has a number of advantages and unique features.

10.1.2 CHAPTER OUTLINE

In this chapter, SPAMM, the work horse tagging pulse sequence, is reviewed in detail along with the DANTE technique, which was invented at approximately the same time as SPAMM. The chapter starts by explaining the effects of the different radio-frequency (RF) and gradient pulses in the SPAMM module on spins dispersion for generating the tagging sinusoidal pattern. The magnetization evolution after the tagging module is also described, including the magnetization relaxation effect on tags fading. Different strategies for enhancing the tagging profile are then discussed, including high-order SPAMM and sinc-modulated tagging. The next section in the chapter addresses a number of technical issues, including the effects of tag spacing and pixel size on tags appearance, magnitude reconstruction and its effect on tagging pattern uniformity, noise effects, and respiratory gating. Different efforts for validating SPAMM are then discussed, including phantom, animal models, and simulation experiments. The simulation section covers the partitions model, SIMTAG, and small-tip-angle approximation. The chapter then covers different SPAMM developments, including cascaded SPAMM, AIR-SPAMM, and phase-sensitive SPAMM. Different pulse sequences that combine SPAMM with velocity encoding are also covered in the chapter, including

SPAMM n' EGGS and SPAMM-PAV. The following sections in the chapter cover SPAMM-based three-dimensional (3D) motion analysis and high-field SPAMM imaging. The last section about SPAMM covers its applications, including tissue deformation and other cardiac and noncardiac applications. Besides SPAMM, the chapter also covers the DANTE tagging technique, starting with its working idea and advantages. Different sequence developments are then reviewed, including double-DANTE, adiabatic DANTE, combined DANTE/phase-contrast (PC), and black-blood DANTE imaging. The chapter then concludes by reviewing the hybrid DANTE/SPAMM sequence. It should be noted that the applications of the SPAMM and DANTE techniques discussed in this chapter are limited to early applications or studies conducted to validate the techniques. For comprehensive coverage of clinical tagging applications, the reader is referred to Chapters 9 and 10 of *Heart Mechanics: Magnetic Resonance Imaging—Advanced Techniques, Clinical Applications, and Future Trends.*

10.2 SPAMM: THE BASICS

SPAMM tagging (Axel and Dougherty 1989b) provides a simple and efficient way for measuring regional heart function parameters, for example, strain, strain rate, and torsion. SPAMM

tagging consists of two nonselective 90° RF pulses interspersed by a modulating gradient in the direction orthogonal to the tag lines, and followed by a spoiler gradient (Figure 10.1a). These four pulses (2 RF pulses and 2 gradients) comprise the tagging preparation module, which is implemented immediately after the detection of the R-wave of the electrocardiogram (ECG). Following tags preparation, a multiphase segmented data acquisition is conducted until the next R-wave, where the tagging–imaging modules are repeated until all data required for constructing the images is acquired. When the SPAMM images acquired at different heart phases are played back in a cine mode, myocardial deformation can be tracked, and measures of regional heart function can be obtained.

10.2.1 THEORY OF SPAMM

Each of the four pulses that comprise the SPAMM tagging module, as shown in Figure 10.1a, has a specific role in generating the tagging pattern. For better understanding of the SPAMM technique, let us track the behavior of nine equidistant magnetization vectors (M_1 to M_9) along the x-axis (the tagging direction, which is perpendicular to the tag lines). We will study the behavior of these vectors at six different

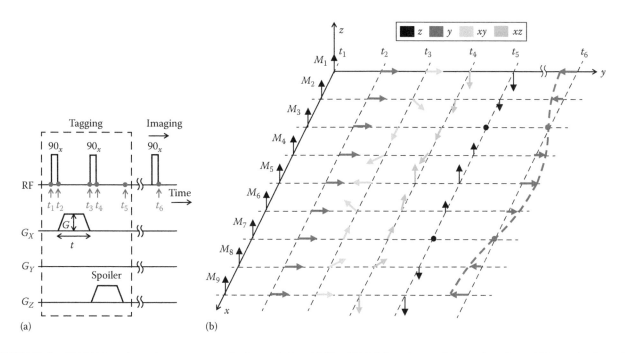

FIGURE 10.1 SPAMM tagging pulse sequence and spins evolution. (a) The SPAMM tagging module consists of two 90° nonselective radio-frequency (RF) pulses, separated by the tagging gradient in the tagging direction (x-direction in this example) and followed by a large spoiler gradient. Only one 90° excitation flip angle in the imaging module is shown in the figure. (b) Spins distribution at timepoints t_1–t_6 before and after the application of each RF pulse. Only nine magnetization vectors M_1–M_9 are shown for clarity. The following color codes are used for spins orientation: black, spins are pointing in the $\pm z$-direction; red, spins are pointing in the $\pm y$-direction; green, spins lie in the x–y plane; and blue, spins lie in the x–z plane. At timepoint t_1 immediately before the application of the first tagging RF pulse, the magnetization is at equilibrium and all spins are pointing in the $+z$-direction. At timepoint t_2 immediately after the implementation of the first 90° tagging RF pulse, all spins are tipped into the transverse plane and are pointing in the $+y$-direction. At timepoint t_3 after the implementation of the tagging gradient, the spins have accumulated different phases based on their x-location, such that they are now dispersed in the x–y plane. The second 90° tagging RF pulse rotates all the spins one more time around the x-axis, such that at timepoint t_4, all spins lie in the x–z plane. The spoiler gradient eliminates all transverse magnetization components (in the x-direction), such that at timepoint t_5, only the longitudinal components are remaining (now all spins point in the $\pm z$-direction and have a sinusoidal pattern along the x-direction). Finally, the 90° imaging RF pulse tips this sinusoidal pattern in the transverse plane, where it is imaged showing the famous tag lines (each sinusoidal period represents two adjacent lines (one bright and one dark)) perpendicular to the x-axis.

timepoints (t_1–t_6), as shown in Figure 10.1a. For this analysis, the followings are assumed: rotating frame of reference, unit-magnitude magnetization vectors, and full magnetization recovery before the R-wave.

10.2.1.1 Magnetization Modulation

At timepoint t_1 immediately before the application of the first tagging RF pulse (= 90°), all magnetization vectors are at equilibrium with unit magnitude in the longitudinal (z) direction (Figure 10.1b). The first RF pulse of the tagging module (applied in the x-direction) tips all the magnetization vectors in the transverse plane. Therefore, at timepoint t_2, all magnetization vectors point in the +y-direction. At this timepoint, the modulating gradient is turned on, which creates a linearly varying weak magnetic field (in the x-direction) that is superimposed on the main magnetic field B_0, and therefore results in increasing spins precession frequency along the x-direction. By the end of the gradient pulse (and immediately before the application of the second tagging RF pulse) at timepoint t_3, the transverse magnetization becomes modulated, that is, different spins accumulate different phase shifts $\left(= \gamma \int G_x \, x \, dt\right)$ based on their location in the x-direction (M_1, located at $x = 0$, experiences zero magnetic field, and thus does not accumulate any phase shift). It should be noted that the spins' phase distribution depends on the area under the gradient pulse, which depends on both the gradient pulse's strength and duration.

10.2.1.2 Magnetization Storage

The second RF pulse of the tagging module (assumed to be applied also in the x-direction) tips the magnetization vectors by another 90° pulse, such that the vectors have the distribution shown at timepoint t_4 in Figure 10.1b (M_3 and M_7 are not affected by the second RF pulse as they already lie in the x-direction). It should be noted that each vector can be represented by its two components in the longitudinal (z) and transverse (x) directions. The (large) spoiler gradient starts at timepoint t_4, which results in dephasing the transverse

magnetization components. By the end of the spoiler gradient at timepoint t_5, the transverse components of the magnetization vectors become totally dephased (nulled), and we are left only with the longitudinal components, which now form a sinusoidal pattern stored in the longitudinal direction until the imaging timepoint t_6, where it is tipped into the transverse direction for readout. The longitudinal magnetization at timepoint t_5 is modulated and can be expressed as

$$M_z(x,t) = M_0 \cos\left(\gamma \int_0^\tau G_x(t) \, x \, dt\right), \qquad (10.1)$$

where
   M_0 is the length of the magnetization vectors at timepoint t_1 before tagging
   τ is the duration of the tagging gradient pulse
   γ is the gyromagnetic ratio

This implementation creates a one-dimensional (1D) tagging pattern in the x-direction, where bright and dark tag lines are represented by the peaks and troughs of the generated sinusoidal pattern. If a tagging grid pattern is required, a second tagging module (RF pulse/modulating gradient/RF pulse/spoiler gradient) is applied in the y-direction immediately after the first tagging module, as shown in Figure 10.2. It should be noted that applying simultaneous x- and y-gradients does not generate a two-dimensional (2D) grid-tagged pattern; it rather results in 1D tagging in an oblique direction, which is determined based on the relative strength of G_x and G_y.

10.2.1.3 Tagging Parameters

The settings of the pulses used in the tagging module determine the shape of the tagging pattern. The modulation magnitude is determined by the tagging flip angles. RF pulses with less than 90° flip angles could be implemented for partial magnetization excitation, which results in reduced tagging contrast, but reserves part of the longitudinal magnetization

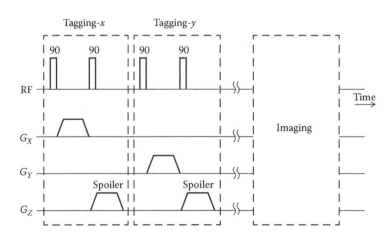

FIGURE 10.2 Two-dimensional (2D) SPAMM. 2D grid tagging is accomplished by consecutive application of the tagging module in the x- and y-directions.

for later modulation during the next cardiac cycles. The orientation of the tag lines is determined by the direction of the applied modulation gradient, and the tagging frequency is determined by the strength and duration of the modulation gradient.

10.2.1.4 Tags Fading

Later at the imaging timepoint t_6, the longitudinal magnetization is recalled for imaging, that is, it is tipped into the transverse plane by the imaging RF pulse (imaging flip angle is assumed to be 90° in our analysis), where the acquired image shows the modulated magnetization as stripes with sinusoidal intensity variation in the tagging direction.

It should be noted that during the time duration between t_5 and t_6, the stored tagged magnetization experiences exponential longitudinal relaxation based on the tissue's T_1 value, which results in reduction of the peak-to-peak tagging contrast, as well as buildup of an additional nontagged magnetization component (also known as the DC component, borrowing the term from "direct current" in electrical engineering), as shown in Figure 10.3. Therefore, the sinusoidal tagging pattern starts with a zero mean (average value) at timepoint t_5, and subsequently develops an overhead DC component, which continues to increase and results in tags fading. At the imaging timepoint t_6, the longitudinal magnetization can be expressed as

$$M_z(x,t) = M_0 \cos\left(\gamma \int_0^\tau G_x(t)\,x\,dt\right) e^{-t/T_1} + M_0\left(1 - e^{-t/T_1}\right).$$
(10.2)

10.2.1.5 Motion Encoding

Since tissue magnetization is a material property, any tissue motion during the time between the SPAMM preparation and subsequent image acquisition results in a corresponding displacement of the tagging pattern in the acquired image.

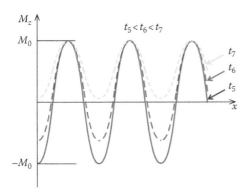

FIGURE 10.3 Tags fading. At timepoint t_5 immediately after tagging preparation (solid blue line), there is a high tagging contrast, ranging from $-M_0$ to $+M_0$. At the imaging timepoint t_6 (dashed red line), the tagging contrast is reduced due to longitudinal magnetization relaxation, which reduces the peak-to-peak signal contrast (AC component) and adds an offset (signal mean or average) DC component. At a later timepoint t_7 in the cardiac cycle (dotted green line), the tagging pattern is shallow. AC, alternating current; DC, direct current.

The value of M_z immediately after the tagging module is applied is given by (assuming 1D tagging and a rectangular gradient pulse)

$$M_z(x,t_5) = M_0(x)\cos(\gamma \tau G_x x) = M_0(x)\cos(\omega_0 x),$$
(10.3)

where
- $\omega_0 = \gamma \tau G_x$ is the frequency of the tagging sinusoid (known as the tagging frequency)
- t_5 is the timepoint immediately after applying the tagging module
- $M_0(x)$ is the equilibrium magnetization value at point x

Due to myocardium deformation during the cardiac cycle, the magnetization vector at a certain location x_0 in the image acquired at timepoint t_6 must have moved from its original location $p(x_0)$ at timepoint t_5, where $p(x_0)$ is known as the reference map. The tagged image, therefore, represents the distribution of the longitudinal magnetization, which is a material property of the tissue, represented as

$$M_z(x_0,t_6) = M_z\big(p(x_0),t_5\big) = M_0\big(p(x_0)\big)\cos\big(\omega_0 p(x_0)\big).$$
(10.4)

This magnetization can be expressed in terms of the tissue displacement u between the imaging and tagging timepoints, which is given by

$$u(x_0,t_6) = p(x_0) - x_0.$$
(10.5)

Using Equations 10.4 and 10.5, the longitudinal magnetization can be rewritten in terms of its displacement:

$$M_z(x_0,t_6) = M_0\big(p(x_0)\big)\cos\big(\omega_0(x_0 + u(x_0,t_6))\big),$$
(10.6)

and therefore it encodes (and shows) tissue displacement. The previously developed equations can be easily expanded into 2D and 3D.

10.2.2 Enhancing the Tagging Profile

The tagging profile affects the accuracy of motion extraction during the image postprocessing stage (Atalar and McVeigh 1994, O'Dell et al. 1995). One limitation of SPAMM tagging is that it produces tag lines with sinusoidal intensity profile, which are more difficult to track than sharper-edged stripes (e.g., as in Zerhouni's magnetization saturation tagging). Therefore, different efforts have been made to enhance the tagging profile, as explained in this section.

10.2.2.1 High-Order SPAMM

The small-tip-angle approximation states that the frequency spectrum (or magnetization profile) of the excitation RF pulse is proportional to the Fourier transform of the time domain pulse sequence (Pauly et al. 2011). Although this approximation has been developed for small flip angles, it is

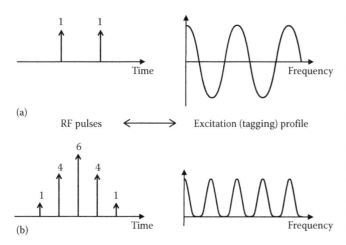

FIGURE 10.4 Binomial SPAMM. (a) 1-1 SPAMM sequence (left) and the corresponding excitation (tagging) profile (right) based on small-tip-angle approximation. (b) 1-4-6-4-1 SPAMM and the corresponding excitation profile. Note the sharper tags profile with higher-order binomials.

still applicable to relatively large flip angles. Therefore, the SPAMM technique described in the previous section (which approximately represents two impulses) generates a sinusoidal tagging profile (Figure 10.4a), resulting in smooth variation of the signal intensity between adjacent bright and dark stripes. In order to create a better tagging profile (closer to the square shape with uniform magnetization excitation and sharp edges), the simple 90°–90° RF pulses in the original tagging module (known as 1-1 SPAMM) are replaced by a composite pulse consisting of simple concatenated RF pulses, or subpulses, whose relative amplitudes are

coefficients of a binomial series (e.g., 1-2-1, 1-3-3-1, 1-4-6-4-1, …), as shown in Figure 10.4 (Axel and Dougherty 1989a). With this broader tagging concept, 1-1 SPAMM could be considered as a special case of binomial SPAMM, where n (the binomial order) = 1.

Basically, the higher the binomial order of the SPAMM sequence, the sharper the resulting tagging profile. The tagging modulation gradients played in-between the tagging RF pulses point in the same direction and have the same strength, and as in 1-1 SPAMM, they control the orientation and frequency of the tag lines. The total flip angle of all tagging RF pulses is kept the same regardless of the binomial order. For example, for a total flip angle of 180°, the flip angle distribution is 90°–90°, 45°–90°–45°, and 22.5°–67.5°–67.5°–22.5° for $n = 1$, 2, and 3, respectively. In practice, the delta Dirac impulse functions shown in Figure 10.4 are replaced by short hard (rectangular) pulses, and instead of changing the pulses' duration, their magnitudes are adjusted based on the binomial coefficients. To avoid perturbing the tagging pattern as a result of local field variation or regional chemical shift differences, the time interval between adjacent tagging RF pulses is kept as short as possible. High-order binomial SPAMM significantly improves the quality of the tag lines, which allows for generating 2D grid tagging patterns. In their original work using binomial SPAMM, Axel and Dougherty (1989a) generated 2D grid tags with two 1-4-6-4-1 tagging modules lasting for 9 ms.

10.2.2.2 Sinc-Modulated RF Pulses

As discussed in the previous section, a high-quality tagging profile is important for achieving accurate strain measurements. Therefore, an ideal tag line would have a rectangular

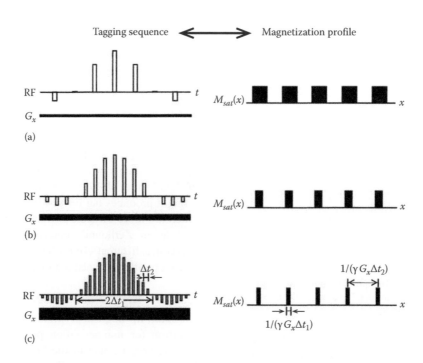

FIGURE 10.5 sinc-Modulated tagging sequences (left) and magnetization profiles (right). Constant gradient is used in all examples. The tags width-to-separation ratios are (a) 1:2, (b) 1:4, and (c) 1:8. (Reproduced from Wu, E.X. et al., *Magn. Reson. Med.*, 48(2), 389, 2002. With permission.)

intensity profile. Building on the high-order SPAMM technique presented in the previous section, Wu et al. (2002) developed a modified SPAMM technique for improving the tagging profile. The developed method is based on modulating the RF pulse train with a sinc function (sinc(x) = sin(x)/x) in the presence of a constant gradient, which according to the small-tip-angle approximation, results in a rectangular tagging profile, where the bandwidth of the sinc function determines the width of the tag line (Figures 10.5 and 10.6). Compared to SPAMM, high-order SPAMM, and DANTE (illustrated later in the chapter),

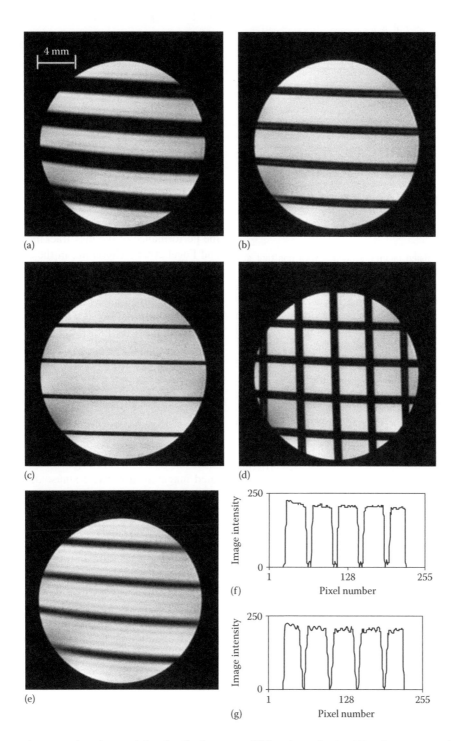

FIGURE 10.6 Phantom images using sinc-modulated radio-frequency (RF) pulse train. (a–c) Tagging patterns of varying tag width-to-separation ratios produced by the sinc-modulated RF pulse trains shown in Figure 10.5a through c, respectively. (d) 2D tagging using the sinc-modulated RF pulse train in figure 5 (b). (e) DANTE tagging equivalent to (b) in terms of tag width and separation. (f, g) Vertical image intensity profiles from images in (b) and (e), respectively. (Reproduced from Wu, E.X. et al., *Magn. Reson. Med.*, 48(2), 389, 2002. With permission.)

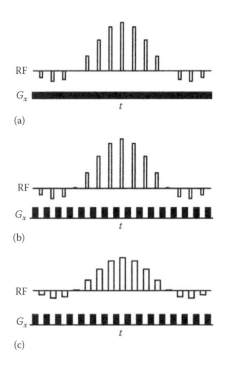

FIGURE 10.7 sinc-Modulated tagging sequence with constant and segmented gradients. (a) sinc-Modulated tagging sequence with a constant gradient. (b) The constant gradient is replaced by gradient segments between the radio-frequency (RF) pulses. (c) The duration of the RF pulses is increased to reduce peak power requirement. (Reproduced from Wu, E.X. et al., *Magn. Reson. Med.*, 48(2), 389, 2002. With permission.)

the developed technique has the flexibility of modifying the ratio between the tagline width and tags separation.

The sinc-modulated tagging pattern could be represented as

$$tag(t) = \text{sinc}(\pi t/\Delta t_1) \times \text{comb}(t, \Delta t_2), \quad (10.7)$$

where
  $\text{sinc}(\pi t/\Delta t_1)$ is the sinc function (with the first zero crossing at $t = \Delta t_1$)
  $\text{comb}(t, \Delta t_2)$ is the comb function with spacing of Δt_2

The tagging profile in the spatial frequency domain can then be approximated by the following convolution (*):

$$M_{tag}(x) = \text{rect}(\gamma G_x \Delta t_1 x) * \text{comb}\left(x, \frac{1}{\gamma G_x \Delta t_2}\right), \quad (10.8)$$

which results in rectangular tags with width = $1/\gamma G_x \Delta t_1$ and separation = $1/\gamma G_x \Delta t_2$.

It should be noted that the RF pulses have a finite width, which may cause an undesirable shading effect in the resulting images (Wu et al. 2002). Assuming the width of the RF pulses is Δt_3, the shading is characterized by modulation with function $\text{sinc}(\pi \gamma G_x \Delta t_3)$. One solution to avoid this shading artifact without modifying the desired rectangular tag profile is to replace the constant gradient G_x by gradient segments in between the tagging RF pulses, as shown in Figure 10.7.

This solution allows for increasing the RF pulse durations to reduce SAR, as well as for equalizing the RF pulse amplitudes to minimize the time required for tags preparation.

10.3 TECHNICAL ISSUES, VALIDATION, AND SIMULATION OF SPAMM

10.3.1 TECHNICAL ISSUES

10.3.1.1 Spatial Resolution and Tagging Appearance

The image spatial resolution (pixel size) relative to tag spacing (distance between adjacent tag lines) is a key issue for determining the appearance of the SPAMM-tagged pattern in the resulting image, especially in children with small anatomy. The ratio of tag-spacing to pixel-size is about 8 in adults, which results in clearly identified intersection points of orthogonal tag lines (Haselgrove and Fogel 2005). However, with reduced ratio (~6), the tagging pattern is less resolved; and for a ratio of 4, the appearance of the tagging pattern changes from a set of parallel lines perpendicular to each other to a checkerboard of white and dark squares (Figures 10.8 and 10.9), which affects the performance of the tags tracking algorithms (Haselgrove and Fogel 2005). Therefore, in the case of small tag-spacing to pixel-size ratios, better analysis results can be obtained by tracking the regions with bright signal in the image rather than tracking the intersection points in the tagging grid. As a general rule, the tag spacing should be less than half the thickness of the heart wall for reliable measurements. It should be also larger than the image pixel size so that the tag lines could be correctly resolved. Nevertheless, these requirements are hard to meet in children, which necessitates a compromise such that tag spacing is always larger than the pixel size.

10.3.1.2 Magnetization Relaxation and Tags Appearance

Immediately after applying the tagging module, the modulated magnetization has a sinusoidal pattern across the tagging direction with zero mean and maximum peak-to-peak (AC component; the term borrowed from "alternating current" in electrical engineering) value of 2, assuming inversion recovery (IR; total tagging flip angle of 180° distributed over the two RF pulses) and unit-magnitude magnetization vectors. The deformation of the tagging pattern is analyzed in the magnitude images, which do not show the magnetization sign. Therefore, the negative lobes of the sinusoidally modulated magnetization are rectified in the magnitude images, resulting in doubling the number of stripes that appear in the image with apparent tagging frequency of $2\omega_0$, as shown in Figure 10.10. With time, longitudinal magnetization relaxation results in reducing the AC component of the tagged magnetization, as well as buildup of a nontagged DC component. Therefore, the resulting magnitude image shows reduced (faded) tagging contrast and uneven tagging pattern, which complicates the analysis process and implementation of tags tracking algorithms. At a later timepoint in the cardiac cycle,

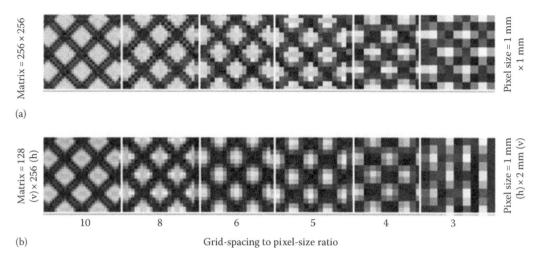

FIGURE 10.8 The effect of changing the grid-spacing to pixel-size ratio on the tagging pattern appearance. The images are obtained using (a) square and (b) rectangular pixels with varying resolution. The tagging pattern can be clearly identified for high grid-spacing to pixel-size ratios; however, when the ratio is decreased to about 4, as needed for studies with small children, the image appears as a checkerboard of white and dark squares. Further, for a given ratio, the rectangular pixels appear more checkerboard-like than the equivalent image obtained with square pixels. h, horizontal; v, vertical. (Reproduced from Haselgrove, J.C. and Fogel, M.A., *J. Cardiovasc. Magn. Reson.*, 7(2), 433, 2005.)

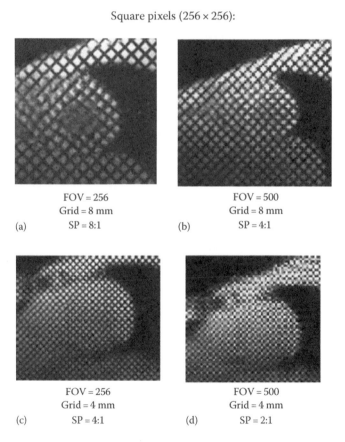

FIGURE 10.9 In vivo SPAMM images with different grid-spacing to pixel-size ratios. A group of parallel stripes perpendicular to each other can be observed for a ratio of (a) 8 or (b, c) 4. However, for a ratio of (d) 2, the tagging pattern shows as a checkerboard. (Reproduced from Haselgrove, J.C. and Fogel, M.A., *J. Cardiovasc. Magn. Reson.*, 7(2), 433, 2005.)

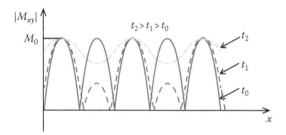

FIGURE 10.10 Tagging profile in magnitude-reconstructed images. Solid blue, dashed red, and dotted green lines show the tagging profile at incrementing timepoints t_0, t_1, and t_2 after tagging preparation. Due to magnitude reconstruction, negative magnetization is rectified and appears positive, which results in doubling the tagging frequency in the beginning of the cardiac cycle, as well as the appearance of nonuniform tagging pattern through the cardiac cycle. Toward the end of the cardiac cycle (timepoint t_2), a great part of longitudinal magnetization recovery has occurred, resulting in shallow, or almost invisible, tagging pattern.

the peaks of the negative sinusoidal lobes reach zero; therefore, the tagging pattern appears with the original tagging frequency ω_0, although the tagging contrast is much less than its original value at the beginning of the cardiac cycle. Finally, when a great part of longitudinal magnetization recovery has occurred toward the end of the cardiac cycle, the tagging pattern can hardly be identified, and the acquired images appear as regular nontagged cine images. It should be noted that the tagging pattern in the blood pool disappears shortly after tagging preparation due to rapid blood flow, which has the effect of improving the blood-to-myocardium contrast.

One solution to avoid the generation of uneven tagging pattern in the magnitude images is to generate the tag lines using saturation recovery (SR) pulses (total tagging flip angle of 90° distributed over the two RF pulses) instead of inversion recovery, that is, replace the 90°–90° RF pulses with 45°–45° pulses. This way, the sinusoidally modulated magnetization always has positive values that range from 0 to 1, albeit with only half the tagging contrast compared to the case of 90°–90° pulses. This strategy facilitates the implementation of the tags tracking algorithms as the tagging pattern always has the same frequency of ω_0 throughout the cardiac cycle.

The visibility of the tagging pattern could be compromised by a number of factors, as follows: (1) B_1 inhomogeneity results in varying degrees of magnetization inversion across the image, leading to varying tag spacing; (2) through-plane motion could result in tagging planes that are not perpendicular to the imaging slice, with the effect of tags blurring, which can be avoided by reducing the slice thickness; (3) rapid myocardial motion could result in aliasing artifacts, which can be alleviated by increasing tag spacing or temporal resolution; and (4) tags fading results in the inability to analyze myocardial motion during diastole, which can be resolved by introducing a "tag delay" after the R-wave of the ECG and before implementation of the tagging module.

10.3.1.3   Noise Effect

The amount of noise in the tagged image has a significant effect on the degree of automation that could be implemented in image analysis as well as the accuracy of the resulting measurements. Especially, with the use of surface coils in cardiac imaging, the noise level may not be the same across the image based on the distance between the coil and the imaged tissue. Several noise suppression algorithms have been compared in tagged images from both patients and healthy volunteers using residual noise and edge strength as measures of the algorithms' performance (Montillo et al. 2003). The results showed that thermal noise variance does not change with position; nevertheless, inhomogeneity correction increases noise variance in deep thoracic regions. The ideal noise suppression technique should remove thermal noise while reserve the tissue edges and other fine details in the image.

10.3.1.4   Respiratory Gating

The adopted respiratory compensation strategy has a clear effect on the quality of the resulting tagged images. Respiratory compensation could be implemented using breath-holding or navigator-echo data acquisition. A SPAMM tagging sequence with respiratory gating has been developed to alleviate tags fading during prolonged breath-hold, which allows access to the whole cardiac cycle (Santa Marta et al. 2006). The developed technique uses Cartesian k-space filling, turbo gradient echo pulses, and both ECG and respiration gating.

10.3.2   SPAMM VALIDATION

10.3.2.1   Phantom Experiments

Controlled phantom experiments are necessary for evaluating the effects of different imaging parameters used in

MRI tagging as well as the accuracy and precision of deformation measurement. As early as 1991, Pipe et al. (1991) conducted an experiment on a rotating phantom to verify the accuracy of motion measurements obtained from cine tagged images.

Measurements from SPAMM tagging have been validated through comparison with an analytic solution (Young et al. 1993). The mathematical model was verified by comparison with optically measured deformation of painted stripes. The displacements of the MRI tags showed excellent agreement with both optical markers and analytic solution. Based on their experiments, Young et al. (1993) showed that SPAMM tagging provides an accurate estimate of deformation measurements. The authors also showed that unbiased estimates of strain can be easily obtained, and that greater accuracy could be achieved using nonhomogeneous finite-element modeling.

Using a hybrid sequence of the SPAMM and DANTE tagging techniques (McVeigh and Atalar 1992; covered later in the chapter), Moore et al. (1994) compared the measurements from tagging to those from photography. The authors measured deformation in a piece of silicon rubber that was cyclically stretched. The results showed that the measurements from the tagged images are accurate and precise.

10.3.2.2   Animal Experiments

MRI tagging has been used to compare measurements of systolic wall thickening to those from sonomicrometry crystals implanted across the myocardial wall in a canine model (Lima et al. 1993). In another study, circumferential myocardial shortening from SPAMM has been compared to measurements from sonomicrometry in a canine model with and without coronary artery ligation (Yeon et al. 2001). The measurements from both techniques correlated well with each other and were similar in the ischemic regions. The results showed that SPAMM can quantify myocardial strain in ischemic and remote myocardium, which allows for distinguishing between normally functioning and ischemic dysfunctional regions.

10.3.3   TAGGING SIMULATION AND ANALYSIS

10.3.3.1   Early Simulation and Analysis Techniques

Computer simulations provide an effective and inexpensive tool for comparing different imaging protocols and tagging analysis algorithms, understanding image characteristics, and optimizing the imaging parameters before testing the protocols on the scanner (Crum et al. 1998). In 1992, Maier et al. (1992a) developed a semiautomatic analysis procedure for evaluating the motion pattern of the left ventricle (LV) in normal volunteers based on SPAMM-tagged images. The developed technique helped in analyzing complicated contraction patterns of the LV. A couple of years later, Reeder and McVeigh (1994) conducted an interesting study that showed the dependency of the tagging contrast on the imaging flip angle and provided criteria for choosing the optimal flip angle. Fourier phase mapping of the tagged images has been used for analyzing different cardiac activation patterns and intramyocardial dynamics (Knollmann et al. 1996). Further, computer simulation of the tagged images has been conducted using connected triangular and tetrahedral elements, which provided structures with known deformations to be used for validating different tagging analysis algorithms (Truscott and Buonocore 2001).

10.3.3.2 Partitions Model

A frequency-domain technique based on the partitions algorithm (Petersson et al. 1993) has been developed to examine different k-space trajectories in simulated tagged images (Crum et al. 1998). In the developed model, the net magnetization occupying a particular position in k-space is labeled as a single partition. The gradient pulses affect the k-space coordinates of the partitions, while the RF pulses change the amplitude of existing partitions and create new ones. The developed model has been used for simulating tagged images, generating ideal intensity profiles from binomial tagging sequences, and studying the effects of k-space undersampling and different k-space filling trajectories on the resulting images.

10.3.3.3 SIMTAG

SIMTAG is a simulation software that has been developed a few years after SPAMM invention for simulating 2D tagged images, noise effects, and object deformation based on mathematical modeling (Crum et al. 1997). SIMTAG has the advantages of flexibility and accessibility, which facilitated its use for comparing different tagging sequences, simulating cardiac tissue displacement, investigating motion-induced artifacts, examining the noise effect on the image, and studying different tissue contrasts.

10.3.3.4 Small-Tip-Angle Approximation

In their seminal paper in 2000, Kerwin and Prince (2000) presented a k-space approximation method for analyzing and designing the tagging sequences. The developed approximation directly relates the pulse sequence to its residual pattern of the longitudinal magnetization M_z, based on k-space approximation of small-tip-angle excitation (Pauly et al. 2011). The extension of the small-tip-angle theory into the z-direction provides an approximate expression for k-space encoding of M_z, analogous to the existing technique for the transverse magnetization. In the case of myocardial tagging, the final tagging pattern is given by,

$$M_z(x) \sim 1 - \frac{1}{2}\gamma^2 \int_k R_p(k) e^{ixk} dk, \qquad (10.9)$$

where $R_p(k)$ is the autocorrelation function of $p(k)$, given by

$$R_p(k) = \int_K p(s)\bar{p}(s-k)ds, \qquad (10.10)$$

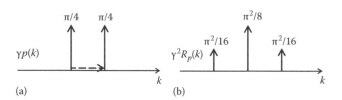

FIGURE 10.11 K-space path and autocorrelation function of 1-1 SPAMM. (a) K-space path $p(k)$ of 1-1 SPAMM with a total tip angle of $\pi/2$ consisting of two impulses. (b) K-space autocorrelation function $R_p(k)$, computed by shifting and multiplying the k-space path, as shown in Equation 10.10, to obtain three impulses.

where the bar above p represents complex conjugate, and $p(k)$ is the 1D path through k-space for a SPAMM sequence with N RF pulses:

$$p(k) = \frac{1}{\gamma}\sum_{i=1}^{N} \theta_i \delta(k - (N-i)\phi), \qquad (10.11)$$

where θ_i is the flip angle of the ith RF pulse, and $\phi = \gamma G$, where G is the size (area) of the modulation gradient pulse. Equation 10.11 shows that the SPAMM path in k-space is a sequence of N equally spaced impulse functions. Figure 10.11 shows an example of a SPAMM path and the generated autocorrelation function.

Equation 10.11 can be used as an approximation of the tagging k-space, which could be implemented for analyzing and designing pulse sequences. The equation shows that the important information needed for approximating a tagging pattern is not the k-space path, but the autocorrelation function of the path. By substituting Equation 10.11 into Equation 10.10, the autocorrelation function $R_p(k)$ can be computed as

$$R_p(k) = \frac{1}{\gamma^2}\sum_{l=1-N}^{N-1}\sum_{i=1}^{N-|l|} \theta_i \theta_{i+|l|} \delta(k - l\phi). \qquad (10.12)$$

By substituting Equation 10.12 into Equation 10.9, the approximate SPAMM pattern is expressed as (tag profiles are shown in Figure 10.12)

$$M_z(x) \sim \sum_{i=0}^{N-1} \alpha_i \cos(i\phi x), \qquad (10.13)$$

where

$$\alpha_i = -\sum_{l=1}^{N-i} \theta_l \times \theta_{l+i}, \quad i = 1,\ldots,N-1, \qquad (10.14)$$

$$\alpha_0 = 1 - \frac{1}{2}\sum_{l=1}^{N} \theta_l^2. \qquad (10.15)$$

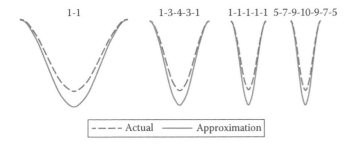

1-1   1-3-4-3-1   1-1-1-1-1 5-7-9-10-9-7-5

- - - - Actual ——— Approximation

FIGURE 10.12 Actual and approximate SPAMM tagging profiles using the small-tip-angle approximation. Comparison of approximated tagging profiles using Equation 10.13 and actual tagging profiles from Bloch equation simulation for four SPAMM sequences. The number and relative amplitudes of RF pulses are denoted above each plot, for a total flip angle of π/2. (Reproduced from Kerwin, W.S. and Prince, J.L., *J. Magn. Reson.*, 142(2), 313, 2000. With permission.)

This tagging k-space approximation showed excellent results for predicting the tagging pattern. Unlike the exact solution, this approximation provides a simple expression of the coefficients of the cosine series. The main finding from this analysis is that the tagging pattern is determined by the autocorrelation function of the k-space path, not by the path itself. Because different paths could be generated with similar autocorrelations, the tagging k-space approximation results in a great deal of flexibility for designing the tagging pulse sequences. More general discussion of the k-space approximation technique is provided in Chapter 12.

10.4 SPAMM DEVELOPMENTS

10.4.1 CASCADED SPAMM

One of the drawbacks of SPAMM tagging is the fading of the tagging pattern throughout the cardiac cycle due to longitudinal magnetization relaxation, which renders the tag lines almost invisible, and thus not analyzable, during late cardiac phases. Practically, while the cardiac cycle duration is about 1 second on average, the tagging pattern lasts for only 0.3–0.5 second with sufficient contrast for reliable tagging analysis. A solution has been provided for alleviating this problem by acquiring a cascaded sequence of SPAMM datasets and integrating them into a volumetric deformable model, thus providing a method for measuring myocardial deformation over the entire cardiac cycle (Park et al. 1999). In order to achieve this goal, sequential sets of SPAMM images are acquired as illustrated in Figure 10.13, such that a new reference set of SPAMM tags is created just before the previous reference tags fade away. This process of cascaded tagging application is repeated until the entire cardiac cycle is covered.

10.4.2 ALTERNATE INVERSION RECOVERY SPAMM

The alternate inversion recovery SPAMM (AIR-SPAMM) technique increases the tagging density and contrast without increasing the scan time (Aletras et al. 2004). AIR-SPAMM requires only a single acquisition and utilizes 180° inversion pulses spaced throughout multiphase data acquisition (Figure 10.14) to keep the recovering magnetization at a

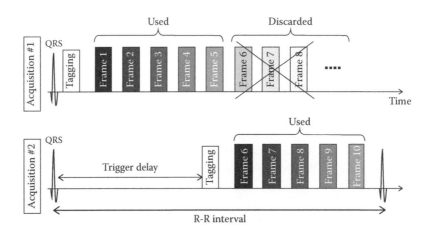

FIGURE 10.13 Cascaded SPAMM. The technique is based on obtaining all timeframes (10 frames in this example) throughout the cardiac cycle in multiple acquisitions (2 acquisitions in this example). In the first acquisition, tagging preparation is performed immediately after the R-wave of the ECG signal, followed by consecutive acquisition of different frames. Only the early frames with sufficient tagging contrast (frames 1–5 in this example) are used for analysis, while the later frames with shallow tagging contrast are discarded. The figure represents the idea of tagline fading as a continuously washed out (lighter) filling color of the textbox, such that the there is a decreasing contrast between the word "frame" in white and the background color. The later frames in the cardiac cycle (frames 6–10 in this example) are acquired in the second acquisition, where tagging preparation takes place after a long trigger delay from the R-wave to ensure tagging contrast remains high until the end of the cardiac cycle. The frames acquired in the second acquisition are cascaded with those acquired in the first acquisition for complete functional analysis of the whole cardiac cycle.

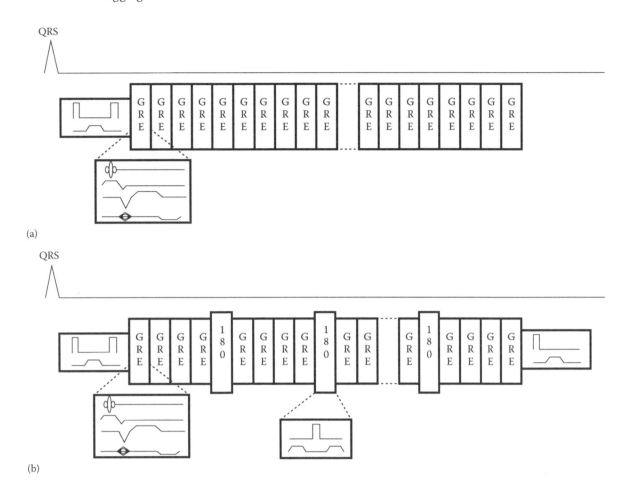

(a)

(b)

FIGURE 10.14 Alternate inversion recovery SPAMM (AIR-SPAMM) pulse sequence. (a) Schematic diagram of conventional SPAMM pulse sequence with gradient echo (GRE) acquisition. Tagging is performed as soon as the R-wave of the ECG signal is detected. (b) Schematic diagram of the AIR-SPAMM pulse sequence with GRE acquisition. The AIR inversion RF pulses are followed by crusher gradient pulse. At the end of the AIR-SPAMM acquisition, the longitudinal magnetization is crushed. (Reproduced from Aletras, A.H. et al., *J. Magn. Reson.*, 166(2), 236, 2004. With permission.)

determined level. Although each inversion pulse conjugates the existing modulated magnetization, the resulting images are not affected by the sign change as magnitude images are reconstructed. Figures 10.15 and 10.16 show phantom images and intensity profile, respectively, of AIR-SPAMM images.

For a 90°–90° SPAMM sequence, the magnetization oscillates sinusoidally between $-M_0$ and $+M_0$, where M_0 is the equilibrium magnetization. To maintain constant tagging contrast, the inversion pulses are applied each τ ms, where τ is a multiple of TRs ($\tau = 8 \times$ TR was used in Aletras et al. (2004). The magnetization at the end of the first τ interval is given by

$$M(\tau) = M_0(1 - e^{-\tau/T_1}) + M_0 \cdot TAG \cdot e^{-\tau/T_1}, \qquad (10.16)$$

where *TAG* is the modulation pattern immediately after applying the tagging module. The next inversion pulse inverts the sign of $M(\tau)$, and therefore at the end of the second τ interval, the magnetization is given by

$$M(2\tau) = M_0\left(1 - 2e^{-\tau/T_1} + e^{-2\tau/T_1}\right) - M_0 \cdot TAG \cdot e^{-2\tau/T_1}. \quad (10.17)$$

which can be approximated by

$$M(2\tau) = -M_0 \cdot TAG \cdot e^{-2\tau/T_1}. \qquad (10.18)$$

It can be shown that in the case of a 90°–90° SPAMM sequence, the inversion pulses result in doubling the tagging frequency without the need to increase the strength of the modulation gradient, which alleviates signal loss from intravoxel dephasing associated with large modulation gradients. On the other hand, in the case of 45°–45° SPAMM sequence, the inversion pulses result in improving the tagging contrast without the need for additional data acquisitions.

10.4.3 Phase-Sensitive SPAMM (REALTAG)

The use of 90°–90° IR scheme provides better tagging contrast than the 45°–45° SR scheme. The improved tagging contrast with IR could be used to achieve higher resolution or more persistent tag lines (less fading) throughout the cardiac cycle. Nevertheless, the problem with IR tagging is that the negative sinusoidal lobes of the modulated magnetization are rectified

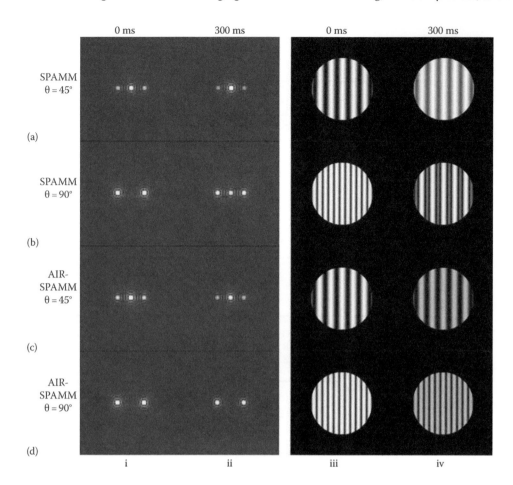

FIGURE 10.15 Simulated k-space and phantom alternate inversion recovery SPAMM (AIR-SPAMM) images. Simulated k-space (columns i and ii) and simulated magnitude phantom images (columns iii and iv) immediately following tagging preparation (columns i and iii) and 300 ms later (columns ii and iv). SPAMM data with θ = 45° and θ = 90° are shown in rows (a) and (b), respectively. Simulated AIR-SPAMM data with θ = 45° and θ = 90° are shown in rows (c) and (d), respectively. (Reproduced from Aletras, A.H. et al., *J. Magn. Reson.*, 166(2), 236, 2004. With permission.)

in the magnitude-reconstructed images, which reduces the tagging contrast (the modulated magnetization ranges from 0 to +1 instead of ranging from −1 to +1) and results in uneven tagging density and spatially variable tagging pattern through the cardiac cycle, leading to complicated tagging analysis.

In 2007, the REALTAG technique was proposed to enable the implementation of IR tagging without the limitations encountered in magnitude reconstruction images (Derbyshire et al. 2007). Figure 10.17 shows a schematic diagram of the phase-sensitive reconstruction process in REALTAG. REALTAG is based on creating phase-sensitive SPAMM images that use information from the phase images to infer the sign of the tagging peaks, and therefore distinguish positive from negative peaks, which restores the enhanced tagging contrast with IR and results in evenly modulated magnetization in the image. REALTAG estimates the phase from a relatively quiescent period in the cardiac cycle (e.g., during diastole), where it generates the phase reference from the central k-space peak; therefore, REALTAG improves the tagging contrast without extending the scan time to obtain a second acquisition (as in CSPAMM), or a separate phase reference scan.

Figure 10.18 shows cardiac REALTAG images at different timepoints in the cardiac cycle. It should be noted that as the cardiac cycle progresses, all tagged magnetization becomes positive, and therefore, the tagging contrast from magnitude reconstruction becomes the same as that from REALTAG reconstruction for the remainder of the cardiac cycle.

10.4.4 3D MOTION ANALYSIS BASED ON SPAMM

Measurement of myocardial deformation in the through-plane direction usually requires an additional acquisition with modified orientation of the tagging grid to acquire motion components perpendicular to the imaging plane. Kuijer et al. (1999) suggested combining 2D SPAMM with through-plane velocity mapping for measuring 3D myocardial deformation, as shown in Figure 10.19 (combing SPAMM with velocity-encoding for simultaneous assessment of myocardial deformation and blood flow is covered in Section 10.5). The 2D tagging grid in the magnitude image is used for measuring in-plane motion, while the simultaneously acquired phase image is used for measuring through-plane motion. A tracking

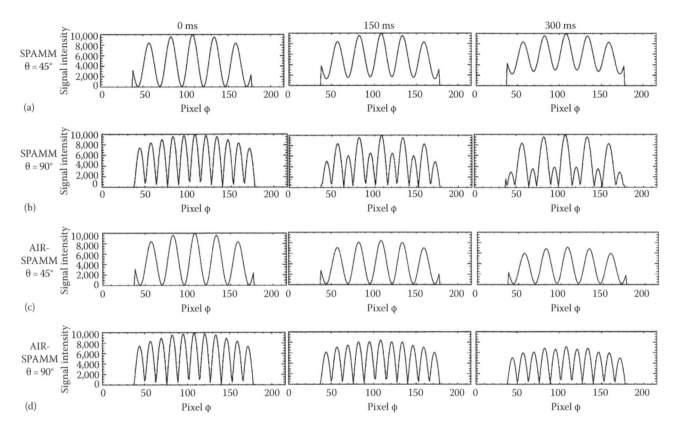

FIGURE 10.16 Alternate inversion recovery SPAMM (AIR-SPAMM) signal intensity profile. Signal intensity profile over three timepoints (0, 150, and 300 ms) for the simulated images shown in Figure 10.15. Note that when using SPAMM with θ = 45° (a), the tag valleys are not consistently at zero over time in contrast to using AIR-SPAMM with θ = 45° (c), where the valleys are always at zero. When SPAMM is used with θ = 90° (b), the magnetization recovery results in variable tag spacing over time for this motionless object. AIR-SPAMM with θ = 90° (d) results in consistent double density tags over time. (Reproduced from Aletras, A.H. et al., *J. Magn. Reson.*, 166(2), 236, 2004. With permission.)

algorithm is used for calculating 3D point-specific motion in the heart based on the measured motion components. The developed technique showed to be competitive to other methods such as 3D tagging or 3D velocity mapping.

10.4.5 HIGH-FIELD SPAMM IMAGING

The quality of SPAMM-tagged images has been evaluated at both 3 T and 1.5 T field strengths (Valeti et al. 2006). The results showed improved image quality at 3 T, mainly due to the doubled signal-to-noise ratio (SNR) and slower myocardial longitudinal relaxation (myocardial T_1 ~ 1150 ms at 3 T versus ~850 ms at 1.5 T), which improve tagging persistence throughout the cardiac cycle.

10.5 COMBINED SPAMM AND VELOCITY ENCODING

10.5.1 SPAMM n' EGGS

10.5.1.1 Pulse Sequence and Image Reconstruction

SPAMM has been combined with phase-contrast (PC) flow imaging for simultaneous and registered measurement of

tissue motion and chamber blood flow in a single-breath-hold scan (Sampath et al. 2008). The resulting technique was called SPAMM n' EGGS (SPAMM acquisitions with encoded gradients for gauging speed), which was introduced by Sampath et al. in 2008. SPAMM n' EGGS is implemented by adding a velocity-encoding bipolar gradient before the readout gradient in the 1-1 SPAMM sequence to record the chamber blood flow (Figure 10.20). To be able to separate the velocity-encoded flow from background phase, the velocity-encoded gradients are turned off during every other heart phase to acquire a reference phase data. The velocity-encoded blood flow can then be calculated using a sliding-window phase-sensitive reconstruction, as shown in Figure 10.21. A modified version of the ramped imaging flip angles, originally presented in (Fischer et al. 1993), is used in the SPAMM n' EGGS technique to achieve an optimal balance between tagging persistence during diastole and early recovery of the flow signal during systole. The imaging flip angles, α_i, are calculated retrospectively based on the last flip angle, α, as follows:

$$\alpha_i = \alpha \tan^{-1}\left(\sin(\alpha_{i+1})e^{-TR/T_1}\right) + (\gamma(n-i))/(n-1), \quad (10.19)$$

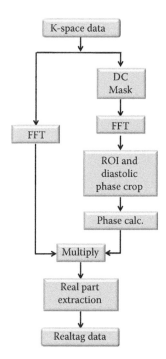

FIGURE 10.17 REALTAG data reconstruction. Schematic diagram of the REALTAG phase-correction procedure. REALTAG estimates the phase from a relatively quiescent period in the cardiac cycle (e.g., during diastole), where it generates the phase reference from the central k-space peak. Phase correction is applied independently to the images for each individual coil before the images are combined. FFT, fast Fourier transform; ROI, region of interest.

where the second term in (10.19) is a ramp-down function with time, n is the number of imaging RF pulses, and γ is the slope of the ramp-down function.

10.5.1.2 Implementation

The SPAMM n' EGGS technique reduces scan time in half (compared to separate acquisitions of tagging and flow images), alleviates temporal and spatial misregistration problems, and results in composite tagged images with colored flow information (Figure 10.22). These features make SPAMM n' EGGS an ideal technique for identifying transient myocardial dysfunction that leads to transvalvular flow abnormalities, for example, in ischemic mitral regurgitation, hypertrophic cardiomyopathy, dilation cardiomyopathy, and LV dyssynchrony. Further, the technique could provide valuable information about the interaction between myocardial contractility and chamber blood flow before and after surgical procedures, for example, mitral valve repair.

The SPAMM n' EGGS technique has been implemented for simultaneously measuring longitudinal strain and transvalvular blood velocity during supine bicycle exercise stress in a wide bore MRI scanner, as shown in Figure 10.23 (Sampath et al. 2011). The advantage of using SPAMM n' EGGS for this application is that transient physiological events are manifested in a correlated fashion in both the tagging and flow images. The study showed the existence of increased diastolic strain rate and peak mitral inflow velocity during exercise, which leads to augmented muscle contractility and ventricular filling efficiency.

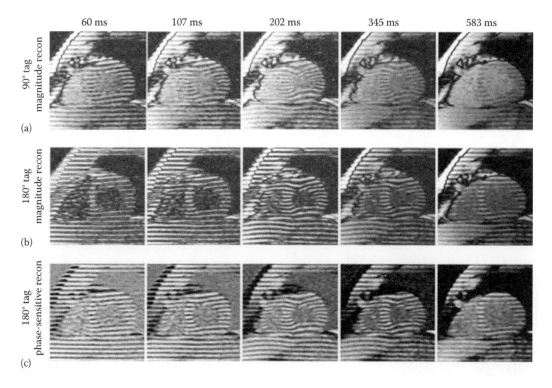

FIGURE 10.18 Comparison of REALTAG images with standard magnitude saturation tags. (a, b) Magnitude-reconstructed images acquired using the 1-1 SPAMM sequence with 90° and 180° total tagging angles, respectively. (c) REALTAG images acquired using 180° 1-1 SPAMM tags and reconstructed with the phase-sensitive method. The 180° tagged images have superior contrast to the 90° tags, and the tagging contrast persists for the duration of the acquisition window. Phase reconstruction provides enhanced tagging contrast compared to magnitude reconstruction. (Reproduced from Derbyshire, J.A. et al., *Magn. Reson. Med.*, 58(1), 206, 2007. With permission.)

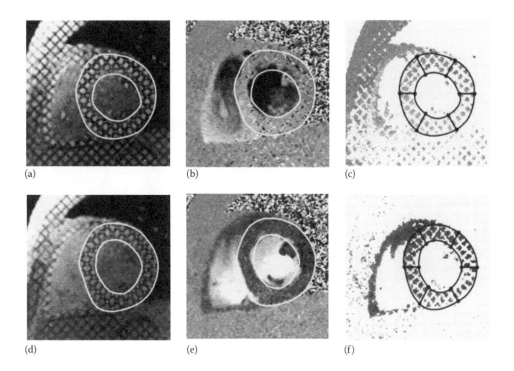

FIGURE 10.19 3D tagging by combining 2D SPAMM and through-plane phase-contrast (PC) imaging. (a) Tagged image at systole (180 ms after the R-wave) with an overlay of manually segmented left ventricle (LV) contours. (b) Corresponding velocity map, represented as a grayscale image. Movement toward the heart base is colored dark. Note the fast flowing blood in a small area between the contours near the septal wall. (c) Velocity map after thresholding and region growing with overlay of 6 segments and 12 nodal points (small dark circles at the intersection of the segments with the LV contours). (d–f) Same as in (a–c), but images are acquired at early-diastole (468 ms after the R-wave). (Reproduced from Kuijer, J.P. et al., *J. Magn. Reson. Imaging*, 9(3), 409, 1999. With permission.)

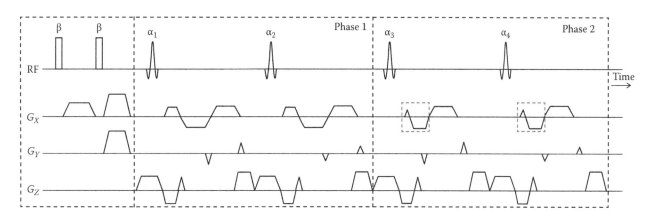

FIGURE 10.20 Diagrammatic representation of the SPAMM n' EGGS pulse sequence. Two views (k-space lines) per cardiac phase are shown for display clarity; actual value typically ranges from 3 to 5. Phase 1 represents the velocity-unencoded (flow-compensated) reference acquisition, while phase 2 represents the velocity-encoded acquisition. The small rectangular boxes in phase 2 highlight the composite gradients obtained by adding the flow-encoding gradients to the existing flow-compensating readout gradients. (Reproduced from Sampath, S. et al., *J. Magn. Reson. Imaging*, 27(4), 809, 2008. With permission.)

10.5.2 SPAMM-PAV

10.5.2.1 Pulse Sequence

The temporal resolution of the SPAMM n' EGGS technique is limited to 40 ms, which makes it difficult to accurately detect rapid mechanical events during early diastole. The SPAMM n' EGGS technique has been modified to achieve high temporal resolution. The modified technique is called SPAMM with polarity alternating velocity-encoding (SPAMM-PAV) (Zhang et al. 2011), which is capable of achieving temporal resolution of 14 ms by playing out the velocity-encoding bipolar gradient pulses with opposite polarity every other heart phase, as shown in Figure 10.24. In addition to doubling the sensitivity for velocity measurement, the applied modification removes the squared gradient terms of the concomitant gradient field for less image artifacts.

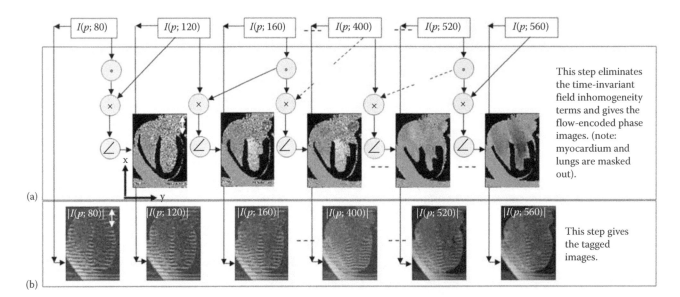

FIGURE 10.21   SPAMM n' EGGS images reconstruction. Schematic diagram of the postprocessing steps used to reconstruct the tagged images and the chamber blood flow images from the reconstructed complex SPAMM n' EGGS images $I(p; t)$, where p and t represent the location and time of acquisition, respectively. (a) Sliding-window phase-sensitive reconstruction is used to isolate the blood flow velocity terms (the unencoded images are used as phase reference). Velocity is measured as the phase angle of the product of one image by the conjugate of the adjacent one, as represented by the mathematical symbols in the figure. (b) The tagged images obtained from magnitude reconstruction. (Reproduced from Sampath, S. et al., *J. Magn. Reson. Imaging*, 27(4), 809, 2008. With permission.)

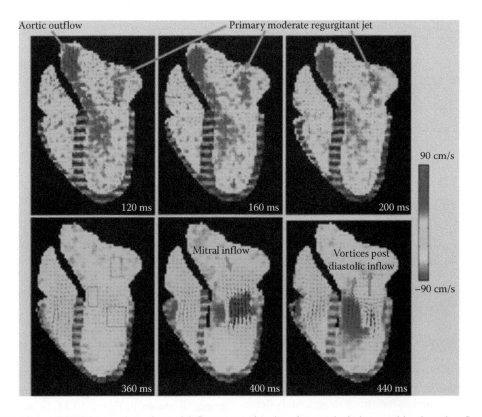

FIGURE 10.22   SPAMM n' EGGS images in a pig model. Representative time frames depicting combined motion-flow data obtained in two short breath-hold acquisitions from a pig with moderate induced ischemic mitral regurgitation. (Reproduced from Sampath, S. et al., *J. Magn. Reson. Imaging*, 27(4), 809, 2008. With permission.)

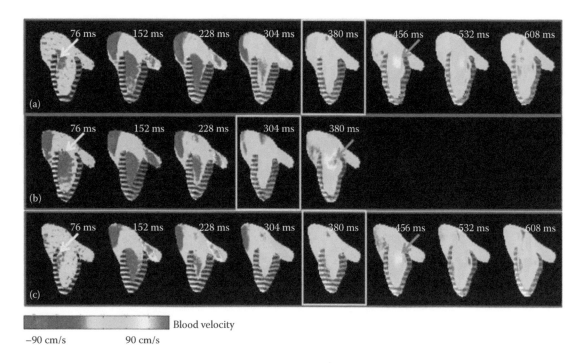

FIGURE 10.23 SPAMM n' EGGS images during rest, stress, and recovery. Combined tagged myocardium and blood velocity maps during (a) rest, (b) exercise stress, and (c) poststress recovery in a normal volunteer using SPAMM n' EGGS. The velocity is color coded, as shown in the color bar. The blood velocity maps show early initiation of aortic flow (yellow arrows) and increased mitral inflow velocities (orange arrows) during stress. The tagged myocardium shows earlier occurrence of end-systolic peak longitudinal shortening during stress (yellow boxes). (Reproduced from Sampath, S. et al., *Magn. Reson. Med.*, 65(1), 51, 2011. With permission.)

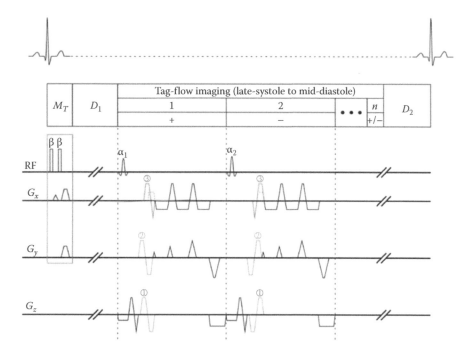

FIGURE 10.24 SPAMM with polarity alternating velocity-encoding (SPAMM-PAV) pulse sequence diagram. 1-1 SPAMM tagging preparation, M_T, is used to encode myocardial displacement. Combined tag-flow images are acquired during early diastole with bipolar gradient pulses sensitive to blood flow played out before each short echo panar imaging (EPI) acquisition (echo train length = 3, with a flyback scheme). The sign of the bipolar gradients are flipped every alternate phase. The figure shows cases when the bipolar gradients are played along the (1) through-plane (solid green), (2) phase-encode (solid blue), and (3) readout (solid red) directions. Note: Case 3 depicts a combined bipolar gradient and read dephaser gradient. In this case, squared concomitant gradient terms are not exactly canceled on the readout axis. The red-dotted readout gradient depicts the isolated read dephaser gradient. D, delay. (Reproduced from Zhang, Z. et al., *Magn. Reson. Med.*, 66(6), 1627, 2011. With permission.)

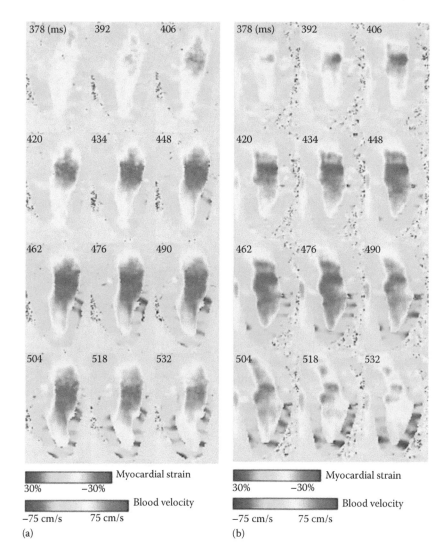

FIGURE 10.25   In vivo SPAMM with polarity alternating velocity-encoding (SPAMM-PAV) images. 2D color-coded combined strain–velocity maps for twelve representative time frames from (a) two-chamber and (b) four-chamber views. Images were obtained from a normal volunteer in a single breath-hold SPAMM-PAV acquisition. (Reproduced from Zhang, Z. et al., *Magn. Reson. Med.*, 66(6), 1627, 2011. With permission.)

10.5.2.2   Implementation

The SPAMM-PAV technique has been tested on eight normal volunteers to compare longitudinal myocardial strain and intracavity pressure difference to the mitral valve inflow velocity (Figure 10.25) (Zhang et al. 2011). The results showed that the apical myocardial regions have higher strain rates than the midventricular and basal regions during the acceleration period of rapid filling (this contractility pattern is reversed during the deceleration filling period), and that apical strain reaches a plateau at peak mitral inflow velocity.

In another study, SPAMM-PAV has been implemented to study LV filling patterns and compare the results to longitudinal myocardial strain in normal volunteers as well as in healthy and infarcted canine models (Zhang et al. 2013). The implemented technique showed high sensitivity for providing direct regional assessment of early-diastolic filling abnormalities, as shown in Figures 10.26 and 10.27.

10.6   SPAMM APPLICATIONS

10.6.1   TISSUE DEFORMATION

SPAMM provides a valuable noninvasive tool for measuring intramyocardial wall motion, separating its components into rigid body motion and deformation, and generating functional images of myocardial contractility (Axel et al. 1992). Shortly after its development, SPAMM has been implemented for measuring different myocardial strain components. For example, in 1991, Clark et al. (1991b) used SPAMM to characterize circumferential myocardial shortening in normal human LV. A few years later, Chai et al. (1997) evaluated longitudinal LV strain from long-axis SPAMM-tagged images.

10.6.2   CLINICAL AND EXPERIMENTAL STUDIES

The SPAMM technique provides a large number of material landmarks, from which different measures of myocardial

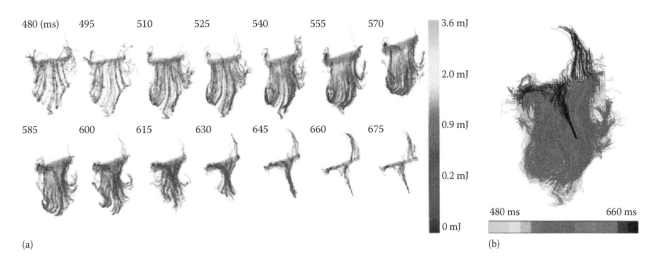

480 (ms)   495   510   525   540   555   570   3.6 mJ

2.0 mJ

585   600   615   630   645   660   675   0.9 mJ

0.2 mJ

0 mJ   480 ms   660 ms

(a)   (b)

FIGURE 10.26 Trajectories of particle traces emitted from the mitral valve plane in a normal volunteer. (a) Time series (row 1, acceleration; row 2, deceleration) of particle traces emitted from the mitral valve plane in a normal volunteer, color-coded to depict instantaneous kinetic energy. The red dots on the pathlines, shown on the top left subfigure, illustrate the position of the emitter particles (released at the first timeframe) at each subsequent timeframe as it propagates into the left ventricle (LV) chamber. A wavefront-like propagation pattern is observed. (b) Overlapped particle trace trajectories of emitter particles released at all timepoints in a normal volunteer. Blood propagating into the LV at an early stage distributes uniformly throughout the LV, while blood entering at later time frames contributes to a more centric filling. (Reproduced from Zhang, R. et al., *Magn. Reson. Med.*, 49(4), 760, 2013. With permission.)

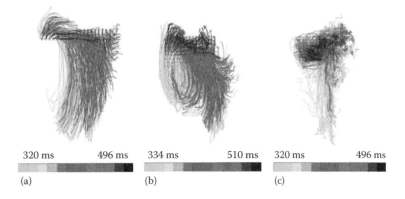

320 ms   496 ms   334 ms   510 ms   320 ms   496 ms

(a)   (b)   (c)

FIGURE 10.27 Overlapped blood flow pathline trajectories in canine. Trajectories in (a) a normal baseline dog, (b) a representative infarcted dog with nominal flow dysfunction, and (c) a representative infarcted dog with severe flow dysfunction. A large vortex is shown around the midbasal region of the septal wall in (b), illustrating a compensatory accentuated filling pattern and nominal flow dysfunction compared to baseline. In (c), the filling pattern is severely impaired, which illustrates shortened centric filling toward the apex and stagnation in the basal regions. (Reproduced from Zhang, R. et al., *Magn. Reson. Med.*, 49(4), 760, 2013. With permission.)

deformation could be obtained. Since its development in 1989, SPAMM has been used in various studies to better understand heart mechanics in healthy and diseased subjects. SPAMM has been implemented for measuring circumferential shortening (Clark et al. 1991b) and diastolic relaxation in normal human subjects (Fogel et al. 2000). It has been also implemented for studying 2D deformation in 12 normal human volunteers (Young et al. 1994a), where the results showed variations in the myocardial deformation measurements among the studied subjects. SPAMM has been also used for evaluating the heart function after coronary artery bypass grafting (CABG) (Maniar et al. 2004), LV reconstruction surgery (Setser et al. 2007), and heart pacing (Prinzen et al. 1999).

SPAMM showed to be an effective tool for identifying ischemia under dobutamine stress (Kuijpers et al. 2003) and studying myocardial contractility during infarction in patients

(Chen et al. 1995) and experimental models (Lima et al. 1995, Kramer et al. 1996, Rogers et al. 1999). SPAMM has been also implemented for evaluating the heart function after reperfusion (Sayad et al. 1998, Verhn et al. 1999). For example, Verhent et al. (1999) used SPAMM to identify regions of myocardial injury in reperfused myocardium, where they found that circumferential shortening in the subendocardial layer is an accurate measure for describing the degree of damage, and that 2D tagging provides a clear discrimination between normal and infarcted tissues.

In the early 1990s, different studies have been conducted for studying myocardial contractility in LV hypertrophy (Maier et al. 1992b, Kramer et al. 1994, Palmon et al. 1994, Young et al. 1994b). Later, SPAMM was implemented for studying aortic stenosis, where it has been shown that ventricular torsion is increased while circumferential shortening is decreased in both children (Delhaas et al. 2004) and adults (Van Der Toorn et al. 2002) with aortic stenosis.

Conducting preclinical studies on small animals, for example, mice, is an important step before starting a clinical study on human subjects. However, in contrast to the human heart, implementing SPAMM in the mouse heart is challenging due to its small size (~5 mm in diameter) and high heart rate (250–650 beats/s), which impose technical difficulties on the imaging sequence to achieve high spatial and temporal resolutions, small tag separation, and short echo time. Nevertheless, mice have been successfully imaged with SPAMM. For example, Zhou et al. developed a high spatial (0.7 mm) and temporal resolution (10 ms) 2D SPAMM sequence for measuring myocardial deformation in the mouse heart (Zhou et al. 2003).

A recent study investigated the test–retest reliability of measuring regional myocardial function with SPAMM tagging (Donekal et al. 2013). Twenty-five participants were scanned twice over about a couple of weeks. The effect of slice orientation on strain measurements was examined by having two volunteers scanned with the SAX plane rotated by 15° out of the true SAX orientation in one of the two scans. The effect of the slice location on tagging measurements was examined by scanning the whole heart in two volunteers. The results showed that SPAMM tagging has excellent interobserver, intraobserver, and interstudy reproducibility for measuring regional heart function, especially circumferential strain and torsion. The reproducibility of circumferential strain and torsion were superior to strain and torsion rates. Radial strain as well as maximal and minimal strains showed higher intra- and interobserver reproducibility than interstudy reproducibility. Finally, the variation in LV circumferential strain due to altered slice orientation was negligible compared to the variation due to change in slice location.

10.6.3 OTHER APPLICATIONS

Besides heart mechanics, SPAMM can be used for studying blood flow (by tracking the tag lines' displacement in the artery lumen), distinguishing blood flow from thrombus, and estimating tissue stiffness (e.g., in tumors) (Axel and Dougherty 1989b). SPAMM can be also used for measuring longitudinal magnetization relaxivity, chemical shift, magnetic field inhomogeneity, B_1 inhomogeneity, and gradient nonlinearity. For example, the time duration the inverted tags take to reach the zero value can be used to calculate T_1. Further, the spatial displacement between the tag lines can be used to estimate chemical shift between different regions. The spacing between the tag lines due to the application of a certain gradient pulse with known shape and duration can be used to calibrate the gradient strength. Finally, nonparallel tag lines (in a stationary tissue) provide an indication of the presence of magnetic field inhomogeneity and/or gradient nonlinearity.

In a study by Wayte and Redpath (1998), SPAMM has been implemented for measuring spatial resolution both in vivo and in vitro using conventional and fast spin echo sequences. The results showed reduced resolution in the phase-encoding direction compared to the frequency-encoding direction. Resolution was reduced below the voxel limit in the phase-encoding direction in tissues with short T_2 in fast spin echo with centric k-space acquisition. The importance of this study is that it showed the capability of using SPAMM as a potential method for determining the appropriate spin echo sequence for a particular application based on the perceived spatial resolution.

A new method (microSPAMM) has been recently presented for achieving super-high-resolution MRI images (Ropele et al. 2010). In addition to FOV shifting, the developed method modulates the longitudinal magnetization with SPAMM for each shift, allowing the acquisition of new and independent k-space data (Figures 10.28 and 10.29).

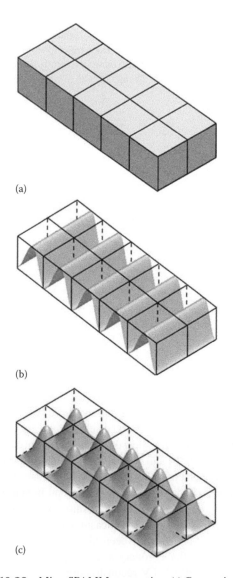

(a)

(b)

(c)

FIGURE 10.28 MicroSPAMM preparation. (a) Conventional MRI, where the entire magnetization within a voxel contributes to the MR signal. (b, c) Residual magnetization after 1D and 2D microSPAMM preparations, respectively. (Reproduced from Ropele, S. et al., *Magn. Reson. Med.*, 64(6), 1671, 2010. With permission.)

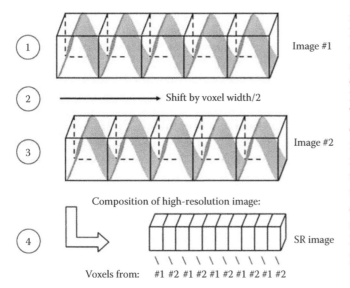

FIGURE 10.29 Super-resolution MR imaging with MicroSPAMM. Image #2 is shifted by half the voxel width in the SPAMM direction compared to image #1. Therefore, both acquisitions provide different regional information based on the magnetization profile. When combined, the two acquisitions provide high-resolution image. (Reproduced from Ropele, S. et al., *Magn. Reson. Med.*, 64(6), 1671, 2010. With permission.)

Resolution improvement can be achieved in up to three dimensions, where the total acquisition time is proportional to the improvement factor for each dimension.

Recently, SPAMM has been used in noncardiovascular clinical applications, including studying motion in the tongue (Parthasarathy et al. 2007), brain (Sabet et al. 2008), eyes (Piccirelli et al. 2009), skeletal muscles (Ceelen et al. 2008), and quasi-static soft tissues (Moerman et al. 2011).

10.7 DANTE

10.7.1 THEORY OF DANTE

The DANTE tagging pulse sequence was introduced in 1990 by Mosher and Smith (1990). DANTE consists of a series of short, hard RF pulses played in the presence of a constant modulation gradient, in contrast to SPAMM where the modulation gradients are played in between the RF pulses. To provide a first approximation of the DANTE tagging profile, the small-tip-angle approximation (Pauly et al. 2011) is considered here, where the excitation spectrum is proportional to the Fourier transform of the pulse sequence in the time domain. The DANTE pulse sequence can be approximated by a train of delta functions multiplied by a rect (box) function, as shown in Figure 10.30. The Fourier transform of the train of delta functions is another train of delta functions, while the Fourier transform of the rect function is a sinc function. As multiplication in the time domain results in convolution in the frequency domain, the DANTE pulse sequence excites a series of sharp sinc peaks, as shown in Figure 10.30. Similar to SPAMM, 2D DANTE is obtained by consecutive application of DANTE preparation on orthogonal directions (Figure 10.31).

10.7.2 DANTE ADVANTAGES

DANTE has the advantage that the width and separation of the tag lines can be easily modified by controlling the pulse sequence parameters, which allows for optimizing the sequence for different clinical applications. The distance between the tag lines is determined by the magnitude of the modulation gradient and the time separation between the RF pulses. Increasing the strength of the modulation gradient or the time separation between the RF pulses results in increased tag line density. However, increasing the total length of the DANTE pulse train results in thinner tag lines (sharper profiles).

DANTE is an efficient and flexible tagging sequence. It has the advantages of improved tagging resolution and reduced eddy currents. The short width of the RF pulses minimizes off-resonance artifacts and allows for excitation in the presence of a continuous modulation gradient. Because the gradients are not rapidly pulsed, smaller eddy currents are generated and the gradient performance (slew rate and stability) is less demanding. Compared to Zerhouni's tagging technique of magnetization saturation, DANTE produces significantly less RF power deposition in the patient; and compared to binomial SPAMM excitation, DANTE can generate sharper tag

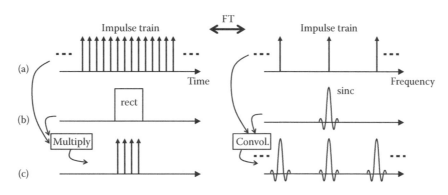

FIGURE 10.30 Quantitative description of the DANTE sequence. A train of impulses (a) is multiplied by the envelope rect function (b), which results in the radio-frequency pulses used in DANTE (c). The right panel shows the Fourier transform of the functions on the left. Multiplication in the time domain is replaced by convolution in the frequency domain.

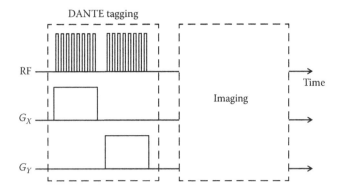

FIGURE 10.31 Two-dimensional DANTE pulse sequence, where two DANTE tags preparation modules are applied in orthogonal directions.

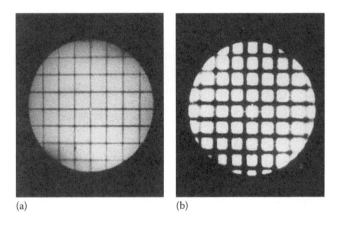

(a)   (b)

FIGURE 10.32 Phantom DANTE- and SPAMM-tagged images. Comparison of DANTE tagging sequence with 1331 SPAMM. A composite 90° flip angle, interpulse delay 0.1 ms and tagging gradient of 20 G/cm were used for both sequences. (a) DANTE tagging sequence with tag thickness of 0.07 mm and tag spacing of 1.2 mm; (b) 1331 SPAMM sequence with tag thickness of 0.53 mm and tag spacing of 1.2 mm. (Reproduced from Mosher, T.J. and Smith, M.B., *Magn. Reson. Med.*, 15(2), 334, 1990. With permission.)

lines with simple control of the tag lines' width and spacing. For example, Figure 10.32 shows the results from comparable DANTE and SPAMM 1-3-3-1 pulse sequences, which resulted in tag thickness of 0.07 and 0.53 mm, respectively (Mosher and Smith 1990).

10.7.3 IMPROVEMENT EFFORTS

Over the years, various efforts have been conducted to improve DANTE imaging from both technical and implementation perspectives. In 1991, Clark et al. (1991a) modified the DANTE pulse sequence to produce selective resonance saturation similar to that produced by continuous wave saturation. The combined DANTE and

continuous wave saturation technique can be used in multisite saturation transfer experiments. In 2002, Salido et al. (2002) studied the effects of phase-encoding order and segments interpolation on the accuracy and quality of the DANTE tags. The authors concluded that the center-out (low-high) phase order and linear interpolation reconstruction provide the highest tag position accuracy and profile quality. In the same year, a modified DANTE sequence was developed using a sinc-modulated RF pulse train to produce sharper tag lines with rectangular profile (Wu et al. 2002; covered in details in Section 10.2.2.2). The DANTE sequence has been also optimized to generate narrow parallel tag lines in a short time duration for in vivo imaging of the rat heart (de Crespigny et al. 1991). In another study (Tsekos et al. 1999), B_1-insensitive DANTE (Tsekos et al. 1995) has been combined with 3D ^{31}P chemical shift imaging (CSI) to study ischemia secondary to coronary occlusion on a closed-chest canine model, where the authors showed that compromised wall motion extends to larger myocardial areas compared to high-energy phosphate deficiencies.

10.7.4 DANTE DEVELOPMENTS

10.7.4.1 Double-DANTE Tagging

The double-DANTE tagging technique by Mosher and Smith (1991) has been developed 1 year after the introduction of DANTE. In double-DANTE tagging, the RF pulse train is phase-modulated to excite the sample at different frequencies, thus increasing the number of tag lines without increasing the total tagging preparation time (Mosher and Smith 1990). As shown in Figure 10.33, alternating the phase of the RF pulses between 0° and 90° generates tag lines at two different frequencies, which results in doubling the tagging density. Similarly, decreasing the phase of the even-numbered RF pulses by 90° generates tag lines at four different frequencies, which results in quadrupling the tagging density.

Double-DANTE tagging has been implemented for mapping the field changes generated by magnetic susceptibility differences (Mosher and Smith 1991). The idea here is to use very small tagging gradients, such that the displacement of the generated tag lines is sensitive to local magnetic field inhomogeneity, which can be used to measure absolute field shifts in the image. One advantage of using double-DANTE tagging in this application is that it can be made very sensitive to B_0 variations (~0.01 parts per million (ppm)) at high spatial resolution. Another advantage is that the absolute field strength can be measured with a single image. Finally, unlike phase-based techniques, random motions do not displace the tag line, and therefore the sequence allows for evaluating the susceptibility effects independent of diffusion. Figure 10.34 shows the effect of adding metallic microspheres to the imaged sample on the resulting tagging grid using double-DANTE imaging.

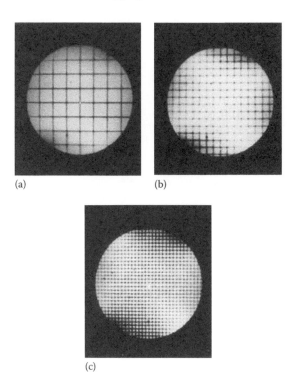

(a) (b)

(c)

FIGURE 10.33 The effects of phase-modulating the DANTE RF pulse train on tags placement. All sequences utilized a 32-pulse DANTE sequence with 0.1 ms interpulse delay and tagging gradient of 20 G/cm. Time required for tags placement was 7 ms/grid for each sequence. (a) No phase modulation generates a 1.2 × 1.2 mm grid. (b) Phase modulation (0°, 90°) generates a 0.6 × 0.6 mm grid. (c) Phase modulation (0°, 180°, 0°, 90°, 0°, 0°, 0°, 270°) generates a 0.3 × 0.3 mm grid. The tag thickness was 0.07 mm for all sequences. (Reproduced from Mosher, T.J. and Smith, M.B., *Magn. Reson. Med.*, 15(2), 334, 1990. With permission.)

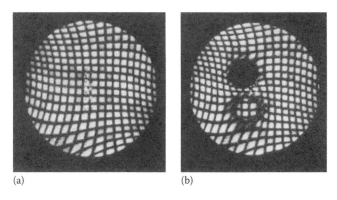

(a) (b)

FIGURE 10.34 The effects of local magnetic field susceptibility on double-DANTE tagging. The taglines are displayed with increasing field strength to the left and bottom of the image. (a) Double-DANTE image obtained in a homogeneous magnetic field. (b) The same image acquired after adding two 18 μL microspheres containing 10 mM $FeCl_3$ (top) and 500 mM $CaCl_2$ (bottom). The local gradients due to magnetic susceptibility differences shift the tag position in the regions of the microspheres. (Reproduced from Mosher, T.J. and Smith, M.B., *Magn. Reson. Med.*, 18(1), 251, 1991. With permission.)

10.7.4.2 Adiabatic DANTE

Adiabatic DANTE sequences have been developed to generate tags with uniform contrast despite the presence of B_1 inhomogeneities (Ke et al. 1992, Tsekos et al. 1995). The adiabatic DANTE sequence showed to produce uniform tagging contrast and sharp tag profile over a sixfold increase in B_1 inhomogeneity (Tsekos et al. 1995), which makes it well suited for surface coil scans. The technique has been implemented, along with ^{31}P spectroscopy, to track LV wall motion and energy metabolism in a canine model of myocardial ischemia (Hendrich et al. 1994).

In their study in 2002, Tsekos et al. (2002) presented a technique for generating sharp myocardial tag lines using the signal intensity minima of the transition zones between 0° and 360° rotation bands. As shown in Figure 10.35, the developed technique uses a sequence of two adiabatic DANTE inversion sequences (P_1 and P_2) applied in the presence of selection gradients S_1 and S_2. Additional gradients (C_1 and C_2) are interleaved with the two pulses to dephase the transverse magnetization. To generate a 2D tagging grid, the sequence given earlier is repeated with the selection gradients applied on the orthogonal direction (Figure 10.35a). The DANTE inversion sequence generates a periodic modulation of M_z composed of bands with unperturbed ($M_z = +M_0$ in zones A, E, and I) and inverted ($M_z = -M_0$ in zones C and G) magnetization. The unperturbed and inverted bands are interleaved in the transition zones (B, D, F, and H). The adiabatic DANTE pulse sequence is generated by segmenting the amplitude, $B_1(t)$, and phase, $\Phi(t)$, modulation functions of the parent adiabatic pulse into N elements using a sawtooth gradient waveform (Tsekos et al. 1995), as shown in Figure 10.36.

10.7.4.3 3D Motion Analysis Based on DANTE

DANTE has been combined with PC imaging for point-specific tracking of myocardial motion along all three axes (Perman et al. 1995). By combining prospective section selection with in-plane DANTE and PC detection of motion perpendicular to the image plane, 3D tissue motion can be analyzed.

10.7.4.4 DANTE and Black-Blood Imaging

DANTE preparation has been recently implemented to improve contrast between the myocardium tissue and flowing blood by producing black-blood images (Li et al. 2012). After DANTE preparation, the magnetization is stored in the longitudinal direction. While static tissues maintain a steady-state condition, flowing spins lose coherence, and therefore do not establish a steady-state condition. Therefore, the longitudinal magnetization of the flowing spins is largely attenuated, resulting in no signal in the resulting image. The developed technique provides a simple, robust, and low-SAR method for improving contrast between blood and myocardium.

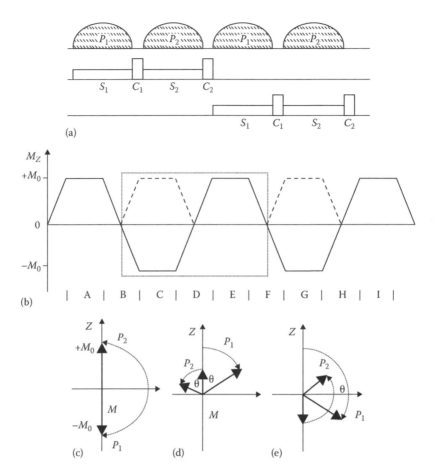

FIGURE 10.35   Adiabatic DANTE pulse sequence and magnetization evolution. (a) Timing diagram of the pulse sequence. (b) Diagrammatic representation of the frequency response of the adiabatic pulses. Illustrations of the magnetization for (c) 180°, (d) 0° < θ < 90°, and (e) 90° < θ < 180° rotations. P_1 and P_2 are adiabatic DANTE inversion pulse sequences, S_1 and S_2 are selective B_0 gradients, and C_1 and C_2 are B_0 gradients to dephase M_{xy}. The frequency profile in (b) depicts a representation of the frequency profile of a single adiabatic DANTE pulse sequence (solid line) and of a tandem (dashed). The dotted box represents the periodic element of the tagging profile. (Reproduced from Tsekos, N.V. et al., *J. Magn. Reson.*, 156(2), 187, 2002. With permission.)

10.8   HYBRID DANTE/SPAMM

A hybrid DANTE/SPAMM sequence has been developed for measuring myocardial deformation in a breath-hold scan (Figure 10.37a) (McVeigh and Atalar 1992). The duration of the tagging sequence was minimized by setting the modulation gradient to a nonzero value during the RF pulses. The developed method provided high-resolution sampling of the tag lines in two orthogonal directions using cross sampling of the k-space (Figure 10.37b). One-dimensional tagging was used instead of a 2D tagging grid to reduce scan time (less phase-encoding k-space views are needed without compromising spatial resolution), reduce motion sensitivity, simplify tagging analysis (parallel tag lines are easier to model), increase tag density (there is no interference between orthogonal tag lines), and improve SNR and tag visualization. Using the developed technique, the authors were able to obtain 3D strain data with temporal resolution of 24 ms from six contiguous slices. The scan lasted for 15 minutes and required 12 breath-holds, each of 16 heartbeats (note that this early study was conducted in 1992). Two cine sequences were obtained for each slice during each breath-hold. A set of parallel tags was oriented perpendicular to the readout direction in the first eight heartbeats; then, an orthogonal set of parallel tags was used in the next eight heartbeats, as shown in Figure 10.38.

10.9   SUMMARY AND KEY POINTS

10.9.1   SUMMARY

Despite its development more than a quarter a century ago, SPAMM tagging is still the mostly used MRI sequence for measuring regional myocardial deformation. Further, it has been the basis for developing advanced tagging sequences. SPAMM has the advantages of simplicity and efficiency, which resulted in its widespread use on various MRI systems from different vendors. Since its introduction in 1989, many technical developments and clinical applications

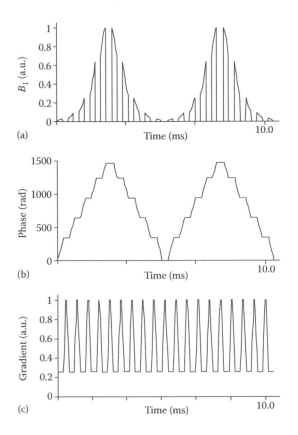

(a)

(b)

(c)

FIGURE 10.36 Adiabatic DANTE inversion sequence. The (a) amplitude $B_1(t)$ and (b) phase $\Phi(t)$ modulation functions of the tandem of two adiabatic DANTE inversion sequences based on hyperbolic secant parent pulses. (c) The corresponding gradient waveform. (Reproduced from Tsekos, N.V. et al., *J. Magn. Reson.*, 156(2), 187, 2002. With permission.)

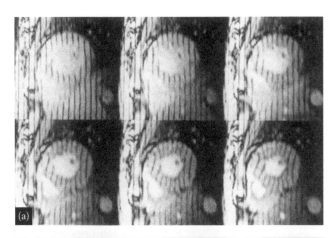

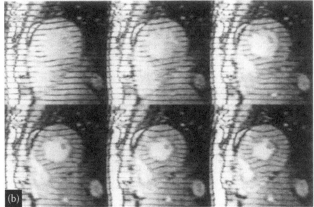

FIGURE 10.38 Hybrid DANTE/SPAMM-tagged images. Six phases of the cardiac cycle imaged in the short-axis orientation with hybrid DANTE/SPAMM with (a) vertical and (b) horizontal tag lines. Temporal resolution is 48 ms. (Reproduced from McVeigh, E.R. and Atalar, E., *Magn. Reson. Med.*, 28(2), 318, 1992. With permission.)

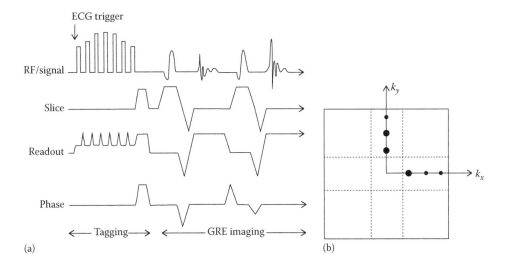

(a)

(b)

FIGURE 10.37 Hybrid DANTE/SPAMM tagging sequence. (a) Pulse sequence. The parallel line tagging pattern is produced by a sequence of rectangular pulses. The gradient producing the dispersion is reduced during the application of the RF pulses to reduce the total required bandwidth, which permits the use of lower amplitude rectangular pulses. (b) The cross pattern used to sample k-space for the final grid-tagged images. The harmonic peaks (black dots) are limited to the regions around the axis. The regions sampled in k-space are enclosed by the dashed lines. The regions obtained through symmetry are in the light dashed lines (left and bottom of k-space). (Reproduced from McVeigh, E.R. and Atalar, E., *Magn. Reson. Med.*, 28(2), 318, 1992. With permission.)

have been conducted using SPAMM. DANTE is another tagging sequence that has its own advantages, although it has not gained much widespread use as SPAMM. DANTE was introduced at almost the same time as SPAMM, it has various similarities with SPAMM, and underwent some technical developments as well. A hybrid DANTE/SPAMM sequence has been developed to combine advantages of both techniques and was used in a number of studies.

10.9.2 KEY POINTS

- In its simplest form, SPAMM tagging consists of two nonselective 90° RF pulses interspersed by a modulating gradient in the direction orthogonal to the tag lines, and followed by a spoiler gradient.
- The orientation of the tag lines is determined by the direction of the applied modulation gradient.
- Longitudinal relaxation results in reduced tagging contrast and the buildup of an additional nontagged magnetization.
- To create a better tagging profile (close to the square shape with uniform excitation and sharp edges), composite RF pulses replace the simple 90°–90° pulses in the original SPAMM tagging module. The higher the binomial order of the composite RF pulse, the sharper the tagging profile.
- sinc-Modulated tagging results in a rectangular tagline profile.
- The image's spatial resolution (pixel size) relative to tag spacing is a key issue in determining the appearance of the SPAMM-tagged pattern.
- As a general rule, the tag spacing should be less than half the thickness of the heart wall for reliable measurements.
- Magnitude reconstruction of the SPAMM images results in nonuniform tagging distribution and frequency through the cardiac cycle.
- The 45°–45° tagging pulse module could be used in SPAMM to avoid creation of negative tags.
- The image's noise affects the quality of the tag lines.
- SPAMM has been validated in phantom experiments, animal models, and tagging simulations.
- Small-tip-angle approximation has been used for analyzing and designing tagging sequences.
- Cascaded SPAMM allows for obtaining a series of cine tagged images through the cardiac cycle with high tagging contrast.
- AIR-SPAMM increases the tagging density and improves the tagging contrast without increasing the scan time.
- Phase-sensitive SPAMM (REALTAG) allows for implementing 90°–90° SPAMM without the limitations of uneven tagging density and spatially variable tagging pattern through the cardiac cycle.
- The SPAMM n' EGGS technique combines SPAMM with PC imaging for simultaneous and registered measurements of tissue motion and chamber blood flow in a single breath-hold scan.
- The SPAMM n' EGGS technique reduces scan time in half (compared to separate acquisitions of tagging and flow images), alleviates temporal and spatial misregistration problems, and results in composite tagged images with colored flow information.
- SPAMM with polarity alternating velocity encoding (SPAMM-PAV) is similar to SPAMM n' EGGS, but results in threefold improvement in temporal resolution.
- Two-dimensional SPAMM can be combined with through-plane phase-encoding velocity mapping for measuring 3D myocardial deformation.
- SPAMM imaging at 3 T is better than that at 1.5 T, mainly due to the doubled SNR and slower myocardial longitudinal relaxation, which improve the tagging persistence throughout the cardiac cycle.
- SPAMM has been implemented in different applications, including tissue deformation, clinical and experimental studies, and noncardiac applications.
- DANTE has the advantages of improved tagging resolution and reduced eddy currents.
- In DANTE, the width and separation of the tag lines can be easily modified by controlling the pulse sequence parameters.
- Different efforts have been conducted to improve the DANTE sequence.
- The double-DANTE sequence increases the number of tag lines without increasing the total tagging preparation time.
- Adiabatic DANTE generates tags with uniform contrast despite the presence of B_1 inhomogeneities.
- DANTE has been combined with PC imaging for point-specific tracking of myocardial motion in 3D.
- DANTE has been used to improve the contrast between static tissue and flowing blood by producing black-blood images.
- The hybrid DANTE/SPAMM sequence allows for measuring myocardial deformation in a breath-hold scan with improved image quality.

REFERENCES

Aletras, A.H., Freidlin, R.Z., Navon, G., and Arai, A.E. (2004). AIR-SPAMM: Alternative inversion recovery spatial modulation of magnetization for myocardial tagging. *J Magn Reson* **166**(2): 236–245.

Atalar, E. and McVeigh, E.R. (1994). Optimization of tag thickness for measuring position with magnetic resonance imaging. *IEEE Trans Med Imaging* **13**(1): 152–160.

Axel, L. and Dougherty, L. (1989a). Heart wall motion: Improved method of spatial modulation of magnetization for MR imaging. *Radiology* **172**(2): 349–350.

Axel, L. and Dougherty, L. (1989b). MR imaging of motion with spatial modulation of magnetization. *Radiology* **171**(3): 841–845.

Axel, L., Goncalves, R.C., and Bloomgarden, D. (1992). Regional heart wall motion: Two-dimensional analysis and functional imaging with MR imaging. *Radiology* **183**(3): 745–750.

Ceelen, K.K., Stekelenburg, A., Mulders, J.L., Strijkers, G.J., Baaijens, F.P., Nicolay, K. and Oomens, C.W. (2008). Validation of a numerical model of skeletal muscle compression with MR tagging: A contribution to pressure ulcer research. *J Biomech Eng* **130**(6): 061015.

Chai, J.W., Chen, Y.T., and Lee, S.K. (1997). MRI assessment of regional heart wall motion in the longitudinal axis sections of left ventricle by spatial modulation of magnetization. *Zhonghua Yi Xue Za Zhi (Taipei)* **60**(1): 13–20.

Chen, M.Y., Tsai, J.W., Chang, M.S., and Yu, B.C. (1995). Assessment of heart wall motion: Modified spatial modulation of magnetization for MR imaging. *Proc Natl Sci Counc Repub China B* **19**(1): 47–53.

Clark, J.F., Harris, G.I., and Dillon, P.F. (1991a). Multisite saturation transfer using DANTE and continuous wave. *Magn Reson Med* **17**(1): 274–278.

Clark, N.R., Reichek, N., Bergey, P., Hoffman, E.A., Brownson, D., Palmon, L., and Axel, L. (1991b). Circumferential myocardial shortening in the normal human left ventricle. Assessment by magnetic resonance imaging using spatial modulation of magnetization. *Circulation* **84**(1): 67–74.

Crum, W.R., Berry, E., Ridgway, J.P., Sivananthan, U.M., Tan, L.B., and Smith, M.A. (1997). Simulation of two-dimensional tagged MRI. *J Magn Reson Imaging* **7**(2): 416–424.

Crum, W.R., Berry, E., Ridgway, J.P., Sivananthan, U.M., Tan, L.B., and Smith, M.A. (1998). Frequency-domain simulation of MR tagging. *J Magn Reson Imaging* **8**(5): 1040–1050.

de Crespigny, A.J., Carpenter, T.A., and Hall, L.D. (1991). Cardiac tagging in the rat using a DANTE sequence. *Magn Reson Med* **21**(1): 151–156.

Delhaas, T., Kotte, J., van der Toorn, A., Snoep, G., Prinzen, F.W., and Arts, T. (2004). Increase in left ventricular torsion-to-shortening ratio in children with valvular aortic stenosis. *Magn Reson Med* **51**(1): 135–139.

Derbyshire, J.A., Sampath, S., and McVeigh, E.R. (2007). Phase-sensitive cardiac tagging–REALTAG. *Magn Reson Med* **58**(1): 206–210.

Donekal, S., Ambale-Venkatesh, B., Berkowitz, S., Wu, C.O., Choi, E.Y., Fernandes, V., Yan, R., Harouni, A.A., Bluemke, D.A., and Lima, J.A. (2013). Inter-study reproducibility of cardiovascular magnetic resonance tagging. *J Cardiovasc Magn Reson* **15**(1): 37.

Fischer, S.E., McKinnon, G.C., Maier, S.E., and Boesiger, P. (1993). Improved myocardial tagging contrast. *Magn Reson Med* **30**(2): 191–200.

Fogel, M.A., Weinberg, P.M., Hubbard, A., and Haselgrove, J. (2000). Diastolic biomechanics in normal infants utilizing MRI tissue tagging. *Circulation* **102**(2): 218–224.

Haselgrove, J.C. and Fogel, M.A. (2005). Application of spatial modulation of magnetization (SPAMM) to children: The effect of image resolution on tagging pattern. *J Cardiovasc Magn Reson* **7**(2): 433–440.

Hendrich, K., Xu, Y., Kim, S.G., and Ugurbil, K. (1994). Surface coil cardiac tagging and 31P spectroscopic localization with B1-insensitive adiabatic pulses. *Magn Reson Med* **31**(5): 541–545.

Ibrahim, El-S.H. (2011). Myocardial tagging by cardiovascular magnetic resonance: Evolution of techniques–pulse sequences, analysis algorithms, and applications. *J Cardiovasc Magn Reson* **13**: 36.

Ke, Y., Shchupp, D.G. and Garwood, M. (1992). Adiabatic DANTE sequences for B1-insensitive narrowband inversion. *J Magn Reson* **96**: 663–669.

Kerwin, W.S. and Prince, J.L. (2000). A k-space analysis of MR tagging. *J Magn Reson* **142**(2): 313–322.

Knollmann, F.D., Maurer, J., Wlodarczyk, W., Bock, J.C., and Felix, R. (1996). Fourier phase mapping of the human heart. The use of spatial modulation of magnetization cine magnetic resonance imaging. *Invest Radiol* **31**(12): 743–748.

Kramer, C.M., Reichek, N., Ferrari, V.A., Theobald, T., Dawson, J., and Axel, L. (1994). Regional heterogeneity of function in hypertrophic cardiomyopathy. *Circulation* **90**(1): 186–194.

Kramer, C.M., Rogers, W.J., Theobald, T.M., Power, T.P., Petruolo, S., and Reichek, N. (1996). Remote noninfarcted region dysfunction soon after first anterior myocardial infarction. A magnetic resonance tagging study. *Circulation* **94**(4): 660–666.

Kuijer, J.P., Marcus, J.T., Gotte, M.J., van Rossum, A.C., and Heethaar, R.M. (1999). Simultaneous MRI tagging and through-plane velocity quantification: A three-dimensional myocardial motion tracking algorithm. *J Magn Reson Imaging* **9**(3): 409–419.

Kuijpers, D., Ho, K.Y., van Dijkman, P.R., Vliegenthart, R., and Oudkerk, M. (2003). Dobutamine cardiovascular magnetic resonance for the detection of myocardial ischemia with the use of myocardial tagging. *Circulation* **107**(12): 1592–1597.

Li, L., Miller, K.L., and Jezzard, P. (2012). DANTE-prepared pulse trains: A novel approach to motion-sensitized and motion-suppressed quantitative magnetic resonance imaging. *Magn Reson Med* **68**(5): 1423–1438.

Lima, J.A., Ferrari, V.A., Reichek, N., Kramer, C.M., Palmon, L., Llaneras, M.R., Tallant, B., Young, A.A., and Axel, L. (1995). Segmental motion and deformation of transmurally infarcted myocardium in acute postinfarct period. *Am J Physiol* **268**(3 Pt 2): H1304–H1312.

Lima, J.A., Jeremy, R., Guier, W., Bouton, S., Zerhouni, E.A., McVeigh, E., Buchalter, M.B., Weisfeldt, M.L., Shapiro, E.P., and Weiss, J.L. (1993). Accurate systolic wall thickening by nuclear magnetic resonance imaging with tissue tagging: Correlation with sonomicrometers in normal and ischemic myocardium. *J Am Coll Cardiol* **21**(7): 1741–1751.

Maier, S.E., Fischer, S.E., McKinnon, G.C., Hess, O.M., Krayenbuehl, H.P., and Boesiger, P. (1992a). Acquisition and evaluation of tagged magnetic resonance images of the human left ventricle. *Comput Med Imaging Graph* **16**(2): 73–80.

Maier, S.E., Fischer, S.E., McKinnon, G.C., Hess, O.M., Krayenbuehl, H.P., and Boesiger, P. (1992b). Evaluation of left ventricular segmental wall motion in hypertrophic cardiomyopathy with myocardial tagging. *Circulation* **86**(6): 1919–1928.

Maniar, H.S., Cupps, B.P., Potter, D.D., Moustakidis, P., Camillo, C.J., Chu, C.M., Pasque, M.K., and Sundt, T.M., 3rd (2004). Ventricular function after coronary artery bypass grafting: Evaluation by magnetic resonance imaging and myocardial strain analysis. *J Thorac Cardiovasc Surg* **128**(1): 76–82.

McVeigh, E.R. and Atalar, E. (1992). Cardiac tagging with breath-hold cine MRI. *Magn Reson Med* **28**(2): 318–327.

Moerman, K.M., Sprengers, A.M., Simms, C.K., Lamerichs, R.M., Stoker, J., and Nederveen, A.J. (2011). Validation of SPAMM tagged MRI based measurement of 3D soft tissue deformation. *Med Phys* **38**(3): 1248–1260.

Montillo, A., Udupa, J., Axel, L., and Metaxas, D. (2003). Interaction between noise suppression and inhomogeneity correction in MRI. *Proceeding SPIE*, San Diego, CA, pp. 1025–1036.

Moore, C.C., Reeder, S.B., and McVeigh, E.R. (1994). Tagged MR imaging in a deforming phantom: Photographic validation. *Radiology* **190**(3): 765–769.

Mosher, T.J. and Smith, M.B. (1990). A DANTE tagging sequence for the evaluation of translational sample motion. *Magn Reson Med* **15**(2): 334–339.

Mosher, T.J. and Smith, M.B. (1991). Magnetic susceptibility measurement using a double-DANTE tagging (DDT) sequence. *Magn Reson Med* **18**(1): 251–255.

O'Dell, W.G., Moore, C.C., Hunter, W.C., Zerhouni, E.A., and McVeigh, E.R. (1995). Three-dimensional myocardial deformations: Calculation with displacement field fitting to tagged MR images. *Radiology* **195**(3): 829–835.

Osman, N.F., Kerwin, W.S., McVeigh, E.R., and Prince, J.L. (1999). Cardiac motion tracking using CINE harmonic phase (HARP) magnetic resonance imaging. *Magn Reson Med* **42**(6): 1048–1060.

Palmon, L.C., Reichek, N., Yeon, S.B., Clark, N.R., Brownson, D., Hoffman, E., and Axel, L. (1994). Intramural myocardial shortening in hypertensive left ventricular hypertrophy with normal pump function. *Circulation* **89**(1): 122–131.

Park, J., Metaxas, D.N., Axel, L., Yuan, Q., and Blom, A.S. (1999). Cascaded MRI-SPAMM for LV motion analysis during a whole cardiac cycle. *Int J Med Inform* **55**(2): 117–126.

Parthasarathy, V., Prince, J.L., Stone, M., Murano, E.Z., and Nessaiver, M. (2007). Measuring tongue motion from tagged cine-MRI using harmonic phase (HARP) processing. *J Acoust Soc Am* **121**(1): 491–504.

Pauly, J., Nishimura, D., and Macovski, A. (2011). A k-space analysis of small-tip-angle excitation. 1989. *J Magn Reson* **213**(2): 544–557.

Perman, W.H., Creswell, L.L., Wyers, S.G., Moulton, M.J., and Pasque, M.K. (1995). Hybrid DANTE and phase-contrast imaging technique for measurement of three-dimensional myocardial wall motion. *J Magn Reson Imaging* **5**(1): 101–106.

Petersson, J.S., Christoffersson, J.O., and Golman, K. (1993). MRI simulation using the k-space formalism. *Magn Reson Imaging* **11**(4): 557–568.

Piccirelli, M., Luechinger, R., Sturm, V., Boesiger, P., Landau, K., and Bergamin, O. (2009). Local deformation of extraocular muscles during eye movement. *Invest Ophthalmol Vis Sci* **50**(11): 5189–5196.

Pipe, J.G., Boes, J.L., and Chenevert, T.L. (1991). Method for measuring three-dimensional motion with tagged MR imaging. *Radiology* **181**(2): 591–595.

Prinzen, F.W., Hunter, W.C., Wyman, B.T., and McVeigh, E.R. (1999). Mapping of regional myocardial strain and work during ventricular pacing: Experimental study using magnetic resonance imaging tagging. *J Am Coll Cardiol* **33**(6): 1735–1742.

Reeder, S.B. and McVeigh, E.R. (1994). Tag contrast in breath-hold CINE cardiac MRI. *Magn Reson Med* **31**(5): 521–525.

Rogers, W.J., Jr., Kramer, C.M., Geskin, G., Hu, Y.L., Theobald, T.M., Vido, D.A., Petruolo, S., and Reichek, N. (1999). Early contrast-enhanced MRI predicts late functional recovery after reperfused myocardial infarction. *Circulation* **99**(6): 744–750.

Ropele, S., Ebner, F., Fazekas, F., and Reishofer, G. (2010). Super-resolution MRI using microscopic spatial modulation of magnetization. *Magn Reson Med* **64**(6): 1671–1675.

Sabet, A.A., Christoforou, E., Zatlin, B., Genin, G.M., and Bayly, P.V. (2008). Deformation of the human brain induced by mild angular head acceleration. *J Biomech* **41**(2): 307–315.

Salido, T.B., Hundley, W.G., Link, K.M., Epstein, F.H., and Hamilton, C.A. (2002). Effects of phase encode order and segment interpolation methods on the quality and accuracy of myocardial tags during assessment of left ventricular contraction. *J Cardiovasc Magn Reson* **4**(2): 245–254.

Sampath, S., Derbyshire, J.A., Ledesma-Carbayo, M.J., and McVeigh, E.R. (2011). Imaging left ventricular tissue mechanics and hemodynamics during supine bicycle exercise using a combined tagging and phase-contrast MRI pulse sequence. *Magn Reson Med* **65**(1): 51–59.

Sampath, S., Kim, J.H., Lederman, R.J., and McVeigh, E.R. (2008). Simultaneous imaging of myocardial motion and chamber blood flow with SPAMM n' EGGS (Spatial Modulation of Magnetization With Encoded Gradients for Gauging Speed). *J Magn Reson Imaging* **27**(4): 809–817.

Santa Marta, C., Ledesma-Carbayo, M.J., Bajo, A., Perez-David, E., Santos, A., and Desco, M. (2006). Respiratory gated SPAMM sequence for magnetic resonance cardiac tagging. *Comp Cardiol* **33**: 61–64.

Sayad, D.E., Willett, D.L., Hundley, W.G., Grayburn, P.A., and Peshock, R.M. (1998). Dobutamine magnetic resonance imaging with myocardial tagging quantitatively predicts improvement in regional function after revascularization. *Am J Cardiol* **82**(9): 1149–1151, A1110.

Setser, R.M., Smedira, N.G., Lieber, M.L., Sabo, E.D., and White, R.D. (2007). Left ventricular torsional mechanics after left ventricular reconstruction surgery for ischemic cardiomyopathy. *J Thorac Cardiovasc Surg* **134**(4): 888–896.

Truscott, K.J. and Buonocore, M.H. (2001). Simulation of tagged MR images with linear tetrahedral solid elements. *J Magn Reson Imaging* **14**(3): 336–340.

Tsekos, N.V., Garwood, M., Merkle, H., Xu, Y., Wilke, N., and Ugurbil, K. (1995). Myocardial tagging with B1 insensitive adiabatic DANTE inversion sequences. *Magn Reson Med* **34**(3): 395–401.

Tsekos, N.V., Garwood, M., and Ugurbil, K. (2002). Tagging of the magnetization with the transition zones of 360 degrees rotations generated by a tandem of two adiabatic DANTE inversion sequences. *J Magn Reson* **156**(2): 187–194.

Tsekos, N.V., Merkle, H., Zhang, Y., Hu, X., and Ugurbil, K. (1999). Anatomical correlation of high energy phosphate and wall motion during occlusion of a coronary artery on the closed-chest canine heart. *Proceedings of the International Society for Magnetic Resonance in Medicine*, Philadelphia, PA.

Valeti, V.U., Chun, W., Potter, D.D., Araoz, P.A., McGee, K.P., Glockner, J.F., and Christian, T.F. (2006). Myocardial tagging and strain analysis at 3 Tesla: Comparison with 1.5 Tesla imaging. *J Magn Reson Imaging* **23**(4): 477–480.

Van Der Toorn, A., Barenbrug, P., Snoep, G., Van Der Veen, F.H., Delhaas, T., Prinzen, F.W., Maessen, J., and Arts, T. (2002). Transmural gradients of cardiac myofiber shortening in aortic valve stenosis patients using MRI tagging. *Am J Physiol Heart Circ Physiol* **283**(4): H1609–H1615.

Verhnet, H., Revel, D., Arteaga, C., Clarysse, P., Sottilini, F., Roux, J.P., and Canet, E. (1999). Predictive value of regional left ventricular circumferential shortening in jeopardized myocardium. A two-dimensional SPAMM cine-MRI study in a canine model. *Invest Radiol* **34**(10): 621–628.

Wayte, S.C. and Redpath, T.W. (1998). Estimating spatial resolution of in vivo MR images using spatial modulation of magnetization. *Magn Reson Imaging* **16**(1): 37–44.

Wu, E.X., Towe, C.W., and Tang, H. (2002). MRI cardiac tagging using a sinc-modulated RF pulse train. *Magn Reson Med* **48**(2): 389–393.

Yeon, S.B., Reichek, N., Tallant, B.A., Lima, J.A., Calhoun, L.P., Clark, N.R., Hoffman, E.A., Ho, K.K., and Axel, L. (2001). Validation of in vivo myocardial strain measurement by magnetic resonance tagging with sonomicrometry. *J Am Coll Cardiol* **38**(2): 555–561.

Young, A.A., Axel, L., Dougherty, L., Bogen, D.K., and Parenteau, C.S. (1993). Validation of tagging with MR imaging to estimate material deformation. *Radiology* **188**(1): 101–108.

Young, A.A., Imai, H., Chang, C.N., and Axel, L. (1994a). Two-dimensional left ventricular deformation during systole using magnetic resonance imaging with spatial modulation of magnetization. *Circulation* **89**(2): 740–752.

Young, A.A., Kramer, C.M., Ferrari, V.A., Axel, L., and Reichek, N. (1994b). Three-dimensional left ventricular deformation in hypertrophic cardiomyopathy. *Circulation* **90**(2): 854–867.

Zerhouni, E.A., Parish, D.M., Rogers, W.J., Yang, A., and Shapiro, E.P. (1988). Human heart: Tagging with MR imaging—A method for noninvasive assessment of myocardial motion. *Radiology* **169**(1): 59–63.

Zhang, Z., Dione, D.P., Brown, P.B., Shapiro, E.M., Sinusas, A.J., and Sampath, S. (2011). Assessment of early diastolic strain-velocity temporal relationships using spatial modulation of magnetization with polarity alternating velocity encoding (SPAMM-PAV). *Magn Reson Med* **66**(6): 1627–1638.

Zhang, Z., Friedman, D., Dione, D.P., Lin, B.A., Duncan, J.S., Sinusas, A.J., and Sampath, S. (2013). Assessment of left ventricular 2D flow pathlines during early diastole using spatial modulation of magnetization with polarity alternating velocity encoding: A study in normal volunteers and canine animals with myocardial infarction. *Magn Reson Med* **70**: 766–775.

Zhou, R., Pickup, S., Glickson, J.D., Scott, C.H., and Ferrari, V.A. (2003). Assessment of global and regional myocardial function in the mouse using cine and tagged MRI. *Magn Reson Med* **49**(4): 760–764.

11 Complementary Spatial Modulation of Magnetization (CSPAMM) Tagging

El-Sayed H. Ibrahim, PhD; Andrew J. Coristine, PhD; Hélène Feliciano, PhD; Davide Piccini, PhD; and Matthias Stuber, PhD

CONTENTS

LIST OF ABBREVIATIONS

Abbreviation	Meaning
1D	One dimensional
2D	Two dimensional
3D	Three dimensional
AoR	Axis of rotation
CAPTOR	Cardiac phase to order reconstruction
CNR	Contrast-to-noise ratio
CRT	Cardiac resynchronization therapy
CSPAMM	Complementary spatial modulation of magnetization
DENSE	Displacement encoding with stimulated echoes
ECG	Electrocardiogram
EPI	Echo planar imaging
EPI-PC	EPI-phase correction
FAST	Fourier analysis of stimulated echoes
FHC	Familial hypertrophic cardiomyopathy
HARP	Harmonic phase
IFC	Inherent fat cancellation
LAX	Long axis
LBBB	Left bundle branch block
LISA	Linearly increasing start-up angles

Abbreviation	Meaning
LV	Left ventricle
MICSR	Magnitude image CSPAMM reconstruction
OCSPAMM	Orthogonal CSPAMM
ORI-CSPAMM	Off-resonance insensitive CSPAMM
PAH	Pulmonary arterial hypertension
PEA	Pulmonary endarterectomy
PPCI	Primary percutaneous coronary intervention
RF	Radiofrequency
RV	Right ventricle
SAX	Short axis
SENC	Strain encoding
SLV	Single LV
SNR	Signal-to-noise ratio
SPAMM	Spatial modulation of magnetization
SPGR	Spoiled gradient echo
SRV	Single RV
SSFP	Steady state with free precession
SSSP	Spectral–spatial selective pulses
STEAM	stimulated echo acquisition mode
STEMI	ST elevation myocardial infarction
Tag-CNR	Tagging contrast-to-noise ratio
TAVI	Transcatheter aortic valve implantation
TF-EPI	Turbo field EPI

11.1 INTRODUCTION

11.1.1 STEFAN FISCHER AND CSPAMM DEVELOPMENT

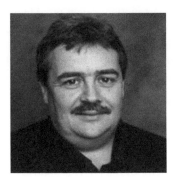

This chapter is dedicated to Stefan Ernst Fischer, PhD, the inventor of CSPAMM. Not only was he a former mentor to the last author of this chapter, but he was also a dear friend for the past two decades. Stefan tragically and unexpectedly passed away while on a business trip to Europe in the summer of 2011. He leaves behind his wife, Elisabeth, as well as his two sons, Ramon and Urs.

Stefan studied electrical engineering at the Swiss Federal Institute of Technology (ETH) in Zurich, Switzerland, where his research was guided by both his passion and talent for engineering. During his PhD study, he developed the complementary spatial modulation of the magnetization (CSPAMM), a myocardial tagging technique that enabled, for the first time, quantitative characterization of both systolic and diastolic myocardial motions (Fischer et al. 1993). He then moved on to address the even more difficult problem of tissue through-plane motion and found a very elegant solution for slice following, which was combined with CSPAMM to create true myocardial motion tracking (Fischer et al. 1994). He then tested the hypothesis that stimulated echo acquisition mode (STEAM) may be used for myocardial tagging since STEAM-modulated information decays exclusively with T_1, making it theoretically very well suited for cardiovascular applications (the myocardial longitudinal relaxation is much slower compared to transverse relaxation [$T_1 \sim 850$ ms and $T_2 \sim 50$ ms at 1.5 T]). When this proved not to be the case, he relentlessly searched for an explanation, which, of course, he found in the end (Fischer et al. 1995). The theoretical and practical implications of Stefan's research laid the foundations for advanced cardiac imaging methods such as strain encoding (SENC) (Osman et al. 2001) and displacement encoding with stimulated echoes (DENSE) (Aletras et al. 1999). While working on these techniques, Stefan also recognized that the accuracy of electrocardiogram (ECG) triggering, a technique on which cardiovascular magnetic resonance (CMR) critically hinges, is adversely affected by the magnetohydrodynamic effect. At that time, MRI scanners were equipped with 3 ECG leads. Stefan recognized that the artifacts originating from the magnetohydrodynamic effect might be avoided by simultaneously analyzing the ECG signal in multiple spatial dimensions, rather than only in a one-dimensional (1D) projection (Fischer et al. 1999). Of course, he was on target and his vector ECG system has now been installed on many vendors' scanners worldwide. With his work on myocardial tagging and vector ECG, he not only took CMR to the next level but also enabled new research and discovery in the field. Not surprisingly, he completed his PhD with the highest honors that the ETH can bestow, the Medal of the ETH Zurich.

Stefan was not only an accomplished engineer and great scientist, but he was also a very successful and gifted teacher. In recognition of his numerous contributions, the Early Career Award session at the 2012 annual meeting of the Society for Cardiovascular Magnetic Resonance (SCMR) in Orlando, FL, was dedicated to the memory of Stefan E. Fischer. Thank you Stefan for your contributions to the field and for teaching so many of us the fundamentals of MRI.

11.1.2 CHAPTER LAYOUT

In this chapter, technical and clinical applications of CSPAMM are covered. The chapter starts by presenting a historical overview of CSPAMM development and the early work of late Dr. Stefan Fischer. The original CSPAMM technique is then described in details along with tagging signal analysis, image construction, data acquisition, and tags fading. Slice through-plane motion and correcting techniques (slice isolation and slice following) are then described. Section 11.5 addresses fast CSPAMM techniques, including combining CSPAMM with echo planar imaging (EPI), turbo field EPI, and spiral data acquisition. Balanced steady-state free precession (SSFP) implementation in CSPAMM is then addressed along with techniques for improving tagging contrast. Section 11.7 addresses magnitude and real-part CSPAMM reconstruction. Two fat suppression techniques that are tailored for CSPAMM, namely the inherent fat cancellation (IFC) and off-resonance insensitive CSPAMM (ORI-CSPAMM), are then described in details. High-resolution CSPAMM and orthogonal CSPAMM (OCSPAMM) are then covered. Section 11.11 covers 3D CSPAMM imaging techniques, including volumetric CSPAMM and accelerated whole-heart imaging. Finally, the chapter covers various CSPAMM applications, including animal studies, ischemic heart disease, left ventricular (LV) torsion, LV hypertrophy, aortic stenosis, pulmonary hypertension, cardiac resynchronization therapy, cardiac electrophysiology, and congenital heart disease.

11.2 CSPAMM AND BEYOND: THE QUEST

11.2.1 THE NEED FOR MRI TAGGING

For many decades, global ventricular heart function has been successfully characterized using echocardiographic methods, as changes in ventricular volume, ejection fraction, and mass have been established as adequate parameters for quantitative assessment of the heart function. With the advent of MRI, supported by advanced hardware and software, it became possible to collect segmented k-space acquisitions triggered to the R-wave of the ECG (Shetty 1988). Using this technology, time-resolved (cine) cross-sectional images could be easily obtained, where the contrast between the ventricular blood pool and myocardium permitted image segmentation and therefore quantitative assessment of ventricular function and mass. Using MRI, acoustic windows are no longer a limitation and plane localization is enabled for any user-specified angulation. While these advantages come at the expense of increased complexity (MRI is hardly a bedside exam), it quickly became clear that a more detailed evaluation of cardiac motion would not only lead to new scientific insight and discovery, but the obtained complementary information might also help guide and monitor treatment as well. On conventional MR images, however, as in

echocardiography, no internal structures of the myocardium are visible (Figure 11.1), and therefore regional myocardial motion parameters cannot be easily obtained. Simultaneously, and with mounting evidence that alterations of the heart mechanics (e.g., the rotational heart motion) might provide useful information (Ingels et al. 1975), there was a clear need for an imaging technology that supports tracking any user-selected point on the myocardium throughout the entire cardiac cycle (Figure 11.2).

11.2.2 TAGS FADING AND CSPAMM

To respond to the need for a technique to evaluate regional myocardial motion, the research teams of Leon Axel and Lawrence Dougherty at UPenn and Elias Zerhouni (who later became the director of the NIH) at Johns Hopkins developed the MRI myocardial tagging technique. Using spatial modulation of magnetization (SPAMM) or selective excitation, stripes or grids of saturated magnetization can be created on the myocardium (Zerhouni et al. 1988, Axel and Dougherty 1989, Ibrahim 2011). On cine images of the heart, the motion and deformation of these taglines could be easily tracked, thereby providing unique and rather unprecedented information about intramyocardial motion of the heart. However, since this modulated magnetization decays not only as a function of time after the modulation or *tagging* procedure, but also due to the radio-frequency (RF) excitations used for imaging, motion of structures internal to the myocardium could only be tracked during the systolic phase of the cardiac cycle. This so-called fading of the taglines precluded simultaneous access to both systolic and diastolic motion patterns of the heart. It was not until Stefan Fischer, in collaboration with Graeme McKinnon in the group of Peter Boesiger, carefully analyzed the background of this tags fading that a solution to the problem was successfully developed, implemented, and tested (Fischer et al. 1993). The technique was called

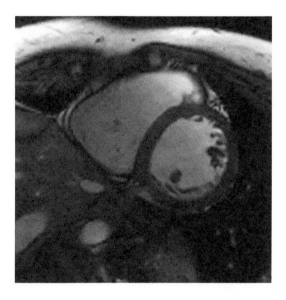

FIGURE 11.1 Example of conventional MRI short-axis image of the heart. No internal structures of the myocardium are visible.

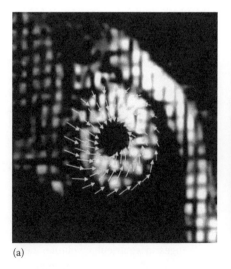

(a)

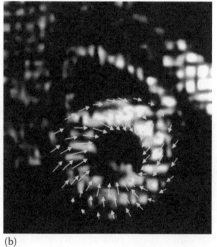

(b)

FIGURE 11.2 Tagging for regional analysis of myocardial deformation. Example of how the tagged images can allow for the visualization of the rotational myocardial movement throughout the cardiac cycle. End-systolic acquisitions are overlaid with the corresponding local trajectories. At the (a) apex, contraction is associated with a counterclockwise rotation (as viewed from apex), whereas at the (b) base, a clockwise rotation is observed. (Reproduced from Stuber, M. et al., *Circulation*, 100(4), 361, 1999b. With permission.)

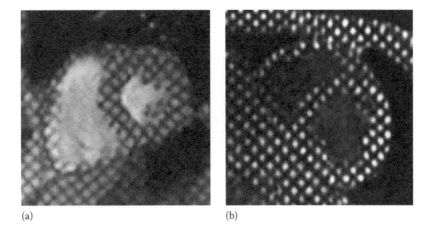

(a)   (b)

FIGURE 11.3 SPAMM versus CSPAMM. Comparison between (a) systolic SPAMM image with a tagging angle of 140° and (b) the corresponding systolic CSPAMM image. (Reproduced from Fischer, S.E. et al., *Magn. Reson. Med.*, 30(2), 191, 1993. With permission.)

complementary SPAMM (CSPAMM). Using CSPAMM, motion parameters from both systolic and diastolic phases of the cardiac cycle could, for the first time, be simultaneously extracted (Figure 11.3).

11.2.3 THROUGH-PLANE MOTION AND SLICE FOLLOWING

It was recognized that the systolic long-axis (LAX) contraction of the heart leads to through-plane displacement of the tissue on two-dimensional (2D) short-axis (SAX) images. This through-plane motion effect is amplified at the basal level of the heart, which inevitably leads to a bias in the extracted motion data because it is not always the case that the same material points are tracked on multiphase cine images (Rogers et al. 1991). As Fischer systematically studied the MRI physics of myocardial tagging, he recognized that a carefully devised extension to CSPAMM could lead to a breakthrough by always visualizing the same material points on SAX images throughout the entire cardiac cycle. In fact, this technique was implemented, tested, and carefully characterized, which led to a slice-following version of CSPAMM enabling "true" myocardial motion tracking and better characterization of regional tissue properties (Fischer et al. 1994).

11.2.4 STIMULATED-ECHO IMAGING

During his studies related to tagging, Fischer hypothesized that stimulated echoes, or STEAM, might be exploited for MRI tissue tagging, simply because the STEAM-modulated signal decays with T_1, and therefore not only offers an opportunity to preserve the tagged information for a relatively long time, but also avoids the subtraction of two images, which is an inherent characteristic of CSPAMM. Fischer thus implemented STEAM tagging and tested it both in moving phantoms and in vivo.

The initial results turned out to be a big disappointment. Although the images were signal starved, what was most confusing was that on the STEAM-modulated images, the heart would always disappear during systole just to reappear

during diastole. While the signal-to-noise ratio (SNR) loss was attributable to the intrinsic 50% signal loss of the STEAM sequence, the periodic disappearance and reappearance of the heart could not be simply explained. It was reassuring, however, that the same effect was observed on cardiac STEAM images in a publication from the group of Jens Frahm, one of the fathers of stimulated echo imaging (Haase et al. 1986). Despite the initial disappointment, Fischer set out to explain what he had observed, and he hypothesized that it was related to systolic tissue contraction, which would shift the modulation frequency along the slice-selection axis. Of course, he was able to prove this hypothesis both theoretically and experimentally (Haase et al. 1986, Fischer et al. 1995).

11.3 CSPAMM: THE ORIGINAL SEQUENCE

11.3.1 TAGGING SIGNAL ANALYSIS

MRI myocardial tagging consists of a magnetization modulation (the tagging module) that is followed by a signal readout module for image formation. This signal readout module is repeated n times to generate a cine series of images, on which the deformation of the heart can be appreciated as a function of time. The tagging module typically occurs immediately after detection of the ECG's R-wave. Line or grid patterns are most commonly used. For signal readout, multiple segmented k-space gradient echo–based imaging approaches can be used, though these will be described later. In any case, to be able to detect the pattern generated by the tagging module of the sequence, the difference between the maxima and minima of the tagged signal should be maximized throughout the entire cardiac cycle. Let us assume that the initial longitudinal magnetization (M_z) is at thermal equilibrium ($M_z = M_0$) before tagging and imaging are performed. Let us also assume that the steady-state magnetization prior to tagging (after each R-wave of the ECG) is always M_{ss} and that the Cartesian coordinate system is defined in terms of (x, y, z). Immediately after application of the tagging module at t_0, the longitudinal component of the SPAMM-modulated magnetization is given by

$$M_z(t_0) = M_{ss} TAG(x,y), \tag{11.1}$$

where $TAG(x,y)$ refers to the modulation function in the xy-plane. The longitudinal magnetization at time t_1 immediately before applying the first imaging RF pulse is

$$M_z(t_1) = (M_{ss}TAG(x,y) - M_0)e^{-t_1/T_1} + M_0, \tag{11.2}$$

where T_1 refers to the longitudinal relaxation time. From Equation 11.2, it becomes evident that the tagged information decays as a function of T_1. Consequently, this equation can be decomposed into two parts, Q_{T1} and Q_{R1}, where Q_{T1} represents the tagged information and Q_{R1} represents the component of the magnetization that recovers as a function of time after tagging, which does not contain any tagged information.

$$Q_{T1} = M_{ss}TAG(x,y)e^{-t_1/T_1}, \tag{11.3}$$

$$Q_{R1} = M_0(1 - e^{-t_1/T_1}). \tag{11.4}$$

After applying the first RF excitation pulse of angle α_1, the longitudinal magnetization is proportional to $\cos(\alpha_1)$. For an imaging sequence in which one RF excitation is used per k-space segment, the Q_{Tk} and Q_{Rk} components at time t_k just before applying the kth RF excitation pulse will thus be

$$Q_{Tk} = M_{ss}TAG(x,y)e^{-t_k/T_1}\prod_{j=1}^{k-1}\cos\alpha_j \tag{11.5}$$

and

$$Q_{Rk} = (Q_{Rk-1}\cos\alpha_{k-1} - M_0)e^{-\Delta t/T1} + M_0, \tag{11.6}$$

where $\Delta t = t_k - t_{k-1}$. Note that new k-space segments must be acquired for each cine frame ($i = 1, \ldots, n$). While Q_{Tk} and Q_{Rk} refer to the longitudinal magnetization, the transverse magnetization after the kth RF excitation pulse is proportional to the signal I_k that is measured. From Equation 11.5, it is evident that the tagged information does not only decay as a function of T_1, but it is also simultaneously scaled by the RF excitations used for the signal readout. After the kth RF excitation, the signal obtained I_k is given by

$$I_k = (Q_{Tk} + Q_{Rk})\sin\alpha_k \tag{11.7}$$

11.3.2   CSPAMM IMAGE CONSTRUCTION

The central idea of CSPAMM entails the separation of Q_{Tk} and Q_{Rk} so that only the tagged component of the magnetization remains, while the relaxing nontagged component can be suppressed. Such a separation can indeed be obtained by acquiring two different images, A and B, in which the tagged information is different (Figure 11.4).

If the steady-state magnetization M_{ss} is equal for both acquisitions, then, $A_k - B_k$ can be written as

$$A_k - B_k \propto \left[TAG_A(x,y) - TAG_B(x,y)\right]e^{-t_k/T_1}\left[\prod_{j=1}^{k-1}\cos\alpha_j\right]\sin\alpha_k. \tag{11.8}$$

In this equation, Q_{Rk} is simply eliminated during subtraction because it does not contain any tagged component, whereas

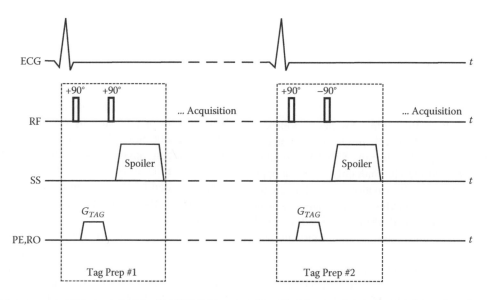

FIGURE 11.4   Pulse sequence diagram of original CSPAMM tagging. Note the change of the polarity of the second tagging RF pulse in the second cardiac cycle. ECG, electrocardiogram; PE, phase encoding; RO, readout; SS, slice selection.

the tagging information is preserved if TAG_A and TAG_B are appropriately chosen. The tagging amplitude is maximized if

$$TAG_A = -TAG_B. \qquad (11.9)$$

In this case, the tagged image will be

$$A_k - B_k \propto 2Q_{Tk}. \qquad (11.10)$$

From a sequence standpoint, such complementary tagging patterns can be fairly easily obtained using two 90° RF pulses interspersed by a gradient that is responsible for modulating the magnetization. By executing the tagging module twice, once with a 90°/90° tagging RF pulse pair and once with a 90°/–90° counterpart, a complementary magnetization modulation is ensured, and the earlier condition is fulfilled. Figure 11.5 shows k-space of CSPAMM and SPAMM tagging. While the earlier considerations mostly provide insight into the tagging part of the technique, they are also closely linked with the imaging part as can be seen in Equation 11.8, which clearly suggests that the tagged signal is affected not only by T_1 recovery but also by the RF excitations of the imaging sequence. In more general terms, the more RF excitations or the higher RF excitation angles, the more the tagged signal

is reduced. Therefore, the choice of an appropriate imaging sequence is crucially important.

11.3.3 Data Acquisition

11.3.3.1 Imaging Sequence and Breath-Hold Time

At the time of original CSPAMM implementation, segmented k-space gradient echo sequences with multiple RF excitations per k-space segment were not readily available, making the choice of the imaging part of the sequence fairly easy. However, on contemporary MRI systems, the appropriate selection of the imaging sequence is important. In the original CSPAMM paper, a simple gradient echo signal readout, in which one k-space line is acquired per RF excitation, was implemented. Considering that two acquisitions are required for CSPAMM, then for a scan matrix of 128 k-space lines, this led to an acquisition time of 2 × 128 RR intervals (cardiac cycles), or more than 4 minutes. Of course, a 4 minute single breath-hold scan is not practical, and so several workarounds were proposed. One of these workarounds included the use of a repetitive breath-hold scheme, where the imaged subjects were asked to breathe in, breathe out, and then hold their breath for 1 second while image data were collected. This was repeated every 4 seconds, which led to an imaging time of more than 10 minutes per slice.

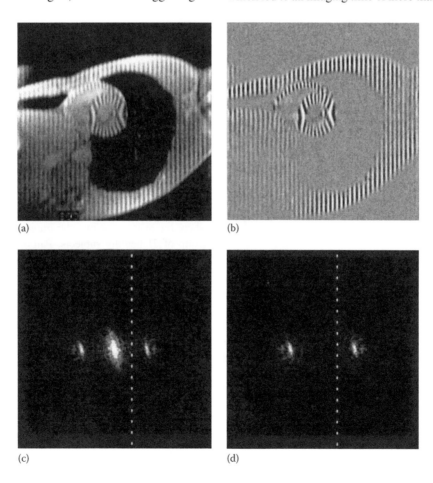

(a)   (b)

(c)   (d)

FIGURE 11.5 (a, c) SPAMM and (b, d) CSPAMM (a, b) images and (c, d) their k-spaces. In contrast to SPAMM, the DC (nonmodulated) signal peak at the k-space center is eliminated in CSPAMM due to the subtraction of two complementary SPAMM images. (Reproduced from Kuijer, J.P. et al., *Magn. Reson. Med.*, 46(5), 993, 2001. With permission.)

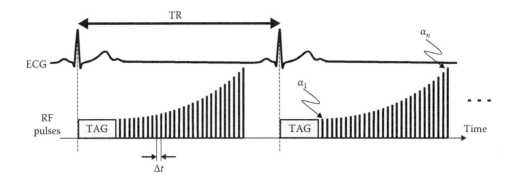

FIGURE 11.6   Ramped imaging flip angles through the cardiac cycle to compensate for tags fading.

11.3.3.2 Ramped Flip Angle

The RF excitation angles must be optimized to satisfy two major boundary conditions: (1) the tagging signal should be constant throughout the entire cardiac cycle (or for each RF excitation during one RR interval); (2) under these constraints, the tagging signal should be maximized. The signal intensity I_{Tk} for the kth RF excitation, which can be described by

$$I_{Tk} \propto M_{ss} TAG(x,y) e^{-t_k/T_1} \left[\prod_{j=1}^{k-1} \cos\alpha_j \right] \sin\alpha_k, \quad (11.11)$$

then needs to satisfy the condition

$$I_{Tk} = I_{Tk-1} \qquad (11.12)$$

to achieve a constant tagging signal intensity. This leads to a series of ramped RF excitation angles $\alpha_1 ... \alpha_n$ (Figure 11.6) that is recursively calculated as

$$\alpha_{k-1} = \tan^{-1}\left[\sin\alpha_k \right] e^{-\Delta t/T_1}. \qquad (11.13)$$

11.3.3.3 Flip Angle Optimization

With an appropriate choice of α_n, I_{Tk} can be maximized. For the aforementioned repetitive breathing pattern, where imaging is only performed every fourth RR interval, an $\alpha_n = 90°$ was used to optimize the signal. However, with more advanced acquisition schemes, where more data are collected in each RR interval, α_n needs to be optimized. This can be done by numerical simulation, in which α_n is gradually changed. The RF excitation series $\alpha_1 ... \alpha_{n-1}$ is determined backwardly according to Equation 11.13, and the resulting signal intensity is then calculated using Equation 11.11. The results can then be plotted graphically and the optimal α_n is determined. As mentioned earlier, this directly relates to the optimal choice of the imaging sequence.

From Equation 11.11, it is evident that fewer excitations lead to a higher signal intensity. This means that the original implementation of CSPAMM, where one single line of k-space is acquired per cine frame and per RR interval, is optimal in terms of signal efficiency, at the expense of scanning time. It is also possible to use a more time-efficient method to cover the k-space (e.g., through the use of EPI [Stuber et al. 1999c] or spiral imaging [Ryf et al. 2004]) while keeping the number of RF excitations unchanged, as will be explained later in the chapter.

11.4 SLICE-FOLLOWING CSPAMM

11.4.1 Tissue Through-Plane Motion

During systole, the heart undergoes longitudinal contraction, in which the base moves toward the apex, before returning back to its original position during diastole (Figure 11.7).

In their study, Rogers et al. (1991) showed that during systole, the LV base, midventricle, and apex move by average displacements of 12.8, 6.9, and 1.6 mm, respectively. This leads to through-plane motion effects on SAX cine images, which are perpendicular to the LAX direction. As a result, the same myocardial tissue is not always visualized in consecutive cine frames. This is accentuated in more basal anatomical levels, where the atria move into the image plane during systole. In a group of 21 healthy subjects, Pattynama et al. (1992) showed that through-plane motion led to systemic underestimation of true myocardial contraction by an average of 16% and 21% at the base and midventricular levels, respectively. While this may be acceptable under certain circumstances, it means that regional tissue characteristics can no longer be reliably characterized and quantified. Therefore, a technique is required that allows for tracking the same tissue during the whole cardiac cycle.

11.4.2 Slice Isolation

One early approach to resolve the heart through-plane motion effect was proposed by Rogers et al. (1991), who developed the *slice isolation* technique. The technique is based on isolating the tissue SAX slice of interest by suppressing the signals from the above and below SAX slices using selective saturation RF pulses applied at end-diastole. A thick imaging plane (thicker than the slice of interest) is then prescribed

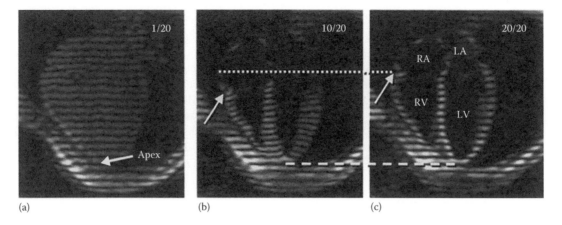

FIGURE 11.7 Longitudinal shortening of the heart during the cardiac cycle. Four-chamber tagged images at (a) end-diastole, (b) systole, and (c) diastole, showing the base movement toward the apex during systole (dotted line and arrows). The apex remains almost at the same position during the cardiac cycle (dashed line). The frame number in the cardiac cycle (out of 20 total frames) is shown on the top-right corner of each image. (Reproduced from Stuber, M. et al., *MAGMA*, 9(1–2), 85, 1999c. With permission.)

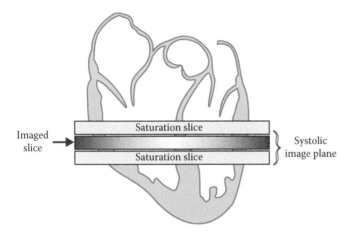

FIGURE 11.8 Slice isolation technique. The magnetization is saturated in two parallel slices adjacent to the imaged slice. The imaging plane is adjusted to include the imaged slice and one of the saturation slices during systole. (Courtesy of Dr. Tamer Basha, Harvard University, Cambridge, MA.)

at end-systole to accommodate the slice displacement in the LAX direction during the cardiac cycle (Figure 11.8).

11.4.3 SLICE FOLLOWING

11.4.3.1 Pulse Sequence

Another alternative of *true myocardial motion tracking* (Figure 11.9) was proposed by Stefan Fischer et al. (1994), which critically builds on the CSPAMM work described earlier. Compared with the slice isolation technique, slice-following CSPAMM does not require any presaturation RF pulses. Therefore, it can be applied in combination with cine imaging. Further, no tissue-dependent optimization is necessary for tissue saturation.

11.4.3.2 Signal Analysis

In a given slice of thickness Δz, the longitudinal magnetization immediately after tagging implementation ($t = 0$) is

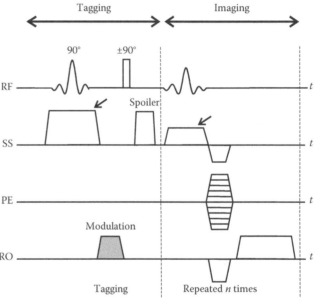

FIGURE 11.9 Slice-following CSPAMM. The sign of the second tagging RF pulse is reversed in the second acquisition. Note the difference in the gradient magnitude (arrows) between tagging and data acquisition, which affects the slice thickness.

given by (the second in-plane dimension, y, is ignored in the following equations for simplicity)

$$M_z(x,z,t=0)=M_{ss}(x,z)TAG(x,z) \quad \text{for } -\Delta z/2 \le z \le \Delta z/2,$$
$$M_z(x,z)=M_{V0}(x,z) \quad \text{for non-tagged magnetization}$$
$$\text{outside the tagged slice.} \quad (11.14)$$

This initial tagged slice will move during the cardiac cycle as described earlier. If, however, the imaged slice is thicker that the tagged slice ($\Delta s > \Delta z$) and encompasses this tagged slice at all times (Figure 11.10), then the signal derived from the entire volume with thickness $\Delta s = a_u - a_l$ can be decomposed into different parts as described earlier in the CSPAMM paragraph. However, because the imaged volume is larger than the tagged volume, the

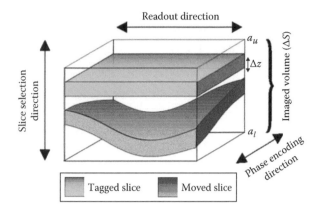

FIGURE 11.10 Graphical description of the slice-following principle. The originally thin tagged slice (shown in green) moves during the cardiac cycle in the slice-selection direction to a new position (shown in purple). A thick slab is imaged to ensure imaging the same tagged slice during the whole cardiac cycle.

signal outside the tagged slice (both above and below), m_{Vk}, substantially contributes to the signal in the imaged slice.

With Q_k being the tagged part of the magnetization and m_{Rk} the relaxing component in the tagged slice (see Q_R defined earlier in the chapter), the acquired signal I_k for a given RF excitation angle α_k can be written as

$$I_k(x) \propto \sin(\alpha_k)\left\{ m_{Rk} + m_{Vk} + \int_{a_l}^{a_u} Q_k(x,z)dz \right\}. \quad (11.15)$$

Note that because the integration in Equation 11.15 is over the thicker imaged slice, then signal from the whole thin tagged slice is always captured despite slice displacement in the through-plane direction. Very similar to the CSPAMM idea mentioned earlier, the unwanted components m_{Rk} and m_{Vk} can be eliminated by subtracting two different images with the signals I_{Ak} and I_{Bk}, for which the periodic tagging pattern has been shifted by 180° (e.g., sin and −sin patterns). The resultant signal will then be

$$I_{Ak}(x) - I_{Bk}(x) \propto 2\sin(\alpha_k)\int_{a_l}^{a_u} Q_k(x,z)dz. \quad (11.16)$$

11.4.3.3 Technical Considerations

As the value in each pixel is proportional to the integral in the z direction, the resultant image is a projection of the shifted and deformed tagged slice onto the x–y plane. As a result, not only is the tag persistence prolonged because of the CSPAMM principle, but also the same tissue will always be visualized in different cine frames. Therefore, the through-plane motion effects are completely avoided. Further, slice-following CSPAMM improves the tagging contrast throughout the whole cardiac cycle because not only the signal from the nontagged tissue is suppressed, but also the signal from the relaxed component of the tagged tissue. However, both CSPAMM and slice-following come at the cost of extra scanning time, which also include disadvantages intrinsic to images subtraction, such as coregistration problems. Nevertheless, with more advanced signal readout strategies, slice-following CSPAMM images with high spatial and temporal resolution can now be easily acquired during a short period of sustained respiration. Another point to be noted is that increasing the width of the imaging slice results in increasing the noise contribution from the nontagged tissues above and below the tagged slice; therefore, the imaging slice thickness should be carefully selected to avoid the through-plane motion effect while maintaining an adequate SNR.

11.4.3.4 Clinical Implementation

Feliciano et al. (2013) from Matthias Stuber's group have recently implemented SSFP CSPAMM for quantitative comparison of strain with and without slice following at different anatomical levels of the heart. The results confirmed the existence of significant differences in quantitative SAX rotation and strain between slice-following and non-slice-following CSPAMM acquisitions (Figure 11.11). Specifically, significant strain underestimation and rotation overestimation at the basal level as well as rotation underestimation at the apical level have been observed during early diastole when through-plane motion was not accounted for using a non-slice-following sequence.

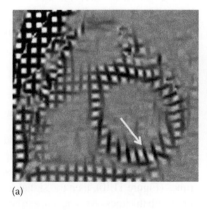
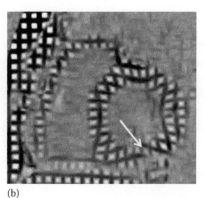

(a)   (b)

FIGURE 11.11 Slice displacement effect on the imaged slice. Significant anatomical difference (arrows) of the imaged basal short-axis slice at end systole (a) without and (b) with the implementation of the slice-following technique with CSPAMM.

11.5 FAST IMAGING WITH CSPAMM

11.5.1 ECHO PLANAR IMAGING

Applications using CSPAMM-like techniques have continued to proliferate—a testament to its utility. In 1999, Stuber et al. (1999c) proposed a segmented EPI slice-following CSPAMM for myocardial tagging (Figure 11.12). Used with an optimized RF excitation scheme (Figure 11.13), this technique enabled the acquisition of as many as 20 systolic and diastolic grid-tagged images per cardiac cycle (Figure 11.14). The developed technique helped reduce scan time from several minutes to about 12 seconds per anatomical level, which allowed for acquiring the images of all cardiac phases for a certain anatomical slice in a single breath-hold; thus avoiding multiple breath-hold acquisitions with

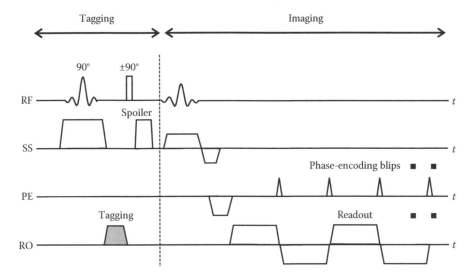

FIGURE 11.12 CSPAMM with echo planar imaging (EPI). The parts of the sequence to the left and right of the vertical dashed line represent magnetization preparation and data acquisition, respectively.

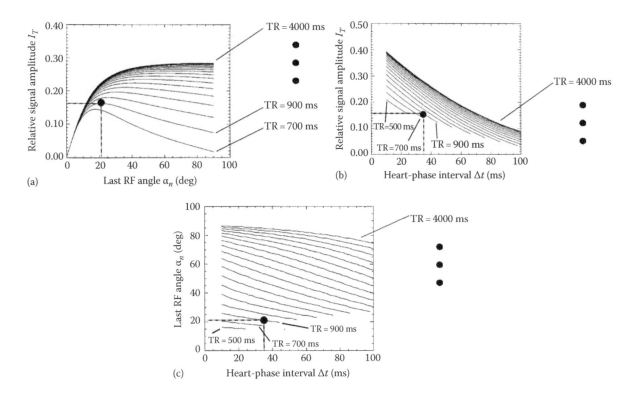

FIGURE 11.13 CSPAMM signal optimization for 20 heart-phase images. (a) Relative signal amplitude derived from the tagged component of the magnetization. The relative signal amplitude is plotted as function of the angle of the last imaging RF pulse (α_n). The data are plotted for a fixed heart-phase interval $\Delta t = 35$ ms taking multiple repetition times (TR) into account. The black dot indicates maximum signal intensity for TR of 900 ms. Maximum signal intensity is ensured if $\alpha_n = 21°$. (b) Maximum relative signal amplitude that can be obtained by an optimized α_n, plotted as a function of Δt and TR. (c) Optimized α_n as a function of Δt and TR. (Reproduced from Stuber, M. et al., *MAGMA*, 9(1–2), 85, 1999c. With permission.)

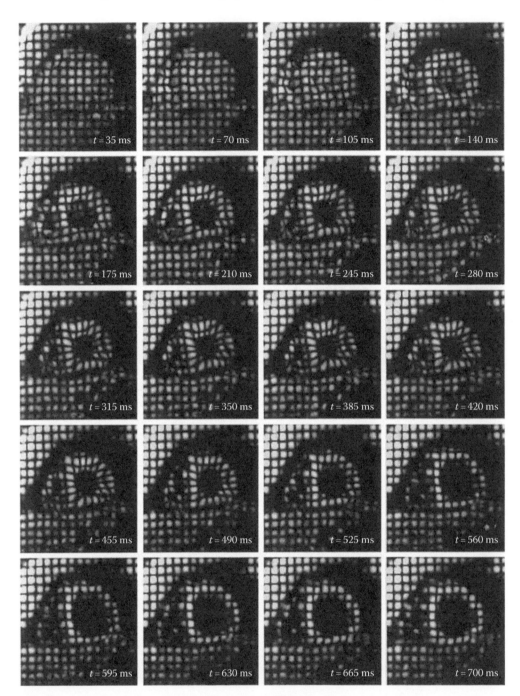

FIGURE 11.14   Twenty phases of the cardiac cycle imaged in an apical short-axis plane of the myocardium. The images are acquired using single breath-hold slice-following CSPAMM myocardial tagging. The acquisition duration = 12 cardiac cycles. The heart-phase interval (temporal resolution) = 35 ms and heart rate = 70 beats/min. (Reproduced from Stuber, M. et al., *MAGMA*, 9(1–2), 85, 1999c. With permission.)

associated sensitivity to artifacts from poor patient compliance or inconsistent depths of end-expiratory breath-holds. Nevertheless, it should be noted that EPI imaging may be susceptible to off-resonance artifacts, and the need for a lengthy echo time (TE) creates the risk of subsequent motion or flow artifacts.

11.5.2   Modified Turbo Field EPI

A modified Turbo Field EPI sequence has been combined with CSPAMM to optimize the scan time and image quality for stress studies (Ryf et al. 2005) (Figure 11.15). The developed sequence included two modifications: (1) introducing a dummy RR interval before data acquisition to avoid measurements before the magnetization reaches the steady-state condition (non-steady-state measurements result in alternating tagline intensity in the final CSPAMM image), and (2) acquiring the EPI reference data in a separate breath-hold before actual data acquisition to reduce scan time and avoid disturbing the steady-state condition. The developed sequence has short scan time and good image quality.

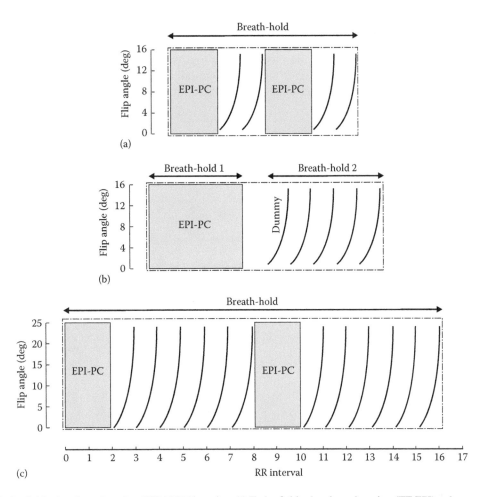

FIGURE 11.15 Turbo field echo planar imaging CSPAMM imaging. (a) Turbo field echo planar imaging (TF-EPI) pulse sequence. (b) Modified TF-EPI sequence. (c) EPI sequence. In order to achieve a constant tagging contrast, the excitation flip angles are ramped. In the modified TF-EPI sequence, EPI-phase correction (EPI-PC) is performed in a separate breath-hold before image acquisition, and a dummy image acquisition, is performed in order to achieve better steady state. This leads to two breath-holds of 4 and 5 RR intervals, respectively. In the (a) TF-EPI and (c) EPI sequences, imaging is intercepted with the EPI-PC. (Reproduced from Ryf, S. et al., *J. Cardiovasc. Magn. Reson.*, 7(4), 693, 2005.)

11.5.3 SPIRAL IMAGING

Spiral imaging provides a very powerful alternative to EPI imaging for signal readout of the tagged myocardium (Figure 11.16). First, spiral imaging provides time-efficient k-space coverage. As a small number of excitation RF pulses are needed, the tagging pattern persists longer, leading to improved tagging contrast (Taylor et al. 2000, Bornert et al. 2001). Second, a short TE is easily obtained, causing flow or motion artifacts to be minimized (Meyer et al. 1992). Third, spiral imaging can be easily combined

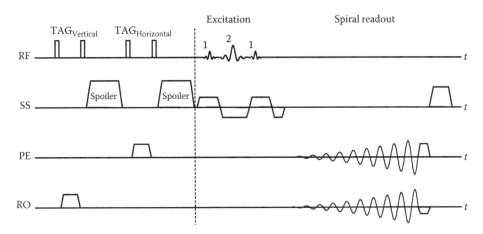

FIGURE 11.16 Grid-tagged CSPAMM with spiral acquisition and spectral–spatial excitation for fat suppression.

with spectral–spatial excitations (Figure 11.16), which leads to an intrinsic fat saturation for each single cine frame. It is also possible to efficiently cover the k-space signal readout in a short amount of time, leading to imaging at a very high temporal resolution (Ryf et al. 2004,

Rutz et al. 2008). Ryf et al. (2004) combined CSPAMM with interleaved spiral imaging, which allowed for acquiring high spatial resolution (4 mm tag separation) or high temporal resolution (77 frames per second) grid-tagged images in a single breath-hold (Figure 11.17).

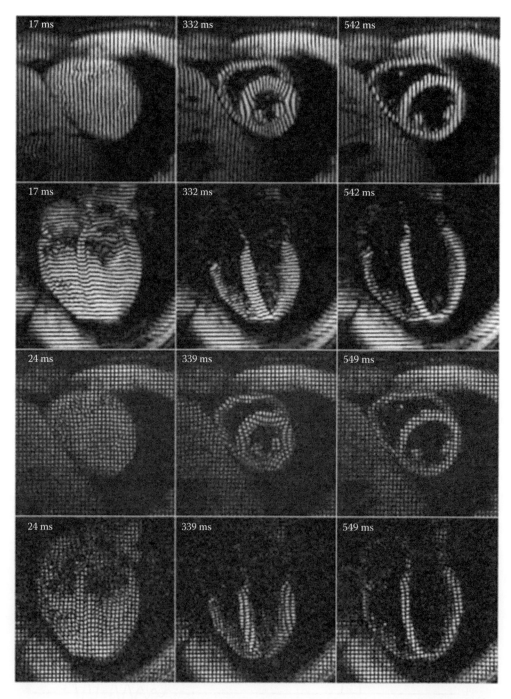

FIGURE 11.17 Midventricular spiral CSPAMM short-axis and long-axis images of line-tagged and grid-tagged myocardium in a healthy subject. The tagline distance is 4 mm and the temporal resolution is 35 ms. The time after the R-wave is indicated on the images. On the grid-tagged, short-axis view, ~50 tagline intersections can be observed. (Reproduced from Ryf, S. et al., *Magn. Reson. Med.*, 51(2), 237, 2004. With permission.)

11.6 CSPAMM WITH SSFP

11.6.1 IMAGING START-UP TECHNIQUES

An SSFP CSPAMM variant has been presented by Zwanenburg et al. (2003). In this approach, the steady-state magnetization is stored in the longitudinal direction using an $\alpha/2$ flip-back RF pulse immediately prior to tagging preparation. Imaging proceeds normally, although excitation is achieved using a series of the linearly increasing start-up angles (LISA) technique (Figure 11.18). Compared to the $\alpha/2$ start-up method (Deimling and Heid 1994), LISA eliminates the artifacts originating from the regions with opposed-phase spins, such as in subcutaneous fat. Compared to spoiled gradient echo (SPGR), LISA-SSFP is twice as fast, with slightly better contrast-to-noise ratio (CNR). Tags also persist longer with LISA-SSFP than with SPGR imaging. As a result, the CSPAMM images could be acquired using SSFP in a single breath-hold.

11.6.2 RAMPED FLIP ANGLES

Ibrahim et al. (2006, Ibrahim and Osman 2004) developed a technique for improving the myocardial tagging contrast in balanced SSFP cine images by optimizing the RF excitation angles to compensate for tags fading during the cardiac cycle. The flip angles are recursively calculated as follows:

$$\alpha_n = \beta_n + \beta_{n-1}; \quad n = 1, 2, \ldots, \tag{11.17}$$

where

$$\beta_0 = \frac{\alpha}{2}, \tag{11.18}$$

$$\beta_n = \sin^{-1}\left(\frac{\sin(\beta_{n-1})}{E_1 \cos^2(\beta_{n-1}) + E_2 \sin^2(\beta_{n-1})}\right), \tag{11.19}$$

α is the first flip angle, $E_1 = e^{-TR/T_1}$, and $E_2 = e^{-TR/T_2}$. In the previous equations, the first flip angle is numerically optimized (in a backward recursive fashion) to maximize SNR throughout the cardiac cycle. The developed ramped flip angle technique led to improving the tagging contrast in SSFP CSPAMM-tagged images. The resulting tagging contrast remained constant during the entire cardiac cycle, approximately doubling that obtained with SPGR (Figures 11.19 and 11.20).

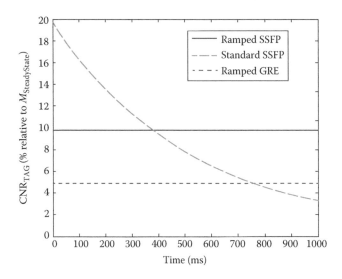

FIGURE 11.19 Numerical simulation of the tagging contrast-to-noise ratio (Tag-CNR) with and without ramped flip angle in steady state with free precession (SSFP) CSPAMM imaging. The following imaging parameters are used: $T_1 = 870$ ms, $T_2 = 55$ ms, TR = 3 ms, TE = TR/2, and RR = 1000 ms. For standard SSFP, the optimum angle = 28°. For the ramped flip angle, the optimal last flip angle = 50°. In standard SSFP, the Tag-CNR decays exponentially with time. However, with the ramped flip angle technique, the Tag-CNR is made constant throughout the whole TRR, with considerable improvement during the late cardiac phases. The constant Tag-CNR obtained with ramped flip angle spoiled gradient echo (SPGR) is shown for reference (the last flip angle = 15°). The Tag-CNR achieved with SPGR is about half of that with SSFP.

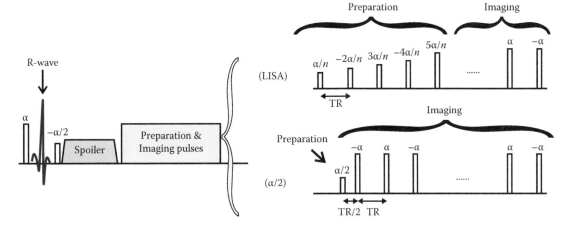

FIGURE 11.18 Steady state with free precession (SSFP) linearly increasing start-up angles (LISA) and $\alpha/2$ magnetization preparation techniques. For either technique, the magnetization is stored in the longitudinal direction after detection of the electrocardiogram R-wave. The remaining transverse magnetization is then spoiled, followed by tagging preparation and image acquisition. (Courtesy of Dr. Tamer Basha, Harvard University, Cambridge, MA.)

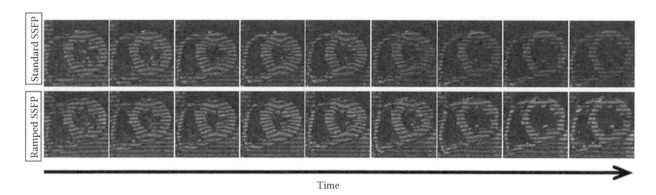

Time

FIGURE 11.20 In vivo results of ramped flip angle steady state with free precession (SSFP) CSPAMM. The first and second rows show standard SSFP and ramped SSFP sequences, respectively. The images are acquired through a 650 ms cardiac cycle. The following imaging parameters are used: $T_1 = 870$ ms, $T_2 = 55$ ms, TR = 3 ms, and TE = TR/2. For standard SSFP, the optimum angle = 28°. For ramped SSFP, the last flip angle = 50°. The figure shows an improved tagging contrast with ramped SSFP compared to standard SSFP, especially during the late phases. With ramped SSFP, the tagging contrast is kept almost constant during the whole cardiac cycle. (Reproduced from Ibrahim, El-S.H. et al., *J. Magn. Reson. Imaging*, 24(5), 1159, 2006. With permission.)

11.7 MAGNITUDE AND REAL-PART CSPAMM RECONSTRUCTION

11.7.1 Magnitude Reconstruction

11.7.1.1 Signal Analysis

The magnitude image CSPAMM reconstruction (MICSR) technique has been developed for improving CSPAMM tagging contrast and persistence (NessAiver and Prince 2003a). By reconstructing only magnitude images, MICSR yields tags with zero mean sinusoidal profiles, which obviates the need for acquiring phase calibration data or applying phase correction algorithms. Let A and B represent the first and second series of images obtained with CSPAMM using +90°/+90° and +90°/−90° tagging pulses, respectively. The signal intensity of CSPAMM, magnitude CSPAMM (|CSPAMM|), and MICSR are then represented as

$$\begin{aligned} \text{CSPAMM} &= A - B = 2M_{ss}\, e^{-t/T_1}\cos(2\pi x/P),\\ |\text{CSPAMM}| &= |A - B| = |\, 2M_{ss}\, e^{-t/T_1}\cos(2\pi x/P)\,|,\\ \text{MICSR} &= |A|^2 - |B|^2 = 4M_{ss}^2(1 - e^{-t/T_1})\, e^{-t/T_1}\cos(2\pi x/P),\end{aligned}$$

$$(11.20)$$

where P is the spatial period of the tagging pattern, and the corresponding contrast behaviors are represented as (Figures 11.21 and 11.22)

$$\begin{aligned} \text{Contrast CSPAMM} &= 4M_{ss}e^{-t/T_1},\\ \text{Contrast}\,|\text{CSPAMM}| &= 2M_{ss}e^{-t/T_1},\\ \text{Contrast MICSR} &= 8M_{ss}^2(1 - e^{-t/T_1})e^{-t/T_1}.\end{aligned}$$

$$(11.21)$$

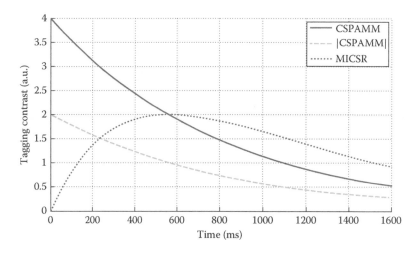

FIGURE 11.21 Tagging contrast in CSPAMM, |CSPAMM|, and magnitude image CSPAMM reconstruction (MICSR). The curves are generated based on Equation 11.21 using $M_0 = 1$ and $T_1 = 800$ ms.

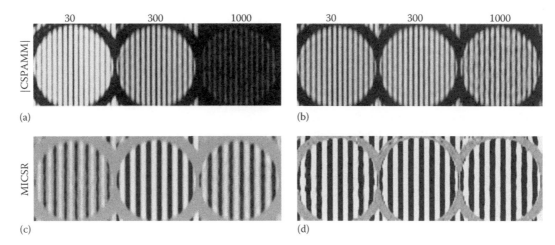

FIGURE 11.22 Magnitude image CSPAMM reconstruction (MICSR) and |CSPAMM| images of a cylinderical phantom with $T_1 = 800$ ms at trigger delays of 30, 300, and 1000 ms. (a) |CSPAMM| images with constant window and level settings demonstrating the change in contrast over time. (b) |CSPAMM| images with the window and level values set differently for each image. (c) MICSR images with a broad threshold ε (see Equation 11.22). (d) MICSR images with narrow ε. (Reproduced from NessAiver, M. and Prince, J.L., *Magn. Reson. Med.*, 50(2), 331, 2003a. With permission.)

11.7.1.2 Optimized Display

Based on the MICSR technique, NessAvier and Prince (2003a,b) developed a method for trinary display of the resulting images, presented by

$$\text{Trinary map} = \begin{cases} +1, & \text{MICSR} \geq \varepsilon \\ \dfrac{\text{MICSR}}{\varepsilon}, & |\text{MICSR}| < \varepsilon \ , \\ -1, & \text{MICSR} \leq -\varepsilon \end{cases} \quad (11.22)$$

which emphasized the tagging persistence and presented a novel way for visualizing myocardial deformation (Figure 11.23).

MICSR showed to have the following advantages: (1) true sinusoidal tagging profile is created as opposed to rectified sinusoids; (2) peak MICSR contrast and CNR are obtained between 200 and 500 ms after the R-wave, corresponding to the period in the cardiac cycle with the largest myocardial deformation (late systole to early diastole); (3) the tagging contrast is higher and persists for a longer

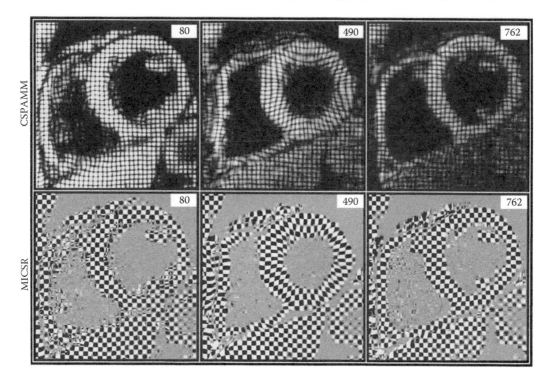

FIGURE 11.23 Representative in vivo CSPAMM and magnitude image CSPAMM reconstruction (images with optimized visualization. Trigger delays of 80, 490, and 762 ms correspond to early-systole, early-diastole, and late-diastole, respectively. (Reproduced from NessAiver, M. and Prince, J.L., *Magn. Reson. Med.*, 50(2), 331, 2003a. With permission.)

period of time than in CSPAMM; and (4) the images are optimized for processing with harmonic phase (HARP) analysis (Osman et al. 1999).

11.7.2 REAL-PART RECONSTRUCTION

Kuijer et al. (2005) presented a technique for improving tagging CNR without increasing the scan time through real-part data reconstruction using an internal phase reference from the tagged images. A simple model of CSPAMM imaging was implemented based on the subtraction of two SPAMM-tagged images I_+ and I_- with inverted tag phases

$$I_+ = (1-b) + b\cos(kx),$$
$$I_- = (1-b) - b\cos(kx), \qquad (11.23)$$
$$I_{CSPAMM} = I_+ - I_- = 2b\cos(kx),$$

where b is the normalized tagging modulation depth, which is related to the total tagging excitation angle α by

$$\alpha = 2\sin^{-1}\left(\sqrt{b}\right). \qquad (11.24)$$

Nevertheless, if we add, instead of subtracting, the two SPAMM images, a phase reference image free of the tagging modulation can be generated

$$I_{sum} = I_+ + I_- = 2(1-b). \qquad (11.25)$$

Choosing $\alpha = 140°$ ($b = 0.88$) results in an artifact-free image with improved tagging contrast. The CNR efficiency of the proposed technique is similar to that of real-part reconstruction with a separate reference scan. However, compared to magnitude image subtraction ($b = 0.5$), the CNR is improved by 70% without increasing the scan time.

11.8 OFF-RESONANCE EFFECTS IN CSPAMM

11.8.1 INHERENT FAT CANCELLATION

11.8.1.1 Pulse Sequence

An efficient fat suppression method (inherent fat cancellation [IFC]) has been developed for CSPAMM imaging (Fahmy et al. 2009), as shown in Figure 11.24. The IFC method makes benefit of the two acquisitions required for CSPAMM imaging by allowing for complementary and in-phase modulations of the water and fat spins, respectively; therefore, in the final CSPAMM image, the tagging contrast of water is increased, while the tagging signal from fat is cancelled. Compared to the spectral–spatial selective pulses (SSSP) fat suppression technique (Delfaut et al. 1999), the IFC method provides fat-suppressed CSPAMM images with high temporal resolution and short TE without increasing the scan time.

11.8.1.2 Signal Analysis

To illustrate the idea of IFC, a SPAMM-tagged image can be written in terms of its different signal peaks in the k-space (Osman et al. 2001)

$$I_{SPAMM}(k) = F^w(k) + F^w(k-k_0)e^{i\theta} + F^w(k+k_0)e^{-i\theta}, \quad (11.26)$$

where

$F(.)$ represents the voxel signal in the k-space
k_0 is the first harmonic frequency
θ is the phase that the magnetization gains during the tagging sequence

Conventional CSPAMM (Figure 11.24a) is based on acquiring and subtracting two SPAMM images that have 180° phase difference (assuming zero phase accumulation)

$$I_{CSPAMM}(k) = 2\left[F^w(k-k_0) + F^w(k+k_0)\right]. \quad (11.27)$$

For a voxel that contains both water and fat contents, the two acquired SPAMM images can be written as

$$I_{SPAMM1}(k) = F^w(k) + F^w(k-k_0) + F^w(k+k_0)$$
$$+ F^f(k) + F^f(k-k_0)e^{i\phi_{cs}} + F^f(k+k_0)e^{-i\phi_{cs}} \quad (11.28)$$

and

$$I_{SPAMM2}(k) = F^w(k) + F^w(k-k_0)e^{i\pi} + F^w(k+k_0)e^{-i\pi}$$
$$+ F^f(k) + F^f(k-k_0)e^{i(\pi+\phi_{cs})} + F^f(k+k_0)e^{-i(\pi+\phi_{cs})}, \quad (11.29)$$

where the first and second images have $\theta = 0°$ and $\theta = 180°$, respectively, and ϕ_{cs} is the phase accrual that develops during the tagging interval t_{tag} due to the chemical shift (resonance frequency difference) between fat and water, given by

$$\phi_{cs} = \gamma B_0 \sigma_{cs} t_{tag}, \qquad (11.30)$$

where

B_0 is the main magnetic field strength
γ is the gyromagnetic ratio
σ_{cs} (= 3.5 ppm) is the water-fat chemical shift

The IFC method is based on reversing the polarity of the tagging gradient in the second SPAMM image (Figure 11.24b), which results in exchanging the location of the tagging components in the k-space; thus, the second SPAMM image is represented as

$$I_{SPAMM2}(k) = F^w(k) + F^w(k+k_0)e^{i\pi} + F^w(k-k_0)e^{-i\pi}$$
$$+ F^f(k) + F^f(k+k_0)e^{i(\pi+\phi_{cs})} + F^f(k-k_0)e^{-i(\pi+\phi_{cs})}, \quad (11.31)$$

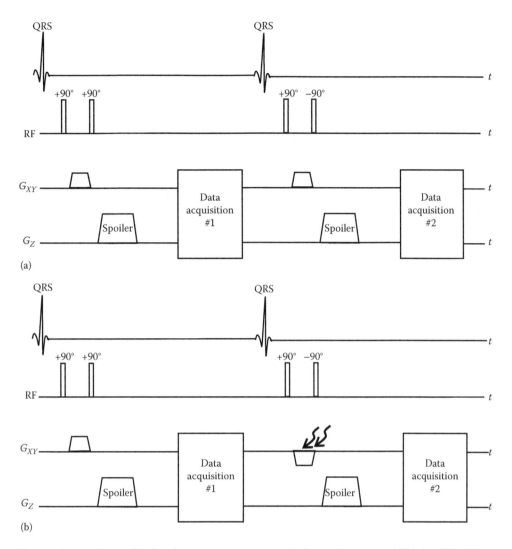

FIGURE 11.24 Inherent fat cancelation (IFC) pulse sequence diagram. (a) Conventional CSPAMM. (b) CSPAMM with IFC, which is similar to the sequence of (a), except for reversing the polarity of the tagging gradient in the second image (arrows) and adjusting the time duration between the two excitation RF pulses, as described in the text.

and therefore the resulting CSPAMM image (obtained by subtracting the two SPAMM images) becomes

$$I_{CSPAMM}(k) = 2\left[F^w(k+k_0)+F^w(k-k_0)\right]$$
$$+ 2\left[F^f(k+k_0)+F^f(k-k_0)\right]\cos(\phi_{cs}), \quad (11.32)$$

in which the fat signal can be suppressed by setting, $\phi_{cs} = \pi/2$ which is achieved by properly modifying the tagging interval t_{tag} in Equation 11.30.

11.8.1.3 In Vivo Results

The IFC technique results in fat-suppressed CSPAMM images (Figure 11.25), while reducing TE (compared to SSSP) from 5 to 1.2 ms and from 2.66 to 0.85 ms at 1.5 and 3.0 T, respectively.

11.8.2 ORI-CSPAMM

Recently, CSPAMM has been combined with Fourier analysis of stimulated echoes (FAST) for quantification of LV systolic and diastolic function (Reyhan and Ennis 2013). The advantage of using CSPAMM is that it provides more easily detectable harmonic peaks later into the cardiac cycle. The developed technique requires a short scan time and provides quantitative assessment of systolic and diastolic LV twist, torsion, twisting rates, time-to-peak twist, duration of untwisting, and ratio of rapid untwist to peak twist.

11.8.2.1 Pulse Sequence

A modified version of CSPAMM, called off-resonance insensitive CSPAMM (ORI-CSPAMM) as shown in Figure 11.26, has been developed and combined with FAST (Reyhan et al. 2014).

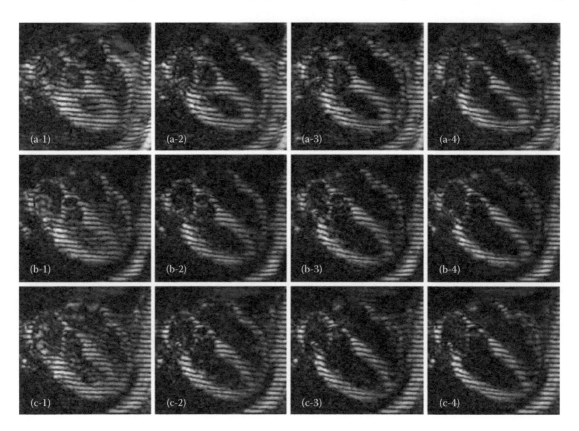

FIGURE 11.25   In vivo CSPAMM images with inherent fat cancelation (IFC) fat suppression. Four-chamber CSPAMM images of a human volunteer's heart acquired on a 3.0 T scanner (a) without fat suppression, (b) using spectral–spatial selective pulses (SSSP) fat suppression, and (c) using IFC fat suppression. (Reproduced from Fahmy, A.S. et al., *Magn. Reson. Med.*, 61(1), 234, 2009. With permission.)

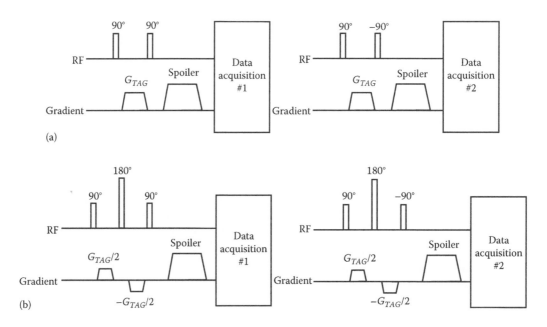

FIGURE 11.26   Off-resonance insensitive CSPAMM (ORI-CSPAMM) pulse sequence. (a) Conventional CSPAMM pulse sequence diagram. (b) ORI-CSPAMM pulse sequence diagram, where the tagging gradient has been divided in two small gradients, separated by a 180° refocusing RF pulse that corrects for off-resonance effects.

11.8.2.2 Signal Analysis

In conventional SPAMM (Figure 11.26a), the phase θ accumulated by the isochromats at position r in the presence of both a magnetic field gradient G and an off-resonant field B_{off} is

$$\theta(r) = \gamma\left(\int_0^\tau \left(G(t) \cdot r + B_{off}(r)\right) dt\right), \qquad (11.33)$$

where
γ is the gyromagnetic ratio
τ is the gradient duration

If the spins are stationary during the time of integration δ, and the off-resonance field is stable in time, then

$$\theta(r) = \gamma\left(M_0 \cdot r + B_{off}(r) \cdot \tau\right), \qquad (11.34)$$

which indicates that the tagging pattern induced by the applied gradient will be spatially shifted in off-resonant tissues, such as fat, relative to on-resonance water.

ORI-SPAMM (Figure 11.26b) is based on refocusing the off-resonance effects by splitting the motion-encoding gradient in half, inserting a hard 180° refocusing pulse in between the two gradients, and inverting the second half of the motion-encoding gradient. The accumulated signal phase immediately before the refocusing pulse is

$$\theta_1(r) = \gamma\left(\frac{M_0}{2} \cdot r + B_{off}(r) \cdot \tau\right). \qquad (11.35)$$

After the application of the refocusing pulse, the sign in Equation 11.35 is reversed. Therefore, the phase accumulated during the interval after the refocusing pulse is

$$\theta_2(r) = \gamma\left(-\frac{M_0}{2} \cdot r + B_{off}(r) \cdot \tau\right). \qquad (11.36)$$

Therefore, the cumulative phase after the spilt refocused motion-encoding gradient is insensitive to off-resonance

$$\theta(r) = -\theta_1(r) + \theta_2(r) = -\gamma\left(M_0 \cdot r\right), \qquad (11.37)$$

which results in that the off-resonance effects during the interval of motion encoding are fully compensated.

11.8.2.3 Phantom and In Vivo Results

ORI-CSPAMM images are shown in Figure 11.27. Similar to the FAST+CSPAMM technique, FAST+ORI-CSPAMM provides an automated method for quantitative assessment

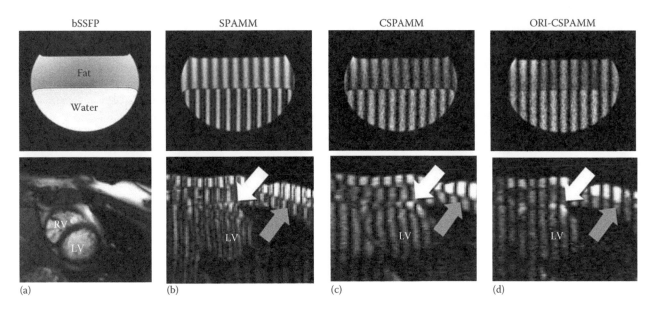

FIGURE 11.27 Off-resonance insensitive CSPAMM (ORI-CSPAMM) images collected from a fat–water phantom and a healthy volunteer. (a) Demonstration of phantom setup and in vivo anatomy. (b) Chemical shift is apparent between water and fat (phantom), between epicardial fat and myocardium (white arrow), and between chest wall fat and muscle (gray arrow) (in vivo) when using conventional 1-1 SPAMM tagging preparation. (c) Chemical shift is apparent between water and fat (phantom), between epicardial fat and myocardium (white arrow), and between chest wall fat and muscle (gray arrow) (in vivo) when using conventional 1-1 CSPAMM tagging preparation. (d) Phantom and in vivo ORI-CSPAMM tag preparation, where the chemical shift-induced tagging pattern displacement is no longer visible due to the additional refocusing RF pulse. (Reproduced from Reyhan, M. et al., *J. Magn. Reson. Imaging*, 39(2), 339, 2014. With permission.)

of LV twist and torsion, but without being affected by off-resonance artifacts. The advantages of implementing ORI-CSPAMM are that it corrects for the off-resonance accrued during tagging preparation and readout, and removes the chemical shift from the tagging pattern. Unlike the fat suppression technique developed by Fahmy et al. (2009), ORI-CSPAMM removes the off-resonance effects from the tagging pattern, while the tag intensity of off-resonant tissues has a residual effect.

11.9 HIGH-RESOLUTION CSPAMM

11.9.1 Signal Analysis

Stuber et al. (1999a) modified CSPAMM imaging to double the tagging resolution (4 mm tag separation in this study) by combining two SPAMM measurements with a 90° phase shift between the two acquisitions. The developed technique is based on modifying the original SPAMM sequence such that the second 90° RF pulse is applied with a phase shift Ψ relative to the first 90° RF pulse (Figure 11.28); therefore, the tagging preparation results in rotating a certain amount of the transverse magnetization back to the longitudinal direction

$$M_z = \begin{bmatrix} -\sin\Psi & \cos\Psi \end{bmatrix} \begin{bmatrix} M_x \\ M_y \end{bmatrix}. \tag{11.38}$$

In the case of tagging with a flip angle, Φ_{tag}, the resulting longitudinal magnetization becomes

$$M_z(r) = -M_{ss}\left[\sin\Psi\sin\left(\Phi_{tag}r\right) - \cos\Psi\cos(\Phi_{tag}r)\right]$$
$$= M_{ss}\cos(\Phi_{tag}r - \Psi), \tag{11.39}$$

which means that the tagging pattern can be shifted to any desired location based on the phase shift, Ψ. If Ψ is set to 90°, then the tagging pattern would be shifted by a quarter cycle between the first (*A*) and second (*B*)

acquisitions of the CSPAMM sequence, such that the modulus images are represented as

$$TAG_A(r) = \left|\cos(\Phi_{tag}r)\right| \tag{11.40}$$

and

$$TAG_B(r) = \left|\sin(\Phi_{tag}r)\right|. \tag{11.41}$$

A tagged image with double the tagging frequency can thus be obtained by simply multiplying the two images TAG_A and TAG_B:

$$TAG_A(r) \times TAG_B(r) = \frac{1}{2}\left|\sin(2\Phi_{tag}r)\right|. \tag{11.42}$$

11.9.2 In Vivo Results

Figure 11.29 shows high-tag-density (4 mm tag separation) CSPAMM images through the cardiac cycle with 35 ms temporal resolution.

11.10 ORTHOGONAL CSPAMM

Orthogonal CSPAMM (OCSPAMM) has been recently introduced to reduce the scan time in half while acquiring grid-tagged CSPAMM images (Wang et al. 2011). If CSPAMM is based on acquiring two separate SPAMM images (which are 180° out of phase with each other) for producing a line-tagged image, then four separate SPAMM acquisitions would be required for producing a 2D grid-tagged CSPAMM image. The OCSPAMM sequence (Figure 11.30) is based on rotating the tag orientation in the second SPAMM acquisition by 90° relative to the first one, such that when the two images are subtracted to produce the final CSPAMM image, the DC signal peak is cancelled (as in conventional CSPAMM), while a 2D grid tagging is obtained, thus producing a CSPAMM grid-tagged image from only 2 SPAMM acquisitions. Figure 11.31 shows k-space construction of OCSPAMM.

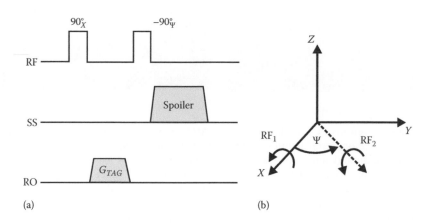

(a)

(b)

FIGURE 11.28 Phase shift addition to tagging. (a) Conventional 1-1 SPAMM sequence modified by the application of a phase shift Ψ between the two 90° tagging RF pulses. (b) The diagram shows the coordinate system of the magnetization, which rotates with the Larmor frequency, and the rotation axis achieved by the two RF pulses.

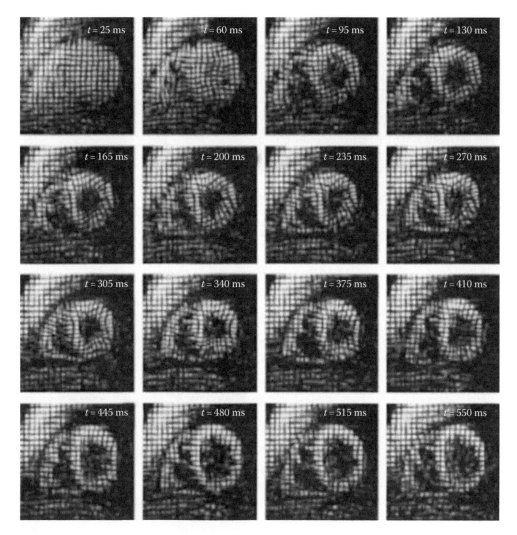

FIGURE 11.29 In vivo high-resolution complementary SPAMM images. Double oblique equatorial acquisition (slice following) of the heart of a healthy volunteer (heartbeat rate = 80). Sixteen heart phases are acquired, with a temporal resolution of 35 ms. The images are the result of the combination of four acquisitions of line-tagged images. The initially modulated tag separation was 8 mm, and the resulting tag separation on the images is 4 mm, based on analysis in Equation 11.42. (Reproduced from Stuber, M. et al., *Magn. Reson. Med.*, 41(3), 639, 1999a. With permission.)

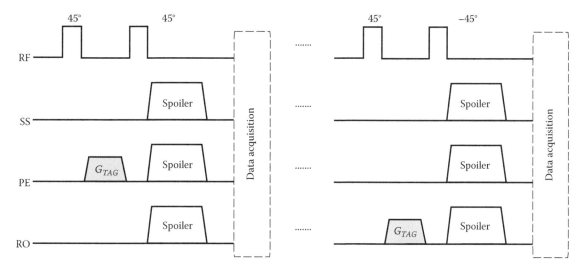

FIGURE 11.30 Sequence diagram for the orthogonal CSPAMM (OCSPAMM) sequence. The first pair of 45° tagging RF pulses, and the tagging gradient in between, creates tags in the *x*-direction. The second pair of 45° tagging RF pulses, and the tagging gradient orthogonal to the first tagging gradient, creates tags in *y*-direction. By subtracting the two tagged images, a 2D grid-tagged CSPAMM image is constructed.

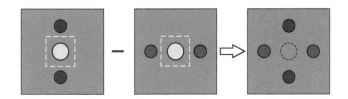

FIGURE 11.31 K-space formation in orthogonal CSPAMM (OCSPAMM). K-space of OCSPAMM (right) is formed by subtracting the k-space of a SPAMM image with tagging in a certain direction (middle) from another SPAMM image with tagging in the orthogonal direction (left). The resulting k-space has no DC signal; it rather has four signal peaks representing a CSPAMM grid-tagged image. (Courtesy of Dr. Tamer Basha, Harvard University, Cambridge, MA.)

11.11 3D CSPAMM

11.11.1 VOLUMETRIC IMAGING

11.11.1.1 Pulse Sequence
Three-dimensional (3D) CSPAMM has been developed to overcome the limitations of generating 3D tagging from multiple LAX and SAX tagged images (Ryf et al. 2002) (Figure 11.32). The sign of the second 90° block pulse is inverted to allow for subtracting the second image from the first image for CSPAMM image construction. Spoiler gradients are applied following each modulation to eliminate the remaining transverse magnetization. The spoiler gradient amplitudes are experimentally optimized to avoid phase coherence.

11.11.1.2 Reconstructed Images
Figures 11.33 and 11.34 show an isosurface-rendered 3D CSPAMM image and extracted LV ring structure, respectively, based on 3D CSPAMM imaging.

11.11.2 ACCELERATED WHOLE-HEART IMAGING

11.11.2.1 Basic Concept
Whole-heart CSPAMM imaging has been introduced in 2008 for accelerated measurement of 3D myocardial motion and deformation in three breath-holds of 18 heartbeats each (Rutz et al. 2008). The acquisitions are performed sequentially, with line tag preparation performed in all orthogonal directions (Figures 11.35 and 11.36). As line tagging is implemented, reduced k-space coverage (orthogonal to the tagging direction) can be achieved to further reduce scan time.

11.11.2.2 Constructed Images and Technique Advantages
A hybrid multishot, segmented EPI sequence has been used for whole-heart CSPAMM imaging. Compared to other techniques, a comparable spatiotemporal acquisition could be acquired approximately four times faster (Figure 11.37). Moreover, as only six harmonic peaks are acquired (rather than eight peaks in lattice tagging), the scan time is inherently reduced by 25%. Further, the developed sequence has the following advantages: (1) shorter period of line tag preparation, (2) improved SNR

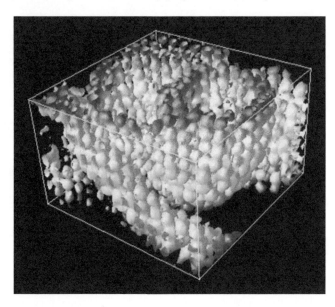

FIGURE 11.33 Isosurface rendering of 3D-CSPAMM. A volume of 128×128 mm^2 is displayed. Tag spacing = 10 mm. (Reproduced from Ryf, S. et al., *J. Magn. Reson. Imaging*, 16(3), 320, 2002. With permission.)

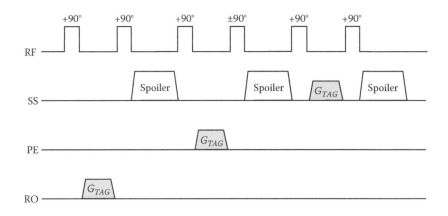

FIGURE 11.32 CSPAMM pulse sequence. The tagging gradients are applied consecutively in three orthogonal directions. Every tagging stage consists of two tagging RF pulses, interspersed by a tagging gradient and followed by a spoiler gradient to remove transverse magnetization. The sign of the second 90° block pulse is inverted to allow for subtracting the second image from the first image for CSPAMM image construction.

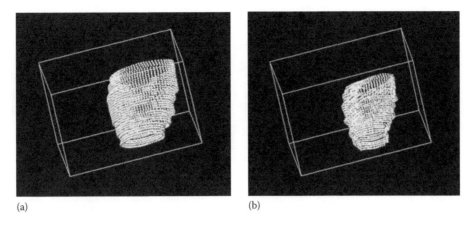

(a)   (b)

FIGURE 11.34 Analysis of in vivo 3D-CSPAMM images. Forty midmyocardial ring structures are placed at (a) end-diastole and tracked until (b) end-systole. (Reproduced from Ryf, S. et al., *J. Magn. Reson. Imaging*, 16(3), 320, 2002. With permission.)

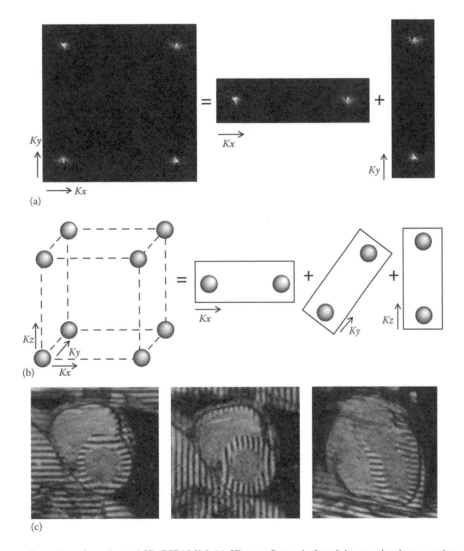

FIGURE 11.35 K-space formation of accelerated 3D CSPAMM. (a) 2D case. Instead of applying tagging in two orthogonal axes in the same scan (k-space on the left; to create a grid-tagged pattern), two 1D tagging scans (2 k-spaces in the middle and right) are conducted consecutively, so that only a small portion of the k-space that includes the signal peaks is acquired each time, instead of acquiring the whole k-space in the case of one acquisition. (b) Extension to 3D case. Instead of applying tagging in three orthogonal directions in the same scan (k-space on the left), three consecutive 1D tagging scans (3 other k-spaces) are conducted consecutively to significantly save data acquisition time. (c) Three orthogonal 1D tagged images. Short-axis slices are tagged in both horizontal and vertical directions in two separate acquisitions, and four-chamber images are tagged in the horizontal direction. (Reproduced from Ibrahim, El-S.H., *J. Cardiovasc. Magn. Reson.*, 13, 36, 2011.)

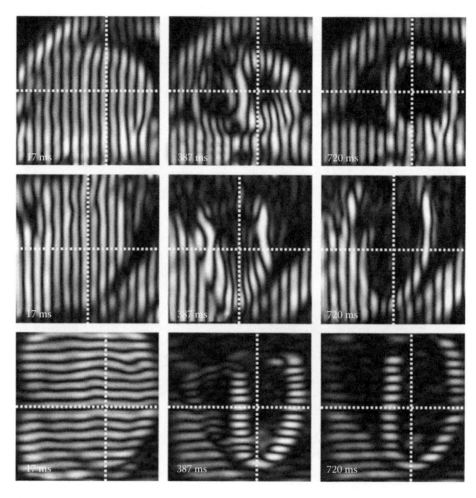

FIGURE 11.36   In vivo accelerated CSPAMM images. Exemplary slices of tagged myocardium of a healthy volunteer for three datasets with orthogonal tagging directions (showed in top, middle, and bottom rows). The 1st (left column; at end-diastole), 11th (middle column; at end-systole), and 20th (right column; last) timeframes are shown. Cut-through planes are indicated with dashed lines. (Reproduced from Rutz, A.K. et al., *Magn. Reson. Med.*, 59(4), 755, 2008. With permission.)

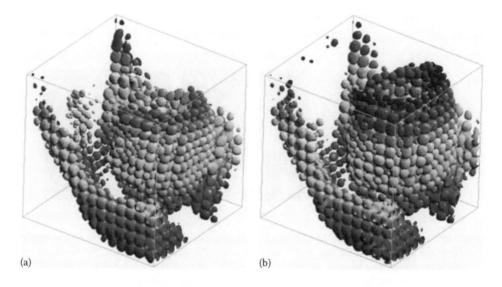

FIGURE 11.37   3D isosurface representations of tagging data composed from three line-tagged datasets showing the left ventricle of a healthy volunteer. Two selected timeframes are shown: (a) timeframe acquired at 387 ms (end-systole) and (b) timeframe acquired at 720 ms (last timeframe) after the electrocardiogram R-wave. (Reproduced from Rutz, A.K. et al., *Magn. Reson. Med.*, 59(4), 755, 2008. With permission.)

with line tagging because the acquired signal is split across two harmonic peaks instead of four or eight peaks in grid or lattice tagging, respectively, and (3) prolonged time between the readout of the two conjugate harmonic peaks.

11.12 APPLICATIONS

Beyond the technical developments addressed earlier in the chapter, CSPAMM has been implemented in a large number of clinical studies and investigations. CSPAMM reproducibility has been studied in normal volunteers, where the results showed good intraobserver, interobserver, and interstudy reproducibility for measuring LV circumferential strain and twist, and less reproducibility for measuring radial strain (Swoboda et al. 2014). Studies for measuring regional LV function are promising, as are those for examining the pattern of right ventricular (RV) contractility. Heart rotation and torsion are equally interesting areas of study, as well as the effect of aging on heart function. Other CSPAMM applications include coronary artery disease, ischemic heart disease, myocardial infarction (MI), hypertrophic cardiomyopathy, interventricular synchrony, valvular diseases, postsurgical cardiac function evaluation, and congenital heart disease. This list is by no means exhaustive, but it illustrates the growing number of clinical applications in which CSPAMM is implemented to study the heart function.

11.12.1 ANIMAL STUDIES

CSPAMM has been implemented for measuring regional function in the mouse heart with the same resolution as in anatomical cine images (Heijman et al. 2004). Scans were

conducted on two healthy mice and two mice with MI on a 6.3T MRI scanner (Figure 11.38).

The feasibility of CSPAMM imaging of rats at 1.5T has been established. In one study (Daire et al. 2008), CSPAMM images were acquired during dobutamine stress. The resulting images showed sufficient image quality for resolving transmural circumferential strain gradient and differentiating between strain measurements at rest and stress with high inter- and intraobserver reproducibility. In another study (Ivancevic et al. 2007), 10 Sprague–Dawley rats, 7 infarcted and 3 normal, were imaged on a clinical 1.5T system. Transmural resolution in myocardial strain measurement was obtained, and decreased myocardial strain was evident in the infarcted regions (Figure 11.39).

The feasibility of CSPAMM imaging in the rat heart after manganese injection has been established. Manganese-enhanced MRI can depict the myocardial areas at risk in models of coronary occlusion reperfusion. However, the manganese relaxation effects may alter the tags by increasing the tags fading. To examine the effect of manganese injection on CSPAMM imaging, Hyacinthe et al. (2008) imaged rats at 1.5T using CSPAMM, before and 15 minutes after $MnCl_2$ injection (Figure 11.40). The results showed increased tagging contrast after manganese injection, which remained comparable to that in control scans despite the faster myocardial relaxation in the presence of manganese.

11.12.2 ISCHEMIC HEART DISEASE

In 2006, Ryf et al. (2006) conducted a study to determine whether postsystolic shortening, measured from CSPAMM

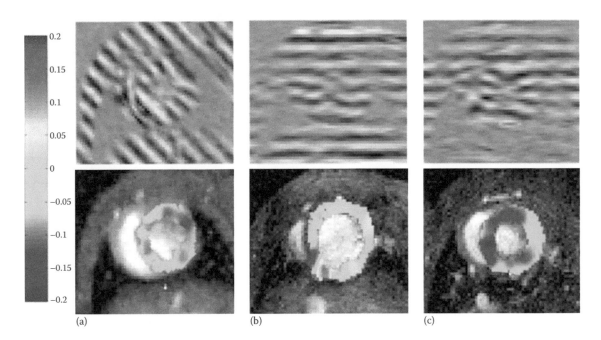

FIGURE 11.38 CSPAMM images of mouse hearts. The top row shows horizontally tagged CSPAMM images of (a) a healthy mouse heart and (b, c) an infarcted mouse heart at end-systole. The slice in (b) was positioned through the infarct region, while the slice in (c) was located remotely above the infarction. The bottom row represents circumferential strain at every tracked point at end-systole. The strain is color-coded according to the color bar on the left. (Reproduced from Heijman, E. et al., *MAGMA*, 17(3–6), 170, 2004. With permission.)

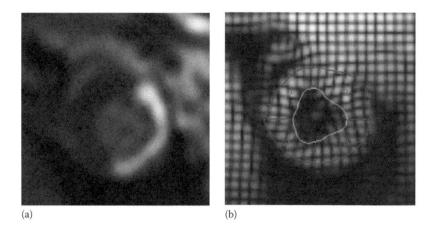

(a)   (b)

FIGURE 11.39   Delayed enhancement and CSPAMM imaging in rat hearts. (a) Late-enhancement image of an infarct in the lateral and anterior sectors of the heart. (b) Sector localization on the corresponding tagged image (1, septal; 2, anterior; 3, lateral; 4, inferior). The hypointense band on the late-enhancement image indicates partial subendocardial sparing, which is consistent with partial preservation of subendocardial function. (Reproduced from Ivancevic, M.K. et al., *Invest. Radiol.*, 42(3), 204, 2007. With permission.)

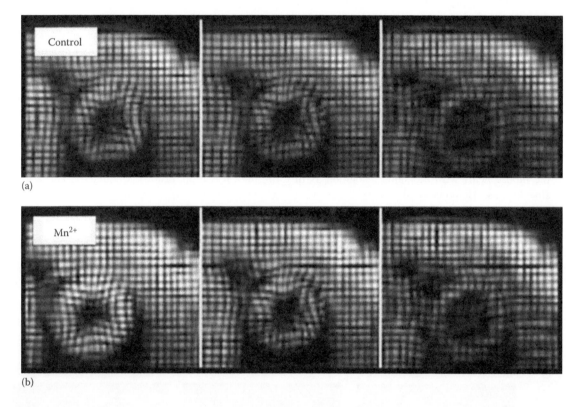

FIGURE 11.40   CSPAMM images at different heart phases (a) before and (b) after intraperitoneal injection of $MnCl_2$. All images have sufficient image quality. (Reproduced from Hyacinthe, J.N. et al., *NMR Biomed.*, 21(1), 15, 2008. With permission.)

images, is a sufficient indicator of myocardial viability. While postsystolic shortening was evidenced in infarcted myocardium and maximal radial displacement was decreased in the scar tissue, there was neither temporal difference in the time-of-maximal radial displacement nor a significant difference in rotation between the infarcted and noninfarcted myocardium. As such, postsystolic shortening alone is not sufficient for diagnosing myocardial viability, as it might be indicative of a recoil effect in which the potential energy stored in the scar tissue is released. These

results imply that circumferential fiber shortening is best suited to characterize regional deformation, whereas radial displacement and rotation are more dependent on tethering effects and are therefore more likely to reflect global chamber mechanics (Figure 11.41).

In a study for evaluating the relationship between the degree of salvage following acute ST elevation myocardial infarction (STEMI) and subsequent reversible contractile dysfunction using MRI, CSPAMM was implemented to measure myocardial strain 1–7 days after primary

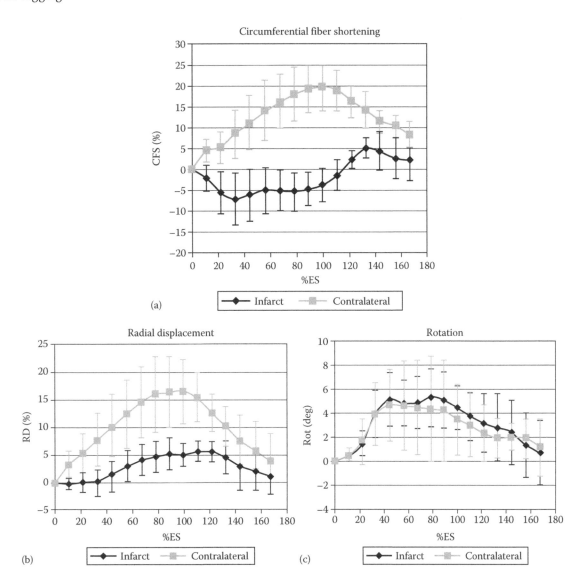

FIGURE 11.41 Deformation parameters of infarcted and contralateral sectors (averaged over all patients) in patients with ischemic heart disease. (a) The infarct region is characterized by an initial stretching and then contraction during diastole (postsystolic shortening). (b) Radial displacement is decreased in the infarct sector compared to the contralateral sector. (c) Rotation does not differ between infarcted and contralateral viable sectors. ES, end-systole. (Reproduced from Ryf, S. et al., *J. Cardiovasc. Magn. Reson.*, 8(3), 445, 2006.)

percutaneous coronary intervention (PPCI) (O'Regan et al. 2013). The results revealed partial peak systolic strain recovery following PPCI even when apparent salvage was less than 25% (Figure 11.42), which implies that late gadolinium enhancement may not be equal to irreversibly injured myocardium, and that salvage assessment performed within the first week of revascularization may underestimate the potential for functional recovery.

11.12.3 LV TORSION

Russel et al. (2008) used CSPAMM to perform an interesting physiological analysis of LV torsion (Figure 11.43) in a group of 12 healthy volunteers. The results showed that displacement of the axis of rotation (Figure 11.44) causes deviation in torsion that is highest in circumferential segments (0.90%) and lowest in transmural layers (0.05%). Circumferentially,

anterolateral torsion was larger than inferior torsion (12.4° vs. 5.0°) and endocardial torsion was smaller than epicardial torsion (7.5° vs. 8.0°). Nevertheless, while the variability in the position of the axis of rotation causes a large variability in circumferential torsion measurements, it has a negligible effect on global measurements. Therefore, analysis in the transmural layers should provide accurate and reliable measurements for studying LV mechanics.

11.12.4 LV HYPERTROPHY

Familial hypertrophic cardiomyopathy (FHC) has been studied using CSPAMM tagging (Ennis et al. 2003). CSPAMM was combined with the cardiac phase to order reconstruction (CAPTOR) technique (Feinstein et al. 1997) for quantifying regional indices of myocardial function throughout the cardiac cycle. The results showed distinct differences in strain

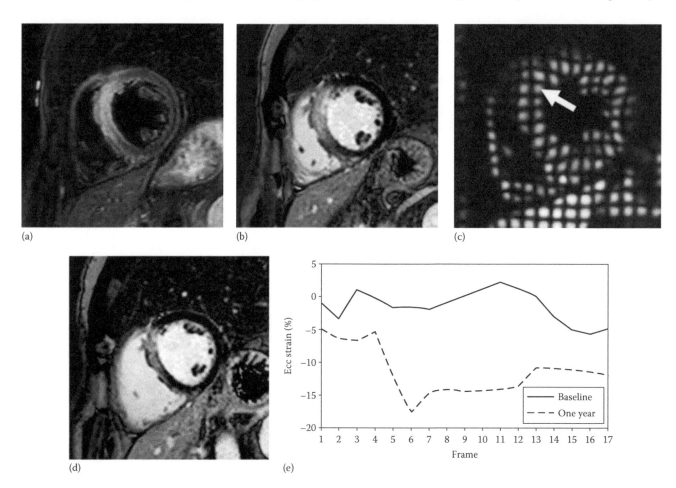

(a)   (b)   (c)

(d)   (e)

FIGURE 11.42 CSPAMM strain assessment in ischemic myocardium. Short-axis MRI images of the left ventricle in a 55-year-old male patient acquired (a–c) at baseline and (d) 1-year follow-up. (a) T2-weighted image showing edema (bright signal) in the anteroseptal wall. (b) Late gadolinium enhancement image showing high signal throughout the ischemic territory. (c) CSPAMM-tagged image (arrow points to area of reduced contractility). (d) Late gadolinium enhancement at 1 year showing a smaller extent of high signal than at baseline. (e) Circumferential strain (Ecc) measured in the anteroseptal midwall (arrow in (c)), demonstrating improved systolic function between baseline and 1-year follow-up, despite apparently poor salvage. (Reproduced from O'Regan, D.P. et al., *Eur. Radiol.*, 1210, 2013. With permission.)

in FHC compared to controls (Figure 11.45). Specifically, while early systolic shortening was similar, the total systolic shortening was significantly reduced in the septal and inferior regions in FHC. Further, early-diastolic strain rate was reduced in all regions and no period of diastasis was observed in FHC. Therefore, the ventricular response to atrial systole could be seen as strain exceeding the end-diastolic reference. As such, diastolic untwisting might be a useful parameter for distinguishing physiological hypertrophy in athletes from pathological hypertrophy in aortic stenosis or hypertrophic cardiomyopathy (Stuber et al. 1999b).

Rutz et al. (2007) studied 29 Fabry patients with and without LV hypertrophy and compared the results to age- and gender-matched healthy volunteers. The results showed that progressive LV hypertrophy, a characteristic of Fabry disease, is associated with an altered myocardial motion pattern. Specifically, longitudinal shortening and circumferential contraction demonstrated reduced peak values with increasing LV mass, and were significantly reduced in Fabry patients with LV hypertrophy. The torsional

deformation and apical rotation were, however, increased in all Fabry patients compared to controls. Therefore, measuring LV rotation and torsion would allow for detecting cardiomyopathy in Fabry patients early before the development of LV hypertrophy.

Torsion analysis from CSPAMM images has been conducted in a study on recessive mutation causing familial hypertrophic cardiomyopathy (Russel et al. 2011). The results showed that the mutation carriers have normal wall thickness, but increased LV torsion with respect to controls, which suggests that healthy carriers may be targets for clinical intervention at a preclinical stage to prevent the onset of future dysfunction.

11.12.5 Valvular Heart Disease

Among some of the early CSPAMM research studies is one that studied the effect of aortic stenosis on alterations in local myocardial motion patterns (Stuber et al. 1999b). This paper, published in *Circulation*, found that diastolic

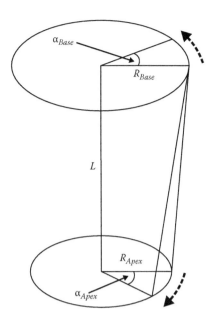

FIGURE 11.43 Myocardial torsion calculation. Twist is defined as ($\alpha_{apex} - \alpha_{base}$). Torsion is defined as ($\alpha_{apex} - \alpha_{base}$). R_m/L, with R_m the mean radius of the basal and apical level. Counterclockwise rotation (as seen from the apex) is represented by a positive flip angle.

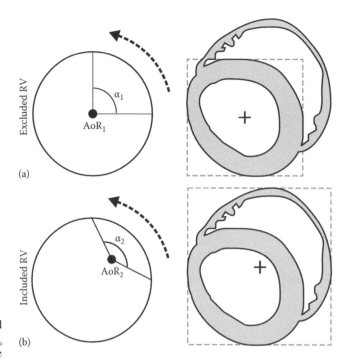

FIGURE 11.44 Displaced axis of rotation results in a different observed rotation angle for the same displacement. Inclusion of the right ventricle mass in the calculation of the axis of rotation (AoR) will move the AoR more toward inferoseptal wall (b), compared to the correct case in (a). (Courtesy of Dr. Tamer Basha, Harvard University, Cambridge, MA.)

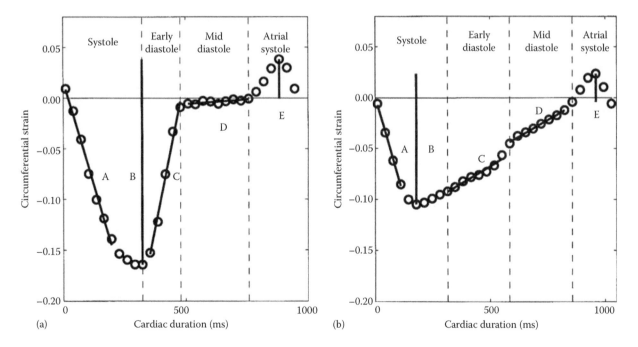

FIGURE 11.45 Left ventricle midwall circumferential strain curve in the inferior wall in a (a) normal subject and (b) hypertrophic cardiomyopathy patient. Indices of cardiac function are shown on the curves: A, systolic strain rate; B, total systolic strain; C, early-diastolic strain rate; D, middiastolic strain rate; and E, lengthening subsequent to atrial systole. Measures B and E were used to calculate the percent lengthening subsequent to atrial systole, defined as E/B. (Reproduced from Ennis, D.B. et al., *Magn. Reson. Med.*, 50(3), 638, 2003. With permission.)

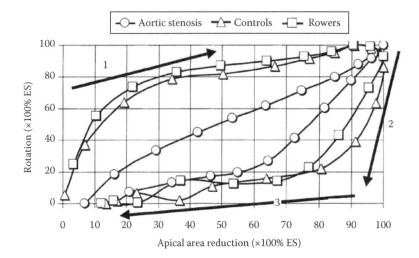

FIGURE 11.46 Left ventricle (LV) rotation-area loop at an apical plane in controls, rowers, and patients with aortic stenosis. The loop is separated into three phases: (1) ejection, (2) isovolumic relaxation, and (3) filling of LV. ES, end-systole. (Reproduced from Stuber, M. et al., *Circulation*, 100(4), 361, 1999b. With permission.)

apical untwisting in patients with pressure overload due to aortic stenosis is delayed compared to healthy controls or athletes who have a similar degree of hypertrophy as the patients (Figure 11.46).

In another study by Nagel et al. (2000), the authors used CSPAMM for studying cardiac torsion and systolic and diastolic wall motion in 12 controls and 13 patients with severe aortic valve stenosis. The results showed that during systole, the normal LV undergoes a clockwise rotation (when viewed from the apex) of −4.4 ± 1.6° at the base and a counterclockwise rotation of +6.8 ± 2.5° at the apex. In patients with aortic valve stenosis, this rotation was found to be reduced at the base and increased at the apex. Further, the overall (normalized) rotation velocity is decreased and maximal torsion is increased in aortic valve stenosis. Together, these results could provide an explanation for the occurrence of diastolic dysfunction in patients with severe pressure overload hypertrophy.

Recently, CSPAMM has been implemented for studying changes in myocardial strain following transcatheter aortic valve implantation (TAVI) (Uddin et al. 2014). TAVI resulted in improved mid-LV circumferential strain and decreased myocardial twist (Figures 11.47 and 11.48). However, while systolic strain rate increased following TAVI, there was no significant change in diastolic strain rate.

11.12.6 Pulmonary Hypertension

Pulmonary arterial hypertension (PAH) has been studied by Marcus et al. (2008) using high temporal resolution (14 ms) CSPAMM. The study showed that PAH is associated with a delay in myocardial peak shortening (Figures 11.49 and 11.50). Further, it was demonstrated that the interventricular delay was caused by an increase in the duration of RV shortening, rather than a delay in the onset of RV shortening,

which was found to be related to septal bowing, decreased LV filling, and decreased stroke volume.

Continuing earlier studies on PAH, Mauritz et al. (2011) implemented CSPAMM to show that the prolonged RV postsystolic isovolumic period in PAH is not a reflection of diastolic dysfunction (Figures 11.51 and 11.52). Although the total postsystolic isovolumic period is longer in the patients than in healthy subjects, the relaxation period is not different. In PAH, the prolonged postsystolic isovolumic period is caused by an additional postsystolic contraction period rather than by an increased relaxation period. Further, the postsystolic contraction period is strongly related to the total postsystolic isovolumic period and is associated with disease severity.

CSPAMM has been implemented for studying postinterventional response in PAH, where 13 consecutive patients with chronic PAH were studied before and 6 months after pulmonary endarterectomy (Mauritz et al. 2012). The results showed that the RV and LV peak strains are resynchronized after the procedure (Figures 11.53 and 11.54). Therefore, the reduction in systolic RV wall stress plays a key role in normalizing interventricular dyssynchrony.

11.12.7 Cardiac Resynchronization Therapy

CSPAMM has been implemented for predicting response to cardiac resynchronization therapy (CRT) (Russel et al. 2007). Two parameters were derived from the tagged images: (1) mechanical dyssynchrony (time difference between regions) and (2) regional heterogeneity (strain difference between regions). The results showed that regional heterogeneity parameters have better correlation with response to CRT than the mechanical dyssynchrony parameters. Therefore, using a heterogeneity-based parameter in addition to the electrocardiogram (ECG)'s QRS width would improve prediction of the response to biventricular pacing.

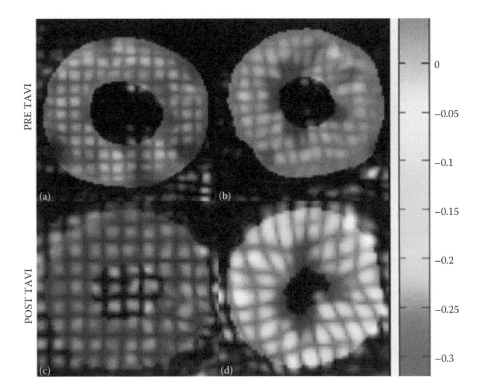

FIGURE 11.47 Example of tag analysis using CSPAMM in patients (a, b) before and (c, d) after transcatheter aortic valve implantation (TAVI). The images are acquired at (a, c) diastole and (b, d) systole. (Reproduced from Uddin, A. et al., *J. Cardiovasc. Magn. Reson.*, 16(Suppl 1), P260, 2014.)

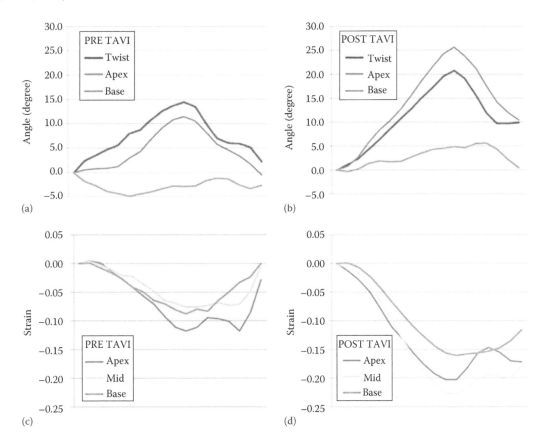

FIGURE 11.48 Change in twist and circumferential strain before and after transcatheter aortic valve implantation (TAVI). (a) Twist pre-TAVI. (b) Twist post-TAVI. (c) Circumferential strain pre-TAVI. (d) Circumferential strain post-TAVI. (Reproduced from Uddin, A. et al., *J. Cardiovasc. Magn. Reson.*, 16(Suppl 1), P260, 2014.)

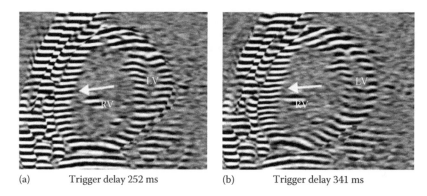

(a)   Trigger delay 252 ms   (b)   Trigger delay 341 ms

FIGURE 11.49 Short-axis tagged images (a) at the time of aortic valve closure at trigger delay and (b) at the time of peak right ventricle (RV) shortening. In the tagged image acquired at peak RV shortening, the distance of the tagging lines in the RV free wall shows further shortening (white arrows), whereas the tagging lines in the left ventricle free wall show relaxation. (Reproduced from Marcus, J.T. et al., *J. Am. Coll. Cardiol.*, 51(7), 750, 2008. With permission.)

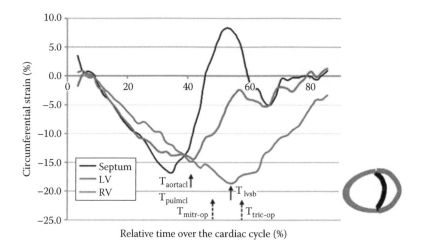

FIGURE 11.50 Circumferential strain over time in pulmonary arterial hypertension (PAH). Circumferential strain curves over time after the electrocardiogram R-wave in the left ventricle (LV) and right ventricle (RV) free walls and septum at a basal level. The LV, RV, and septum start simultaneously with shortening (negative strain), but the RV reaches its peak later than the LV by 12% of the cardiac cycle time. The closure times of the aortic ($T_{aortacl}$) and pulmonary (T_{pulmcl}) valves are coincident with peak LV shortening. The time-of-maximal leftward septal bowing (T_{lvsb}) is coincident with septal stretching (positive strain) and with peak RV shortening. The opening times of the mitral ($T_{mitr-op}$) and tricuspid ($T_{tric-op}$) valves indicate the onset times of LV and RV filling. (Reproduced from Marcus, J.T. et al., *J. Am. Coll. Cardiol.*, 51(7), 750, 2008. With permission.)

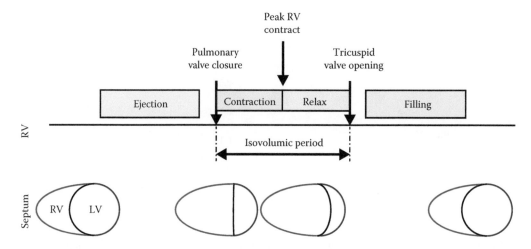

FIGURE 11.51 Postsystolic isovolumic period and septal deformation in pulmonary arterial hypertension (PAH). The isovolumic period consists of contraction and relaxation periods.

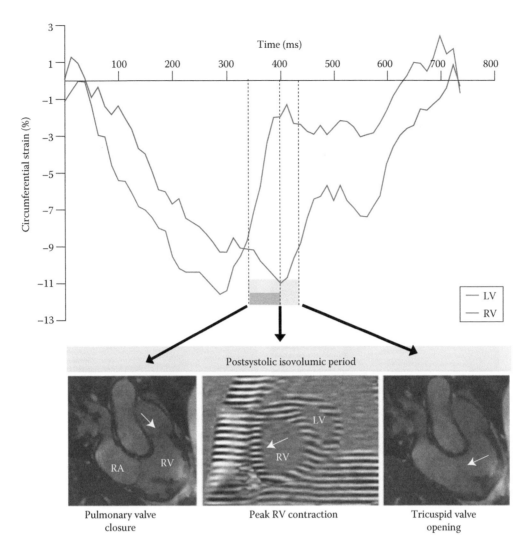

FIGURE 11.52 MRI-derived circumferential strain, cine, and tagged images of a patient with pulmonary arterial hypertension (PAH). Circumferential strain curves of the left ventricle (LV) and right ventricle (RV) during the cardiac cycle. The images show RV two-chamber cine images at the time of pulmonary valve closure (left; arrow) and tricuspid valve opening (right; arrow), as well as short-axis-tagged image (middle) at the time of peak RV contraction (arrow). The RV strain curve shows that, after pulmonary valve closure (341 ms), the RV wall continues its active contraction, reaching its peak at 399 ms and thus giving a postsystolic contraction period of 58 ms. The isovolumic relaxation starts after RV peak contraction (399 ms) until tricuspid valve opening (431 ms) giving an isovolumic relaxation period of 32 ms. The RR interval is 767 ms. (Reproduced from Mauritz, G.J. et al., *Heart*, 97(6), 473, 2011. With permission.)

Russel et al. (2009a) used CSPAMM in another study on 34 CRT candidates and 12 controls to study regional heart function. The results showed a significantly higher correlation between basal and apical rotations in acute responders than in nonresponders and controls (Figure 11.55). The sensitivity and specificity were 82% and 83%, respectively, for predicting acute responders. As the apical rotation is inverted in most patients, the loss of opposite base-apex rotation could be used as a reliable marker for predicting acute responders in CRT-eligible patients.

Circumferential strain computed from CSPAMM-tagged images has been compared to LV volume obtained with real-time 3D echocardiography in CRT candidates (Russel et al. 2009b). MRI is advantageous to echocardiography for measuring strain due to the limitations of the acoustic window and angle of the ultrasound beam in echocardiography. The study results revealed high cross-correlations between regional MRI-derived LV strain and echo-derived LV volume (Figure 11.56). However, regional differences in time delay between the curves were found, resulting in differences in the quantification of mechanical dyssynchrony. This could be attributed to the poor correlation between regions with little or positive circumferential strain and the accompanying regional volume curves. Therefore, both modalities might represent different measures of mechanical dyssynchrony (Russel et al. 2009b).

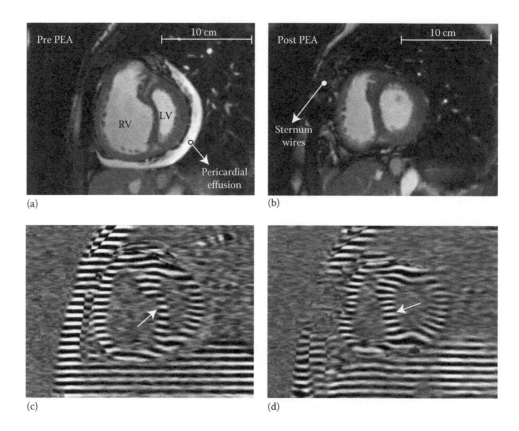

FIGURE 11.53 Pulmonary arterial hypertension (PAH) before and after pulmonary endarterectomy (PEA) examined with cine and CSPAMM tagged images. Short-axis (a, b) cine and (c, d) tagged images at the time of peak RV shortening in a patient with chronic thromboembolic pulmonary hypertension (a, c) before and (b, d) after PEA. Leftward ventricular septal bowing, as present before PEA, recovers 6 months after PEA (white arrows in (c, d)). (Reproduced from Mauritz, G.J. et al., *J. Cardiovasc. Magn. Reson.*, 14, 5, 2012.)

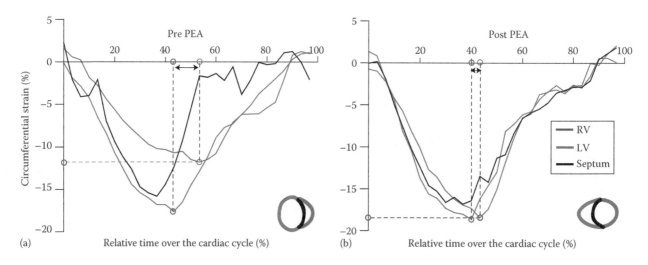

FIGURE 11.54 Circumferential strain curves over time after the electrocardiogram R-wave in the left ventricle (LV) and right ventricle (RV) free walls and the septum in a pulmonary hypertension patient (a) pre- and (b) postpulmonary endarterectomy (PEA). Pre-PEA: the LV, RV, and septum start simultaneously with shortening (negative strain), but the RV reaches its peak later than the LV and the RV peak strain is lower. Post-PEA: the left-right synchrony and RV peak strain have recovered. (Reproduced from Mauritz, G.J. et al., *J. Cardiovasc. Magn. Reson.*, 14, 5, 2012.)

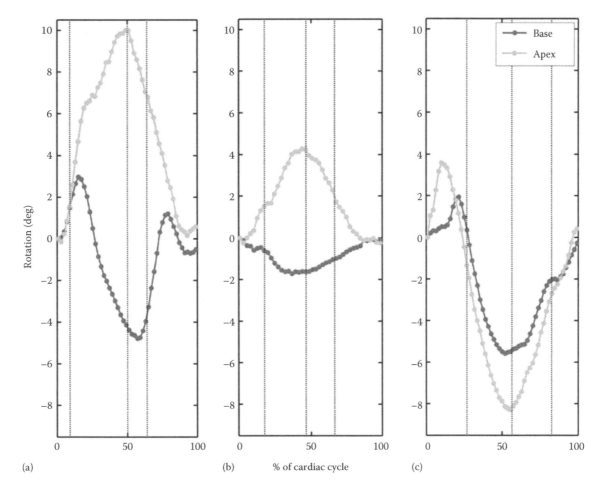

FIGURE 11.55 Basal and apical rotation curves in (a) healthy subject, (b) cardiac resynchronization therapy (CRT) nonresponder, and (c) CRT responder. Positive rotation is represented counterclockwise when viewed from the apex. It can be seen that although the amount of rotation is impaired, the CRT nonresponder shows normal rotational directions, whereas in the CRT responder, apical rotation is inverted. Vertical black dotted lines indicate aortic valve opening, aortic valve closure, and mitral valve opening, respectively. (Reproduced from Russel, I.K. et al., *J. Card. Fail.*, 15(8), 717, 2009a. With permission.)

11.12.8 LEFT BUNDLE BRANCH BLOCK

Recently, CSPAMM has been implemented for measuring circumferential strain in cardiomyopathy with and without left bundle branch block (LBBB) (Han et al. 2010). The results showed that the strength of myocardial contraction is significantly reduced in cardiomyopathic patients regardless of the conduction pattern (Figure 11.57). Further, there existed an association between LBBB and dyskinesis of the antero-septum or the entire septum in some patients with systolic dysfunction. Therefore, identifying different patterns of mechanical contraction in LBBB may be important for selecting patients for CRT.

11.12.9 CONGENITAL HEART DISEASE

CSPAMM has been implemented for measuring global and regional rotation and torsion in normal subjects and asymptomatic single LV (SLV) and single RV (SRV) patients after total cavo-pulmonary connection (Krishnamurthy et al. 2014) (Figure 11.58 and Table 11.1). The SLV and SRV patients showed a significantly impaired rotation compared to normal subjects, with SRV patients more severely affected. In single-ventricular patients, basal rotation was more impaired compared to apical rotation, suggesting a detrimental effect of the hypoplastic chamber connected to the base.

Another study has been conducted to compare circumferential and longitudinal strain in normal subjects and asymptomatic children with SLV and SRV hearts (Noel 2014). The results demonstrated significant differences in strain in SLV and SRV compared to normal hearts. Septal circumferential strain was significantly reduced in single-ventricle patients, with progressive reduction from apex to base, while lateral strain was normal (Figure 11.59).

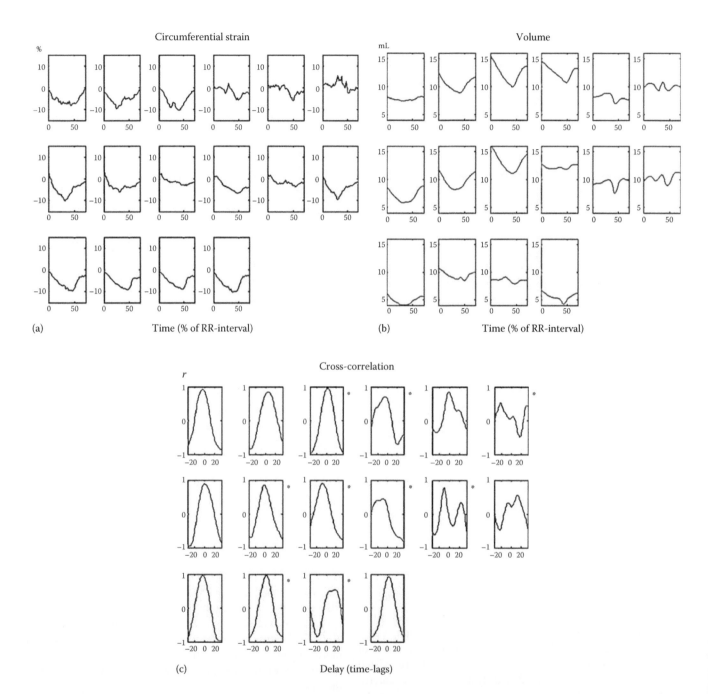

FIGURE 11.56 (a) Circumferential train, (b) volume, and (c) cross-correlation curves of all segments in a cardiac resynchronization therapy candidate. From top to bottom: base, mid, and apex. From left to right: inferoseptal, anteroseptal, anterior, anterolateral, inferolateral, and inferior segments (apex: septal, anterior, lateral, inferior). In the cross-correlation curves, a positive peak cross-correlation value depicts that the strain curve reached its peak before the volume curve. Cross-correlation curves marked with * indicate a segment with delayed contrast enhancement. (Reproduced from Russel, I.K. et al., *Int. J. Cardiovasc. Imaging*, 25(1), 1, 2009b.)

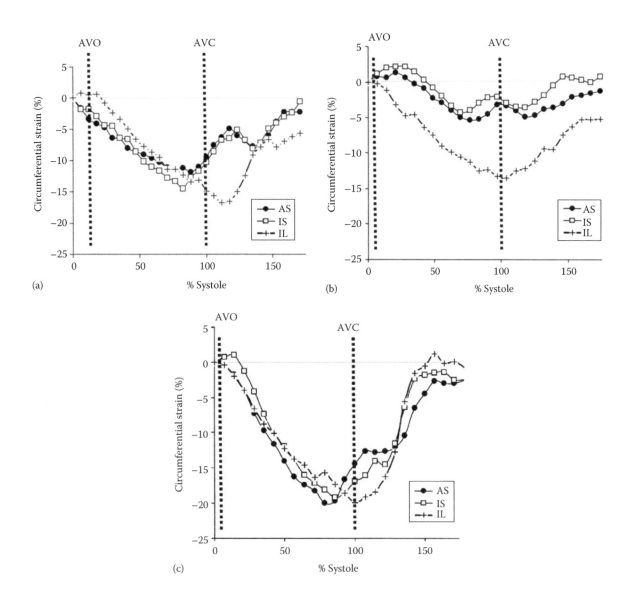

FIGURE 11.57 Septal circumferential strain patterns in patients with non–left bundle branch block (non-LBBB) and a healthy subject. All subjects had normal contraction patterns with maximum negative circumferential strain reached in the septum earlier than in the infer-olateral wall. (a) A patient with interventricular conduction delay and QRS duration of 146 ms. (b) A patient with normal QRS duration of 98 ms. (c) A healthy subject with normal QRS duration of 98 ms. AS, anteroseptum; AVC, aortic valve closure; AVO, aortic valve opening; IL, inferolateral wall; IS, inferoseptum. (Reproduced from Han, Y. et al., *J. Cardiovasc. Magn. Reson.*, 12, 2, 2010.)

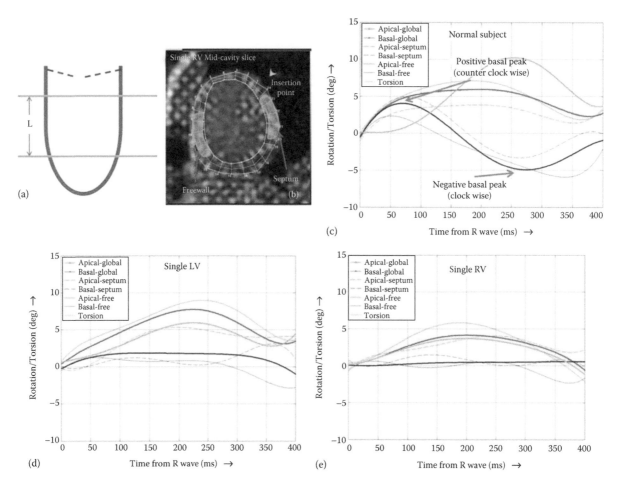

FIGURE 11.58   Myocardial rotation in patients with single ventricle. (a) Schematic showing short-axis acquisition of CSPAMM images at the basal and apical levels of the systemic ventricle. (b) CSPAMM image of a single RV patient at the midcavity location is showed with the myo-cardium segmented, indicating the insertion point, septum, and free wall. Representative plots of rotation (global, septal wall, and free wall) in (c) normal subject, (d) patient with systemic single left ventricle (LV), and (e) systemic single right ventricle (RV). All positive values represent counterclockwise rotation when looked from apex. Note the presence of substantial positive and negative peaks in the basal rotation of a normal subject (c), which are significantly diminished in case of patients with systemic single LV and RV (d, e), leading to a decreased peak torsion. (Reproduced from Krishnamurthy, R. et al., *J. Cardiovasc. Magn. Reson.*, 16(Suppl 1), P122, 2014.)

TABLE 11.1
Peak Rotation of Short-Axis Slices in Normal Subjects and in Patients with Systemic Single Ventricle

| | Peak Rotation (°), (+) Counterclockwise, (−) Clockwise | | | | | | | | | | |
| | Global | | | Septum | | | Free Wall | | | Peak Torsion (°) | Normalized Peak Torsion (°/cm) |
	Apical	Basal (+)	Basal (−)	Apical	Basal (+)	Basal (−)	Apical	Basal (+)	Basal (−)		
Normal	5.8	3.8	−5.4	7.8	3.7	−7.8	5.4	3.3	−5.9	9.9	2.6
SLV	4.7	0.8	−3.9	4.0	2.2	−5.5	5.5	1.2	−5.2	7.4	2.1
SRV	3.0	0.4	−1.6	5.4	2.7	−0.8	3.4	0.1	−5.1	3.9	1.2
% Change (normal vs. SLV)	18.4	79.0	27.7	47.9	41.5	29.8	−1.7	63.2	11.4	24.5	19.9
% Change (normal vs. SRV)	57.9	90.0	70.4	30.7	27	89.7	37.1	96.7	13.6	60.6	53.8

Source: Reproduced from Krishnamurthy, R. et al., *J. Cardiovasc. Magn. Reson.*, 16(Suppl 1), P122, 2014.
SLV, single left ventricle; SRV, single right ventricle.

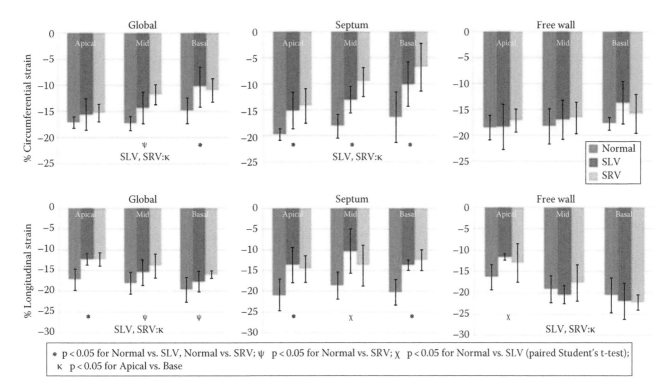

FIGURE 11.59 Bar plots showing longitudinal and circumferential strain values in a pediatric population with systemic single ventricles. There is a significant reduction in strain values. The septum is the most affected region with negligible differences observed in the free wall. Also, there is a significant difference observed from apex to base globally in both the single systemic ventricle patients, while the free wall longitudinal strain shows a significant increase. SLV, single left ventricle; SRV, single right ventricle. (Reproduced from Noel, C. et al., *J. Cardiovasc. Magn. Reson.*, 16(Suppl 1), P111, 2014.)

11.13 SUMMARY AND KEY POINTS

11.13.1 SUMMARY

CSPAMM tagging provides accurate quantification of regional myocardial function that cannot be easily obtained with alternative techniques. The many CSPAMM developments described in this chapter do not exist solely as academic pursuits. A great number of these advances have been developed to answer specific scientific questions in selected patient populations. In other cases, these developments have been exploited to better understand certain heart diseases and improve clinical care. In this context, CSPAMM with its inherent ability to visualize both systolic and diastolic myocardial motion with or without true myocardial motion tracking will continue to play a very important role in advancing regional heart function evaluation with MRI.

11.13.2 KEY POINTS

- On conventional MR images, no internal structures of the myocardium are visible, and therefore regional myocardial motion parameters cannot be easily obtained.
- MRI tagging creates virtual markers on the myocardium, which allows for analyzing intramyocardial tissue deformation.

- Compared to SPAMM, CSPAMM provides higher and more persistent tagging contrast.
- CSPAMM is based on acquiring two consecutive SPAMM images with different tagging polarity, such that when the two images are subtracted, the signal component from the nontagged magnetization is eliminated, while that from the tagged magnetization is doubled.
- The imaging flip angles could be ramped through the cardiac cycle to compensate for tags fading, secondary to longitudinal relaxation and the repetitive application of imaging RF pulses.
- The slice-following technique compensates for the heart through-plane motion, to ensure that the same myocardial tissue is imaged throughout the whole cardiac cycle.
- Slice following is based on tagging a thin slice and then imaging a thicker slice that encompasses the thin tagged slice. Certain technical and clinical precautions should be taken into consideration for accurate and reproducible results.
- CSPAMM tagging could be combined with fast data acquisition techniques (e.g., EPI and spiral imaging) to shorten scan time.
- CSPAMM can be combined with SSFP imaging for improved tagging contrast.

- Magnitude and real-time CSPAMM reconstruction techniques result in improved tagging contrast and persistence through the cardiac cycle.
- Special fat suppression techniques have been developed for eliminating off-resonance effects in CSPAMM, including IFC and ORI-CSPAMM. These techniques allow for high-quality and efficient CSPAMM imaging.
- High-resolution CSPAMM results in doubling the tagging resolution at the cost of increased scan time.
- Orthogonal CSPAMM provides grid-tagged CSPAMM images without additional scan time.
- 3D CSPAMM is based on repeating the tagging modulation in all three spatial directions.
- Accelerated whole-heart imaging is based on acquiring the k-space in multiple 1D tagging steps along orthogonal directions.
- CSPAMM has been used in many applications, including animal studies, ischemic heart disease, LV torsion, LV hypertrophy, valvular heart disease, pulmonary hypertension, cardiac resynchronization therapy, cardiac electrophysiology, and congenital heart disease.

ACKNOWLEDGMENT

The author thanks Dr. Tamer Basha from Harvard University for his help with the line-art figure design.

REFERENCES

Aletras, A. H., Ding, S., Balaban, R. S., and Wen, H. (1999). DENSE: Displacement encoding with stimulated echoes in cardiac functional MRI. *J Magn Reson* 137(1): 247–252.

Axel, L. and Dougherty, L. (1989). MR imaging of motion with spatial modulation of magnetization. *Radiology* 171(3): 841–845.

Bornert, P., Stuber, M., Botnar, R. M., Kissinger, K. V., Koken, P., Spuentrup, E., and Manning, W. J. (2001). Direct comparison of 3D spiral vs. Cartesian gradient-echo coronary magnetic resonance angiography. *Magn Reson Med* 46(4): 789–794.

Daire, J. L., Jacob, J. P., Hyacinthe, J. N., Croisille, P., Montet-Abou, K., Richter, S., Botsikas, D., Lepetit-Coiffe, M., Morel, D., and Vallee, J. P. (2008). Cine and tagged cardiovascular magnetic resonance imaging in normal rat at 1.5 T: A rest and stress study. *J Cardiovasc Magn Reson* 10: 48.

Deimling, M. and Heid, O. (1994). Magnetization prepared true FISP imaging. *Proceedings of the International Society of Magnetic Resonance in Medicine*. San Francisco, CA.

Delfaut, E. M., Beltran, J., Johnson, G., Rousseau, J., Marchandise, X., and Cotten, A. (1999). Fat suppression in MR imaging: Techniques and pitfalls. *Radiographics* 19(2): 373–382.

Ennis, D. B., Epstein, F. H., Kellman, P., Fananapazir, L., McVeigh, E. R., and Arai, A. E. (2003). Assessment of regional systolic and diastolic dysfunction in familial hypertrophic cardiomyopathy using MR tagging. *Magn Reson Med* 50(3): 638–642.

Fahmy, A. S., Basha, T. A., and Osman, N. F. (2009). Inherent fat cancellation in complementary spatial modulation of magnetization. *Magn Reson Med* 61(1): 234–238.

Feinstein, J. A., Epstein, F. H., Arai, A. E., Foo, T. K., Hartley, M. R., Balaban, R. S., and Wolff, S. D. (1997). Using cardiac phase to order reconstruction (CAPTOR): A method to improve diastolic images. *J Magn Reson Imaging* 7(5): 794–798.

Feliciano, H., Piccini, D., Kuijer, J. P., and Stuber, M. (2013). A quantitative comparison between slice-followed and non-slice-followed 3T bSSFP CSPAMM myocardial motion tracking. *Proceedings of the International Society of Magnetic Resonance in Medicine*, p. 1380. Salt Lake City, UT.

Fischer, S. E., McKinnon, G. C., Maier, S. E., and Boesiger, P. (1993). Improved myocardial tagging contrast. *Magn Reson Med* 30(2): 191–200.

Fischer, S. E., McKinnon, G. C., Scheidegger, M. B., Prins, W., Meier, D., and Boesiger, P. (1994). True myocardial motion tracking. *Magn Reson Med* 31(4): 401–413.

Fischer, S. E., Stuber, M., Scheidegger, M. B., and Boesiger, P. (1995). Limitations of stimulated echo acquisition mode (STEAM) techniques in cardiac applications. *Magn Reson Med* 34(1): 80–91.

Fischer, S. E., Wickline, S. A., and Lorenz, C. H. (1999). Novel real-time R-wave detection algorithm based on the vectorcardiogram for accurate gated magnetic resonance acquisitions. *Magn Reson Med* 42(2): 361–370.

Haase, A., Frahm, J., Matthaei, D., Hanicke, W., Bomsdorf, H., Kunz, D., and Tischler, R. (1986). MR imaging using stimulated echoes (STEAM). *Radiology* 160(3): 787–790.

Han, Y., Chan, J., Haber, I., Peters, D. C., Zimetbaum, P. J., Manning, W. J., and Yeon, S. B. (2010). Circumferential myocardial strain in cardiomyopathy with and without left bundle branch block. *J Cardiovasc Magn Reson* 12: 2.

Heijman, E., Strijkers, G. J., Habets, J., Janssen, B., and Nicolay, K. (2004). Magnetic resonance imaging of regional cardiac function in the mouse. *MAGMA* 17(3–6): 170–178.

Hyacinthe, J. N., Ivancevic, M. K., Daire, J. L., and Vallee, J. P. (2008). Feasibility of complementary spatial modulation of magnetization tagging in the rat heart after manganese injection. *NMR Biomed* 21(1): 15–21.

Ibrahim, El-S. H., Stuber, M., Schär, M., and Osman, N. F. (2006). Improved myocardial tagging contrast in cine balanced SSFP images. *J Magn Reson Imaging* 24(5): 1159–1167.

Ibrahim, El-S. H. (2011). Myocardial tagging by cardiovascular magnetic resonance: Evolution of techniques–pulse sequences, analysis algorithms, and applications. *J Cardiovasc Magn Reson* 13: 36.

Ibrahim, El-S. H. and Osman, N. F. (2004). A technique for improving tag contrast persistence in SSFP MRI imaging using adaptive flip angle. *Proceedings of the IEEE ISBI*, pp. 1051–1054. Arlington, VA.

Ingels, N. B., Jr., Daughters, G. T., 2nd, Stinson, E. B., and Alderman, E. L. (1975). Measurement of midwall myocardial dynamics in intact man by radiography of surgically implanted markers. *Circulation* 52(5): 859–867.

Ivancevic, M. K., Daire, J. L., Hyacinthe, J. N., Crelier, G., Kozerke, S., Montet-Abou, K., Gunes-Tatar, I., Morel, D. R., and Vallee, J. P. (2007). High-resolution complementary spatial modulation of magnetization (CSPAMM) rat heart tagging on a 1.5 Tesla clinical magnetic resonance system: A preliminary feasibility study. *Invest Radiol* 42(3): 204–210.

Krishnamurthy, R., Noel, C., Pednekar, A., Atweh, L. A., and Krishnamurthy, R. (2014). Comparison of myocardial rotation and torsion in asymptomatic children with single RV, single LV and normal hearts. *J Cardiovasc Magn Reson* 16(Suppl 1): P122.

Kuijer, J. P., Jansen, E., Marcus, J. T., van Rossum, A. C., and Heethaar, R. M. (2001). Improved harmonic phase myocardial strain maps. *Magn Reson Med* 46(5): 993–999.

Kuijer, J. P., Zwanenburg, J. J., Marcus, J. T., and Hofman, M. B. (2005). CSPAMM real-part reconstruction using an internal phase reference. *Proceedings of the International Society of Magnetic Resonance in Medicine*. Miami, FL.

Marcus, J. T., Gan, C. T., Zwanenburg, J. J., Boonstra, A., Allaart, C. P., Gotte, M. J., and Vonk-Noordegraaf, A. (2008). Interventricular mechanical asynchrony in pulmonary arterial hypertension: Left-to-right delay in peak shortening is related to right ventricular overload and left ventricular underfilling. *J Am Coll Cardiol* **51**(7): 750–757.

Mauritz, G. J., Marcus, J. T., Westerhof, N., Postmus, P. E., and Vonk-Noordegraaf, A. (2011). Prolonged right ventricular post-systolic isovolumic period in pulmonary arterial hypertension is not a reflection of diastolic dysfunction. *Heart* **97**(6): 473–478.

Mauritz, G. J., Vonk-Noordegraaf, A., Kind, T., Surie, S., Kloek, J. J., Bresser, P., Saouti, N., Bosboom, J., Westerhof, N., and Marcus, J. T. (2012). Pulmonary endarterectomy normalizes interventricular dyssynchrony and right ventricular systolic wall stress. *J Cardiovasc Magn Reson* **14**: 5.

Meyer, C. H., Hu, B. S., Nishimura, D. G., and Macovski, A. (1992). Fast spiral coronary artery imaging. *Magn Reson Med* **28**(2): 202–213.

Nagel, E., Stuber, M., Burkhard, B., Fischer, S. E., Scheidegger, M. B., Boesiger, P., and Hess, O. M. (2000). Cardiac rotation and relaxation in patients with aortic valve stenosis. *Eur Heart J* **21**(7): 582–589.

NessAiver, M. and Prince, J. L. (2003a). Magnitude image CSPAMM reconstruction (MICSR). *Magn Reson Med* **50**(2): 331–342.

NessAiver, M. and Prince, J. L. (2003b). Visualization of myocardial motion using MICSR trinary checkerboard display. *Inf Process Med Imaging* **18**: 573–585.

Noel, C., Krishnamurthy, R., Pednekar, A., Chu, D., and Krishnamurthy, R. (2014). Prospective comparison of circumferential and longitudinal strain in asymptomatic children with single left ventricle, single right ventricle and normal hearts. *J Cardiovasc Magn Reson* **16**(Suppl 1): P111.

O'Regan, D. P., Ariff, B., Baksi, A. J., Gordon, F., Durighel, G., and Cook, S. A. (2013). Salvage assessment with cardiac MRI following acute myocardial infarction underestimates potential for recovery of systolic strain. *Eur Radiol* **23**(5): 1210–1217.

Osman, N. F., Kerwin, W. S., McVeigh, E. R., and Prince, J. L. (1999). Cardiac motion tracking using CINE harmonic phase (HARP) magnetic resonance imaging. *Magn Reson Med* **42**(6): 1048–1060.

Osman, N. F., Sampath, S., Atalar, E., and Prince, J. L. (2001). Imaging longitudinal cardiac strain on short-axis images using strain-encoded MRI. *Magn Reson Med* **46**(2): 324–334.

Pattynama, P. M., Doornbos, J., Hermans, J., van der Wall, E. E., and de Roos, A. (1992). Magnetic resonance evaluation of regional left ventricular function. Effect of through-plane motion. *Invest Radiol* **27**(9): 681–685.

Reyhan, M. and Ennis, D. B. (2013). Quantitative assessment of systolic and diastolic left ventricular twist using Fourier Analysis of Stimulated echoes (FAST) and CSPAMM. *J Magn Reson Imaging* **37**(3): 678–683.

Reyhan, M., Natsuaki, Y., and Ennis, D. B. (2014). Off-resonance insensitive complementary SPAtial Modulation of Magnetization (ORI-CSPAMM) for quantification of left ventricular twist. *J Magn Reson Imaging* **39**(2): 339–345.

Rogers, W. J., Jr., Shapiro, E. P., Weiss, J. L., Buchalter, M. B., Rademakers, F. E., Weisfeldt, M. L., and Zerhouni, E. A. (1991). Quantification of and correction for left ventricular systolic long-axis shortening by magnetic resonance tissue tagging and slice isolation. *Circulation* **84**(2): 721–731.

Russel, I. K., Brouwer, W. P., Germans, T., Knaapen, P., Marcus, J. T., van der Velden, J., Gotte, M. J., and van Rossum, A. C. (2011). Increased left ventricular torsion in hypertrophic cardiomyopathy mutation carriers with normal wall thickness. *J Cardiovasc Magn Reson* **13**: 3.

Russel, I. K., Gotte, M. J., de Roest, G. J., Marcus, J. T., Tecelao, S. R., Allaart, C. P., de Cock, C. C., Heethaar, R. M., and van Rossum, A. C. (2009a). Loss of opposite left ventricular basal and apical rotation predicts acute response to cardiac resynchronization therapy and is associated with long-term reversed remodeling. *J Card Fail* **15**(8): 717–725.

Russel, I. K., Gotte, M. J., Kuijer, J. P., and Marcus, J. T. (2008). Regional assessment of left ventricular torsion by CMR tagging. *J Cardiovasc Magn Reson* **10**: 26.

Russel, I. K., van Dijk, J., Kleijn, S. A., Germans, T., de Roest, G., Marcus, J. T., Kamp, O., Gotte, M. J., and van Rossum, A. C. (2009b). Relation between three-dimensional echocardiography derived left ventricular volume and MRI derived circumferential strain in patients eligible for cardiac resynchronization therapy. *Int J Cardiovasc Imaging* **25**(1): 1–11.

Russel, I. K., Zwanenburg, J. J., Germans, T., Marcus, J. T., Allaart, C. P., de Cock, C. C., Gotte, M. J., and van Rossum, A. C. (2007). Mechanical dyssynchrony or myocardial shortening as MRI predictor of response to biventricular pacing? *J Magn Reson Imaging* **26**(6): 1452–1460.

Rutz, A. K., Juli, C. F., Ryf, S., Widmer, U., Kozerke, S., Eckhardt, B. P., and Boesiger, P. (2007). Altered myocardial motion pattern in Fabry patients assessed with CMR-tagging. *J Cardiovasc Magn Reson* **9**(6): 891–898.

Rutz, A. K., Ryf, S., Plein, S., Boesiger, P., and Kozerke, S. (2008). Accelerated whole-heart 3D CSPAMM for myocardial motion quantification. *Magn Reson Med* **59**(4): 755–763.

Ryf, S., Kissinger, K. V., Spiegel, M. A., Bornert, P., Manning, W. J., Boesiger, P., and Stuber, M. (2004). Spiral MR myocardial tagging. *Magn Reson Med* **51**(2): 237–242.

Ryf, S., Rutz, A. K., Boesiger, P., and Schwitter, J. (2006). Is post-systolic shortening a reliable indicator of myocardial viability? An MR tagging and late-enhancement study. *J Cardiovasc Magn Reson* **8**(3): 445–451.

Ryf, S., Schwitter, J., Spiegel, M. A., Rutz, A. K., Luechinger, R., Crelier, G. R., and Boesiger, P. (2005). Accelerated tagging for the assessment of left ventricular myocardial contraction under physical stress. *J Cardiovasc Magn Reson* **7**(4): 693–703.

Ryf, S., Spiegel, M. A., Gerber, M., and Boesiger, P. (2002). Myocardial tagging with 3D-CSPAMM. *J Magn Reson Imaging* **16**(3): 320–325.

Shetty, A. N. (1988). Suppression of radiofrequency interference in cardiac gated MRI: A simple design. *Magn Reson Med* **8**(1): 84–88.

Stuber, M., Fischer, S. E., Scheidegger, M. B., and Boesiger, P. (1999a). Toward high-resolution myocardial tagging. *Magn Reson Med* **41**(3): 639–643.

Stuber, M., Scheidegger, M. B., Fischer, S. E., Nagel, E., Steinemann, F., Hess, O. M., and Boesiger, P. (1999b). Alterations in the local myocardial motion pattern in patients suffering from pressure overload due to aortic stenosis. *Circulation* **100**(4): 361–368.

Stuber, M., Spiegel, M. A., Fischer, S. E., Scheidegger, M. B., Danias, P. G., Pedersen, E. M., and Boesiger, P. (1999c). Single breath-hold slice-following CSPAMM myocardial tagging. *MAGMA* **9**(1–2): 85–91.

Swoboda, P. P., Larghat, A., Zaman, A., Fairbairn, T. A., Motwani, M., Greenwood, J. P., and Plein, S. (2014). Reproducibility of myocardial strain and left ventricular twist measured using complementary spatial modulation of magnetization. *J Magn Reson Imaging* **39**(4): 887–894.

Taylor, A. M., Keegan, J., Jhooti, P., Gatehouse, P. D., Firmin, D. N., and Pennell, D. J. (2000). A comparison between segmented k-space FLASH and interleaved spiral MR coronary angiography sequences. *J Magn Reson Imaging* **11**(4): 394–400.

Uddin, A., Fairbairn, T. A., Swoboda, P. P., Kidambi, A., Motwani, M., Ripley, D. P., Musa, T. A., McDiarmid, A. K., Plein, S., and Greenwood, J. P. (2014). CMR evaluation of change in myocardial strain following transcatheter aortic valve implantation. *J Cardiovasc Magn Reson* **16**(Suppl 1): P260.

Wang, H., Kadbi, M., Kotys, M., Ersoy, M., Chatzimavroudis, G. P., Setser, R. M., Alshaher, M., Fischer, S. E., and Amini, A. A. (2011). Orthogonal CSPAMM (OCSPAMM) MR tagging for imaging ventricular wall motion. *Conf Proc IEEE Eng Med Biol Soc* **2011**: 535–538.

Zerhouni, E. A., Parish, D. M., Rogers, W. J., Yang, A., and Shapiro, E. P. (1988). Human heart: Tagging with MR imaging—a method for noninvasive assessment of myocardial motion. *Radiology* **169**(1): 59–63.

Zwanenburg, J. J., Kuijer, J. P., Marcus, J. T., and Heethaar, R. M. (2003). Steady-state free precession with myocardial tagging: CSPAMM in a single breathhold. *Magn Reson Med* **49**(4): 722–730.

12 Special Myocardial Tagging Patterns

Abbas Nasiraei-Moghaddam, PhD; Daniel B. Ennis, PhD; and El-Sayed H. Ibrahim, PhD

CONTENTS

LIST OF ABBREVIATIONS

Abbreviation	Meaning
1D	One dimensional
2D	Two dimensional
BPF	Band-pass filter
BW	Bandwidth
CAP	Cardiac Atlas Project
CHD	Congenital heart disease
CIRCOME	Circumferential compression encoding
CMP	Cardiomyopathy
CNR	Contrast-to-noise ratio
CRLB	Cramer–Rao lower bound
CRT	Complementary radial tagging
CSPAMM	Complementary SPAMM
CST	Central section theorem
CT	Computed tomography
DANTE	Delay alternating with nutations for tailored excitation
DC	Direct current
ECG	Electrocardiogram
FIR	Finite impulse response
FOV	Field of view
FT	Fourier transform
GRE	Gradient echo
HARP	Harmonic phase
LAX	Long axis
L-DANTE	Localized DANTE
LSE	Least-squares estimation
L-SPAMM	Localized SPAMM
LV	Left ventricle

M-SPAMM	Multirate SPAMM
PFT	Polar Fourier transform
RF	Radiofrequency
SAR	Specific absorption rate
SAX	Short axis
SE	Spin echo
SNR	Signal-to-noise ratio
SPAMM	Spatial modulation of magnetization
STAG	Striped tags
TE	Echo time
TR	Repetition time
VTAG	Variable-density tagging

12.1 INTRODUCTION

12.1.1 IMPORTANCE OF SPECIAL MYOCARDIAL TAGGING PATTERNS

MRI tagging is a unique technique that provides the opportunity to noninvasively tag the myocardium in a predefined pattern prior to imaging (Zerhouni et al. 1988, Axel and Dougherty 1989, Ibrahim 2011). The tagging pattern spatially labels the myocardium, and as the heart deforms, the tagging pattern deforms accordingly. The motion of the tagging pattern can be observed in the subsequently acquired time-resolved (cine) images. The full potential of this tool, however, is not fulfilled unless the tagging pattern matches both the myocardial geometry and motion. The geometry of healthy and unhealthy hearts are largely circular (in short-axis (SAX) views), where the underlying motion pattern can be compactly described in a polar coordinate system. Specifically, it is apparent in a SAX view that the heart grossly contracts in the circumferential direction and thickens in the radial direction.

Several attempts have been made to customize the tagging pattern to the gross geometry and motion pattern of the heart. Some investigators (Chandra and Yang 1996, Ikonomidou and Sergiadis 2002) tried to limit tagging only to the location of the heart itself in order to avoid obstructing nearby anatomical details. This so-called "localized" tagging technique has been reported for the localized spatial modulation of magnetization (L-SPAMM) and localized delay alternating with nutations for tailored excitation (L-DANTE) techniques (Chandra and Yang 1996). Other investigators (McVeigh and Bolster 1998) spatially customized the spacing of the parallel taglines. This approach takes advantage of the fact that during myocardial contraction some parts of the heart experience contraction, while others experience stretching. Therefore, by considering the expected deformation within different regions of the myocardium, a tagging pattern can be generated that best captures the underlying deformation. This type of tagging, which is called variable-density tagging (VTAG), is the second category of the special patterns that will be discussed in this chapter.

Other investigators described techniques for producing tagging spots, rather than lines (Kerwin and Prince 2000). This approach produces more discrete features to be tracked with less obstruction of the underlying anatomy. Another category of the tagging methods aims to closely match the gross geometry of the heart, which is described best in the pseudo-cylindrical coordinate system. This category of the tagging methods includes radial tagging (Zerhouni et al. 1988, Bosmans et al. 1996), ring-tags (Spiegel et al. 2003), and, most recently, circular tagging (Nasiraei-Moghaddam and Finn 2014). These methods closely match the annular geometry of the heart and directly measure the polar deformation of the heart as it contracts and relaxes.

The main challenges for producing the aforementioned special myocardial tagging patterns are the quality of the tagging pattern and the efficiency of the corresponding sequence (i.e., the time required to generate an acceptable pattern). In fact, these two challenges are very closely related. Creating an ideal tagging pattern may require a lengthy combination of radiofrequency (RF) pulses and gradients, which last for tens of milliseconds. Therefore, a compromise has to be made so that the tagging pattern is acceptable and can be generated in a short period of time. Typically, it is required to complete the generation of the tagging pattern in a few milliseconds. For capturing myocardial motion, this usually means generating the tagging pattern immediately after the detection of the R-wave of the electrocardiogram (ECG) signal and before the onset of any measurable heart motion.

Tailoring the desirable tagging pattern can be easily understood through selective excitation, wherein the location of the tagged (i.e., saturated) spins is selectively controlled. This is the approach that was adopted for first implementation of cardiac tagging, which generated radial tags (Zerhouni et al. 1988). A similar approach has been also used to generate ring-tags (Spiegel et al. 2003). This approach generates the tagging pattern at a single discrete curved line without exciting or saturating nearby structures. Repeating this process for each

spatial location generates additional taglines. The efficiency of this approach, however, is poor as it can only generate a very limited number of tags sequentially.

Methods that impart a broader excitation and simultaneously tag multiple regions result in higher efficiency, which means that more taglines can be generated in a shorter preparation time. Nevertheless, this efficiency is achieved at the cost of more complex sequence design. Therefore, depending on the application at hand, we may trade simplicity for efficiency if required.

12.1.2 Chapter Layout

In this chapter, we explore and compare different techniques for generating specialized myocardial tagging patterns. The chapter starts by briefly reviewing basics of magnetization excitation as well as basic tagging techniques: SPAMM (Axel and Dougherty 1989), DANTE (Mosher and Smith 1990), and complementary SPAMM (CSPAMM) (Fischer et al. 1993), which will serve as the starting point toward covering nonconventional tagging patterns in the rest of the chapter. The chapter then covers localized and variable-density tagging. The localized tagging techniques covered in the chapter include tagging with multispectral RF pulses (McVeigh and Zerhouni 1991), L-SPAMM (Chandra and Yang 1996, Ikonomidou and Sergiadis 2002), and L-DANTE (Chandra and Yang 1996). For variable-density tagging (McVeigh and Bolster 1998), the chapter discusses the technique's importance and implementation, mathematical analysis, and pulse sequence design. The weighted path k-space analysis approach (Kerwin and Prince 2000) is then described along with its implementation in the cases of SPAMM and variable-density tagging. The multirate SPAMM (M-SPAMM) technique (Ikonomidou and Sergiadis 2003) is then discussed at the end of this section. Techniques for creating optimal tags profile and thickness are then discussed.

The chapter then reviews the first implementation of radial tagging as presented by Zerhouni et al. (1988), followed by the striped tags (STAG) technique (Bolster et al. 1990). The RingTag technique (Spiegel et al. 2003) is then described along with some technical remarks. The next section provides an overview of polar tagging (Nasiraei-Moghaddam and Finn 2014), including its advantages, limitations, and examples of different clinical applications. This part of the chapter addresses the two components of polar tagging: circular tagging and radial tagging. The circular tagging section starts by discussing the initial approach to create this tagline pattern, followed by description of the polar tagging basic idea and detailed mathematical analysis of the magnetization excitation process. This section also discusses the technique's implementation and validation, as well as its different versions, including nonuniform circular tagging, inline circular density maps, real-time circular tagging, polar harmonic phase (polar HARP), and high-resolution circular tagging. The radial tagging section describes the approach for creating this tagging pattern from the polar tagging perspective. The circumferential compression encoding (CIRCOME) technique (Moghaddam and Finn 2008a) is then described for measuring circumferential strain from radially tagged images. The CIRCOME technique's basic idea, implementation, performance, and validation are discussed. The creation of nonuniform radial tagging pattern is also discussed, followed by discussion of the optimal radial tag profile and the complementary radial tagging (CRT) technique (Wang et al. 2015). It should be noted that almost all clinical applications of special tagging patterns are discussed in its chapter; not in the clinical application chapters in the end of the book. This is related to the novelty of these techniques and their current limited implementation, as described later in the chapter, which make it more appropriate to group the technique's applications in this chapter rather than merging them with the more established techniques in Chapters 9 and 10 of *Heart Mechanics: Magnetic Resonance Imaging—Advanced Techniques, Clinical Applications, and Future Trends.*

12.2 BASICS OF MAGNETIZATION EXCITATION

Neglecting the relaxation effect, the Bloch equation in the rotating frame of reference can be written in the matrix form as

$$\begin{bmatrix} \dot{M}_x \\ \dot{M}_y \\ \dot{M}_z \end{bmatrix} = \gamma \begin{bmatrix} 0 & \vec{G}\cdot\vec{r} & -B_{1y} \\ -\vec{G}\cdot\vec{r} & 0 & B_{1x} \\ B_{1y} & -B_{1x} & 0 \end{bmatrix} \begin{bmatrix} M_x \\ M_y \\ M_z \end{bmatrix}, \quad (12.1)$$

where

- M_x, M_y, and M_z are the magnetization components in the three physical directions
- $\dot{M}_x$, $\dot{M}_y$, and $\dot{M}_z$ are the magnetization derivatives with respect to time
- γ is the gyromagnetic ratio
- $\vec{r}$ is the position of the spin relative to the magnet isocenter
- $\vec{G}$ is the applied gradient field vector
- B_{1x} and B_{1y} are the components of the applied RF field

Both the gradient and RF field can be functions of time. Equation 12.1 describes how the bulk observable magnetization vector evolves with time in a nonlinear fashion. Analytic solutions exist for simple cases, but Bloch equation simulation may be required to understand the magnetizations history and final state.

It has been shown that for small tip angles, where the magnitude of M_z is almost constant, the amount of excitation can be estimated from the Fourier transform (FT) of the B_1 field (Pauly et al. 2011) as follows:

$$M_{xy}(\vec{r}) \approx i\gamma M_0 \int_0^T B_1(t) e^{i\vec{r}\cdot\vec{k}(t)} dt, \quad (12.2)$$

where the spatial frequency, $\vec{k}$, is defined as

$$\vec{k}(t) = -\gamma \int_t^T \vec{G}(s) ds. \quad (12.3)$$

According to this definition, $\vec{k}(t)$ is the location of the spin system in the k-space at time t, where the gradient field drives the system to the k-space center at the end of the pulse period ($t = T$). In other words, as a consequence of the changing gradient fields and B_1 modulation during the excitation, the spins can be excited at specific spatial frequencies in the k-space to generate the desired tagging pattern. The FT of this k-space characterizes the resultant M_{xy}, which is closely related to M_z, giving rise to the tagging pattern in the acquired image. Inversely, to generate a specific tagging pattern, we should first determine the desired M_z, and consequently M_{xy}, then apply inverse FT to it in order to get the values for the excitation k-space. Subsequently, we can design the tagging sequence (amplitude and timing of the gradient and RF pulses) in a way that fills up the k-space with the calculated values. The method for designing the sequence, however, remains challenging due to the nonlinearity of the Bloch equations, especially if the small tip angle approximation is not applicable.

As will be shown in this chapter, a good portion of the sequence development of specialized tagging patterns is based on the principles of k-space excitation. It is important, however, to consider two issues when utilizing this technique. First, we should note that the small tip angle approximation is based on the "quasi-static" assumption since the rate of change of M_z is assumed to be negligible compared to that of M_{xy}. Since the quasi-static condition should not be assumed for all specialized tagging pattern sequences, this approximation is not always appropriate. The second issue with this technique is the difference between M_{xy} and M_z, as the FT method relates M_{xy} to the B_1, while the tagging preparation concerns M_z.

12.3 BRIEF REVIEW OF BASIC TAGGING SEQUENCES*

12.3.1 SPAMM

Spatial modulation of magnetization (SPAMM) has been widely used for myocardial tagging since its invention in the late 1980s until the current day (Axel and Dougherty 1989). In its simplest form, SPAMM is based on wrapping the magnetization in a periodic fashion through space by applying only two equal-strength nonselective RF pulses separated by a "wrapping" gradient (Figure 12.1). The first RF pulse tips the magnetization into the transverse plane where all spins are initially in-phase. A gradient pulse immediately follows along the desired tagging direction. This gradient has the effect of wrapping (modulating) the transverse magnetization in a sinusoidal fashion along the gradient direction through incremental phase shifting of the spins in this direction. It should be noted that the larger the gradient pulse, the higher the tagging frequency. The modulated magnetization is then restored back to the longitudinal position by the second tagging RF pulse. In its simplest form, 90° RF

---
* Based on similar sections in a review article by the senior author: Ibrahim, El-S.H. (2011). Myocardial tagging by cardiovascular magnetic resonance: Evolution of techniques–pulse sequences, analysis algorithms, and applications. *J Cardiovasc Magn Reson* **13**: 36.

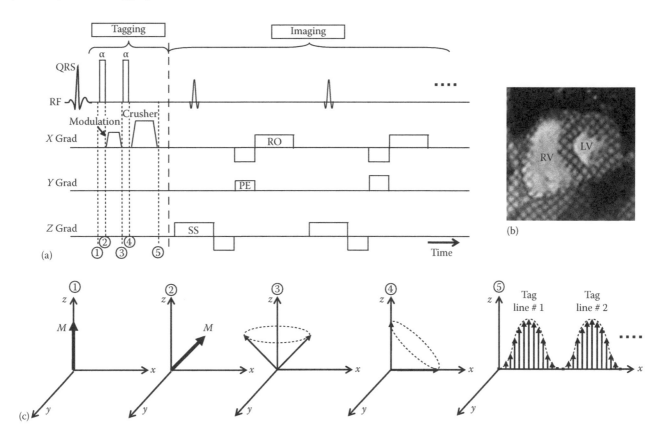

FIGURE 12.1 SPAMM tagging. (a) SPAMM pulse sequence. The tagging part consists of only two nonselective RF pulses (usually, 90° each), separated by the tagging gradient in the tagging direction, and followed by a large crusher gradient. The imaging part shows conventional Cartesian k-space acquisition (RO = readout, PE = phase encoding, SS = slice selection). This sequence creates parallel taglines orthogonal to the x-axis. (b) Example of a SPAMM grid-tagged image showing left ventricle (LV) and right ventricle (RV). Note that this grid pattern needs the application of an extra tagging stage (in the orthogonal direction) next to the first one and before imaging takes place. Note also that the dark myocardium between the taglines is not completely black due to longitudinal relaxation. (c) Illustration of spins evolution during different time points in the tagging stage as follows: immediately before tagging application (time point 1), the magnetization (M) is at equilibrium state in the longitudinal direction. Immediately after the application of the first RF pulse (time point 2), the magnetization is tipped into the transverse direction by certain flip angle (45° RF pulses are assumed here for illustration). The tagging gradient then follows, which disperses the spins in the tagging direction (x-direction in this case), such that by the end of the gradient pulse (time point 3), the spins are modulated by incremental phase shifts along the x-axis (the figure shows all vectors emerging from the origin just for simplicity). The second tagging RF pulse tips the resulting modulated magnetization by another 45° into the transverse direction to result in spins modulated as shown at time point (4). A crusher gradient immediately follows to eliminate transverse magnetization components, leaving only the longitudinal magnetization, which show a sinusoidal pattern along the x-axis with values ranging from 0 to M. (Reproduced from Ibrahim, El-S.H., *J. Cardiovasc. Magn. Reson.*, 13, 36, 2011.)

pulses are used to modulate the whole magnetization, that is, use the whole dynamic range of magnetization modulation from $-M_0$ to $+M_0$ (assuming the magnetization is at thermal equilibrium before tagging). Alternatively, RF pulses with <90° flip angles could be used for partial modulation, that is, leaving part of the longitudinal magnetization intact for later use. A large "spoiler" or "crusher" gradient follows the second RF pulse to eliminate any remaining transverse magnetization before image acquisition. If grid tagging is required, a second tagging module (RF pulse, modulating gradient, RF pulse, spoiler gradient) immediately follows the first module with the modulating gradient applied in the direction orthogonal to that in the first module. Data acquisition (the imaging stage) occurs at a later time point to explore tissue deformation. In its simplest form, the imaging stage consists of a series of slice-selective RF pulses, each followed

by phase-encoding and readout gradients for k-space filling (Cartesian k-space acquisition). It should be understood that the imaging stage is separate from the tagging stage and that the tagging pattern experiences deformation based on tissue displacement during the time in between the two stages (tagging and imaging).

12.3.2 DANTE

One year after SPAMM was introduced, Mosher and Smith (1990) presented a similar tagging technique, called delay alternating with nutations for tailored excitation (DANTE), which generates a high-density pattern of thin tags. The technique applies a train of RF pulses in the presence of a continuous gradient to create taglines in the gradient direction (Figure 12.2). The flexibility of adjusting the tags spacing

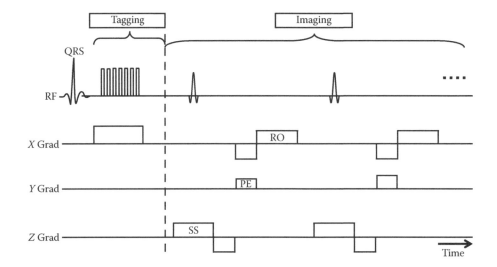

FIGURE 12.2   DANTE pulse sequence. The tagging module contains a series of hard (nonselective) RF pulses run simultaneously with an accompanying gradient in the tagging direction (1D tagging is shown here). The imaging stage follows after tagging. The figure shows conventional Cartesian k-space acquisition. PE, phase encoding; RO, readout; SS, slice following. (Reproduced from Ibrahim, El-S.H., *J. Cardiovasc. Magn. Reson.*, 13, 36, 2011.)

and thickness are added advantages of the DANTE sequence. DANTE tagging underwent some developments. In 1995, Tsekos et al. (1995) developed an improved DANTE technique with B_1-insensitive adiabatic inversion sequence to generate tags with uniform contrast across the myocardium. Later, Salido et al. (2002) studied the effects of phase-encoding order and segments interpolation on the quality and accuracy of the DANTE tags. In the same year, Wu et al. (2002) developed a DANTE sequence using sinc-modulated RF pulse train in the presence of constant gradient to improve the tags profile, where the proposed technique produced rectangular tags profile and offered easier control of the tag's width-to-separation ratio.

12.3.3 CSPAMM

One limitation of the SPAMM and DANTE tagging techniques is the fading of the tagging pattern through the cardiac cycle due to longitudinal magnetization relaxation. The loss of tagging contrast toward the end of the cardiac cycle results in unrecognizable tagging pattern, which precludes the analysis of diastolic heart phases. It was not until 1993 when Fischer et al. (1993) introduced an improved tagging technique, named complementary SPAMM (CSPAMM), to resolve this problem. To grasp the idea behind CSPAMM, it is necessary to understand the magnetization evolution with time in the CSPAMM tagging sequence (Figure 12.3). Immediately after applying the tagging sequence, the whole magnetization is tagged or modulated (90° RF pulses are assumed) and stored in the longitudinal direction. With time, the magnetization experiences longitudinal relaxation, trying to reach the equilibrium state. This has two effects on the stored tagging pattern: (1) introducing a growing nontagged magnetization offset (we call it here the DC component,

borrowing the term "direct current (DC)" from electrical engineering) and (2) reducing the magnitude of the tagged component (the peak-to-peak difference of the sinusoidal tagged magnetization, called alternating current (AC) component). Thus, during the imaging stage, the excited magnetization has two components: tagged (or AC) and non-tagged (or DC), with the DC overhead impairing the visibility of the (already fading) tagged component. It should be noted that the multiple application of the imaging RF pulses also results in reducing the tagged magnetization component (each RF pulse consumes a part of the tagged magnetization stored in the longitudinal direction).

The solution provided in CSPAMM consists of two parts: (1) eliminating the nontagged (DC) magnetization and (2) enhancing the tagged magnetization to counteract the fading process. To eliminate the nontagged magnetization, two consecutive scans are acquired with exactly the same parameters, except for the polarity of one of the tagging RF pulses. The 90°/90° RF pulses in the first scan modulate the magnetization with a positive sinusoidal pattern, whereas the 90°/−90° RF pulses in the second scan produce a negative sinusoidal pattern. It should be noted that the DC magnetization component is the same at corresponding time points in both scans. Therefore, the overhead DC magnetization can be eliminated by simply subtracting the images in the first scan from the corresponding images (at the same heart phases) in the second scan. This subtraction also has the effect of improving the image signal-to-noise ratio (SNR) by 40% as two acquisitions with independent noise terms are added together. To resolve the second problem of the fading tagging contrast, the concept of "ramped flip angle" is implemented. Basically, during the imaging stage, the flip angles of the RF pulses determine how much magnetization is tipped into the transverse plane for data acquisition. Thus, increasing the imaging flip angles

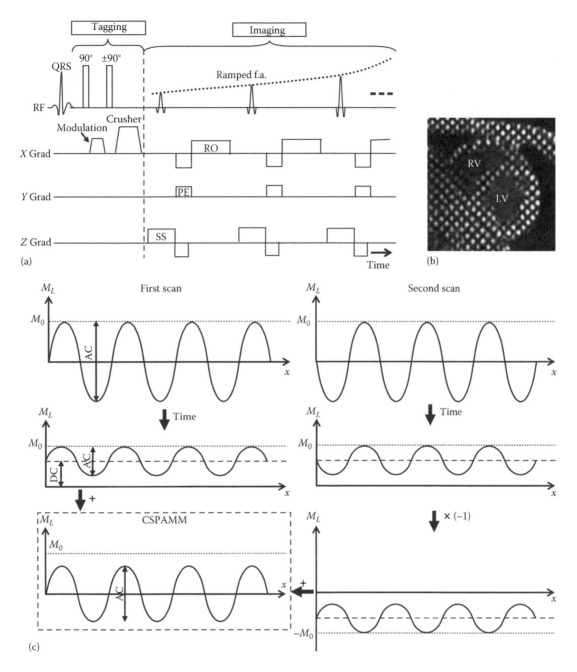

FIGURE 12.3   CSPAMM tagging. Pulse sequence and magnetization analysis. (a) CSPAMM pulse sequence. The sequence includes consecutive running of two SPAMM sequences, with the polarity of the second tagging RF pulse changed in the second SPAMM acquisition. Notice also the ramped flip angles of the imaging RF pulses to compensate for tags fading. (b) Example of a CSPAMM grid-tagged image. Notice that nontagged tissues appear black due to the elimination of the offset DC signal. (c) The concept of magnetization subtraction in CSPAMM. Two scans are acquired as shown in the pulse sequence, which results in positive and negative sinusoidal tagging patterns from the first and second scans, respectively. With time, the tagging patterns experience longitudinal relaxation, trying to reach equilibrium (M_0). This relaxation has two effects on the tagging pattern: the peak-to-peak (AC) magnitude is decreased; and the tagging pattern starts to have a nonzero average (DC component added to it). However, the DC component is the same in both SPAMM scans. Thus, at any time point, when the two acquired images are subtracted, the DC component cancels out and the peak-to-peak magnitude of the tagged component is doubled. (Reproduced from Ibrahim, El-S.H., *J. Cardiovasc. Magn. Reson.*, 13, 36, 2011.)

through the cardiac cycle compensates for the fading tagging contrast because more percentage of the available longitudinal magnetization is used at later heart phases. In their work, Fischer et al. (1993) introduced a recursive formula for calculating the imaging flip angles based on the tissue T_1 time constant and flip angle of the next RF pulse.

12.4 LOCALIZED TAGGING

12.4.1 TAGGING WITH MULTISPECTRAL RF PULSES

The invention of SPAMM (Axel and Dougherty 1989), shortly after the tagging concept was presented by Zerhouni et al. (1988), introduced the concept of motion encoding through the generation of nonselective parallel tagging planes. This tagging concept, which is now widely spread, generates parallel saturated planes throughout the object, usually in a manner that intersects the imaging plane perpendicularly. While tagging is a powerful tool for deformation analysis of moving objects, it has a limited benefit within the stationary regions and, in fact, it can obscure some anatomical structures. One objective of specialized tagging patterns is therefore to limit the tags to the region of interest while retain the other advantages of the tagging method. One approach to achieve this goal has been described by McVeigh and Zerhouni (1991), who used a multispectral RF pulses in the tagging sequence, as shown in Figure 12.4, to generate orthogonal saturation bands that tag only a small region of the heart, albeit still saturating some tissues distant from the heart. As pointed out by Chandra and Yang (1996), such localized tagging techniques may have other advantages too. For example, these techniques would be useful for optimizing the tagging contrast locally without using excessive RF power or losing anatomical information elsewhere in the imaging plane, which is useful in some applications, for example, measuring small motion or mapping susceptibility differences.

12.4.2 LOCALIZED SPAMM (L-SPAMM)

In 1996, Chandra and Yang (1996) suggested a variant of the SPAMM technique, called localized SPAMM (L-SPAMM), in which the tagging RF pulses are slice-selective, thereby generating the tagging pattern only within a selected part of the imaging plane. As shown in Figure 12.5, the implementation of this tagging pattern requires band-limited RF pulses (which are longer than the nonselective hard pulses used in conventional SPAMM) applied simultaneously with a readout gradient field to excite only the desired region in a certain direction (shown for the readout direction in Figure 12.5). The choice of the location and width of the region to be tagged are determined by the frequency of the RF pulses and magnitude of the gradient field, respectively. The undesirable effect of selective excitation is the phase dispersion of the excited spins. To counteract this effect, either a preemphasis or a refocusing gradient is applied for each excitation. This, however, further prolongs the tagging preparation sequence.

Figures 12.6 and 12.7 show numerical simulation and phantom experiment results of the L-SPAMM technique. The suggested tagging sequence requires about 15 ms in its simplest form, whereas conventional SPAMM tags can be generated in 3–5 ms. In a more complex form, more than one region of interest can be selected for tagging, and therefore longer preparation duration might be needed. Nevertheless, long preparation times are not desirable for myocardial tagging because of the rapid heart motion at early systole.

12.4.3 LOCALIZED DANTE (L-DANTE)

Chandra and Yang (1996) proposed a localized DANTE (L-DANTE) sequence (Figure 12.8), which is identical to the conventional DANTE tagging sequence, except that it uses longer RF pulses. The long RF pulses have the effect of imposing sinc modulation in the frequency space, which

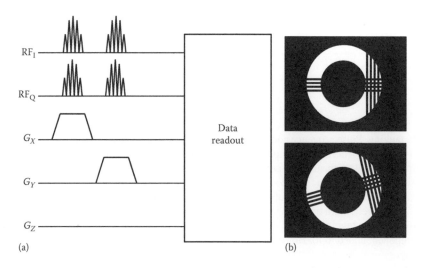

FIGURE 12.4 Tagging with multispectral RF pulses. (a) Pulse sequence. The sinc-Hamming envelope of the tagging pulses is modulated with discrete sideband frequencies to simultaneously tag a set of parallel planes. Two multispectral pulses with orthogonal gradients are shown. (b) An illustration of the resulting 4×4 tagging grid in a rotating phantom.

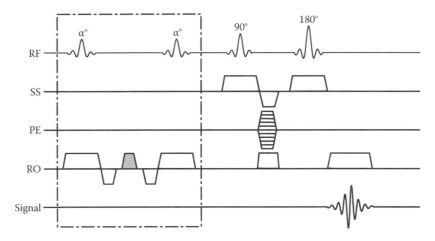

FIGURE 12.5 Localized SPAMM pulse sequence. The pulse sequence is similar to conventional 1-1 SPAMM, except that the tagging RF pulses are slice-selective, which are run with associated gradients. The selective pulses modulate the spins in a predefined excitation area within the imaging plane, which is determined by the bandwidth of the RF pulse and strength of the gradient.

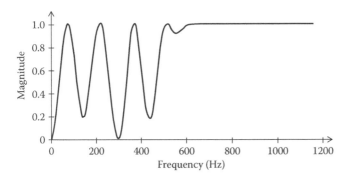

FIGURE 12.6 Simulated frequency response of the longitudinal magnetization generated by localized SPAMM using 2 sinc functions.

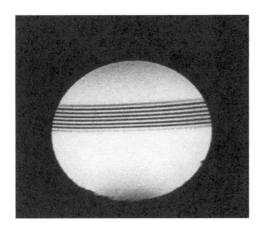

FIGURE 12.7 Localized SPAMM-tagged phantom image. The modulation parameters are as described in Figure 12.6. (Reproduced from Chandra, S. and Yang, Y., *J. Magn. Reson. B*, 111(3), 285, 1996. With permission.)

confines the excitation within a predefined region in the imaging plane. In other words, the spins receive the full power needed to achieve the desired flip angle only at the fundamental frequency, while the flip angles are modulated by the sinc function at all other harmonics. Besides the sinc function, several other functions can be imposed on DANTE excitation, with variations in power distribution between the excitation harmonics. Therefore, the developed L-DANTE sequence can be described as an intermediate case between conventional DANTE and single-frequency continuous wave excitation. The duration of the L-DANTE tagging preparation period is longer than that in SPAMM, but still acceptable for cardiac tagging. Figures 12.9 and 12.10 show numerical simulation and phantom experiment results of the L-DANTE technique.

12.4.4 Localized SPAMM: Rotational Approach

In 2002, Ikonomidou and Sergiadis (2002) presented a mathematical analysis of 1-1 SPAMM tagging using the rotational operator (Le Roux 1988, Shinnar et al. 1989, Pauly et al. 1991). In this approach, the effect of the RF pulse and gradient field on spin rotation is described as follows:

$$\begin{bmatrix} M_{xy}^+ \\ \bar{M}_{xy}^+ \\ M_z^+ \end{bmatrix} = \begin{bmatrix} (\bar{\alpha})^2 & -\beta^2 & 2\bar{\alpha}\beta \\ -(\bar{\beta})^2 & \alpha^2 & 2\alpha\bar{\beta} \\ -\bar{\alpha}\bar{\beta} & -\alpha\beta & \alpha\bar{\alpha} - \beta\bar{\beta} \end{bmatrix} \begin{bmatrix} M_{xy}^- \\ \bar{M}_{xy}^- \\ M_z^- \end{bmatrix}, \quad (12.4)$$

where

$$M_{xy} = M_x + i M_y, \quad (12.5)$$

and the negative and positive superscripts denote the state of the magnetization before and after rotation, respectively, and α and β are the Cayley–Klein parameters that

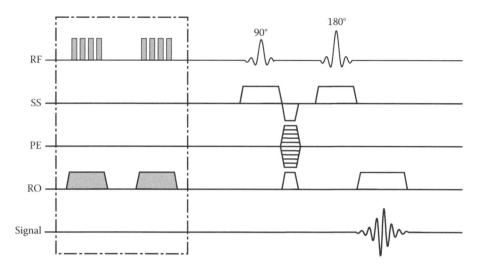

FIGURE 12.8 Localized DANTE pulse sequence. The sequence is similar to the conventional DANTE sequence, except that the RF pulses are slightly longer. Two RF trains are shown to illustrate the possibility of tagging two different regions in the image plane. Spin echo imaging is shown in this sequence.

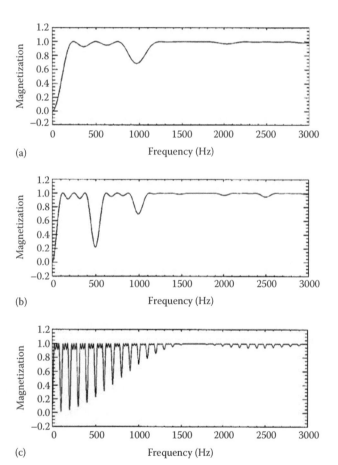

FIGURE 12.9 Simulated frequency response of the longitudinal magnetization generated by localized DANTE tagging. The figure shows implementation of (a) 1, (b) 2, and (c) 10 ms interpulse delay. The pulse width = 600 μs; number of RF pulses = 4; and DANTE gradient strength =1.0 Gauss/cm. (Reproduced from Chandra, S. and Yang, Y., *J. Magn. Reson. B*, 111(3), 285, 1996. With permission.)

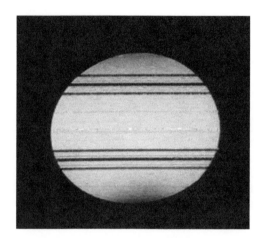

FIGURE 12.10 Localized DANTE-tagged phantom image. The tagging parameters are the same as described in Figure 12.9. (Reproduced from Chandra, S. and Yang, Y., *J. Magn. Reson. B*, 111(3), 285, 1996. With permission.)

characterize the rotation (the bar above the variable represents its complex conjugate). These two parameters are calculated from two polynomials A and B of order N as follows:

$$\alpha = z^{N/2}A(z^{-1}),$$ (12.6)

$$\beta = z^{N/2}B(z^{-1}),$$ (12.7)

$$z = \exp(i\gamma G \Delta t),$$ (12.8)

where

γ is the gyromagnetic ratio
G is the gradient's amplitude in the x-direction
x is the spin's position along the gradient's axis
Δt is the analysis time step
z represents the rotation during each time step due to the presence of the gradient

After the second pulse, the longitudinal magnetization (i.e., $M_z^{(2)}$), can be expressed as

$$M_z^{(2)} = -\bar{\alpha}\bar{\beta}M_{xy}^{(1)+} - \alpha\beta\overline{M_{xy}^{(1)+}} + \left(\alpha\bar{\alpha} - \beta\bar{\beta}\right)M_z^{(1)}$$

$$= -2\mathrm{Re}\left[\bar{\alpha}\bar{\beta}M_{xy}^{(1)+}\right] + \left(|A|^2 - |B|^2\right)M_z^{(1)}$$

$$= -4|A|^2|B|^2 M_0 \,\mathrm{Re}[\exp(-i\gamma GxT - 2i\,\mathrm{Arg}(A))z^{-n}]$$

$$+ \left(|A|^2 - |B|^2\right)^2 M_0$$

$$= -4|A|^2|B|^2 M_0 \,\cos[\gamma Gx\,(n\Delta t + T) + 2\,\mathrm{Arg}(A)]$$

$$+ \left(|A|^2 - |B|^2\right)^2 M_0 \qquad (12.9)$$

where

T is the duration of the gradient pulse
Re and Arg represent the real part and angle of the complex variable, respectively

Substituting

$$|A| = \frac{\cos\pi}{8}, \qquad (12.10)$$

$$|B| = \frac{\sin\pi}{8} \qquad (12.11)$$

for the regions to be modulated, and having

$$|A| = 1, \qquad (12.12)$$

$$|B| = 0 \qquad (12.13)$$

for the regions not to be modulated results in a $\pi/4$ flip angle in the tagged regions (for a $\pi/4 - \pi/4$ tagging sequence) and a zero flip angle elsewhere. Assuming a constant gradient throughout the tagging sequence, we get an L-SPAMM pattern (Ikonomidou and Sergiadis 2002):

$$M_z^{(2)} \cong \begin{cases} \left(-\sin^2\left(\pi/4\right)\cos\left[\gamma Gx\left(T + T_P\right)\right]\right. \\ \left. + \cos^2\left(\pi/4\right)\right)M_0; \text{ inside ROI} \\ M_0; \text{ outside ROI} \end{cases} \qquad (12.14)$$

where T_P is the duration of the RF pulse. The key concept here is that the phase component is canceled out in the case of two identical pulses; therefore, the preemphasis and refocusing gradients are not needed, which allows for minimizing the time duration of the tagging preparation sequence. A sample RF pulse (with a constant gradient) along with its excitation profile and sample image are shown in Figure 12.11. In this example, the total tag preparation time is 2.24 ms, which

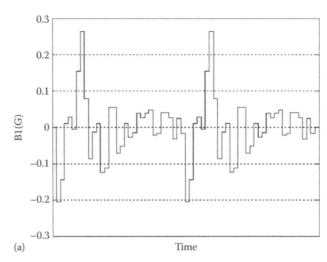

(a)

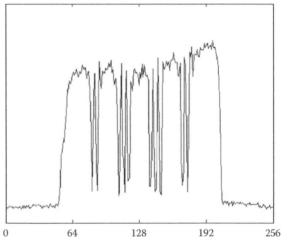

(b)

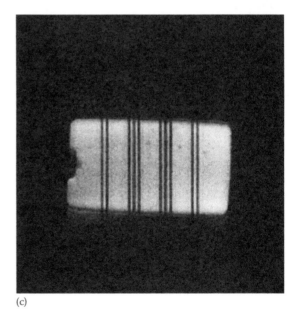

(c)

FIGURE 12.11 The rotational approach of localized SPAMM. (a) Excitation pulse shape. (b) Experimental tagging profile produced using the pulse in (a). (c) Phantom image acquired with the pulse in (a). (Reproduced from Ikonomidou, V.N. and Sergiadis, G.D., *J. Magn. Reson.*, 157(2), 218, 2002. With permission.)

creates localized tagging at four separate locations (two independent regions and a mirror-symmetric counterpart). This approach not only removes the refocusing gradients from the sequence but also allows for using nonrefocusable pulses, for example, minimum-phase and maximum-phase pulses (Ikonomidou and Sergiadis 2002).

In the same paper, Ikonomidou and Sergiadis (2002) also explained how to move the entire tagging pattern by adding a phase difference to each of the pulses, thereby permitting flexible positioning of the taglines. In summary, the principal contribution of the rotational analysis is the demonstration of the conditions under which a uniform gradient field could be used to generate spatially localized tags. This effect is similar to the variable-density tagging (VTAG) pattern approach (McVeigh and Bolster 1998), described in the following section.

12.5 VARIABLE-DENSITY TAGGING

12.5.1 IMPORTANCE AND IMPLEMENTATION

The cardiac geometry and motion are most easily described and measured in the polar coordinate system. Nevertheless, Cartesian tagging methods, for example, SPAMM, have been used more widely due to the relative simplicity with which they can be generated. An interesting consequence of the heart's polar geometry and deformation is that the appearance of the uniformly spaced Cartesian tags becomes heterogeneously deformed at end-systole. Specifically, in some regions, the parallel taglines get closer together as a result of myocardial circumferential shortening (negative circumferential strain), whereas in other regions, they get further separated because of wall thickening (positive radial strain).

McVeigh and Bolster (1998) showed that the distance between the taglines during the cardiac cycle can be chosen to match the geometry and contraction of the heart in order to resolve myocardial deformation more precisely. For example, increased tag spacing may result in too few taglines across the myocardial wall, which negatively affects precise measurement of radial wall thickening. If, however, the taglines are too closely spaced, then they appear blurred during contraction as the increased tag density exceeds the spatial resolution capability for clearly identifying individual taglines. Because some part of the heart thickens in one Cartesian direction, while another part contracts in the same direction (e.g., during systole, the lateral and septal left ventricle (LV) walls experience thickening and contraction in the horizontal and vertical directions, respectively, while the anterior and inferior walls experience contraction and thickening in the horizontal and vertical directions, respectively), it is not possible to obtain a uniform tagline separation pattern that is optimally sensitive to both circumferential shortening and radial thickening. McVeigh and Bolster (1998) suggested the VTAG technique to address and reduce this shortcoming.

The VTAG technique customizes the separation of adjacent parallel taglines to match the expected motion of specific

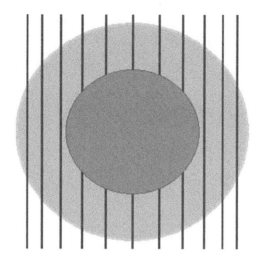

FIGURE 12.12 Variable-density tagging (VTAG) pattern. The figure shows 11 vertical taglines placed across the LV. The tagline separation in the upper and lower parts of the heart (where circumferential strain will cause myocardial contraction) is larger than those in the right and left parts (where radial strain will cause myocardial thickening). This variable tagging pattern can be adjusted based on individual heart dimensions.

myocardial regions. In regions where the tagline separation increases during systole (radial thickening), the taglines are placed closer to each other at the beginning of the cardiac cycle. Alternatively, in regions where the tagline separation decreases during systole (circumferential shortening), the taglines are placed farther apart so they remain detectable after contraction. Figure 12.12 schematically illustrates one such period of the tagline positions overlaid on a SAX view of the myocardium. Practically, a tagline separation of at least 4 pixels is required for accurate resolving of the tags location (McVeigh and Gao 1994), although this depends on the slice thickness. Accordingly, the initial tag separation in the circumferential direction (anterior and inferior regions) must be chosen large enough (e.g., 5–6 pixels apart), such that they maintain a tag separation of at least 4 pixels at end-systole. On the other hand, the initial tag separation in the radial direction (septal and lateral regions) can be set at 4 pixels because the tag separation will increase through systole. The general approach in VTAG is to extend the SPAMM technique to generate a tagging pattern with a much longer period that consists of several, almost a dozen of, spatially dependent tags.

12.5.2 MATHEMATICAL ANALYSIS

Based on the FT concept, explained briefly in the beginning of the chapter, the tagging pattern and k-space excitation are related by FT. The first step in VTAG design is to generate the Fourier coefficients of the tagging pattern and then use these coefficients to construct the corresponding RF pulse train. Let us assume that the desired tagging pattern is represented by the convolution $f(x) * g(x)$, where $g(x)$ is the tag profile and $f(x)$ is a symmetric distribution of impulses, given by (McVeigh and Bolster 1998)

$$f(x) = \delta(x) + \sum_{j=1}^{J}\left(\delta(x-x_j) + \delta(x+x_j)\right), \quad (12.15)$$

where $\delta(x)$ is the delta Dirac impulse function. If the width of the desired tagging pattern $f(x)$ is $2L$, then the periodic representation of $f(x)$ can be written as

$$\tilde{f}(x+m2L) = f(x), \quad (12.16)$$

where m is an integer and $-L < x \leq L$. The resulting Fourier series coefficients for the periodic function $\tilde{f}(x)$ are

$$a_0 = \frac{1}{2L}(2J+1), \quad (12.17)$$

$$a_n = \frac{1}{L}\left(1 + 2\sum_{j=1}^{J}\cos\left(\frac{n\pi x_j}{L}\right)\right), \quad n=1,\ldots,\infty, \quad (12.18)$$

where

x_j is the position of an individual tagline with respect to the center of the tagging pattern

L is the length of one side of the symmetric tagging pattern

The Fourier series for $\tilde{f}(x)$ can then be written as

$$\tilde{f}(x) = a_0 + \sum_{n=1}^{\infty} a_n \cos\left(\frac{n\pi x}{L}\right), \quad (12.19)$$

where the coefficients a_n are the relative amplitudes used in the RF pulse train.

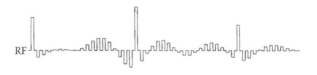

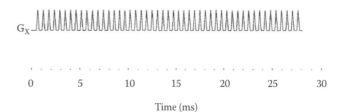

FIGURE 12.13 Example of a VTAG pulse sequence. The sequence consists of 50 RF pulses, which generate tag separations of 5,4,3,3,3,3 pixels. (Reproduced from McVeigh, E.R. and Bolster, B.D., *Magn. Reson. Med.*, 39(4), 657, 1998. With permission.)

12.5.3 PULSE SEQUENCE

Figure 12.13 shows a sample pulse sequence used for VTAG (McVeigh and Bolster 1998). The signal in the first row shows the RF pulse, while the second row represents the gradient field, which is zero whenever the RF pulse is not zero. Therefore, the effect of each small subpulse in the RF pulse train is essentially concentrated at one point in the k-space as a delta function. Figure 12.14 shows SAX images acquired with conventional tagging and VTAG techniques.

As is apparent from Figure 12.13, dozens of RF and gradient subpulses are required to generate the VTAG pattern, which results in a long tag preparation duration as a consequence of the limited slew rate of the gradient fields. Therefore, about 20–30 ms is needed to generate the VTAG pattern, which is much longer than the time required for

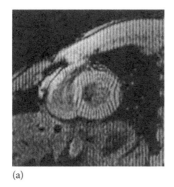
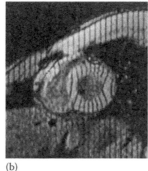
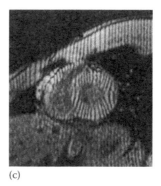

(a)   (b)   (c)

FIGURE 12.14 A comparison between a VTAG image and two standard line tagged images. (a) The VTAG image has a 5-pixels tag separation between the center tagline and its closest neighbors, a 4-pixels separation for the next tag, and 3-pixels for the remaining tags. (b) Standard tagged image with fixed 5-pixels tag separation does not sample the radial thickening (septal and lateral regions) with high spatial resolution. (c) Standard tagged image with fixed 3-pixels tag separation does not resolve the individual tags in the circumferential shortening (anterior and inferior) regions. The VTAG pattern properly samples all regions in the same image. (Reproduced from McVeigh, E.R. and Bolster, B.D., *Magn. Reson. Med.*, 39(4), 657, 1998. With permission.)

generating a constant-separation tagging pattern. One idea to reduce the long RF pulse train is through removing the low amplitude pulses and combining adjacent gradient pulses into a single pulse. Also, the implementation of the sequence on scanners with enhanced gradient systems would reduce the duration of the tag preparation sequence.

12.5.4 K-Space Analysis of MRI Tagging

12.5.4.1 Weighted Path

In 2000, Kerwin and Prince (2000) presented a method for k-space analysis of MRI tagging through relating the tagging pulse sequence directly to the residual pattern of the longitudinal magnetization caused by the pulse sequence. This analysis is an extension of the aforementioned FT analysis for calculation of the transverse magnetization, and therefore, in the same way, it depends on the small tip angle approximation (Pauly et al. 2011). The simplified (shortened) VTAG sequence is one of the examples Kerwin and Prince presented as an application of this analysis method. Here, we derive a modified version of that analysis, which gives us insights about the tagging process as well as the limitations of this analysis.

Referring to Equation 12.2, the profile of the transverse magnetization after applying the tagging sequence can be written as a function of the RF field, $B_1(t)$. Defining a "weighted path" can help with understanding the FT relation between the tagging profile and RF field by removing the time-dependent terms from that equation. The weighted path is defined as follows:

$$wp\left(\vec{k}\right)=\int_0^T B_1(t)\delta\left(\vec{k}(t)-\vec{k}\right)dt, \quad (12.20)$$

where

$\vec{k}$ can be any point in the k-space (with dimensionality up to three)

$\vec{k}(t)$ is a function of the present time as described in Equation 12.3

It is important to note that $\vec{k}(t)$ is equal to zero, by definition, at the end of excitation time ($t = T$). The weighted path $wp(\vec{k})$ describes the effect of the RF pulse on k-space excitation regardless of the moment when it was applied. Since the gradient field is limited, $wp(\vec{k})$ is always in the form of a continuous path. In the two-dimensional (2D) case, one can imagine that this weighted path is sketched by a pen, which is moved around the k-space by the applied gradients and ends up at the center of the k-space. The weighted path (imprint) of the pen on the paper will be stronger if it moves slower (lower-amplitude gradient fields) or if more ink flows out of the pen (stronger RF pulse). A zero-amplitude gradient while the RF pulse is being applied, therefore, resembles a drop of ink on the stationary paper and

is represented as a delta function in $wp(\vec{k})$. For any case, this path is terminated at the origin of the k-space when the excitation finishes ($t = T$).

Substituting Equation 12.20 into 12.2 results in the following expression, which shows the FT relation between the weighted path and transverse magnetization:

$$M_{xy}\left(\vec{r}\right)\approx i\gamma M_0\int_K wp\left(\vec{k}\right)e^{i\vec{r}\cdot\vec{k}}d\vec{k}. \quad (12.21)$$

Note that in this equation $\vec{k}$ is not a function of time anymore. Although this equation gives a clear image of how the transverse magnetization, M_{xy}, is formed by the sequence, the generated tagging pattern is determined by the profile of the longitudinal magnetization, M_z. Kerwin and Prince (2000) used the Bloch equation (Equation 12.1) to find M_z based on M_{xy} and the applied RF and gradient pulses. Herein, we prefer to use the direct relation between the magnetization components, assuming that the total magnitude remains fixed during the excitation. This assumption is a reasonable approximation when the tagging preparation duration is short relative to the relaxation parameters of the tissue being investigated. For simplicity, we normalize the magnetization components by M_0. Therefore,

$$M_z^2 = 1-\left|M_{xy}\right|^2$$

$$= 1-M_{xy}\cdot\overline{M_{xy}} =$$

$$= 1-\gamma^2\int_K wp\left(\vec{k}\right)e^{i\vec{r}\cdot\vec{k}}d\vec{k}\cdot\int_K \overline{wp(\vec{k'})}e^{-i\vec{r}\cdot\vec{k'}}d\vec{k'}, \quad (12.22)$$

where the bar above a symbol represents its complex conjugate. By combining the two integrals in Equation 12.22 and defining the new spatial frequency $\vec{k''}=\vec{k}-\vec{k'}$ instead of $\vec{k'}$, we may rewrite the aforementioned equation as follows:

$$M_z^2 = 1-\gamma^2\int_K\int_K wp(\vec{k})\overline{wp(\vec{k}-\vec{k''})}d\vec{k}\cdot e^{i\vec{r}\cdot\vec{k''}}d\vec{k''}. \quad (12.23)$$

Considering the fact that the autocorrelation function of the weighted path is

$$R_{wp}\left(\vec{k''}\right)=\int_K wp\left(\vec{k}\right)\overline{wp(\vec{k}-\vec{k''})}d\vec{k}, \quad (12.24)$$

then Equation 12.23 can be written as

$$\left(M_z\left(\vec{r}\right)\right)^2 = 1-\gamma^2\int_K R_{wp}\left(\vec{k}\right)\cdot e^{i\vec{r}\cdot\vec{k}}d\vec{k} = 1-\gamma^2\cdot FT\left\{R_{wp}\left(\vec{k}\right)\right\}.$$

$$(12.25)$$

This equation shows how the FT of the autocorrelation function of the weighted path is related to M_z^2. For small M_{xy}, we may use the following approximation:

$$M_z = \sqrt{1 - M_{xy} \cdot \overline{M_{xy}}} \approx 1 - \frac{1}{2}|M_{xy}| \, |\overline{M_{xy}}| \approx 1 - \frac{1}{2}\gamma^2 \cdot FT\left\{R_{wp}\left(\vec{k}\right)\right\}. \tag{12.26}$$

Though derived differently, Equation 12.26 is the same equation defined by Kerwin and Prince (2000). It should be noted that the last assumption of M_{xy} being small is not accurate enough for most tagging applications where full saturation of the taglines enhances the tagging contrast.

12.5.4.2 Example 1: SPAMM Tagging

Herein, we study the simple example of 1-1 SPAMM (with two 45° pulses), which has been also examined by Kerwin and Prince, who formulated the weighted path for the SPAMM sequence as

$$wp\left(\vec{k}\right) = \frac{1}{\gamma}\sum_{m=1}^{N}\theta_m\delta\left(\vec{k} - (N-m)\vec{\Phi}\right), \tag{12.27}$$

where each θ_m represents the angle of excitation in one of the SPAMM RF pulses, and

$$\vec{\Phi} = \gamma\vec{G}. \tag{12.28}$$

The weighted path, wp, as well as its autocorrelation function are shown in Figure 12.15. This figure illustrates the simulated tag profile generated by this approximation in comparison to the exact simulation.

According to Equation 12.26, the tagging pattern is given by

$$M_z \approx 1 - \frac{1}{2}\frac{\pi^2}{8}\left(1 + \cos\left(\vec{r}\cdot\vec{\Phi}\right)\right). \tag{12.29}$$

Equation 12.29 shows a contrast of about 1.23 in the M_z between the dark and bright lines, but we know that in 1-1 SPAMM with two 45° pulses this contrast is limited to 1.0, when the magnetization is normalized by M_0. This 23% overestimation in tagging contrast is shown in the simulation in Figure 12.15 as well as all other SPAMM simulations in the original work by Kerwin and Prince. The reason for this overestimation is that Equation 12.27 is only good for small angles where $\sin(\theta_m) \approx \theta_m$ (the angle θ_m is represented in radians), which is not the case in conventional tagging. Regardless of the contrast overestimation, this tagging analysis method is powerful for determining the magnetization pattern generated from a certain tagging sequence. Furthermore, it can be used to design the pulse sequence for a desired tagging pattern.

12.5.4.3 Example 2: Variable-Density Tagging

Among the examples given in the original k-space analysis paper (Kerwin and Prince 2000), we choose the case of VTAG to show how this analysis method can be used to generate an efficient pulse sequence for a variable-density tagging pattern. Figure 12.16 shows the weighted path as well as its autocorrelation function for the sequence shown in Figure 12.13 with separations of 5, 4, 3, 3, 3, 3, 3, and 3 pixels.

Using spectral decomposition, a short weighted path with fewer spectral peaks (15 instead of 50) can be generated, which has almost the same autocorrelation function as the long sequence (Figure 12.17). This resulted in the design of a simpler sequence for the same VTAG pattern, which is considerably shorter in time.

Figure 12.18 illustrates the generated tagging pattern using the shortened sequence in comparison to the pattern generated by the sequence in Figure 12.13. The comparison shows that despite a subtle contrast mismatch, the overall patterns match very well for the two sequences. We would like to remind the reader that both designs are based on the small tip angle and quasi-static assumptions. The mathematical principle outlined in the k-space analysis of MRI tagging provides an attractive method for designing time-efficient tagging sequences.

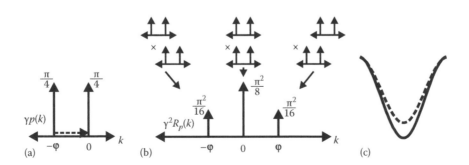

FIGURE 12.15 Simulation of 1–1 SPAMM sequence (total flip angle of $\pi/2$) using k-space analysis. (a) The k-space path consists of two impulses. (b) The k-space autocorrelation function, computed by shifting and multiplying the k-space path, as shown in the figure. (c) Actual (dashed line) and simulated (solid line) tag profiles base on the weighted path analysis.

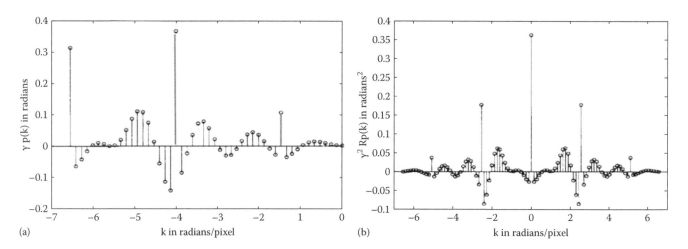

FIGURE 12.16   Analysis of the 5, 4, 3, 3, 3, 3, 3, 3 VTAG pattern in Figure 12.13 using k-space analysis technique. (a) The k-space path. (b) The autocorrelation function of the k-space path. (Reproduced from Kerwin, W.S. and Prince, J.L., *J. Magn. Reson.*, 142(2), 313, 2000. With permission.)

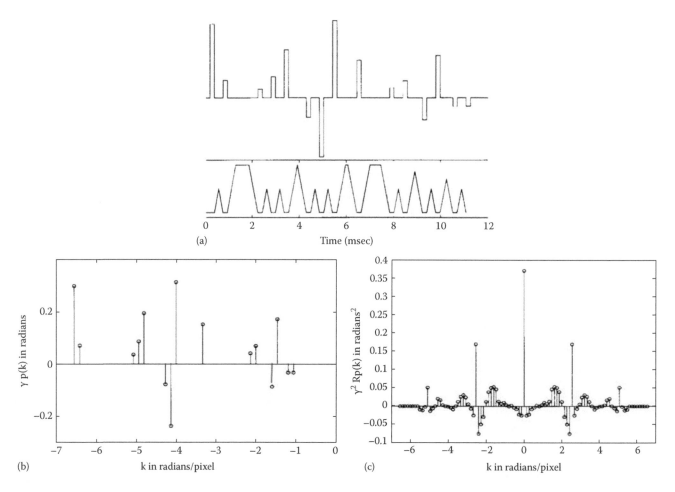

FIGURE 12.17   Shorter pulse sequence for 5, 4, 3, 3, 3, 3, 3, 3 VTAG generation. (a) The shorter pulse sequence, (b) The corresponding k-space path has little resemblance to that in Figure 12.16a. (b) The autocorrelation function of the path is nearly identical to that in Figure 12.16b. (Reproduced from Kerwin, W.S. and Prince, J.L., *J. Magn. Reson.*, 142(2), 313, 2000. With permission.)

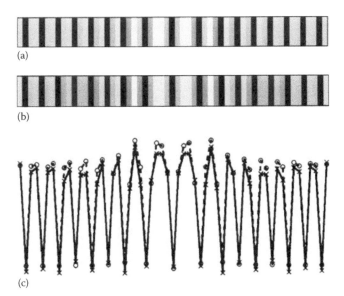

(a)

(b)

(c)

FIGURE 12.18 Comparison of simulated pixel intensities and profiles for the standard (a; and 'o' symbols in (c)) and short (b; and 'x' symbols in (c)) VTAG pulse sequences in Figures 12.13 and 12.17. (Reproduced from Kerwin, W.S. and Prince, J.L., *J. Magn. Reson.*, 142(2), 313, 2000. With permission.)

12.5.5 Multirate SPAMM Tagging (M-SPAMM)

12.5.5.1 Mathematical Analysis

Following the implementation of the L-SPAMM tagging technique, Ikonomidou and Sergiadis extended it into the M-SPAMM (Figure 12.19) by combining L-SPAMM with variable-density tagging through a Shinnar–Le Roux pulse design algorithm (Ikonomidou and Sergiadis 2003). The method uses finite impulse response (FIR) filters wherein the modulus of the filter is used to select the areas in which the tagging takes place, while the phase of the filter is used to manipulate the density of the taglines.

The M-SPAMM technique is in essence the same as the L-SPAMM technique, described previously in Section 12.4.4. The main difference, however, is in the last part of the phase expression of the cosine term in Equation 12.9. In contrast to L-SPAMM, identical linear-phase pulses or a pair of minimum- and maximum-phase pulses are no longer used to

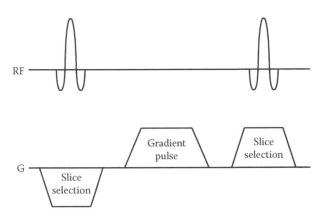

RF

Gradient pulse

Slice selection

G

Slice selection

FIGURE 12.19 M-SPAMM pulse sequence.

cancel out the phase. Rather, multiband filters that have piecewise linear phases with a different slope for each passband are used. Assuming the sequence consists of two pulses with different passband regions, then for the higher-order passband region the system behaves exactly the same as the original L-SPAMM technique. For the lower-order region, however, the phase difference between the two pulses changes the tagline density in that region. In more details, the developed method takes advantage of the filters' phase in order to modify the tagline density. Based on the analysis in Equation 12.4 and Equations 12.6 through 12.8, let B be a multiband filter with piecewise linear phase, which has different slope in each passband. Such filters can be designed as sums of FIR bandpass filters (BPFs) of different orders. For the analysis here, let

$$B = B_A + B_B, \tag{12.30}$$

where B_A and B_B are linear-phase band-pass FIR filters with different passbands, which have orders of $N_A - 1$ and $N_B - 1$, respectively. Further, let us assume that $N_A > N_B$ and

$$(N_A - N_B)\Delta t = T_\Delta. \tag{12.31}$$

Since the overall pulse duration corresponds to the length of filter B_A, in its passbands the tagging pattern is given by

$$M_z = -4|A|^2|B|^2 \cos\left(\gamma GxT\right)M_0 + \left(|A|^2 - |B|^2\right)^2 M_0. \tag{12.32}$$

Nevertheless, the tagline density in the passbands of B_B will be affected by its lesser order than B_A, which is given by (after taking the limit that $\Delta t \to 0$)

$$M_z = -4|A|^2|B|^2 \cos\left[i\gamma Gx\left(T - T_\Delta\right)\right]M_0 + \left(|A|^2 - |B|^2\right)^2 M_0. \tag{12.33}$$

Equations 12.32 and 12.33 mean that in the passbands of B_A, the tagline density corresponds to the gradient pulse's duration T, while in the passbands of B_B, it corresponds to $T - T_\Delta$, that is, the gradient pulse duration minus the duration difference between the pulses resulting from B_A and B_B. This means that the resulting tagging pattern is not only restricted to specified areas of the image as in L-SPAMM, but also the tagline density varies between these areas, resulting in a multirate tagging pattern (Ikonomidou and Sergiadis 2003).

12.5.5.2 Implementation

As a multirate tagging example, Ikonomidou and Sergiadis (2003) produced the 3–3–3–3–4–5–5–4–3–3–3–3 tagging pattern originally proposed by McVeigh and Bolster (1998), which is symmetric with respect to the on-resonance point. If the on-resonance point corresponds to pixel 0, then the taglines should be positioned at pixels 0, 5, 9, 12, 15, 18, and 21. The desired pattern can be divided into two areas, one of periodicity 5, comprising tags at pixels 0 and 5, and one of periodicity 3, comprising tags at pixels 9–21. The number of pixels in the positive frequency range is chosen = 30 (the common multiple of 3 and 5 that is greater than 21), $N_A = 61$, and $N_B = 53$. The tagging sequence duration is 7.6 ms, plus approximately 2 ms for gradient switching. One advantage of the developed multirate tagging technique is that it allows for using gradient pulses of different signs, which results in transferring the pulse's phase to the magnetization distribution and makes the final tagline distribution independent of the pulse duration.

12.6 TAGS' PROFILE AND THICKNESS OPTIMIZATION

12.6.1 RECTANGULAR TAG PROFILE

In 2002, Wu et al. (2002) provided a modified tagging sequence for improved tagging profile. In the developed sequence, a sinc-modulated RF pulse train is used in the presence of a constant gradient. The RF pulse train creates a rectangular tag profile, while the bandwidth (BW) of the sinc envelope controls the tagline thickness. Compared to the DANTE and SPAMM sequences, the developed sequence has sharper taglines with the capability of changing the tag-thickness to tag-separation ratio. These advantages allow for better tags tracking and accurate quantification of myocardial displacement.

Mathematically, the resulting tagging pattern can be approximated as (Figure 12.20; Δt_3 is minimal; * represents convolution)

$$M_{sat}(x) = \left(\text{rect}(\gamma G_x \Delta t_1 x) * \text{comb}\left(x, \frac{1}{\gamma G_x \Delta t_2}\right) \right)$$
$$\times \text{sinc}(\pi x \gamma G_x \Delta t_3), \quad (12.34)$$

where

sinc$(\pi t/\Delta t_1)$ is the sinc function with the first zero-crossing at Δt_1
comb$(t,\Delta t_2)$ is the comb function with spacing of Δt_2
Δt_3 is the duration of individual rectangular RF pulses

To improve the sequence utility for practical implementation, the constant gradient G_x can be replaced by gradient pulses implemented between the RF pulses without affecting the saturation profile (Figure 12.21). Figure 12.22 shows an example of a phantom with sinc-modulated tagging.

12.6.2 OPTIMAL TAG PROFILE

Although several tagging techniques have been developed, identifying the tagging pattern that minimizes the tags tracking error is of a great importance. In 2003, Nguyen et al. (2003) conducted a study to investigate the optimal tag profile for myocardial motion estimation. Herein, the tag motion tracking problem was formulated as a nonlinear least-squares problem, for which an expression for the Cramer–Rao lower bound (CRLB) of the average estimation error variance was found. Using this measure, the authors searched the class of band-limited signals to determine the tag shape that minimizes the CRLB. Under some simplifying assumption, it has been showed that the optimal tag profile has a sinusoidal pattern, which results in a significantly reduced average estimation error variance compared to other commonly used tag profiles. Further, the results showed that the higher the tagging frequency the less sensitive the resulting measurements to noise. It should be noted that these conclusions are applicable to a large group of tagging and tracking approaches as the CRLB is independent of the estimation method.

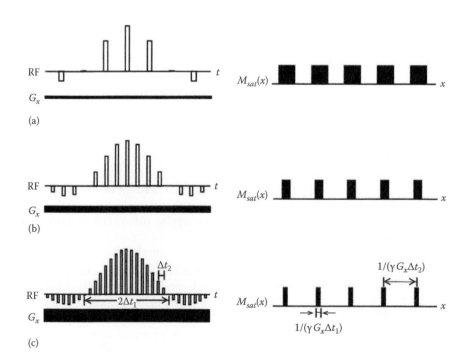

FIGURE 12.20 Illustration of sinc-modulated RF pulse trains in the presence of a constant gradient and approximate magnetization saturation profiles. The tags' width-to-separation ratios are (a) 1:2, (b) 1:4, and (c) 1:8. (Reproduced from Wu, E.X. et al., *Magn. Reson. Med.*, 48(2), 389, 2002. With permission.)

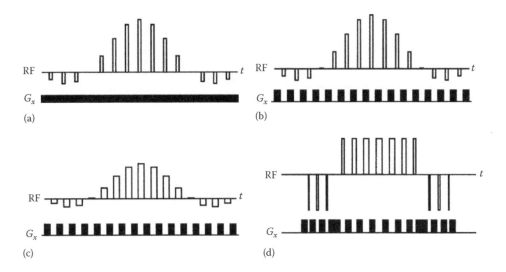

FIGURE 12.21 Sinc-modulated RF pulse train and equivalent combination of RF pulse train and gradient. (a) Sinc-modulated RF pulse train with a constant gradient. (b) The constant gradient is replaced by gradient segments between the RF pulses. (c) Widened RF pulses are used to reduce the peak power requirement. (d) Equalized RF amplitudes are used to reduce the overall pulse train duration. (Reproduced from Wu, E.X. et al., *Magn. Reson. Med.*, 48(2), 389, 2002. With permission.)

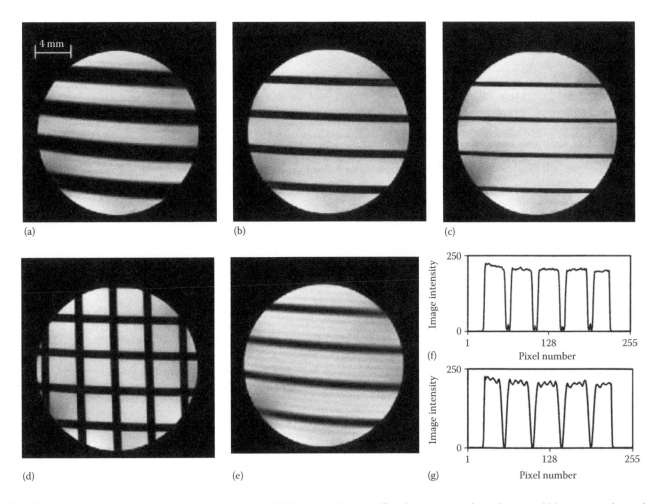

FIGURE 12.22 Phantom images using sinc-modulated RF pulse train. (a–c) Tagging patterns of varying tag width-to-separation ratios produced by the sinc-modulated RF pulse trains shown in Figure 12.20a through c, respectively. (d) 2D tagging using the sinc-modulated RF pulse train in Figure 12.20b. (e) DANTE tagging equivalent to that shown in (b) in terms of tag width and separation. (f,g) Vertical image intensity profiles from images in (b) and (e), respectively, showing improved tag profile of the sinc-modulated tagging. (Reproduced from Wu, E.X. et al., *Magn. Reson. Med.*, 48(2), 389, 2002. With permission.)

12.6.3 Optimal Tag Thickness

In an early study on optimality of the tag thickness and its effect on tagging analysis, Atalar and McVeigh (1994) showed that, based on a least-squares estimation (LSE) algorithm, it is possible to define the tagline position with a precision on the order of one tenth of the pixel size. The conducted analysis was based on calculating the CRLB for the tag position estimation error as a function of the tagline thickness, tag profile shape, and line spread function. The results showed that the tag thickness that minimizes the tag position estimation error is between 0.8 and 1.5 pixels, depending on the shape of the tag profile and line spread function. Further, if optimal tag thickness is used, the tag position can be estimated with an error less than 0.9/contrast-to-noise ratio (CNR) (in pixels). Based on these results, the following guidelines have been suggested for designing the tagging pattern: (1) the tag thickness should be slightly larger than the optimal thickness, for example, 2 pixels wide, to avoid the tag thickness from becoming less than the optimal thickness during myocardial contraction; (2) the taglines should be placed perpendicular to the direction with the highest resolution in the image; and (3) the tag spacing should be as small as possible to generate highly accurate strain field, although the tagline center estimation may be affected by the Gibbs artifact, depending on the tag profile.

12.7 RADIAL TAGGING: FIRST IMPLEMENTATION*

12.7.1 Basic Idea and Pulse Sequence

The first tagged MRI image, performed by Zerhouni et al. (1988), showed taglines oriented in multiple radial directions intersecting a SAX view of the heart. The ability to noninvasively image myocardial twist was considered as a unique advantage of that method, which allowed for non-invasive imaging of cardiac mechanics. Figure 12.23 illustrates the concept of the tagging technique developed by Zerhouni et al.

As shown in Figure 12.24, each tagline is generated by one spatially selective RF pulse that saturates the magnetization in a thin tag plane that orthogonally intersects the imaging plane showing a SAX views of the heart. The location of the perturbed magnetization (hypointense signal) appears as radially oriented stripes in the image, as shown in Figure 12.25. For cardiac studies, a number of radial taglines are prescribed to intersect in the middle of the LV cavity. The number of taglines is very limited in this method as all the taglines need to be generated immediately after detection of the ECG R-wave and before significant cardiac motion, which is hard to achieve for a large number of taglines because each tagline needs a separate RF pulse (along with its associated gradients) to create it.

---

* Radial tagging will be revisited with more details later in the chapter in Section 12.12 as one implementation of polar tagging.

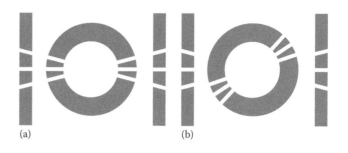

FIGURE 12.23 Tagging by magnetization saturation. The illustration shows three radial taglines generated with three inversion pulses. (a) Representation of the phantom immediately after tags generation. (b) Representation of the phantom later after tagging, where the rotating disk shows rotated taglines, while the fixed poles on the left and right show unchanged position of the taglines.

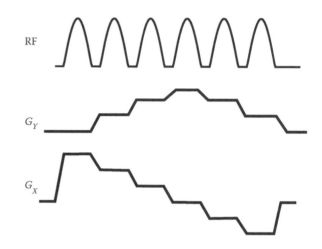

FIGURE 12.24 Generation of six radial taglines with six slice-selective inversion pulses.

12.7.2 Practical Considerations and Implementation

It should be noted that with radial tagging, the measurement of radial strain is heavily dependent on proper identification of the myocardial borders. As errors in the segmentation of the myocardial contours are usually greater than those in tags tracking, strain calculation, particularly in the radial direction, are better based solely on segmentation of the taglines to avoid significant measurement errors (Bazille et al. 1994).

A few years after the invention of the tagging technique, Bosmans et al. (1996) combined radial tagging with gradient echo (GRE) imaging and compared the results to spin echo (SE) imaging. Further, the authors studied the effects of flow-compensating gradients, excitation flip angles, and flip angles of the saturation pulses on the resulting MR signal both with simulations and in vivo experiments. The results showed that GRE imaging with flow-compensating gradients is robust for myocardial tagging implementation. Further, using optimized flip angles and saturation bands significantly improves the taglines identification, as they persist for most of the cardiac cycle.

In 2001, Dong et al. (2001) used radial tagging for assessing LV relaxation by measuring the untwisting, or recoil,

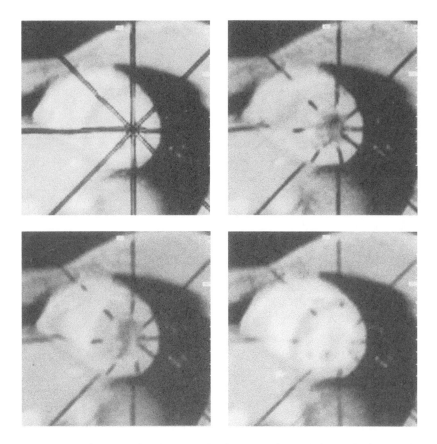

FIGURE 12.25 In vivo radially tagged images using the magnetization saturation technique. The images (from top left to bottom right) show different frames through the cardiac cycle. Note the movement and fading of the taglines through the cardiac cycle. (Reproduced from Bosmans, H. et al., *MAGMA*, 4(2), 123, 1996. With permission.)

rate as a measure of the isovolumic relaxation time constant (τ) measured by echocardiography. The results showed close correlation between the two measures ($R = -0.86$), which shows that the recoil rate, determined by MRI tagging, provides an isovolumic-phase, preload-independent measure of LV relaxation. Therefore, this parameter would be useful for studying diastolic function in conditions that affect the filling rates, for example, aging, hypertension, and congestive heart failure.

12.8 STRIPED TAGS (STAG)

In an early effort for creating polar tags, Bolster et al. (1990) developed the striped tags (STAG) technique to perform tagging in polar coordinates. The radial taglines obtained with the magnetization saturation technique developed by Zerhouni et al. (1988) (Figure 12.26a) are excellent for measuring circumferential strain (on SAX slices); however, this technique is not useful for measuring radial strain. Although the tagging

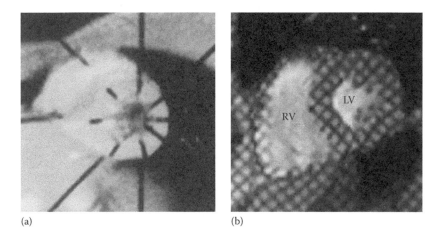

(a)   (b)

FIGURE 12.26   (a) Radial tagging using magnetization saturation. (b) SPAMM tagging in a SAX image.

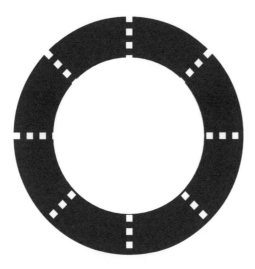

FIGURE 12.27 Illustration of the STAG tagging technique in a SAX LV view. STAG generates dotted radial lines suitable for measuring both circumferential and radial strains from the same set of SAX images.

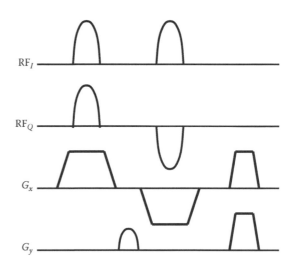

FIGURE 12.28 The STAG pulse sequence. The sequence combines the features of localized tagging (localized RF pulses) and SPAMM (modulation gradient in between the two RF pulses). RF_I and RF_Q represent the in-phase and quadrature-phase components of the RF pulse, respectively.

grid created with SPAMM tagging (Axel and Dougherty 1989) (Figure 12.26b) allows for some assessment of the radial strain, the resulting tagline intersections do not occur at the same depth at different locations in the myocardium, which makes direct comparison of transmural thickening not straightforward. Further, the interference patterns of the tagline intersections at high resolution complicate the tagging analysis. As shown in Figure 12.27, the STAG method is a hybrid magnetization saturation/modulation technique. It uses the polar coordinate system, such that about four radial collinear reference points (beads) are placed across the myocardial wall at different angles in the SAX view. This provides good resolution for measuring both radial and circumferential strains.

Similar to SPAMM, the STAG sequence spatially modulates the magnetization, except that this happens for selected locations (Figure 12.28). In STAG, the two 90° nonselective tagging RF pulses used in SPAMM are switched into slice-selective pulses applied perpendicular to the imaging plane. After applying the first 90° RF pulse, a gradient is applied parallel to the imaging plane and orthogonal to the first slice-selection gradient. This gradient is used to create a linear phase shift of the transverse magnetization as a function of the distance along the tag plane excited with the first RF pulse. The second 90° RF pulse then tips the transverse magnetization back to the longitudinal direction, which results in linear phase shift along the tag section and shows as a sinusoidal variation of the longitudinal magnetization along that tagline. Finally, spoiler gradients are applied to eliminate any remaining transverse magnetization. This sequence is repeated as many times as needed to create radial STAG lines (that intersect at the center of the LV cavity in a SAX view) before image acquisition takes place. Again, similar to the original tagging sequence based on selective excitation, a limited number of taglines can be created in order not to miss capturing the heart motion during early systole.

It should be noted that the gradient used during the tagging RF pulses causes a spin dephasing across the section that defines the tagged plane. Therefore, a pair of self-refocusing RF pulses are used in the STAG sequence, such that the dephasing caused by the gradient used with the first RF pulse is refocused by reversing the sign of the gradient used with the second RF pulse. To avoid having the second RF pulse excites a plane different from the one excited by the first RF pulse (in case the excited plane is not exactly at the center of the gradient), the quadrature channel of the second RF pulse (RF_Q) is reversed (Figure 12.28) such that the phase applied to the second RF pulse counteracts the effect of the reversed gradient, causing the same plane to be excited by both RF pulses.

12.9 RINGTAGS*

12.9.1 BASIC IDEA AND PULSE SEQUENCE

The nearly circular shape of the LV in SAX views makes it useful to have the taglines curved to match the apparent annular geometry, especially for estimates of transmural gradients in wall thickening (radial strain). This is particularly important as conventional line or grid tagging allows only for measurement of midwall displacement to a limited extent due to the relatively low spatial resolution of the tagging pattern compared to the wall thickness. This observation necessitated the development of tagging methods that could produce nonlinear or curved taglines.

One approach to generate curved taglines is to use a continuous and long RF pulse that selectively excites the spins within the object over an on-resonance excitation plane while the applied gradient fields are simultaneously moving the plane. This results is a single saturated (or inverted) convex tagline that can be created within (or near) a specific

---

* Circular tagging will be revisited with more details in the Section 12.11 as one implementation of polar tagging.

anatomical landmark, such as the endocardium, epicardium, or mid-myocardium. This approach has been adopted by Spiegel et al. (2003) who developed the RingTag technique. The principle of RingTag (Figure 12.29) includes the implementation of a continuous RF pulse together with a selection gradient. If the RF pulse is applied with an off-center frequency, Δf, the saturation band is shifted by Δx, measured as follows:

$$\Delta x = \frac{2\pi \vec{G}}{\gamma G^2} \cdot \Delta f, \qquad (12.35)$$

where

γ is the gyromagnetic ratio
$\vec{G}$ is the gradient specifying the displacement direction

RingTag becomes more effective when it is combined with radial or other types of tagging so that all components of myocardial motion can be estimated from the same SAX image. This combination was employed by Spiegel et al. (2003) for assessing the myocardial centerline, which can be useful, for example, for distinguishing the epicardial and endocardial wall thickening contributions. In general, components of the gradient field must work in consort to move the effective tagging plane around the image space. Simultaneously, the RF amplitude must be modulated to excite the spins, and an offset frequency must be applied to shift the on-resonance plane (saturation line) away from the isocenter of the magnet. Without this offset frequency, the on-resonance rotating plane always passes through the isocenter because the gradient fields are always zero at that point. In other words, the direction of the gradient field only determines the direction of the saturation plane, but the distance of this plane from the isocenter of the magnet is determined by the frequency offset in the RF pulse. The pulse sequence diagram and simulation of the RingTag technique are illustrated in Figure 12.30. Figure 12.31 shows a SAX image tagged with the RingTag technique along with the tag profile.

12.9.2 Technical Remarks

It is important to note that the area outside of the desired RingTag pattern is also affected by this method since the saturation line passes through these areas and partially saturates them too, as shown in Figure 12.30. The only difference between the spins outside the tagline and those on the tagline is the magnitude of excitation (i.e., saturation), which depends on both the duration during which the spins are on-resonance and the amplitude of the RF pulse. As a result, if the gradient field rotates uniformly, as is the case with the sequence shown in Figure 12.30, then the resulting tagging contrast depends on the amount of tagline curvature. The reason for this phenomenon is that larger curvature corresponds to a greater angle of rotation, which is directly proportional to the amount of time the curve takes to be traversed, or equivalently the duration of its excitation. Hence, for a constant RF amplitude, the magnitude of spin saturation is lesser in regions where the rate of rotation is slower (lower curvature). Similarly, we expect the contrast between the tagline and the regions inside the curve to be greater compared to the contrast with neighboring points outside the curve (Figure 12.31) as the internal points have a shorter, if any, on-resonance period. Another remark about the RingTag technique is that the generated tagline is strictly convex, as can be seen in Figure 12.32, that is, concave taglines cannot be generated. This, however, is not a limitation, in general, for cardiac motion encoding because the heart is nearly always convex for a wide range of pathophysiologic circumstances.

The flexibility of the RingTag technique for generating any convex tagging curve is appealing and the pulse sequence

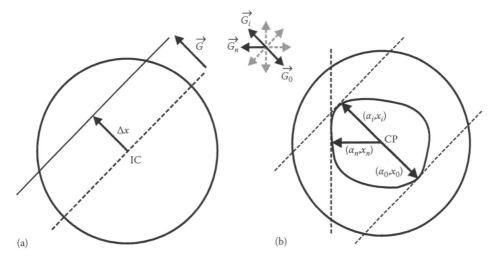

FIGURE 12.29 Principle of generating the RingTag. A saturation line is shifted outside the isocenter (IC) by applying an RF pulse with an off-center frequency Δf, which shifts the line by Δx. (a) The shift direction is defined by the selection gradient G. (b) If the selection gradient G is temporally rotated around a chosen center point (CP), the saturation band follows a convex contour by varying the off-center frequency, which results in a circular tagline.

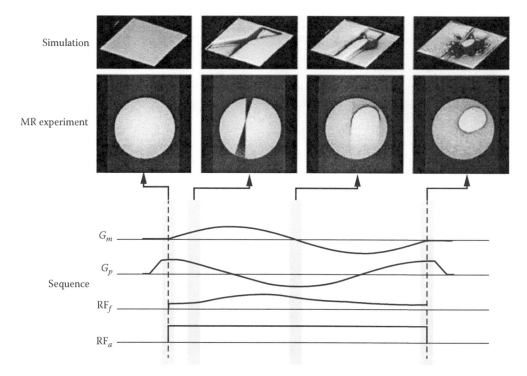

FIGURE 12.30 RingTag generation steps and pulse sequence. Sinusoidal-driven gradients (G_m and G_p along the readout and phase-encoding directions, respectively) define the direction of shifted saturation band whereby the distance is given by the offset frequency (RF_f) of the RF pulse with constant amplitude (RF_a). The generation of the RingTag saturation structure visualized by simulation (top row) and measurements in a phantom (middle row). Simulation was performed by numerically solving the Bloch equations, and the temporally resolved phantom images were generated by individual measurements with a partly applied RingTag pulse each. Four time points in the evolution of the RingTag saturation structure are shown in the MRI sequence (bottom). (Reproduced from Spiegel, M.A. et al., *Invest. Radiol.*, 38(10), 669, 2003. With permission.)

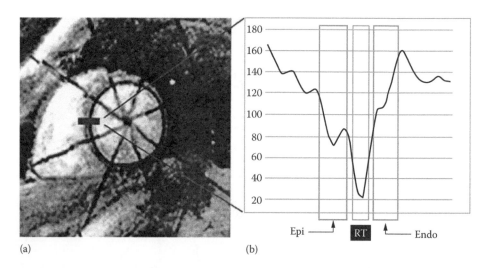

FIGURE 12.31 Intensity profile (b) through the RingTag saturation band in (a). The figure shows low signal intensity from the RingTag (RT) with a steep inner intensity gradient toward the endocardium (Endo) and a more flattened profile in the outer region toward the epicardium (Epi). (Reproduced from Spiegel, M.A. et al., *Invest. Radiol.*, 38(10), 669, 2003. With permission.)

design is innovative, but its applications have been limited. This arises as a consequence of the complexity of designing the gradient and RF waveforms on a patient-specific basis, the convexity limitation, and the time needed to generate useful tagging patterns. Nevertheless, as quantification of motion in regions outside the heart becomes more widely adopted, RingTag may be an attractive option.

12.10 POLAR TAGGING

Polar tagging is the general term we will use for all patterns that generate the taglines in the circular (Section 12.11) and radial (Section 12.12) directions around the center of the heart (Moghaddam et al. 2011c, Khan 2013, Nasiraei-Moghaddam and Finn 2014), as shown in Figure 12.33. Neither the tagline

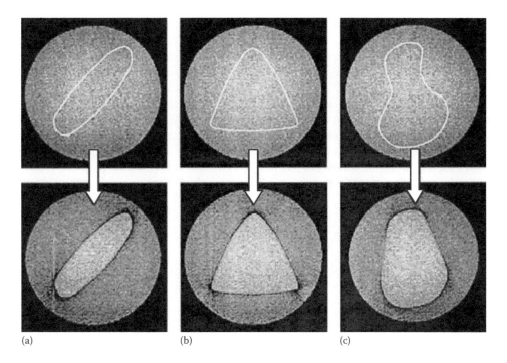

FIGURE 12.32 Demonstration of the generation of irregular RingTag shapes. The length of prescribed and tagged contours differed minimally by 0.5% and 0.4% for (a) and (b), respectively. This demonstrates that the inner intensity gradient in the image detects the ring contour even at regions with lower ring suppression (regions with short residence time of the saturation pulse). At regions with small curvature radius, the slopes were enhanced up to a factor of 1.9 and 2.9 for contours (a) and (b), respectively. The RingTag production is limited to rings; concave shapes show canceling of parts of the predefined saturation band (c). (Reproduced from Spiegel, M.A. et al., *Invest. Radiol.*, 38(10), 669, 2003. With permission.)

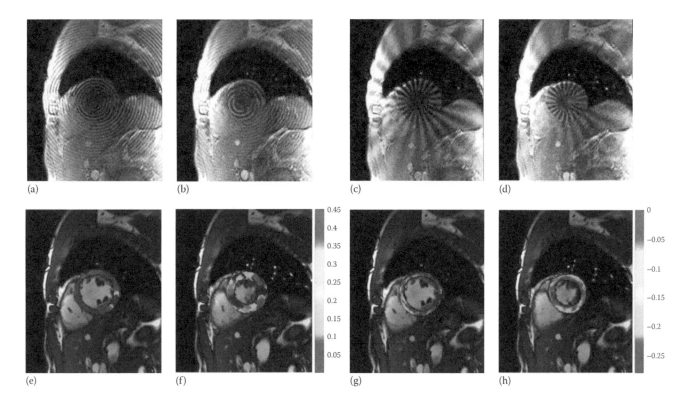

FIGURE 12.33 Polar tagging. Top row: Representative (a, c) diastolic and (b, d) systolic SAX images showing (a, b) circular and (c, d) radial tagging in a healthy volunteer. Bottom row: The calculated (e, f) radial and (g, h) circumferential strain maps of the corresponding cardiac phases in the top row, superimposed on corresponding SSFP cine images of the myocardium. The limited density of the circular taglines and broken lines in the 4 o' clock region caused an error in the estimation of radial strain in that region, as shown in (f). (Reproduced from Nasiraei-Moghaddam, A. and Finn, J.P., *Magn. Reson. Med.*, 71(5), 1750, 2014. With permission.)

density nor their curvature needs to be constant, though we focus mostly on uniform polar patterns and then generalize the concept to other related patterns. Both the geometry and motion of the myocardium in the SAX view are better described in the polar coordinate system compared to the Cartesian system. In fact, standard analysis of the grid-tagged data in a SAX view results in computing radial and circumferential strain components because the Cartesian strain components are spatially heterogeneous and difficult to interpret. Therefore, polar coordinate tagging is advantageous to the common grid and line patterns for both intuitive visualization and deformation analysis. Specifically, polar tagging is useful for the assessment of conditions where changes in radial or circumferential strain have direct diagnostic or prognostic implications, for example, in patients with congenital heart disease (CHD) where strain imaging can detect preclinical conditions (Khan et al. 2014). Further, the polar tagging patterns facilitate the implementation of certain algorithms for automated processing of the tagged image in the frequency domain (Moghaddam and Finn 2008a,b), as discussed in Section 12.13.

Radial tagging as in its first implementation discussed in Section 12.7 was not widely used due to a number of factors, including high specific absorption rate (SAR) from tight radial excitations as well as long tag preparation time that prohibits strain measurement during early systole and results in nonsimultaneous application of the taglines. On the other hand, circular tagging has rarely been studied in the literature, as discussed in Section 12.9. Recently, Moghaddam (Moghaddam and Gharib (2011b), Moghaddam et al. (2011c), and Nasiraei Moghaddam (2012)) developed a new approach for polar tagging based on off-resonance excitation, proposed different versions of the technique that suit various applications, and evaluated clinical implementations in some preliminary studies. One advantage of the developed technique is that the RF energy for radial tagging is much less than that used in the previous implementation of radial tagging with magnetization saturation or inversion pulses (Zerhouni et al. 1988), despite the shorter tags preparation time in the proposed technique. The less SAR could be attributed to the fact that the proposed tags preparation sequence incorporates off-resonance excitation, which plays a significant role in decreasing the energy absorbed in the imaged object.

12.11   CIRCULAR TAGGING

12.11.1   INITIAL APPROACH

The first polar tagging pattern that we describe is the circular tagging pattern, in which a quasiperiodic pattern of concentric dark circles is generated in the image. Looking from the center of the image, which can be easily chosen to be at the LV center, an almost sinusoidal alteration of the brightness is observable in all directions. If such a pattern is generated in a simple homogeneous phantom where there exists no other structure, we would expect a strong representation of a single spatial frequency in all directions to be apparent in the k-space. It may cross our minds that regardless of the k-space center that represents the average image intensity, the spectrum of this image

has significant values only for a particular spatial frequency, but in all directions. This gives rise to a centered circular pattern of high signal intensity in the k-space, which corresponds to the sinusoidally alternating pattern in the image. To investigate the accuracy of this idea, we first examine it rigorously through a mathematical approach.

A single spatial frequency that is uniformly distributed in all directions can be mathematically modeled as a circular one-dimensional (1D) delta function around the center of the k-space:

$$S(k,\varphi) = \frac{\delta(k - k_0)}{(2\pi k)}, \qquad (12.36)$$

where
k and φ represent the magnitude and phase of the complex spatial frequency, respectively
k_0 represents the single dominant spatial frequency mentioned earlier

The division by $2\pi k$ is used for normalization purposes. Because of the angular symmetry of this function, its FT, $I(r, \theta)$, is calculated through its 1D Hankel transform, H, which is known to be the zero-order Bessel function of the first kind, J_0, as follows:

$$I(r,\theta) = H\{S(k,\varphi)\} = 2\pi \int_0^\infty S(k)J_0(rk)kdk = J_0(r/r_0), \quad (12.37)$$

where J_0 is the zero-order Bessel function of the first kind, and

$$r_0 = \frac{1}{k_0}. \qquad (12.38)$$

It is worth noting that the zeros of this Bessel function are separated by a distance of almost π, which means that the signal alteration is very close to the periodicity of a sinusoidal function (Figure 12.34). The envelope of this function decreases slowly (slower than $1/r$), and therefore looks almost constant after the first few periods. We may then conclude that such a pattern is close enough to what we want for a circular tagging pattern. This approach also helps quantifying the maximum achievable modulation contrast.

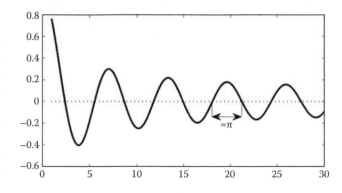

FIGURE 12.34   Approximation of the tag profile in circular tagging.

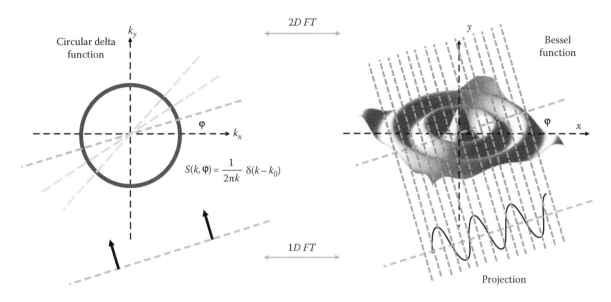

FIGURE 12.35 The application of the central section theorem for circular tagging.

In reality, the image intensity is always positive and therefore a spectral peak (DC component) is always present at the center of the k-space. We may ignore this central peak in our current analysis, but eventually the magnitude ratio of the circular delta function to the central peak determines the contrast of the generated tags, which is a principal determinant of the tags quality. Having accepted Equation 12.36 as the proper k-space representation of a circular tagging pattern, we can then use the central section theorem (CST) to gain insight about how we can design the pulse sequence to generate such a pattern. According to CST, each radial section in the Fourier domain (equivalent to the k-space in our discussion) equals the FT of the projection of the magnetization pattern in a direction perpendicular to that radial section. This theorem infers that the projection of such a pattern, described by the Bessel function, in any direction results in a perfect sinusoidal function, the familiar tagging pattern generated by 1-1 SPAMM (Figure 12.35). Inspired by image reconstruction in computed tomography (CT), if we exploit the back-projection technique we may generate the Bessel function-based circular pattern from these sinusoidal projections.* This suggests then, that the superposition of several 1-1 SPAMM preparations, which are applied evenly in all directions, would result in the desired circular tagging pattern. A higher number of SPAMM preparations will generate a smoother circular pattern. In the limit for a very large number of directionally oriented SPAMM preparations, each with small effective excitations, a very smooth circular tagging pattern can be produced.

There are, however, two major difficulties in implementing this idea. First of all, we need to complete the entire tagging preparation sequence within a short period of time (<10–20 ms) at the beginning of the cardiac cycle to limit blurring of the tagging pattern due to cardiac motion and to avoid missing significant cardiac motion events during early systole. Therefore, we cannot afford to apply 1-1 SPAMM (~5–10 ms, including the spoiling gradient) in many directions. While this consideration is helpful, a more significant problem is the nonlinearity of the Bloch equation, which limits the validity of the superposition concept to small excitations (small tip angle approximation) (Pauly et al. 2011) as discussed earlier in Section 12.2.

12.11.2 BASIC IDEA

To overcome the aforementioned problems, an alternative approach is needed in order to implement the circular tagging preparation sequence (Moghaddam et al. 2011c, Nasiraei-Moghaddam and Finn 2014). In this approach, an on-resonance rotating plane limits the directional excitation to a thin slab perpendicular to the slice of interest, thereby excluding other spins from the excitation, which resolves the superposition problem. The pattern becomes sinusoidal and not Bessel function anymore. Assuming the RF pulse is tuned to the Larmor frequency before the in-plane gradients are played, then the resonance frequency offset, $\Delta\omega$, at position $\vec{r}$ caused by the sine wave gradient field $G(t)$, is given by

$$\Delta\omega(\vec{r},t) = \gamma G_0 r \cos\left(\varphi_G(t) - \varphi_r\right), \qquad (12.39)$$

$$\varphi_G(t) = \frac{\pi}{2} + \frac{2\pi t}{T_p}, \quad \frac{-T_p}{2} < t < \frac{T_p}{2}, \qquad (12.40)$$

where

G_0, φ_G, and T_p are the magnitude, phase, and period, respectively, of the gradient

(r, φ_r) are the in-plane coordinates of the spins in the polar coordinate system

At each time point, t, the on-resonance spins (when $\Delta\omega = 0$) are located in a plane perpendicular to $\vec{G}(G_0, \varphi_G)$.

---

* The image reconstruction in CT is based on filtered back-projection rather than simple back-projection. In our current case, we have only one significant spatial frequency in any direction and so the result of filtered back-projection is the same as back-projection.

This on-resonance plane is perpendicular to the imaging plane and rotates around the magnet isocenter in a complete circle during the time period T_p. Therefore, every point in the imaging plane experiences the on-resonance condition at two time points, T_{on1} and T_{on1}, where

$$T_{on2} = T_{on1} + T_p/2, \qquad (12.41)$$

as shown in Figure 12.36. The resonance condition is assumed to span a short period of time around each of these two time points, where each ray in the imaging plane experiences a half-circle sine wave gradient between T_{on1} and T_{on2}. This extra gradient is similar to the tagging gradient used in the SPAMM sequence and therefore results in a periodic modulation of the magnetization over that ray. Nevertheless, in contrast to SPAMM where the excitation occurs simultaneously for all spins in the imaging plane, in the proposed sequence the time of the first excitation, T_{on1}, is a function of φ_r, which results in a curved tagging pattern. This results in a pattern of equispaced coaxial cylinders whose intersection with the imaging plane results in a pattern of co-centered circles. The magnitude of the applied gradients determines the density of the created circles. A common characteristic between the developed method for circular tagging and the RingTag method (Spiegel et al. 2003), described earlier in Section 12.9, is that the gradient field changes to rotate the on-resonance plane while the RF magnetic field is being applied. Nevertheless, although RingTag selectively excites the on-resonance spins over a single-curved line, the proposed method generates multiple circular taglines simultaneously. Figure 12.36 shows the extra gradient for points on one specific ray. A similar profile exists for any other ray as well. Since we need to repeat this excitation for all neighboring rays sequentially, the total RF pulse is in the form of a constant continuous RF pulse. In the next section, we conduct a more detailed explanation of the excitation process.

12.11.3 EXCITATION PROCESS

12.11.3.1 Mathematical Formulation

In the previous sections of the chapter, we described tagging methods that can be analyzed well enough through quasi-static excitation of the spins using FT analysis. Here, we are going to relax that constraint in the analysis of the polar tagging sequences, which will allow for decreasing the energy required for high-density tagging. In this formulation, the magnetization relaxation times are ignored, and therefore the magnitude of the magnetization is considered constant during the excitation. This leaves us with two parameters for analysis: θ, the angle with the longitudinal direction (the direction of the constant magnetic field, equivalent to the magnetization direction at equilibrium); and φ, the phase in the transverse plane (Figure 12.37). The magnetization vector (M_x, M_y, M_z) is written based on these two angles as follows (Nasiraei-Moghaddam and Finn 2014):

$$M_x = M \sin\theta \cos\varphi, \qquad (12.42)$$

$$M_y = M \sin\theta \sin\varphi, \qquad (12.43)$$

$$M_z = M \cos\theta. \qquad (12.44)$$

As discussed earlier (see Equation 12.1), the Bloch equation (without relaxation) can be written in matrix form as follows:

$$\begin{bmatrix} \dot{M}_x \\ \dot{M}_y \\ \dot{M}_z \end{bmatrix} = \gamma \begin{bmatrix} 0 & \vec{G}\cdot\vec{r} & -B_{1y} \\ -\vec{G}\cdot\vec{r} & 0 & B_{1x} \\ B_{1y} & -B_{1x} & 0 \end{bmatrix} \begin{bmatrix} M_x \\ M_y \\ M_z \end{bmatrix}. \qquad (12.45)$$

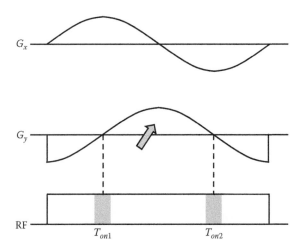

FIGURE 12.36 Schematic of the preparation sequence for circular tagging in the x–y plane. G_x and G_y generate a rotating excitation plane perpendicular to the x–y plane. The RF pulse envelope has a constant magnitude during the excitation. A sample spin located on the x-axis will be on resonance at two time points (T_{on1} and T_{on2}). The extra gradient between these two time points (arrow) is similar to the modulating gradient in SPAMM tagging, which results in a periodic pattern in each direction.

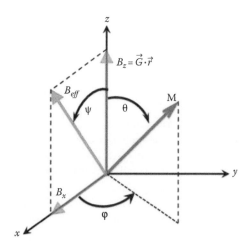

FIGURE 12.37 The effective magnetic field and its components in the rotating frame. The figure shows a representative magnetization vector, M, during the excitation period. The angle θ between M and the z axis quantifies the amount of excitation, analogous to an imaging excitation flip angle.

For the M_z component, this reduces to

$$\dot{M}_z = -\gamma B_{1x} M_y = -\gamma B_{1x} M \sin\theta \sin\varphi, \quad (12.46)$$

assuming that $B_{1y} = 0$ for simplicity. If we then take the derivative of M_z from Equation 12.44, we obtain the following:

$$M_z = M\cos\theta \quad \Rightarrow \quad \dot{M}_z = -M\sin\theta \cdot \dot{\theta}. \quad (12.47)$$

Based on Equations 12.46 and 12.47, this reveals the corresponding part of the Bloch equation in the spherical coordinates as

$$\dot{\theta} = \gamma B_{1x} \sin\varphi. \quad (12.48)$$

The time rate of change of the other variable, φ, is obtained by first dividing M_y by M_x in Equations 12.42 and 12.43:

$$\tan\varphi = \frac{M_y}{M_x}. \quad (12.49)$$

from which we can infer that

$$\left(1 + \tan^2\varphi\right) = \frac{M_x^2 + M_y^2}{M_x^2} = \frac{M_{xy}^2}{M_x^2}. \quad (12.50)$$

Alternately, we can take the derivative of Equation 12.49, which results in

$$(1 + \tan^2\varphi)\dot{\varphi} = \frac{M_x\dot{M}_y - \dot{M}_x M_y}{M_x^2}. \quad (12.51)$$

By combining Equations 12.50 and 12.51, we obtain

$$\dot{\varphi} = \frac{M_x\dot{M}_y - \dot{M}_x M_y}{M_{xy}^2}. \quad (12.52)$$

Finally, by substituting Equations 12.42 through 12.45, we obtain

$$\dot{\varphi} = -\gamma \vec{G} \cdot \vec{r} + \gamma B_{1x} \cot\theta\cos\varphi$$

$$= \gamma B_{1x}\left(-\cot\psi + \cot\theta\cos\varphi\right). \quad (12.53)$$

This result, together with Equation 12.48, represents the Bloch equation in the spherical coordinate system in the form of a set of nonlinear autonomous ordinary differential equations with no simple analytical solution.

12.11.3.2 Adiabatic Excitation

The polar tagging sequences, including both radial and circular tagging, are based on generating a rotating excitation plane perpendicular to the imaging plane, which brings the spins on-resonance sequentially as it rotates around the center of the image. To generate radial tags, the on-resonance

excitation plane goes half a circle around the center. However, to generate circular tags, the on-resonance excitation plane rotates full circle, and therefore each spin is on-resonance at two time points, as previously described (Figure 12.36). At each of these two time points, the effective magnetic field, defined in the rotating frame of reference, passes through the transverse plane, and therefore the transverse rotation of the spins switches between clockwise and counterclockwise directions. This transfer may take place through two different mechanisms. One is the adiabatic mechanism in which the speed of rotation around the effective magnetic field, B_{eff}, is significantly greater than the speed of rotation of B_{eff} itself. In this mechanism, the direction of net magnetization follows the direction of B_{eff} and can flip completely with it. This kind of excitation, however, is not suitable for circular tagging since the excitation at the second time point effectively nulls the first one by returning the magnetization close to its equilibrium condition. In contrast, in the second mechanism, the magnetization fails to follow B_{eff} around the on-resonance moment, which results in the "turning condition" (described in the next section). The difference between these two mechanisms is illustrated in Figure 12.38. A considerable excitation during the turning condition is the key for producing an effective circular tagging sequence.

12.11.3.3 Turning Condition

In adiabatic rotation, there is no turning in the path of the spins. Considering φ as a function of time, when B_{eff} goes from the positive z-direction to the negative z-direction, there will be a local maximum for this function in the vicinity of t_{on}. That is, the second derivative of the function is negative ($\ddot{\varphi} < 0$) when the first derivative is nulled ($\dot{\varphi} = 0$) (see Figure 12.38) (Nasiraei-Moghaddam and Finn 2014). In contrast, the turning condition is characterized by a local minimum of φ (the second derivative is positive ($\ddot{\varphi} > 0$) when $\dot{\varphi} = 0$) since the spins' direction of rotation changes from clockwise to counterclockwise. This turning, however, may get reversed again, as shown in Figure 12.38. For an incomplete turning, the local minimum of φ is followed by a local maximum again. Therefore, in order to guarantee a complete turning, one should make sure that $\ddot{\varphi}$ remains positive as $\dot{\varphi}$ is close to zero.

Using Equation 12.53, we take the second derivative of φ to obtain the following:

$$\ddot{\varphi} = \gamma B_{1x}\left(-(1+\cot^2\theta)\cos\varphi \cdot \dot{\theta} - \cot\theta\sin\varphi \cdot \dot{\varphi} + (1+\cot^2\psi)\dot{\psi}\right), \quad (12.54)$$

where the angles are defined in Figure 12.37. Substituting $\dot{\varphi}$ and $\dot{\theta}$ from Equation 12.53 and Equation 12.48 into Equation 12.54, $\ddot{\varphi} > 0$ results in the following condition:

$$\frac{\dot{\psi}}{\gamma B_{1x}} > \sin^2\psi\left[\cot\theta \cdot \sin\varphi(\cot\theta \cdot \cos\varphi - \cot\psi)\right.$$

$$\left. + \cos\varphi \cdot \sin\varphi(1 + \cot^2\theta)\right]. \quad (12.55)$$

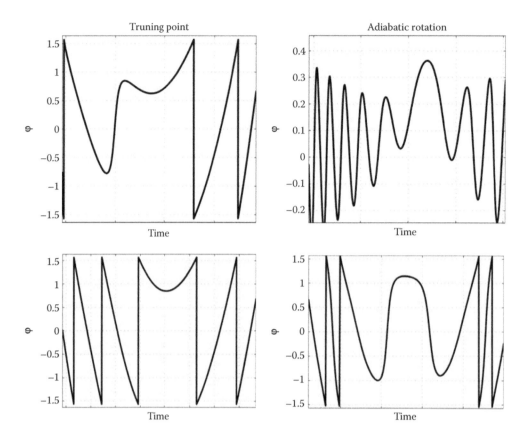

FIGURE 12.38 The typical changes of angle φ around the first excitation time point (T_{on1}) compared to adiabatic excitation. In the first row, the starting point of the magnetization was the equilibrium position (in the z-direction), whereas in the second row the starting point was offset by 45°. In the left column, the direction of rotation (shown by gradient of φ) changes suddenly from clockwise to counterclockwise. In the adiabatic condition, this change happens smoothly. (Reproduced from Nasiraei-Moghaddam, A. and Finn, J.P., *Magn. Reson. Med.*, 71(5), 1750, 2014. With permission.)

Using Equation 12.48, this condition can be rewritten as follows:

$$\frac{\dot{\psi}}{\dot{\theta}} > \sin^2\psi \left[\cot\theta (\cot\theta \cdot \cos\varphi - \cot\psi) + \cos\varphi (1 + \cot^2\theta) \right],$$
$$(12.56)$$

which implies that $\ddot{\varphi} > 0$ is associated with having a rapid change in the direction of the effective magnetic field, quantified by $\dot{\psi}$ compared to B_{1x}, and also changes in flip angle, θ. Considering Equations 12.53 and 12.55, when $\dot{\varphi} = 0$, this can be reduced to one of the following forms:

$$\frac{\dot{\psi}}{\gamma B_{1x}} > \sin^2\psi \cdot \cos\varphi \cdot \sin\varphi \, (1 + \cot^2\theta)$$

$$\Rightarrow \frac{\dot{\psi}}{\gamma B_{1x}} > \sin\psi \sin\varphi \, (\sin\psi \cos\varphi + \cos\psi \cot\theta). \quad (12.57)$$

$$\frac{\dot{\psi}}{\gamma B_{1x}} > (\sin^2\psi \cdot \sin 2\varphi + \sin 2\psi \cdot \sin\varphi \cdot \cot\theta)/2. \quad (12.58)$$

Considering that each of the sine functions has a maximum amplitude of one, a sufficient condition to meet Equation 12.58 is obtained when

$$\frac{\dot{\psi}}{\gamma |B_{1x}|} > 0.5 (1 + \cot\theta). \quad (12.59)$$

This condition only concerns the moment at which $\dot{\varphi} \to 0$ and it does not indicate a particular value for $\dot{\psi}$ since θ and its cotangent are not determined. Fortunately, the $\cot\theta$ term is minimum at the most critical turning condition when $\theta \sim 90°$ and the turning has not taken place yet. Hence, this implies that in order to have a turning point for small values of θ, a faster change in ψ is required. In particular, for $\theta > 45°$, Equation 12.59 shows that the condition $\dot{\psi}/\gamma |B_{1x}| > 1$ is sufficient at the time of turning. Figure 12.39 shows that Equation 12.59 is valid for a limited period of time around t_{on} when $\dot{\psi}$ spikes over $\gamma/|B_{1x}|$ (Nasiraei-Moghaddam and Finn 2014). It should be noted, however, that in addition to the magnitude of $\dot{\psi}/\gamma |B_{1x}|$, the length of the aforementioned period of time (t_{turn}) is also important. The duration t_{turn} should be long enough to complete the turning since for a very short

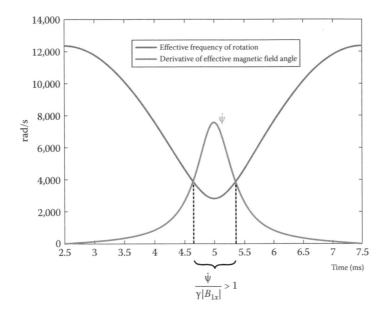

FIGURE 12.39 The effective frequency of spins rotation (the V-shaped plot) compared to the time derivative of the effective magnetic field angle. The figure shows that these two processes take place at comparable rates only in a small fraction of time (in the neighborhood of T_{on}) in the excitation period.

t_{turn} the turning may get started but be reversed later on. From a design perspective, it is important to have a quantitative estimation of how long t_{turn} should be to guarantee a complete turning. Here, we show that if in particular φ reaches 90°, then the turning will necessarily be completed (will not be reversed).

Suppose that φ increases ($\dot{\varphi} > 0$) until it passes 90° when $\psi \geq 90°$ (corresponding to $t \geq t_{on}$). Reversing the turning would require that $\dot{\varphi}$ decreases until it becomes zero. That is, $\dot{\varphi} \to 0$ while $\ddot{\varphi}$ is negative. This condition is not possible according to Equation 12.55, as explained by the following equations:

$$\varphi \geq 90° \Rightarrow 2\varphi \geq 180°$$
$$\Rightarrow \sin(2\varphi) \leq 0$$
$$\Rightarrow A = \sin^2(\psi)\sin(2\varphi)\left(1 + \cot^2\theta\right) \leq 0. \quad (12.60)$$

On the other hand,

$$\dot{\varphi} = \cot\theta \cdot \cos\varphi - \cot\psi; \quad \dot{\varphi} \to 0. \quad (12.61)$$

Therefore,

$$\sin^2\psi \cdot \cot\theta \cdot \sin\varphi(\cot\theta \cdot \cos\varphi - \cot\psi) + A/2 \leq 0. \quad (12.62)$$

This means that the right-hand side of Equation 12.56 is negative, while we know that the left-hand side is positive. Therefore, Equation 12.56 holds, which in turn guarantees that $\ddot{\varphi}$ is positive. In summary, $\varphi \geq 90°$ during t_{turn}, when the $\dot{\psi} \geq \gamma B_{1x}$ condition is maintained, acts as a sufficient condition for the turning to get completed and the desired excitation is imparted.

It is worth noting that $\dot{\psi}$ is a characteristic of the sequence and not the position or orientation of the spins, hence

$$\dot{\psi} = \frac{G_0\, r\cos(\omega_G t')\, \omega_G B_{1x}}{\left(G_0\, r\sin(\omega_G t')\right)^2 + B_{1x}^2} = \cot(\omega_G t') \cdot \cos\psi \cdot \sin\psi \cdot \omega_G,$$

$$(12.63)$$

where t' and ω_G represent $(T_{on1}-t)$ and $2\pi/T_p$, respectively. This shows that $\dot{\psi}$ is only a function of the sequence parameters and, of course, r, the distance from the isocenter. Therefore, we need to maintain the condition, $\dot{\psi} \geq \gamma B_{1x}$, for the smallest radius (r) for which tagging is required.

Figure 12.40 shows the evolution of in-plane phase and transverse magnetization in circular tagging, while Figure 12.41 shows circular tagged phantom and in vivo images, as well as the resulting k-space. It is interesting to note that one limitation that circular tagging shares with line tagging is the limited thickness of the myocardium, which may make it challenging to place a sufficient number of circular tags inside the myocardial wall.

12.11.4 Nonuniform Circular Tagging

As the circular symmetry of the LV shape in the SAX view does not exist in some pathological conditions, an elliptical tagging pattern may be more suitable than circular tagging for the assessment of radial strain in these conditions. Further, such capability would allow for more efficient measurement of other strain components from long-axis (LAX) tagged images. Oval taglines are obtained by setting nonequal amplitudes to the gradient pulses that form the rotating excitation plane, as

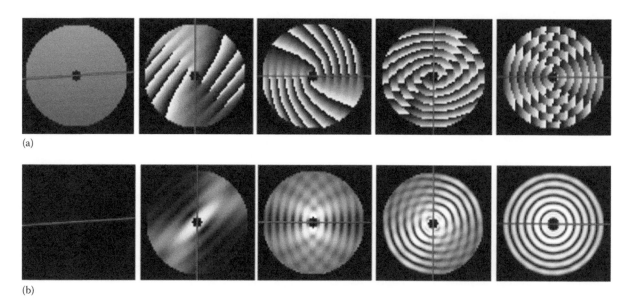

(a)

(b)

FIGURE 12.40   The evolution of the (a) in-plane phase, φ, and (b) transverse magnetization, M_{xy}, in a uniform phantom during the circular tagging sequence. Neglecting the phase wraps, an almost linear phase change is seen over any radial direction at the end of the preparation (top right). The red line shows the position of the perpendicular on-resonance plane. The panels show the situation at the beginning (left) and every quarter of the cycle as the on-resonance plane rotates counterclockwise until the circular tagging is completed (right). (Reproduced from Nasiraei-Moghaddam, A. and Finn, J.P., *Magn. Reson. Med.*, 71(5), 1750, 2014. With permission.)

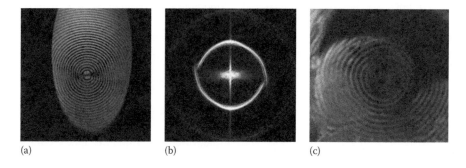

(a)   (b)   (c)

FIGURE 12.41   Circular tagging in the image space and k-space. (a) Circular tagging on a phantom. (b) K-space of the image in (a). (c) Circular tagging on a healthy volunteer. The effect of circular tagging is well separated in k-space. (Reproduced from Moghaddam, A.N. et al., *J. Cardiovasc. Magn. Reson.*, 13(Suppl 1), O27, 2011c.)

shown in Figures 12.42 and 12.43 (Moayed and Moghaddam 2014). For example, the amplitude of the G_x gradient should be selected larger than that of the G_y gradient to create a vertically oval tagging pattern. In general, the gradient amplitudes could be set based on the relationship between the large and small diameters of an oval-shaped heart to generate taglines tangent to the heart wall.

12.12   RADIAL TAGGING

12.12.1   ALTERNATE IMPLEMENTATION*

Tagging in the radial direction was the first type of tagging developed and applied in the heart, as discussed earlier in the chapter (Zerhouni et al. 1988). The pattern we describe in this

section features two characteristics that are different from the first radial tagging implementation. One feature is the density of the taglines, which can be much higher than earlier versions. The second feature is the width of taglines that increases with radius. These two characteristics, which are helpful for processing the tagged images, stem from a different approach for the implementation of this tagging sequence (Moghaddam and Finn 2010a, Nasiraei-Moghaddam and Finn 2014). Figure 12.44 shows these two sequences side by side to better show their similarities and differences (Moghaddam et al. 2010b). A rotating excitation plane with an alternating RF pulse, as shown in Figure 12.44a and represented by the following equations, results in an off-resonance type of excitation around the effective magnetic field (Figure 12.45), which generates a radial tagging pattern:

$$B_1(t) = B_1 \sin(2\pi f_c t) \sin(\pi t N / T_g), \qquad (12.64)$$

---

* We had the "first implementation" of this method covered earlier in the chapter in Section 12.7.

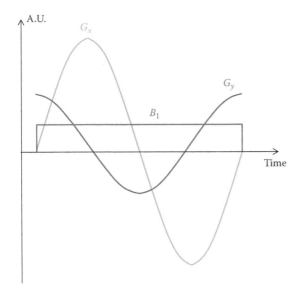

FIGURE 12.42 The pulse sequence diagram for elliptical tagging. Note that the tagging gradients have different scales.

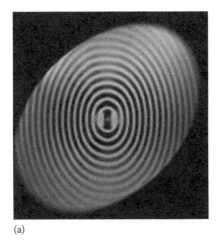

(a)

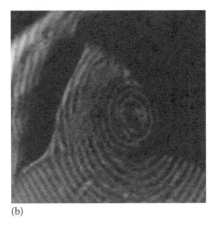

(b)

FIGURE 12.43 Implemented oval shape tagging pattern in (a) a phantom and (b) a cardiac patient. (Reproduced from Moayed, V. and Moghaddam, A.N., *J. Cardiovasc. Magn. Reson.*, 16(Suppl 1), P31, 2014.)

$$G_x = G_0 \sin\left(\pi t / T_g\right), \tag{12.65}$$

$$G_y = G_0 \cos\left(\pi t / T_g\right), \tag{12.66}$$

where the parameters in the aforementioned equations are defined in Figure 12.44a and f_c is the RF carrier frequency. The magnetization for the central part of the rotational excitation slab remains in the longitudinal direction when the envelope of the RF pulse crosses zero. Therefore, each zero-crossing of the RF pulse results in a bright radial tagline in the tagged image, that is, the number of the zero-crossings of the RF pulse determines the density of the radial taglines.

At first glance, the new sequence (Figure 12.44a) looks nothing more than a continuous version of the old one (Figure 12.44b). The continuity is of course the main reason for the second characteristic (increase of the tagline width with radius). For the first characteristic (higher density of the taglines), however, the reason is not so simple. As a matter of fact, each lobe of the RF pulse is not responsible for creating a single tagline, but rather it contributes to the formation of the adjacent taglines as well, as illustrated in Figure 12.46. This means that tagging can take place using less RF energy, and therefore the number and density of the taglines can be increased. In the new approach, we no longer use conventional spatially selective RF pulses. Figure 12.46 shows the trajectory of the tip of a single spin from different viewpoints during the excitation with this RF pulse. It is clearly different from selective excitation. In this example, only one-third of the excitation takes place during the RF signal lobe in which the on-resonance condition happens. If the magnitude of the gradient field increases, the share of the on-resonance lobe in the excitation process goes up, but the overall excitation decreases unless the B_1 magnitude also increases to make it up. This means we get closer to the selective regime, which is less energy efficient.

In contrast to the original radial implementation (Zerhouni et al. 1988), which is very confined, the new version of radial tagging spans a spectrum from almost selective excitation (large gradient fields and large RF pulses) to highly nonselective excitation. We should be cautious when using the word "nonselective" in this context since this term usually reminds us of very short hard RF pulses that excite a large portion of the body. This is not what we mean here. The RF pulses used with the newly developed sequence are very wide in time and very narrow in the frequency domain. Their function, however, differs from conventional selective pulses because of the time-varying gradient that changes the selected region for on-resonance excitation. Therefore, the excitation does not take place on a selective regime. More accurately, the "nonselective" term here is an attribute of the excitation rather than the RF pulse itself.

The quantification of the excitation in radial tagging, when it is highly nonselective, can be explained based on the approach used for circular tagging. By applying the duality concept, radial tagging could be implemented by exploiting a different interference effect: instead of being on-resonance twice with a single frequency, the spins can be on-resonance only

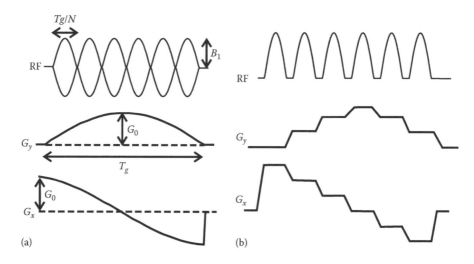

FIGURE 12.44   (a) New and (b) conventional pulse sequences for radial tagging.

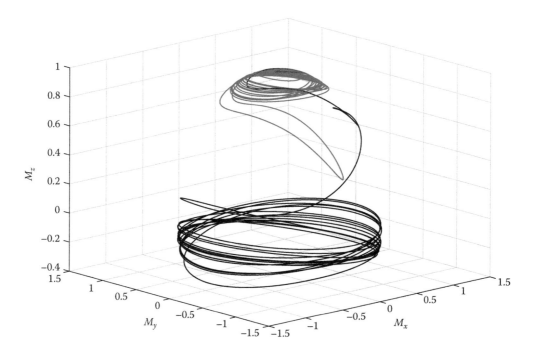

FIGURE 12.45   Simulated path of the magnetization tip in the rotating frame for two precessing spins with different locations in radial tagging (red path for bright band and black path for dark band).

once, but with different frequencies (Nasiraei-Moghaddam and Finn 2014). Here, the gradient field generates a rotating on-resonance plane that traverses half a circle in the presence of two constant RF pulses with slightly different frequencies, $f_c - f_1$ and $f_c + f_1$, such that on-resonance excitations take place at two time points, as shown in Figure 12.47. This dual sequence results in the dual pattern of circular tagging, that is, radial tagging. Physically, the two RF pulses can be generated by a single RF pulse with a sinusoidal envelope of frequency f_1, modulated by frequency f_c, as follows:

$$\cos 2\pi f_1 t \cdot \sin 2\pi f_c t = \frac{1}{2}\left(\sin 2\pi\left(f_c + f_1\right)t + \sin 2\pi\left(f_c - f_1\right)t\right).$$

$$(12.67)$$

Equation 12.67 and Figure 12.47 show that each spin is on-resonance at two time points shortly before and after the rotating plane passes through its location. Each of these resonances occurs with a constant B_{1x} as we had for the circular tagging. Therefore, the same excitation, described for the first t_{on} in the circular case, occurs twice. These two excitations around one t_{on} replace the two separate on-resonance excitations we had for circular tagging. They may interfere constructively or destructively depending on the azimuthal angle of the spins' position in the imaging plane. If the two hypothetical RF pulses arrive with opposed phases, those spins do not get excited at all. In contrast, the points on rays that see the RF pulses in-phase are excited most. This means that as the excitation plane rotates, the rays that are on-resonance at the time of zero-crossings of

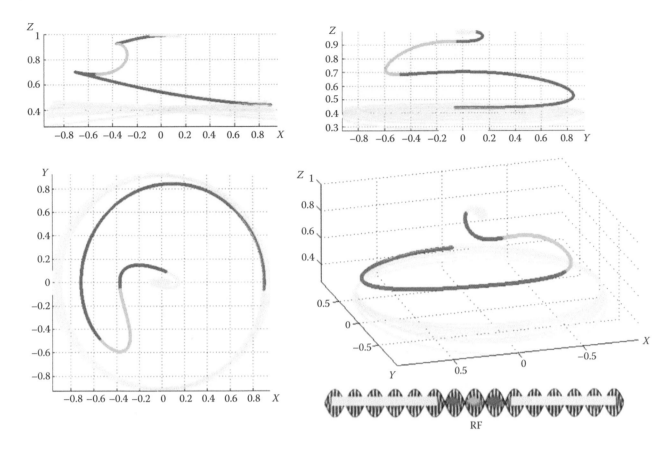

FIGURE 12.46 The path of a spin during radial tagging from different points of view. The following parameters were used: $B_1 = 2$ μT, $G_0 = 2$ mT/m, $r = 4$ cm, number of taglines = 15, and tagging time = 25 ms. The figure shows that the on-resonance lobe (shown in green) is responsible for only one-third of the excitation. The contributions of the pre- and postadjacent lobes are particularly significant.

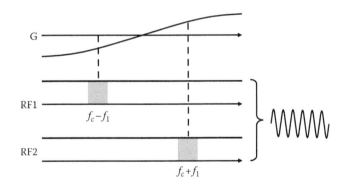

FIGURE 12.47 The radial tagging sequence as the dual version of the circular tagging process. The gradient field generates a rotating on-resonance plane that traverses half a circle in the imaging plane. Two constant RF pulses with slightly different central frequencies are used, such that their combination generates a sinusoidal envelope.

fan shape, which facilitates image postprocessing in the Fourier domain, for example, with the CIRCOME method (Moghaddam et al. 2007, Moghaddam and Finn 2008a,b), as described later in the chapter in Section 12.13.3. It should be noted that the tagline widening itself is useful as it causes the taglines to fade faster with distance from the tags' center, which results in less obscuring of the surrounding tissues. Figure 12.48 shows an example of radially tagged SAX image at end-diastole and end-systole.

12.12.2 Nonuniform Radial Tagging

There are a few derivatives of the polar tagging in which the on-resonance rotating plane does not rotate uniformly, similar to the nonuniform circular tagging discussed earlier. For the radial case, the taglines are not distributed evenly in the radial direction, whereas for the circular case, the curvature of the taglines do not remain constant. These derivations can be useful for evaluating some focal points on the myocardium wall or more generally for evaluating the wall motion in oblique slices of the heart when it has an oval shape. Some of these derivations are shown in Figure 12.49. None of these tagging preparation sequences takes more than 10 ms to generate.

the sine waveform acquire no excitation, while the rays that see the maximum of the sine wave are excited most, that is, an alternating radial pattern is produced for the residual longitudinal magnetization. The amount of modulation, however, decreases as the distance from the center of image increases. Further, the thickness of the radial tags grows radially in a

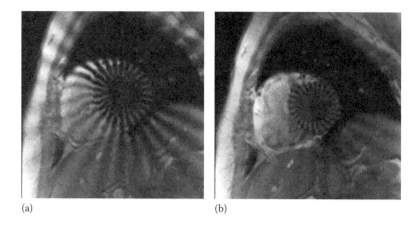

FIGURE 12.48 Radially tagged SAX LV slice at (a) diastolic and (b) systolic frames.

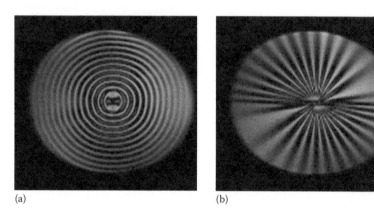

FIGURE 12.49 Nonuniform (a) circular and (b) radial tagging.

12.12.3 COMPLEMENTARY RADIAL TAGGING (CTR)

12.12.3.1 Basic Idea and Implementation

Similar to the CSPAMM tagging technique (Fischer et al. 1993) developed for conventionally tagged images, Wang et al. (2015) developed the complementary radial tagging (CRT) technique for improved radial tagging contrast. The CRT technique acquires two sets of radially tagged images with phase shift in the tagging pattern between the two sets. By subtracting the two sets of tagged images and implementing ramped flip angles imaging, a constant tagging contrast could be achieved throughout the cardiac cycle.

It is more convenient to express the radial tagging profile in the polar coordinate system, where the tagged image (I_{total}) consists of both tagged (I_{tag}) and untagged (I_{image}) components:

$$I_{total}(r,\theta,t) = I_{image}(r,\theta,t) + I_{tag}(r,\theta,t), \quad (12.68)$$

where the tag center is the origin, r is the radius, θ is the polar angle, and t is the time. The subtraction of two sets of tagged images eliminates the relaxed nontagged components and generates CRT images that contain only the tagging information:

$$I_{total,1}(r,\theta,t) - I_{total,2}(r,\theta,t) = I_{tag,1}(r,\theta,t) - I_{tag,2}(r,\theta,t). \quad (12.69)$$

The two sets of tagged images are acquired with the same RF pulse, but with sinusoidal gradients of different phases, where the phase shift (φ) between the gradients is given by

$$\varphi = \frac{\pi}{2N_{tag}}, \quad (12.70)$$

and N_{tag} is the number of taglines. If the phase shift φ is adjusted such that the tagging profiles in the two images have similar, but rotated, tagging patterns, represented as

$$I_{tag,1}(r,\theta,t) = I_{tag,2}(r,\theta+\varphi,t) \approx -I_{tag,2}(r,\theta,t), \quad (12.71)$$

then the two tagging profiles have opposite signs, and the tagging contrast is, therefore, doubled after subtraction:

$$I_{total,1}(r,\theta,t) - I_{total,2}(r,\theta,t) \approx 2I_{tag,2}(r,\theta,t). \quad (12.72)$$

By further applying ramped imaging flip angles similar to CSPAMM imaging, the resulting CRT images have a constant tagging contrast during the whole cardiac cycle.

In Wang et al. (2015), the authors used five half-sinusoid lobes in the tagging RF pulse to generate 10 radial lines in each set of images and a total of 20 CRT radial lines after

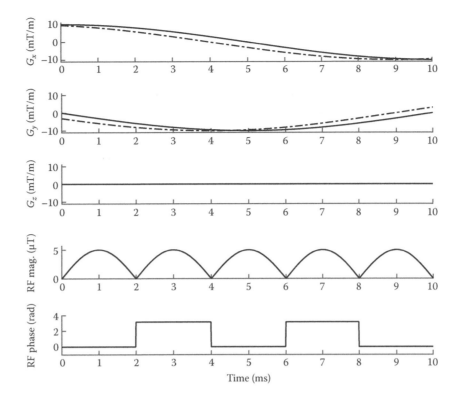

FIGURE 12.50 RF pulse (magnitude and phase) and gradient waveforms for the CRT pulse sequence. The sinusoidal-shaped gradients generate one set of radial tags (solid line), while the phase-shifted *x*- and *y*- gradients (dashed line) generate the complementary set of radial tags. The five sinusoidal lobes in the RF pulse create five radial taglines and 10 radial tags intersections with the LV wall, which double after CRT image subtraction.

image subtraction (Figure 12.50). It should be noted that the same number of RF lobes results in doubling the tagline density in CRT compared to the original radial tagging in (Nasiraei-Moghaddam and Finn 2014). Figure 12.51 shows CRT images versus conventional radially tagged images.

In summary, the CRT method generates an enhanced radial tagging contrast, which allows for accurate measurement of the LV rotational mechanics, especially at mid-diastasis and late diastole.

12.12.3.2 Alternative CRT Implementation

As an extension of the previous work by Wang et al. (2015), the same authors (Wang et al. 2014) developed an improved CRT technique, in which instead of using a single RF waveform and two phase-shifted gradient waveforms as in conventional CRT imaging, two different sinusoidal RF pulses are used with the same gradients (Figure 12.52) to generate the two radial tagging patterns.

The two RF pulses have the same magnitude with a phase difference of $\pi/2$, which generates two sets of inverted tagging patterns (Equation 12.73) and results in an enhanced tagging pattern after image subtraction (Equation 12.74) (Wang et al. 2014):

$$I_{tag,2}(r,\theta) = I_{tag,1}\left(r,\theta+\frac{\pi}{2}\right) \approx -I_{tag,1}(r,\theta). \quad (12.73)$$

$$I_{total,1}(r,\theta) - I_{total,2}(r,\theta) \approx 2I_{tag,1}(r,\theta). \quad (12.74)$$

Figure 12.53a shows a CRT image acquired using a single RF pulse envelope and two different gradients, while Figure 12.53b shows the image acquired with the improved CRT technique using different RF pulses with phase shifts, but the same gradients.

12.13 ANALYSIS METHODS SPECIFIC TO POLAR-TAGGED IMAGES

12.13.1 Polar HARP

The harmonic phase (HARP) concept (Osman et al., 1999) has been extended to the polar coordinate system. In the easiest form, and inspired by Figure 12.41a and b, we may assume that the spectral peaks of SPAMM have been spread over a circle for circular tagging. Therefore, by applying a half-circular BPF in k-space (Figure 12.54), the magnitude and phase images of the fundamental frequency in the circularly tagged image can be obtained. Using HARP analysis, tissue displacement in the direction normal to the taglines is calculated based on tracking the location of the pixels with the same phase in consecutive timeframes (Babaee and Moghaddam 2012). Figure 12.55 shows an unwrapped phase image of the circularly tagged image in Figure 12.54. The figure also shows the phase difference between the original and deformed images. This phase difference can be used to evaluate displacement in the radial direction.

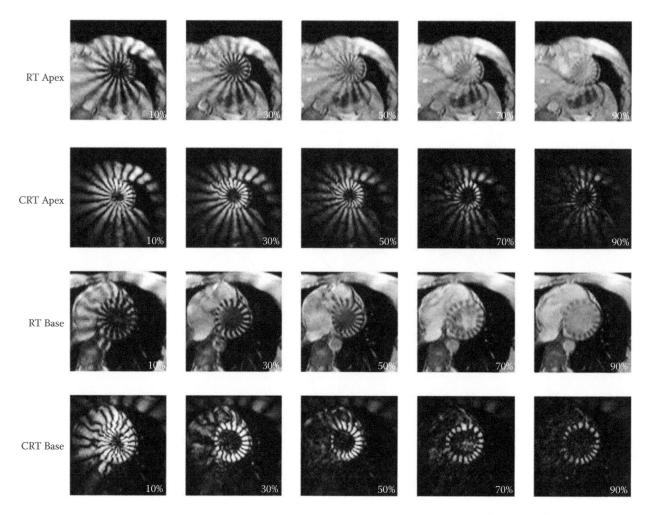

FIGURE 12.51 Comparison between radially tagged (RT) images and complementary (CRT) images in a healthy human subject. For RT and CRT images, apical and basal LV images in the SAX view are annotated as RT Apex, CRT Apex, RT Base, and CRT Base, respectively. The taglines fade in the RT images, but retain higher contrast in the CRT images, especially at later cardiac phases. The acquisition time as percentage of the cardiac cycle length (RR period) is shown on each image. (Reproduced from Wang, Z. et al., *Magn. Reson. Med.*, 73(4), 1432, 2015. With permission.)

12.13.2 High-Resolution Circular Tagging

High-density tagging facilitates the postprocessing step required for strain quantification and improves the measurements' accuracy. In this context, the polar HARP technique (Babaee and Moghaddam 2012), which determines the position of the polar tags from the reconstructed phase image, has been extended to increase the resolution and density of the circular tags during reconstruction (Aghaeifar et al. 2013a,b). Specifically, successive directional filters are used to decrease distortion in the angle images. The density of the taglines is then increased by multiplying the phase of the resulting angle images. To accommodate for the enhanced tagline density, the image resolution is increased by zero padding the k-space. These enhancement steps have been successfully implemented for matrices up to 1640 × 1920 pixels in size with increased reconstruction time of less than a second for each image frame (Figure 12.56; Aghaeifar et al. 2013a).

Figure 12.57 illustrates the processing steps of the improved polar HARP technique (Aghaeifar et al. 2013b). Based on the HARP theory of operation, the first step in tags reconstruction is the isolation of the spectral peaks corresponding to the

circular tags. As the circular tags are represented by an augmented crown around the k-space center, a narrow 2D half Gaussian BPF is used to extract this information from the k-space (Babaee and Moghaddam 2012). It should be noted that because of the conjugate symmetry of the k-space, using a full-circle Gaussian filter generates no phase for real objects. The 2D Gaussian filter is represented as

$$g(k_x, k_y) = \frac{1}{2\pi\sigma} e^{\frac{\left(\sqrt{k_x^2 + k_y^2} - R_{max}\right)^2}{2\sigma^2}} \qquad (12.75)$$

where R_{max} (see Figure 12.58) is the radius corresponding to the maximum energy density, E_i, defined as the average of the absolute magnitudes at a specific radius r_i

$$E_i = \frac{\sum f(k_x, k_y)}{2\pi r_i} \Bigg|_{\sqrt{k_x^2 + k_y^2} = r_i}, \qquad (12.76)$$

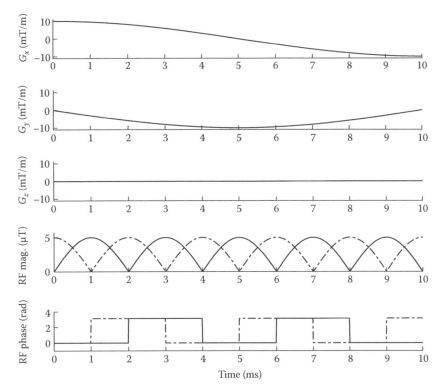

FIGURE 12.52 Alternative complementary radial tagging (CRT) pulse sequence diagram using two different sinusoidal RF pulses with the same gradients. Two RF pulses (solid and dashed lines) generate the two sets of radial tagged images with a phase difference.

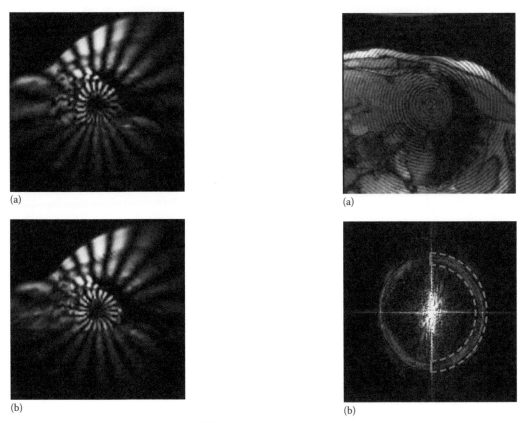

FIGURE 12.53 In vivo complementary radial tagging (CRT) images acquired using (a) single RF pulse and different gradients, and (b) two RF pulses with the same gradients. (Reproduced from Wang, Z. et al., *Proceedings of the International Society of Magnetic Resonance in Medicine*, p. 4232, 2014. With permission.)

FIGURE 12.54 (a) A circularly tagged image of a healthy volunteer and (b) its corresponding k-space. The half-circular band-pass filter is shown in (b). (Reproduced from Babaee, N. and Moghaddam, A.N., *J. Cardiovasc. Magn. Reson.*, 14(Suppl 1), W15, 2012.)

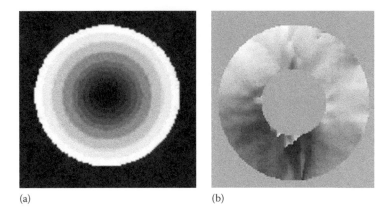

(a)   (b)

FIGURE 12.55 (a) An unwrapped phase image that contains the myocardium in Figure 12.54. (b) The phase difference between the original and deformed images. (Reproduced from Babaee, N. and Moghaddam, A.N., *J. Cardiovasc. Magn. Reson.*, 14(Suppl 1), W15, 2012.)

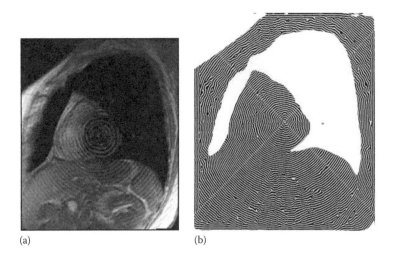

(a)   (b)

FIGURE 12.56 (a) Regular and (b) high-density circularly tagged images.

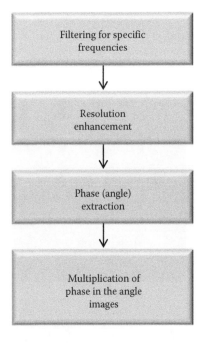

FIGURE 12.57 Algorithm for generating high-density circular tagged images.

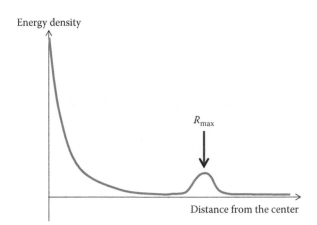

FIGURE 12.58 The first peak in the energy density function represents R_{max}.

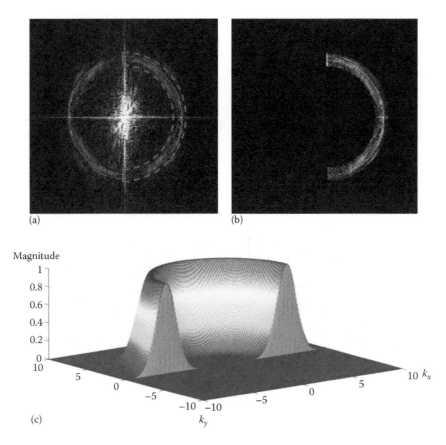

FIGURE 12.59 Polar HARP, where the k-space is filtered using a 2D half-Gaussian band-pass filter. (a) Frequency domain of a circularly tagged phantom. (b) The result of applying the Gaussian filer in k-space. (c) Gaussian band-pass filter.

where $f(k_x, k_y)$ is the absolute magnitude value in the k-space. The resulting k-space image after applying the Gaussian filter (Figure 12.59) is given by

$$P(k_x, k_y) = g(k_x, k_y) \times I(k_x, k_y), \qquad (12.77)$$

$$-\frac{\pi}{2} < \varphi < \frac{\pi}{2} \bigg| \varphi = \tan^{-1}\frac{k_y}{k_x}. \qquad (12.78)$$

where I represents the circularly tagged image. To acquire the phase corresponding to the taglines, angle images are produced, wherein the phase angle is wrapped between $-\pi$ and $+\pi$. To improve the tagline density, the phase image is multiplied by factor n and the cosine of resulting phase image is calculated:

$$-\pi < \theta < \pi, \quad P = P_0, \qquad (12.79)$$

$$-n\pi < n\theta < n\pi, \quad P = P_0, \qquad (12.80)$$

$$-1 < \cos(n\theta) < 1, \quad P = nP_0, \qquad (12.81)$$

where

P in the previous equations represents the tagline density
P_0 is the tagline density in the original image

In practice, tag increment factors up to 6 have been successfully examined (Aghaeifar et al. 2013b). Since the size of the

k-space matrix is not sufficient for presenting the effect of the multiplied phase in the images, the image resolution needs to be increased, for example, using k-space zero filling.

12.13.3 CIRCOME

12.13.3.1 Basic Idea

Circumferential strain is a major index of the cardiac function as it measures myocardial contractility. Calculating strain from conventional MRI-tagged images typically includes two steps: (1) measuring the displacement field, which is a time-consuming postprocessing step, and (2) performing spatial differentiation on the displacement field, which is a noise-sensitive process. Circumferential compression encoding (CIRCOME) is a novel technique for noninvasive and quick measurement of circumferential strain (Moghaddam et al. 2007, Moghaddam and Finn 2008a,b). CIRCOME directly uses the frequency information in the k-space of radially tagged images to measure circumferential strain. Therefore, it avoids explicit measurement of the displacement field and does not require spatial differentiation to calculate strain. Furthermore, CIRCOME has the potential to simultaneously encode circumferential myocardial contraction in several SAX slices and in real-time, which allows for robust measurement of global circumferential strain.

In MRI tagging, the distance of a point from the k-space center corresponds to the tagging frequency, whereas its angle shows the tags' direction (Moghaddam and Finn 2008a) (Figure 12.60). Specifically, in the case of radial tagging, symmetrical distribution of spatial frequency in the image results in a circle in the k-space with a constant magnitude (Figure 12.61). However, if the distribution of that spatial frequency is not symmetric, its effect would still be focused on the same circle, but not uniformly anymore.

The CIRCOME algorithm consists of three steps (Moghaddam and Finn 2008a):

1. Acquisition of a ring-shaped crown region in the k-space
2. Reconstruction of a circumferentially compression-weighted image by applying narrow circular band-pass filters in the k-space
3. Calculation of circumferential strain

12.13.3.2 Circular Band-Pass Filtering of K-Space

Figure 12.62a shows a radially tagged SAX image, while Figure 12.62b shows the resulting reconstructed image of a specific circular region of the k-space of the image in Figure 12.62a. Figure 12.62b demonstrates only part of the tissue structure with the level of compression associated with the extracted k-space data. Regions with different degrees of radial taglines compression can be obtained through circular band-pass filtering of the k-space (Moghaddam and Finn 2008a) (Figure 12.63). These regions become more specific with more selective filters (i.e., thinner circle or smaller filters' BW in the k-space). A functional image encoded by the level of radial taglines compression can be obtained through sequential scanning of the whole k-space by circular BPFs and weighing of each recovered region with the corresponding frequency. Figure 12.64 shows the result of this procedure in the case of a slight deformation in a simulated image.

12.13.3.3 Calculation of Circumferential Strain

Circumferential strain, defined as the percentage change in tissue length, can be calculated from the k-space information because the circumferential length at a certain point is inversely proportional to the spatial frequency that

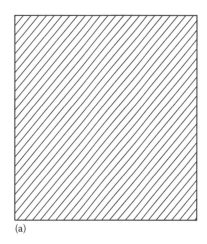

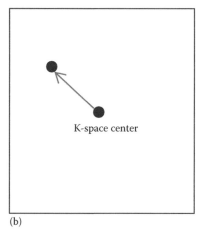

(a)   (b)

FIGURE 12.60   Relationship between taglines in the image domain and representation in the k-space. (a) Tagged image. (b) A point in the k-space and the vector that connects it to the k-space origin. The length of this vector and its direction determine the frequency and direction, respectively, of the taglines in the image.

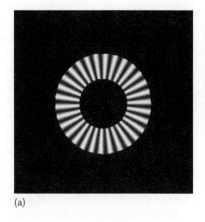

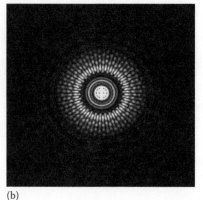

(a)   (b)

FIGURE 12.61   (a) Magnetization modulation resulting from radial tagging in a circular phantom. (b) Fourier domain of the simulated image in (a).

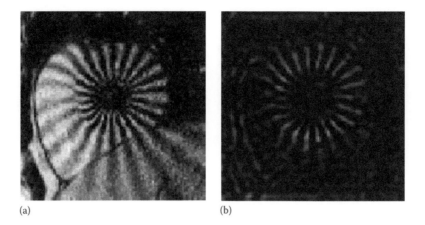

FIGURE 12.62 Radial tagging and circular band-pass filtering. (a) A short-axis image of a healthy heart with radial taglines. (b) Reconstruction of the image in (a) using a narrow circular band-pass filter in the Fourier domain. The reconstructed image mainly contains the LV and some noise in the background.

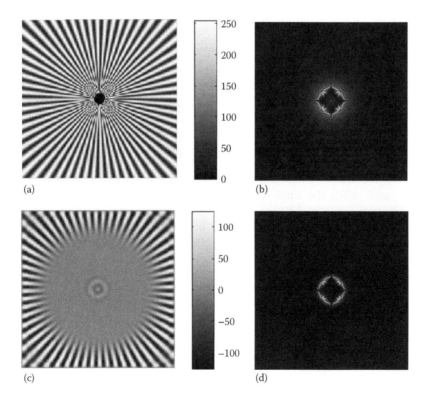

FIGURE 12.63 (a) A sample image with radial tagging, (b) its spatial frequencies in k-space, (c) filtered image that shows the region with a tagline density level in a specific range, and (d) band-pass filtered k-space of the image in (c).

corresponds to the radial density of the taglines at that point, that is, circumferential strain can be calculated as

$$\varepsilon = \frac{L'}{L} - 1$$
$$= \frac{k}{k'} - 1, \tag{12.82}$$

where $L(k)$ and $L'(k')$ represent the tissue length (corresponding spatial frequency of the radial taglines) before and after

deformation, respectively. Global circumferential strain can then be determined by simply measuring the shift of the average circumferential frequency between two timeframes. Further, regional circumferential strain can be measured by comparing the frequency between corresponding regions before and after deformation. Therefore, the CIRCOME technique allows for automatic calculation of circumferential strain without the need for applying time-consuming tissue tracking techniques or differentiation operations (Moghaddam and Finn 2008a).

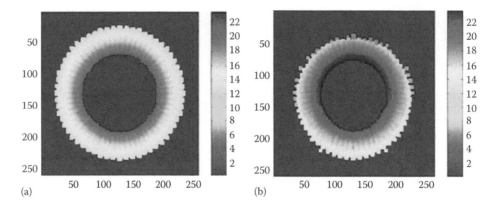

FIGURE 12.64   (a) Circumferential frequency of the radially tagged image in Figure 12.61(a), where the level of compression is shown with color coding. (b) Contraction of the higher half of the circle is obvious in the colored image. (Reproduced from Moghaddam, A.N. et al., CIRcumferential COMpression Encoding (CIRCOME), *Proceedings of the International Society for Magnetic Resonance in Medicine*, Berlin, Germany, 2007, p. 2515. With permission.)

12.13.3.4 Technique's Efficiency and Validation

The performance of the CIRCOME technique has been compared to HARP analysis (Moghaddam et al. 2011a). Circumferential strain has been measured in five healthy volunteers and a single-ventricle patient. The imaging parameters were as follows: 30 radial taglines across the whole LV, field of view (FOV) = 250 mm, slice thickness = 5 mm, echo time (TE)/repetition time (TR) = 4.6/87 ms, BW = 250 Hz/pixel, and imaging flip angle = 15°. In general, the CIRCOME and HARP global circumferential strain measurements showed good agreement. The global circumferential strain in the five healthy volunteers was in the normal physiological range, while the single-ventricle patient had a maximum absolute strain of 27%, as shown in Figure 12.65. Regional strain measurements from HARP showed spatial variations, especially between the LV free wall and the septum. On the other hand, the overall strain calculated using CIRCOME was similar to the average strain for these segments, which shows that circumferential strain measurements from CIRCOME are comparable to those from HARP.

12.13.3.5 Parameters Affecting CIRCOME

Various parameters, including tagline fading, eccentricity of the radial taglines' center and their density, spatial resolution, and SNR, affect the accuracy of circumferential strain measurement with the CIRCOME technique, as shown in the simulations in Figures 12.66 and 12.67 (Moghaddam and Finn 2008a). The tagline fading (Figure 12.66b), as a consequence of longitudinal magnetization relaxation during the cardiac cycle, affects the efficiency of the CIRCOME technique. Nevertheless, higher tagline density could help differentiate between the taglines and confounding anatomy in the k-space. In general, the CIRCOME algorithm should be designed to be robust against changes in the circular peaks generated by the radial taglines.

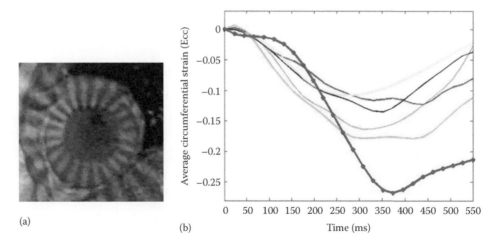

FIGURE 12.65   Radial tagging in congenital heart disease. (a) A radially tagged image of a single-ventricle patient overlaid by the density weighted image of the taglines. (b) Strain estimation for normal versus a single-ventricle patient data (bold line with dots). The circumferential strain is significantly higher in the single-ventricle patient compared to normal subjects at all levels. (Reproduced from Moghaddam, A.N. et al., Left ventricular strain through Radial Tagging: Efficiency and validity, *Proceedings of the International Society for Magnetic Resonance in Medicine*, Montreal, Quebec, Canada, 2011a, p. 3368. With permission.)

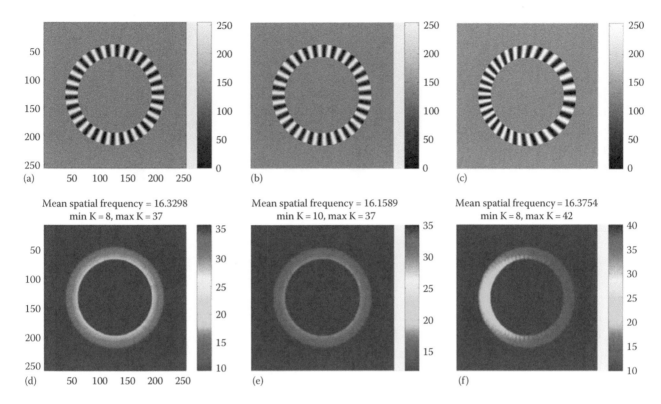

FIGURE 12.66 Simulated radially tagged images of a SAX slice of the LV are shown in the top row, followed by their corresponding color-coded CIRCOME images in the bottom row, which show the effects of radial taglines fading and eccentricity on the resulting images. (a, d) Original images. (b, e) The effect of tagline fading. (c, f) The effect of eccentricity. The color scales are different depending on the detectible spatial frequencies.

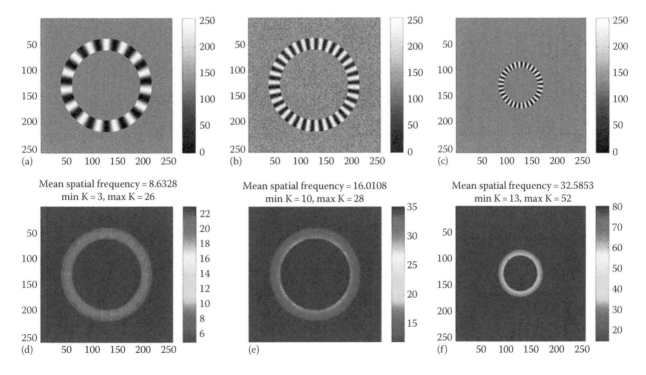

FIGURE 12.67 Simulated radially tagged images of a SAX slice of the LV are shown in the top row, followed by their corresponding color-coded CIRCOME images in the bottom row, which show the effects of sparse tagging, noise, and resolution. (a, d) Sparse tagging. (b, e) The effect of noise with a standard deviation of 10% of the maximum signal. (c, f) The effect of lower resolutions. Scales of coloring are different depending on the detectible spatial frequencies.

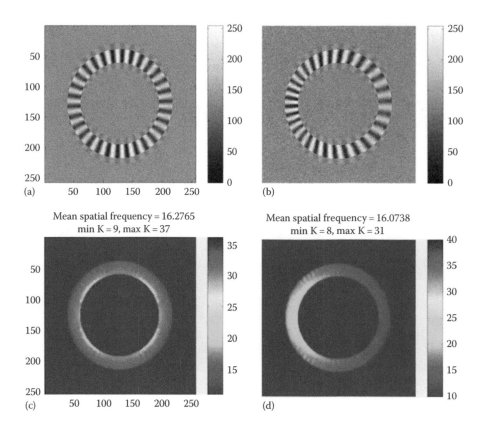

FIGURE 12.68   (a, b) Simulated radially tagged images of an LV SAX slice, and (c, d) their corresponding color-coded CIRCOME, which show the effects of (a, c) motion and (b, d) combined motion, sparsity, noise, and tags fading.

Ideally, the intersection point of the radial taglines should be at the center of the LV cavity in SAX views. Nevertheless, this condition is not always fulfilled, where the eccentricity in the center of the taglines results in a wider range of distribution of the tagline density (Figure 12.66f). This in turn increases the BW of the circular ring in the k-space over which the tagged information is encoded and decreases the relative strength of each associated spatial frequency in this BW. The former effect results in increased processing time of the implemented algorithm, while the latter leads to decreased accuracy in identifying the taglines from other structures with the same spatial frequency.

The sparser the radial taglines the harder to separate them from confounding anatomy based on the k-space filtering approach in CIRCOME. In Figure 12.67a, the angular frequency of the taglines is half of that in the original image, which brings the corresponding spatial frequency closer to the center of k-space, as shown in Figure 12.67d, and makes it more difficult to isolate the tagging pattern from static tissues. Figure 12.67b, e shows the effect of increased noise on the tagged image. Finally, Figure 12.67c, f shows the effect of reduced spatial resolution on the tagged image, where the central angular frequency of the taglines and associated BW are inversely proportional to the pixel size.

Figure 12.68 illustrates the robustness of the CIRCOME technique in a variety of imperfect imaging conditions (motion in Figure 12.68a, c and combined effects of motion, eccentricity, noise, and tags fading in Figure 12.68b, d). It has been shown that the error in strain measurement using CIRCOME does not exceed 10% of the maximum strain (Moghaddam and Finn 2008a). In particular, the technique showed to be less affected by eccentricity of the taglines center. However, the tagline sparsity caused the most significant error.

12.14   TOWARD REAL-TIME STRAIN IMAGING WITH POLAR TAGGING

12.14.1   INLINE CIRCULAR DENSITY MAPS

Despite the advantages of cardiac tagging, offline processing remains a major limitation in clinical applications. Fortunately, polar tagging has features that help with online processing. Using CIRCOME, Aghaeifar et al. (2014) developed a fast reconstruction technique for inline generation of radial strain maps from circular tagged images, such that the results are immediately available on the scanner console. As the circular tags are represented by a localized annulus in k-space (Figure 12.69), myocardial contraction, which increases the compression of the underlying tagging pattern, leads to widening of the annular ring in the frequency domain. Therefore, strain can be evaluated simply by finding the most prevalent spatial frequency of each annular region in the k-space, which shows the local tagging density in this region. A density map of radial strain (Figure 12.70) can thus be generated by implementing a series of narrow band-pass ring-shaped filters in k-space and cross-correlating the reconstructed images with the original one.

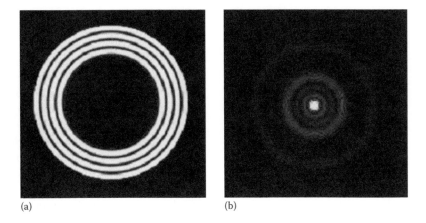

(a)   (b)

FIGURE 12.69 Relation between (a) circular tags in image domain and (b) corresponding result in the k-space domain. Circular tags are represented as an augmented crown around the center in the k-space.

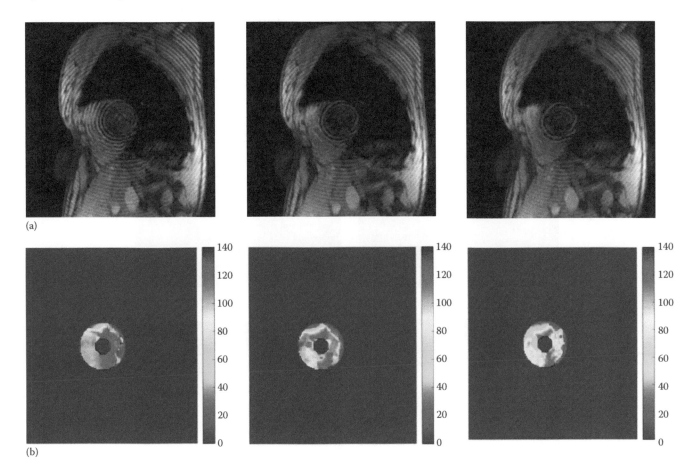

(a)

(b)

FIGURE 12.70 (a) Three consecutive frames of circularly tagged images through the cardiac cycle and (b) their corresponding density maps. The red areas in the density maps represent higher density of the taglines in these areas.

12.14.2 REAL-TIME CIRCULAR TAGGING

In an effort to accelerate strain maps reconstruction, Golshani et al. (2014) investigated the feasibility of real-time data acquisition in radial strain imaging from circularly tagged images. The idea of the developed technique is to selectively sample the k-space with a set of concentric ring acquisitions, then reconstruct the image using an algorithm based on Hankel Transform. Figure 12.71 shows an example of selective k-space sampling, where 21 concentric circles (out of total 192 circles) are chosen for acquisition, resulting in 89% saving in data acquisition time. The 21 circles include 4 circles in the central k-space region that

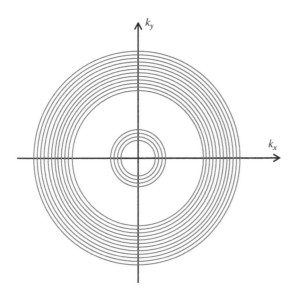

FIGURE 12.71 Real-time circular tagging. The k-space selected for the final reconstruction from partial ring acquisitions in the k-space.

capture the image contrast, and 17 circles that span the spatial frequency range of the circular tagging pattern. Figure 12.72 shows images reconstructed with different acceleration factors, where the general shape and quality of the taglines have been maintained. With acquisitions of 30%, 11%, and 8% of the full k-space data, the correlation coefficients between the resulting reconstructed images and the original image acquired with all k-space data were 0.99, 0.92, and 0.86, respectively. Nevertheless, some deviations can be observed in the tagging pattern when the data acquisition goes all the way down to 8% (Figure 12.72e). To evaluate the quality of the resulting images, the cross-correlation coefficients between these images and the original image, which is reconstructed from the entire k-space data, have been measured. This study shows the capability of acquiring more than nine frames per second of tagged images using the developed technique, which would allow for fast and efficient strain imaging with potential applications in stress and dynamic imaging.

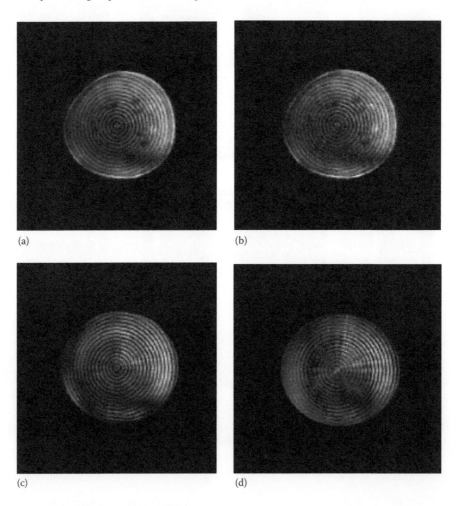

(a)　(b)　(c)　(d)

FIGURE 12.72 Image quality with partial k-space acquisition in circular tagging. (a) Image reconstructed by the proposed algorithm using the entire k-space data. (b) Image reconstructed from 30% of k-space data. (c) Image reconstructed from 11% of k-space data. (d) Image reconstructed from 8% of k-space. As can be seen, the quality of taglines in the last image is degraded, where the correlation coefficient value is reduced as well.

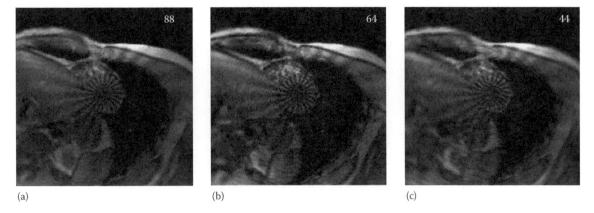

FIGURE 12.73 Partial data acquisition and image reconstruction of radially tagged images using (a) 88, (b) 64, and (c) 40 radial spokes in the k-space.

12.14.3 REAL-TIME RADIAL TAGGING

Most recently, Golshani et al. (2015) developed a similar technique for fast acquisition and reconstruction of the radially tagged images using polar Fourier transform (PFT)—a Hankel-based transform for reconstruction of nonuniform distributed data on polar grids. The developed technique showed high robustness against reduction of the number of acquired radial spokes. Figure 12.73 illustrates this robustness in a volunteer, where the images are reconstructed using different number of radial spokes. The technique allowed for reducing the imaging time by two thirds with no degradation of the quality of the tagged myocardium in the images.

12.15 CLINICAL APPLICATIONS OF POLAR TAGGING

A number of preliminary studies have been recently conducted to illustrate the clinical importance of polar tagging. In 2013, Kaveh et al. (2013) used radially tagged images for fast and reliable quantification of the LV twist, defined as the difference between apical and basal rotations, directly in the image domain without the need for complicated postprocessing. In other studies by Khan et al. (2013, 2014), the authors evaluated polar tagging for measuring radial and circumferential strain in healthy volunteers, patients with CHD, and patients with cardiomyopathy (CMP). Comparative visual assessment of polar versus conventional grid tagging was performed by two observers for each of the six mid-ventricular segments (based on AHA 17-segment model), and scores were assigned for the overall tags quality, strain, confidence in the findings, and ease of interpretation. Further, quantitative analysis of global and segmental strain was performed using a semiautomated tool. The results showed that the healthy volunteers had the highest scores for tags quality, strain, and confidence and ease of interpretation, followed by the CHD and CMP patients.

Nevertheless, the scores for the tags quality and confidence in strain assessment were not significantly different among conventional grid tagging (5–7 mm tag separation), circular tagging (5 mm tag separation), and radial tagging (18° tag separation). For ease of interpretation, however, polar tagging was significantly superior to conventional grid tagging. Figures 12.74 through 12.76 show polar-tagged images in a healthy volunteer, CHD patient, and CMP patient, respectively.

Recently, Kaveh et al. (2014) used radial tagging (22 taglines per circle) to investigate the regional rotation pattern of the LV mid-ventricular wall in healthy subjects and patients with CMP. The results showed that mid-ventricular rotation and rotation rate were decreased in the CMP patients relative to the healthy subjects in most circumferential segments (Figure 12.77). Further, the homogeneity of the regional rotations was significantly higher in the healthy subjects compared to the patients, as shown in Figure 12.78.

Circular tagging allows for directly measuring radial strain, as shown in Figure 12.79. Immediately after applying the circular tags, which takes only about 10 ms, the spatial frequency in the k-space is constant for all points. As described in the CIRCOME method, the spatial frequency of each point in the deformed image can be determined by sequential band-pass filtering of the k-space. Radial strain is then measured from the relative change in spatial frequency between the initial and deformed states (Haftekhanaki et al. 2012).

For further validation, circular tagging has been compared to HARP analysis for measuring radial strain (Figure 12.80), where the results showed general agreement between the two techniques, despite a slight measurement underestimation by HARP (Haftekhanaki et al. 2012). Nevertheless, as no tag tracking or differentiation operation is needed in circular tagging, the technique is associated with reduced computational cost and increased measurement accuracy.

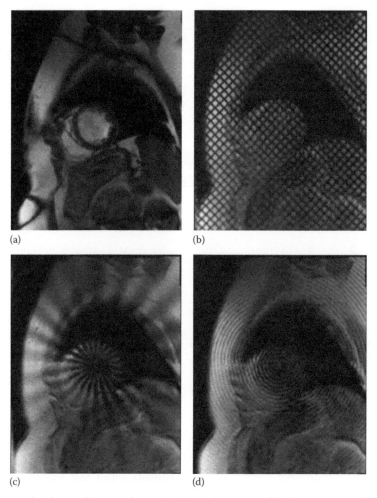

(a)

(b)

(c)

(d)

FIGURE 12.74   Polar and conventional tagged images from a healthy volunteer. (a) Cine image in a mid-ventricular slice. (b) Cartesian grid tagging pattern. (c) Radial tagging pattern. (d) Circular tagging pattern.

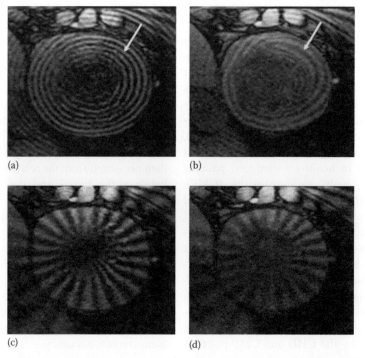

(a)

(b)

(c)

(d)

FIGURE 12.75   (a, b) Circular- and (c, d) radial-tagged images from a patient with single functional ventricle acquired during (a, c) diastole and (b, d) systole. Some morphological changes can be directly observed in the images with no processing (arrows).

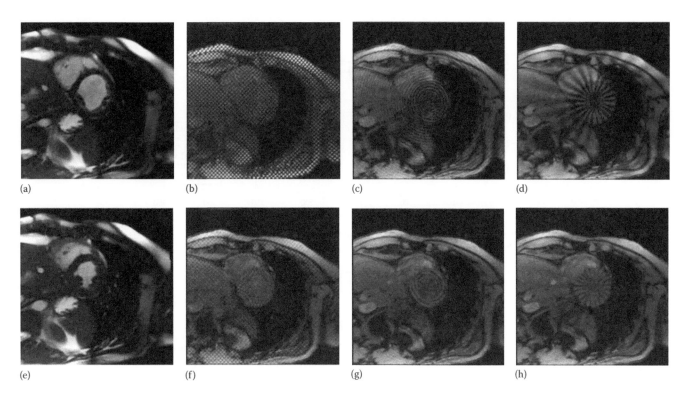

FIGURE 12.76 Polar-tagged images from a cardiomyopathic patient. The patient has infarction affecting the septum and a global ejection fraction of 20%. (a–d) Diastolic and (e–h) systolic images showing diminished strain (radial strain 7.8%; circumferential strain −6.9%).

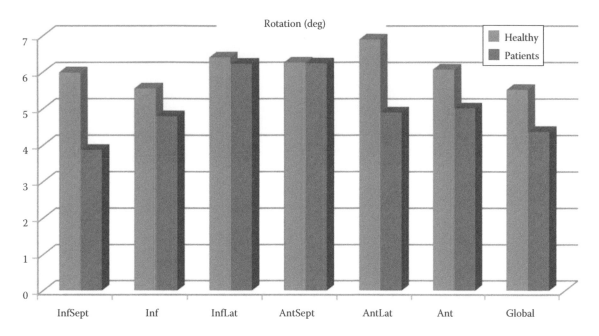

FIGURE 12.77 Segmental and global peak rotation differences between healthy and cardiomyopathic patients as determined by radial tagging.

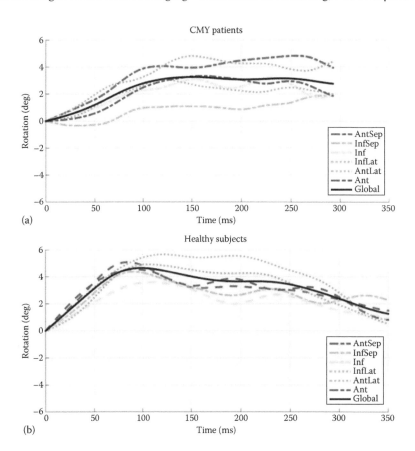

FIGURE 12.78 Mean regional and global rotation of the LV mid-ventricle in (a) nine cardiomyopathic patients and (b) 12 healthy subjects, as determined by radial tagging.

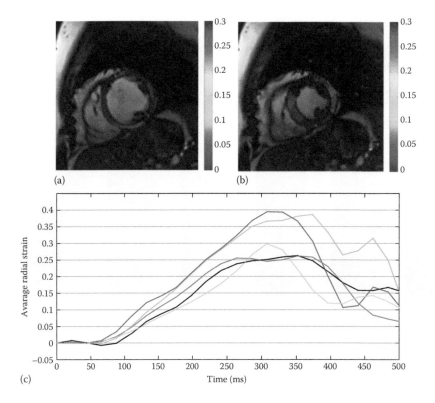

FIGURE 12.79 Radial strain from circular tagging. The radial strain map on a per-pixel basis overlaid on the SSFP image of a healthy volunteer at (a) diastole and (b) systole. (c) Global radial strain estimation over the cardiac cycle for five normal volunteers in the mid-LV, calculated using the CIRCOME method.

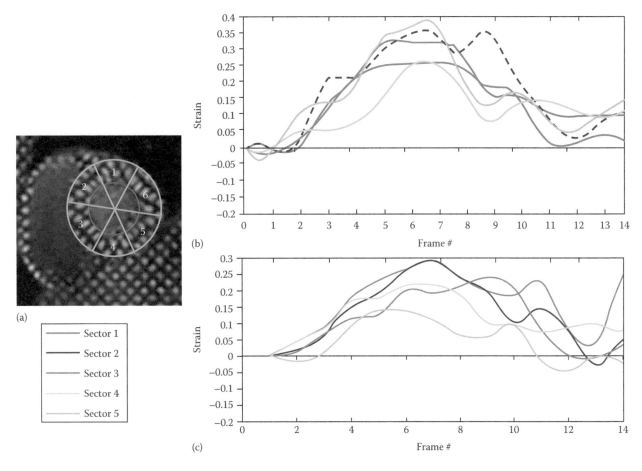

FIGURE 12.80 Circular tagging versus HARP analysis. (a) An LV mid-ventricle short-axis slice with grid taglines and standard segments. Global radial strain estimated over the cardiac cycle for different segments, calculated by (b) the circular compression encoding (CIRCOME) technique and (c) HARP analysis. (Reproduced from Haftekhanaki, M. et al., Measuring the radial component of left ventricular strain with circular tagging, Feasibility and initial results, *Proceedings of the International Society for Magnetic Resonance in Medicine*, Melbourne, Victoria, Australia, 2012, p. 3794. With permission.)

12.16 SUMMARY AND KEY POINTS

12.16.1 SUMMARY

Magnetic resonance tagging is a powerful technique for encoding certain patterns in the imaged object. The potential clinical importance of tagging the heart for quantifying its motion has resulted in a tremendous amount of time and energy spent designing tagging patterns that avail themselves to capturing the cardiac motion most effectively.

Cartesian tagging patterns, though not the first patterns invented, quickly became the clinical and research standard for encoding spatial magnetization saturation patterns to evaluate motion of the beating heart. Cartesian tagging patterns, in particular using the SPAMM technique, can be generated very quickly and have remained the most common and accepted way for generating cardiac tagged images.

A great amount of knowledge has been gained by evaluating methods that can generate other Cartesian tagging patterns with nonuniform spacing and in localized regions, but to date, these techniques have not seen widespread adoption. Recently, non-Cartesian tagging patterns have been revisited.

The earliest work of Zerhouni et al., which first established the field of myocardial tagging, has led to new discoveries about more efficient and effective ways for generating tagging patterns that are more matched to the natural geometry of the heart in the SAX view.

More recently, a coherent mathematical framework has been developed for describing both radial and circular tagging patterns, which can be generated in a short time duration, such that it is practical to use them for cardiac motion imaging. Future work will establish the importance of the polar tagging methods and potential clinical applications.

12.16.2 KEY POINTS

- The SPAMM technique has been the most widely used tagging sequence since its invention in the late 1980s until the current day.
- In its simplest form, SPAMM is based on wrapping the magnetization in a periodic fashion through space by applying only two equal-strength nonselective RF pulses separated by a wrapping gradient.

- DANTE applies a train of RF pulses in the presence of a continuous gradient to create a high-density pattern of thin tags.
- CSPAMM enhances the tagging contrast and eliminates tags fading. The tagging contrast is enhanced through the acquisition of two datasets of images with opposite tagging patterns, which when subtracted result in improved tagging contrast. Tags fading is eliminated using ramped imaging flip angles through the cardiac cycle.
- Localized tagging limits the tags to the region of interest; therefore, it eliminates anatomical obstruction in the nontagged regions.
- Using multispectral RF pulses in the tagging sequence leads to the generation of orthogonal saturation bands that tag only a small region of the heart, albeit still saturating some tissues distant from the heart.
- In L-SPAMM, the tagging RF pulses are slice-selective, thereby generating the tagging pattern only within a selected part of the imaging plane.
- The location and width of the region to be tagged in L-SPAMM are determined, respectively, by the frequency of the RF pulses and magnitude of the gradient field.
- Tags preparation in L-SPAMM requires about 15 ms versus 3–5 ms in conventional SPAMM.
- L-DANTE is identical to the conventional DANTE sequence, except that it uses longer RF pulses, which have the effect of imposing sinc modulation in the frequency space and confining the excitation within a predefined region in the imaging plane.
- L-DANTE can be considered as an intermediate case between conventional DANTE and single-frequency continuous wave excitation.
- The duration of the L-DANTE tagging preparation period is about 10 ms, which is longer than that in conventional SPAMM.
- Because some parts of the heart thicken in one Cartesian direction, while other parts contract in the same direction, it is not possible to obtain a uniform tagline separation pattern that is optimally sensitive to both circumferential shortening and radial thickening.
- The general approach in VTAG is to extend the SPAMM technique to generate a tagging pattern with a much longer period (20–30 ms) that consists of several, almost a dozen of, spatially dependent tags.
- In VTAG, the taglines are placed closer to each other at the beginning of the cardiac cycle in the regions where the tagline separation increases during systole (radial thickening). Alternatively, in regions where the tagline separation decreases during systole (circumferential shortening), the taglines are placed farther apart so they remain detectable at end-systole.

- K-space analysis of the tagging sequences is based on relating the tagging pulse sequence directly to the residual pattern of the longitudinal magnetization caused by the pulse sequence.
- Using the weighted path concept in k-space analysis allows for understanding the FT relation between the tagging profile and RF field by removing the time-dependency factors.
- Using the small tip angle assumption results in simulation errors in the k-space analysis of the tagging patterns as this condition is not fulfilled in conventional tagging techniques.
- Using spectral decomposition, a short weighted path with fewer spectral peaks can be generated, which allows for designing a simpler and shorter sequence for the same tagging pattern.
- M-SPAMM combines L-SPAMM with variable-density tagging by using FIR filters, wherein the modulus of the filter is used to select the areas in which the tagging takes place, while the phase of the filter is used to manipulate the density of the taglines.
- The main challenges for producing special non-Cartesian tagging patterns are the quality of the tagging pattern and efficiency of the corresponding pulse sequence.
- The principles of k-space excitation have been used for the development of most specialized tagging patterns.
- The first tagging technique, developed by Zerhouni et al., generated taglines in multiple radial directions using a series of selective inversion pulses before image acquisition.
- The initial implementation of radial tagging using selective magnetization saturation has a number of limitations, including long tag preparation time and high SAR.
- The STAG technique is a hybrid magnetization saturation/modulation technique, which combines the advantages of both approaches and allows for efficiently measuring both circumferential and radial strains from the same set of SAX tagged images.
- STAG uses the polar coordinate system, such that about four radial collinear reference points (beads) are placed across the myocardial wall at different angles in the SAX view.
- Similar to SPAMM, the STAG sequence spatially modulates the magnetization, except that this happens for selected locations, as the two 90° nonselective tagging RF pulses used in SPAMM are switched in STAG into slice-selective pulses applied perpendicular to the imaging plane.
- Rectangular tag profiles can be created by using a sinc-modulated RF pulse train in the presence of a constant gradient, where the BW of the sinc envelope controls the tag thickness. This allows for generating sharper taglines with the capability of changing the tag-thickness to tag-separation ratio.

- The sinusoidal function showed to be the optimal tagging profile for myocardial motion estimation.
- It has been shown that the tag thickness that minimizes the tag position estimation error is between 0.8 and 1.5 pixels, depending on the shape of the tag profile and line spread function.
- For generating the optimal tagging pattern, the tag thickness should be slightly larger than the optimal thickness, the taglines should be placed perpendicular to the direction with the highest resolution in the image, and the tag spacing should be as small as possible.
- The nearly circular shape of the LV in SAX views makes it useful to have the taglines curved to match its apparent annular geometry, especially for estimating transmural gradients in wall thickening, which is the idea of the RingTag technique.
- Curved taglines are generated in RingTag by using a continuous and long RF pulse that selectively excites the spins within the object over an on-resonance excitation plane while the applied gradient fields are simultaneously moving the plane.
- RingTag becomes more effective when it is combined with radial or other types of tagging, such that all components of myocardial motion can be observed or estimated from the same set of SAX tagged images.
- Polar tagging represents all patterns that generate the taglines in the radial or circular directions around the center of the heart.
- Both the geometry and motion of the myocardium in the SAX view are better described in the polar coordinate system compared to the Cartesian system.
- One advantage of polar tagging is that the RF energy for radial tagging is much less than that used in the conventional implementation of radial tagging with magnetization saturation or inversion pulses, despite the shorter tagging time in polar tagging.
- Limitations of polar tagging include the need for placing the center of the polar tagging pattern at the center of the LV cavity, and the limited thickness of the myocardium, which may make it challenging to place a sufficient number of circular tags inside the myocardial wall.
- In circular tagging, an on-resonance rotating frame limits the directional excitation to a thin slab perpendicular to the slice of interest, thereby excluding other spins from the excitation.
- A common characteristic of circular tagging and RingTag is that in both techniques the gradient field changes to rotate the on-resonance plane while the RF magnetic field is being applied. Nevertheless, although RingTag selectively excites the on-resonance spins over a single-curved line, circular tagging generates multiple circular taglines simultaneously.
- Circular tagging allows for directly measuring radial strain by calculating the relative change in the spatial

- frequency between the initial and deformed circular tags.
- Circular tagging has been compared to HARP for measuring radial strain, where the results showed general agreement between the two techniques, despite a slight measurement underestimation by HARP.
- As the circular symmetry of the LV shape in the SAX view does not exist in some pathological conditions, an elliptical tagging pattern may be more suitable than circular tagging for assessment of radial strain in these conditions.
- Oval taglines are obtained by setting nonequal amplitudes to the gradient pulses that form the rotating excitation plane in circular tagging.
- As the circular tags are represented by a localized annulus in the k-space, myocardial contraction leads to widening of the annular ring in the frequency domain. Therefore, strain can be evaluated simply by finding the most prevalent spatial frequency of each annular region in the k-space.
- Polar HARP applies a half-circular BPF in the k-space to obtain the magnitude and phase images of the fundamental frequency in the circularly tagged image, based on which tissue displacement in the direction normal to the taglines is calculated using HARP analysis.
- Polar HARP can be extended to increase the resolution and density of the circular tags by using successive directional filters and multiplying the phase of the resulting angle images.
- Compared to the original radial tagging technique, the radial implementation of polar tagging provides higher tagline density, where the width of taglines increases with radius.
- In the radial implementation of polar tagging, each lobe of the RF pulse is not responsible for creating a single tagline; it rather contributes to the formation of the adjacent taglines as well.
- By applying the duality concept to circular tagging, radial tagging could be implemented by exploiting a different interference effect.
- Calculating strain from conventional tagged images includes two steps that are not needed in polar tagging: (1) measuring the displacement field, which is a time-consuming postprocessing step, and (2) performing spatial differentiation on the displacement field, which is a noise-sensitive process.
- The CIRCOME technique allows for noninvasive and quick measurement of circumferential strain by directly using the frequency information in the k-space of radially tagged images. Therefore, it avoids explicit measurement of the displacement field and does not require spatial differentiation to calculate strain.
- The CIRCOME technique can simultaneously encode circumferential myocardial compression in

several SAX slices and in real time, which allows for robust measurement of global circumferential strain.

- Regions with different degrees of radial taglines compression can be obtained through circular BPF of the k-space. These regions become more specific with more selective filters, that is, thinner circle or smaller filters' BW in the k-space.

- Circumferential strain measured with CIRCOME showed good agreement with HARP.

- Various parameters, including tagline fading, eccentricity of the radial taglines' center and their density, spatial resolution, and SNR, affect the accuracy of circumferential strain measurement with the CIRCOME technique. However, the CIRCOME technique showed good robustness in a variety of imperfect imaging conditions.

- In nonuniform radial tagging, the taglines are not distributed evenly in the radial direction, which is useful for evaluating some focal points on the myocardium wall, or more generally for evaluating the wall motion in oblique slices of the heart when it has an oval shape.

- Similar to CSPAMM, the complementary radial tagging (CRT) technique improves the radial tagging contrast through acquiring two sets of radially tagged images, which upon subtraction eliminate the untagged signal and retain only the tagged component. Further, ramped imaging flip angles is used to maintain constant tagging contrast through the cardiac cycle.

- Real-time circular tagging is implemented by selectively sampling the k-space with a set of concentric ring acquisitions, then reconstructing the image using a modified filtered back-projection algorithm.

- Real-time radial tagging is implemented by partial radial acquisition of the k-space.

ACKNOWLEDGMENT

The authors thank Dr. Elham Mohammadi from Amirkabir University in Iran for help with polar tagging figures preparation.

REFERENCES

Aghaeifar, A., Babaee, N., and Moghaddam, A. N. (2013a). High resolution high density CMR circular tagging. *J Cardiovasc Magn Reson* **15**(Suppl 1): P88.

Aghaeifar, A., Babaee, N., Moghaddam, A. N., and Ayatollahi, A. (2013b). High resolution tagging pattern in the polar coordinate system: A reconstruction based approach. *Proceedings of the 21st Iranian Conference on Electrical Engineering (ICEE)*, pp. 1–5. Mashhad, Iran.

Aghaeifar, A., Moghaddam, A. N., and Finn, J. P. (2014). Inline generation of tagline density maps for radial strain quantification from circular MR tagging. *Proceedings of the International Society of Magnetic Resonance in Medicine*, p. 5022. Milan, Italy.

Atalar, E. and McVeigh, E. R. (1994). Optimization of tag thickness for measuring position with magnetic resonance imaging. *IEEE Trans Med Imaging* **13**(1): 152–160.

Axel, L. and Dougherty, L. (1989). MR imaging of motion with spatial modulation of magnetization. *Radiology* **171**(3): 841–845.

Babaee, N. and Moghaddam, A. N. (2012). Polar HARP for the polar CMR tagging. *J Cardiovasc Magn Reson* **14**(Suppl 1): W15.

Bazille, A., Guttman, M. A., McVeigh, E. R., and Zerhouni, E. A. (1994). Impact of semiautomated versus manual image segmentation errors on myocardial strain calculation by magnetic resonance tagging. *Invest Radiol* **29**(4): 427–433.

Bolster, B. D., Jr., McVeigh, E. R., and Zerhouni, E. A. (1990). Myocardial tagging in polar coordinates with use of striped tags. *Radiology* **177**(3): 769–772.

Bosmans, H., Bogaert, J., Rademakers, F., Marchal, G., Laub, G., Verschakelen, J., and Baert, A. L. (1996). Left ventricular radial tagging acquisition using gradient-recalled-echo techniques: Sequence optimization. *MAGMA* **4**(2): 123–133.

Chandra, S. and Yang, Y. (1996). Simulations and demonstrations of localized tagging experiments. *J Magn Reson B* **111**(3): 285–288.

Dong, S. J., Hees, P. S., Siu, C. O., Weiss, J. L., and Shapiro, E. P. (2001). MRI assessment of LV relaxation by untwisting rate: A new isovolumic phase measure of tau. *Am J Physiol Heart Circ Physiol* **281**(5): H2002–H2009.

Fischer, S. E., McKinnon, G. C., Maier, S. E., and Boesiger, P. (1993). Improved myocardial tagging contrast. *Magn Reson Med* **30**(2): 191–200.

Golshani, S., Moghaddam, A. N., Wu, H. H., and Finn, J. P. (2014). Circular tagging with concentric data acquisition: Can we go real-time? *Proceedings of the International Society of Magnetic Resonance in Medicine*, p. 5312. Milan, Italy.

Golshani, S. and Nasiraei Moghaddam, A. (2015). Efficient radial tagging: Undersampled radial acquisition with polar Fourier transform reconstruction. *Proceedings of the International Society of Magnetic Resonance in Medicine*, p. 4471. Toronto, Ontario, Canada.

Haftekhanaki, M., Moghaddam, A. N., Abd-Elmoniem, K., and Finn, J. P. (2012). Measuring the radial component of left ventricular strain with circular tagging: Feasibility and initial results. *Proceedings of the International Society of Magnetic Resonance in Medicine*, p. 3794. Melbourne, Victoria, Australia.

Ibrahim, El-S. H. (2011). Myocardial tagging by cardiovascular magnetic resonance: Evolution of techniques–pulse sequences, analysis algorithms, and applications. *J Cardiovasc Magn Reson* **13**: 36.

Ikonomidou, V. N. and Sergiadis, G. D. (2002). A rotational approach to localized SPAMM 1–1 tagging. *J Magn Reson* **157**(2): 218–222.

Ikonomidou, V. N. and Sergiadis, G. D. (2003). Multirate SPAMM tagging. *IEEE Trans Biomed Eng* **50**(9): 1045–1051.

Kaveh, R., Moghaddam, A. N., Khan, S. N., and Finn, J. P. (2013). Twist measurement of the left ventricle through radial tagging. *J Cardiovasc Magn Reson* **15**(Suppl 1): E48.

Kaveh, R., Moghaddam, A. N., Khan, S. N., and Finn, J. P. (2014). Regional rotation of the left ventricle in healthy and cardiomyopathic subjects measured with radial myocardial tagging. *J Cardiovasc Magn Reson* **16**(Suppl 1): P24.

Kerwin, W. S. and Prince, J. L. (2000). A k-space analysis of MR tagging. *J Magn Reson* **142**(2): 313–322.

Khan, S. N., Moghaddam, A. N., Kaveh, R., Nsair, A., Bhatia, M., and Finn, J. P. (2013). Myocardial tagging in the polar coordinate system; initial clinical results. *Proceedings of the International Society of Magnetic Resonance in Medicine*, p. 487. Salt Lake City, UT.

Khan, S. N., Moghaddam, A. N., Kaveh, R., Plotnik, A., Lehrman, E., Nsair, A., and Finn, J. P. (2014). Myocardial tagging in the polar coordinate system; early clinical experience. *J Cardiovasc Magn Reson* **16**(Suppl 1): P387.

Le Roux, P. (1988). Exact synthesis of radiofrequency waveforms. *Proceedings of the International Society of Magnetic Resonance in Medicine*, p. 1048. San Francisco, CA.

McVeigh, E. R. and Bolster, B. D., Jr. (1998). Improved sampling of myocardial motion with variable separation tagging. *Magn Reson Med* **39**(4): 657–661.

McVeigh, E. R. and Gao, L. (1994). Resolution and SNR requirements for detecting transmural gradients in myocardial wall thickening with MR tagging. *Radiology* **193**(P): 199.

McVeigh, E. R. and Zerhouni, E. A. (1991). Noninvasive measurement of transmural gradients in myocardial strain with MR imaging. *Radiology* **180**(3): 677–683.

Moayed, V. and Moghaddam, A. N. (2014). Non-uniform polar tagging. *J Cardiovasc Magn Reson* **16**(Suppl 1): P31.

Moghaddam, A. N., Abd-Elmoniem, K., Heidari, G., Ruehm, S., and Finn, J. P. (2011a). Left ventricular strain through Radial Tagging: Efficiency and validity. *Proceedings of the International Society of Magnetic Resonance in Medicine*, p. 3368. Montreal, Quebec, Canada.

Moghaddam, A. N. and Finn, J. (2010a). Measuring the myocardial angular information through the Radial Tagging. *Proceedings of the International Society of Magnetic Resonance in Medicine*, p. 3572. Stockholm, Sweden.

Moghaddam, A. N. and Finn, J. P. (2008a). Accelerated circumferential strain quantification of the left ventricle using CIRCOME: Simulation and factor analysis. *Proceedings of the SPIE*, pp. 1–8. San Diego, CA.

Moghaddam, A. N. and Finn, P. (2008b). Circumferential strain encoding of the left ventricle using CIRCOME: Sequence, algorithm and factor analysis. *J Cardiovasc Magn Reson* **10**(Suppl 1): A199.

Moghaddam, A. N., Finn, P., and Gharib, M. (2007). CIRcumferential COMpression Encoding (CIRCOME). *Proceedings of the International Society of Magnetic Resonance in Medicine*, p. 2515. Berlin, Germany.

Moghaddam, A. N. and Gharib, M. (2011b). Method for obtaining strain from radially-tagged magnetic resonance imaging (MRI). O. G. o. t. U. S. P. a. T. O. Patents. California Institute of Technology, Pasadena, CA. US 08073523.

Moghaddam, A. N., Natsuaki, Y., and Finn, J. (2010b). Radial Tagging of MR images: A continuous RF excitation approach. *Proceedings of the International Society of Magnetic Resonance in Medicine*, p. 766. Stockholm, Sweden.

Moghaddam, A. N., Natsuaki, Y., and Finn, J. P. (2011c). CMR tagging in the polar coordinate system. *J Cardiovasc Magn Reson* **13**(Suppl 1): O27.

Mosher, T. J. and Smith, M. B. (1990). A DANTE tagging sequence for the evaluation of translational sample motion. *Magn Reson Med* **15**(2): 334–339.

Nasiraei-Moghaddam, A. (2012). Pattern generating method of altered magnetization in target volume of object involves shaping alternating gradient signal to generate rotating on-resonance

excitation plane. USA, UNIV CALIFORNIA(REGC-C). WO2012106574-A2; WO2012106574-A3; US2013320978-A1; EP2670302-A2.

Nasiraei-Moghaddam, A. and Finn, J. P. (2014). Tagging of cardiac magnetic resonance images in the polar coordinate system: Physical principles and practical implementation. *Magn Reson Med* **71**(5): 1750–1759.

Nguyen, T. D., Reeves, S. J., and Denney, T. S. (2003). On the optimality of magnetic resonance tag patterns for heart wall motion estimation. *IEEE Trans Imag Process* **12**: 524–532.

Osman, N. F., Kerwin, W. S., McVeigh, E. R., and Prince, J. L. (1999). Cardiac motion tracking using CINE harmonic phase (HARP) magnetic resonance imaging. *Magn Reson Med* **42**(6): 1048–1060.

Pauly, J., Le Roux, P., Nishimura, D., and Macovski, A. (1991). Parameter relations for the Shinnar-Le Roux selective excitation pulse design algorithm [NMR imaging]. *IEEE Trans Med Imaging* **10**(1): 53–65.

Pauly, J., Nishimura, D., and Macovski, A. (2011). A k-space analysis of small-tip-angle excitation. 1989. *J Magn Reson* **213**(2): 544–557.

Salido, T. B., Hundley, W. G., Link, K. M., Epstein, F. H., and Hamilton, C. A. (2002). Effects of phase encode order and segment interpolation methods on the quality and accuracy of myocardial tags during assessment of left ventricular contraction. *J Cardiovasc Magn Reson* **4**(2): 245–254.

Shinnar, M., Eleff, S., Subramanian, H., and Leigh, J. S. (1989). The synthesis of pulse sequences yielding arbitrary magnetization vectors. *Magn Reson Med* **12**(1): 74–80.

Spiegel, M. A., Luechinger, R., Schwitter, J., and Boesiger, P. (2003). RingTag: Ring-shaped tagging for myocardial centerline assessment. *Invest Radiol* **38**(10): 669–678.

Tsekos, N. V., Garwood, M., Merkle, H., Xu, Y., Wilke, N., and Ugurbil, K. (1995). Myocardial tagging with B1 insensitive adiabatic DANTE inversion sequences. *Magn Reson Med* **34**(3): 395–401.

Wang, Z., Moghaddam, A. N., Zou, Y., Srinivasan, S., Finn, J. P., and Ennis, D. B. (2014). Improved myocardial contrast using novel complementary radial MR tagging technique. *Proceedings of the International Society of Magnetic Resonance in Medicine*, p. 4232. Milan, Italy.

Wang, Z., Nasiraei-Moghaddam, A., Reyhan, M. L., Srinivasan, S., Finn, J. P., and Ennis, D. B. (2015). Complementary radial tagging for improved myocardial tagging contrast. *Magn Reson Med* **73**(4): 1432–1440.

Wu, E. X., Towe, C. W., and Tang, H. (2002). MRI cardiac tagging using a sinc-modulated RF pulse train. *Magn Reson Med* **48**(2): 389–393.

Zerhouni, E. A., Parish, D. M., Rogers, W. J., Yang, A., and Shapiro, E. P. (1988). Human heart: Tagging with MR imaging--a method for noninvasive assessment of myocardial motion. *Radiology* **169**(1): 59–63.

13 Advanced Magnetic Resonance Imaging Techniques for Measuring Heart Mechanics

El-Sayed H. Ibrahim, PhD

CONTENTS

LIST OF ABBREVIATIONS

Abbreviation	Meaning
1D	One dimensional
2D	Two dimensional
3D	Three dimensional
ATFM	Active trajectory field model
BPF	Band-pass filter
bSSFP	Balanced steady state with free precession
C-SENC	Composite SENC
CANSEL	Cosine and sine modulation to eliminate echoes
CRT	Cardiac resynchronization therapy
CSPAMM	Complementary SPAMM
DANTE	Delays alternating with nutations for tailored excitation
DC	Direct current
DENSE	Displacement encoding with stimulated echoes
DHE	Delayed hyperenhancement
DWI	Diffusion-weighted imaging
EPI	Echo planar imaging
FEM	Finite-element modeling
FID	Free induction decay
FOV	Field of view
FT	Fourier transform
Gd	Gadolinium
HARP	Harmonic phase
HFnEF	Heart failure with normal ejection fraction
HT	High tuning
LAX	Long axis
LPF	Low-pass filter
LT	Low tuning
LV	Left ventricle
MESA	Multi-Ethnic Study of Atherosclerosis
meta-DENSE	Mixed echo train acquisition DENSE
MI	Myocardial infarction
NT	No tuning
PC	Phase contrast
RF	Radiofrequency
ROI	Region of interest
SAX	Short axis
SENC	Strain encoding
SENSE	Sensitivity encoding
SNR	Signal-to-noise ratio
SPAMM	Spatial modulation of magnetization
STEAM	Stimulated echo acquisition mode
sf-fast-SENC	Slice-following fast-SENC
sf-SENC	Slice-following SENC
TPM	Tissue phase mapping
TruHARP	Total removal of unwanted harmonic peaks
venc	Velocity encoding

13.1 INTRODUCTION

13.1.1 ADVANCED TECHNIQUES FOR MEASURING HEART MECHANICS: AN OVERVIEW

Although conventional MRI tagging, especially spatial modulation of magnetization (SPAMM), remains the most established technique for evaluating regional heart function, various other advanced, and more complicated, techniques have been developed over the past 17 years or so. These techniques provide more information about the heart mechanics with better visualization schemes and more accurate results. These techniques are harmonic phase (HARP) imaging, displacement encoding with stimulated echoes (DENSE), strain encoding (SENC), tissue phase mapping (TPM), and magnetic resonance elastography (MRE). These techniques represent the state of the art in heart mechanics analysis with MRI. They have been implemented in different research and clinical trials with promising results, which makes them constitute the future trend in the field.

13.1.2 CHAPTER LAYOUT

This chapter is based on, and is an extension of, the review article by the author in *JCMR* (Ibrahim 2011). Many of the figures in this chapter are reproduced from those in the review article. The chapter provides a brief overview of the HARP, DENSE, SENC, TPM, and MRE techniques along with key developments of each of them. It should be noted that this chapter is by no means a comprehensive coverage of these techniques, as each of them requires one or more chapters for adequate coverage, which is the purpose of *Heart Mechanics: Magnetic Resonance Imaging—Advanced Techniques, Clinical Applications, and Future Trends*.

This chapter starts by illustrating the concept behind the HARP technique, followed by a description of the original sequence developed by Osman et al. (1999) at Johns Hopkins University in 1999. Key sequence developments and techniques for improving tagline tracking, increasing signal-to-noise ratio (SNR), and reducing scan time in HARP imaging are then covered. The chapter then covers the DENSE technique, starting with the original sequence developed by Aletras et al. (1999b) and followed by a description of the different signal echoes contributing to the DENSE image. Different sequence developments are then covered along with echo combination and echo suppression techniques. The fast-DENSE and three-dimensional (3D) DENSE techniques are then covered, followed by a brief review of the studies conducted to evaluate the technique's performance, generate composite cardiac information from DENSE, and improve DENSE image processing. The chapter then covers the SENC technique, starting with the original technique developed by Osman et al. (2001), and followed by different sequence development stages, including slice-following SENC, fast-SENC, and slice-following fast-SENC. The chapter then covers the composite SENC (C-SENC) technique, followed by 3D techniques. TPM MRI is then covered, starting with the technique's basic concept and pulse sequence, and followed by different sequence development and data analysis methods. The chapter then describes a number of techniques for generating composite information based on TPM imaging, followed by different applications of the technique. Finally, the chapter covers MRE, including basic technique, technical developments, and clinical applications.

13.2 HARP ANALYSIS

13.2.1 FOURIER SPACE OF THE TAGGED IMAGES

A standard SPAMM-tagged image can be mathematically expressed as the amplitude modulation of the underlying image by a truncated cosine series function. As a result, the magnitude of the Fourier transform (FT) of a SPAMM-tagged image comprises multiple spectral peaks. The number of generated spectral peaks depends on the number of radiofrequency (RF) pulses used to generate the modulated tagged images. Typically, if n RF pulses are used in the tagging preparation sequence, then $2n+1$ spectral peaks are observed in the k-space: one signal peak (the direct current (DC) peak) located in the k-space center and $2n$ harmonic peaks that are off-centered. The orientation and location of the harmonic peaks in reference to the DC peak depend on the orientation and magnitude of the tagging modulation gradient, respectively.

13.2.2 ORIGINAL SEQUENCE

The HARP technique was developed in 1999 by Nael Osman in Jerry Prince's lab at Johns Hopkins University (Osman et al. 1999, 2000, Osman and Prince 2000). HARP is sometimes mistaken as a new tagging *acquisition* technique, which is not true as HARP is a tagging *analysis* technique. In contrast to the previously developed tagging analysis techniques that depend on directly tracking the taglines' displacement in the image space, HARP tracks the signal phase in the k-space of the tagged image, with tremendous reduction in analysis time.

13.2.2.1 Harmonic Phase Image

The first step of constructing the HARP image is to generate a phase image by extracting (using a band-pass filter [BPF]) the first harmonic peak in the k-space of the tagged image (Figure 13.1). It should be noted that the Fourier spectrum of the harmonic peaks is determined by the tagging frequency, spectrum of the underlying image, and expected tissue motion. Besides the phase image, a magnitude image is generated by applying a low-pass filter (LPF) to the image's k-space. The magnitude image does not show the tag lines; it rather shows an anatomical black-blood image of the heart. By multiplying the magnitude and phase images, the harmonic phase image is constructed, which looks very similar to the original tagged image. The signal intensity in the harmonic phase image reflects the magnetization phase, which is a material property of the tissue.

13.2.2.2 Tissue Tracking

The basic underlying principle of HARP analysis is that the HARP (ϕ) of a material point (p) is an imposed material property that is invariant in time (t), that is,

$$\phi(p_{m+1}, t_{m+1}) = \phi(p_m, t_m), \tag{13.1}$$

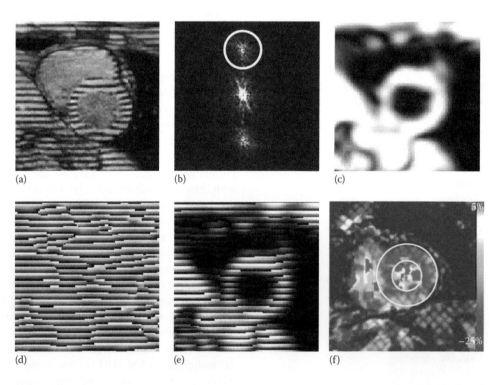

(a) (b) (c)

(d) (e) (f)

FIGURE 13.1 The harmonic phase (HARP) technique. Constructing the HARP image. (a) Original spatial modulation of magnetization (SPAMM)-tagged image. (b) K-space of the tagged image. HARP applies a spatial band-pass filter (BPF) to extract only the first harmonic peak (inside the circle). (c) Magnitude image extracted by applying a low-pass filter (LPF) to the k-space in (b). The image shows the underlying anatomical structure (with the blood signal suppressed) in the tagged image. (d) Phase image extracted by applying a BPF to the k-space in (b). (e) Multiplying the magnitude and phase images results in the harmonic phase image with modulation pattern very similar to that in the original tagged image. (f) An example of a grid-tagged image analyzed with HARP, showing color-coded myocardial circumferential strain. (Reproduced from Ibrahim, El-S.H., *J. Cardiovasc. Magn. Reson.*, 13, 36, 2011.)

where the subscript refers to the frame number in the set of cine tagged images. Thus, by tracking the harmonic phase of each pixel over time, one can track the pixel's position, and therefore determine tissue displacement over time. A neighborhood search is typically performed to find the pixel's position p_{m+1} at time t_{m+1} that has the same harmonic phase (within a small error bar) as that of pixel p_m at time t_m. This step is repeated for successive timeframe to obtain the motion pathline for each selected point in the tagged myocardium.

The simplicity and robustness of the HARP technique resulted in reducing the tagging analysis time by at least an order of magnitude, which facilitated analyzing large volumes of data in a relatively short time. HARP has been validated against conventional tag analysis techniques (Garot et al. 2000) and demonstrated high degrees of robustness and reproducibility, as shown in the results from the Multi-Ethnic Study of Atherosclerosis (MESA) study (Castillo et al. 2005) and several other studies (Kraitchman et al. 2003, Phatak et al. 2009).

13.2.3 Technique Development

13.2.3.1 Eliminating Spectral Signal Interference

The interference from the adjacent signal peaks in the tagged image may result in image artifacts and inaccurate results from the HARP analysis. Nevertheless, there are different approaches to reduce or eliminate these spectral interferences, for example, by changing the pulse sequence parameters (e.g., to spread the signal peaks) (Kuijer et al. 2006), reducing the size of the applied BPF, using inversion recovery to null the signal from certain peaks, or adding through-plane dephasing gradients in the pulse sequence. However, these approaches have limitations: reducing SNR, compromising spatial resolution, or prohibiting cine imaging. Another approach to reduce spectral interference is to use composite SPAMM (CSPAMM) tagging (Fischer et al. 1993, Kuijer et al. 2001) instead of SPAMM. As the DC signal is naturally suppressed in CSPAMM, then filters with wider bandwidth and more flexible cutoff points can be used in the HARP implementation without including signal from the DC peak. Therefore, HARP implementation on CSPAMM-tagged images results in fewer tracking errors than when implemented on SPAMM-tagged images.

13.2.3.2 TruHARP

Another technique for reducing the spectral interference in HARP analysis is called total removal of unwanted harmonic peaks (TruHARP) (Agarwal et al. 2010). TruHARP requires a single breath-hold scan to acquire five tagged images with specific gradient orientations and phase cycling schemes, such that the DC and first harmonic (and its conjugate) peaks are extracted by combining the resulting images in a certain way. So, in this sense, TruHARP can be considered as an extension of CSPAMM.

13.2.3.3 Harmonic Peak Combination

It is a conventional practice to extract one of the harmonic peaks in HARP analysis. The amplitude modulation operation in the tagging process divides the total harmonic energy equally on both sides of the DC peak. Thus, the energy is divided equally into each of the two symmetric harmonic peaks. By extracting only one of the harmonic peaks, SNR is automatically reduced by 50%. One idea to improve the HARP performance is to combine the positive and negative harmonic peaks in the tagged images before conducting the HARP analysis (Ryf et al. 2004). This modification has the effects of correcting for the phase errors and improving SNR, which results in eliminating phase distortion artifacts in the images and improving reproducibility of strain measurements.

13.2.3.4 Extended HARP

As in any two-dimensional (2D) imaging technique, HARP suffers from tissue through-plane motion, which results in that the same tissue does not show in the imaging plane during the whole cardiac cycle, especially in short-axis (SAX) planes where the conical shape of the left ventricle (LV) contributes to this phenomenon. To address this issue, an extended HARP technique has been developed to measure strain in the myocardial regions that appear only during the systolic phase of the cardiac cycle (Tecelao et al. 2006). The accuracy of the developed technique has been quantified based on mathematical modeling of myocardial deformation using Hilbert Transform.

13.2.3.5 Phase Manipulation

Bilgen (2010) developed a technique for improving tagline detection with HARP using special phase manipulation. The developed technique is based on applying a special combination of wrapped phases to the harmonic phase images to create images with unique intensity patterns that can be exploited for automatic tagline detection. The developed technique allows for strain measurement at higher spatial resolution and in a multiscale fashion.

13.2.4 Improving Tagline Tracking

13.2.4.1 Tagline Regeneration

In addition to the HARP developments that stemmed from k-space perspective, other developments were created to improve motion tracking based on the image space. In 2004, Osman and Prince (2004) developed a method for regenerating the taglines using HARP. The synthesized taglines showed crisp profile than the original taglines with a sinusoidal profile.

13.2.4.2 HARP with Spatial Continuity

In another development, HARP was combined with active contour models to improve tagline detection, especially at low SNR levels where tracking errors are expected (Khalifa et al. 2005). Other developments have been made that followed similar reasoning lines. For example, Liu and Prince (2010) presented a refined HARP technique that includes a spatial continuity condition for the sake of minimizing motion estimation errors that may result from large tissue deformation, through-plane motion, or at the myocardium boundaries. Specifically, an optimal tracking scheme has been implemented to start from a certain seed point and move to each point in the image based on the shortest-path principle, which encourages the search to stay within the same tissue region as the seed point. The proposed method resulted in minimal motion tracking errors and showed to be robust and fast.

13.2.5 IMPROVING SNR

Tagline deformation in the reference (first) timeframe results in an additional phase value in the phase images, which leads to significant underestimation of ventricular contraction. In this context, HARP can be used to restore the undeformed taglines in the reference timeframe for accurate motion quantification (Li and Yu 2010). In this case, the fact that the locations of the off-center spectral peaks are dependent on the tagging frequency is exploited, such that a single point of the spectral peak could be used to fully recover the undeformed taglines.

13.2.6 REDUCING SCAN TIME

13.2.6.1 FastHARP

In HARP analysis, a region around the harmonic peak in the k-space is filtered out using BPF to create the harmonic phase image. Keeping this in mind, the image acquisition time can be significantly decreased by acquiring a smaller region in k-space around the harmonic peak of interest. In other words, the first stage of the filtering process can take place during image acquisition. This approach of directly acquiring the harmonic images has been described by Sampath et al. (2003) and is referred to as the fastHARP technique. The fastHARP technique depends on combined implementation of multicoil data acquisition, echo planar imaging (EPI), and fast data processing on a computer unit next to the scanner. In the developed technique, alternating horizontally and vertically tagged images are acquired on consecutive heartbeats. The corresponding images from consecutive heartbeats are then combined and processed to generate grid-tagged images at a rate of four images per second. Using the fastHARP technique, a complete set of one-dimensional (1D) cine SPAMM-tagged images was acquired during each heartbeat with temporal resolution of 40 ms using a free-breathing single-shot EPI sequence.

13.2.6.2 Real-Time HARP

In parallel with the development of the fastHARP technique, a real-time reconstruction and strain visualization method was developed to keep pace with real-time data acquisition (Abd-Elmoniem 2007b). The key innovation in the developed method is the implementation of localized reconstruction (restricted to the LV) using chirp FT customized to fast 2D data reconstruction. As in Sampath's work (Sampath et al. 2003), horizontal and vertical tagging are applied alternatively in consecutive heartbeats, and then combined together to update strain calculations every heartbeat. However, instead of acquiring the whole k-space and extracting the spectral peak of

interest using a BPF as in conventional HARP, the developed technique acquires only a small region of the k-space around the spectral peak of interest, which significantly reduces the data acquisition time. Another key addition in the developed technique is the implementation of a custom-designed chirp inverse FT algorithm with a priori designed lookup tables to reconstruct only a small region of interest (ROI) around the heart, which helps accelerate the image display rate.

13.2.7 3D IMAGING

13.2.7.1 HARP with 3D CSPAMM

The efforts to improve the HARP technique are not restricted to reducing scan time or processing time only; they rather extend to allow for 3D strain analysis. For example, in 2002, Ryf et al. (2002) and Haber and Westin (2002) proposed 3D myocardial motion analysis techniques based on extensions of 2D HARP. Ryf et al. (2002) extended HARP analysis to 3D CSPAMM-tagged images, while Haber and Westin (2002) derived a 3D finite-element model for estimating myocardial 3D motion from multiple 2D tagged images.

13.2.7.2 3D HARP

Later in 2005, the 3D HARP technique was developed as a straightforward extension of 2D HARP for fast and semiautomatic tracking of myocardial 3D motion (Pan et al. 2005). In 3D HARP, a parallel set of SAX grid-tagged images and a radial set of long-axis (LAX) images with horizontal taglines are combined to construct a 3D mesh around the LV (Figure 13.2). Motion tracking is automatically conducted

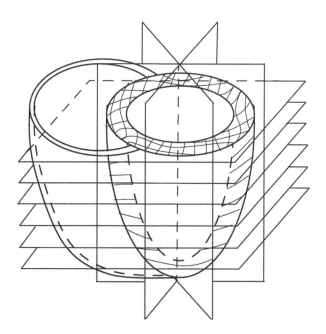

FIGURE 13.2 Three-dimensional strain analysis with HARP. Two series of tagged images are acquired: (1) a stack of parallel short-axis grid-tagged images to measure in-plane (circumferential and radial) strain and (2) a radial set of long-axis line-tagged images to measure through-plane (longitudinal) strain. (Reproduced from Ibrahim, El-S.H., *J. Cardiovasc. Magn. Reson.*, 13, 36, 2011.)

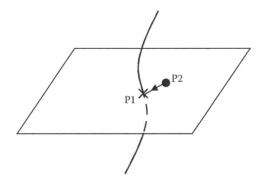

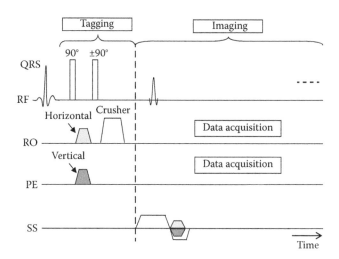

FIGURE 13.3 Three-dimensional (3D) harmonic phase (HARP). The HARP concept is extended to 3D to track myocardial deformation. The intersection of the tagline with the image plane, point P1, is linked to the nearest point on the next frame (point P2) with the same characteristic phase.

FIGURE 13.4 The zHARP pulse sequence. The pulse sequence is based on complementary SPAMM (CSPAMM) tagging. Two CSPAMM images are acquired with horizontal and vertical taglines to obtain in-plane strain. Through-plane strain is obtained by adding positive (light gray) and negative (dark gray) z-gradients after the slice-election pulse of the horizontally and vertically tagged images, respectively. (Reproduced from Ibrahim, El-S.H., *J. Cardiovasc. Magn. Reson.*, 13, 36, 2011.)

using a 3D version of the phase-invariance concept implemented in HARP. Further, the phase of each material point in all timeframes is checked against its initial value to minimize error accumulation through the cardiac cycle (Figure 13.3). The 3D HARP technique compared well with other validated techniques and provided complete 3D motion analysis of the LV in about 10 min.

13.2.7.3 zHARP

The zHARP technique was developed in 2005 for 3D strain quantification from a single image plane using tagging and phase encoding for measuring in-plane and through-plane strain components, respectively, without increasing the scan time (Abd-Elmoniem et al. 2005, 2007a). The zHARP technique is based on slice-following CSPAMM (Fischer et al. 1994). The acquisition of the first set of the CSPAMM-tagged images (two SPAMM scans with horizontal taglines) is modified by adding a small z-encoding gradient to the slice-selection refocusing pulse, as shown in Figure 13.4, to encode through-plane motion. Another z-encoding gradient with an opposite polarity is added to the second set of CSPAMM images (two SPAMM scans with vertical taglines). The horizontal and vertical taglines provide in-plane motion information, while the added z-encoding gradients resolve motion in the through-plane direction. As CSPAMM tagging is implemented, susceptibility and field-inhomogeneity artifacts are eliminated after image subtraction. The in-plane and through-plane motion components are extracted by applying HARP to the positive and negative harmonic peaks (a total of four harmonic peaks) and solving the resulting set of equations. zHARP has the advantage of producing 3D motion information in the slice of interest in a short scan time (four short breath-holds) and without the need to acquire orthogonal sets of tagged images.

13.2.7.4 Multislice zHARP

The zHARP technique has been extended into a multislice technique for rapid 3D strain tensor quantification (Abd-Elmoniem et al. 2008). To achieve this goal, a stack of SAX zHARP images is acquired and processed to derive an array

of 3D strain tensors without the need to image slices with multiple orientations or use numerical interpolation. Multislice zHARP allows for 3D strain quantification in the whole heart in less than 20 s. It should be noted that the idea of combining tagging and phase encoding or velocity encoding, for simultaneous acquisition of in-plane and through-plane myocardial motion information, has been previously provided by Perman et al. (1995) and Kuijer et al. (1999).

13.2.7.5 Improved HARP Motion Analysis

Two techniques have been presented to improve 3D motion analysis with HARP (Chuang et al. 2010, Venkatesh et al. 2010). In the first technique (Venkatesh et al. 2010), a new method of phase unwrapping has been developed to allow for accurate measurement of 3D strain in the entire LV. Specifically, phase residues in the HARP images are used to automatically detect phase inconsistencies in the wrapped-phase images. With the proposed technique, tagged images covering multiple slices are acquired every breath-hold, which allows for strain measurement in the whole heart in a short time and with high accuracy. The second technique for improving 3D motion analysis with HARP has been developed by Chuang et al. (2010) to increase the motion detection sensitivity and reduce susceptibility to noise by combining tagging, automated material point tracking, and finite-element modeling (FEM).

13.3 DENSE

13.3.1 ORIGINAL SEQUENCE

In DENSE, intramyocardial motion is measured by encoding tissue displacement in the phase of a stimulated

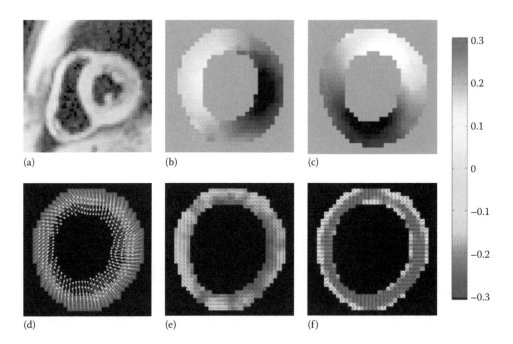

FIGURE 13.5 End-systolic cine DENSE data of a normal subject acquired in a single breath-hold with 22 cardiac phases. (a) Magnitude image. (b) Phase image encoded with displacement in the left–right direction. (c) Phase image encoded with displacement in the up–down direction. (d) Two-dimensional end-diastole to end-systole displacement map. (e) Second principal strain map. (f) First principal strain map. (Reproduced from Epstein, F.H., *J. Nucl. Cardiol.*, 14, 729, 2007. With permission.)

echo and displaying the displacement-encoded phase on a pixel-by-pixel basis (Aletras et al. 1999b; Figure 13.5).

13.3.1.1 DENSE and STEAM

DENSE evolved as a stimulated echo acquisition mode (STEAM) pulse sequence (Haase et al. 1986) with additional displacement encodings (Figure 13.6), in contrast to HARP, which stemmed from the tagging perspective. Actually, although HARP and DENSE have been separately developed and were presented as evolving from different perspectives, they have more similarities than differences, and they represent two approaches to phase-based strain analysis (Kuijer et al. 2006).

13.3.1.2 Displacement Encoding in DENSE

The DENSE technique is based on the STEAM pulse sequence, which has been used in various imaging applications. As a STEAM-based sequence, DENSE consists of three stages for magnetization modulation, mixing, and demodulation. During the modulation part of the sequence, the longitudinal magnetization is tipped into the transverse plane, encoded with a displacement-encoding gradient, and then stored back in the longitudinal direction until imaging takes place. The advantage of storing the magnetization in the longitudinal direction is that it allows for less magnetization relaxation (myocardial T1 is much larger than T2; e.g., 850 and 50 ms, respectively, at 1.5 T), and therefore higher tagging contrast through the cardiac cycle. Later, during the imaging stage (data acquisition or signal readout), the modulated magnetization is excited (tipped into the transverse plane) and decoded using a gradient

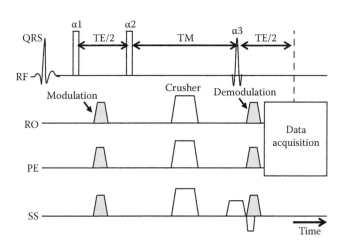

FIGURE 13.6 The DENSE pulse sequence. Displacement encoding (modulation) and decoding (demodulation) gradients are added after the first and third RF pulses, respectively. Both gradients have equal magnitudes, and they are applied in the direction where displacement information is to be obtained (in all three directions in this example). During the mixing time (TM) between modulation and demodulation, large crusher gradients are applied to dephase any transverse magnetization, such that the modulated magnetization is stored in the longitudinal direction, where it experiences only longitudinal relaxation. The time between the first and second RF pulses is equal to the time between the third RF pulse and data acquisition = half the echo time (TE/2). PE, phase encoding; RO, readout; SS, slice selection. (Reproduced from Ibrahim, El-S.H., *J. Cardiovasc. Magn. Reson.*, 13, 36, 2011.)

with the same magnitude as that of the encoding gradient. The effect of the displacement-decoding gradients in DENSE is to shift the stimulated echo to the center of the k-space. This operation does not affect the amplitude modulation of the DENSE magnitude-reconstructed images compared to those in SPAMM (except for removing the tagging pattern from the image). However, it causes the phase of the stimulated echo to be directly proportional to tissue displacement. Stationary spins are perfectly rewound and have zero net phase accumulation. However, spins that have moved in the gradient's direction during the mixing time accumulate phase due to their different spatial positions in between modulation and demodulation. By acquiring a second reference DENSE image and subtracting the two phase images, displacement information in the gradient's direction can be deciphered. For 3D motion analysis, four DENSE images are required (one reference image and three images encoded in three orthogonal directions).

13.3.1.3 DENSE Advantages

The DENSE images can be processed to reveal motion information on the pixel level by displaying a small vector at each pixel location. The vector's orientation and length represent the motion direction and magnitude, respectively (Figure 13.7).

One advantage of the DENSE technique is that it is a black-blood sequence (due to the disturbance of the modulated magnetization in the blood pool during the mixing period), which facilitates myocardial segmentation in the resulting images. From a k-space perspective, the demodulated DENSE images have the displacement-encoded echo centered at the k-space center, while other echoes are shifted or suppressed with the goal of sampling the displacement-encoded echo at high spatial resolution. Numerical simulations and in vivo experiments have been conducted to validate DENSE accuracy

(Feng et al. 2009), and the sequence has been successfully implemented in several studies (Ashikaga et al. 2005, Aletras et al. 2006, Spottiswoode et al. 2008a). Strain measurements by DENSE showed to be highly reproducible and quantitatively equivalent to those obtained from conventional myocardial tagging sequences.

13.3.2 DIFFERENT SIGNAL ECHOES IN DENSE

Three echoes can be distinguished in DENSE as follows: stimulated (displacement-encoded) echo, complex conjugate of the stimulated echo (antiecho), and T1 relaxation echo (nonmodulated DC echo) (Figure 13.8). Notice that both the stimulated echo and complex conjugate echo are multiplied by a factor of 0.5. Therefore, the magnitude of the DENSE data is only one-half of that of the unmodulated MRI data, an inherent limitation of STEAM imaging. Only the phase of the displacement-encoded echo is directly related to tissue displacement. Therefore, it is usually the case that only the stimulated echo is sampled in DENSE since, otherwise, the additionally sampled echoes interfere with the stimulated echo and cause errors in tissue motion estimation. Nevertheless, recent techniques have been developed to improve SNR or eliminate the artifacts by correlatively adding different echoes or suppressing unwanted echoes, respectively, as described later in Sections 13.3.4 and 13.3.5.

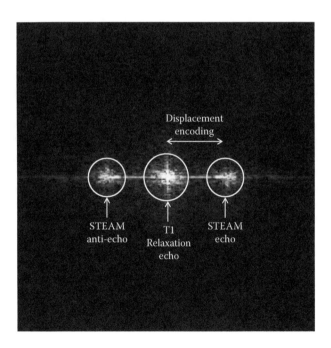

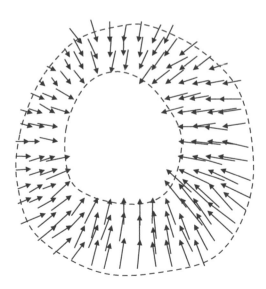

FIGURE 13.7 DENSE tissue displacement map. An example of a DENSE image of the left ventricle, where representative vectors are drawn at each pixel, with the vector's magnitude and direction representing the displacement value and orientation, respectively.

FIGURE 13.8 K-space showing different echoes in DENSE. Three echoes are generated in DENSE: stimulated echo, stimulated anti-echo, and T1 relaxation echo. Only the stimulated echo contains the displacement information of interest, while the other echoes are to be suppressed. The higher the displacement-encoding frequency, the larger the separation between the stimulated echo and T1 relaxation echo, which results in that the displacement-encoded image is not corrupted by undesired signals. (Reproduced from Ibrahim, El-S.H., *J. Cardiovasc. Magn. Reson.*, 13, 36, 2011.)

Suppressing the unwanted echoes (antiecho and T1 relaxation echo) can be achieved by applying a large displacement-encoding gradient such that the spatial frequencies of the unwanted echoes are shifted beyond the frequency range detected during data acquisition. It should be noted that shifting the longitudinal relaxation echo outside the sampled region in k-space requires the implementation of considerably large displacement-encoding gradients to ensure that the spatial frequency of the T1 relaxation echo is greater than the frequency range detected during data acquisition. Nevertheless, in practice, large displacement-encoding gradients may cause magnetization dephasing and signal loss of the desired stimulated echo when imaging contracting tissues like the myocardium. More practical techniques for suppressing the T1 relaxation echo include using inversion recovery, CSPAMM, or other phase cycling techniques. Inversion recovery suppresses the echo only at a certain timepoint and thus is not applicable to cine DENSE imaging. Subtracting data from complementary acquisitions, as in CSPAMM, suppresses the T1 relaxation echo independently of the acquisition time and longitudinal relaxation rate; however, this approach requires two acquisitions and can result in incomplete echo suppression in the case of variable heart rate between the two acquisitions. Recent advances in phase cycling techniques showed the capability of isolating the stimulated echo from the artifact-generating echoes; however, the number of data acquisitions in this case should be at least equal to the number of echoes, which results in long scan time.

13.3.3   Sequence Development

13.3.3.1   Cine DENSE

When introduced in 1999, the DENSE data were acquired at a single cardiac phase, usually at end-systole. A navigator-guided non-breath-hold approach has been proposed in 2003 to acquire multiphase DENSE data (Pai and Wen 2003). In this sequence, two navigator echoes are applied before and after the DENSE sequence. A single breath-hold conventional cine DENSE technique has been proposed in the following year (Buonocore 2004, Kim et al. 2004b). The arrangement of the sequence modules for this cine DENSE method is illustrated in Figure 13.9, where the displacement-encoding module is applied immediately after the electrocardiogram (ECG) R-wave trigger, followed by multiphase readout modules.

13.3.3.2   Multipoint and Balanced Displacement Encoding

The DENSE sequence typically encodes displacement in two or three orthogonal directions and acquires an additional phase reference image without displacement encoding. This approach has been extended by Bennett et al. (2006), who proposed a variant displacement-encoding strategy for 2D DENSE imaging. Later, Zhong et al. (2009) presented a general framework for designing and analyzing displacement-encoding and displacement-decoding processes and used this framework to develop specific strategies for both simple and balanced multipoint displacement encoding (Figure 13.10). The advantage of this strategy is that it provides reduced phase noise variance for a given displacement-encoding frequency and eliminates the direction bias in phase noise. Compared to the simple multipoint method, the balanced multipoint method reduces the phase noise covariances by over 99% and almost eliminates the direction bias, although that these advantages may come at the expense of increased phase wrapping.

13.3.4   Meta-DENSE and Echo Combination

13.3.4.1   Meta-DENSE

The mixed echo train acquisition DENSE (meta-DENSE) method is a modified DENSE technique, which results in fast data acquisition and high spatial resolution (Aletras and Wen 2001). In meta-DENSE, a modified fast spin-echo readout is implemented to ensure that any contributions from the local stimulated echoes are added coherently. Further, inversion recovery is implemented to eliminate the unencoded signals, and the gradient waveforms are balanced between consecutive inversion pulses to ensure successful artifact removal. The meta-DENSE technique allows for longer readout periods than in conventional cine DENSE because the T2* transverse relaxation is replaced by T2 relaxation.

In a further development to suppress the antiecho signal in DENSE, meta-DENSE has been combined with RF phase cycling (Aletras and Arai 2004). In the modified sequence, both real and imaginary magnetization components are acquired in successive acquisitions and combined to construct the whole position-encoded complex signal. The improvement in image quality obtained by suppressing both the T1 relaxation echo using inversion recovery and the antiecho

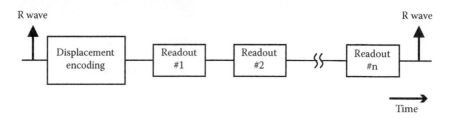

FIGURE 13.9   Schematic diagram of cine DENSE imaging. Displacement encoding is applied immediately after the detection of the R-wave of the electrocardiogram, followed by a sequence of readouts at different heart phases.

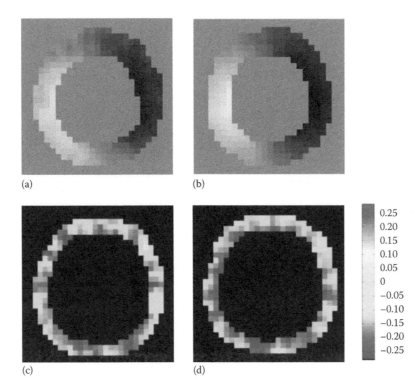

FIGURE 13.10 (a, b) Short-axis end-diastolic DENSE phase (in x-direction) images and (c, d) the corresponding circumferential strain maps in a healthy volunteer using (a, c) simple and (b, d) balanced 3-point displacement encodings. (Reproduced from Zhong, X. et al., *Magn. Reson. Med.*, 61(4), 981, 2009. With permission.)

signal using RF phase cycling results in strain maps with significantly reduced artifacts.

13.3.4.2 Echo Combination

Although the phases of both the stimulated echo and complex conjugate echo contain information about tissue displacement, typically only the stimulated echo is used for DENSE post-processing. Kim et al. (2004a) and Kim and Kellman (2007) proposed an echo combination technique to coherently combine the stimulated echo with the complex conjugate echo, so that the displacement-encoded information can be extracted from the combined data for improved SNR (Figure 13.11). The advantages of the echo combination DENSE technique

include enhanced SNR, improved data acquisition efficiency, and elimination of phase errors due to interscan motion and imaging variations.

Because echo combination is based on extracting a pair of subsampled modulated images, which have uncorrelated noise, and adding them together, SNR is enhanced in the resulting combined image. In CSPAMM-modulated images, the two subsampled images are extracted by splitting the raw data matrix into positive and negative parts (Kim et al. 2004a). The two images are separately reconstructed using inverse FT and then added together. The resulting averaged image is used to retrieve motion information as in conventional DENSE. This echo combination technique results in

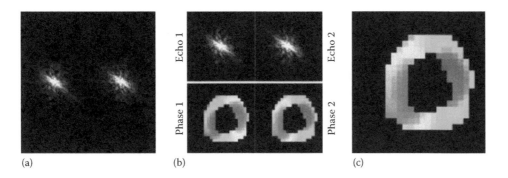

FIGURE 13.11 Echo combination reconstruction in DENSE. (a) Two echoes are positioned at opposite sides of the k-space of the complementary SPAMM (CSPAMM) image. (b) The CSPAMM k-space is divided into two smaller k-spaces, and the two subsampled k-spaces are separately reconstructed. (c) The resulting image after combining the two subsampled phase images (the phase difference is divided by two). (Reproduced from Kim, D. and Kellman, P., *NMR Biomed.*, 20(6), 591, 2007. With permission.)

SNR improvement ranging from 14% to 34% throughout the cardiac cycle (Kim et al. 2004a). It should be noted that DENSE echo combination is similar to the signal peak combination idea previously described for HARP in Section 12.2.3 (Ryf et al. 2004), although that both techniques have been separately developed in 2004.

13.3.5   ECHO SUPPRESSION

13.3.5.1   CANSEL

Epstein and Gilson (2004) extended the CSPAMM method to use cosine and sine modulation to eliminate (CANSEL) both the T1 relaxation echo and complex conjugate echo without the need for using a large displacement-encoding frequency. CANSEL results in improved SNR for accurate measurement of through-plane and in-plane tissue displacements. However, CANSEL is associated with long scan time due to the required multiple data acquisitions.

13.3.5.2   Through-Plane Dephasing with CSPAMM

Another approach to suppress the artifact-generating echoes in DENSE is to implement through-plane dephasing gradients in addition to CSPAMM modulation (Zhong et al. 2006). The advantage of this approach is that it selectively dephases the unwanted echoes without significantly affecting the stimulated echo. Further, the implementation of this technique is independent of the tissue T1 value and displacement-encoding frequency, and it does not require additional acquisitions. It should be noted, however, that the induced through-plane spatial frequency must be constrained when imaging the heart to avoid signal loss due to cardiac deformation. Another limitation of this technique is that through-plane dephasing cannot be used when displacement encoding is applied in the through-plane direction or when volumetric 3D DENSE imaging is conducted.

13.3.6   REDUCING SCAN TIME

13.3.6.1   Fast-DENSE

The fast-DENSE technique was developed in 1999 as a single breath-hold sequence for measuring myocardial strain in a single slice (Aletras et al. 1999a). In fast-DENSE, a multishot segmented k-space EPI sampling scheme is implemented to reduce scan time. The technique requires minimal user intervention, and the resulting measurements have sufficient resolution to reveal transmural strain variation across the LV wall. Another single breath-hold, high-spatial-resolution, 2D cine DENSE technique was developed in 2004 by Kim et al. (2004b). In this technique, three cine data sets are acquired in each encoding direction: a phase reference data set and two complementary displacement-encoded data sets. Displacement encoding is implemented in two orthogonal directions by swapping the readout and phase-encoding directions. The complementary data sets are used to suppress T1 relaxation artifacts. The fast-DENSE technique resulted in significant reduction in scan time, which allowed for acquiring each cine data set in only three heartbeats.

13.3.6.2   DENSE with SENSE

Parallel imaging can be combined with DENSE to accelerate data acquisition. For example, DENSE has been combined with the sensitivity-encoding (SENSE) technique (Pruessmann et al. 1999) to reduce total breath-hold time (Aletras et al. 2005). In DENSE with SENSE, a single nonencoded low-resolution B_1 map is acquired for reconstructing all three complex images (two orthogonal directions plus a reference), which allows for shorter scan time compared to when separate maps are acquired for each of the three DENSE images. Further, this SENSE acceleration scheme does not change the strain noise level compared to unaccelerated scans. DENSE with SENSE allows for obtaining high-quality strain maps within an appropriate scan time for clinical use (Aletras et al. 2005).

In another approach to improve SNR and data acquisition efficiency, DENSE has been combined with SENSE, echo combination reconstruction, and balanced steady state with free precession (bSSFP) 3.0 T imaging (Kim and Kellman 2007). The implementation of parallel imaging allows for accelerating the DENSE cine acquisition rate by a factor of two, resulting in a total acquisition time of 12 heartbeats. The combined implementation of bSSFP, echo combination, and 3.0 T field strength allows for increasing SNR and compensating for the losses associated with parallel readout.

13.3.6.3   High-Resolution DENSE

Zhong and Yu (2010) developed a 2D multiphase DENSE method for direct quantification of Lagrangian strain and implemented their method for imaging the mouse heart under dobutamine stimulation. The developed method allowed for direct cardiac strain quantification at both baseline and high workload with high spatial (0.56 mm) and temporal (<10 ms) resolutions.

13.3.7   3D DENSE

A method has been developed for 3D tracking of myocardial motion using slice-following cine DENSE (Spottiswoode et al. 2008b). This method allows for obtaining true 3D frame-to-frame motion trajectories of the material points initially lying inside the imaging plane, as well as quantifying myocardial through-plane tissue rotation.

Navigator-echo volumetric cine DENSE imaging with spiral acquisition is another option for measuring 3D myocardial strain (Spottiswoode et al. 2008b). The navigator-echo technique allows for free-breathing imaging, and spiral 3D acquisition (stack of parallel 2D spirals) allows for TE minimization, SNR improvement, and efficient data sampling. Balanced displacement-encoding is implemented to improve SNR, while fat suppression and three-point phase cycling are implemented to reduce artifacts from unwanted signals. Nevertheless, a limitation of this sequence is its long scan time, which could limit the sequence's clinical applicability.

Multislice DENSE imaging can be implemented by position encoding the whole heart during the modulation stage, followed by multiple position decodings of different slices (Sigfridsson et al. 2010). Displacement encodings are applied in three oblique directions with interleaved phase cycling to subtract the background phase error. In one implementation, a total of three slices have been acquired using three EPI excitations each, in an 18-heartbeat single breath-hold scan.

Nasiraei-Moghaddam and Gharib (2009) acquired 10 slices of SAX DENSE data from normal volunteers, with the displacement-encoding applied in three orthogonal directions, which allowed for identifying connected regions within the LV myocardium. In another study, Hess et al. (2009) presented an alternative method for estimating 3D strain by calculating the full 3D strain tensor for an entire slice of myocardial tissue using both cine DENSE and SENC imaging.

13.3.8 TECHNIQUE EVALUATION

In DENSE, the phase of the stimulated echo is influenced by off-resonance and B_0 inhomogeneity in addition to the encoded displacement. If the phase shifts from sources other than the encoded displacement are not accounted for, they lead to errors in the measured tissue motion. Therefore, multiple measurements need to be acquired in DENSE to cancel out the undesired phase shifts and retrieve only the phase pertaining to tissue motion. A study has been conducted, which showed that the accuracy of DENSE imaging can be severely affected by the unencoded free induction decay (FID) and off-resonance signals (Haraldsson et al. 2011). Nevertheless, phase alteration can be used to distinguish the phases in the FID and stimulated echo signals, which makes any influence of the FID easier to identify compared to normal situations where the phases of these signal components are correlative.

Other factors, including the flip angle implementation strategy, field strength, and spatial variation of the receiver coil sensitivity, influence SNR of the resulting DENSE images with different trade-offs. The field strength and receiver coil sensitivity influence SNR with the same order of magnitude, whereas the flip angle strategy can have a larger effect on SNR (Sigfridsson et al. 2011). Therefore, careful choice of the imaging hardware and imaging protocol is important for achieving sufficient SNR for accurate analysis of the DENSE images.

13.3.9 COMPOSITE DATA ACQUISITION

13.3.9.1 Strain and Viability

The DENSE sequence can be modified for simultaneous acquisition of myocardial displacement-encoding and contrast delayed-enhancement information from the same raw data by acquiring two complementary DENSE images (Gilson et al. 2004). Myocardial displacement information is obtained from the phase-reconstructed image after subtracting the complementary DENSE acquisitions, while contrast-enhancement information is obtained from the T1-weighted magnitude-reconstructed image after adding the two DENSE acquisitions. One advantage of the developed technique is that the resulting strain maps are perfectly registered with the gadolinium (Gd)-enhanced images, which reduces misregistration errors associated with separate acquisitions of strain and delayed-enhancement images. The proposed technique

may be useful for studying the mechanisms underlying regional myocardial dysfunction in patients with myocardial infarction (MI). It should be noted that other approaches have been previously reported for simultaneously measuring myocardial function and viability information (Osman et al. 1999, Sampath et al. 2003). The method in Osman et al. (1999) employed magnetization transfer to improve the contrast between normal and Gd-enhanced regions, while the method in Sampath et al. (2003) implemented spin locking for the same purpose. See also Section 13.4.3. for a similar technique in SENC.

13.3.9.2 Strain and Perfusion

DENSE could be used for simultaneous measurement of myocardial strain and perfusion (Le et al. 2010). The fact that the DENSE images are T1-weighted makes their contrast affected by Gd accumulation inside the tissue. In this setting, a single-shot multislice sequence is implemented, where the DENSE images are repeatedly acquired every other heartbeat over 3–4 min, covering the first-pass and initial washout of the contrast agent. The perfusion and strain information are obtained from the DENSE magnitude and phase data, respectively. The simultaneous measurement of myocardial perfusion and strain allows for reducing scan time while correlating the perfusion and function information.

13.3.10 DENSE IMAGE PROCESSING

A computationally efficient and reliable technique has been developed for processing the DENSE images (Spottiswoode et al. 2007). The developed technique is based on spatiotemporal phase unwrapping of the cine DENSE images, followed by material point tracking and temporal fitting of the motion trajectories. The technique improves motion tracking by fitting curves to the temporal evolution of the trajectories. The resulting improvement in the intramyocardial strain measurements is appreciated in the strain histograms, as well as from identifying regions of myocardial dysfunction in images of patients with MI.

FEM can be implemented to reconstruct and visualize myocardial dynamic displacement and strain fields from DENSE images (Liu et al. 2009). The continuous displacement field in the model is mathematically described based on discrete DENSE vectors using a minimization method with smoothness regularization. This DENSE postprocessing technique is stable and can be used to obtain a patient-specific 3D model of cardiac mechanics. However, FEM suffers from nonspecific parameterization and exhaustive computations.

Different efforts have been made to avoid the implementation of FEM in DENSE analysis (Gilliam et al. 2009, Spottiswoode et al. 2009). In one study, Gilliam et al. (2009) developed an automated motion recovery technique, termed active trajectory field model (ATFM), for analyzing the DENSE images. The developed deformable model exploits both image information and prior knowledge about cardiac motion for automatic recovery of cardiac motion from noisy images. The effectiveness of the ATFM technique has been demonstrated by measuring myocardial motion in murine SAX DENSE images both before and after MI. In another study, Spottiswoode et al. (2009) presented a 2D semiautomatic segmentation method that implemented tissue tracking based on the motion encoding into the phase of the cine DENSE images. The required user interaction is reduced to manual demarcation of the myocardium in a single frame. The proposed method has several advantages: the segmentation parameters are based on practical physiological limits; the contours are calculated in the first few cardiac phases, which have poor blood/myocardium contrast; and the method's implementation is independent of the shape of the delineated tissue, which makes it applicable to both SAX and LAX images.

13.4 SENC

13.4.1 Original Sequence

13.4.1.1 SENC Advantages

SENC MRI is a relatively new imaging technique that generates images whose pixel intensities are directly related to the amount of tissue strain (Osman et al. 2001; Figure 13.12). SENC is similar to DENSE in that it is based on a STEAM pulse sequence. However, in contrast to DENSE, the strain information in SENC is obtained from the magnitude images. SENC has the advantages of measuring strain with high-resolution (on the pixel level) and using simple postprocessing. A color-coded image is obtained that shows through-plane strain. From the applications point of view, SENC is used not only to image myocardial strain, but also to generate black-blood cine images of the heart that can be used to accurately estimate global heart function. In addition, recent work showed that SENC is effective for detecting stiff masses (Osman 2003).

13.4.1.2 SENC and Tagging

SENC evolved from a tagging perspective, not from a STEAM perspective as in DENSE. Nevertheless, in contrast to conventional tagging sequences, tagging in SENC is applied in the through-plane direction using a modulation gradient in the z-direction, which creates a parallel stack of magnetization-saturated planes that lie inside, and parallel to, the imaging plane, as shown in Figure 13.13. During the cardiac cycle, these parallel tagged planes move closer to each other or further apart based on tissue contraction or stretching in the through-plane direction, respectively, which affects the tagging (modulation) frequency.

13.4.1.3 Low-Tuning and High-Tuning Images

The data acquisition part of the SENC pulse sequence is preceded by regular slice excitation played in combination with a demodulation gradient played in the z-direction. In SENC MRI literatures, the demodulation gradient is usually referred to as the "tuning gradient." Usually, two images are acquired with different tunings, which are referred to

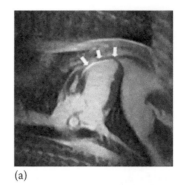

(a)

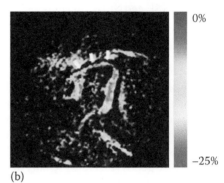

0%

−25%

(b)

FIGURE 13.12 Comparison of strain encoding (SENC) functional images with a delayed-enhancement image. All images were acquired at end systole. (a) Delayed-enhancement image acquired 15 min after gadolinium injection, with hyperenhanced nonviable infarcted myocardium (arrows). (b) Conventional SENC functional image showing dysfunction (arrows) in the infarcted myocardium. (Reproduced from Pan, L. et al., *Magn. Reson. Med.*, 55(2), 386, 2006. With permission.)

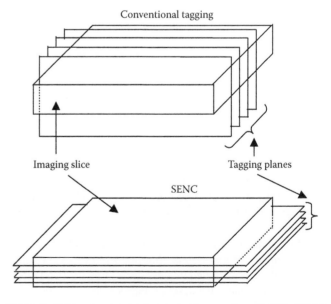

FIGURE 13.13 Tagging planes in strain encoding (SENC). SENC uses tagging as in conventional spatial modulation of magnetization (SPAMM). However, the tag planes are applied parallel to, and lie inside, the imaging slice; thus, through-plane strain is measured.

as the low-tuning (LT) and high-tuning (HT) images. The LT image is usually acquired at the same applied modulation frequency to capture signals from static (noncontracting) tissues. On the other hand, the HT image is acquired at a higher frequency (calculated based on slice thickness, applied modulation frequency, and expected tissue strain) to capture signals from contracting tissues. It is clear from Figure 13.14 that only static tissues (e.g., chest wall and liver) are visible throughout all the cardiac phases in the LT images, whereas contracting myocardium disappears gradually during systole. On the other hand, the myocardial signal intensity increases with tissue contraction in the HT images. Therefore, by adding the counterpart images (acquired at the same timeframe) from the LT and HT data sets, a black-blood cine set of images is generated, which is usually referred to as the "anatomy" images (Ibrahim et al. 2008a).

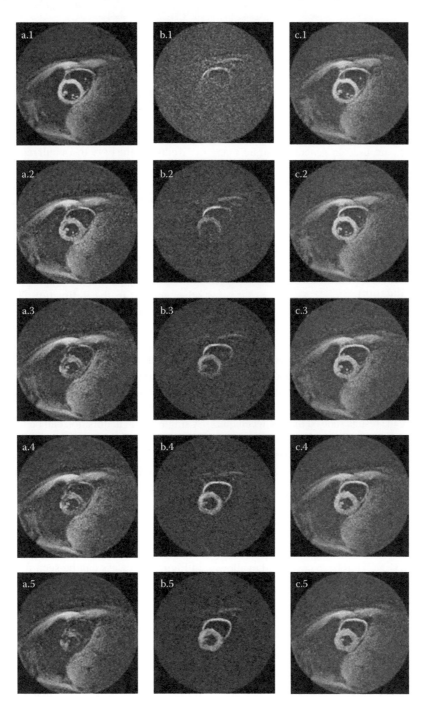

FIGURE 13.14 Short-axis images of a healthy volunteer's heart acquired using strain encoding with different tunings. The images from top to bottom represent different cardiac phases from end-diastole (top) to end-systole (bottom). The (a) left and (b) middle columns show low-tuning (LT) and high-tuning (HT) images, respectively. (c) The right column shows the anatomy images resulting from combining the corresponding LT and HT images. Note myocardium disappearance and appearance in the LT and HT images, respectively, during systole. (Reproduced from Fahmy, A.S. et al., *Magn. Reson. Med.*, 55(2), 404, 2006. With permission.)

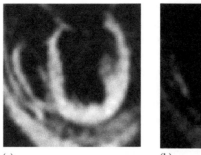 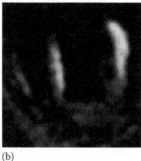 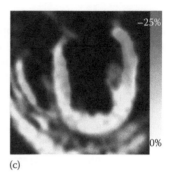

(a)   (b)   (c)

FIGURE 13.15   Strain encoding (SENC) image constructed from low-tuning (LT) and high-tuning (HT) images. (a) An LT image show-ing noncontracting tissues. (b) An HT image showing contracting tissues. (c) The LT and HT images are combined to show a color-coded strain image (multiplied by the anatomical image to suppress signals from blood and background). Note that this four-chamber slice shows through-plane strain (circumferential strain in this case), and note the big noncontacting apical region. (Reproduced from Ibrahim, El-S.H., *J. Cardiovasc. Magn. Reson.*, 13, 36, 2011.)

The LT and HT images are used to generate a strain map (Figure 13.15) using a simple mathematical operation. Due to the image noise, the estimated strain of the pixels in the blood pool or background is erroneous, which causes the reconstructed color map not to be plausibly visible. A solution to this problem can be achieved by using the anatomy image to mask the colored strain map, where the low intensity of the anatomy image suppresses the appearance of the background noise, as shown in Figure 13.15c.

13.4.1.4   Technique Validation

Because SENC measures through-plane strain, the SAX and LAX images show myocardial longitudinal and circumferential strain, respectively. Similar to DENSE, SENC is a black-blood sequence because of the destruction of the tagging pattern in the blood pool during the time in between modulation and data acqui-sition. SENC has been validated against conventional tagging techniques for measuring both systolic and diastolic LV strain (Neizel et al. 2009a), where the results showed that the technique is robust, accurate, and reproducible. The sequence has been suc-cessfully implemented in several clinical studies (Hamdan et al. 2008, 2009, Korosoglou et al. 2008, 2009, 2010, Youssef et al. 2008, Neizel et al. 2009b, Shehata et al. 2010, Koos et al. 2013).

13.4.2   Sequence Development

13.4.2.1   Slice-Following SENC

Slice-following SENC (sf-SENC) has been developed to allow for measuring strain in the same myocardial tissue throughout the cardiac cycle despite through-plane tissue displacement (Fahmy et al. 2006). Similar to slice-following CSPAMM, sf-SENC is based on tagging a thin slice (in the z-direction), followed by imaging a thicker slice during data acquisition.

13.4.2.2   Fast-SENC

In another SENC development, Pan et al. (2006) presented the fast-SENC technique, which is a real-time version of SENC (Figure 13.16). Three modifications have been implemented to allow SENC imaging in a single heartbeat: (1) reduced field of view (FOV) using selective excitation; (2) spiral data acqui-sition; and (3) interleaved LT and HT tunings.

Reducing the FOV to a small region around the heart allows for fast acquisition of the k-space. That is, sparse traversing of the k-space, and hence shorter acquisition times, is possible without introducing fold-over artifacts. This modification is particularly suited for cardiac imaging as the heart occupies only a small region inside the chest. To be able to reduce the FOV without introducing aliasing artifacts, the nonselective tagging (modulating) RF pulses in SENC are replaced by slice-selective pulses, one applied in the x-direction and the other applied in the y-direction. Therefore, the only modu-lated region is the cuboid resulting from the intersection of the two excited slices, as shown in Figure 13.17 (appears as a small square ROI around the heart when looking from the z-direction). This allows for reducing the acquisition matrix without affecting spatial resolution.

Replacing Cartesian k-space acquisition by spiral acqui-sition (Figure 13.18) significantly reduces the scan time. A single-spiral acquisition can be implemented to reduce scan time to a single heartbeat. Nevertheless, spiral data acquisition is usually implemented using interleaved short spirals instead of using one long spiral in order to reduce off-resonance arti-facts, especially at high field strengths.

In conventional SENC, two sets of images (LT and HT) are acquired in two separate scans, from which strain images are constructed. An alternative approach is to acquire only one set of images with interleaved LT and HT tunings, as shown in Figure 13.19. As can be seen from the figure, each pair of adjacent images is combined to construct a SENC image, such that there is no apparent effect on temporal resolution.

The fast-SENC technique allows for real-time strain imag-ing, which is necessary in certain applications, for example, during stress tests, dynamic imaging, or interventional MRI imaging. Korosoglou et al. (2008) evaluated the fast-SENC technique at 3.0 T and showed that the information obtained from fast-SENC is equal to that obtained from conventional tagging with prolonged breath-holds.

13.4.2.3   Slice-Following Fast-SENC

Ibrahim et al. (2007b) combined the features of slice-following and real-time imaging by developing the

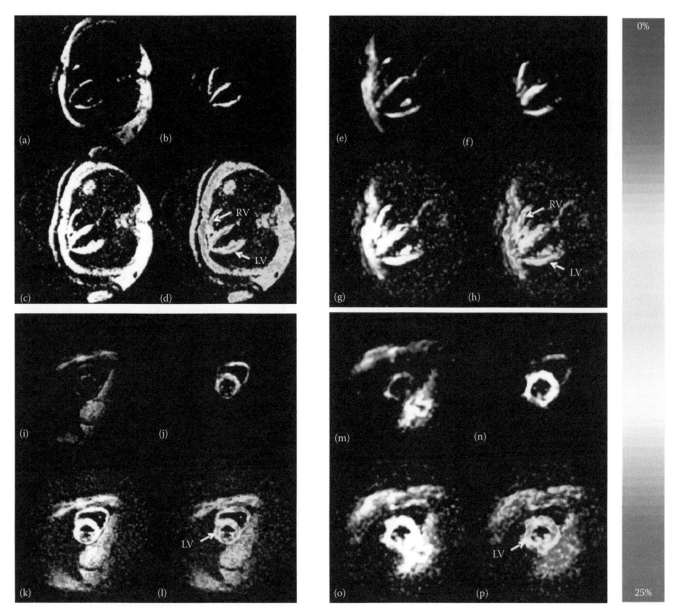

FIGURE 13.16 Long-axis (LAX) (top panels) and short-axis (SAX) (bottom panels) end-systolic strain encoding (SENC) (left panels) and fast-SENC (right panels) images of a normal human subject. The conventional SENC images are acquired during two breath-holds with 12 heartbeats each. The fast-SENC images are acquired in one heartbeat. The four images of each group are (a, e, i, m) low-tuning, (b, f, j, n) high-tuning, (c, g, k, o) anatomical, and (d, h, l, p) strain images. The LAX images show circumferential strain, whereas the SAX images show longitudinal strain. (Reproduced from Pan, L. et al., *Magn. Reson. Med.*, 55(2), 386, 2006. With permission.)

slice-following fast-SENC (sf-fast-SENC) technique. To be able to combine the two features, the tagged region has to be limited in all three directions. It has to have limited expansions in the x- and y-directions to allow for using a reduced FOV, which is necessary for real-time imaging. Further, the tagged region has to have a limited thickness in the z-direction, which is necessary for applying the slice-following technique. To fulfill these requirements, the first tagging RF pulse in SENC is replaced by a 2D cylindrical excitation pulse in the x–y plane, and the second tagging RF pulse is replaced by a slice-selective pulse in the z-direction (Figure 13.20). Therefore, the only

tagged part is the disk-shaped region (which contains the heart) resulting from the intersection of the excited cylinder and orthogonal plane. During data acquisition, a thick slice (with reduced FOV) is excited to encompass the tagged region despite displacement in the z-direction. Similar to fast-SENC, interleaved LT and HT acquisition and spiral imaging are implemented to reduce scan time to one heartbeat. The sf-fast-SENC technique has been tested on volunteers, where the results showed differences between the strain measurements with and without slice-following, especially in basal slices and during systole (Figure 13.21).

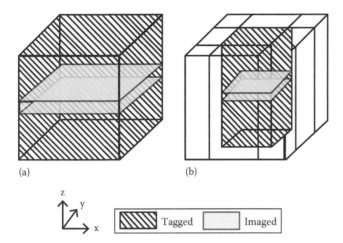

FIGURE 13.17 (a) Nonselective excitation in strain encoding (SENC) and (b) selective excitation in fast-SENC. In SENC, the whole body is tagged; thus, large field of view (FOV) imaging is required. In fast-SENC, tagging is restricted to the intersection of the two orthogonal slabs, which allows for using a small imaging FOV without introducing fold-over artifacts.

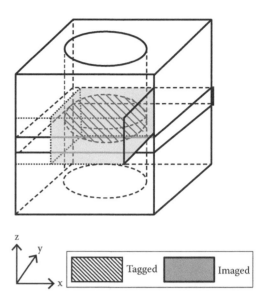

FIGURE 13.20 Selective excitation in slice-following fast-SENC. Tagging is restricted to a disk-shaped thin region (shown hashed in the figure), which is the intersection of a 2D cylindrically excited region and an orthogonal refocusing slice. A thick slice with reduced FOV (shown gray in the figure) is then used for imaging.

13.4.3 COMPOSITE SENC (C-SENC)

Another contribution by Ibrahim et al. (2007a,c, 2008b) is the C-SENC technique, which acquires both myocardial functional and viability information in one scan. It should be noted that the idea in C-SENC is similar to that developed by Gilson et al. (2004) for DENSE (see Section 13.3.9).

In C-SENC, the SENC sequence is modified to acquire a third image (besides the LT and HT images), as shown in Figure 13.22. This third image is acquired without any tunings (thus called the no-tuning (NT) image) to capture the nontagged signal at the k-space center (Figure 13.23). The NT image is a saturation-recovery T1-weighted image because it captures the signal from the longitudinally relaxing magnetization.

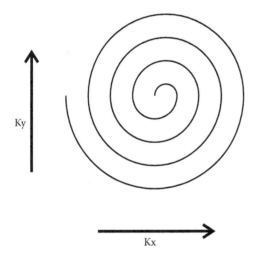

FIGURE 13.18 Spiral k-space acquisition.

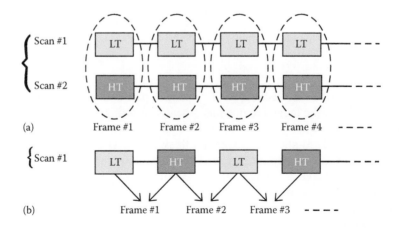

FIGURE 13.19 Interleaved-tuning acquisition in strain encoding (SENC). (a) In conventional SENC, two scans are required to capture the low-tuning (LT) and high-tuning (HT) images at different heart phases. (b) In interleaved-tuning acquisition, the LT and HT tunings are applied alternatively in one scan only. Each pair of adjacent images is combined to construct a SENC image.

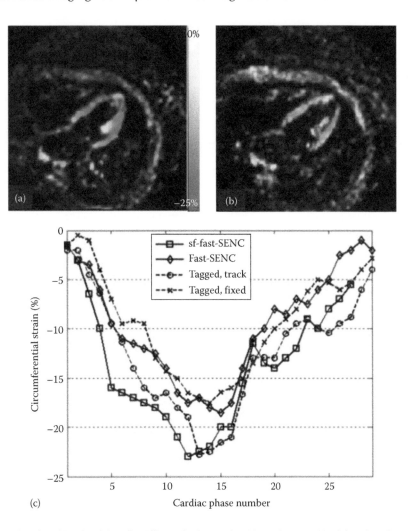

FIGURE 13.21 Slice-following fast-SENC (sf-fast-SENC) results from a healthy volunteer. (a) sf-fast-SENC circumferential strain image acquired at 330 ms after the R-wave. (b) The corresponding fast-SENC strain image. (c) Strain curves for a region of interest (ROI) on the septal wall of left ventricle throughout the cardiac cycle. Strain values are calculated from the sf-fast-SENC and fast-SENC images, as well as from the orthogonal short-axis spatial modulation of magnetization (SPAMM)-tagged images for the same ROI. The curves show differences between the values computed from sf-fast-SENC and fast-SENC images, especially at end-systole. In addition, there is a similarity between the strain values computed from the SENC images and those computed from the orthogonal SPAMM-tagged images. (Reproduced from Ibrahim, El-S.H. et al., *J. Magn. Reson. Imaging*, 26(6), 1461, 2007b. With permission.)

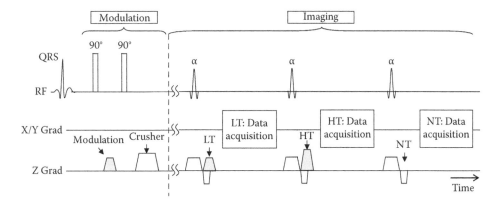

FIGURE 13.22 Composite strain encoding (C-SENC) pulse sequence. The sequence is similar to conventional SENC with the exception that an additional image (no tuning, NT) is acquired without any tuning. HT, high tuning; LT, low tuning.

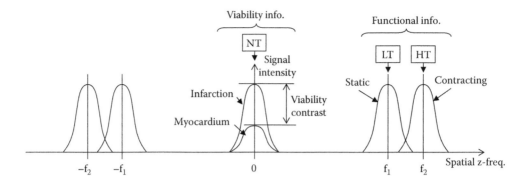

FIGURE 13.23 Different signal peaks acquired in composite strain encoding (C-SENC). The low-tuning (LT) and high-tuning (HT) signal peaks result from noncontracting and contracting tissues, respectively. At zero frequency, another signal peak (the DC peak) arises from relaxed magnetization. Infarcted myocardium shows larger signal intensity than normal myocardium 10–15 min after gadolinium injection due to the contrast agent preferential accumulation in the infarcted tissue. NT, no tuning.

When C-SENC is applied 10–15 min after gadolinium injection, the infarcted myocardium appears bright due to shortened T1, secondary to contrast accumulation in the infarcted region, in contrast to the darker viable myocardium. In C-SENC, strain information is obtained from the LT and HT images as in conventional SENC while viability information is obtained from the NT image. When the three images are combined together, a composite image is constructed, which shows both myocardial function and viability information (Figure 13.24).

C-SENC imaging has many advantages over conventional imaging: (1) the scan time is reduced in half as only a single scan is required to obtain both functional and viability information instead of separate scans for SENC and delayed hyperenhancement (DHE) imaging; (2) the misregistration problems are alleviate as the LT, HT, and NT images are virtually acquired at the same timepoint; (3) simple postprocessing is required to construct the color-coded composite image; and (4) the resulting image has black-blood contrast for accurate identification of the endocardial border. Nevertheless, despite of its several advantages, C-SENC has some limitations: (1) the composite image is acquired at a single phase in the cardiac cycle, and (2) the myocardium-infarction contrast is suboptimal to that obtained in inversion recovery DHE imaging. Nevertheless, these points can be addressed by applying further modifications to the SENC

pulse sequence. For example, Basha et al. (2009) combined SENC with bSSFP imaging. The results showed that the implementation of bSSFP imaging results in more accurate results than with spoiled gradient sequences.

13.4.4 3D Strain Imaging Using SENC

13.4.4.1 SENC with HARP

SENC has been combined with HARP for measuring 3D myocardial strain in a single SAX slice (Sampath et al. 2009; Figure 13.25). In-plane circumferential and radial strain components are calculated from the HARP images, while through-plane longitudinal strain is calculated from the SENC images. The developed pulse sequence requires only six heartbeats. Two series of HARP images with horizontal and vertical taglines are acquired in the first and second heartbeats, respectively. Two additional series of HARP reference images (at the k-space center) are acquired in the third and fourth heartbeats. Finally, two SENC images with different tunings are acquired in the last two heartbeats. It should be noted that a 3D strain tensor cannot be calculated using the proposed technique as longitudinal shear components are missing. However, multiple SAX slices could be acquired with the proposed technique in a single breath-hold of multiple six-heartbeat length (as many as the number of imaged slices).

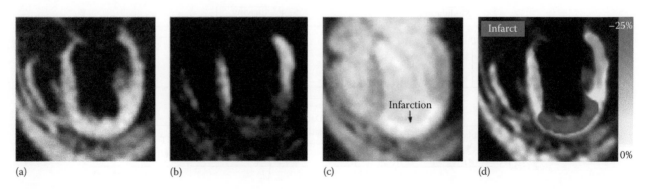

FIGURE 13.24 Composite strain encoding (C-SENC) image formation. (a) Low-tuning (LT) image showing noncontracting tissue. (b) High-tuning (HT) image showing contracting myocardium. (c) No-tuning (NT) image showing contrast between normal (gray) and infarcted (bright) myocardium. (d) The C-SENC image is formed by combining functional information (represented in degrees of red) obtained from the LT and HT images with viability information (represented in blue) obtained from the NT image. All images are obtained at end-systole. (Reproduced from Ibrahim, El-S.H., *J. Cardiovasc. Magn. Reson.*, 13, 36, 2011.)

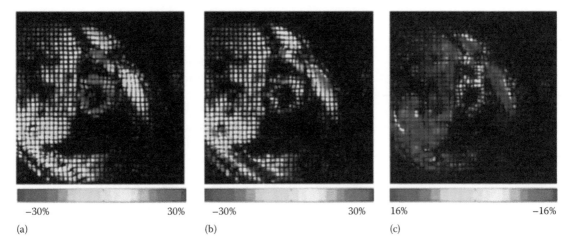

−30% 30%	−30% 30%	16% −16%
(a)	(b)	(c)

FIGURE 13.25 Color-coded (a) circumferential, (b) radial, and (c) longitudinal strain images in a short-axis slice at end-systole. The tagging grid is shown overlaid on the strain maps. In-plane and through-plane strain components are measured using HARP and SENC, respectively. (Reproduced from Sampath, S. et al., *Magn. Reson. Imaging*, 27(1), 55, 2009. With permission.)

13.4.4.2 SENC with DENSE

SENC has been combined with DENSE for measuring 3D strain in a single slice (Hess et al. 2009). The proposed method combines the advantages of DENSE (high spatial resolution and simple postprocessing) with SENC's capability of measuring through-plane motion in a single acquisition. In the developed method, 2D DNESE is implemented for measuring in-plane strain in two adjacent slices stacked on top of each other while SENC is implemented for measuring through-plane strain in the two slices in order to calculate a 3D strain tensor (the scan requires five breath-holds). It should be noted that the implementation of SENC for measuring through-plane motion is faster than imaging two separate slices with DENSE using through-plane encodings.

13.5 TISSUE PHASE MAPPING

13.5.1 Basic Concept

Tissue phase mapping (TPM) imaging, also known as phase-contrast (PC) imaging, is based on the fact that the generated MR signal is composed of both magnitude and phase. By adding a bipolar gradient to the imaging pulse sequence, the spins moving in the gradient's direction accumulate phase that is directly proportional to their velocity. Therefore, the measurement of the MR signal phase allows for quantifying motion of the moving spins. A reference data set (acquired without adding any bipolar gradients) is also obtained to subtract background phase from the generated TPM images. By adding bipolar gradients in the readout, phase-encoding, and slice-selection directions, 3D motion can be quantified (Figure 13.26).

13.5.2 Pulse Sequence

The TPM pulse sequence includes bipolar gradient pulses in the directions where velocity is to be measured (Figure 13.27). The reference image is usually acquired using an RF-spoiled nonencoded gradient-echo sequence. The velocity-encoding (venc) setting in the imaging parameters should be carefully determined to avoid aliasing (resulting from using too small venc value) and unnecessary noise (resulting from using too large venc value). Since velocity encoding in all three dimensions requires four scans, TPM imaging is characterized by a relatively long scan time.

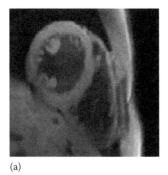 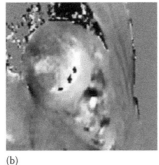 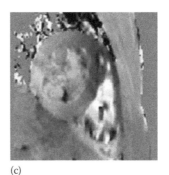 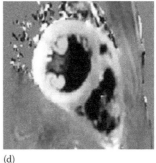

(a) (b) (c) (d)

FIGURE 13.26 Tissue phase mapping (TPM) velocity images of the heart. (a) Anatomical image. TPM images showing velocity in the (b) anterior–posterior, (c) foot–head, and (d) left–right directions, respectively.

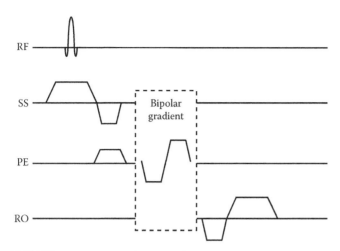

FIGURE 13.27 Tissue phase mapping pulse sequence, where bipolar gradients (shown in a dashed square) are added in the directions where velocity is to be encoded. PE, phase encoding; RO, readout; SS, slice selection.

13.5.3 Sequence Development

The signal from the blood pool is usually saturated by implementing black-blood techniques to avoid the artifacts resulting from fast-flowing blood. Navigator-echo-based respiratory control could be implemented to improve temporal and spatial resolutions (Ehman and Felmlee 1989). The resolution could be also improved using view sharing techniques and parallel imaging. Specifically, kt-BLAST (Lutz et al. 2011) and kt-GRAPPA (Jung et al. 2008) reconstructions have been implemented in TPM imaging and resulted in acceleration factors of 4 and 6, respectively.

13.5.4 Data Analysis

The information obtained from the TPM velocity maps has been used to generate velocity curves throughout the cardiac cycle in different SAX segments (Notomi et al. 2005). The results revealed pronounced regional differences in the myocardial motion pattern (Figure 13.28).

Foll et al. (2009) developed a multisegment, multislice visualization model to compare regional myocardial function between different subject groups. In the developed visualization model, in-plane and through-plane velocity components are represented by vectors and color code, respectively, as shown in Figure 13.29.

13.5.5 Combined TPM and Tagging

TPM imaging has been combined with delays alternating with nutations for tailored excitation (DANTE) tagging (Mosher and Smith 1990) for measuring through-plane and in-plane motion components, respectively.

13.5.6 Applications

13.5.6.1 Strain Rate Measurement
TPM imaging has been implemented for measuring myocardial strain rate. Kvitting et al. (2004) used time-resolved 3D TPM imaging for quantifying myocardial strain with a temporal resolution of 108 ms. In another study, Selskog et al. (2002) measured 3D strain rate using TPM imaging and presented a method for visualizing the whole 3D strain rate tensor. The results showed that the main direction of strain rate is nonplanar and varies from region to region in the myocardium.

13.5.6.2 Acceleration Phase Mapping
Recently, TPM imaging has been used for measuring regional myocardial acceleration using a tripolar gradient that refocuses the velocity-induced phase shifts (Staehle et al. 2011).

13.5.6.3 Age and Gender Differences
In a comprehensive study on 58 volunteers from different age groups, the results from TPM imaging showed that aging is associated with decreased and prolonged diastolic longitudinal and radial velocities, as well as reduced longitudinal velocities and apical rotation (Foll et al. 2010).

13.5.6.4 Ischemic Heart Disease
Karwatowski et al. (1994) used TPM MRI for studying global and regional longitudinal motion patterns in ischemic heart disease with and without MI. The results demonstrated significantly lower mean diastolic peak velocities in patients with coronary artery disease without infarction than in controls. In another study on patients with MI, Markl et al. (1999) showed that the longitudinal and radial velocities are better than circumferential velocities for identifying regional wall motion variation.

13.5.6.5 Cardiac Dyssynchrony
Foll et al. (2011) implemented TP for evaluating age-related LV dyssynchrony of the myocardium radial and longitudinal motion components. In another study by Markl et al. (2002), the velocities from 24 segments in a single slice were correlated with the velocity averaged over the entire LV. The results from that study showed that the myocardial radial velocity curves could be used as a reference for representing intact ventricular contractility. Delfino et al. (2008) used TPM imaging for studying patients with heart failure evaluated for cardiac resynchronization therapy (CRT), where the results showed significantly lower peak velocity and delayed time-to-peak velocity in the lateral wall in the patients compared to controls.

13.6 MR ELASTOGRAPHY

MR elastography (MRE) is a relatively recent noninvasive imaging approach that provides in vivo data about biomechanical properties of tissue (Figure 13.30). The general concept of MRE is to transmit low-frequency mechanical waves into the object and image those waves using MRI motion-sensitized sequences. This allows for solving locally for the stress–strain relationship to obtain the complex-valued shear modulus. Many different technical realizations exist, which all probe tissue characteristics in the frequency domain. Despite the challenges of applying MRE in the heart, MRE has a large potential for revealing intrinsic myocardial mechanical properties based on studying the stress–strain relationship.

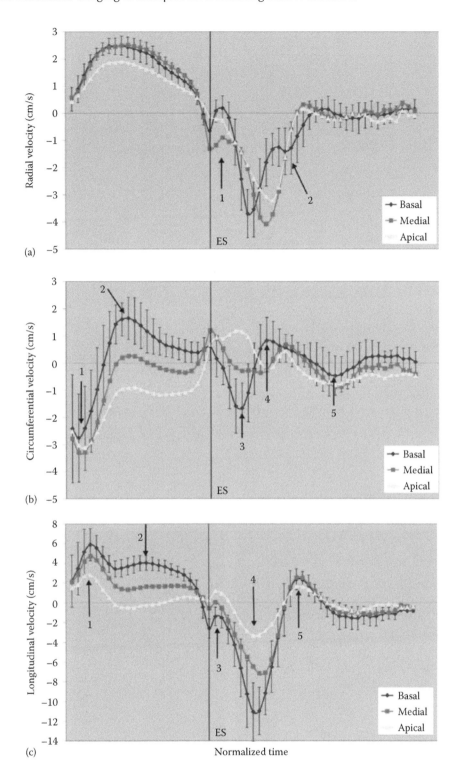

FIGURE 13.28 Time curves showing (a) radial, (b) circumferential, and (c) longitudinal myocardial velocities in volunteers. Each graph shows data comparison in basal, midventricular, and apical short-axis slices. ES, end-systole. (Reproduced from Jung, B. et al., *J. Magn. Reson. Imaging*, 24, 1033, 2006. With permission.)

13.6.1 Different Approaches to MRE

Generally, there are two different approaches to MRE: dynamic MRE, where periodic excitation is used, and static MRE, which measures the difference in spin location before and after an applied static compression.

13.6.1.1 Static MRE

At low frequencies, the loss effects vanish and we are in the so-called rubbery plateau where the stiffness attains a constant value (Verdier 2003). This represents mathematically the "serial limit" of the different microscopic stiffnesses of

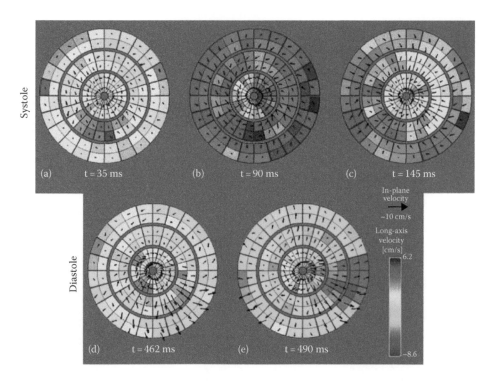

FIGURE 13.29   Distribution of regional myocardial velocities for (a–c) three systolic and (d, e) two diastolic timeframes within the cardiac cycle in a patient with dilated cardiomyopathy. (Reproduced from Foll, D. et al., *J. Magn. Reson. Imaging*, 29(5), 1043, 2009. With permission.)

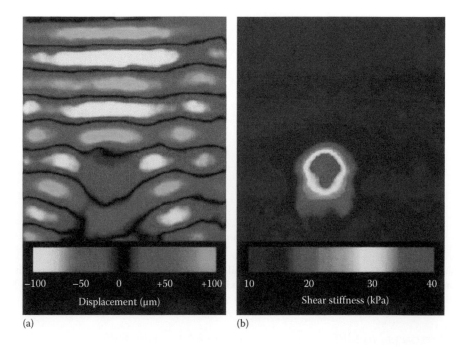

FIGURE 13.30   Magnetic resonance elastography (MRE) in an object with diameter comparable to wavelength. (a) Shear waves propagating in a phantom with an embedded 1.5cm-diameter cylinder of stiffer gel. Shear waves at 300 Hz were applied at the top margin of the gel block, with transverse motion oriented orthogonal to the plane of the image. (b) The elastogram clearly depicts the object, even though it is relatively small compared to the wavelength. (Reproduced from Manduca, A. et al., *Med. Image Anal.*, 5(4), 237, 2001. With permission.)

the material and is denoted as static elastography (Chenevert et al. 1998). The advantage of this method is that the complex shear modulus is real valued. Static MRE is very sensitive to motion, for example, physiological motion from breathing; therefore, in general, quantification using this approach is not feasible and thus this method remains qualitative.

13.6.1.2 Dynamic MRE

The general concept of dynamic MRE consists of three steps. Initially, a mechanical transducer is attached to the object/patient to generate stationary monochromatic low-frequency vibrations (~50 Hz) in order to ensure a temporal steady-state condition. The second step consists of applying a suitable motion-sensitized MRI sequence. This sequence is phase-locked to the mechanical vibration in order to provide MRI phase images, which are modulated by the local tissue displacement at certain timepoints during the oscillatory cycle. The third step requires solving the propagation equation of a monochromatic mechanical wave in a linear isotropic viscoelastic material. The MRE experiment can be repeated at different vibration frequencies in order to obtain unbiased information about the dispersion properties of the material (Kruse et al. 2000, Sinkus et al. 2007).

13.6.2 MRE Pulse Sequences

The overall concept of the MRE sequence is similar to the classical MR diffusion-weighted imaging (DWI) sequence. However, the main difference between MRE and DWI is that in MRE the pulse sequence timing is actively controlled based on the externally generated excitation waves; however, in DWI the imaging sequence passively records the random motion of the water molecules.

13.6.2.1 Basic MRE Sequence

A typical spin-echo-based MRE sequence is generally used in MRE, although other sequences, for example, gradient echo, bSSFP, and DENSE, have been used. In a basic MRE sequence, a shot is defined as the combination of one magnetization RF excitation, magnetization encoding, and corresponding data readout, independent of the sequence details (Figure 13.31). The shot time duration needs to be an integer multiple of the mechanical vibration frequency in order to allow the motion-sensitizing gradients to probe the mechanical vibration during each shot at exactly the same instance of the mechanical wave's oscillatory cycle (Sinkus et al. 2000). This well-known method of phase locking allows for measuring the motion-encoded phase signal at many time points, which are normally beyond the temporal resolution of the technique (Suga et al. 2003).

13.6.2.2 Motion Encoding

The gradient channel on which the motion-encoding gradient is applied determines which component of the displacement vector is measured. Thus, independent of the sequence details, the phase signal of the final MRI image is directly proportional to the value of the corresponding wave component at a given phase of the oscillatory cycle. The image sensitivity to nonsynchronous motion can be minimized by nulling the individual moments of the gradient waveform, that is, using balanced gradients.

13.6.2.3 Motion Estimation

The MRE acquisition protocol can be shifted relative to the phase of the mechanical vibration in order to capture motion during another state of the oscillatory cycle. Thereby, snapshots of the moving wave can be measured at different timepoints during the oscillatory cycle. Theoretically, only two snapshots are necessary for the estimation of amplitude and phase; however, more advanced encoding methods can be implemented to increase the image SNR by simultaneously acquiring data in several directions (Wang et al. 2008).

13.6.3 Reconstruction of Elasticity Maps

In case of dynamic elastography, there are in general three different approaches to obtain local maps for the complex shear modulus

1. Local frequency estimation approach (Manduca et al. 2001) using directional filtering and BPFs to suppress contributions from noise and compressional waves (Manduca et al. 2003).
2. Indirect approach (Van Houten et al. 1999), that is, simulating the expected displacement field within a small ROI using the propagation equation based on an initial guess for the distribution of the viscoelastic parameters and iteratively updating the guess by minimizing the error between the simulated and measured displacement data.
3. Direct approach, that is, solving the propagation equation locally while assuming local homogeneity (Sinkus et al. 2000).

13.6.4 Validation of MRE Data

Reconstructed MRE shear moduli data have been extensively compared to FEM simulations (Sinkus et al. 2000, Litwiller et al. 2010), phantom data (Ringleb et al. 2005, Sinkus et al. 2005), and data obtained from rheometers (Hamhaber et al. 2003, Vappou et al. 2007, Chatelin et al. 2011). Overall, there is a very good agreement for the real part of the shear modulus, but to a lesser extent for the imaginary part, as expected from theoretical considerations. FEM can also be used for exploring the effects of various factors, including the boundary conditions, frequencies, geometry, and amount of tissue preloading on the measured shear stiffness (Chen et al. 2006, Clarke et al. 2011).

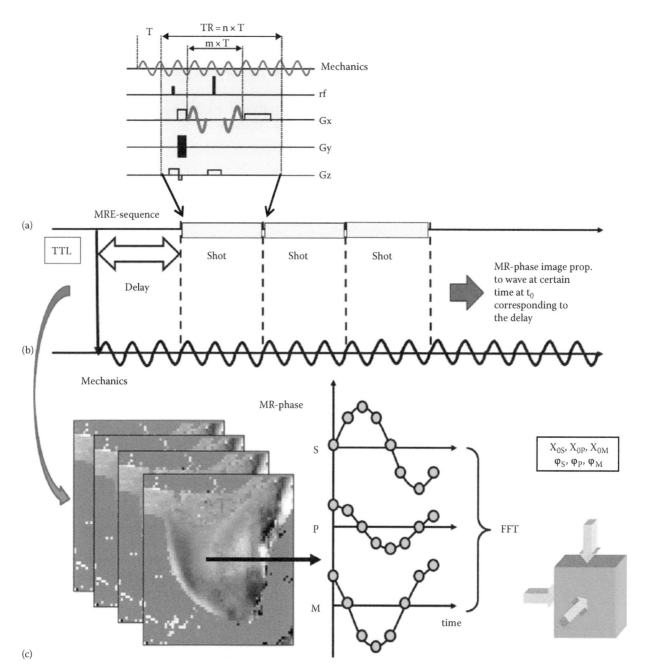

FIGURE 13.31 Schematic representation of the data acquisition chain and subsequent calculation of the complex-valued displacement vector. (a) A motion-sensitized MR sequence consisting of the repetition of "shots" (yellow area), which have a fixed and known phase relation with the mechanical vibration. (b) The MR system triggers, via a trigger delay (TTL) signal, the beginning of the mechanical vibration. After a predefined delay, the magnetic resonance elastography sequence acquires, in a phase-locked manner, an image (phase image, ϕ) of the mechanical wave for a fixed, but arbitrary (and unknown), timepoint of the oscillatory cycle. (c) Repetition of the acquisition with a modified delay allows for sampling one entire oscillatory cycle. Repetition of the entire procedure with the motion-sensitized gradients attached to the S/P/M (z/y/x) gradient channels allows for calculating—after applying a temporal Fourier transform for each pixel—the complex-valued displacement vector (X) of the wave.

13.6.5 CARDIAC MRE

Symptoms of congestive heart failure while maintaining a normal ventricular ejection fraction represent between 35% and 55% of the heart failure patients. Previously denoted as diastolic heart failure, it is currently referred to as heart failure with normal ejection fraction (HFnEF) or HF with preserved EF. HFnEF, or the "stiff heart syndrome," is a diastolic dysfunction that is most likely related to changes in the myocardial compliance and, hence, an alteration of its viscoelastic properties (Kitzman et al. 2001).

13.6.5.1 Myocardial Diastolic Viscoelastic Properties with MRI

Initial measurements of the regional viscoelastic diastolic properties of the LV myocardium were obtained ex vivo using MRI methods based on DENSE imaging and PC velocity mapping (Wen et al. 2005), wherein a simple model of the myocardial wall was used assuming tissue incompressibility and Hookean elastic material.

13.6.5.2 Cardiac MRE Pulse Sequences

Adapting the MRE sequences to the heart raises several distinct challenges. First, the echo time must be rather short in order to cope with the short T2 and T2* of the myocardium; second, due to the viscosity strongly increase with frequency, it is rather difficult for the generated waves to reach the heart using externally applied mechanical drivers with high frequencies (>100 Hz). Therefore, dedicated imaging sequences have to be used in cardiac MRE in order to cope with these constraints (Rump et al. 2007, Robert et al. 2009).

13.6.5.3 Cardiac and Stiffness Changes during the Cardiac Cycle

Figure 13.32 presents two in-plane motion amplitudes, A_x and A_y, for the LV acquired in a SAX slice at one instance of the cardiac cycle for three different MRE acquisition conditions: vibration is active and motion-encoding is active, vibration is inactive and motion-encoding is active, and vibration is active and motion-encoding is inactive.

13.6.5.4 Shell Phantom of the Heart

To model the wave propagation in the heart and gain initial experience in cardiac MRE, Kolipaka et al. (2009) designed a simplified spherical shell phantom of the heart. Here, the equation of motion used is based on Hamilton's variational principle (Junger and Fiet 1972) and contains higher-order spatial derivatives. This MRE model uses either a dedicated thin-shell model in order to convert the shear waves into intrinsic material parameters (Kolipaka et al. 2010, 2011) or uses the slope of the phase of the wave displacements to provide local wave speed information (Kolipaka et al. 2012). Initial results in a pig model (Figure 13.33) compared the stiffness–volume diagrams to invasively measured pressure data, where the results showed good visual agreement.

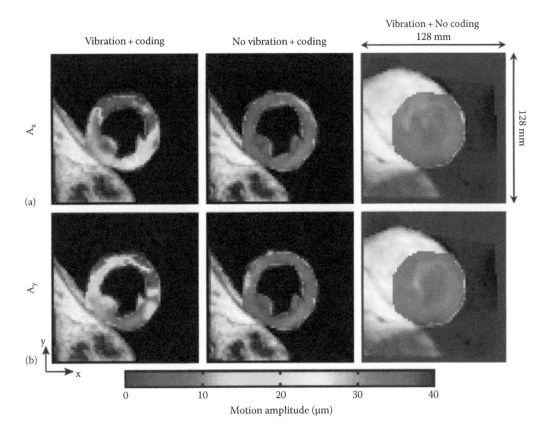

FIGURE 13.32 Cardiac stiffness changes during the cardiac cycle. In-plane motion amplitude (in micrometers) estimated from displacement-encoding (DENSE) magnetic resonance elastography (MRE) acquisitions in a volunteer: (a) motion along the x-direction and (b) motion amplitude along the y-direction. The left, middle, and right columns correspond to conventional (both vibrational excitation and motion encoding), no vibrational excitation, and no motion encoding DENSE MRE acquisitions. (Reproduced from Robert, B. et al., *Magn. Reson. Med.*, 62(5), 1155, 2009. With permission.)

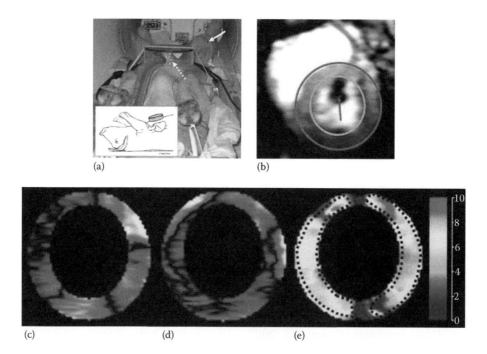

(a)   (b)

(c)   (d)   (e)

FIGURE 13.33 In vivo MR elastography (MRE) in a pig's heart. (a) Example of the experimental setup indicating the location of the pneumatic driver (dotted arrow) and catheter (solid arrow) in a pig model. (b) Short-axis magnitude image during diastole, with contours delineating the left ventricle (LV) myocardium and an arrow in the blood pool indicating the pressure sensor. (c, d) MRE wave images of the LV myocardium showing one offset of the radial and circumferential displacements, respectively. (e) The corresponding stiffness map obtained from the spherical shell analysis at a pressure of 8.61 mmHg, with mean stiffness in the region of interest of 6.4 ± 1.1 kPa. (Reproduced from Kolipaka, A. et al., *Magn. Reson. Med.*, 64(3), 862, 2010. With permission.)

13.7 SUMMARY AND KEY POINTS

13.7.1 SUMMARY

Advanced MRI techniques for measuring myocardial deformation, namely HARP, DENSE, SENC, TPM, and MRE imaging, provide fast, high-resolution, and intuitive means for evaluating and visualizing regional myocardial contractility patterns. Each of these techniques has been developed over time, which resulted in various versions suitable for implementation in different imaging situations. Further, hybrid techniques have been developed for obtaining composite or multidimensional information about the heart function. Although some of these techniques made their way into commercial products, most of them are still in the development phase. It should be noted that this chapter provides only a brief overview of these techniques for completeness of this book. No mathematical formulation, pulse sequence analysis, or comprehensive coverage of the different developments for each of these techniques is covered in this chapter. Actually, such a comprehensive coverage requires almost a whole book by itself. Therefore, *Heart Mechanics: Magnetic Resonance Imaging. Advanced Techniques, Clinical Applications, and Future Trends* is dedicated to covering these advanced techniques along with other state-of-the-art topics in heart mechanics with MRI, including MRI tagging data acquisition strategies (imaging sequences) and their effects on the resulting tagged images, mathematical techniques and algorithms for analyzing the tagged images, and various clinical applications of myocardial tagging. In *Heart Mechanics: Magnetic Resonance Imaging—Advanced Techniques, Clinical Applications, and Future Trends,* we investigate the relationships, similarities, and differences between these different techniques along with the advantages and limitations of each of them, as well as provide a comprehensive coverage of different clinical applications of the techniques covered in the book.

13.7.2 KEY POINTS

- HARP is a tagging *analysis*, not *acquisition*, technique.
- HARP tracks the taglines by studying the phase signal in the phase constructed images, which is totally different from conventional tagging analysis techniques that track the tagline displacement in the magnitude constructed images.
- The basic underlying principle in HARP tracking is that the harmonic phase of a material point is an imposed material property that is invariant in time.
- The simplicity and robustness of HARP resulted in reducing tag analysis time by at least an order of magnitude, which facilitated analyzing large volumes of tagged data in a reasonable short time.
- The implementation of the HARP technique on CSPAMM-tagged images results in fewer tracking errors than when implemented on SPAMM-tagged images.
- By extracting only one of the harmonic peaks in HARP analysis, SNR is reduced by 50%.

- The image acquisition time can be significantly decreased by acquiring a smaller region in k-space around the harmonic peak of interest for HARP analysis, which is the concept behind the fastHARP technique.
- The zHARP technique allows for 3D strain quantification from a single image plane using tagging and phase-encoding for measuring in-plane and through-plane strain components, respectively.
- DENSE measures intramyocardial motion by encoding the tissue displacement into the phase of the stimulated echo and displaying the displacement-encoded phase on a pixel-by-pixel basis.
- DENSE evolved as a STEAM pulse sequence with displacement encoding, in contrast to HARP, which has been developed based on MRI tagging.
- As a STEAM-based sequence, DENSE consists of three stages: magnetization modulation, mixing, and demodulation.
- The DENSE images can be processed to reveal motion information on the pixel level by displaying a small vector at each pixel location. The vector's orientation and length represent the motion direction and magnitude, respectively.
- Three signal echoes can be distinguished in DENSE: stimulated (displacement-encoded) echo, complex conjugate of the stimulated echo (antiecho), and T1 relaxation echo (nonmodulated DC echo). Only the phase of the displacement-encoded echo is directly related to tissue displacement.
- Suppressing the unwanted echoes (antiecho and T1 relaxation echo) can be implemented to eliminate artifacts and improve image quality in DENSE.
- Alternatively, different echoes could be combined in a specific coherent fashion to improve SNR in DENSE.
- DENSE scan time can be reduced by combining the sequence with EPI acquisition or parallel imaging techniques.
- Both myocardial displacement and viability contrast-enhancement information could be obtained simultaneously by acquiring and combining two complementary DENSE images.
- SENC is similar to DENSE in that it is based on a STEAM sequence. However, in contrast to DENSE, the strain information in SENC is obtained from the magnitude images.
- SENC has the advantages of measuring strain with high resolution (on the pixel level) using simple postprocessing that results in a color-coded image showing through-plane strain.
- In contrast to conventional tagging sequences, tagging in SENC is applied in the through-plane direction, which creates a stack of magnetization-saturated planes that lie inside, and parallel to, the imaging plane. Therefore, SENC measures through-plane strain in contrast to in-plane strain measured in conventional tagging techniques.

- The C-SENC technique acquires both myocardial functional and viability information in the same scan, which reduces the scan time in half and alleviates misregistration problems.
- SENC has been combined with HARP for measuring myocardial 3D motion in a single SAX slice, where in-plane circumferential and radial strain components are calculated from the HARP images, while through-plane longitudinal strain is calculated from the SENC images.
- SENC has been combined with DENSE for measuring 3D strain in a single slice, where the developed technique combines the advantages of both SENC and DENSE.
- TPM MRI is based on the fact that the generated MR signal is composed of both magnitude and phase. Therefore, by adding a bipolar gradient to the imaging pulse sequence, the spins moving in the gradient's direction accumulate phase that is directly proportional to their velocity.
- A reference data set (acquired without adding the bipolar gradient) is required in TPM MRI to subtract background phase from the generated TPM images.
- The venc setting in the TPM imaging parameters should be carefully determined to avoid aliasing as well as unnecessary noise in the resulting images.
- Black-blood techniques are usually implemented with TPM imaging to avoid the artifacts generated from the fast-flowing blood.
- TPM MRI has been combined with tagging for measuring both through-plane and in-plane motion components.
- The relationship between the applied stress and resulting strain is governed by the viscoelastic mechanical properties of tissues, which can be measured using MRE.
- The dynamic MRE approach is the one most commonly used within the MR community, where a single mechanical frequency is typically used for excitation and the wave propagation process is imaged and analyzed in the steady-state regime.
- In case of dynamic MRE, there are in general three different approaches to obtain local maps for the complex shear modulus: local frequency estimation, indirect approach, and direct approach. All approaches have advantages and limitations.
- MRE, with its ability to solve for the local stress-strain relationship can provide a real solution for characterizing the myocardial biomechanical properties.
- The myocardial stiffness can be used in the domain of cardiac MRE for estimating the internal pressure within the LV, assuming that the baseline elasticity of the myocardium is known.
- Adapting the MRE sequences to the heart is challenging due to the myocardium short T2 and significantly increasing viscosity with frequency, besides other motion heart challenges.

REFERENCES

Abd-Elmoniem, K.Z., Osman, N.F., Prince, J.L., and Stuber, M. (2007a). Three-dimensional magnetic resonance myocardial motion tracking from a single image plane. *Magn Reson Med* **58**(1): 92–102.

Abd-Elmoniem, K.Z., Sampath, S., Osman, N.F., and Prince, J.L. (2007b). Real-time monitoring of cardiac regional function using fastHARP MRI and region-of-interest reconstruction. *IEEE Trans Biomed Eng* **54**(9): 1650–1656.

Abd-Elmoniem, K.Z., Stuber, M., Osman, N.F., and Prince, J.L. (2005). ZHARP: Three-dimensional motion tracking from a single image plane. *Inf Process Med Imaging* **19**: 639–651.

Abd-Elmoniem, K.Z., Stuber, M., and Prince, J.L. (2008). Direct three-dimensional myocardial strain tensor quantification and tracking using zHARP. *Med Image Anal* **12**(6): 778–786.

Agarwal, H.K., Prince, J.L., and Abd-Elmoniem, K.Z. (2010). Total removal of unwanted harmonic peaks (TruHARP) MRI for single breath-hold high-resolution myocardial motion and strain quantification. *Magn Reson Med* **64**(2): 574–585.

Aletras, A.H. and Arai, A.E. (2004). meta-DENSE complex acquisition for reduced intravoxel dephasing. *J Magn Reson* **169**(2): 246–249.

Aletras, A.H., Balaban, R.S., and Wen, H. (1999a). High-resolution strain analysis of the human heart with fast-DENSE. *J Magn Reson* **140**(1): 41–57.

Aletras, A.H., Ding, S., Balaban, R.S., and Wen, H. (1999b). DENSE: Displacement encoding with stimulated echoes in cardiac functional MRI. *J Magn Reson* **137**(1): 247–252.

Aletras, A.H., Ingkanisorn, W.P., Mancini, C., and Arai, A.E. (2005). DENSE with SENSE. *J Magn Reson* **176**(1): 99–106.

Aletras, A.H., Tilak, G.S., Natanzon, A., Hsu, L.Y., Gonzalez, F.M., Hoyt, R.F., Jr., and Arai, A.E. (2006). Retrospective determination of the area at risk for reperfused acute myocardial infarction with T2-weighted cardiac magnetic resonance imaging: Histopathological and displacement encoding with stimulated echoes (DENSE) functional validations. *Circulation* **113**(15): 1865–1870.

Aletras, A.H. and Wen, H. (2001). Mixed echo train acquisition displacement encoding with stimulated echoes: An optimized DENSE method for in vivo functional imaging of the human heart. *Magn Reson Med* **46**(3): 523–534.

Ashikaga, H., Mickelsen, S.R., Ennis, D.B., Rodriguez, I., Kellman, P., Wen, H., and McVeigh, E.R. (2005). Electromechanical analysis of infarct border zone in chronic myocardial infarction. *Am J Physiol Heart Circ Physiol* **289**(3): H1099–H1105.

Basha, T.A., Ibrahim, El-S.H., Weiss, R.G., and Osman, N.F. (2009). Cine cardiac imaging using black-blood steady-state free precession (BB-SSFP) at 3T. *J Magn Reson Imaging* **30**(1): 94–103.

Bennett, E., Spottiswoode, B., Lorenz, C.H., and Wen, H. (2006). Optimal combination of phase cycling and gradient spoiling in DENSE displacement mapping. *Proceedings of the International Society of Magnetic Resonance in Medicine*, Seattle, WA.

Bilgen, M. (2010). Harmonic phase interference for the detection of tag line crossings and beyond in homogeneous strain analysis of cardiac tagged MRI data. *Australas Phys Eng Sci Med* **33**(4): 357–366.

Buonocore, M.H. (2004). Latest pulse sequence for displacement-encoded MR imaging incorporates essential technical improvements for multiphase measurement of intramyocardial strain. *Radiology* **230**(3): 615–617.

Castillo, E., Osman, N.F., Rosen, B.D., El-Shehaby, I., Pan, L., Jerosch-Herold, M., Lai, S., Bluemke, D.A., and Lima, J.A. (2005). Quantitative assessment of regional myocardial function with MR-tagging in a multi-center study: Interobserver and intraobserver agreement of fast strain analysis with Harmonic Phase (HARP) MRI. *J Cardiovasc Magn Reson* **7**(5): 783–791.

Chatelin, S., Oudry, J., Perichon, N., Sandrin, L., Allemann, P., Soler, L., and Willinger, R. (2011). In vivo liver tissue mechanical properties by Transient Elastography: Comparison with Dynamic Mechanical Analysis. *Biorheology* **48**(2): 75–88.

Chen, Q., Ringleb, S.I., Manduca, A., Ehman, R.L., and An, K.N. (2006). Differential effects of pre-tension on shear wave propagation in elastic media with different boundary conditions as measured by magnetic resonance elastography and finite element modeling. *J Biomech* **39**(8): 1428–1434.

Chenevert, T.L., Skovoroda, A.R., O'Donnell, M., and Emelianov, S.Y. (1998). Elasticity reconstructive imaging by means of stimulated echo MRI. *Magn Reson Med* **39**(3): 482–490.

Chuang, J.S., Zemljic-Harpf, A., Ross, R.S., Frank, L.R., McCulloch, A.D., and Omens, J.H. (2010). Determination of three-dimensional ventricular strain distributions in gene-targeted mice using tagged MRI. *Magn Reson Med* **64**(5): 1281–1288.

Clarke, E.C., Cheng, S., Green, M., Sinkus, R., and Bilston, L.E. (2011). Using static preload with magnetic resonance elastography to estimate large strain viscoelastic properties of bovine liver. *J Biomech* **44**(13): 2461–2465.

Delfino, J.G., Fornwalt, B.K., Eisner, R.L., Leon, A.R., and Oshinski, J.N. (2008). Cross-correlation delay to quantify myocardial dyssynchrony from phase contrast magnetic resonance (PCMR) velocity data. *J Magn Reson Imaging* **28**(5): 1086–1091.

Ehman, R.L. and Felmlee, J.P. (1989). Adaptive technique for high-definition MR imaging of moving structures. *Radiology* **173**(1): 255–263.

Epstein, F.H. (2007). MRI of left ventricular function. *J Nucl Cardiol* **14**: 729–744.

Epstein, F.H. and Gilson, W.D. (2004). Displacement-encoded cardiac MRI using cosine and sine modulation to eliminate (CANSEL) artifact-generating echoes. *Magn Reson Med* **52**(4): 774–781.

Fahmy, A.S., Pan, L., Stuber, M., and Osman, N.F. (2006). Correction of through-plane deformation artifacts in stimulated echo acquisition mode cardiac imaging. *Magn Reson Med* **55**(2): 404–412.

Feng, L., Donnino, R., Babb, J., Axel, L., and Kim, D. (2009). Numerical and in vivo validation of fast cine displacement-encoded with stimulated echoes (DENSE) MRI for quantification of regional cardiac function. *Magn Reson Med* **62**(3): 682–690.

Fischer, S.E., McKinnon, G.C., Maier, S.E., and Boesiger, P. (1993). Improved myocardial tagging contrast. *Magn Reson Med* **30**(2): 191–200.

Fischer, S.E., McKinnon, G.C., Scheidegger, M.B., Prins, W., Meier, D., and Boesiger, P. (1994). True myocardial motion tracking. *Magn Reson Med* **31**(4): 401–413.

Foll, D., Jung, B., Germann, E., Hennig, J., Bode, C., and Markl, M. (2011). Magnetic resonance tissue phase mapping: Analysis of age-related and pathologically altered left ventricular radial and long-axis dyssynchrony. *J Magn Reson Imaging* **34**(3): 518–525.

Foll, D., Jung, B., Schilli, E., Staehle, F., Geibel, A., Hennig, J., Bode, C., and Markl, M. (2010). Magnetic resonance tissue phase mapping of myocardial motion: New insight in age and gender. *Circ Cardiovasc Imaging* **3**(1): 54–64.

Foll, D., Jung, B., Staehle, F., Schilli, E., Bode, C., Hennig, J., and Markl, M. (2009). Visualization of multidirectional regional left ventricular dynamics by high-temporal-resolution tissue phase mapping. *J Magn Reson Imaging* **29**(5): 1043–1052.

Garot, J., Bluemke, D.A., Osman, N.F., Rochitte, C.E., McVeigh, E.R., Zerhouni, E.A., Prince, J.L., and Lima, J.A. (2000). Fast determination of regional myocardial strain fields from tagged cardiac images using harmonic phase MRI. *Circulation* **101**(9): 981–988.

Gilliam, A.D., Epstein, F.H., and Acton, S.T. (2009). Cardiac motion recovery via active trajectory field models. *IEEE Trans Inf Technol Biomed* **13**(2): 226–235.

Gilson, W.D., Yang, Z., French, B.A., and Epstein, F.H. (2004). Complementary displacement-encoded MRI for contrast-enhanced infarct detection and quantification of myocardial function in mice. *Magn Reson Med* **51**(4): 744–752.

Haase, A., Frahm, J., Matthaei, D., Hanicke, W., Bomsdorf, H., Kunz, D., and Tischler, R. (1986). MR imaging using stimulated echoes (STEAM). *Radiology* **160**(3): 787–790.

Haber, I. and Westin, C.F. (2002). Model-based 3D tracking of cardiac motion in HARP images. *Proceedings of the International Society for Magnetic Resonance in Medicine*, Honolulu, HI.

Hamdan, A., Thouet, T., Kelle, S., Paetsch, I., Gebker, R., Wellnhofer, E., Schnackenburg, B., Fahmy, A.S., Osman, N.F., and Fleck, E. (2008). Regional right ventricular function and timing of contraction in healthy volunteers evaluated by strain-encoded MRI. *J Magn Reson Imaging* **28**(6): 1379–1385.

Hamdan, A., Thouet, T., Kelle, S., Wellnhofer, E., Paetsch, I., Gebker, R., Schnackenburg, B. et al. (2009). Strain-encoded MRI to evaluate normal left ventricular function and timing of contraction at 3.0 Tesla. *J Magn Reson Imaging* **29**(4): 799–808.

Hamhaber, U., Grieshaber, F.A., Nagel, J.H., and Klose, U. (2003). Comparison of quantitative shear wave MR-elastography with mechanical compression tests. *Magn Reson Med* **49**(1): 71–77.

Haraldsson, H., Sigfridsson, A., Sakuma, H., Engvall, J., and Ebbers, T. (2011). Influence of the FID and off-resonance effects in dense MRI. *Magn Reson Med* **65**(4): 1103–1111.

Hess, A.T., Zhong, X., Spottiswoode, B.S., Epstein, F.H., and Meintjes, E.M. (2009). Myocardial 3D strain calculation by combining cine displacement encoding with stimulated echoes (DENSE) and cine strain encoding (SENC) imaging. *Magn Reson Med* **62**(1): 77–84.

Ibrahim, El-S.H. (2011). Myocardial tagging by cardiovascular magnetic resonance: Evolution of techniques—Pulse sequences, analysis algorithms, and applications. *J Cardiovasc Magn Reson* **13**: 36.

Ibrahim, El-S.H., Spooner, A.E., Stuber, M., Weiss, R.G., and Osman, N.F. (2007a). Free-breathing combined functional and viability MRI cardiac imaging. *J Cardiovasc Magn Reson* **9**: 229–231.

Ibrahim, El-S.H., Stuber, M., Fahmy, A.S., Abd-Elmoniem, K.Z., Sasano, T., Abraham, M.R., and Osman, N.F. (2007b). Real-time MR imaging of myocardial regional function using strain-encoding (SENC) with tissue through-plane motion tracking. *J Magn Reson Imaging* **26**(6): 1461–1470.

Ibrahim, El-S.H., Stuber, M., Kraitchman, D.L., Weiss, R.G., and Osman, N.F. (2007c). Combined functional and viability cardiac MR imaging in a single breathhold. *Magn Reson Med* **58**(4): 843–849.

Ibrahim, El-S.H., Weiss, R.G., Stuber, M., Kraitchman, D.L., Pan, L., Spooner, A.E., and Osman, N.F. (2008a). Stimulated-echo acquisition mode (STEAM) MRI for black-blood delayed hyperenhanced myocardial imaging. *J Magn Reson Imaging* **27**(1): 229–238.

Ibrahim, El-S.H., Weiss, R.G., Stuber, M., Spooner, A.E., and Osman, N.F. (2008b). Identification of different heart tissues from MRI C-SENC images using an unsupervised multi-stage fuzzy clustering technique. *J Magn Reson Imaging* **28**(2): 519–526.

Jung, B., Foll, D., Bottler, P., Peterson, S., Hennig, J., and Markl, M. (2006). Detailed analysis of myocardial motion in volunteers and patients using high-temporal-resolution MR tissue phase mapping. *J Magn Reson Imaging* **24**: 1033–1039.

Jung, B., Honal, M., Ullmann, P., Hennig, J., and Markl, M. (2008). Highly k-t-space-accelerated phase-contrast MRI. *Magn Reson Med* **60**(5): 1169–1177.

Junger, C.M. and Fiet, D. (1972). The in vacuo vibrations of shells. In: *Sound, Structures and Their Interaction*. Cambridge, MA: MIT Press.

Karwatowski, S.P., Mohiaddin, R., Yang, G.Z., Firmin, D.N., Sutton, M.S., Underwood, S.R., and Longmore, D.B. (1994). Assessment of regional left ventricular long-axis motion with MR velocity mapping in healthy subjects. *J Magn Reson Imaging* **4**(2): 151–155.

Khalifa, A., Youssef, A.B., and Osman, N. (2005). Improved harmonic phase (HARP) method for motion tracking a tagged cardiac MR images. *Conf Proc IEEE Eng Med Biol Soc* **4**: 4298–4301.

Kim, D., Epstein, F.H., Gilson, W.D., and Axel, L. (2004a). Increasing the signal-to-noise ratio in DENSE MRI by combining displacement-encoded echoes. *Magn Reson Med* **52**(1): 188–192.

Kim, D., Gilson, W.D., Kramer, C.M., and Epstein, F.H. (2004b). Myocardial tissue tracking with two-dimensional cine displacement-encoded MR imaging: Development and initial evaluation. *Radiology* **230**(3): 862–871.

Kim, D. and Kellman, P. (2007). Improved cine displacement-encoded MRI using balanced steady-state free precession and time-adaptive sensitivity encoding parallel imaging at 3 T. *NMR Biomed* **20**(6): 591–601.

Kitzman, D.W., Gardin, J.M., Gottdiener, J.S., Arnold, A., Boineau, R., Aurigemma, G., Marino, E.K., Lyles, M., Cushman, M., and Enright, P.L. (2001). Importance of heart failure with preserved systolic function in patients > or = 65 years of age. CHS Research Group. Cardiovascular Health Study. *Am J Cardiol* **87**(4): 413–419.

Kolipaka, A., Aggarwal, S., McGee, K., Anavekar, N., Manduca, A., Ehman, R., and Araoz, P. (2012). Magnetic resonance elastography as a method to estimate myocardial contractility. *J Magn Reson Imaging* **36**(1): 120–127.

Kolipaka, A., Araoz, P., McGee, K., Manduca, A., and Ehman, R. (2010). Magnetic resonance elastography as a method for the assessment of effective myocardial stiffness throughout the cardiac cycle. *Magn Reson Med* **64**(3): 862–870.

Kolipaka, A., McGee, K.P., Araoz, P.A., Glaser, K.J., Manduca, A., and Ehman, R.L. (2009). Evaluation of a rapid, multiphase MRE sequence in a heart-simulating phantom. *Magn Reson Med* **62**(3): 691–698.

Kolipaka, A., McGee, K.P., Manduca, A., Anavekar, N., Ehman, R.L., and Araoz, P.A. (2011). In vivo assessment of MR elastography-derived effective end-diastolic myocardial stiffness under different loading conditions. *J Magn Reson Imaging* **33**(5): 1224–1228.

Koos, R., Altiok, E., Doetsch, J., Neizel, M., Krombach, G., Marx, N., and Hoffmann, R. (2013). Layer-specific strain-encoded MRI for the evaluation of left ventricular function and infarct transmurality in patients with chronic coronary artery disease. *Int J Cardiol* **166**(1): 85–89.

Korosoglou, G., Lehrke, S., Wochele, A., Hoerig, B., Lossnitzer, D., Steen, H., Giannitsis, E., Osman, N.F., and Katus, H.A. (2010). Strain-encoded CMR for the detection of inducible ischemia during intermediate stress. *JACC Cardiovasc Imaging* **3**(4): 361–371.

Korosoglou, G., Lossnitzer, D., Schellberg, D., Lewien, A., Wochele, A., Schaeufele, T., Neizel, M. et al. (2009). Strain-encoded cardiac MRI as an adjunct for dobutamine stress testing: Incremental value to conventional wall motion analysis. *Circ Cardiovasc Imaging* **2**(2): 132–140.

Korosoglou, G., Youssef, A.A., Bilchick, K.C., Ibrahim, El-S.H., Lardo, A.C., Lai, S., and Osman, N.F. (2008). Real-time fast strain-encoded magnetic resonance imaging to evaluate regional myocardial function at 3.0 Tesla: Comparison to conventional tagging. *J Magn Reson Imaging* **27**(5): 1012–1018.

Kraitchman, D.L., Sampath, S., Castillo, E., Derbyshire, J.A., Boston, R.C., Bluemke, D.A., Gerber, B.L., Prince, J.L., and Osman, N.F. (2003). Quantitative ischemia detection during cardiac magnetic resonance stress testing by use of FastHARP. *Circulation* **107**(15): 2025–2030.

Kruse, S.A., Smith, J.A., Lawrence, A.J., Dresner, M.A., Manduca, A., Greenleaf, J.F., and Ehman, R.L. (2000). Tissue characterization using magnetic resonance elastography: Preliminary results. *Phys Med Biol* **45**: 1579–1590.

Kuijer, J.P., Hofman, M.B., Zwanenburg, J.J., Marcus, J.T., van Rossum, A.C., and Heethaar, R.M. (2006). DENSE and HARP: Two views on the same technique of phase-based strain imaging. *J Magn Reson Imaging* **24**(6): 1432–1438.

Kuijer, J.P., Jansen, E., Marcus, J.T., van Rossum, A.C., and Heethaar, R.M. (2001). Improved harmonic phase myocardial strain maps. *Magn Reson Med* **46**(5): 993–999.

Kuijer, J.P., Marcus, J.T., Gotte, M.J., van Rossum, A.C., and Heethaar, R.M. (1999). Simultaneous MRI tagging and through-plane velocity quantification: A three-dimensional myocardial motion tracking algorithm. *J Magn Reson Imaging* **9**(3): 409–419.

Kvitting, J.P., Ebbers, T., Engvall, J., Sutherland, G.R., Wranne, B., and Wigstrom, L. (2004). Three-directional myocardial motion assessed using 3D phase contrast MRI. *J Cardiovasc Magn Reson* **6**(3): 627–636.

Le, Y., Stein, A., Berry, C., Kellman, P., Bennett, E.E., Taylor, J., Lucas, K. et al. (2010). Simultaneous myocardial strain and dark-blood perfusion imaging using a displacement-encoded MRI pulse sequence. *Magn Reson Med* **64**(3): 787–798.

Li, W. and Yu, X. (2010). Quantification of myocardial strain at early systole in mouse heart: Restoration of undeformed tagging grid with single-point HARP. *J Magn Reson Imaging* **32**(3): 608–614.

Litwiller, D.V., Lee, S.J., Kolipaka, A., Mariappan, Y.K., Glaser, K.J., Pulido, J.S., and Ehman, R.L. (2010). MR elastography of the ex vivo bovine globe. *J Magn Reson Imaging* **32**(1): 44–51.

Liu, X. and Prince, J.L. (2010). Shortest path refinement for motion estimation from tagged MR images. *IEEE Trans Med Imaging* **29**(8): 1560–1572.

Liu, Y., Wen, H., Gorman, R.C., Pilla, J.J., Gorman, J.H., 3rd, Buckberg, G., Teague, S.D., and Kassab, G.S. (2009). Reconstruction of myocardial tissue motion and strain fields from displacement-encoded MR imaging. *Am J Physiol Heart Circ Physiol* **297**(3): H1151–H1162.

Lutz, A., Bornstedt, A., Manzke, R., Etyngier, P., Nienhaus, G.U., Rottbauer, W., and Rasche, V. (2011). Acceleration of tissue phase mapping with sensitivity encoding at 3T. *J Cardiovasc Magn Reson* **13**: 59.

Manduca, A., Lake, D.S., Kruse, S.A., and Ehman, R.L. (2003). Spatio-temporal directional filtering for improved inversion of MR elastography images. *Med Image Anal* **7**(4): 465–473.

Manduca, A., Oliphant, T.E., Dresner, M.A., Mahowald, J.L., Kruse, S.A., Amromin, E., Felmlee, J.P., Greenleaf, J.F., and Ehman, R.L. (2001). Magnetic resonance elastography: Non-invasive mapping of tissue elasticity. *Med Image Anal* **5**(4): 237–254.

Markl, M., Schneider, B., and Hennig, J. (2002). Fast phase contrast cardiac magnetic resonance imaging: Improved assessment and analysis of left ventricular wall motion. *J Magn Reson Imaging* **15**(6): 642–653.

Markl, M., Schneider, B., Hennig, J., Peschl, S., Winterer, J., Krause, T., and Laubenberger, J. (1999). Cardiac phase contrast gradient echo MRI: Measurement of myocardial wall motion in healthy volunteers and patients. *Int J Card Imaging* **15**(6): 441–452.

Mosher, T.J. and Smith, M.B. (1990). A DANTE tagging sequence for the evaluation of translational sample motion. *Magn Reson Med* **15**(2): 334–339.

Nasiraei-Moghaddam, A. and Gharib, M. (2009). Evidence for the existence of a functional helical myocardial band. *Am J Physiol Heart Circ Physiol* **296**(1): H127–H131.

Neizel, M., Lossnitzer, D., Korosoglou, G., Schaufele, T., Lewien, A., Steen, H., Katus, H.A., Osman, N.F., and Giannitsis, E. (2009a). Strain-encoded (SENC) magnetic resonance imaging to evaluate regional heterogeneity of myocardial strain in healthy volunteers: Comparison with conventional tagging. *J Magn Reson Imaging* **29**(1): 99–105.

Neizel, M., Lossnitzer, D., Korosoglou, G., Schaufele, T., Peykarjou, H., Steen, H., Ocklenburg, C., Giannitsis, E., Katus, H.A., and Osman, N.F. (2009b). Strain-encoded MRI for evaluation of left ventricular function and transmurality in acute myocardial infarction. *Circ Cardiovasc Imaging* **2**(2): 116–122.

Notomi, Y., Setser, R.M., Shiota, T., Martin-Miklovic, M.G., Weaver, J.A., Popovic, Z.B., Yamada, H., Greenberg, N.L., White, R.D., and Thomas, J.D. (2005). Assessment of left ventricular torsional deformation by Doppler tissue imaging: Validation study with tagged magnetic resonance imaging. *Circulation* **111**(9): 1141–1147.

Osman, N.F. (2003). Detecting stiff masses using strain-encoded (SENC) imaging. *Magn Reson Med* **49**(3): 605–608.

Osman, N.F., Kerwin, W.S., McVeigh, E.R., and Prince, J.L. (1999). Cardiac motion tracking using CINE harmonic phase (HARP) magnetic resonance imaging. *Magn Reson Med* **42**(6): 1048–1060.

Osman, N.F., McVeigh, E.R., and Prince, J.L. (2000). Imaging heart motion using harmonic phase MRI. *IEEE Trans Med Imaging* **19**(3): 186–202.

Osman, N.F. and Prince, J.L. (2000). Visualizing myocardial function using HARP MRI. *Phys Med Biol* **45**(6): 1665–1682.

Osman, N.F. and Prince, J.L. (2004). Regenerating MR tagged images using harmonic phase (HARP) methods. *IEEE Trans Biomed Eng* **51**(8): 1428–1433.

Osman, N.F., Sampath, S., Atalar, E., and Prince, J.L. (2001). Imaging longitudinal cardiac strain on short-axis images using strain-encoded MRI. *Magn Reson Med* **46**(2): 324–334.

Pai, V.M. and Wen, H. (2003). Rapid-motion-perception based cardiac navigators: Using the high flow blood volume as a marker for the position of the heart. *J Cardiovasc Magn Reson* **5**(4): 531–543.

Pan, L., Prince, J.L., Lima, J.A., and Osman, N.F. (2005). Fast tracking of cardiac motion using 3D-HARP. *IEEE Trans Biomed Eng* **52**(8): 1425–1435.

Pan, L., Stuber, M., Kraitchman, D.L., Fritzges, D.L., Gilson, W.D., and Osman, N.F. (2006). Real-time imaging of regional myocardial function using fast-SENC. *Magn Reson Med* **55**(2): 386–395.

Perman, W.H., Creswell, L.L., Wyers, S.G., Moulton, M.J., and Pasque, M.K. (1995). Hybrid DANTE and phase-contrast imaging technique for measurement of three-dimensional myocardial wall motion. *J Magn Reson Imaging* **5**(1): 101–106.

Phatak, N.S., Maas, S.A., Veress, A.I., Pack, N.A., Di Bella, E.V., and Weiss, J.A. (2009). Strain measurement in the left ventricle during systole with deformable image registration. *Med Image Anal* **13**(2): 354–361.

Pruessmann, K.P., Weiger, M., Scheidegger, M.B., and Boesiger, P. (1999). SENSE: Sensitivity encoding for fast MRI. *Magn Reson Med* **42**(5): 952–962.

Ringleb, S.I., Chen, Q., Lake, D.S., Manduca, A., Ehman, R.L., and An, K.N. (2005). Quantitative shear wave magnetic resonance elastography: Comparison to a dynamic shear material test. *Magn Reson Med* **53**(5): 1197–1201.

Robert, B., Sinkus, R., Gennisson, J.L., and Fink, M. (2009). Application of DENSE-MR-elastography to the human heart. *Magn Reson Med* **62**(5): 1155–1163.

Rump, J., Klatt, D., Braun, J., Warmuth, C., and Sack, I. (2007). Fractional encoding of harmonic motions in MR elastography. *Magn Reson Med* **57**(2): 388–395.

Ryf, S., Spiegel, M.A., Gerber, M., and Boesiger, P. (2002). Myocardial tagging with 3D-CSPAMM. *J Magn Reson Imaging* **16**(3): 320–325.

Ryf, S., Tsao, J., Schwitter, J., Stuessi, A., and Boesiger, P. (2004). Peak-combination HARP: A method to correct for phase errors in HARP. *J Magn Reson Imaging* **20**(5): 874–880.

Sampath, S., Derbyshire, J.A., Atalar, E., Osman, N.F., and Prince, J.L. (2003). Real-time imaging of two-dimensional cardiac strain using a harmonic phase magnetic resonance imaging (HARP-MRI) pulse sequence. *Magn Reson Med* **50**(1): 154–163.

Sampath, S., Osman, N.F., and Prince, J.L. (2009). A combined harmonic phase and strain-encoded pulse sequence for measuring three-dimensional strain. *Magn Reson Imaging* **27**(1): 55–61.

Selskog, P., Heiberg, E., Ebbers, T., Wigstrom, L., and Karlsson, M. (2002). Kinematics of the heart: Strain-rate imaging from time-resolved three-dimensional phase contrast MRI. *IEEE Trans Med Imaging* **21**(9): 1105–1109.

Shehata, M.L., Basha, T.A., Tantawy, W.H., Lima, J.A., Vogel-Claussen, J., Bluemke, D.A., Hassoun, P.M., and Osman, N.F. (2010). Real-time single-heartbeat fast strain-encoded imaging of right ventricular regional function: Normal versus chronic pulmonary hypertension. *Magn Reson Med* **64**(1): 98–106.

Sigfridsson, A., Haraldsson, H., Ebbers, T., Knutsson, H., and Sakuma, H. (2010). Single-breath-hold multiple-slice DENSE MRI. *Magn Reson Med* **63**(5): 1411–1414.

Sigfridsson, A., Haraldsson, H., Ebbers, T., Knutsson, H., and Sakuma, H. (2011). In vivo SNR in DENSE MRI; temporal and regional effects of field strength, receiver coil sensitivity and flip angle strategies. *Magn Reson Imaging* **29**(2): 202–208.

Sinkus, R., Lorenzen, J., Schrader, D., Lorenzen, M., Dargatz, M., and Holz, D. (2000). High-resolution tensor MR elastography for breast tumour detection. *Phys Med Biol* **45**(6): 1649–1664.

Sinkus, R., Siegmann, K., Xydeas, T., Tanter, M., Claussen, C., and Fink, M. (2007). MR elastography of breast lesions: Understanding the solid/liquid duality can improve the specificity of contrast-enhanced MR mammography. *Magn Reson Med* **58**(6): 1135–1144.

Sinkus, R., Tanter, M., Xydeas, T., Catheline, S., Bercoff, J., and Fink, M. (2005). Viscoelastic shear properties of in vivo breast lesions measured by MR elastography. *Magn Reson Imaging* **23**(2): 159–165.

Spottiswoode, B., Russell, J.B., Moosa, S., Meintjes, E.M., Epstein, F.H., and Mayosi, B.M. (2008a). Abnormal diastolic and systolic septal motion following pericardiectomy demonstrated by cine DENSE MRI. *Cardiovasc J Afr* **19**(4): 208–209.

Spottiswoode, B.S., Zhong, X., Hess, A.T., Kramer, C.M., Meintjes, E.M., Mayosi, B.M., and Epstein, F.H. (2007). Tracking myocardial motion from cine DENSE images using spatiotemporal phase unwrapping and temporal fitting. *IEEE Trans Med Imaging* **26**(1): 15–30.

Spottiswoode, B.S., Zhong, X., Lorenz, C.H., Mayosi, B.M., Meintjes, E.M., and Epstein, F.H. (2008b). 3D myocardial tissue tracking with slice followed cine DENSE MRI. *J Magn Reson Imaging* **27**(5): 1019–1027.

Spottiswoode, B.S., Zhong, X., Lorenz, C.H., Mayosi, B.M., Meintjes, E.M., and Epstein, F.H. (2009). Motion-guided segmentation for cine DENSE MRI. *Med Image Anal* **13**(1): 105–115.

Staehle, F., Jung, B.A., Bauer, S., Leupold, J., Bock, J., Lorenz, R., Foll, D., and Markl, M. (2011). Three-directional acceleration phase mapping of myocardial function. *Magn Reson Med* **65**(5): 1335–1345.

Suga, M., Matsuda, T., Minato, K., Oshiro, O., Chihara, K., Okamoto, J., Takizawa, O., Komori, M., and Takahashi, T. (2003). Measurement of in vivo local shear modulus using MR elastography multiple-phase patchwork offsets. *IEEE Trans Biomed Eng* **50**(7): 908–915.

Tecelao, S.R., Zwanenburg, J.J., Kuijer, J.P., and Marcus, J.T. (2006). Extended harmonic phase tracking of myocardial motion: Improved coverage of myocardium and its effect on strain results. *J Magn Reson Imaging* **23**(5): 682–690.

Van Houten, E.E., Paulsen, K.D., Miga, M.I., Kennedy, F.E., and Weaver, J.B. (1999). An overlapping subzone technique for MR-based elastic property reconstruction. *Magn Reson Med* **42**(4): 779–786.

Vappou, J., Breton, E., Choquet, P., Goetz, C., Willinger, R., and Constantinesco, A. (2007). Magnetic resonance elastography compared with rotational rheometry for in vitro brain tissue viscoelasticity measurement. *MAGMA* **20**(5–6): 273–278.

Venkatesh, B.A., Gupta, H., Lloyd, S.G., Dell 'Italia, L., and Denney, T.S., Jr. (2010). 3D left ventricular strain from unwrapped harmonic phase measurements. *J Magn Reson Imaging* **31**(4): 854–862.

Verdier, C. (2003). Rheological properties of living materials. From cells to tissues. *J Theor Med* **5**(2): 25.

Wang, H., Weaver, J.B., Doyley, M.M., Kennedy, F.E., and Paulsen, K.D. (2008). Optimized motion estimation for MRE data with reduced motion encodes. *Phys Med Biol* **53**(8): 2181–2196.

Wen, H., Bennett, E., Epstein, N., and Plehn, J. (2005). Magnetic resonance imaging assessment of myocardial elastic modulus and viscosity using displacement imaging and phase-contrast velocity mapping. *Magn Reson Med* **54**(3): 538–548.

Youssef, A., Ibrahim, El-S.H., Korosoglou, G., Abraham, M.R., Weiss, R.G., and Osman, N.F. (2008). Strain-encoding cardiovascular magnetic resonance for assessment of right-ventricular regional function. *J Cardiovasc Magn Reson* **10**: 33.

Zhong, J. and Yu, X. (2010). Strain and torsion quantification in mouse hearts under dobutamine stimulation using 2D multiphase MR DENSE. *Magn Reson Med* **64**(5): 1315–1322.

Zhong, X., Helm, P.A., and Epstein, F.H. (2009). Balanced multipoint displacement encoding for DENSE MRI. *Magn Reson Med* **61**(4): 981–988.

Zhong, X., Spottiswoode, B.S., Cowart, E.A., Gilson, W.D., and Epstein, F.H. (2006). Selective suppression of artifact-generating echoes in cine DENSE using through-plane dephasing. *Magn Reson Med* **56**(5): 1126–1131.

Index

For Product Safety Concerns and Information please contact
our EU representative GPSR@taylorandfrancis.com Taylor & Francis
Verlag GmbH, Kaufingerstraße 24, 80331 München, Germany

T - #0158 - 160425 - C0 - 279/216/33 - PB - 9780367871178 - Gloss Lamination